Mosby's
**Nursing
Drug
Reference**

Mosby's

Nursing
Drug
Reference

Linda Skidmore-Roth, R.N., M.S.N., N.P.

Formerly, New Mexico State University,
Nursing Faculty, Las Cruces, New Mexico;
El Paso Community College, El Paso, Texas

The C. V. Mosby Company

St. Louis • Washington, D.C. • Toronto   1988

Editor: Don Ladig
Assistant editor: Robin Carter
Project manager: Teri Merchant
Production editors: Deborah Vogel, Robert A. Kelly
Design: Liz Fett

A NOTE TO THE READER:

The author and publisher of *Mosby's Nursing Drug Reference* have diligently verified the medications and nursing considerations discussed for accuracy and compatibility with officially accepted standards at the time of publication. With continual advancements in pharmacology, our knowledge base in this field continues to expand. Therefore, we recommend that the reader always check product information for changes in dose and contraindications before administering any drug. This is critical when dealing with new or rarely used medications.

The C.V. Mosby Company
11830 Westline Industrial Drive, St. Louis, Missouri 63146

Library of Congress Cataloging-in-Publication Data

Skidmore-Roth, Linda.
    Mosby's nursing drug reference.

    Includes bibliographies and index.
    1. Drugs—Prescribing—Handbooks, manuals, etc.
2. Nursing—Handbooks, manuals, etc.   I.   Title.
II.   Title: Nursing drug reference. [DNLM: 1.   Drugs—
handbooks.   2.   Drugs—nurses' instruction. QV 39 S628m]
RM138.S59   1988   615'.14   87-31245
ISBN 0-8016-5037-2

GW/D/D   9   8   7   6   5   4   3   2   01/A/080

Clinical pharmacology consultants

Carmen Aceves-Blumenthal, M.S.
Assistant Professor, Southeastern College of Pharmaceutical Sciences, North Miami Beach, Florida

Danial E. Baker, Pharm.D.
Assistant Professor, Washington State University, Pullman, Washington

R. Keith Campbell, Pharm.D.
Professor, Washington State University, Pullman, Washington

Catherine Celestin, Pharm.D.
Assistant Professor, Southeastern College of Pharmaceutical Sciences, North Miami Beach, Florida

Bruce D. Clayton, Pharm.D.
Professor, University of Arkansas, Little Rock, Arkansas

Edward H. Clouse, Ph.D.
Associate Professor, Southeastern College of Pharmaceutical Sciences, North Miami Beach, Florida

David E. Domann, M.S., F.A.S.C.P.
Consultant Pharmacist, Atchison, Kansas

Patricia A. Howard, B.S., R.Ph.
Clinical Instructor, University of Kansas Medical Center, Kansas City, Kansas

Judith K. Marquis, Ph.D.
Assistant Professor, Boston University School of Medicine, Boston, Massachusetts

Bozena B. Michniak, Ph.D., M.P.S.
Assistant Professor, University of South Carolina, Columbia, South Carolina

John Murski, B.S., R.Ph.
Pharmacology Consultant, Newtown, Pennsylvania

Keith M. Olsen, Pharm.D.
Assistant Professor, University of Arkansas, Little Rock, Arkansas

Roberta J. Secrest, Ph.D., Pharm.D., R.Ph.
Post-Doctoral Scientist, Eli Lilly and Company, Indianapolis, Indiana

Kay See-Lasley, M.S.
Pharmacology Consultant, Lawrence, Kansas

Carol Walsh, Ph.D.
Associate Professor, Boston University School of Medicine, Boston, Massachusetts

Lynn Roger Willis, Ph.D.
Professor, Indianapolis University, School of Medicine, Indianapolis, Indiana

Clinical nursing consultants

Marie B. Andrews, R.N., B.S.N., M.S.N.
Lecturer, Texas Woman's University, Houston, Texas

Ruth Bowen, R.N., M.S.
Lecturer, Texas Woman's University, Denton, Texas

Mary Lou Cheatham, R.N., B.S.N., M.S.N.
Associate Professor, Ball State University, Muncie, Indiana

Barbara H. Goodkin, R.N., M.S.
Instructor, Washtenaw Community College, Ann Arbor, Michigan

Patricia Hong, R.N., M.A.
Instructor, Anchorage Community College, Anchorage, Alaska

Joan M. Jenks, R.N., M.S.N.
Assistant Professor, Thomas Jefferson University, Philadelphia, Pennsylvania

Andrew T. McPhee, B.S.
Instructor, Windham Regional Technical School, Willimantic, Connecticut

Marylou Medlin, R.N., B.S.N., M.N.
Instructor, Charity Hospital School of Nursing, New Orleans, Louisiana

Maureen J. Osis, R.N., M.N.
Clinical Nurse Specialist, Calgary, Alberta

Michele Poradzisz, R.N., M.S.
Instructor, De Paul University, Chicago, Illinois

Roberta Ronayne, R.N., B.Sc.N., M.Sc.
Assistant Professor, University of Ottawa, Ottawa, Ontario

Regina Stroud, R.N., M.S.
Instructor, Rancho Santiago College, Santa Ana, California

Richard E. Watters, R.N., B.Sc., B.Ed.
Instructor, Grande Prairie Regional College, Grande Prairie, Alberta

Patsy R. Wigodsky, B.S.N., M.S.N.
Associate Professor, Methodist College of Nursing, Omaha, Nebraska

To my husband, Allen,
who has been nonthreatened
by my success and supportive
in everything I have aspired to do.

Preface

Although drug references abound, few are available that are truly portable and geared specifically for clinical use by the practicing nurse or student. The guiding principle throughout the development of this reference has been to provide the user with a book that allows easy access to drug information, and nursing considerations that specifically tell the nurse what to do in terms that are consistent with the nursing process. Every detail—down to the choice of paper, typeface, cover, binding, use of color, and appendixes—has been carefully chosen with the user in mind.

Over 1100 generic and 5000 trade medications, alphabetized by generic name, are included. Trade names are given for all medications commonly used in the United States and Canada. Drugs available only in Canada are identified by an asterisk.

The following information is provided, wherever possible, for safe and effective administration of each drug:

Pronunciations: Pronunciations are provided to help the nursing student master the more complex generic names.

Functional and chemical classifications: All known broad functional and chemical classifications are given. These classifications allow the nurse to see similarities and dissimilarities among drugs in the same functional but different chemical classes.

Controlled-substance schedule: Schedules are included for the United States (I, II, III, IV, V) and Canada (F, G).

Action: Major pharmacologic properties are described in concise terms. Action is discussed to the cellular level when the information is available.

Side effects and adverse reactions: Grouped by body system, common side effects are italicized and life-threatening reactions are in bold italic type. This feature allows the nurse to instantly identify common and life-threatening reactions.

Dosages and routes: All available and approved dosages and routes are given for adult, pediatric, and geriatric patients.

Available forms: All available forms—including tablets, capsules, extended-release, injectables (IV, IM, SC), solutions, creams, ointments, lotions, gels, shampoos, elixirs, suspensions, suppositories, sprays, aerosols, and lozenges—are provided.

Contraindications: Contraindications are instances in which a medication should absolutely not be given. When the FDA has assigned pregnancy safety category D and X, it appears here.

Precautions: Special precautionary steps are given here, including FDA pregnancy safety categories A, B, and C.

Pharmacokinetics: Metabolism, distribution, and elimination are provided for all dosage forms, if known.

Interactions and incompatibilities: This section includes confirmed drug, food, and smoking interactions. The reaction is listed first, and then the drug or nutrient causing that interaction.

Nursing considerations: Nursing considerations, which are highlighted in blue, are divided and organized to foster use of the nursing process in drug administration: Assess, Administer, Perform/Provide, Evaluate, and Teach Patient/Family. Nursing considerations are consistently grouped under these headings to help the nurse group interventions that can be used for planning nursing care.

Laboratory test interferences: When known, laboratory test interferences are provided.

Treatment of overdose: Drugs and treatment for overdoses are provided for appropriate drugs.

The following appendixes are included to further enhance the usability of this reference: abbreviations, measurement conversions, bibliography, and combination products. A compatibility chart for commonly used IV medications has been printed on the inside front cover for quick access, and a controlled substance chart, the FDA pregnancy categories, and a nomogram have been printed on the inside back cover for quick access.

I am indebted to the nursing and pharmacology consultants who reviewed the manuscript and thank them for their criticism and encouragement. I would also like to thank Don Ladig and Robin Carter, my editors, whose active encouragement and enthusiasm have made this book better than it might otherwise have been. I am likewise grateful to Teri Merchant, Elizabeth Fett, and Audrey Rhoades. I, along with the publisher, welcome comments from users of *Mosby's Nursing Drug Reference* so that we may continue to provide current and useful information in future editions.

Linda Skidmore-Roth

Contents

absorbable gelatin

Gelfoam

Func. class.: Hemostatic
Chem. class.: Purified gelatin solution

Action: Absorbs blood, provides area for clot formation, healthy tissue growth
Uses: Hemostatis during surgery, decubitus ulcers
Dosage and routes:
• *Adult:* TOP hold in place for 15 sec after saturating with isotonic NaCL injection or thrombin solution
Decubitus ulcer
• *Adult:* TOP place into ulcer, may add more as needed, not to be removed
Available forms include: Sponge, pack, cone, powder
Side effects/adverse reactions: None reported
Contraindications: Hypersensitivity, frank infection, abnormal bleeding, postpartum bleeding
Precautions: Neonates/infants, hepatic disease
Pharmacokinetics:
IMPLANT: Absorbed in 4-6 wk
Interactions/incompatibilities: None known
NURSING CONSIDERATIONS
Administer:
• By lightly packing, do not overpack foam
• Dry, hold for 10-15 sec, remove
• Moist, place in sterile saline or thrombin solution, squeeze after removing, blot before applying
• After debridement of decubiti unless dressing change qd; do not remove sponge, may add more sponges over top of old ones
Perform/provide:
• Discard unused portion; do not resterilize

Evaluate:
• Infection: fever, redness, inflammation
Teach patient/family:
• That foam is absorbed in 4-6 wk, does not need to be removed

acebutolol

(ase-bute'-oh-lole)
Sectral
Func. class.: Antihypertensive
Chem. class.: Nonselective β-blocker

Action: Competitively blocks stimulation of β-adrenergic receptor within vascular smooth muscle; produces chronotropic, inotropic activity (decreases rate of SA node discharge, increases recovery time), slows conduction of AV node, decreases heart rate, which decreases O_2 consumption in myocardium; also, decreases renin-aldosterone-angiotensin system at high doses, inhibits β-2 receptors in bronchial system (high doses)
Uses: Mild to moderate hypertension, sinus tachycardia, persistent atrial extrasystoles, tachydysrhythmias, prophylaxis of angina pectoris
Dosage and routes:
Hypertension
• *Adult:* PO 400 mg qd or in 2 divided doses, may be increased to desired response
Ventricular dysrhythmia
• *Adult:* PO until dose 200 mg bid, may increase gradually, usual range 600-1200 mg daily
Available forms include: Caps 200, 400 mg
Side effects/adverse reactions:
CV: Profound hypotension, bradycardia, CHF, cold extremities, postural hypotension, 2nd or 3rd degree heart block
CNS: Insomnia, fatigue, dizziness,

---

italics = common side effects   **bold italic** = life threatening reactions

mental changes, memory loss, hallucinations, depression, lethargy, drowsiness, strange dreams, catatonia

GI: Nausea, diarrhea, vomiting, ***mesenteric arterial thrombosis, ischemic colitis***

INTEG: Rash, fever, alopecia

HEMA: Agranulocytosis, thrombocytopenia, purpura

EENT: Sore throat, dry burning eyes

GU: Impotence

ENDO: Increased hypoglycemic response to insulin

*RESP: **Bronchospasm,*** dyspnea, wheezing

Contraindications: Hypersensitivity to β-blockers, cardiogenic shock, heart block (2nd, 3rd degree), sinus bradycardia, CHF, cardiac failure

Precautions: Major surgery, pregnancy (B), lactation, diabetes mellitus, renal disease, thyroid disease, COPD, asthma, well compensated heart failure, CAD

Pharmacokinetics:

PO: Peak 2-4 hr; half-life 6-7 hr, excreted unchanged in urine, protein binding 5%-15%

Interactions/incompatibilities:

• Increased hypotension, bradycardia: reserpine, hydralazine, methyldopa, prazosin, anticholinergics

• Decreased antihypertensive effects: indomethacin

• Increased hypoglycemic effect: insulin

• Decreased bronchodilation: theophyllines

NURSING CONSIDERATIONS

Assess:

• I&O, weight daily

• B/P, pulse q4h; note rate, rhythm, quality

• Apical/radial pulse before administration; notify physician of any significant changes

• Baselines in renal, liver function tests before therapy begins

Administer:

• PO ac, hs, tablet may be crushed or swallowed whole

• Reduced dosage in renal dysfunction

Perform/provide:

• Storage protected from light, moisture; placed in cool environment

Evaluate:

• Therapeutic response: decreased B/P after 1-2 wk

• Edema in feet, legs daily

• Skin turgor, dryness of mucous membranes for hydration status

Teach patient/family:

• Not to discontinue drug abruptly, taper over 2 wk, may cause precipitate angina

• Not to use OTC products containing α-adrenergic stimulants (such as nasal decongestants, OTC cold preparations) unless directed by physician

• To report bradycardia, dizziness, confusion, depression, fever

• To take pulse at home, advise when to notify physician

• To avoid alcohol, smoking, sodium intake

• To comply with weight control, dietary adjustments, modified exercise program

• To carry Medic Alert ID to identify drug that you are taking, allergies

• To avoid hazardous activities if dizziness is present

• To report symptoms of CHF: difficult breathing, especially on exertion or when lying down, night cough, swelling of extremities

Lab test interferences:

Interference: Glucose/insulin tolerance tests

Treatment of overdose: Lavage, IV atropine for bradycardia, IV theophylline for bronchospasm, digitalis, O_2, diuretic for cardiac failure, hemodialysis, IV glucose for hyperglycemia, IV diazepam (or phenytoin) for seizures

acetaminophen

(a-seat-a-mee'noe-fen)

Aceta, Actamin, Anapap, Atasol,* Campain,* Dapa, Datril, Liquiprin, Panadol, Parten, Pedric, Robigesic,* Rounax,* Tempra, Tylenol, Valadol, Valcrin

Func. class.: Nonnarcotic analgesic

Chem. class.: Nonsalicylate, para aminophenol derivative

Action: Blocks pain impulses in CNS that occur in response to inhibition of prostaglandin synthesis; antipyretic action results from inhibition of hypothalamic heat-regulating center.

Uses: Mild to moderate pain or fever

Dosage and routes:

• *Adult and child >10 yr:* PO 325-650 mg q4h prn, not to exceed 4 g/day; REC: 325-650 mg q4h prn, not to exceed 4 g/day

• *Child 0-3 mo:* 40 mg/dose

• *Child 4-11 mo:* 80 mg/dose

• *Child <1 yr:* PO/REC 15-60 mg/dose all q4-6h, not to exceed 65 mg/kg/day

• *Child 1-2 yr:* PO/REC 60 mg/dose

• *Child 2-3 yr:* PO/REC 120 mg/dose

• *Child 3-4 yr:* PO/REC 180 mg/dose

• *Child 4-5 yr:* PO/REC 240 mg/dose

• *Child 5-10 yr:* PO/REC 325 mg/dose

Available forms include: Rectal supp 120, 125, 325, 650 mg; chewable tab 80 mg; caps 325, 500, 650 mg; elix 120, 160, 325 mg/5 ml; liq 160 mg/5 ml; sol 100 mg/1 ml, 120 mg/2.5 ml

Side effects/adverse reactions:

*SYST: **Anaphylaxis***

*HEMA: **Leukopenia, neutropenia, hemolytic anemia** (long-term use), **thrombocytopenia, pancytopenia***

CNS: Stimulation, drowsiness

GI: Nausea, vomiting, abdominal pain, ***hepatotoxicity***

INTEG: Rash, urticaria, angioedema

TOXICITY: Cyanosis, anemia, neutropenia, jaundice, pancytopenia, CNS stimulation, delirium then vascular collapse, convulsions, coma, death

Contraindications: Hypersensitivity

Precautions: Anemia, hepatic disease, renal disease, chronic alcoholism, pregnancy

Pharmacokinetics:

PO: Onset 10-30 min, peak ½-2 hr, duration 4-6 hr

REC: Onset slow, duration 4-6 hr Metabolized by liver, excreted by kidneys, crosses placenta, excreted in breast milk, half-life 1-4 hr

Interactions/incompatibilities:

• Increased effects of: anticoagulants, chloramphenicol

• Decreased effects of this drug: cholestyramine, oral contraceptives, narcotics, anticholinergics

• Increased effect of this drug: diflunisal, caffeine, alcohol

NURSING CONSIDERATIONS

Assess:

• Liver function studies: AST, ALT, bilirubin, creatinine if patient is on long-term therapy

• Renal function studies: BUN, urine creatinine if patient is on long-term therapy

• Blood studies: CBC, pro-time if patient is on long-term therapy

• I&O ratio; decreasing output may indicate renal failure (long-term therapy)

Administer:

• To patient crushed or whole;

---

italics = common side effects   ***bold italic*** = life threatening reactions

chewable tablets may be chewed
• With food or milk to decrease gastric symptoms
Evaluate:
• Therapeutic response: absence of pain, fever
• Hepatotoxicity: dark urine, clay-colored stools, yellowing of skin, sclera, itching, abdominal pain, fever, diarrhea if patient is on long-term therapy
• Allergic reactions: rash, urticaria; if these occur, drug may need to be discontinued
• Renal dysfunction: decreased urine output
Teach patient/family:
• Not to exceed recommend dosage; acute poisoning may result
• To read label on other OTC drugs; many contain acetaminophen
Treatment of overdose: Drug level q4h, gastric lavage, administer acetylcysteine

---

acetazolamide/ acetazolamide sodium

(a-set-a-zole′a-mide)
Cetazol, Diamox, Hydrazol/Diamox Parenteral

Func. class.: Diuretic; carbonic anhydrase inhibitor
Chem. class.: Sulfonamide derivative

Action: Inhibits carbonic anhydrase activity in proximal renal tubules to decrease reabsorption of water, sodium; decreases carbonic anhydrase in CNS, increasing seizure threshold; able to decrease aqueous humor in eye, which lowers intraocular pressure
Uses: Open-angle glaucoma, narrow-angle glaucoma, epilepsy (petit mal, grand mal, mixed), edema in CHF, drug-induced edema, acute mountain sickness

Dosage and routes:
Closed-angle glaucoma
• *Adult:* PO/IM/IV 250 mg q4h, or 250 mg bid, to be used for short-term therapy
Open-angle glaucoma
• *Adult:* PO/IM/IV 250 mg-1g/day in divided doses for amounts over 250 mg
Edema
• *Adult:* IM/IV 250-375 mg/day in AM
• *Child:* IM/IV 5 mg/kg/day in AM
Seizures
• *Adult:* PO/IM/IV 8-30 mg/kg/day, usual range 375-1000 mg/day
• *Child:* PO/IM/IV 8-30 mg/kg/day in divided doses tid or qid, or 300-900 mg/m²/day, not to exceed 1.5 g/day
Mountain sickness
• *Adult:* PO 250 mg q8-12h
Available forms include: Tabs 125 g, 250 mg; caps sust rel 500 mg; inj IM/IV 500 mg
Side effects/adverse reactions:
GU: Frequency, hypokalemia, polyuria, uremia, glucosuria, hematuria, decreased libido, impotence
CNS: Drowsiness, paresthesia, anxiety, depression, headache, dizziness, confusion, stimulation, fatigue, convulsions
GI: Nausea, vomiting, anorexia, constipation, diarrhea, melena, weight loss, hepatic insufficiency
EENT: Myopia, tinnitus
INTEG: Rash, pruritus, urticaria, fever
ENDO: Hypoglycemia
HEMA: Hyperchloremia, aplastic anemia, hemolytic anemia, leukopenia, agranulocytosis, thrombocytopenia, purpura, pancytopenia
Contraindications: Hypersensitivity to sulfonamides, severe renal disease, severe hepatic disease,

---

electrolyte imbalances (hyponatremia, hypokalemia), hypochloremic acidosis, Addison's disease, long-term use in narrow-angle glaucoma
Precautions: Hypercalciuria, pregnancy, COPD
Pharmacokinetics:
PO: Onset ½-1 hr, peak 2-4 hr, duration 6-12 hr
PO—SUS REL: Onset 2 hr, peak 8-12 hr, duration 18-24 hr
IV: Onset 2 min, peak 15 min, duration 4-5 hr
65% absorbed if fasting (oral), 75% absorbed if given with food; half-life 2½-5½ hr; excreted unchanged by kidneys (80% within 24 hr), crosses placenta
Interactions/incompatibilities:
• Increased action of: amphetamines, procainamide, quinidine, tricyclics
• Decreased effects of: salicylates, lithium, barbiturates, methotrexate, chlorpropamide
• Hypokalemia: with other diuretics, corticosteroids, amphotericin B
NURSING CONSIDERATIONS
Assess:
• Weight daily, I&O daily to determine fluid loss; effect of drug may be decreased if used qd
• Rate, depth, rhythm of respiration, effect of exertion
• B/P lying, standing; postural hypotension may occur
• Electrolytes: potassium, sodium, chloride; include BUN, blood sugar, CBC, serum creatinine, blood pH, ABGs
Administer:
• PO or IV if possible, IM administration is painful
• In AM to avoid interference with sleep if using drug as diuretic
• Potassium replacement if potassium is less than 3.0
• With food if nausea occurs; absorption may be decreased slightly

Evaluate:
• Therapeutic response: improvement in edema of feet, legs, sacral area daily if medication is being used in CHF; or decrease in aqueous humor if medication is being used in glaucoma
• Improvement in CVP q8h
• Signs of metabolic acidosis: drowsiness, restlessness
• Signs of hypokalemia: postural hypotension, malaise, fatigue, tachycardia, leg cramps, weakness
• Rashes, temperature elevation qd
• Confusion, especially in elderly; take safety precautions if needed
Teach patient/family:
• To increase fluid intake 2-3 L/day unless contraindicated; to rise slowly from lying or sitting position
• To notify physician if sore throat, unusual bleeding, bruising, paresthesias, tremors, flank pain, or skin rash occurs
• To avoid hazardous activities if drowsiness occurs
Lab test interferences:
False positive: Urinary protein
Treatment of overdose: Lavage if taken orally, monitor electrolytes, administer dextrose in saline

---

acetic acid

Domeboro Otic, VoSol Otic, Bofofair Otic, Birotic
Func. class.: Otic
Chem. class.: Weak acid

Action: Provides antibacterial action to decrease ear infection
Uses: Prevention of swimmer's ear, ear canal infection (external)
Dosage and routes:
• *Adult and child:* INSTILL 3-6 gtts tid-qid or use saturated wick for 24 hr, then use instillation
Swimmer's ear
• *Adult and child:* INSTILL 2 gtts bid

Available forms include: Sol 2%
Side effects/adverse reactions:
EENT: Itching, irritation in ear
INTEG: Rash, urticaria
Contraindications: Hypersensitivity, perforated eardrum
Pharmacokinetics: Not known
Interactions/incompatibilities:
None known
NURSING CONSIDERATIONS
Administer:
• After removing impacted cerumen by irrigation
• After cleaning stopper with alcohol
• After restraining child if necessary
• Warming solution to body temperature
Evaluate:
• Therapeutic response: decreased ear pain
• For redness, swelling, pain in ear, which indicates superimposed infection
Teach patient/family:
• Method of instillation, using aseptic technique including not touching dropper to ear
• That dizziness may occur after instillation

---

acetohexamide

(a-seat-oh-hex′a-mide)
Dimelor,* Dymelor
Func. class.: Antidiabetic
Chem. class.: Sulfonylurea (1st generation)

Action: Causes functioning β-cells in pancreas to synthesize, release insulin, leading to drop in blood glucose levels; stimulation of insulin results in increased insulin binding; not effective if patient lacks functioning β-cells
Uses: Stable adult-onset diabetes mellitus (type II)

Dosage and routes:
• *Adult:* PO 250 mg-1.5 g/day; usually given before breakfast, unless large dose is required, then dose is divided in two
Available forms include: Tabs 250 mg scored
Side effects/adverse reactions:
CNS: Headache, weakness
GI: Nausea, vomiting, diarrhea, *hepatotoxicity, jaundice*
HEMA: Leukopenia, thrombocytopenia, agranulocytosis, aplastic anemia, increased AST, ALT, alk phosphatase
INTEG: Rash, allergic reactions, pruritus, urticaria, eczema, photosensitivity, erythema
ENDO: Hypoglycemia
Contraindications: Hypersensitivity to sulfonylureas, juvenile or brittle diabetes, renal disease, hepatic disease
Precautions: Pregnancy (C), elderly, cardiac disease, thyroid disease, severe hypoglycemic reactions
Pharmacokinetics:
PO: Completely absorbed by GI route, onset 1 hr, peak 2-4 hr, duration 12-24 hr, half-life 1-1½ hr, metabolized in liver, excreted in urine, (metabolites, unchanged drug) breast milk
Interactions/incompatibilities:
• Adverse effects: oral anticoagulants, hydantoins, salicylates, sulfonamides, nonsteroidal antiinflammatories
• Increased effects of this drug: insulin, MAOIs
• Decreased action of this drug: calcium channel blockers, corticosteroids, oral contraceptives, thiazide diuretics, thyroid preparations, estrogens

NURSING CONSIDERATIONS
Administer:
• Drug 30 min before meals
Perform/provide:
• Storage in tight container in cool environment
Evaluate:
• Therapeutic response: decrease in polyuria, polydipsia, polyphagia, clear sensorium, absence of dizziness, stable gait
• Hypoglycemic/hyperglycemic reaction that can occur soon after meals
Teach patient/family:
• To check for symptoms of cholestatic jaundice: dark urine, pruritus, yellow sclera; if these occur physician should be notified
• To use capillary blood glucose test while on this drug
• To test urine glucose levels with Chemstrip approximately 2 hr after each meal
• Symptoms of hypo/hyperglycemia, what to do about each
• Drug must be continued on daily basis; explain consequence of discontinuing drug abruptly
• To take drug in morning to prevent hypoglycemic reactions at night
• To avoid OTC medications unless prescribed by physician
• That diabetes is life-long illness; that this drug is not cure
• That all food included in diet plan must be eaten in order to prevent hypoglycemia
• To carry Medic-Alert ID for emergency purposes
Treatment of overdose: 10%-50% glucose solution

acetohydroxamic acid
(a-set-oh-hye-drox-am'ic)
Lithostat
Func. class.: Ammonia detoxicant, reversible urease inhibitor
Chem. class.: Hydroxylamine, ethyl acetate compound

Action: Inhibits bacterial enzyme urease, which decreases conversion of urea to ammonia, preventing formation of renal stones, decreasing growth of already existing stones
Uses: Renal calculi
Dosage and routes:
• *Adult:* PO 250 mg tid-qid q6-8h when stomach is empty, not to exceed 1.5 g/day
• *Child:* PO 10 mg/kg/day in 2-3 divided doses
Available forms include: Tabs 250 mg
Side effects/adverse reactions:
*HEMA: **Hemolytic anemia, reticulocytosis, thrombocytopenia***
CNS: Headache, depression, restlessness, anxiety, nervousness
GI: Nausea, vomiting, anorexia, malaise, diarrhea, constipation
INTEG: Rash on face, arms, alopecia
CV: Phlebitis, deep vein thrombosis, pulmonary embolism, palpitation
Contraindications: Hypersensitivity, severe renal disease, lactation, nonurease-producing organisms, pregnancy
Precautions: Deep vein thrombosis, hepatic disease
Pharmacokinetics:
PO: Peak 15-60 min, half-life 3½-10 hr, metabolized, excreted in urine as unchanged drug (15%-60%)
Interactions/incompatibilities:
• Decreased absorption of both

drugs: iron preparations
• Rash: alcohol
NURSING CONSIDERATIONS
Assess:
• I&O ratio; observe for decrease in urinary output
• CBC, platelets, reticulocytes before, during therapy (q3 mo)
Administer:
• On empty stomach only, to facilitate absorption
Perform/provide:
• Storage in tight container at room temperature
Evaluate:
• Therapeutic response: decrease in stone formation on x-ray, decreased pain in kidney region, absence of hematuria
Teach patient/family:
• To avoid alcohol, OTC preparations that contain alcohol; skin rashes have occurred
• To report any pain, redness, or hard area, usually in legs
• Stress patient compliance with medical regimen; bone marrow depression may occur

---

acetophenazine maleate

(a-set-oh-fen′a-zeen)
Tindal
Func. class.: Antipsychotic/neuroleptic
Chem. class.: Phenothiazine, piperazine

Action: Depresses cerebral cortex, hypothalamus, limbic system, which control activity, aggression; blocks neurotransmission produced by dopamine at synapse; exhibits strong α-adrenergic, anticholinergic blocking action; mechanism for antipsychotic effects is unclear
Uses: Psychotic reactions, schizophrenia, mania in bipolar depression

Dosage and routes:
• *Adult:* PO 20 mg tid or qid, hospitalized patients may be on 8-120 mg qd in divided doses, max dosage 600 mg qd
• *Child:* PO 0.8-1.6 mg/kg/day in divided doses tid, not to exceed 80 mg/day outpatient, 120 mg/day inpatient
Available forms include: Tabs 20 mg
Side effects/adverse reactions:
RESP: **Laryngospasm,** dyspnea, *respiratory depression*
CNS: Extrapyramidal symptoms: pseudoparkinsonism, akathisia, dystonia, tardive dyskinesia, seizures, *headache*
HEMA: Anemia, leukopenia, leukocytosis, **agranulocytosis**
INTEG: Rash, photosensitivity, dermatitis
EENT: Blurred vision, glaucoma
GI: Dry mouth, nausea, vomiting, anorexia, constipation, diarrhea, jaundice, weight gain
GU: Urinary retention, urinary frequency, enuresis, impotence, amenorrhea, gynecomastia
CV: Orthostatic hypotension, hypertension, **cardiac arrest,** ECG changes, **tachycardia**
Contraindications: Hypersensitivity, circulatory collapse, liver damage, cerebral arteriosclerosis, coronary disease, severe hypertension/hypotension, blood dyscrasias, coma, child <12 years, brain damage, bone marrow depression, alcohol and barbiturate withdrawal states
Precautions: Pregnancy, lactation, seizure disorders, hypertension, hepatic disease, cardiac disease
Pharmacokinetics:
PO: Onset erratic, peak 2-4 hr; duration may be detected for up to 6 mo after last dose; metabolized by liver, excreted in urine (metabolites), crosses placenta, enters

breast milk; 95% bound to plasma proteins; elimination half-life 10-20 hr

Interactions/incompatibilities:
• Oversedation: other CNS depressants, alcohol, barbiturate anesthetics
• Toxicity: epinephrine
• Decreased absorption: aluminum hydroxide or magnesium hydroxide antacids
• Decreased effects of: lithium, levodopa
• Increased effects of both drugs: β-adrenergic blockers, alcohol
• Increased anticholinergic effects: anticholinergics

NURSING CONSIDERATIONS

Assess:
• Swallowing of PO medication; check for hoarding or giving of medication to other patients
• I&O ratio; palpate bladder if low urinary output occurs
• Bilirubin, CBC, liver function studies monthly
• Urinalysis is recommended before and during prolonged therapy

Administer:
• Antiparkinsonian agent; to be used if EPS occur

Perform/provide:
• Decreased noise input by dimming lights, avoiding loud noises
• Supervised ambulation until stabilized on medication; do not involve in strenuous exercise program because fainting is possible; patient should not stand still for long periods of time
• Increased fluids to prevent constipation
• Sips of water, candy, gum for dry mouth
• Storage in tight, light-resistant container in cool environment

Evaluate:
• Therapeutic response: decrease in emotional excitement, hallucinations, delusions, paranoia, reorganization of patterns of thought, speech
• Affect, orientation, LOC, reflexes, gait, coordination, sleep pattern disturbances
• B/P standing and lying, include pulse and respirations; take these q4h during initial treatment; establish baseline before starting treatment; report drops of 30 mm Hg
• Dizziness, faintness, palpitations, tachycardia on rising
• EPS, including akathisia (inability to sit still, no pattern to movements), tardive dyskinesia (bizarre movements of the jaw, mouth, tongue, extremities), pseudoparkinsonism (rigidity, tremors, pill rolling, shuffling gait)
• Skin turgor daily
• Constipation, urinary retention daily; if these occur, increase bulk, water in diet

Teach patient/family:
• That orthostatic hypotension occurs often, and to rise from sitting or lying position gradually
• To avoid hot tubs, hot showers, or tub baths since hypotension may occur
• To avoid abrupt withdrawal of this drug or EPS may result; drug should be withdrawn slowly
• To avoid OTC preparations (cough, hayfever, cold) unless approved by physician since serious drug interactions may occur; avoid use with alcohol or CNS depressants, increased drowsiness may occur
• To use sunscreen during sun exposure to prevent burns
• Regarding compliance with drug regimen
• About EPS and necessity for meticulous oral hygiene since oral candidiasis may occur
• To report sore throat, malaise, fever, bleeding, mouth sores; if these occur, CBC should be drawn and

---

italics = common side effects   ***bold italic*** = life threatening reactions

drug discontinued

• In hot weather, heat stroke may occur; take extra precautions to stay cool

• Urine may turn pink or reddish-brown

Lab test interferences:

Increase: Liver function tests, cardiac enzymes, cholesterol, blood glucose, prolactin, bilirubin, PBI, cholinesterase, ^{131}I

Decrease: Hormones (blood, urine)

False positive: Pregnancy tests, PKU

False negative: Urinary steroids, 17-OHCS

Treatment of overdose: Lavage, if orally injested, provide an airway; *do not induce vomiting*

---

acetylcholine chloride

(a-se-teel-koe'leen)

Miochol direct-acting

Func. class.: Miotic, cholinergic

Chem. class.: Quaternary ammonium compound

Action: Intense, immediate miosis (pupil constriction) by causing contraction of sphincter muscle of iris

Uses: Anterior segment surgery; cataract removal keratoplasty, peripheral iridectomy or cyclodialysis

Dosage and routes:

• *Adult and child:* INSTILL 0.5-2 ml of a 1% sol in anterior chamber of eye (instillation by physician)

Available forms include: Sol 1:100; powder

Side effects/adverse reactions:

CV: Hypotension, bradycardia

EENT: Blurred vision, lens opacities

Contraindications: Hypersensitivity, when miosis is undesirable

Precautions: Acute cardiac failure, bronchial asthma

Pharmacokinetics:

INSTILL: Miosis occurs immediately, duration 10 min

Interactions/incompatibilities:

None known

NURSING CONSIDERATIONS

Administer:

• Check vial for percentage of solution

• Check label for expiration date

• After shaking vial to mix drug to clear solution, push stopper to mix solvent with powder; do not use if stopper cannot be forced down

• After cleaning stopper with alcohol or other germicidial

• IV atropine 0.6-0.8 mg for systemic reactions

Perform/provide:

• Used reconstituted solution immediately; discard unused portion

Teach patient/family:

• To report change in vision, blurring or loss of sight, trouble breathing, sweating, flushing

---

acetylcysteine

(a-se-til-sis'tay-een)

Airbron,* Mucomyst, Parrolex

Func. class.: Mucolytic

Chem. class.: Amino acid L-cysteine

Action: Decreases viscosity of secretions by breaking disulfide links of mucoproteins; increases hepatic glutathione, which is necessary to inactivate toxic metabolites in acetaminophen overdose

Uses: Acetaminophen toxicity, bronchitis, pneumonia, cystic fibrosis, emphysema, atelectasis, tuberculosis, complications of thoracic, cardiovascular surgery, diagnosis in bronchial lab tests

Dosage and routes:

• *Adult and child:* INSTILL 1-2 ml (10%-20% sol) q1-4h prn or 3-5 ml (20% sol) or 6-10 ml (10% sol) by mouthpiece tid or qid

• *Adult and child:* PO 140 mg/kg, then 70 mg/kg q4h × 17 doses to total of 1330 mg/kg

Available forms include: Sol 10%, 20%

Side effects/adverse reactions:

CNS: Dizziness, drowsiness, headache, fever, chills

GI: Nausea, stomatitis, constipation, vomiting, anorexia, ***hepatotoxicity***

EENT: Rhinorrhea, tooth damage

CV: Hypotension

INTEG: Urticaria, rash, fever, clamminess

*RESP: **Bronchospasm,*** burning, hemoptysis, chest tightness

Contraindications: Hypersensitivity, increased intracranial pressure, status asthmaticus

Precautions: Hypothyroidism, Addison's disease, CNS depression, brain tumor, asthma, hepatic disease, renal disease, COPD, psychosis, alcoholism, convulsive disorders, lactation

Pharmacokinetics:

INH/INSTILL: Onset 1 min, duration 5-10 min, metabolized by liver, excreted in urine

Interactions/incompatibilities:

• Do not use with iron, copper, rubber

• Do not mix with antibiotics: tetracycline, chlortetracycline, oxytetracycline, erythromycin, lactobionate, amphotericin-B, sodium ampicillin, iodized oil, chymotrypsin, trypsin, hydrogen peroxide

NURSING CONSIDERATIONS

Assess:

• VS, cardiac status including checking for dysrhythmias, increased rate, palpitations

• ABGs for increased CO_2 retention in asthma patients

• Antidotal use: liver function tests, acetaminophen levels; inform

physician if dose is vomited or vomiting is persistent

Administer:

• Store in refrigerator: use within 96 hr of opening

• Before meals ½-1 hr for better absorption, to decrease nausea

• 20% solutions diluted with NS over water for injection; may give 10% solution undiluted

• Only after patient clears airway by deep breathing, coughing

• Antidotal use: give within 24 hr; give with cola or soft drink to disguise taste; can be given with H_2O through tubes; use within 1 hr

• By syringe 2-3 doses of 1-2 ml of 20% or 2-4 ml of 10% solution

• Decreased dose to elderly patients; their metabolism may be slowed

• Gum, hard candy, frequent rinsing of mouth for dryness of oral cavity

• Only if suction machine is available

Perform/provide:

• Storage in refrigerator after opening

• Assistance with inhaled dose: bronchodilator if bronchospasm occurs

• Mechanical suction if cough insufficient to remove excess bronchial secretions

Evaluate:

• Therapeutic response: absence of purulent secretions when coughing

• Cough: type, frequency, character including sputum

• Rate, rhythm of respirations, increased dyspnea; discontinue if bronchospasm occurs

• Antidotal use: hepatic encephalopathy

Teach patient/family:

• Avoid driving or other hazardous activities until patient is stabilized on this medication

• Avoid alcohol, other CNS de-

pressants; will enhance sedating properties of this drug
• That unpleasant odor will decrease after repeated use
• That discoloration of solution after bottle is opened does not impair its effectiveness
• Avoid smoking, smoke-filled rooms, perfume, dust, environmental pollutants, cleaners

activated charcoal

Arm-a-char, Charcoaide, Charcocaps, Charcodote, Charcotabs, Digestalin

Func. class.: Antiflatulent/antidote

Action: Binds poisons, increases adsorption in GI tract
Uses: Flatulence, poisoning, dyspepsia, distention, deodorant in wounds, diarrhea
Dosage and routes:
Poisoning
• *Adult and child:* PO 5-10 × weight of substance ingested, minimum dose 30 g/250 ml of water
Flatulence/dyspepsia
• *Adult:* PO 600 mg-5 g tid-qid
Available forms include: Powder; liq 12.5, 25, 40 g; caps 260 mg; tabs 325, 650 mg
Side effects/adverse reactions:
GI: Nausea, black stools, vomiting, constipation, diarrhea
Contraindications: Hypersensitivity to this drug, unconsciousness/semiconsciousness, poisoning of cyanide, mineral acids, alkalies
Pharmacokinetics:
PO: Not metabolized, excreted in feces
Interactions/incompatibilities:
• Decreased effectiveness of both drugs: ipecac, laxatives
• Do not mix with dairy products

NURSING CONSIDERATIONS
Assess:
• Respiration, pulse, B/P to determine charcoal effectiveness if taken for barbiturate/narcotic poisoning
Administer:
• After inducing vomiting first
• After mixing with water or fruit juice to form thick syrup; do not use dairy products to mix charcoal
• Repeat dose if vomiting occurs soon after dose
• After spacing at least 1 hr before or after other drugs, or absorption will be decreased
• <3 days
Evaluate:
• Therapeutic response: LOC, alert (poisoning)
Teach patient/family:
• That stools will be black

acyclovir (topical)
(ay-sye'kloe-ver)
Zovirax
Func. class.: Local antiinfective
Chem. class.: Antiviral

Action: Interferes with viral DNA replication
Uses: Simple mucocutaneous herpes simplex, initial herpes genitalis
Dosage and routes:
• *Adult and child:* TOP apply to all lesions q3h × 1 wk
Available forms include: Top oint 5%
Side effects/adverse reactions:
INTEG: Rash, urticaria, stinging, burning
Contraindications: Hypersensitivity
Precautions: Pregnancy (C), lactation
Interactions/incompatibilities:
None known

NURSING CONSIDERATIONS
Administer:
• Enough medication to completely cover lesions
• After cleansing with soap, water before each application, dry well
Perform/provide:
• Storage at room temperature in dry place
Evaluate:
• Allergic reaction: burning, stinging, swelling, redness
• Therapeutic response: decrease in size, number of lesions
Teach patient/family:
• To apply with glove to prevent further infection
• To avoid use of OTC creams, ointments, lotions unless directed by physician
• To use medical asepsis (hand washing) before, after each application

acyclovir sodium
(ay-sye-kloe-ver)
Zovirax
Func. class.: Antiviral
Chem. class.: Acylic purine nucleoside analog

Action: Interferes with DNA synthesis needed for viral replication
Uses: Mucocutaneous herpes simplex virus, herpes genitalis (HSV-1, HSV-2)
Dosage and routes:
Herpes simplex
• *Adult and child >12 yr:* IV INF 5 mg/kg over 1 hr q8h × 1 wk
• *Child <12 yr:* IV INF 250 mg/m² over 1 hr q8h × 1 wk
Genital herpes
• *Adult:* PO 200 mg q4h while awake for 5 days to 6 mo depending whether initial, recurrent, or chronic
Available forms include: Caps 200 mg; inj IV 500 mg, oint (see topical listings)
Side effects/adverse reactions:
CNS: Tremors, confusion, lethargy, hallucinations, convulsions, dizziness, *headache*
HEMA: Anemia, increased bleeding time, ***bone marrow depression, granulocytopenia, thrombocytopenia, leukopenia, megaloblastic anemia***
GI: Nausea, vomiting, diarrhea, increased ALT, AST, abdominal pain, glossitis, colitis
GU: Oliguria, proteinuria, hematuria, *vaginitis, moniliasis,* ***glomerulonephritis, acute renal failure***
INTEG: Rash, urticaria, pruritus, phlebitis at IV site
Contraindications: Hypersensitivity, herpes zoster in immunosuppressed individual
Precautions: Lactation, hepatic disease, renal disease, electrolyte imbalance, dehydration, pregnancy (C)
Pharmacokinetics:
IV: Peak 1 hr, half-life 20 min-3 hr, (terminal), metabolized by liver, excreted by kidneys as unchanged drug (95%), crosses placenta
Interactions/incompatibilities:
• Increased neurotoxocity, nephrotoxicity: aminoglycosides, amphotericin, interferon, probenecid, methotrexate
NURSING CONSIDERATIONS
Assess:
• I&O ratio; report hematuria, oliguria, fatigue, weakness; may indicate nephrotoxicity; check for protein in urine during treatment
• Any patient with compromised renal system, since drug is excreted slowly in poor renal system function; toxicity may occur rapidly
• Liver studies: AST, ALT
• Blood studies: WBC, RBC, Hct, Hgb, bleeding time; blood dyscra-

sias may occur; drug should be discontinued

• Renal studies: urinalysis, protein, BUN, creatinine, CrCl

• C&S before drug therapy; drug may be taken as soon as culture is taken; repeat C&S after treatment

Administer:

• After reconstituting with 10 ml sterile water/500 mg of drug; shake, use within 12 hr; give over at least 1 hr to prevent nephrotoxicity

Perform/provide:

• Storage at room temperature for up to 12 hr after reconstitution

• Adequate intake of fluids (2000 ml) to prevent deposit in kidneys

Evaluate:

• Therapeutic response: absence of itching, painful lesions

• Bowel pattern before, during treatment; if severe abdominal pain with bleeding occurs, drug should be discontinued

• Skin eruptions: rash, urticaria, itching

• Allergies before treatment, reaction of each medication; place allergies on chart, Kardex in bright red letters; notify all people giving drugs

Teach patient/family:

• That drug may be taken orally before infection occurs; drug should be taken when itching or pain occurs, usually before eruptions

• That partners need to be told that patient has herpes; they could become infected

• That drug does not cure infection, just controls symptoms

• To report sore throat, fever, fatigue; could indicate superimposed infection

• That drug must be taken in equal intervals around clock to maintain blood levels for 10 days

• To notify physician of side effects of bruising, bleeding, fatigue,

malaise; may indicate blood dyscrasias

---

albumin, normal serum 5%/25%

(al-byoo'min)

Albuminar 5%, Albutein 5%, Buminate 5%, Plasbumin 5%, Albuminar 25%, Albumisol 25%, Buminate 25%, Plasbumin 25%

Func. class.: Blood derivative
Chem. class.: Placental human plasma

Action: Exerts oncotic pressure on tissue fluids, which expands volume of circulating blood

Uses: Burns, hyperbilirubinemia, shock, hypoproteinemia, varicella zoster infections

Dosage and routes:

Burns

• *Adult:* IV dose to maintain plasma albumin at 30-50 g/L

Shock

• *Adult:* IV 500 ml of 5% sol q30 min, as needed

• *Child:* ¼-½ adult dose in non-emergencies

Hypoproteinemia

• *Adult:* IV 1000-2000 ml of 5% sol qd, not to exceed 5-10 ml/min or 25-100 g of 25% sol qd, not to exceed 3 ml/min, titrated to patient response

Hyperbilirubinemia/erythoblastosis fetalis

• *Infant:* IV 1 g of 25% sol/kg before transfusion

Available forms include: Inj IV 50, 250 mg/ml

Side effects/adverse reactions:

GI: Nausea, vomiting, increased salivation

INTEG: Rash, urticaria

CNS: Fever, chills, flushing, headache

RESP: Altered respirations

CV: Fluid overload, hypotension,

erratic pulse, tachycardia

Contraindications: Hypersensitivity, congestive heart failure, severe anemia

Precautions: Decreased salt intake, decreased cardiac reserve, lack of albumin deficiency, hepatic disease, renal disease

Pharmacokinetics: In hyponutrition states metabolized as protein/energy source.

Interactions/incompatibilities: None known

NURSING CONSIDERATIONS

Assess:

• Blood studies Hct, Hgb; if serum declines, dyspnea, hypoxemia can result

• Decreased B/P, erratic pulse, respiration

• I&O ratio: urinary output may decrease

• CVP, pulmonary wedge pressure will increase if overload occurs

Administer:

• IV slowly, to prevent fluid overload; dilute with NS for injection or D₅W; may be given undiluted; use infusion pump

• Within 4 hr of opening

Perform/provide:

• Adequate hydration before administration

• Check type of albumin, some stored at room temperature, some need to be refrigerated

Evaluate:

• Therapeutic response: increased B/P, decreased edema, increased serum albumin

• Allergy: fever, rash, itching, chills, flushing, urticaria, nausea, vomiting, hypotension, requires discontinuation of infusion, use of new lot if therapy reinstituted

• CVP reading: distended neck veins indicate circulatory overload; shortness of breath, anxiety, insomnia, expiratory rales, frothy blood-tinged cough, cyanosis indicate pulmonary overload

Lab test interferences:

False increase: Alk phosphatase

---

albuterol

(al-byoo′ter-ole)

Proventil, Ventolin

Func. class.: Adrenergic β-2 agonist

Action: Causes increased contractility and heart rate by acting on β-receptors in heart; also, acts on α-receptors causing vasoconstriction in blood vessels when larger doses are administered, causing vasodilation in renal, intracerebral, coronary dopaminergic receptors

Uses: Prevention of exercise-induced asthma, bronchospasm

Dosage and routes:

Asthma

• *Adult:* INH 2 puffs 15 min before exercising

Bronchospasm

• *Adult:* INH 1-2 puffs q4-6h PO 2-4 mg tid-qid, not to exceed 8 mg

Available forms include: Aerosol 90 μg/actuation; tabs 2, 4 mg; syr 2 mg/ml

Side effects/adverse reactions:

CNS: Tremors, anxiety, insomnia, headache, dizziness, stimulation, restlessness, hallucinations

EENT: Dry nose, irritation of nose and throat

CV: Palpitations, tachycardia, hypertension, angina, hypotension

GI: Heartburn, nausea, vomiting

MS: Muscle cramps

RESP: Bronchospasm

Contraindications: Hypersensitivity to sympathomimetics

Precautions: Lactation, pregnancy, cardiac disorders, hyperthyroidism, diabetes mellitus

Pharmacokinetics:

PO: Onset ½ hr, peak 2½ hr, du-

ration 4-6 hr, half-life 2½ hr
INH: Onset 5-15 min, peak ½-2 hr, duration 3-6 hr, half-life 4 hr
Metabolized in the liver, excreted in urine, crosses placenta, breast milk, blood-brain barrier
Interactions/incompatibilities:
• Increased action of: aerosol bronchodilators
• Increased action of this drug: tricyclic antidepressants, MAOIs
• May inhibit action of this drug: other β-blockers
NURSING CONSIDERATIONS
Assess:
• Respiratory function: vital capacity, forced expiratory volume, ABGs
Administer:
• After shaking, exhale, place mouthpiece in mouth, inhale slowly, hold breath, remove, exhale slowly
• Gum, sips of water for dry mouth
Perform/provide:
• Storage in light-resistant container, do not expose to temperatures over 86° F
Evaluate:
• Therapeutic response: absence of dyspnea, wheezing after 1 hr
Teach patient/family:
• Not to use OTC medications, extra stimulation may occur
• Use of inhaler, review package insert with patient
• To avoid getting aerosol in eyes
• To wash inhaler in warm water qd and dry
• On all aspects of drug; avoid smoking, smoke-filled rooms, persons with respiratory infections
Treatment of overdose: Administer a β1-adrenergic blocker

allopurinol
(al-oh-pure′i-nole)
Lopurin, Zyloprim, Zurinol
Func. class.: Antigout drug
Chem. class.: Enzyme inhibitor

Action: Decreases uric acid levels by inhibiting conversion of xanthine oxidase to uric acid
Uses: Gout, hyperuricemia, impaired renal function, recurrent calcium oxalate calculi
Dosage and routes:
Gout/hyperuricemia
• *Adult:* PO 200-600 mg qd depending on severity
• *Child 6-10 yr:* 300 mg qd
• *Child <6 yr:* 150 mg qd
Impaired renal function
• *Adult:* PO 200 mg qd in adequate CrCl
Recurrent calculi
• *Adult:* PO 200-300 mg qd
Uric acid nephropathy prevention
• *Adult:* PO 600-800 mg qd × 2-3 days
Available forms include: Tabs 100, 300 mg
Side effects/adverse reactions:
*HEMA: **Agranulocytosis, thrombocytopenia, aplastic anemia, pancytopenia***
CNS: Headache, drowsiness, neuritis, dizziness
GI: Nausea, vomiting, anorexia, malaise, metallic taste, cramps, peptic ulcer
EENT: Retinopathy, cataracts
INTEG: Stomatitis, fever, chills, dermatitis, pruritus, purpura, erythema
Contraindications: Hypersensitivity
Precautions: Pregnancy, lactation, renal disease, hepatic disease
Pharmacokinetics:
PO: Peak 2-4 hr; excreted in feces,

urine, half-life 2-3 hr, terminal half-life 18-30 hr

Interactions/incompatibilities:
• Increased action: oral anticoagulants, chlorpropamide, cyclophosphamide, hydantoin, theophylline, vidarabine, thiazide diuretics
• Decreased effects of: probenecid
• Rash: ampicillin, amoxicillin

NURSING CONSIDERATIONS
Assess:
• Uric acid levels q2 wk; uric acid levels should be 6 mg/dl
• CBC, AST, BUN, creatinine before starting treatment, monthly
• I&O ratio; increase fluids to prevent stone formation

Administer:
• With meals, to prevent GI symptoms
• A few days before antineoplastic therapy

Evaluate:
• Therapeutic response: decreased pain in joints, decreased stone formation in kidney
• Nutritional status: discourage organ meat, sardines, salmon, legumes, gravies (high purine foods)

Teach patient/family:
• To report skin rash, stomatitis, malaise, fever, aching; drug should be d/c'd
• To avoid hazardous activities if drowsiness or dizziness occurs
• To avoid alcohol, caffeine; will increase uric acid levels
• Avoid large doses of vitamin C; kidney stone formation may occur

Lab test interferences:
Increase: AST/ALT, alk phosphatase
Decrease: Hct/Hgb, leukocytes

alprazolam

(al-pray'zoe-lam)
Xanax
Func. class.: Antianxiety
Chem. class.: Benzodiazepine

Controlled Substance Schedule IV
Action: Depresses subcortical levels of CNS, including limbic system, reticular formation
Uses: Anxiety, panic disorders, anxiety with depressive symptoms
Dosage and routes:
• *Adult:* PO 0.25-0.5 mg tid, not to exceed 4 mg in divided doses/day
• *Geriatric:* PO 0.25 mg bid-tid
Available forms include: Tab 0.25, 0.5, 1 mg
Side effects/adverse reactions:
CNS: Dizziness, drowsiness, confusion, headache, anxiety, tremors, stimulation, fatigue, depression, insomnia, hallucinations
GI: Constipation, dry mouth, nausea, vomiting, anorexia, diarrhea
INTEG: Rash, dermatitis, itching
CV: Orthostatic hypotension, **ECG changes, tachycardia,** hypotension
EENT: Blurred vision, tinnitus, mydriasis
Contraindications: Hypersensitivity to benzodiazepines, narrow-angle glaucoma, psychosis, pregnancy (D), child <18 yr
Precautions: Elderly, debilitated, hepatic disease, renal disease
Pharmacokinetics:
PO: Onset 30 min, peak 1-2 hr, duration 4-6 hr, therapeutic response 2-3 days, metabolized by liver, excreted by kidneys, crosses placenta, breast milk, half-life 12-15 hr
Interactions/incompatibilities:
• Increased CNS depressants: an-

---

ticonvulsants, alcohol

• Decreased action of this drug: disulfiram, cimetidine

• Decreased action of: levodopa

NURSING CONSIDERATIONS

Assess:

• B/P (lying, standing), pulse; if systolic B/P drops 20 mm Hg, hold drug, notify physician

• Blood studies: CBC during long-term therapy; blood dyscrasias have occurred rarely

• Hepatic studies: AST, ALT, bilirubin, creatinine, LDH, alk phosphatase

• I&O; may indicate renal dysfunction

Administer:

• With food or milk for GI symptoms

• Crushed if patient is unable to swallow medication whole

• Sugarless gum, hard candy, frequent sips of water for dry mouth

Perform/provide:

• Assistance with ambulation during beginning therapy; drowsiness/dizziness occurs

• Safety measures, including side-rails

• Check to see PO medication has been swallowed

Evaluate:

• Therapeutic response: decreased anxiety, restlessness, sleeplessness

• Mental status: mood, sensorium, affect, sleeping pattern, drowsiness, dizziness

• Physical dependency, withdrawal symptoms: headache, nausea, vomiting, muscle pain, weakness after long-term use

• Suicidal tendencies

Teach patient/family:

• That drug may be taken with food

• Not to be used for everyday stress or longer than 4 mo, unless directed by physician

• Avoid OTC preparations unless approved by physician

• To avoid driving, activities that require alertness, since drowsiness may occur

• To avoid alcohol ingestion or other psychotropic medications, unless prescribed by physician

• Not to discontinue medication abruptly after long-term use

• To rise slowly or fainting may occur

• That drowsiness might worsen at beginning of treatment

Lab test interferences:

Increase: AST/ALT, serum bilirubin

False increase: 17-OHCS

Decrease: RAIU

Treatment of overdose: Lavage, VS, supportive care

---

alprostadil

(al-pros′ta-dil)

Prostin VR Pediatric

Func. class.: Hormone

Chem. class.: Prostaglandin

Action: Relaxes smooth muscles of ductus arteriosus; results in increased O_2 content throughout body

Uses: Patent ductus arteriosus (palliative treatment)

Dosage and routes:

• *Infants:* IV INF 0.1 µg/kg/min, until desired response, then reduce to lowest effective amount, not to exceed 0.4 µg/kg/min

Available forms include: Inj IV 500 µg/ml

Side effects/adverse reactions:

RESP: Apnea

HEMA: DIC (disseminated intravascular clotting), *thrombocytopenia*

CNS: Fever, convulsions, lethargy

GI: Diarrhea, regurgitation

GU: Oliguria, hematuria, *anuria*

INTEG: Rash on face, arms, alopecia, flushing

CV: Bradycardia, tachycardia, hy-

potension, **CHF,** ventricular fibril-lation, shock

Contraindications: Hypersensitiv-ity, respiratory distress syndrome (RDS)

Precautions: Bleeding disorders

Pharmacokinetics:

PO: 15-30 min, metabolized in lungs, up to 80%, excreted in urine (metabolites)

Interactions/incompatibilities:

None known

NURSING CONSIDERATIONS

Assess:

• ABGs, arterial pH, arterial pres-sure, continuous ECG; if arterial pressure decreases, reduce or stop drug

Administer:

• Only with emergency equipment available

• After diluting with NS or D_5W injection

Perform/provide:

• Refrigeration for drug; discard all mixed unused portion

Evaluate:

• Apnea and bradycardia; if these occur, discontinue drug

• Therapeutic response: increased PO_2 (cyanotic heart disease)

• Increased pH, B/P, output, de-creased ratio of PA to AP (restricted systemic blood flow)

Teach patient/family:

• To report change in urine pat-terns, difficulty breathing, or rash

---

aluminum acetate

Burow's Solution, Buro-Sol, mod-ified Burow's solution, Bluboro, Domeboro

Func. class.: Astringent
Chem. class.: Aluminum product

Action: Maintains skin acidity, which is protective to skin surface
Uses: Skin irritation, inflamma-tion, athlete's foot, insect bites,

poison ivy, eczema, acne, rash, bruises, pruritus (anal)

Dosage and routes:

• *Adult and child:* TOP apply for 15-30 min, q4-8h (1:10-40); Gar-gle use 1:10 sol prn

Available forms include: Topical solution

Side effects/adverse reactions:

INTEG: Irritation, increasing in-flammation

Contraindications: Tight, occlu-sive dressing

Interactions/incompatibilities:

• Inhibits action of topical colla-genase ointment

• Soap decreases action

NURSING CONSIDERATIONS

Administer:

• 1 pk/1 pt water

Perform/provide:

• Wet dressings using only loose fitting dressing

Evaluate:

• Area of body to receive topical application, irritation, rash, breaks, dryness

Teach patient/family:

• To discontinue use if irritation occurs

• To avoid using near eye area

• To retain otic preparation for 2-3 min

---

aluminum carbonate gel

Basaljel

Func. class.: Antacid
Chem. class.: Aluminum product

Action: Neutralizes gastric acidity, binds phosphates in GI tract, these phosphates are excreted

Uses: Urinary antacid, phosphate stones (prevention)

Dosage and routes:

Urinary phosphate stones

• *Adult:* SUSP 5-10 ml as needed; EXTRA STREN SUSP 2.5-5 ml as needed; PO 1-2 as needed

---

Antacid
• *Adult:* SUSP 15-30 ml in water or juice 1 hr pc, hs; EXTRA STREN SUSP 5-15 ml in water or juice 1 hr pc, hs; PO 2-6 1 hr pc, hs

Available forms include: Caps 500, 608 mg; tabs 500, 608 mg; susp 400/5 ml; extra stren susp 1000/ml

Side effects/adverse reactions:

GI: Constipation, anorexia, obstruction, fecal impaction

META: Hypophosphatemia, hypercalciuria

Contraindications: Hypersensitivity to this drug or aluminum products

Precautions: Elderly, fluid restriction, decreased GI motility, GI obstruction, dehydration, renal disease, sodium-restricted diets

Pharmacokinetics:

PO: Excreted in feces

Interactions/incompatibilities:

• Decreased effectiveness of: tetracyclines, ketoconazole

• Decreased absorption of: anticholinergics, chlordiazepoxide, cimetidine, corticosteroids, iron salts, phenothiazines, phenytoin, fat-soluble vitamins, digitalis

NURSING CONSIDERATIONS

Administer:

• Laxatives, or stool softeners if constipation occurs

Evaluate:

• Therapeutic response: absence of pain, decreased acidity

• Hypophosphatemia: anorexia, weakness, fatigue, bone pain, hyporeflexia

• Constipation, may need to switch to magnesium antacid

• Phosphate levels, urinary pH, Ca^+, electrolytes

Teach patient/family:

• Increase fluids to 2000 ml/day unless contraindicated

• Avoid phosphate foods (most dairy products, eggs, fruits, carbonated beverages) during drug therapy

• Add cheese, corn, pasta, plums, prunes, lentils after drug is discontinued

---

aluminum hydroxide

ALternaGel, Alu-Cap, Al-U-Creme, Alugel,* Aluminett, Amphojel, Basaljel,* Dialume, Hydroxal, No-Co-Gel, Nutrajel

Func. class.: Antacid
Chem. class.: Aluminum product

Action: Neutralizes gastric acidity, binds phosphates in GI tract, these phosphates are excreted

Uses: Antacid, hyperphosphatemia in chronic renal failure

Dosage and routes:

• *Adult:* SUSP 5-10 ml 1 hr pc, hs; PO 600 mg 1 hr pc, hs, chewed with milk or water

Hyperphosphatemia in renal failure

• *Adult:* SUSP 500 mg-2 g bid-qid

Available forms include: Caps 475, 500 mg; tabs 300, 500 mg; chewable tabs 600 mg; susp (4%) 600 mg/5 ml; liq 600 mg/5 ml

Side effects/adverse reactions:

GI: Constipation, anorexia, *obstruction,* fecal impaction

META: Hypophosphatemia, hypercalciuria

Contraindications: Hypersensitivity to this drug or aluminum products

Precautions: Elderly, fluid restriction, decreased GI motility, GI obstruction, dehydration, renal disease, sodium-restricted diets

Pharmacokinetics:

PO: Onset 20-40 min, excreted in feces

Interactions/incompatibilities:

• Decreased effectiveness of: tetracyclines

NURSING CONSIDERATIONS
Assess:
• Phosphate levels since drug is bound in GI system
Administer:
• Laxatives, or stool softeners if constipation occurs
• After shaking liquid
Evaluate:
• Therapeutic response: absence of pain, decreased acidity
• Hypophosphatemia: anorexia, weakness, fatigue, bone pain, hyporeflexia
• Constipation, increase bulk in diet if needed
• Phosphate levels, urinary pH, Ca^+, electrolytes
Teach patient/family:
• Increase fluids to 2000 ml/day unless contraindicated
• Avoid phosphate foods (most dairy products, eggs, fruits, carbonated beverages) during drug therapy
• Add cheese, corn, pasta, plums, prunes, lentils after drug is discontinued

---

aluminum phosphate
Phosphaljel
Func. class.: Antacid
Chem. class.: Aluminum products

Action: Neutralizes gastric acidity, binds phosphates in GI tract, these phosphates are excreted
Uses: Antacid
Dosage and routes:
• *Adult:* SUSP 5-10 ml 1 hr pc, hs
Available forms include: Susp 233 mg/5 ml
Side effects/adverse reactions:
GI: Constipation, anorexia, ***obstruction,*** fecal impaction
META: Hyperphosphatemia
Contraindications: Hypersensitivity to this drug or aluminum products

Precautions: Elderly, fluid restriction, decreased GI motility, GI obstruction, dehydration, renal disease, sodium-restricted diets
Pharmacokinetics:
PO: Onset 20-40 min, excreted in feces
Interactions/incompatibilities:
• Decreased effectiveness of: tetracyclines
NURSING CONSIDERATIONS
Administer:
• Laxatives, or stool softeners if constipation occurs
• After shaking solution
Evaluate:
• Therapeutic response: absence of pain, decreased acidity
• Constipation, increase bulk in diet if needed or alternate with magnesium antacids
• Phosphate levels, urinary pH, Ca^+, electrolytes
Teach patient/family:
• Increase fluids to 2000 ml unless contraindicated
• Not to switch antacids unless directed by physician

---

amantadine HCl
(a-man'ta-deen)
Symmetrel
Func. class.: Antiviral, antiparkinsonian agent
Chem. class.: Tricyclic amine

Action: Prevents uncoating of nucleic acid in viral cell, preventing penetration of virus to host
Uses: Prophylaxis or treatment of influenza type A, extrapyramidal reactions, parkinsonism, respiratory tract infections
Dosage and routes:
Influenza type A
• *Adult and child >9 yr:* PO 200 mg/day in single dose or divided bid
• *Child 1-9 yr:* PO 4.4-8.8 mg/kg/

---

day divided bid-tid, not to exceed 150 mg/day

Extrapyramidal reaction/parkinsonism

• *Adult:* PO 100 mg bid, up to 400 mg/day in EPS; give for 1 wk then 100 mg as needed in parkinsonism

Available forms include: Caps 100 mg; syr 50 mg/5 ml

Side effects/adverse reactions:

CNS: Headache, dizziness, drowsiness, fatigue, anxiety, psychosis, depression, hallucinations, tremors, convulsions

CV: Orthostatic hypotension, *CHF*

INTEG: Photosensitivity, dermatitis

EENT: Blurred vision

HEMA: Leukopenia

GI: Nausea, vomiting, constipation, dry mouth

GU: Frequency, retention

Contraindications: Hypersensitivity, lactation, child <1 yr, pregnancy (C)

Precautions: Epilepsy, CHF, orthostatic hypotension, psychiatric disorders, hepatic disease, renal disease

Pharmacokinetics:

PO: Onset 48 hr, half-life 24 hr, not metabolized, excreted in urine (90%) unchanged, crosses placenta, excreted in breast milk

Interactions/incompatibilities:

• Increased anticholingeric response: atropine, other anticholinergics

• Increased CNS stimulation: CNS stimulants

NURSING CONSIDERATIONS

Assess:

• I&O ratio; report frequency, hesitancy

Administer:

• Before exposure to influenza; continue for 10 days after contact

• At least 4 hr before hs to prevent insomnia

• After meals for better absorption, to decrease GI symptoms

• In divided doses to prevent CNS disturbances: headache, dizziness, fatigue, drowsiness

Perform/provide:

• Storage in tight, dry container

Evaluate:

• Therapeutic response: absence of temperature, malaise, cough, dyspnea in infection; tremors, shuffling, gait in Parkinson's disease

• Bowel pattern before, during treatment

• Skin eruptions, photosensitivity after administration of drug

• Respiratory status: rate, character, wheezing, tightness in chest

• Allergies before initiation of treatment, reaction of each medication; place allergies on chart, Kardex in bright red letters; notify all people giving drugs

Teach patient/family:

• Change body position slowly to prevent orthostatic hypotension

• Aspects of drug therapy: need to report dyspnea, weight gain, dizziness, poor concentration, dysuria, behavioral changes

• To avoid hazardous activities if dizziness occurs

• To take drug exactly as prescribed; parkinsonian crisis may occur if drug is discontinued abruptly

Treatment of overdose: Withdraw drug, maintain airway, administer epinephrine, aminophylline, O_2, IV corticosteroids

---

ambenonium chloride

(am-be-noe'nee-um)
Mytelase caplets

Func. class.: Cholinergics

Chem. class.: Synthetic quarternary ammonium compound

Action: Inhibits destruction of acetylcholine, which increases concentration at sites where acetylcholine is released; this facilitates transmission of impulses across myoneural junction

Uses: Myasthenia gravis when other drugs cannot be used

Dosage and routes:

• *Adult:* PO 5 mg q3-4h, then gradually increased q1-2 days, usually 5-25 mg is sufficient

Available forms include: Tabs 10 mg

Side effects/adverse reactions:

INTEG: Rash, urticaria

CNS: Dizziness, headache, sweating, confusion, weakness, *convulsions,* incoordination, *paralysis*

GI: Nausea, diarrhea, vomiting, cramps

CV: Tachycardia

GU: Frequency, incontinence

RESP: Respiratory depression, bronchospasm, constriction

EENT: Miosis, blurred vision, lacrimation

Contraindications: Bradycardia, hypotension, obstruction of intestine, renal system

Precautions: Seizure disorders, bronchial asthma, coronary occlusion, hyperthyroidism, dysrhythmias, peptic ulcer, megacolon, poor GI motility

Pharmacokinetics:

PO: Onset 2-30 min, duration 3-8 hr

Interactions/incompatibilities:

• Decreased action of this drug: aminoglycosides, anesthetics, antidysrhythmics, mecamylamine, polymyxin, quinidine

• Increased action of: neuromuscular blockers

NURSING CONSIDERATIONS

Assess:

• VS, respiration q8h

• I&O ratio; check for urinary retention or incontinence

Administer:

• Only with atropine sulfate available for cholinergic crisis

• Only after all other cholinergics have been discontinued

• Increased doses if tolerance occurs

• With food or milk to decrease GI symptoms; may decrease action of this drug

• Larger doses after exercise or fatigue

• On empty stomach for better absorption

Perform/provide:

• Storage at room temperature

Evaluate:

• Therapeutic response: increased muscle strength, improved gait, absence of labored breathing (if severe)

• Bradycardia, hypotension, bronchospasm, headache, dizziness, convulsions, respiratory depression; drug should be discontinued if toxicity occurs

• Muscle strength: hand grasp

Teach patient/family:

• To take drug exactly as prescribed

• That drug is not a cure, it only relieves symptoms

• All aspects of drug: action, side effects, dose, when to notify physician

• To wear Medic Alert ID specifying myasthenia gravis, drugs taken

---

amcinonide

(am-sin'oh-nide)

Cyclocort

Func. class.: Topical corticosteroid

Chem. class.: Synthetic fluorinated agent, group II potency

Action: Possesses antipruritic, antiinflammatory actions

Uses: Psoriasis, eczema, contact dermatitis, pruritus

Dosage and routes:

• *Adult and child:* Apply to affected area bid-tid, rub completely into skin

Available forms include: Cream 0.1%; oint 0.1%

Side effects/adverse reactions:

INTEG: Burning, dryness, itching, irritation, acne, folliculitis, hypertrichosis, perioral dermatitis, hypopigmentation, atrophy, striae, miliaria, allergic contact dermatitis, secondary infection

Contraindications: Hypersensitivity to corticosteroids, fungal infections

Precautions: Pregnancy (C), lactation, viral infections, bacterial infections

Interactions/incompatibilities: None known

NURSING CONSIDERATIONS

Assess:

• Temperature, worsening of rash; if fever develops drug should be discontinued

Administer:

• Only to affected areas; do not get in eyes

• Medication, then cover with occlusive dressing (only if prescribed), seal to normal skin, change q12h

• Only to dermatoses; do not use on weeping, denuded, or infected area

Perform/provide:

• Cleansing before application of drug

• Treatment for a few days after area has cleared

• Storage at room temperature

Evaluate:

• Therapeutic response: absence of severe itching, patches on skin, flaking

Teach patient/family:

• To avoid sunlight on affected area; burns may occur

• If local irritation or fever develops, discontinue drug, notify physician

amdinocillin

(am-din-oh-sill'in)
Coactin

Func. class.: Broad spectrum antibiotic

Chem. class.: Penicillin-Misc. B-Lactam

Action: Interferes with cell wall replication of susceptible organisms; the cell wall, rendered osmotically unstable, swells, bursts from osmotic pressure

Uses: Gram-negative organisms (*Serratia, Citrobacter, Enterobacter, Shigella, Salmonella, Klebsiella, E. coli);* in combination with other antibiotics *(P. mirabilis, P. morganii, Providencia)*

Dosage and routes:

• *Adult:* IM/IV 10 mg/kg q4-6h

Available forms include: Powder for inj IM, IV 500 mg, 1 g

Side effects/adverse reactions:

HEMA: Anemia, increased bleeding time, *bone marrow depression, granulocytopenia*

GI:Nausea, vomiting, diarrhea, increased AST, ALT, abdominal pain, glossitis, colitis

GU: Oliguria, proteinuria, hematuria, *vaginitis, moniliasis, glomerulonephritis*

CNS: Lethargy, hallucinations, anxiety, depression, twitching, *coma, convulsions*

META: Hyperkalemia, hypokalemia, alkalosis, hypernatremia

Contraindications: Hypersensitivity to penicillins; neonates

Precautions: Hypersensitivity to cephalosporins, allergies, renal disease, hepatic disease, myasthenia gravis, pregnancy (B)

Interactions/incompatibilities:

• Decreased antimicrobial effectiveness of this drug: tetracyclines, erythromycins

• Increased penicillin concentrations when used with: aspirin, probenicid
Pharmacokinetics:
IM: Peak 24-45 min
IV: Peak 2-3 hr
NURSING CONSIDERATIONS
Assess:
• I&O ratio; report hematuria, oliguria since penicillin in high doses is nephrotoxic
• Any patient with a compromised renal system since drug is excreted slowly in poor renal system function; toxicity may occur rapidly
• Liver studies: AST, ALT
• Blood studies: WBC, RBC, H&H, bleeding time
• Renal studies: urinalysis, protein, blood
• Culture, sensitivity before drug therapy; drug may be taken as soon as culture is taken
• On empty stomach for best absorption
Administer:
• IV, check site for inflammation, extravasation
• Drug after C&S completed
Perform/provide:
• Adrenaline, suction, tracheostomy set, endotracheal intubation equipment on the unit
• Adequate intake of fluids (2000 ml) during diarrhea episodes
• Scratch test to assess allergy after securing order from physician; usually done when penicillin is only drug of choice
• Storage of reconstituted solution at room temperature for 24 hr or 3 days refrigerated
Evaluate:
• Therapeutic effectiveness: absence of temperature, draining wounds
• Bowel pattern before, during treatment
• Skin eruptions after administra-

tion of penicillin to 1 wk after discontinuing drug
• Respiratory status: rate, character, wheezing, tightness in chest
• Allergies before initiation of treatment, reaction of each medication; place allergies on chart, Kardex in bright red
Teach patient/family:
• Aspects of drug therapy: need to complete entire course of medication to ensure organism death (10-14 days); culture may be taken after completed course of medication
• To report sore throat, fever, fatigue (could indicate a superimposed infection)
• To wear or carry a Medic Alert ID if allergic to penicillins
• To notify nurse of diarrhea stools
Lab test interferences:
False positive: Urine glucose, urine protein
Decrease: Uric acid
Treatment of overdose: Withdraw drug, maintain airway, administer epinephrine, aminophylline, O_2, IV corticosteroids for anaphylaxis

---

amikacin sulfate
(am-i-kay'sin)
Amikin
Func. class.: Antibiotic
Chem. class.: Aminoglycoside

Action: Interferes with protein synthesis in bacterial cell by binding to ribosomal subunit, which causes misreading of genetic code; inaccurate peptide sequence forms in protein chain, causing bacterial death
Uses: Severe systemic infections of CNS, respiratory, GI, urinary tract, bone, skin, soft tissues caused by *P. aeruginosa, E. coli, Enterobacter, Acinetobacter, Providencia, Citrobacter, Staphylococcus, Serratia, Proteus*

Dosage and routes:
Severe systemic infections
• *Adult and child:* IV INF 15 mg/kg/day in 2-3 divided doses q8-12h in 100-200 ml D_5W over 30-60 min, not to exceed 1.5 g; decreased doses are needed in poor renal function as determined by blood levels, renal function studies; IM 15 mg/kg/day in divided doses q8-12h
• *Neonates:* IV INF 10 mg/kg initially, then 7.5 mg/kg q12h in D_5W over 1-2 hr
Severe urinary tract infections
• *Adults:* IM 250 mg bid
• *Adults with poor renal function:* 7.5 mg/kg initially, then increased as determined by blood levels, renal function studies
Available forms include: Inj IM, IV 50, 250 mg/ml
Side effects/adverse reactions:
GU: Oliguria, hematuria, renal damage, azotemia, failure, nephrotoxicity
CNS: Confusion, depression, numbness, tremors, *convulsions,* muscle twitching, *neurotoxicity*
EENT: Ototoxicity, deafness, visual disturbances
HEMA: Agranulocytosis, thrombocytopenia, leukopenia, eosinophilia, anemia
GI: Nausea, vomiting, anorexia, increased ALT, AST, bilirubin, hepatomegaly, *hepatic necrosis,* splenomegaly, diarrhea, steatorrhea
CV: Hypotension
INTEG: Rash, burning, urticaria, photosensitivity, dermatitis
Contraindications: Mild to moderate infections, severe renal disease, hypersensitivity
Precautions: Neonates, mild renal disease, pregnancy (D), myasthenia gravis, lactation, hearing deficits, Parkinson's disease, elderly
Pharmacokinetics:
IM: Onset rapid, peak 1-2 hr

IV: Onset immediate, peak 1-2 hr
Plasma half-life 2-3 hr; not metabolized, excreted unchanged in urine, crosses placental barrier
Interactions/incompatibilities:
• Increased ototoxicity, neurotoxicity, nephrotoxicity: other aminoglycosides, amphotericin B, polymyxin, vancomycin, ethacrynic acid, furosemide, mannitol, methoxyflurane, cisplatin, cephalosporins
• Decreased effects of: parenteral penicillins, digoxin, vitamin B_{12}
• Do not mix in solution or syringe: carbenicillin, ticarcillin, amphotericin B, cephalothin, erythromycin, heparin
NURSING CONSIDERATIONS
Assess:
• Weight before treatment; calculation of dosage is usually done based on ideal body weight, but may be calculated on actual body weight
• I&O ratio, urinalysis daily for proteinuria, cells, casts; report sudden change in urine output
• VS during infusion, watch for hypotension, change in pulse
• IV site for thrombophlebitis including pain, redness, swelling q30 min, change site if needed; apply warm compresses to discontinued site
• Serum peak, drawn at 30-60 min after IV infusion or 60 min after IM injection, trough level drawn just before next dose; blood level should be 2-4 times bacteriostatic level
• Urine pH if drug is used for UTI; urine should be kept alkaline
Administer:
• IM injection in large muscle mass, rotate injection sites
• Drug in evenly spaced doses to maintain blood level
• Bicarbonate to alkalinize urine if

ordered for UTI, as drug is most active in alkaline environment

Perform/provide:

• Adequate fluids of 2-3 L/day unless contraindicated to prevent irritation of tubules

• Flush of IV line with NS or D_5W after infusion

• Supervised ambulation, other safety measures with vestibular dysfunction

Evaluate:

• Therapeutic effect: absence of fever, draining wounds, negative C&S after treatment

• Renal impairment by securing urine for CrCl testing, BUN, serum creatinine; lower dosage should be given in renal impairment (CrCl <80 ml/min)

• Deafness by audiometric testing, ringing, roaring in ears, vertigo; assess hearing before, during, after treatment

• Dehydration: high sp gr, decrease in skin turgor, dry mucous membranes, dark urine

• Overgrowth of infection including increased temperature, malaise, redness, pain, swelling, perineal itching, diarrhea, stomatitis, change in cough, sputum

• C&S before starting treatment to identify organism

• Vestibular dysfunction: nausea, vomiting, dizziness, headache; drug should be discontinued if severe

• Injection sites for redness, swelling, abscesses; use warm compresses at site

Teach patient/family:

• To report headache, dizziness, symptoms for overgrowth of infection, renal impairment

• To report loss of hearing, ringing, roaring in ears or feeling of fullness in head

Treatment of overdose: Hemodialysis, monitor serum levels of drug

amiloride HCl

(a-mill′oh-ride)
Midamor
Func. class.: Potassium-sparing diuretic
Chem. class.: Pyrazine

Action: Acts primarily on distal tubule, secondarily by inhibiting reabsorption of sodium, potassium

Uses: Edema in CHF in combination with other diuretics, for hypertension

Dosage and routes:

• *Adult:* PO 5 mg qd, may be increased to 10-20 mg qd if needed

Available forms include: Tab 5 mg

Side effects/adverse reactions:

GU: Polyuria, gynecomastia, ejaculatory problems, dysuria, frequency, impotence

ELECT: Hypochloremic alkalosis, hypomagnesemia, hyperuricemia, hypocalcemia, hyponatremia, hyperkalemia

CNS: Headache, dizziness, fatigue, weakness, headache, paresthesias

GI: Nausea, diarrhea, dry mouth, vomiting, anorexia, cramps, constipation, pancreatitis, dry mouth, abdominal pain

EENT: Loss of hearing, tinnitus, blurred vision, nasal congestion, increased intraocular pressure

INTEG: Rash, pruritus, photosensitivity, alopecia, urticaria

MS: Cramps

*HEMA: **Thrombocytopenia, agranulocytosis, leukopenia, neutropenia, anemia***

CV: Orthostatic hypotension

Contraindications: Anuria

Precautions: Dehydration, ascites, hepatic disease, severe renal disease, pregnancy (B)

Pharmacokinetics:

PO: Onset 2 hr, peak 6-10 hr, duration 24 hr; excreted in urine, feces, crosses placenta, excreted in breast milk, half-life 6-9 hr

Interactions/incompatibilities:

• Enhanced action of: antihypertensives, lithium

• Hyperkalemia: other potassium-sparing diuretics, potassium products

NURSING CONSIDERATIONS

Assess:

• Weight, I&O daily to determine fluid loss; effect of drug may be decreased if used qd

• Rate, depth, rhythm of respiration, effect of exertion

• B/P lying, standing; postural hypotension may occur

• Electrolytes: potassium, sodium, chloride; include BUN, CBC, serum creatinine, blood pH, ABGs

Administer:

• In AM to avoid interference with sleep if using drug as a diuretic

• With food, if nausea occurs, absorption may be decreased slightly

Evaluate:

• Improvement in edema of feet, legs, sacral area daily if medication is being used in CHF

• Improvement in CVP q8h

• Signs of metabolic acidosis: drowsiness, restlessness

• Rashes, temperature elevation qd

• Confusion especially in elderly; take safety precautions if needed

Teach patient/family:

• To increase fluid intake 2-3 L/day unless contraindicated; to rise slowly from lying or sitting position

• Adverse reactions: muscle cramps, weakness, nausea, dizziness

• Take with food or milk for GI symptoms

• Take early in day to prevent nocturia

• Avoid potassium-rich foods: oranges, bananas

Lab test interferences:

Interfere: GTT

Treatment of overdose: Lavage if taken orally, monitor electrolytes, administer sodium bicarbonate for $K^+ >6.5$ mEq/L

amino acid injection

(a-mee'noe)

FreAmine HBC, HepatAmine

Func. class.: Caloric

Action: Needed for anabolism to maintain structure, decrease catabolism, promote healing

Uses: Hepatic encephalopathy, cirrhosis, hepatitis, nutritional support in cancer

Dosage and routes:

• *Adult:* IV 80-120 g/day; 500 ml of amino acids/500 ml $D_{50}W$ given over 24 hr

Available forms include: Inj IV many strengths, types

Side effects/adverse reactions:

CNS: Dizziness, headache, confusion, loss of consciousness

CV: Hypertension, *CHF, pulmonary edema*

GI: Nausea, vomiting, liver fat deposits, abdominal pain

GU: Glycosuria, osmotic diuresis

ENDO: Hyperglycemia, rebound hypoglycemia, electrolyte imbalances, hyperosmolar syndrome, hyperosmolar hyperglycemic nonketotic syndrome, alkalosis, acidosis, hypophosphatemia, hyperammonemia, dehydration, hypocalcemia

INTEG: Chills, flushing, warm feeling, rash, urticaria, extravasation necrosis, phlebitis at injection site

Contraindications: Hypersensitivity, severe electrolyte imbalances, anuria, severe liver damage, maple syrup urine disease

Precautions: Renal disease, pregnancy (C), children, diabetes mellitus, CHF

Interactions/incompatibilities:
None known
NURSING CONSIDERATIONS
Assess:
• Electrolytes (K, Na, Ca, Cl, Mg), blood glucose, ammonia, phosphate
• Renal, liver function studies: BUN, creatinine, ALT, AST, bilirubin
• Injection site for extravasation: redness along vein, edema at site, necrosis, pain, hard tender area; site should be changed immediately
• Monitor respiratory function q4h: auscultate lung fields bilaterally for rales, respirations, quality, rate, rhythm
• Monitor temperature q4h for increased fever, indicating infection; if infection suspected, infusion is discontinued, tubing bottle cultured
• Urine glucose q6h using Tes-Tape, Clinistix, Keto-Diastix, which are not affected by infusion substances
Administer:
• Total parenteral nutrition only mixed with dextrose to promote protein synthesis
• Immediately after mixing in pharmacy under strict aseptic technique using laminar flowhood, use infusion pump, in-line filter
• Using careful monitoring technique; do not speed up infusion; pulmonary edema, glucose overload will result
Perform/provide
• Storage depends on type of solution; consult manufacturer
• Changing dressing on IV site to prevent infection q24-48h
Evaluate:
• Hyperammonemia: nausea, vomiting, malaise, tremors, anorexia, convulsions
• Therapeutic response: weight gain, decrease in jaundice in liver disorders

Teach patient/family
• Reason for use of TPN
• If chills, sweating are experienced, they should be reported at once

---

amino acid solution
Aminosyn, FreAmine III, Novamine, Travsol
Func. class.: Caloric

Action: Needed for anabolism to maintain structure, decrease catabolism, promote healing
Uses: Hepatic encephalopathy, cirrhosis, hepatitis, nutritional support in cancer
Dosage and routes:
• *Adult:* IV 1-1.5 g/kg/day titrated to patient's needs
• *Child:* IV 2-3 g/kg/day titrated to patient's needs
Available forms include: Inj IV many types, strengths
Side effects/adverse reactions:
CNS: Dizziness, headache, confusion, loss of consciousness
CV: Hypertension, *CHF, pulmonary edema*
GI: Nausea, vomiting, liver fat deposits, abdominal pain
GU: Glycosuria, osmotic diuresis
ENDO: Hyperglycemia, rebound hypoglycemia, electrolyte imbalances, hyperosmolar syndrome, hyperosmolar hyperglycemic nonketotic syndrome, alkalosis, acidosis, hypophosphatemia, hyperammonemia, dehydration, hypocalcemia
INTEG: Chills, flushing, warm feeling, rash, urticaria, extravasation, necrosis, phlebitis at injection site
Contraindications: Hypersensitivity, severe electrolyte imbalances, anuria, severe liver damage, maple syrup urine disease
Precautions: Renal disease, preg-

nancy (C), children, diabetes mellitus, CHF

Interactions/incompatibilities:
None known

NURSING CONSIDERATIONS
Assess:
• Electrolytes (K, Na, Ca, Cl, Mg), blood glucose, ammonia, phosphate
• Renal, liver function studies: BUN, creatinine, ALT, AST, bilirubin
• Injection site for extravasation: redness along vein, edema at site, necrosis, pain, hard tender area; site should be changed immediately
• Monitor respiratory function q4h: auscultate lung fields bilaterally for rales, respirations, quality, rate, rhythm
• Monitor temperature q4h for increased fever, indicating infection; if infection suspected, infusion is discontinued, tubing, bottle cultured
• Urine glucose q6h using Tes-Tape, Clinistix, Keto-Diastix, which are not affected by infusion substances

Administer:
• Total parenteral nutrition only mixed with dextrose to promote protein synthesis
• Immediately after mixing in pharmacy under strict aseptic technique using laminar flowhood, use infusion pump, in-line filter
• Using careful monitoring technique; do not speed up infusion; pulmonary edema, glucose overload will result

Perform/provide
• Storage depends on type of solution; consult manufacturer
• Changing dressing on IV site to prevent infection q24-48h

Evaluate:
• Hyperammonemia: nausea, vomiting, malaise, tremors, anorexia, convulsions

• Therapeutic response: weight gain, decrease in jaundice in liver disorders

Teach patient/family
• Reason for use of TPN
• If chills, sweating are experienced, they should be reported at once

---

aminocaproic acid

(a-mee-noe-ka-proe'ik)
Amicar, EACA

Func. class.: Hemostatic
Chem. class.: Synthetic monoaminocarboxylic acid

Action: Inhibits activation of profibrinolysin without inhibiting lysis of profibinolysin clot

Uses: Hemorrhage from hyperfibrinolysis, adjunctive therapy in hemophilia

Dosage and routes:
• *Adult:* PO/IV 5 g loading dose, then 1-1.25 g q1h if needed, not to exceed 30 g/day

Available forms include: Inj IV 250 mg/ml; tab 500 mg; syr 250 mg/ml

Side effects/adverse reactions:
GU: Dysuria, frequency, oliguria, *renal failure,* ejaculatory failure
GI: Nausea, vomiting, abdominal cramps, diarrhea
INTEG: Rash
CNS:Headache, dizziness, malaise, fatigue, hallucinations, delirium, psychosis, *convulsions*
HEMA: Thrombosis
CV: Dysrhythmias, orthostatic hypotension, bradycardia, myopathy
EENT: Tinnitus, nasal congestion, conjunctival suffusion

Contraindications: Hypersensitivity, frank infection, abnormal bleeding, postpartum bleeding, severe renal disease, DIC, upper urinary tract bleeding

Precautions: Neonates/infants,

mild or moderate renal disease, hepatic disease, thrombosis, cardiac disease, pregnancy (C)

Pharmacokinetics:
PO/IV: Peak 2 hr, excreted by kidneys as unmetabolized drug

Interactions/incompatibilities:
Increased coagulation: estrogens, anticoagulants (oral)

NURSING CONSIDERATIONS
Assess:
• I&O, if urinary output decreases, notify physician and stop drug
• Blood studies: coagulation factors, platelets, protamine coagulation test for extravascular clotting, thrombopheblitis
• B/P, pulse for increase
• Drug level: 0.13 mg/ml is required to decrease fibrinolysis
• Creatine phosphokinase, urinalysis

Administer:
• Give IV loading dose 30 min to avoid hypotension
• IV push slowly, with plastic syringe only
• After dilution with NS, D₅W, LR

Perform/provide:
• Storage in tight container in cool environment

Evaluate:
• Allergy: fever, rash, itching, jaundice
• Myopathy: if weakness, fever, myoglobinemia, or oliguria; discontinue drug
• Bleeding: mucous membrane, epistaxis, eccyhmosis, petechiae, hematuria, hematemesis

Teach patient/family:
• To report any signs of bleeding (gums, under skin, urine, stools, emesis) or myopathy
• To change position slowly to decrease orthostatic hypotension
• Proper administration for 8-10 days following dental procedure in hemophilia

Lab test interferences:
Increased: K⁺, CPK

---

aminoglutethimide
(a-meen-noe-gloo-te-th'i-mide)
Cytadren
Func. class.: Antineoplastic, adrenal steroid inhibitor
Chem. class.: Hormone

Action: Acts by inhibiting DNA, RNA, protein synthesis; is derived from *Streptomyces verticillus;* replication is decreased by binding to DNA, which causes strand splitting; phase specific in G_2 and M phases

Uses: Metastatic breast cancer, adrenal cancer, suppression of adrenal function in Cushing's syndrome

Dosage and routes:
• *Adult:* PO 250 mg qid at 6 hr intervals, may increase by 250 mg/day q1-2 wk, not to exceed 2 g/day

Available forms include: Tabs 250 mg

Side effects/adverse reactions:
*HEMA: **Thrombocytopenia, leukopenia, myelosuppression, anemia***
*GI: Nausea, vomiting, anorexia, **hepatotoxicity***
INTEG: Rash, pruritus, hirsutism
CV: Hypotension, tachycardia
CNS: Dizziness, headache

Contraindications: Hypersensitivity, hypothyroidism, pregnancy (D)

Precautions: Renal disease, hepatic disease, respiratory disease

Pharmacokinetics: Half-life 13 hr, metabolized in liver, excreted in urine, crosses placenta

Interactions/incompatibilities:
• Aminoglutethimide accelerates metabolism of dexamethasone; therefore if needed give hydrocortisone

NURSING CONSIDERATIONS
Assess:
• CBC, differential, platelet count weekly; withhold drug if WBC is <4000 or platelet count is <75,000; notify physician of these results
• Renal function studies: BUN, serum uric acid, urine CrCl, electrolytes before, during therapy
• I&O ratio; report fall in urine output of 30 ml/hr
• Monitor temperature q4h; may indicate beginning infection
• Liver function tests before, during therapy (bilirubin, AST, ALT, LDH) as needed or monthly
• RBC, Hct, Hgb, since these may be decreased

Administer:
• Medications by oral route if possible; avoid IM, SC, IV routes to prevent infections
• Antacid before oral agent; give drug after evening meal before bedtime
• Antiemetic 30-60 min before giving drug to prevent vomiting
• Antibiotics for prophylaxis of infection
• Local or systemic drugs for infection

Perform/provide:
• Strict medical asepsis, protective isolation if WBC levels are low
• Special skin care
• Liquid diet, including cola, Jello; dry toast or crackers may be added if patient is not nauseated or vomiting
• Nutritious diet with iron and vitamin supplements as ordered

Evaluate:
• Bleeding: hematuria, guaiac, bruising, petechiae, mucosa or orifices q8h
• Food preferences; list likes, dislikes
• Edema in feet, joint, stomach pain, shaking
• Inflammation of mucosa, breaks in skin
• Yellowing of skin, sclera, dark urine, clay-colored stools, itchy skin, abdominal pain, fever, diarrhea
• Symptoms indicating severe allergic reaction: rash, pruritus, urticaria, purpuric skin lesions, itching, flushing

Teach patient/family:
• To report any complaints, side effects to nurse or physician
• That masculinization can occur, is reversible after discontinuing treatment

---

aminophylline (theophylline ethylenediamine)
(am-in-off'i-lin)
Corophyllin,* Lixaminol, Phyllocontin, Somophyllin-DF

Func. class.: Spasmolytic
Chem. class.: Xanthine, ethylenediamide

Action: Relaxes smooth muscle of respiratory system by blocking phosphodiesterase, which increases cyclic AMP
Uses: Bronchial asthma, bronchospasm, Cheyne-Stokes respirations
Dosage and routes:
• *Adult:* PO 500 mg, then 250-500 mg q6-8h; CONT IV 0.3-0.9 mg/kg/hr (maintenance); RECT 500 mg q6-8h
• *Child:* PO 7.5 mg/kg, then 3-6 mg/kg q6-8h; IV 7.5 mg/kg, then 3-6 mg/kg q6-8h injected over 5 min, do not exceed 25 mg/min; may give loading dose of 5.6 mg/kg over ½ hr; CONT IV 1 mg/kg/hr (maintenance)

Available forms include: Inj IV, IM, rectal supp 250, 500 mg; rectal sol 300 mg/5 ml; elix 250 mg/5 ml; oral liq 105 mg/5 ml; tabs 100,

200 mg, tabs con-rel 225 mg; tabs sust-rel 300 mg

Side effects/adverse reactions:

CNS: Anxiety, restlessness, insomnia, dizziness, convulsions, headache, light-headedness

CV: Palpitations, sinus tachycardia, hypotension

GI: Nausea, vomiting, anorexia, diarrhea, bitter taste, dyspepsia, anal irritation (suppositories)

RESP: Increased rate

INTEG: Flushing, urticaria

Contraindications: Hypersensitivity to xanthines, tachydysrhythmias

Precautions: Elderly, CHF, cor pulmonale, hepatic disease, active peptic ulcer disease, diabetes mellitus, hyperthyroidism, hypertension, children

Pharmacokinetics:

IV: Peak 30 min

Interactions/incompatibilities:

• Do not mix in syringe with other drugs

• Increased action of this drug: cimetidine, propranolol, erythromycin, troleandomycin

• May increase effects of: anticoagulants

• Cardiotoxicity: β-blockade

NURSING CONSIDERATIONS

Assess:

• Theophylline blood levels (therapeutic level is 10-20 μg/ml); toxicity may occur with small increase above 20 μg/ml

• Monitor I&O; diuresis occurs, dehydration may result in elderly or children

• Whether theophylline was given recently

Administer:

• PO after meals to decrease GI symptoms; absorption may be affected

• IV after diluting in D_5W to decrease burning sensation at injection site; only clear solutions

• Avoid IM injection; pain occurs

Evaluate:

• Therapeutic response: decreased dyspnea, respiratory rate, rhythm

• Respiratory rate, rhythm, depth; auscultate lung fields bilaterally; notify physician of abnormalities

• Allergic reactions: rash, urticaria; if these occur, drug should be discontinued

Teach patient/family

• To check OTC medications, current prescription medications for ephedrine; will increase CNS stimulation

• To avoid hazardous activities; dizziness may occur

• On all aspects of drug therapy: dosage, routes, side effects, when to notify the physician

• If GI upset occurs, to take drug with 8 oz water; avoid food, since absorption may be decreased

• To remain in bed 15-20 min after rectal suppository is inserted to avoid removal

---

amiodarone HCl

(a-mee′-oh-da-rone)

Cordarone

Func. class.: Antidysrhythmic (Class III)

Chem. class.: Iodinated benzofuran derivative

Action: Increases SAN conduction, repolarization because of noncompetitive α-, β-adrenergic inhibition; also increases refractory period

Uses: Severe ventricular tachycardia, cardioversion, ventricular fibrillation

Dosage and routes:

• *Adult:* Loading dose 800-1600 mg 1-3 wk; then 600-800 mg 1 mo; maintenance 200-400 mg

Available forms include: Tabs 200 mg

Side effects/adverse reactions:

CNS: Headache, dizziness, involuntary movement, confusion, psychosis, anxiety, tremors, depression, hallucinations

GI: Nausea, vomiting, diarrhea, abdominal pain, anorexia, constipation, *hepatotoxicity*

CV: Hypotension, bradycardia, angina, PVCs, *sinus arrest, cardiogenic shock*

INTEG: Rash, photosensitivity

EENT: Blurred vision, halos, photophobia

ENDO: Hyperthyroidism or hypothyroidism

MS: Weakness, pain in extremities

RESP: Pulmonary fibrosis

Precautions: Goiter, Hashimoto's thyroiditis, sinus node dysfunction, AV block, 2, 3 electrolyte imbalances

Pharmacokinetics:

PO: Onset 1-3 wk, peak 2-10 hr; half-life 53 days; metabolized by liver, excreted by kidneys

Interactions/incompatibilities:

• Bradycardia: β-blockers, calcium channel blockers

• Increased effects of: digitalis

• Tachycardia: quinidine, disopyramide

• Increased anticoagulant effects: warfarin

• Bradycardia, arrest: lidocaine

NURSING CONSIDERATIONS

Assess:

• I&O ratio; electrolytes: K, Na, Cl

• Liver function studies: AST, ALT, bilirubin, alk phosphatase

• ECG continuously to determine drug effectiveness, check for PVCs, other dysrhythmias

• For dehydration or hypovolemia

• B/P continuously for hypotension, hypertension

Administer:

• Reduced dosage slowly with ECG monitoring

• By IV, but change should be made as soon as possible (PO)

Evaluate:

• For rebound hypertension after 1-2 hr

• CNS symptoms: confusion, psychosis, numbness, depression, involuntary movements; if these occur drug should be discontinued

• Hypothyroidism: lethargy, dizziness, constipation, enlarged thyroid gland, edema of extremities, cool, pale skin

• Hyperthyroidism: restlessness, tachycardia, eyelid puffiness, weight loss, frequent urination, menstrual irregularities, dyspnea, warm, moist skin

• Pulmonary toxicity: dyspnea, fatigue, cough, fever, chest pain; drug should be discontinued

• Cardiac rate, respiration: rate, rhythm, character, chest pain

Teach patient/family:

• Aspects of drug therapy: action, side effects, dosage, route, when to notify physician

• To use sunscreen or stay out of sun to prevent burns

• To report side effects immediately

• That skin discoloration is reversible

• That dark glasses may be needed for photophobia

Treatment of overdose: O_2, artificial ventilation, ECG, administer dopamine for circulatory depression, administer diazepam or thiopental for convulsions

---

amitriptyline HCl

(a-mee-trip'ti-leen)
Amitril, Elavil, Emitrip, Endep, Enovil, Levate,* Meravil,* Novotriptyn,* Rolavil*

Func. class.: Antidepressant—tricyclic
Chem. class.: Tertiary amine

Action: Blocks reuptake of norepinephrine, serotonin into nerve endings, increasing action of norepinephrine, serotonin in nerve cells

Uses: Endogenous depression

Dosage and routes:
• *Adult:* PO 50-100 mg hs, may increase to 200 mg qd, not to exceed 300 mg/day; IM 20-30 mg qid, or 80-120 mg hs
• *Adolescent/geriatric:* PO 30 mg/day in divided doses, may be increased to 150 mg/day

Available forms include: Tabs 10, 25, 50, 75, 100, 150 mg; inj IM 10 mg/ml

Side effects/adverse reactions:
*HEMA: **Agranulocytosis, thrombocytopenia, eosinophilia, leukopenia***
CNS: Dizziness, drowsiness, confusion, headache, anxiety, tremors, stimulation, weakness, insomnia, nightmares, EPS (elderly), increased psychiatric symptoms
GI: Diarrhea, dry mouth, nausea, vomiting, ***paralytic ileus,*** increased appetite, cramps, epigastric distress, jaundice, ***hepatitis,*** stomatitis
GU: Retention
INTEG: Rash, urticaria, sweating, pruritus, photosensitivity
*CV: Orthostatic hypotension, **ECG changes, tachycardia, hypertension,*** palpations
EENT: Blurred vision, tinnitus, mydriasis, ophthalmoplegia

Contraindications: Hypersensitivity to tricyclic antidepressants, recovery phase of myocardial infarction

Precautions: Suicidal patients, convulsive disorders, prostatic hypertrophy, schizophrenia, psychotic, severe depression, increased intraocular pressure, narrow-angle glaucoma, urinary retention, cardiac disease, hepatic disease/renal disease, hyperthyroidism, electroshock therapy, elective surgery, child <12 yr, pregnancy (C)

Pharmacokinetics:
PO/IM: Onset 45 min, peak 2-12 hr, therapeutic response 2-3 wk; metabolized by liver, excreted in urine/feces, crosses placenta, excreted in breast milk, half-life 10-50 hr

Interactions/incompatibilities:
• Decreased effects of: guanethidine, clonidine, indirect acting sympathomimetics (ephedrine)
• Increased effects of: direct acting sympathomimetics (epinephrine), alcohol, barbiturates, benzodiazepines, CNS depressants
• Hyperpyretic crisis, convulsions, hypertensive episode: MAOI (pargyline [Eutonyl])

NURSING CONSIDERATIONS

Assess:
• B/P (lying, standing), pulse q4h; if systolic B/P drops 20 mm Hg hold drug, notify physician; take vital signs q4h in patients with cardiovascular disease
• Blood studies: CBC, leukocytes, differential, cardiac enzymes if patient is receiving long-term therapy
• Hepatic studies: AST, ALT, bilirubin, creatinine
• Weight qwk, appetite may increase with drug
• ECG for flattening of T wave, bundle branch block, AV block, dysrhythmias in cardiac patients

---

italics = common side effects   ***bold italic*** = life threatening reactions

Administer:
• Increased fluids, bulk in diet if constipation, urinary retention occur
• With food or milk for GI symptoms
• Crushed if patient is unable to swallow medication whole
• Dosage hs if over-sedation occurs during day; may take entire dose hs; elderly may not tolerate once/day dosing
• Gum, hard candy, or frequent sips of water for dry mouth

Perform/provide:
• Storage at room temperature, do not freeze
• Assistance with ambulation during beginning therapy since drowsiness/dizziness occurs
• Safety measure including siderails primarily in elderly
• Checking to see PO medication swallowed

Evaluate:
• EPS primarily in elderly: rigidity, dystonia, akathisia
• Mental status: mood, sensorium, affect, suicidal tendencies; increase in psychiatric symptoms: depression, panic
• Urinary retention, constipation; constipation is more likely to occur in children
• Withdrawal symptoms: headache, nausea, vomiting, muscle pain, weakness; do not usually occur unless drug was discontinued abruptly
• Alcohol consumption; if alcohol is consumed, hold dose until morning

Teach patient/family:
• That therapeutic effects may take 2-3 wk
• Use caution in driving or other activities requiring alertness because of drowsiness, dizziness, blurred vision

• To avoid alcohol ingestion, other CNS depressants
• Not to discontinue medication quickly after long-term use, may cause nausea, headache, malaise
• To wear sunscreen or large hat since photosensitivity occurs

Lab test interferences:
Increase: Serum bilirubin, blood glucose, alk phosphatase
Decrease: VMA, 5-HIAA
False increase: Urinary catecholamines

Treatment of overdose: ECG monitoring, induce emesis, lavage, activated charcoal, administer anticonvulsant

ammonia, aromatic spirits

Func. class.: Respiratory stimulants
Chem. class.: Aromatic hydroalcoholic solution of ammonia

Action: Stimulates medulla (respiratory, vasomotor areas) by irritation of sensory receptors in mucosa of nasal passages, esophagus, stomach

Uses: To treat, prevent fainting

Dosage and routes:
• *Adult and child:* INH prn; PO 2-4 ml diluted in water
Available forms include: Inh 0.33, 0.4 ml; sol

Side effects/adverse reactions:
None known

Pharmacokinetics:
Not known

Interactions/incompatibilities:
None known

NURSING CONSIDERATIONS
Assess:
• Vital signs, B/P after administration of inhalant

Administer:
• By inhalation, do not place pack-

ets in pockets, may open, cause caustic burns

• Orally by diluting 2-4 ml in >30 ml of water

Perform/provide:

• Storage protected from light at room temperature

Evaluate:

• Cause of fainting

---

ammonium chloride

Func. class.: Acidifier
Chem. class.: Ammonium

Action: Lowers urinary pH, liberates hydrogen and chloride ions in blood and extracellular fluid with decreased pH and correction of alkalosis

Uses: Alkalosis (metabolic), systemic and urinary acidifer, expectorant, diuretic

Dosage and routes:

Alkalosis

• *Adult and child:* IV INF 0.9-1.3 ml/min of a 2.14% sol, not to exceed 2 ml/min

Acidifier

• *Adult:* PO 4-12 g/day in divided doses

• *Child:* PO 75 mg/kg/day in divided doses

Expectorant

• *Adult:* PO 250-500 mg q2-4h as needed

Available forms include: Tabs 500 mg, 1 g; inj IV 0.4, 5 mEq/ml

Side effects/adverse reactions:

CNS: Drowsiness, headache, confusion, stimulation, tremors, *twitching, hyperreflexia, tetany, EEG changes*

CV: Bradycardia, dysrhythmias, bounding pulse

GU: Glycosuria, thirst

GI: Gastric irritation, nausea, vomiting, anorexia, diarrhea

INTEG: Rash, pain at infusion site

META: Acidosis, hypokalemia, hy-perchloremia, hyperglycemia

RESP: **Apnea,** irregular respirations, hyperventilation

Contraindications: Hypersensitivity, severe hepatic disease, severe renal disease

Precautions: Severe respiratory disease, cardiac edema, infants, pregnancy (C), children

Pharmacokinetics:

PO: Absorbed in 3-6 hr; metabolized in liver, excreted in urine and feces

Interactions/incompatibilities:

• Increased toxicity: PAS

• Decreased effects of: amphetamines, tricyclic antidepressants

NURSING CONSIDERATIONS

Assess:

• Respiratory rate, rhythm, depth, notify physician of abnormalities that may indicate acidosis

• Electrolytes and CO_2, chloride before and during treatment

• Urine pH, urinary output, urine glucose, specific gravity during beginning treatment

• I&O ratio, report large increases or decreases

Administer:

• PO with meals if GI symptoms occur

• IV slowly to avoid pain at infusion site and toxicity

• After diluting solutions to 2.14% (IV)

• With water for expectorant

Evaluate:

• For CNS symptoms: confusion, twitching, hyperreflexia, stimulation, headache that may indicate ammonia toxicity

Teach patient/family:

• To increase potassium in diet: bananas, oranges, cantelope, honeydew, spinach, potatoes, dry fruit

Lab test interferences:

Increase: Blood ammonia, AST/ALT

---

italics = common side effects   **bold italic** = life threatening reactions

Decrease: Serum magnesium, urine urobilinogen

---

amobarbital/amobarbital sodium

(am-oh-bar'bi-tal)

Amytal, Isobec/Amytal sodium

Func. class.: Sedative/hypnotic-barbiturate (intermediate acting)

Chem. class.: Amylobarbitone

Controlled Substance Schedule II (USA), Schedule G (Canada)

Action: Depresses activity in brain cells primarily in reticular activating system in brainstem, also selectively depresses neurons in posterior hypothalamus, limbic structures; able to decrease seizure activity by inhibition of epileptic activity in CNS

Uses: Sedation, preanesthetic sedation, insomnia, anticonvulsant, adjunct in psychiatry, hypnotic

Dosage and routes:

Preanesthetic sedation

• *Adult and child:* PO/IM 200 mg 1-2 hr preoperatively

Sedation

• *Adult:* PO 30-50 mg bid or tid, may be from 15-120 mg bid-qid

• *Child:* PO 2 mg/kg/day in 4 divided doses

Anticonvulsant/psychiatry

• *Adult:* IV 65-500 mg given over several min, not to exceed 100 mg/min; not to exceed 1 g

• *Child* <6 yr: IV/IM 3-5 mg/kg over several min

Insomnia

• *Adult:* PO/IM 65-200 mg hs, not to exceed 5 ml in one site

• *Child:* IM 3-5 mg/kg at hs, not to exceed 5 ml in one site

Available forms include: Tabs 30, 50, 100 mg; caps 65, 200 mg; powder for inj IM, IV 250, 500 mg/vial

Side effects/adverse reactions:

CNS: Lethargy, drowsiness, hangover, dizziness, stimulation in the elderly and children, lightheadedness, physical dependence, CNS depression, mental depression, slurred speech

GI: Nausea, vomiting, diarrhea, constipation

INTEG: Rash, urticaria, pain, abscesses at injection site, angioedema, thrombophlebitis, *Stevens-Johnson syndrome*

CV: Hypotension, bradycardia

RESP: Depression, apnea, *laryngospasm, bronchospasm*

HEMA: Agranulocytosis, thrombocytopenia, megaloblastic anemia (long-term treatment)

Contraindications: Hypersensitivity to barbiturates, respiratory depression, addiction to barbiturates, severe liver impairment, porphyria

Precautions: Anemia, pregnancy (B), lactation, hepatic disease, renal disease, hypertension, elderly, acute/chronic pain

Pharmacokinetics:

PO: Onset 10-30 min, duration 6-8 hr

IV: Onset 5 min, duration 3-6 hr

Metabolized by liver, excreted by kidneys (inactive metabolites), crosses placenta, highly protein bound, excreted in breast milk, half-life 16-40 hr

Interactions/incompatibilities:

• Increased CNS depression: alcohol, MAOIs, sedative, narcotics

• Decreased effect of: oral anticoagulants, corticosteroids, griseofulvin, quinidine

• Increased half-life of: doxycycline

NURSING CONSIDERATIONS

Assess:

• VS q30 min after parenteral route for 2 hr

• Blood studies: Hct, Hgb, RBCs,

---

serum folate, vitamin D (if on long-term therapy); pro-time in patients receiving anticoagulants
• Hepatic studies: AST, ALT, bilirubin; if increased, drug is usually discontinued

Administer:
• After removal of cigarettes, to prevent fires
• IM injection in deep large muscle mass to prevent tissue sloughing, abscesses
• After trying conservative measures for insomnia
• After mixing with sterile water for injection; inject within 30 min of preparation
• IV only with resuscitative equipment available, administer at <100 mg/min (only by qualified personnel)
• ½-1 hr before hs for sleeplessness
• On empty stomach for best absorption

Perform/provide:
• Assistance with ambulation after receiving dose
• Safety measures: siderails, nightlight, callbell within easy reach
• Checking to see PO medication swallowed

Evaluate:
• Therapeutic response: ability to sleep at night, decreased amount of early morning awakening if taking drug for insomnia, or decrease in number, severity of seizures if taking drug for seizure disorder
• Mental status: mood, sensorium, affect, memory (long, short)
• Physical dependency: more frequent requests for medication, shakes, anxiety
• Barbiturate toxicity: hypotension; pulmonary constriction; cold, clammy skin; cyanosis of lips; insomnia; nausea; vomiting; hallucinations; delirium; weakness; mild symptoms may occur in 8-12 hr without drug

• Respiratory dysfunction: respiratory depression, character, rate, rhythm; hold drug if respirations are <12 /min or if pupils are dilated
• Blood dyscrasias: fever, sore throat, bruising, rash, jaundice, epistaxis

Teach patient/family:
• That hangover is common
• That drug is indicated only for short-term treatment of insomnia and is probably ineffective after 2 wk
• That physical dependency may result when used for extended periods of time (45-90 days depending on dose)
• To avoid driving or other activities requiring alertness
• To avoid alcohol ingestion or CNS depressants; serious CNS depression may result
• Not to discontinue medication quickly after long-term use; drug should be tapered over 1 wk
• To tell all prescribers that a barbiturate is being taken
• That withdrawal insomnia may occur after short-term use; do not start using drug again, insomnia will improve in 1-3 nights
• That effects may take 2 nights for benefits to be noticed
• Alternate measures to improve sleep: reading, exercise several hours before hs, warm bath, warm milk, TV, self-hypnosis, deep breathing

Lab test interferences:
False increase: Sulfobromophthalein

Treatment of overdose: Lavage, activated charcoal, warming blanket, vital signs, hemodialysis, alkalinize urine

---

italics = common side effects   ***bold italic*** = life threatening reactions

amoxapine

(a-mox'a-peen)
Asendin

Func. class.: Antidepressant—tricyclic
Chem. class.: Dibenzoxazepine derivative—secondary amine

Action: Blocks reuptake of norepinephrine, serotonin into nerve endings, increasing action of norepinephrine, serotonin in nerve cells

Uses: Depression

Dosage and routes:

• *Adult:* PO 50 mg tid, may increase to 100 mg tid on 3rd day of therapy; not to exceed 300 mg/day unless lower doses have been given for at least 2 wk, may be given daily dose hs, not to exceed 600 mg/day in hospitalized patients

Available forms include: Tabs 10, 25, 50, 75, 100, 150 mg

Side effects/adverse reactions:

HEMA: Agranulocytosis, thrombocytopenia, eosinophilia, leukopenia

CNS: Dizziness, drowsiness, confusion, headache, anxiety, tremors, stimulation, weakness, insomnia, nightmares, EPS (elderly), increased psychiatric symptoms, paresthesia

GI: Diarrhea, dry mouth, nausea, vomiting, *paralytic ileus,* increased appetite, cramps, epigastric distress, jaundice, *hepatitis,* stomatitis

GU: Retention, *acute renal failure*

INTEG: Rash, urticaria, sweating, pruritus, photosensitivity

CV: Orthostatic hypotension, ECG changes, tachycardia, hypertension, palpitations

EENT: Blurred vision, tinnitus, mydriasis, ophthalmoplegia

Contraindications: Hypersensitivity to tricyclic antidepressants, recovery phase of myocardial infarction, convulsive disorders, prostatic hypertrophy

Precautions: Suicidal patients, severe depression, increased intraocular pressure, narrow-angle glaucoma, urinary retention, cardiac disease, hepatic disease, hyperthyroidism, electroshock therapy, elective surgery, elderly, pregnancy (C)

Pharmacokinetics:

PO: Steady state 2-7 days; metabolized by liver, excreted by kidneys, crosses placenta, half-life 8 hr

Interactions/incompatibilities:

• Decreased effects of: guanethidine, clonidine, indirect acting sympathomimetics (ephedrine)

• Increased effects of: direct acting sympathomimetics (epinephrine), alcohol, barbiturates, benzodiazepines, CNS depressants

• Hyperpyretic crisis, convulsions, hypertensive episode: MAOI (pargyline [Eutonyl])

NURSING CONSIDERATIONS

Assess:

• B/P (lying, standing), pulse q4h; if systolic B/P drops 20 mm Hg hold drug, notify physician; take vital signs q4h in patients with cardiovascular disease

• Blood studies: CBC, leukocytes, differential, cardiac enzymes if patient is receiving long-term therapy

• Hepatic studies: AST, ALT, bilirubin, creatinine

• Weight qwk, appetite may increase with drug

• ECG for flattening of T wave, bundle branch block, AV block, dysrhythmias in cardiac patients

Administer:

• Increased fluids, bulk in diet if constipation, urinary retention occur

• With food or milk for GI symptoms

• Crushed if patient is unable to swallow medication whole

• Dosage hs if over-sedation occurs during day; may take entire dose hs; elderly may not tolerate once/day dosing

• Gum, hard candy, or frequent sips of water for dry mouth

Perform/provide:

• Storage at room temperature, do not freeze

• Assistance with ambulation during beginning therapy since drowsiness/dizziness occurs

• Safety measures including siderails primarily in elderly

• Checking to see PO medication swallowed

Evaluate:

• EPS primarily in elderly: rigidity, dystonia, akathisia

• Mental status: mood, sensorium, affect, suicidal tendencies, increase in psychiatric symptoms: depression, panic

• Urinary retention, constipation; constipation is more likely to occur in children

• Withdrawal symptoms: headache, nausea, vomiting, muscle pain, weakness; do not usually occur unless drug was discontinued abruptly

• Alcohol consumption; if alcohol is consumed, hold dose until morning

Teach patient/family:

• That therapeutic effects may take 2-3 wk

• Use caution in driving or other activities requiring alertness because of drowsiness, dizziness, blurred vision

• To avoid alcohol ingestion, other CNS depressants

• Not to discontinue medication quickly after long-term use, may cause nausea, headache, malaise

• To wear sunscreen or large hat since photosensitivity occurs

Lab test interferences:

Increase: Serum bilirubin, blood glucose, alk phosphatase

False increase: Urinary catecholamines

Decrease: VMA, 5-HIAA

Treatment of overdose: ECG monitoring, induce emesis, lavage, activated charcoal, administer anticonvulsant

---

amoxicillin/clavulanate potassium

(a-mox-i-sill′in)

Augmentin, Clavulin*

Func. class.: Broad spectrum antibiotic

Chem. class.: Aminopenicillin-B lactase inhibitor

Action: Interferes with cell wall replication of susceptible organisms; the cell wall, rendered osmotically unstable, swells, and bursts from osmotic pressure

Uses: Sinus infections, mastoiditis, meningitis, pneumonia, urinary tract infections; effective for strains of *E. coli, P. mirabilis, H. influenzae, S. faecalis, S. pneumoniae,* and lactase-producing organisms

Dosage and routes:

• *Adult:* PO 250-500 mg q8h depending on severity of infection

• *Child:* PO 20-40 mg/kg/day in divided doses q8h

Available forms include: Tabs 250, 500 mg; chew tabs 125 mg; powder for oral susp 125, 250 mg/5 ml

Side effects/adverse reactions:

HEMA: Anemia, increased bleeding time, ***bone marrow depression, granulocytopenia, leukopenia, eosinophilia***

GI:Nausea, diarrhea, vomiting, increased AST, ALT, abdominal pain, glossitis, colitis

---

italics = common side effects   ***bold italic*** = life threatening reactions

GU: Oliguria, proteinuria, hematuria, *vaginitis, moniliasis,* **glomerulonephritis**

CNS: Lethargy, hallucinations, anxiety, depression, twitching, **coma, convulsions**

META: Hyperkalemia, hypokalemia, alkalosis, hypernatremia

Contraindications: Hypersensitivity to penicillins; neonates

Precautions: Pregnancy, hypersensitivity to cephalosporins

Interactions/incompatibilities:

• Decreased antimicrobial effectiveness of this drug: tetracyclines, erythromycins

• Increased penicillin concentrations when used with: aspirin, probenicid

Pharmacokinetics:

PO: Peak 2 hr, duration 6-8 hr; half-life 1-1⅓ hr, metabolized in liver, excreted in urine, crosses placenta, enters breast milk

NURSING CONSIDERATIONS

Assess:

• I&O ratio; report hematuria, oliguria since penicillin in high doses is nephrotoxic

• Any patient with a compromised renal system, since drug is excreted slowly in poor renal system function; toxicity may occur rapidly

• Liver studies: AST, ALT

• Blood studies: WBC, RBC, H&H, bleeding time

• Renal studies: urinalysis, protein, blood

• Culture, sensitivity before drug therapy; drug may be taken as soon as culture is taken

Administer:

• After C&S completed

• On empty stomach for best absorption

Perform/provide:

• Adrenaline, suction, tracheostomy set, endotracheal intubation equipment on unit

• Adequate intake of fluids (2000 ml) during diarrhea episodes

• Scratch test to assess allergy after securing order from physician; usually done when penicillin is only drug of choice

• Storage in tight container

Evaluate:

• For therapeutic effectiveness: absence of temperature, draining wounds

• Bowel pattern before, during treatment

• Skin eruptions after administration of penicillin to 1 wk after discontinuing drug

• Respiratory status: rate, character, wheezing, tightness in chest

• Allergies before initiation of treatment, reaction of each medication; place allergies on chart, Kardex in bright red

Teach patient/family:

• To take oral penicillin on empty stomach with full glass of water

• Aspects of drug therapy: need to complete entire course of medication to ensure organism death (10-14 days); culture may be taken after completed course of medication

• To report sore throat, fever, fatigue (could indicate a superimposed infection)

• That drug must be taken in equal intervals around the clock to maintain blood levels

• To wear or carry a Medic Alert ID if allergic to penicillins

• To notify nurse of diarrhea stools

Lab test interferences:

False positive: Urine glucose, urine protein

Decrease: Uric acid

Treatment of overdose: Withdraw drug, maintain airway, administer epinephrine, aminophylline, O_2, IV corticosteroids for anaphylaxis

amoxicillin trihydrate

(a-mox-i-sill'in)

Amoxican,* Amoxil, Apo-Amoxi,* Larotid, Polymox, Robamox, Sumox, Trimox, Utimox, Wymox

Func. class.: Broad spectrum antibiotic

Chem. class.: Aminopenicillin

Action: Interferes with cell wall replication of susceptible organisms; the cell wall, rendered osmotically unstable, swells, and bursts from osmotic pressure

Uses: Effective for gram-positive cocci *(S. aureus, S. pyogenes, S. faecalis, S. pneumoniae)*, gram-negative cocci *(N. gonorrhoeae, N. meningitidis, E. coli)*, gram-positive bacilli *(C. diphtheriae, L. monocytogenes)*, gram-negative bacilli *(H. influenzae, P. mirabilis, Salmonella)*

Dosage and routes:
Systemic infections
• *Adult:* PO 750 mg-1.5 g qd in divided doses q8h
• *Child:* PO 20-40 mg/kg/day in divided doses q8h

Gonorrhea/urinary tract infections
• *Adult:* PO 3 g given with 1 g Probenecid as a single dose

Available forms include: Caps 250, 500 mg; chew tabs 125, 250 mg; powder for oral susp 50, 125, 250 mg/5 ml

Side effects/adverse reactions:
HEMA: Anemia, increased bleeding time, *bone marrow depression, granulocytopenia*
GI: Nausea, vomiting, diarrhea, increased AST, ALT, abdominal pain, glossitis, colitis
GU: Oliguria, proteinuria, hematuria, *vaginitis, moniliasis, glomerulonephritis*
CNS: Lethargy, hallucinations, anxiety, depression, twitching, *coma, convulsions*
META: Hyperkalemia, hypokalemia, alkalosis, hypernatremia
Contraindications: Hypersensitivity to penicillins; neonates
Precautions: Pregnancy, hypersensitivity to cephalosporins
Interactions/incompatibilities:
• Decreased antimicrobial effectiveness of this drug: tetracyclines, erythromycins
• Increased penicillin concentrations when used with: aspirin, probenicid
Pharmacokinetics:
PO: Peak 2 hr, duration 6-8 hr; half-life 1-1⅓ hr, metabolized in liver, excreted in urine, crosses placenta, enters breast milk

NURSING CONSIDERATIONS
Assess:
• I&O ratio; report hematuria, oliguria since penicillin in high doses is nephrotoxic
• Any patient with a compromised renal system, since drug is excreted slowly in poor renal system function; toxicity may occur rapidly
• Liver studies: AST, ALT
• Blood studies: WBC, RBC, H&H, bleeding time
• Renal studies: urinalysis, protein, blood
• Culture, sensitivity before drug therapy; drug may be taken as soon as culture is taken
Administer:
• After C&S completed
Perform/provide:
• Adrenaline, suction, tracheostomy set, endotracheal intubation equipment on unit
• Adequate intake of fluids (2000 ml) during diarrhea episodes
• Scratch test to assess allergy after securing order from physician; usually done when penicillin is only drug of choice
• Storage in tight container; after

---

italics = common side effects   ***bold italic*** = life threatening reactions

reconstituting or oral suspension should be refrigerated or stored at room temperature for 2 wk

Evaluate:

• Therapeutic effectiveness: absence of temperature, draining wounds

• Bowel pattern before, during treatment

• Skin eruptions after administration of penicillin to 1 wk after discontinuing drug

• Respiratory status: rate, character, wheezing, tightness in the chest

• Allergies before initiation of treatment, reaction of each medication; place allergies on chart, Kardex in bright red

Teach patient/family:

• To take oral penicillin on empty stomach with full glass of water

• Aspects of drug therapy: need to complete entire course of medication to ensure organism death (10-14 days); culture may be taken after completed course of medication

• To report sore throat, fever, fatigue (could indicate a superimposed infection)

• That drug must be taken in equal intervals around the clock to maintain blood levels

• To wear or carry a Medic Alert ID if allergic to penicillins

• To notify nurse of diarrhea stools

Lab test interferences:

False positive: Urine glucose, urine protein

Decrease: Uric acid

Treatment of overdose: Withdraw drug, maintain airway, administer epinephrine, aminophylline, O_2, IV corticosteroids for anaphylaxis

amphetamine sulfate

(am-fet'a-meen)

Racemic Amphetamine Sulfate

Func. class.: Cerebral stimulant
Chem. class.: Amphetamine

Controlled Substance Schedule II

Action: Increases release of norepinephrine, dopamine in cerebral cortex to reticular activating system

Uses: Narcolepsy, exogenous obesity, attention deficit disorder, hyperkinetic syndrome

Dosage and routes:

Narcolepsy

• *Adult:* PO 5-60 mg qd in divided doses

• *Child >12 yr:* PO 10 mg qd increasing by 10 mg/wk

• *Child 6-12 yr:* PO 5 mg qd increasing by 5 mg/wk

Attention deficit disorder

• *Child >6 yr:* PO 5 mg qd-bid increasing by 5 mg/wk

• *Child 3-6 yr:* PO 2.5 mg qd increasing by 2.5 mg/wk

Obesity

• *Adult:* PO 5-10 mg 30 min before meals

Available forms include: Tabs 5, 10 mg; sus rel caps 15 mg

Side effects/adverse reactions:

CNS: Hyperactivity, insomnia, restlessness, talkativeness, dizziness, headache, chills, stimulation, dysphoria, irritability, aggressiveness

GI: Nausea, vomiting, anorexia, dry mouth, diarrhea, constipation, weight loss, metallic taste, cramps

GU: Impotence, change in libido

CV: Palpitations, tachycardia, hypertension, hypotension

INTEG: Urticaria

Contraindications: Hypersensitivity to sympathomimetic amines, hyperthyroidism, hypertension, glaucoma hypertrophy, severe arteriosclerosis, nephritis, angina pectoris, parkinsonism, drug abuse, cardiovascular disease, anxiety

Precautions: Gilles de la Tourette's disorder, pregnancy, lactation, child <3 yr, diabetes mellitus, elderly

Pharmacokinetics:
PO: Onset 30 min, peak 1-3 hr, duration 4-20 hr, metabolized by liver, excreted by kidneys, crosses placenta, breast milk, half-life 10-30 hr

Interactions/incompatibilities:
• Hypertensive crisis: MAOIs or within 14 days of MAOIs
• Increased effect of this drug: acetazolamide, antacids, sodium bicarbonate, ascorbic acid, ammonium chloride, phenothiazines, haloperidol
• Decreased effects of this drug: barbiturates
• Decreased effects of: guanethidine, other antihypertensives

NURSING CONSIDERATIONS
Assess:
• VS, B/P since this drug may reverse antihypertensives; check patients with cardiac disease more often
• CBC, urinalysis, in diabetes: blood sugar, urine sugar; insulin changes may need to be made since eating will decrease
• Height, growth rate in children, growth rate may be decreased

Administer:
• At least 6 hr before hs to avoid sleeplessness
• For obesity only if patient is on weight reduction program that includes dietary changes, exercise; patient will develop tolerance, and weight loss won't occur without additional methods
• Gum, hard candy, frequent sips of water for dry mouth
• If drug is for obesity, 1 hr before meals

Perform/provide:
• Check to see PO medication has been swallowed

Evaluate:
• Mental status: mood, sensorium, affect, stimulation, insomnia; aggressiveness may occur
• Physical dependency; should not be used for extended time; dose should be discontinued gradually
• Withdrawal symptoms: headache, nausea, vomiting, muscle pain, weakness
• Drug tolerance will develop after long-term use
• Dosage should not be increased if tolerance develops

Teach patient/family:
• To decrease caffeine consumption (coffee, tea, cola, chocolate) which may increase irritability, stimulation
• Avoid OTC preparations unless approved by physician
• To taper off drug over several weeks, or depression, increased sleeping, lethargy may occur
• To avoid alcohol ingestion
• To avoid hazardous activities until patient is stabilized on medication
• To get needed rest, patients will feel more tired at end of day

Treatment of overdose: Administer fluids, hemodialysis, peritoneal dialysis, antihypertensives for increased B/P; ammonium Cl for increased excretion

---

amphotericin B
(am-foe-ter′i-sin)
Fungizone
Func. class.: Antifungal
Chem. class.: Amphoteric polyene macrolide

Action: Increases cell membrane permeability in susceptible organisms by binding sterols; decreases

K, Na, and nutrients in cell

Uses: Histoplasmosis, blastomycosis, coccidioidomycosis, cryptococcosis, aspergillosis, phycomycosis, candidiasis, sporotrichosis causing severe meningitis, septicemia, skin infections

Dosage and routes:

• *Adult and child:* IV INF 1 mg/250 ml D₅W (0.1 mg/ml) over 2-4 hr or 0.25 mg/kg/day over 6 hr; may be increased gradually up to 1 mg/kg/day, not to exceed 1.5 mg/kg; TOP apply to area, rub in bid-qid; INTRAARTERIAL 5-15 mg into joint spaces

Available forms include: Powder for inj 50 mg; top cream, lotion, oint 3%

Side effects/adverse reactions:

EENT: Tinnitus, deafness, diplopia, blurred vision

INTEG: Burning, irritation, necrosis at injection site, flushing, dermatitis, skin rash (topical route)

CNS: Headache, fever, chills, peripheral nerve pain, paresthesias, peripheral neuropathy, *convulsions,* dizziness

GU: Hypokalemia, axotemia, hyposthenuria, *renal tubular acidosis,* nephrocalcinosis, *permanent renal impairment, anuria, oliguria*

GI: Nausea, vomiting, anorexia, diarrhea, cramps, hemorrhagic gastroenteritis, acute liver failure

MS: Arthralgia, myalgia, generalized pain, weakness

HEMA: Normochromic, normocytic anemia, *thrombocytopenia, agranulocytosis, leukopenia, eosinophilia,* hypokalemia, hyponatremia, hypomagnesemia

Contraindications: Hypersensitivity, severe bone marrow depression

Precautions: Renal disease

Pharmacokinetics:

IV: Peak 1-2 hr, initial half-life 24 hr, metabolized in liver, excreted in urine (metabolites), breast milk, highly bound to plasma proteins; penetrates poorly CSF, bronchial secretions, aqueous humor, muscle, bone

Interactions/incompatibilities:

• Increased nephrotoxicity: other nephrotoxic antibiotics (aminoglycosides, cisplatin, vancomycin, cyclosporine, polymixin B)

• Increased hypokalemia: corticosteroids, digitalis, skeletal muscle relaxants

• Antagonism: miconazole

• Do not mix in sodium solutions or diluent with preservatives

NURSING CONSIDERATIONS

Assess:

• VS q15-30 min during first infusion; note changes in pulse, B/P

• I&O ratio; watch for decreasing urinary output, change in sp gr; discontinue drug to prevent permanent damage to renal tubules

• Blood studies: CBC, K, Na, Ca, Mg q2 wk

• Drug level during treatment

• Weight weekly; if weight increases over 2 lb/wk, edema is present, renal damage should be considered

Administer:

• After diluting with 10 ml sterile water (no preservatives), then dilute with 500 ml of solution to concentration of 0.1 mg/ml

• IV using in-line filter (mean pore diameter >1 μm) using distal veins, check for extravasation, necrosis q8h

• Drug only after C&S confirms organism, drug needed to treat condition; make sure drug is used in life-threatening infections

• Topical using loose dressing; wash clothing after therapy

Perform/provide:

• Protection from light during infusion, cover with foil

• Symptomatic treatment as ordered for adverse reactions: aspirin, antihistamines, antiemetics, antispasmodics

• Storage, protected from moisture and light; diluted solution is stable for 24 hr

Evaluate:

• Therapeutic response: decreased fever, malaise, rash, negative C&S for infecting organism

• For renal toxicity: increasing BUN, serum creatinine; if BUN is >40 mg/dl or if serum creatinine >3 mg/dl, drug may be discontinued or dosage reduced

• For hepatotoxicity: increasing AST, ALT, alk phosphatase, bilirubin

• For allergic reaction: dermatitis, rash; drug should be discontinued, antihistamines (mild reaction) or epinephrine (severe reaction) administered

• For hypokalemia: anorexia, drowsiness, weakness, decreased reflexes, dizziness, increased urinary output, increased thirst, paresthesias

• For ototoxicity: tinnitus (ringing, roaring in ears) vertigo, loss of hearing (rare)

Teach patient/family:

• That long-term therapy may be needed to clear infection (2 wk-3 mo depending on type of infection)

• Proper hygiene for topical applications: handwashing techniques, nail care, washing of articles that come in contact with infected areas; change linens qd

---

amphotericin B (topical)

(am-foe-ter'i-sin)
Fungizone
Func. class.: Local antiinfective
Chem. class.: Antifungal (polyene)

Action: Interferes with fungal DNA replication; binds sterols in fungal cell membrane, which increases permeability, leaking of cell nutrients

Uses: Cutaneous, mucocutaneous infections caused by candida

Dosage and routes:

• *Adult and child:* TOP bid-qid for 7-21 days or longer if needed

Available forms include: Cream, lotion, oint 3%

Side effects/adverse reactions:

INTEG: Rash, urticaria, stinging, burning, dry skin, pruritus, contact dermatitis

Contraindications: Hypersensitivity

Precautions: Pregnancy, lactation

Interactions/incompatibilities: None known

NURSING CONSIDERATIONS

Administer:

• Enough medication to completely cover lesions

• After cleansing with soap, water before each application, dry well (if ordered)

Perform/provide:

• Storage at room temperature in dry place

Evaluate:

• Allergic reaction: burning, stinging, swelling, redness

• Therapeutic response: decrease in size, number of lesions

Teach patient/family:

• To apply with glove to prevent further infection

• To avoid use of OTC creams, ointments, lotions unless directed by physician

• To use medical asepsis (hand washing) before, after each application to prevent further infection

• Not to cover with occlusive dressing

---

italics = common side effects   **bold italic** = life threatening reactions

ampicillin/ampicillin sodium/ampicillin trihydrate

(am-pi-sill'in)

Amcap, Amcill, Ampicin, Ampi-lean,* D-Amp, NovoAmpicillin,* Penbritin,* Pfizerpen A, Principen, Roampicillin, Supen, Omnipen-N, Pen A/N, Polycillin-N, Totacillin-N, Omnipen

Func. class.: Broad spectrum antibiotic

Chem. class.: Aminopenicillin

Action: Interferes with cell wall replication of susceptible organisms; the cell wall, rendered osmotically unstable, swells, bursts from osmotic pressure

Uses: Effective for gram-positive cocci *(S. aureus, S. pyogenes, S. faecalis, S. pneumoniae),* gram-negative cocci *(N. gonorrhoeae, N. meningitidis),* gram-negative bacilli *(H. influenzae, P. mirabilis, Salmonella, Shigella, L. monocytogenes),* gram-positive bacilli

Dosage and routes:
Systemic infections
• *Adult:* PO 1-2 g qd in divided doses q6h; IV/IM 2-8 g qd in divided doses q4-6h
• *Child:* PO 50-100 mg/kg/day in divided doses q6h; IV/IM 100-200 mg/kg/day in divided doses q6h
Meningitis
• *Adult:* IV 8-14 g/day in divided doses q3-4h × 3 days
• *Child:* IV 200-300 mg/kg/day in divided doses q3-4h × 3 days
Gonorrhea
• *Adult:* PO 3.5 g given with 1 g Probenecid as a single dose
Available forms include: Powder for inj IV, IM 125, 250, 500 mg, 1, 2, 10 g; IV inf 500 mg, 1, 2 g;

caps 250, 500 mg; powder for oral susp 100, 125, 250, 500 mg/5 ml
Side effects/adverse reactions:
HEMA: Anemia, increased bleeding time, *bone marrow depression, granulocytopenia*
GI: Nausea, vomiting, diarrhea, increased AST, ALT, abdominal pain, glossitis, colitis
GU: Oliguria, proteinuria, hematuria, *vaginitis, moniliasis, glomerulonephritis*
CNS: Lethargy, hallucinations, anxiety, depression, twitching, *coma, convulsions*
Contraindications: Hypersensitivity to penicillins
Precautions: Pregnancy; hypersensitivity to cephalosporins; neonates
Pharmacokinetics:
PO: Peak 2 hr
IV: Peak 5 min
IM: Peak 1 hr
Half-life 50-110 min; metabolized in liver, excreted in urine, bile, breast milk, crosses placenta
Interactions/incompatibilities:
• Decreased antimicrobial effectiveness of this drug: tetracyclines, erythromycins
• Increased penicillin concentrations when used with: aspirin, probenicid
NURSING CONSIDERATIONS
Assess:
• I&O ratio; report hematuria, oliguria since penicillin in high doses is nephrotoxic
• Any patient with compromised renal system, since drug is excreted slowly in poor renal system function; toxicity may occur rapidly
• Liver studies: AST, ALT
• Blood studies: WBC, RBC, H&H, bleeding time
• Renal studies: urinalysis, protein, blood
• Culture, sensitivity before drug

---

therapy; drug may be taken as soon as culture is taken

Administer:
• After C&S completed
• On empty stomach for best absorption

Perform/provide:
• Adrenaline, suction, tracheostomy set, endotracheal intubation equipment on unit
• Adequate intake of fluids (2000 ml) during diarrhea episodes
• Scratch test to assess allergy after securing order from physician; usually done when penicillin is only drug of choice
• Storage in tight container; after reconstituting or oral suspension should be refrigerated or stored at room temperature for 2 wk

Evaluate:
• Therapeutic effectiveness: absence of temperature, draining wounds
• Bowel pattern before, during treatment
• Skin eruptions after administration of penicillin to 1 wk after discontinuing drug
• Respiratory status: rate, character, wheezing, tightness in chest
• Allergies before initiation of treatment; reaction of each medication; place allergies on chart, Kardex in bright red

Teach patient/family:
• To take oral penicillin on empty stomach with full glass of water
• Aspects of drug therapy: need to complete entire course of medication to ensure organism death (10-14 days); culture may be taken after completed course of medication
• To report sore throat, fever, fatigue (could indicate superimposed infection)
• That drug must be taken in equal intervals around the clock to maintain blood levels
• To wear or carry a Medic Alert ID if allergic to penicillins
• To notify nurse of diarrhea stools

Lab test interferences:
False positive: Urine glucose, urine protein
Decrease: Uric acid

Treatment of overdose: Withdraw drug, maintain airway, administer epinephrine, aminophylline, O_2, IV corticosteroids for anaphylaxis

amrinone lactate
(am'ri-none)
Inocor

Func. class.: Cardiac inotropic agent
Chem. class.: Bipyrimidine derivative

Action: Positive inotropic agent with vasodilator properties; reduces preload and afterload by direct relaxation on vascular smooth muscle
Uses: Short-term management of CHF that has not responded to other medication; can be used with digitalis

Dosage and routes:
• *Adult:* IV BOL 0.75 mg/kg given over 2-3 min; start infusion of 5-10 μg/kg/min; may give another bolus ½ hr after start of therapy, not to exceed 10 mg/kg total daily use
Available forms include: Inj 5 mg/ml

Side effects/adverse reactions:
*HEMA: **Thrombocytopenia***
CV: Dysrhythmias, hypotension, headache, chest pain
GI: Nausea, vomiting, anorexia, abdominal pain, ***hepatotoxicity,*** ascites, jaundice, hiccups
INTEG: Allergic reactions, burning at injection site
*ENDO: **Nephrogenic diabetes insipidus***

RESP: Pleuritis, ***pulmonary densities, hypoxemia***

Contraindications: Hypersensitivity to this drug or bisulfites, severe aortic disease, severe pulmonic valvular disease, acute myocardial infarction

Precautions: Lactation, pregnancy (C), children, renal disease, hepatic disease

Pharmacokinetics:

IV: Onset 2-5 min, peak 10 min, duration variable; half-life 4-6 hr, metabolized in liver, excreted in urine as metabolites 60%-90%

Interactions/incompatibilities:

• Excessive hypotension: disopyramide

NURSING CONSIDERATIONS

Assess:

• B/P and pulse q5 min during infusion; if B/P drops 30 mm Hg, stop infusion and call physician

• Electrolytes: potassium, sodium, chloride, calcium; renal function studies: BUN, creatinine; blood studies: platelet count

• ALT, AST, bilirubin daily

• I&O ratio and weight qd, diuresis should increase with continuing therapy

• If platelets are <150,000/mm³ drug is usually discontinued and another drug started

Administer:

• Do not mix with glucose solutions directly, chemical reaction occurs over 24 hr; precipitate forms if amrinone and furosemide come in contact

• Into running dextrose infusion through Y connector or directly into tubing; dilute with normal saline to concentration of 1-3 mg/ml, do not mix with glucose for long-term infusion

• By infusion pump for doses other than bolus

• Potassium supplements if ordered for potassium levels <3.0

Evaluate:

• Extravasation, change site q48h

• Therapeutic response: increased cardiac output, decreased PCWP, adequate CVP, decreased dyspnea, fatigue, edema

Treatment of overdose: Discontinue drug

---

amyl nitrate

(am'il)

Func. class.: Coronary vasodilator

Chem. class.: Nitrate

Action: Relaxes vascular smooth muscle, may dilate coronary blood vessels, resulting in reduced venous return, decreased cardiac output; reduces preload, afterload, which decreases left ventricular end diastolic pressure, systemic vascular resistance

Uses: Angina, coronary constriction, cyanide poisoning, biliary colic, bronchospasm

Dosage and routes:

Angina

• ***Adult:*** INH 0.18-0.3 ml as needed, 1-6 inhalations

Cyanide poisoning

• ***Adult:*** INH 0.3 ml ampule inhaled 15 sec until preparation of sodium nitrite infusion is ready

Available forms include: Inh pearls 0.18, 0.3 ml

Side effects/adverse reactions:

*CV: Postural hypotension, **tachycardia, cardiovascular collapse***

RESP: Respiratory depression, apnea

CNS: Headache, dizziness, weakness

GI: Nausea, vomiting, abdominal pain

INTEG: Flushing, pallor, sweating

Contraindications: Hypersensitivity to nitrites, pregnancy, severe anemia, acute myocardial infarction, increased intracranial pres-

---

sure, hypertension
Precautions: Lactation, children, drug abuse, glaucoma, head injury, cerebral hemorrhage, hypotension
Pharmacokinetics:
INH: Onset 30 sec, duration 3-5 min; metabolized by liver, ⅓ excreted in urine, half-life 1-4 min
Interactions/incompatibilities:
• Increased hypotension: alcohol, β-blockers, antihypertensive narcotics, tricyclics
• Decreased effects: sympathomimetics
NURSING CONSIDERATIONS
Assess:
• B/P, pulse during treatment until stable
Administer:
• After wrapping, crushing ampule to avoid cuts
• Ordered analgesic if headache develops
• To patient who is sitting or lying down during treatment; keep head low, use deep breaths, which will decrease dizziness
• Drug, and have patient rest for 15 min
Perform/provide:
• Storage in light-resistant area in cool environment
Evaluate:
• Therapeutic response: relief of chest pain (angina) or increased ease of breathing (bronchospasm)
• For drug tolerance: the need for more medication for each attack
• For postural hypotension, headache during treatment, which are common side effects because of vasodilation
Teach patient/family:
• To keep a record of angina attacks, and what aggravates condition
• That medication may explode in presence of flame
• To take several deep breaths despite foul odor

• To make position changes slowly to prevent orthostatic hypotension
• To keep drug out of reach of children and in secure place, as there is high abuse potential

---

anisotropine methylbromide

(an-iss-oh-troe′peen)
Valpin 50
Func. class.: Gastrointestinal anticholinergic
Chem. class.: Synthetic quaternary ammonium compound

Action: Inhibits muscarinic actions of acetylcholine at postganglionic parasympathetic neuroeffector sites
Uses: Treatment of peptic ulcer disease in combination with other drugs
Dosage and routes:
• *Adult:* PO 50 mg tid, titrated to patient response
Available forms include: Tabs 50 mg
Side effects/adverse reactions:
CNS: Confusion, stimulation in elderly, headache, insomnia, dizziness, drowsiness, anxiety, weakness, hallucination
GI: Dry mouth, constipation, paralytic ileus, heartburn, nausea, vomiting, dysphagia, absence of taste
GU: Hesitancy, retention, impotence
CV: Palpitations, tachycardia
EENT: Blurred vision, photophobia, mydriasis, cycloplegia, increased ocular tension
INTEG: Urticaria, rash, pruritus, anhidrosis, fever, allergic reactions
Contraindications: Hypersensitivity to anticholinergics, narrow-angle glaucoma, GI obstruction, myasthenia gravis, paralytic ileus, GI atony, toxic megacolon
Precautions: Hyperthyroidism,

coronary artery disease, dysrhythmias, CHF, ulcerative colitis, hypertension, hiatal hernia, hepatic disease, renal disease

Pharmacokinetics:

PO: Onset 1-2 hr, duration 4-6 hr, metabolized by liver, excreted in urine

Interactions/incompatibilities:

• Increased anticholinergic effect: amantadine, tricyclic antidepressants, MAOIs

• Increased effect of: nitrofurantoin

• Decreased effect of: phenothiazines, levodopa

NURSING CONSIDERATIONS

Assess:

• VS, cardiac status: checking for dysrhythmias, increased rate, palpitations

• I&O ratio; check for urinary retention or hesitancy

Administer:

• ½-1 hr ac for better absorption

• Decreased dose to elderly patients; their metabolism may be slowed

• Gum, hard candy, frequent rinsing of mouth for dryness of oral cavity

Perform/provide:

• Storage at room temperature

• Increased fluids, bulk, exercise to patient's lifestyle to decrease constipation

Evaluate:

• Therapeutic response: absence of epigastric pain, bleeding, nausea, vomiting

• GI complaints: pain, bleeding (frank or occult), nausea, vomiting, anorexia

Teach patient/family:

• Avoid driving or other hazardous activities until stabilized on medication

• Avoid alcohol or other CNS depressants; will enhance sedating properties of this drug

• To avoid hot environments,

stroke may occur, drug suppresses perspiration

• To use sunglasses when outside to prevent photophobia

Treatment of overdose: Induce emesis if conscious, or gastric lavage, use cold packs for hyperthermia, if severe may use physostigmine (controversial)

---

anthralin

(an'thra-lin)

Anthra-Derm, Lasan, Drithocreme

Func. class.: Antipsoriatic/antieczema medication

Action: Inhibits epidermal cell replication by decreasing mitosis by halting nucleic protein synthesis

Uses: Psoriasis, eczema, chronic dermatitis

Dosage and routes:

• *Adult and child:* TOP apply to affected area qd or bid

Available forms include: Top cream 0.1%, 0.2%, 0.25%, 0.4%, 0.5%, 1%; top oint 0.1%, 0.25%, 0.4%, 0.5%, 1%

Side effects/adverse reactions:

INTEG: Rash on normal skin, folliculitis, discoloration of nails, hair, skin

GU: Renal irritation, toxicity

Contraindications: Hypersensitivity, renal disease, inflamed skin, child, lactation

Precautions: Erythema, pregnancy (C)

Pharmacokinetics:

TOP: Absorption poor, absorbed amount excreted in urine

Interactions/incompatibilities: None known

NURSING CONSIDERATIONS

Assess:

• Urinalysis qwk, for albumin, casts

Administer:

• Cover with dressing or paper tape

to avoid staining clothing

• After putting on gloves to protect healthy skin, wash after application

• After covering healthy skin with a protectant such as petrolatum or zinc oxide to prevent damage to adjacent tissues

• For 2-4 wk as needed

• To scalp after olive oil or mineral oil is applied to head, remove scales using comb

• At hs, leave on required time (10 min-12 hr)

Perform/provide:

• Removal of gauze bandage, cream by applying mineral oil before cleaning area; if area is not cleaned, maceration may occur

• Storage in tight covered container at room temperature

Evaluate:

• Therapeutic response: decreased itching, redness, dry scaly area

• Area of the body involved, including time involved, what helps or aggravates condition

Teach patient/family:

• To avoid application on normal skin or getting cream in eyes or mucous membranes

• That skin, nails, hair may turn brown-yellow color if applied to these areas

• To discontinue use if rash, irritation, folliculitis develops

---

antihemophilic factor (AHF)

(an-tee-hee-moe-fill'ik)

Antihemophilic Globulin, H.T. Factorate, Hemofil, Hemofil T, Humafac, Koate, Profilate, Koate H.T., Koate H.S.

Func. class.: Hemostatic
Chem. class.: Factor VIII

Action: Necessary for conversion of prothrombin to thrombin in clotting

Uses: Hemophilia A, patients with acquired circulating factor VIII inhibitors

Dosage and routes: Depends on severity of deficiency

• *Adult and child:* IV 10-20 U/kg q8-24 h; INF 10-20 ml/3 min

Available forms include: Inj IV (number of units noted on label)

Side effects/adverse reactions:

GI: Nausea, vomiting, abdominal cramps, jaundice, *viral hepatitis*

INTEG: Rash, flushing, *urticaria*

CNS: Headache, dizziness, malaise, paresthesia, *lethargy, chills, fever, flushing*

HEMA: **Thrombosis, hemolysis, AIDS**

CV: Hypotension, tachycardia

RESP: **Bronchospasm**

EENT: Visual disturbances

Contraindications: Hypersensitivity

Precautions: Neonates/infants, hepatic disease, blood types A, B, AB

Pharmacokinetics:

IV: Half-life 4 hr, terminal 15 hr

Interactions/incompatibilities: None known

NURSING CONSIDERATIONS

Assess:

• Blood studies (coagulation factors assay by % normal: 5% prevents spontaneous hemorrhage, 30%-50% for surgery, 80%-100% for severe hemorrhage)

• Pulse: discontinue infusion if significant increase

• Hct, Coombs' with blood types A, B, AB

• Test for factor VIII inhibitors before starting treatment, may require concomitant antiinhibitor coagulant complex therapy

Administer:

• After rotating gently to mix

• IV slowly, plastic syringe to reconstitute, administer; adheres to glass

---

italics = common side effects   ***bold italic*** = life threatening reactions

• After dilution with warm NS, D₅W, LR

Perform/provide:

• Storage in refrigerator, do not freeze

Evaluate:

• Therapeutic response

• Allergy: fever, rash, itching, jaundice; give Benadryl, continue therapy if reaction is mild

• Blood group of patient, donors (if applicable; most factor VIII not from specific blood group donors)

• Bleeding: ankles, knees, elbows, other joints

Teach patient/family:

• To report any signs of bleeding: gums, under skin, urine, stools, emesis

• To avoid salicylates (increase bleeding tendencies)

• To prepare, administer factor VIII concentrates at first danger sign

• Signs of viral hepatitis

• That immunization for hepatitis B may be given first

---

apomorphine HCl

(a-poe-mor'feen)

Func. class.: Emetic, dopamine agonist

Chem. class.: Morphine, hydrochloric acid

Controlled Substance Schedule II

Action: Acts centrally by stimulating chemoreceptor trigger zone, which in turn acts on vomiting center

Uses: In poisoning/drug overdose to induce vomiting promptly (10-15 min); is almost 100% effective

Dosage and routes:

• *Adult:* IM/SC 2-10 mg then 200-300 ml evaporated milk or water

• *Child >1 yr:* IM/SC 0.07 mg/kg then 16 oz evaporated milk or water

• *Child <1 yr:* IM/SC 0.07 mg/kg then 8 oz evaporated milk or water

Available forms include: Tabs (parenteral) 6 mg

Side effects/adverse reactions:

CNS: Euphoria, depression, restlessness, tremor, muscle weakness

GI: Nausea, anorexia, dry mouth, diarrhea, constipation, weight loss, metallic taste, cramps, salivation

CV: Circulatory failure, tachycardia, irregular rapid pulse, decreased B/P

RESP: Respiratory depression

Contraindications: Hypersensitivity to narcotics, respiratory depression, corrosive poisoning, coma, shock, narcosis from CNS depressants

Precautions: Children, cardiac decompensation, elderly

Pharmacokinetics:

PO: Onset 10-15 min

SC: Onset 1-2 min, metabolized by liver, excreted by kidneys

Interactions/incompatibilities:

• Incompatible with iodides, iron preparations, tannins, oxidizing agents

NURSING CONSIDERATIONS

Assess:

• Vital signs, B/P; check patients with cardiac disease more often

Administer:

• Drug then evaporated milk or water (200-300 ml for adult) to increase absorption of poison, facilitate emetic action of drug

• Dopamine antagonists to reverse emetic effect of this drug

• Activated charcoal if this drug doesn't work; may begin lavage after 10-15 min

Perform/provide:

• Only clear solutions; do not expose to light or air

Evaluate:

• Type of poisoning; do not administer if petroleum products or caus-

tic substances have been ingested: kerosene, gasoline, lye, Drano
• Respiratory status before, during, after administration of emetic, check rate, rhythm, character; respiratory depression can occur rapidly with elderly or debilitated patients; record B/P, pulse; check for odor of alcohol on breath, clothes

aprobarbital

(a-proe-bar'bi-tal)
Alurate
Func. class.: Sedative/hypnotic-barbiturate
Chem. class.: Barbitone (intermediate acting)

Controlled Substance Schedule III (USA), Schedule G (Canada)
Action: Depresses activity in brain cells primarily in reticular activating system in brainstem, also selectively depresses neurons in posterior hypothalamus, limbic structures
Uses: Sedation, insomnia
Dosage and routes:
Sedation
• *Adult:* PO 15-40 mg tid or qid; use reduced dose in geriatrics
Insomnia
• *Adult:* PO 40-160 mg qhs, use reduced dose in geriatrics
Available forms include: Elix 40 mg/5 ml
Side effects/adverse reactions:
CNS: Lethargy, drowsiness, hangover, dizziness, confusion, convulsion, stimulation in elderly, lightheadedness
GI: Nausea, vomiting
INTEG: Rash, urticaria, angioedema, *Stevens-Johnson syndrome*
Contraindications: Hypersensitivity to barbiturates, respiratory disease, porphyria, addiction to barbiturates

Precautions: Hypertension, hepatic disease, renal disease, pregnancy (D)
Pharmacokinetics:
PO: Onset 1 hr, peak 3 hr, duration 6-8 hr; metabolized by liver, excreted by kidneys (up to 50% in unchanged form); half-life 27 hr
Interactions/incompatibilities:
• Increased CNS depression: alcohol, MAOIs, sedative, narcotics
• Decreased effect of: oral anticoagulants, corticosteroids, griseofulvin, quinidine
• Increased half-life of: doxycycline
NURSING CONSIDERATIONS
Assess:
• Blood studies: Hct, Hgb, RBCs, serum folate (if on long-term therapy); pro-time in patients receiving anticoagulants
• Hepatic studies: AST, ALT, bilirubin; if increased, the drug is usually discontinued
Administer:
• After removal of cigarettes, to prevent fires
• After trying conservative measures for insomnia
• ½-1 hr before hs for sleeplessness
• On empty stomach for best absorption
Perform/provide:
• Assistance with ambulation after receiving dose
• Safety measures: siderails, nightlight, callbell within easy reach
Evaluate:
• Therapeutic response: ability to sleep at night, decreased amount of early morning awakening if taking drug for insomnia
• Mental status: mood, sensorium, affect, memory (long, short)
• Physical dependency: more frequent requests for medication, shakes, anxiety
• Barbiturate toxicity: hypotension; pulmonary constriction; cold,

---

italics = common side effects   ***bold italic*** = life threatening reactions

clammy skin; cyanosis of the lips; insomnia; nausea; vomiting; hallucinations; delirium; weakness; mild symptoms may occur in 8-12 hr without drug

• Respiratory dysfunction: respiratory depression, character, rate, rhythm; hold drug if respirations are <12 /min or if pupils are dilated

• Blood dyscrasias: fever, sore throat, bruising, rash, jaundice, epistaxis

Teach patient/family:

• That hangover is common

• That drug is indicated only for short-term treatment of insomnia and is probably ineffective after 2 wk

• That physical dependency may result when used for extended periods of time (45-90 days depending on dose)

• To avoid driving or other activities requiring alertness

• To avoid alcohol ingestion or CNS depressants; serious CNS depression may result

• Not to discontinue medication quickly after long-term use; drug should be tapered over 1-2 wk

• To tell all prescribers that barbiturate is being taken

• That withdrawal insomnia may occur after short-term use; do not start using drug again, insomnia will improve in 1-3 nights

• That effects may take 2 nights for benefits to be noticed

• Alternate measures to improve sleep: reading, exercise several hours before hs, warm bath, warm milk, TV, self-hypnosis, deep breathing

Lab test interferences:

False increase: Sulfobromophthalein

Treatment of overdose: Lavage, activated charcoal, warming blanket, vital signs, hemodialysis, alkalinize urine

---

ascorbic acid (vitamin C)

(a-skor'bic)

Ascorbicap, Ascorbineed, Best-C, Cecon, Cenolate, Cetane, Cevalin, Cevi-Bid, Ce-Vi-Sol, Cevita, Redoxon,* Solucap C, Vitacee, Viterra C

Func. class.: Vitamin C, water-soluble vitamin

Action: Needed for wound healing, collagen synthesis, antioxidant, carbohydrate metabolism

Uses: Vitamin C deficiency, scurvy, delays wound and bone healing, chronic disease, urine acidification, prior to gastrectomy

Dosage and routes:

Scurvy

• *Adult:* PO/SC/IM/IV 100 mg-2 g qd, then 50 mg or more qd

• *Child:* PO/SC/IM/IV 100-300 mg qd, then 35 mg or more qd

Wound healing/chronic disease/fracture

• *Adult:* SC/IM/IV/PO 200-500 mg qd

• *Child:* SC/IM/IV/PO 100-200 mg added doses

Urine acidification

• *Adult:* 4-12 g qd in divided doses

Available forms include: Tabs 25, 50, 100, 250, 500, 1000, 1500 mg; tabs effervescent 1000 mg; tabs chewable 100, 250, 500 mg; tabs timed release 500, 750, 1000, 1500 mg; caps timed release 500 mg; crys 4 g/tsp; powd 4 g/tsp; liq 35 mg/0.6 ml; sol 100 mg/ml; syr 20 mg/ml, 500 mg/5 ml; inj SC, IM, IV 100, 250, 500 mg/ml

Side effects/adverse reactions:

CNS: Headache, insomnia, dizziness, fatigue, flushing

GI: Nausea, vomiting, diarrhea, anorexia, heartburn, cramps

GU: Polyuria, urine acidification, oxalate or urate renal stones

HEMA: Hemolytic anemia in patients with G-6-PD

Contraindications: None significant

Precautions: Gout, pregnancy

Pharmacokinetics:

PO, INJ: Metabolized in liver, unused amounts excreted in urine (unchanged) and metabolites, crosses placenta, breast milk

Interactions/incompatibilities:

• Increased effects of: salicylates, oral contraceptives

• Increased side effects of: PAS, digitalis, sulfonamides

• Decreased effects of: phenothiazines, disulfiram, amphetamines

NURSING CONSIDERATIONS

Assess:

• I&O ratio

• Ascorbic acid levels throughout treatment if continued deficiency is suspected

Evaluate:

• Therapeutic response: absence of anorexia, irritability, pallor, joint pain, hyperkeratosis, petechiae, poor wound healing

• Nutritional status: citrus fruits, vegetables

• Injection sites for inflammation

Teach patient/family

• Necessary foods to be included in diet

• That if oral contraceptives are taken, increased levels of vitamin C are needed

• That smoking decreases vitamin C levels

Lab test interferences:

• False positive, negatives in glucose tests

asparaginase (L-asparaginase)

(a-spar'a-gin-ase)
Elspar, Kidrolase

Func. class.: Antineoplastic
Chem. class.: E. coli enzyme

Action: Indirectly inhibits protein synthesis in tumor cells; without amino acid, DNA, RNA synthesis is halted

Uses: Acute lymphocytic leukemia in combination with other antineoplastics

Dosage and routes:

In combination

• *Adult:* IV 1000 IU/kg/day × 10 days given over 30 min; IM 6000 IU/m²/day

Sole induction

• *Adult:* IV 200 IU/kg/day × 28 days

Available forms include: Inj 10,000 IU

Side effects/adverse reactions:

*HEMA: **Thrombocytopenia, leukopenia, myelosuppression, anemia***

*GI: Nausea, vomiting, anorexia, cramps, stomatitis, **hepatotoxicity,*** pancreatitis

GU: Urinary retention, ***renal failure,*** glycosuria, polyuria, azotemia

INTEG: Rash, urticaria, chills, fever

ENDO: Hyperglycemia

*RESP: **Fibrosis, pulmonary infiltrate***

CV: Chest pain

CNS: Neuritis, dizziness, headache, coma, depression, fatigue, confusion, hallucinations

Contraindications: Hypersensitivity, infants, pregnancy (1st trimester), lactation, pancreatitis

Precautions: Renal disease, hepatic disease

Pharmacokinetics: Half-life 4-9 hr, terminal 1.4-1.8 hr

Interactions/incompatibilities:
• May decrease action of methotrexate
• Do not use with radiation
• May increase toxicity when used with vincristine, prednisone
• Synergism may result when used in combination with cytarabine, azauridine

NURSING CONSIDERATIONS
Assess:
• CBC, differential, platelet count weekly; withhold drug if WBC is <4000 or platelet count is <75,000; notify physician of these results
• Pulmonary function tests, chest X-ray studies before, during therapy; chest X-ray film should be obtained q2 wk during treatment
• Renal function studies: BUN, serum uric acid, urine CrCl, electrolytes before, during therapy
• I&O ratio; report fall in urine output of 30/ml/hr
• Monitor temperature q4h; may indicate beginning infection
• Liver function tests before, during therapy (bilirubin, AST, ALT, LDH) as needed or monthly
• RBC, Hct, Hgb since these may be decreased
• Serum, urine glucose levels

Administer:
• Medications by oral route if possible; avoid IM, SC, IV routes to prevent infections
• Antiemetic 30-60 min before giving drug to prevent vomiting
• Allopurinol or sodium bicarbonate to maintain uric acid levels, alkalinization of urine
• Antibiotics for prophylaxis of infection
• IV infusion using 21-, 23-, 25-gauge needle; administer by slow IV infusion
• Topical or systemic analgesics for pain
• Local or systemic drugs for infection
• Transfusion for anemia
• Antispasmodic

Perform/provide:
• Strict medical asepsis, protective isolation if WBC levels are low
• Special skin care
• Deep-breathing exercises with patient 3-4 × day; place in semi-Fowler's position
• Liquid diet: cola, Jell-O; dry toast or crackers may be added if patient is not nauseated or vomiting
• Increase fluid intake to 2-3 L/day to prevent urate deposits, calculi formation
• Diet low in purines: organ meats (kidney, liver), dried beans, peas to maintain alkaline urine
• Rinsing of mouth 3-4 × day with water, hydrogen peroxide
• Brushing of teeth 2-3 × day with soft brush or cotton-tipped applicators for stomatitis; use unwaxed dental floss
• Warm compresses at injection site for inflammation
• Nutritious diet with iron, vitamin supplements
• HOB increased to facilitate breathing

Evaluate:
• Bleeding: hematuria, guaiac, bruising or petechiae, mucosa or orifices q8h
• Dyspnea, rales, unproductive cough, chest pain, tachypnea fatigue, increased pulse, pallor, lethargy, or swelling around eyes or lips
• Food preferences; list likes, dislikes
• Edema in feet, joint pain, stomach pain, shaking
• Inflammation of mucosa, breaks in skin
• Yellowing of skin and sclera, dark urine, clay-colored stools,

itchy skin, abdominal pain, fever, diarrhea

• Buccal cavity q8h for dryness, sores or ulceration, white patches, oral pain, bleeding, dysphagia

• Local irritation, pain, burning, discoloration at injection site

• Symptoms indicating severe allergic reaction: rash, pruritus, urticaria, purpuric skin lesions, itching, flushing

• Frequency of stools, characteristics: cramping, acidosis; signs of dehydration: rapid respirations, poor skin turgor, decreased urine output, dry skin, restlessness, weakness

Teach patient/family:

• Of protective isolation precautions

• To report any complaints or side effects to nurse or physician

• To report any changes in breathing or coughing

• To avoid foods with citric acid, hot or rough texture

Lab test interferences:

Decrease: Thyroid function tests

---

aspirin

(as′pir-in)

Ancasal,* ASA, Aspirin,* Ecotrin, Empirin, Entrophen,* Novasen,* Sal-Adult,* Sal-Infant,* Supasa*

Func. class.: Nonnarcotic analgesic

Chem. class.: Salicylate

Action: Acts by blocking pain impulses in CNS that occur in response to inhibition of prostaglandin synthesis; antipyretic action results from inhibition of hypothalamic heat-regulating center

Uses: Mild to moderate pain or fever including arthritis, thromboembolic disorders, transient ischemic attacks in men

Dosage and routes:
Arthritis

• *Adult:* PO 2.6-5.2 g/day in divided doses

• *Child:* PO 90-130 mg/kg/day in divided doses

Pain/fever

• *Adult:* PO/REC 325-650 mg q4h prn, not to exceed 4 g/day

• *Child:* PO/REC 40-100 mg/kg/day in divided doses q4-6h prn

Thromboembolic disorders

• *Adult:* PO 325-650 mg/day or bid

Transient ischemic attacks in men

• *Adult:* PO 650 mg bid or 325 mg qid

Available forms include: Tabs 65, 81, 325, 500, 650, 950 mg; chewable tabs 81 mg; caps 325, 500 mg; tabs controlled-release 800 mg; tabs time-release 650 mg; supp 60, 120, 130, 195, 200, 300, 325, 600, 650 mg, 1.2 g; cream

Side effects/adverse reactions:

*HEMA: **Thrombocytopenia, agranulocytosis, leukopenia, neutropenia, hemolytic anemia,*** increased pro-time

CNS: Stimulation, drowsiness, dizziness, confusion, convulsion, headache, flushing, hallucinations, coma

GI: Nausea, vomiting, GI bleeding, diarrhea, heartburn, anorexia, ***hepatitis***

INTEG: Rash, urticaria, bruising

EENT: Tinnitus, hearing loss

CV: Rapid pulse, pulmonary edema

RESP: Wheezing, hyperpnea

ENDO: Hypoglycemia, hyponatremia, hypokalemia

Contraindications: Hypersensitivity to salicylates, GI bleeding, bleeding disorders, children < 3 yr, pregnancy, lactation, vitamin K deficiency

Precautions: Anemia, hepatic disease, renal disease, Hodgkin's disease

---

italics = common side effects   ***bold italic*** = life threatening reactions

Pharmacokinetics:

PO: Onset 15-30 min, peak 1-2 hr, duration 4-6 hr

REC: Onset slow, duration 4-6 hr
Metabolized by liver, excreted by kidneys, crosses placenta, excreted in breast milk, half-life 1-3½ hr

Interactions/incompatibilities:

• Decreased effects of this drug: antacids, steroids, urinary alkalizers

• Increased blood loss: alcohol, heparin

• Increased effects of: anticoagulants, insulin, methotrexate

• Decreased effects of: probenecid, spironolactone, sulfinpyrazone, sulfonylamides

• Toxic effects: PABA

• Decreased blood sugar levels: salicylates

NURSING CONSIDERATIONS

Assess:

• Liver function studies: AST, ALT, bilirubin, creatinine if patient is on long-term therapy

• Renal function studies: BUN, urine creatinine if patient is on long-term therapy

• Blood studies: CBC, Hct, Hgb, pro-time if patient is on long-term therapy

• I&O ratio; decreasing output may indicate renal failure (long-term therapy)

Administer:

• To patient crushed or whole; chewable tablets may be chewed

• With food or milk to decrease gastric symptoms; give 30 min before or 2 hr after meals

Perform/provide:

• Repositioning to decrease pain

• Cool cloth for fever

Evaluate:

• Hepatotoxicity: dark urine, clay-colored stools, yellowing of skin, sclera, itching, abdominal pain, fever, diarrhea if patient is on long-term therapy

• Allergic reactions: rash, urticaria; if these occur, drug may need to be discontinued

• Renal dysfunction: decreased urine output

• Ototoxicity: tinnitus, ringing, roaring in ears; audiometric testing needed before, after long-term therapy

• Visual changes: blurring, halos, corneal, retinal damage

• Edema in feet, ankles, legs

• Prior drug history; there are many drug interactions

Teach patient/family:

• To report any symptoms of hepatotoxicity, renal toxicity, visual changes, ototoxicity, allergic reactions (long-term therapy)

• Not to exceed recommended dosage; acute poisoning may result

• To read label on other OTC drugs; many contain aspirin

• That the therapeutic response takes 2 wk (arthritis)

• To avoid alcohol ingestion; GI bleeding may occur

Lab test interferences:

Increase: Coagulation studies, liver function studies, serum uric acid, amylase, CO_2, urinary protein

Decrease: Serum potassium, PBI, cholesterol

Interfere: Urine catecholamines, pregnancy test

Treatment of overdose: Lavage, activated charcoal, monitor electrolytes, VS

atenolol

(a-ten'oh-lole)
Tenormin

Func. class.: Antihypertensive
Chem. class.: β-Blocker, β-1, 2 blocker (high doses)

Action: Competitively blocks stimulation of β-adrenergic receptor within vascular smooth muscle;

produces negative chronotropic, inotropic activity (decreases rate of SA node discharge, increases recovery time), slows conduction of AV node, decreases heart rate, decreases O_2 consumption in myocardium; also, decreases renin-aldosterone-angiotensin system at high doses, inhibits β-2 receptors in bronchial system

Uses: Mild to moderate hypertension, prophylaxis of angina pectoris

Dosage and routes:

• *Adult:* PO 50 mg qd, increasing ql-2 wk to 200 mg qd

Available forms include: Tabs 50, 100 mg

Side effects/adverse reactions:

CV: Profound hypotension, bradycardia, CHF, cold extremities, postural hypotension, 2nd or 3rd degree heart block

CNS: Insomnia, fatigue, dizziness, mental changes, memory loss, hallucinations, depression, lethargy, drowsiness, strange dreams, catatonia

GI: Nausea, diarrhea, vomiting, *mesenteric arterial thrombosis, ischemic colitis*

INTEG: Rash, fever, alopecia

HEMA: Agranulocytosis, thrombocytopenia, purpura

EENT: Sore throat, dry burning eyes

GU: Impotence

ENDO: Increased hypoglycemic response to insulin

RESP: Bronchospasm, dyspnea, wheezing

Contraindications: Hypersensitivity to β-blockers, cardiogenic shock, heart block (2nd, 3rd degree), sinus bradycardia, CHF, cardiac failure

Precautions: Major surgery, pregnancy (C), lactation, diabetes mellitus, renal disease, thyroid disease, COPD, asthma, well compensated heart failure, CAD

Pharmacokinetics:

PO: Peak 2-4 hr; half-life 6-7 hr, excreted unchanged in urine, protein binding 5%-15%

Interactions/incompatibilities:

• Increased hypotension, bradycardia: reserpine, hydralazine, methyldopa, prazosin, anticholinergics, digoxin

• Decreased antihypertensive effects: indomethacin

• Increased hypoglycemic effect: insulin

• Decreased bronchodilation: theophyllines

NURSING CONSIDERATIONS

Assess:

• I&O, weight daily

• B/P, pulse q4h; note rate, rhythm, quality

• Apical/radial pulse before administration; notify physician of any significant changes

• Baselines in renal, liver function tests before therapy begins

Administer:

• PO ac, hs, tablet may be crushed or swallowed whole

• Reduced dosage in renal dysfunction

Perform/provide:

• Storage protected from light, moisture; placed in cool environment

Evaluate:

• Therapeutic response: decreased B/P after 1-2 wk

• Edema in feet, legs daily

• Skin turgor, dryness of mucous membranes for hydration status

Teach patient/family:

• Not to discontinue drug abruptly, taper over 2 wk

• Not to use OTC products unless directed by physician

• To report bradycardia, dizziness, confusion, depression, fever

• To take pulse at home, advise when to notify physician

---

italics = common side effects   ***bold italic*** = life threatening reactions

• To avoid alcohol, smoking, sodium intake

• To comply with weight control, dietary adjustments, modified exercise program

• To carry Medic Alert ID to identify drug that you are taking, allergies

• To avoid hazardous activities if dizziness is present

Lab test interferences:

Interference: Glucose/insulin tolerance tests

Treatment of overdose: Lavage, IV atropine for bradycardia, IV theophylline for bronchospasm, digitalis, O_2, diuretic for cardiac failure, hemodialysis

---

atracurium besylate

(a-tra-cyoor'ee-um)
Tracrium

Func. class.: Neuromuscular blocker (nondepolarizing)
Chem. class.: Biquaternary nonchlorine diester

Action: Inhibits transmission of nerve impulses by binding with cholinergic receptor sites, antagonizing action of acetylcholine

Uses: Facilitation of endotracheal intubation, skeletal muscle relaxation during mechanical ventilation, surgery, or general anesthesia

Dosage and routes:

• *Adult:* IV BOL 0.4-0.5 mg/kg, then 0.08-0.10 mg/kg 20-45 min after 1st dose if needed for prolonged procedures

Available forms include: Inj IV 10 mg/ml

Side effects/adverse reactions:

CV: Bradycardia, tachycardia, increase, decrease B/P

*RESP: Prolonged apnea, **bronchospasm, cyanosis, respiratory depression***

EENT: Increased secretions

INTEG: Rash, flushing, pruritus, urticaria

Contraindications: Hypersensitivity

Precautions: Pregnancy, cardiac disease, lactation, children <2 yr, electrolyte imbalances, dehydration, neuromuscular disease, respiratory disease

Pharmacokinetics:

IV: Onset 2 min, duration 20-60 min; half-life 2 min, 29 min (terminal), excreted in urine, feces (metabolites), crosses placenta

Interactions/incompatibilities:

• Increased neuromuscular blockade: aminoglycosides, clindamycin, lincomycin, quinidine, local anesthetics, polymyxin antibiotics, lithium, narcotic analgesics, thiazides, enflurane, isoflurane

• Dysrhythmias: theophylline

• Do not mix with barbiturates in solution or syringe

NURSING CONSIDERATIONS

Assess:

• For electrolyte imbalances (K, Mg), may lead to increased action of this drug

• Vital signs (B/P, pulse, respirations, airway) until fully recovered; rate, depth, pattern of respirations, strength of hand grip

• I&O ratio; check for urinary retention, frequency, hesitancy

Administer:

• Using nerve stimulator by anesthesiologist to determine neuromuscular blockade

• Anticholinesterase to reverse neuromuscular blockade

• By slow IV over 1-2 min (only by qualified person, usually an anesthesiologist)

• Only slightly discolored solution

Perform/provide:

• Storage in light-resistant area

• Reassurance if communication is difficult during recovery from neuromuscular blockade

---

Evaluate:

• Therapeutic response: paralysis of jaw, eyelid, head, neck, rest of body

• Recovery: decreased paralysis of face, diaphragm, leg, arm, rest of body

• Allergic reactions: rash, fever, respiratory distress, pruritus; drug should be discontinued

Treatment of overdose: Edrophonium or neostigmine, atropine, monitor VS; may require mechanical ventilation

---

atropine sulfate

(a′troe-peen)

Func. class.: Anticholinergic-para sympatholytic

Chem. class.: Belladonna alkaloid

Action: Blocks acetylcholine at parasympathetic neuroeffector sites; antagonizes histamine, serotonin; increases cardiac output, heart rate by blocking vasal stimulation in heart

Uses: Bradycardia, bradydysrhythmia, anticholinesterase insecticide poisoning, blocking cardiac vagal reflexes, decreasing secretions before surgery, antispasmodic with GU, biliary surgery

Dosage and routes:

Bradycardia/bradydysrhythmias

• *Adult:* IV BOL 0.5-1 mg, repeat in 5 min, not to exceed 2 mg

• *Child:* IV BOL 0.01 mg/kg up to 0.4 mg or 0.3 mg/m², may repeat q4-6h

Insecticide poisoning

• *Adult and child:* IM/IV 2 mg qh until muscarinic symptoms disappear, may need 6 mg qh

Available forms include: Inj 0.05, 0.1, 0.3, 0.4, 0.5, 0.8, 1 mg/ml

Side effects/adverse reactions:

GU: Retention, hesitancy, impotence, dysuria

CNS: Headache, dizziness, involuntary movement, confusion, psychosis, anxiety, coma

GI: Dry mouth, Nausea, vomiting, diarrhea, abdominal pain, anorexia, constipation, paralytic ileus, abdominal distention

CV: Hypotension, paradoxical bradycardia, angina, PVCs, hypertension, tachycardia, ectopic ventricular beats

INTEG: Rash, urticaria, contact dermatitis, dry skin, flushing

EENT: Blurred vision, photophobia, glaucoma, eye pain, conjunctivitis

Contraindications: Hypersensitivity to belladonna alkaloids, angle-closure glaucoma, GI obstructions, myasthenia gravis, thyrotoxicosis, ulcerative colitis, prostatic hypertrophy

Precautions: Pregnancy, renal disease, lactation, CHF, tachydysrhythmias, hyperthyroidism, COPD, hepatic disease, child <6 yr

Pharmacokinetics:

IV: Peak 2-4 min

IM: Peak 30 min

Half-life 2-3 hr, excreted unchanged by kidneys (70%-90% in 24 hr); metabolized in liver, crosses placenta, excreted in breast milk

Interactions/incompatibilities:

• Decreased effects of: phenothiazines, levodopa

• Increased side effects: methotrimeprazine

• Increased effects of: anticholinergics, antidepressants, antivirals, MAOIs

• Incompatible with all drugs in solution or syringe (except analgesics)

NURSING CONSIDERATIONS

Assess:

• I&O ratio; check for urinary retention, daily output

• ECG for hypertension, ectopic

ventricular beats, PVC
• For bowel sounds, check for constipation
Administer:
• Increased bulk, water in diet if constipation occurs
• Frequent mouth rinsing, gum or candy for dry mouth
Perform/provide:
• Sugarless hard candy, gum, frequent rinsing of mouth for dryness
Evaluate:
• Respiratory status: rate, rhythm, cyanosis, wheezing, dyspnea, engorged neck veins
• Increased intraocular pressure: eye pain, nausea, vomiting, blurred vision, increased tearing
• Cardiac rate: rhythm, character, B/P continuously
• Allergic reaction: rash, urticaria
Teach patient/family:
• To avoid hazardous activities if dizziness occurs
• To report blurred vision, chest pain, allergic reactions
• Increased risks of prostration if prolonged exposure to increased temperatures
• Avoid OTC drugs used for colds, hay fever, etc.
Treatment of overdose: O_2, artificial ventilation, ECG, administer dopamine for circulatory depression, administer diazepam or thiopental for convulsions

atropine sulfate (optic)

(a'troe-peen)
Atropisol, BufOpto Atropine, Isopto Atropine
Func. class.: Mydriatic
Chem. class.: Belladonna alkaloid

Action: Blocks response of iris sphincter muscle, muscle of accommodation of ciliary body to cholinergic stimulation, resulting in dilation, paralysis of accommodation
Uses: Iritis, cycloplegic refraction
Dosage and routes:
• *Adult:* INSTILL SOL 1-2 gtts of a 1% sol qd-tid for iritis or 1 hr before refracting (cycloplegic refraction); INSTILL OINT 2-3 × / day
• *Child:* INSTILL SOL 1-2 gtts of a 0.5% sol qd-tid for iritis or bid × 1-3 days before exam (cycloplegic refraction); INSTILL OINT qd-bid 2-3 days before exam
Available forms include: Oint 0.5%, 1%; sol 0.5%, 1%, 2%, 3%
Side effects/adverse reactions:
SYST: Tachycardia, confusion, fever, flushing, dry skin, dry mouth, abdominal discomfort (infants: bladder distention, irregular pulse, respiratory depression)
Contraindications: Hypersensitivity, infants <3 mo, local or systemic glaucoma, conjunctivitis
Pharmacokinetics:
INSTILL: Peak 30-40 min (mydriasis), 60-180 min (cycloplegia), duration 6-12 days
Interactions/incompatibilities:
None known
NURSING CONSIDERATIONS
Evaluate:
• Therapeutic response: decrease in inflammation (iritis) or cycloplegic refraction
• Eye pain, discontinue use if pain occurs
Teach patient/family:
• To report change in vision, blurring or loss of sight, trouble breathing, sweating, flushing
• Method of instillation: pressure on lacrimal sac for 1 min, do not touch dropper to eye
• That blurred vision will decrease with repeated use of drug
• Not to do hazardous things until able to see

- Wait 5 min to use other drops
- Do not blink more than usual

---

auranofin

(aur-an-oo-fin)
Ridaura

Func. class.: Gold salt
Chem. class.: Active gold compound (2%)

Action: Antiinflammatory action unknown, may decrease phagocytosis, lysosomal activity or decrease prostaglandin synthesis; decreases concentration of rheumatoid factor, immunoglobulins
Uses: Rheumatoid arthritis
Dosage and routes:
- *Adult:* PO 6 mg qd or 3 mg bid, may increase to 9 mg/day after 3 mo
Available forms include: Caps 3 mg
Side effects/adverse reactions:
*HEMA: **Thrombocytopenia, agranulocytosis, aplastic anemia,** leukopenia, eosinophilia*
INTEG: Rash, pruritus, dermatitis, exfoliative dermatitis
GI: Diarrhea, abdominal cramping, stomatitis, nausea, vomiting, enterocolitis, anorexia, flatulence, metallic taste, dyspepsia jaundice, increased AST, ALT, glossitis, gingivitis
GU: Proteinuria, hematuria
*RESP: **Interstitial pneumonitis, fibrosis***
Contraindications: Hypersensitivity to gold, necrotizing enterocolitis, bone marrow aplasia, child <6 yr, lactation, pregnancy (C), pulmonary fibrosis, exfoliative dermatitis, blood dyscrasias
Precautions: Elderly, CHF, diabetes mellitus, allergic conditions, ulcerative colitis, renal disease, liver disease

Pharmacokinetics:
PO: Absorbed by GI tract, peak 2 hr, steady state 8-16 wk, excreted in urine, feces
Interactions/incompatibilities:
None known
NURSING CONSIDERATIONS
Assess:
- Respiratory status: dyspnea, wheezing; if respiratory problems occur, drug should be discontinued
- I&O ratio
- Urine: hematuria, proteinuria, increased BUN, creatinine, may require decrease in dosage
- Platelet counts q mo, drug should be discontinued if <100,000/mm^3
- Hepatic test: ALT, AST, alk phosphatase, HCL as ordered for diarrhea
Administer:
- bid or may give as single dose q am
Evaluate:
- Therapeutic response: ability to move joints with less pain
- Diarrhea stools; if severe, drug should be discontinued
- Allergy: rash, dermatitis, pruritus; drug should be discontinued if any of these occur
- Gold toxicity: decreased Hgb, WBC <4000/mm^3, granulocytes <1500/mm^3, platelets <150,000/mm^3, severe diarrhea, stomatitis, hematuria, rash, itching, proteinuria
Teach patient/family
- That drug must be taken as prescribed to be useful
- That diarrhea is common, but if blood appears in stools or urine notify physician at once
- To report skin conditions, stomatitis, fatigue, jaundice; may indicate blood dyscrasias
- That therapeutic effect may take 3-4 mo
- To use dilute hydrogen peroxide for mild stomatitis, avoid hot spicy

---

italics = common side effects   ***bold italic*** = life threatening reactions

foods, food with high acidic content; use soft toothbrush, rinse more frequently

Lab test interferences:
False positive: TB test

---

aurothioglucose/gold sodium thiomalate

(aur-oh-thye-oh-gloo'kose)
Solganal/Myochrysine

Func. class.: Gold salts
Chem. class.: Active gold compound

Action: Antiinflammatory action unknown; may decrease phagocytosis, lysosomal activity, prostaglandin synthesis.

Uses: Rheumatoid arthritis, psoriatic arthritis

Dosage and routes:
• *Adult:* IM 10 mg, then 25 mg q wk × 2-3 wk, then 50 mg/wk until total of 1 g is administered, then 25-50 mg q3-4 wk if there is improvement without toxicity (aurothioglucose)
• *Adult:* IM 10 mg, then 25 mg after 1 wk, then 50 mg q wk for total of 14-20 doses, then 50 mg q2 wk × 4, then 50 mg q3 wk × 4, then 50 mg q mo for maintenance (gold sodium thiomalate)
• *Child 6-12 yr:* IM 1 mg/kg/ wk × 20 wk, or ¼ of adult dose (aurothioglucose)
• *Child:* IM 1 mg/kg/wk × 20 wk, then q3-4 wk if improvement without toxicity (gold sodium thiomalate)

Available forms include: IM inj 50 mg/ml

Side effects/adverse reactions:
EENT: Iritis, corneal ulcers
HEMA: Thrombocytopenia, agranulocytosis, aplastic anemia, leukopenia, eosinophilia
INTEG: Rash, pruritus, dermatitis, exfoliative dermatitis, angioedema

GI: Stomatitis, nausea, vomiting, metallic taste, jaundice, *hepatitis*
GU: Proteinuria, hematuria, nephrosis, tubular necrosis
RESP: Interstitial pneumonitis
CNS: Dizziness, syncope
CV: Bradycardia
SYST: Anaphylaxis

Contraindications: Hypersensitivity to gold, systemic lupus erythematosus, uncontrolled diabetes mellitus, marked hypertension, CHF, pregnancy (C), lactation, renal disease, liver disease

Precautions: Decrease tolerance in elderly, children, blood dyscrasias

Pharmacokinetics:
PO: Absorbed by GI tract, peak 2 hr, steady state 8-16 wk, excreted in urine, feces

Interactions/incompatibilities:
• Increased risk blood dyscrasias: antimalarials, cytotoxic agents, immunosuppressants, oxyphenbutazone, phenylbutazone, penicillamine

NURSING CONSIDERATIONS
Assess:
• Respiratory status: dyspnea, wheezing; if respiratory problems occur, drug should be discontinued
• I&O ratio
• Urine: hematuria, proteinuria, increased BUN, creatinine, may require decrease in dosage
• Platelet counts q mo, drug should be discontinued if <100,000/mm³
• Hepatic test: ALT, AST, alk phosphatase, HCL as ordered for diarrhea

Administer:
• bid or may give as single dose q AM

Evaluate:
• Therapeutic response: ability to move joints with less pain
• Diarrhea stools; if severe, drug should be discontinued
• Allergy: rash, dermatitis, pruritus; drug should be discontinued if

any of these occur
• Gold toxicity: decreased Hgb, WBC <4000/mm³, granulocytes <1500/mm³, platelets <150,000/mm³, severe diarrhea, stomatitis, hematuria, rash, itching, proteinuria

Teach patient/family
• That drug must be taken as prescribed to be useful
• That diarrhea is common, but if blood appears in stools or urine, notify physician at once
• To report skin conditions, stomatitis, fatigue, jaundice, which may indicate blood dyscrasias
• That therapeutic effect may take 3-4 months
• To use dilute hydrogen peroxide for mild stomatitis, avoid hot spicy foods or food with high acidic content; use soft toothbrush, rinse more frequently

Lab test interferences:
False positive: TB test

---

azatadine maleate

(a-za′ta-deen)
Optimine
Func. class.: Antihistamine
Chem. class.: Piperidine H₁-receptor antagonist

Action: Acts on blood vessels, GI, respiratory system by competing with histamine for H₁-receptor site; decreases allergic response by blocking histamine

Uses: Allergy symptoms, rhinitis, chronic urticaria

Dosage and routes:
• *Adult:* PO 1-2 mg bid, not to exceed 4 mg/day

Available forms include: Tabs 1 mg

Side effects/adverse reactions:
CNS: Dizziness, drowsiness, poor coordination, fatigue, anxiety, euphoria, confusion, paresthesia, neuritis, sweating, chills
CV: Hypotension, palpitations, tachycardia
RESP: Increased thick secretions, wheezing, chest tightness
*HEMA: **Thrombocytopenia, agranulocytosis, hemolytic anemia***
GI: Dry mouth, nausea, vomiting, anorexia, constipation, diarrhea
INTEG: Rash, urticaria, photosensitivity
GU: Retention, dysuria, frequency, impotence
EENT: Blurred vision, dilated pupils, tinnitus, nasal stuffiness, dry nose, throat, mouth

Contraindications: Hypersensitivity to H₁-receptor antagonist, acute asthma attack, lower respiratory tract disease, child <12 yr

Precautions: Increased intraocular pressure, renal disease, cardiac disease, hypertension, bronchial asthma, seizure disorder, stenosed peptic ulcers, hyperthyroidism, prostatic hypertrophy, bladder neck obstruction, pregnancy (B)

Pharmacokinetics:
PO: Peak 4 hr; metabolized in liver, excreted by kidneys, crosses placenta, crosses blood-brain barrier, minimally bound to plasma proteins, half-life 9-12 hr

Interactions/incompatibilities:
• Increased CNS depression: barbiturates, narcotics, hypnotics, tricyclic antidepressants, alcohol
• Decreased effect of: oral anticoagulants, heparin
• Increased effect of this drug: MAOIs

NURSING CONSIDERATIONS
Assess:
• I&O ratio; be alert for urinary retention, frequency, dysuria; drug should be discontinued if these occur
• CBC during long-term therapy

Administer:
• Coffee, tea, cola (caffeine) to de-

---

crease drowsiness
• With meals if GI symptoms occur; absorption may slightly decrease

Perform/provide:
• Hard candy, gum, frequent rinsing of mouth for dryness
• Storage in tight container at room temperature

Evaluate:
• Therapeutic response: absence of running or congested nose, or rashes
• Blood dyscrasias: thrombocytopenia, agranulocytosis; these occur rarely
• Respiratory status: rate, rhythm, increase in bronchial secretions, wheezing, chest tightness
• Cardiac status: palpitations, increased pulse, hypotension

Teach patient/family:
• All aspects of drug use; to notify physician if confusion, sedation, or hypotension occurs
• To avoid driving or other hazardous activities if drowsiness occurs
• To avoid concurrent use of alcohol or other CNS depressants

Lab test interferences:
False negative: Skin allergy tests
Treatment of overdose: Administer ipecac syrup or lavage, diazepam, vasopressors, barbiturates (short-acting)

---

azathioprine

(ay-za-thye'oh-preen)
Imuran

Func. class.: Immunosuppressant
Chem. class.: Purine analog

Action: Produces immunosuppression by inhibiting purine synthesis in cells
Uses: Renal transplants to prevent rejection, refractory rheumatoid arthritis

Dosage and routes:
Prevention of rejection
• *Adult and child:* PO 3-5 mg/kg/day, then maintenance of at least 1-2 mg/kg/day
Refractory rheumatoid arthritis
• *Adult:* PO 1/mg/kg/day, may increase dose after 2 mo by 0.5 mg/kg/day, not to exceed 2.5 mg/kg/day
Available forms include: Tabs 50 mg; inj IV 100 mg
Side effects/adverse reactions:
GI: Nausea, vomiting, stomatitis, esophagitis, *pancreatitis, hepatotoxicity, jaundice*
HEMA: **Leukopenia, thrombocytopenia, anemia, pancytopenia**
INTEG: Rash
MS: Arthralgia, muscle wasting
Contraindications: Hypersensitivity
Precautions: Severe renal disease, severe hepatic disease
Pharmacokinetics: Metabolized in liver, excreted in urine (active metabolite), crosses placenta
Interactions/incompatibilities:
• Increased action of this drug: allopurinol

NURSING CONSIDERATIONS
Assess:
• Blood studies: Hgb, WBC, platelets during treatment monthly; if leukocytes are <3000/mm^3 drug should be discontinued
• Liver function studies: alk phosphatase, AST, ALT, bilirubin
Administer:
• For several days before transplant surgery
• All medications PO if possible, avoiding IM injections since bleeding may occur
• With meals for GI upset
Evaluate:
• Hepatotoxicity: dark urine, jaundice, itching, light-colored stools; drug should be discontinued

---

Teach patient/family:
• That therapeutic response may take 3-4 mo in rheumatoid arthritis
• To report fever, chills, sore throat, fatigue since serious infections may occur
• To use contraceptive measures during treatment, for 12 wk after ending therapy

---

azlocillin sodium

(az-loe-sill'in)

Azlin

Func. class.: Broad spectrum antibiotic

Chem. class.: Extended spectrum penicillin

Action: Interferes with cell wall replication of susceptible organisms; The cell wall, rendered osmotically unstable, swells, bursts from osmotic pressure

Uses: Lower respiratory infections, skin, bone, bacterial septicemia, urinary tract infections, yaws; effective for gram-positive cocci *(S. aureus, S. pyogenes, S. faecalis)*, gram-positive bacilli *(C. perfringens, C. tetani)*, gram-negative bacilli *(Bacteroides, P. aeruginosa, E. coli), H. influenzae, P. mirabilis*

Dosage and routes:
• *Adult:* IV 200-350 mg/kg/day in 4-6 divided doses, max 24 g
Cystic fibrosis
• *Child:* IV 75 mg/kg q4h max 24 g
Available forms include: Powder for inj 2, 3, 4 g

Side effects/adverse reactions:
HEMA: Anemia, increased bleeding time, *bone marrow depression, granulocytopenia*
GI:Nausea, vomiting, diarrhea, increased AST, ALT, abdominal pain, glossitis, colitis
GU: Oliguria, proteinuria, hematuria, *vaginitis, moniliasis, glomerulonephritis*
CNS: Lethargy, hallucinations, anxiety, depression, twitching, *coma, convulsions*
META: Hyperkalemia, hypokalemia, alkalosis, hypernatremia

Contraindications: Hypersensitivity to penicillins

Precautions: Pregnancy (B), hypersensitivity to cephalosporins, neonates

Pharmacokinetics: Half-life 55-70 min, metabolized in liver, excreted in urine, bile, breast milk (small amount), crosses placenta

Interactions/incompatibilities:
• Decreased antimicrobial effectiveness of this drug: tetracyclines, erythromycins
• Increased penicillin concentrations when used with: aspirin, probenicid

NURSING CONSIDERATIONS

Assess:
• I&O ratio; report hematuria, oliguria since penicillin in high doses is nephrotoxic
• Any patient with compromised renal system, since drug is excreted slowly in poor renal system function; toxicity may occur rapidly
• Liver studies: AST, ALT
• Blood studies: WBC, RBC, H&H, bleeding time
• Renal studies: urinalysis, protein, blood
• Culture, sensitivity before drug therapy; drug may be taken as soon as culture is taken

Administer:
• After C&S completed
• Slowly (IV) over 5 min to prevent chest discomfort

Perform/provide:
• Adrenaline, suction, tracheostomy set, endotracheal intubation equipment on unit
• Adequate intake of fluids (2000 ml) during diarrhea episodes

---

italics = common side effects   ***bold italic*** = life threatening reactions

• Scratch test to assess allergy after securing order from physician; usually done when penicillin is only drug of choice

• Storage in cool environment; solution is stable for 24 hr at room temperature

Evaluate:

• For therapeutic effectiveness: absence of temperature, draining wounds

• Bowel pattern before, during treatment

• Skin eruptions after administration of penicillin to 1 wk after discontinuing drug

• Respiratory status: rate, character, wheezing, tightness in chest

• Allergies before initiation of treatment; reaction of each medication; place allergies on chart, Kardex in bright red

Teach patient/family:

• Culture may be taken after completed course of medication

• To report sore throat, fever, fatigue (could indicate superimposed infection)

• To wear or carry a Medic Alert ID if allergic to penicillins

• To notify nurse of diarrhea stools

Lab test interferences:

False positive: Urine glucose, urine protein

Decrease: Uric acid

Treatment of overdose: Withdraw drug, maintain airway, administer epinephrine, aminophylline, O_2, IV corticosteroids for anaphylaxis

---

bacampicillin HCl

(ba-kam-pi-sill'in)

Penglobe,* Spectrobid

Func. class.: Broad spectrum antibiotic

Chem. class.: Aminopenicillin

Action: Interferes with cell wall replication of susceptible organisms; the cell wall, rendered osmotically unstable, swells, bursts from osmotic pressure

Uses: Respiratory tract infections, skin urinary tract infections; effective for gram-positive cocci *(S. faecalis, S. pneumoniae),* gram-negative cocci *(N. gonorrhoeae),* gram-negative bacilli *(E. coli, H. influenzae, P. mirabilis)*

Dosage and routes:

• *Adult:* PO 400-800 mg q12h

• *Child:* PO 25-50 mg/kg/day in divided doses q12h

Available forms include: Tabs 400 mg; powder for oral susp 125 mg/5 ml

Side effects/adverse reactions:

HEMA: Anemia, increased bleeding time, *bone marrow depression, granulocytopenia*

GI: Nausea, vomiting, diarrhea, increased AST, ALT, abdominal pain, glossitis, colitis

GU: Oliguria, proteinuria, hematuria, *vaginitis, moniliasis, glomerulonephritis*

CNS: Lethargy, hallucinations, anxiety, depression, twitching, *coma, convulsions*

META: Hyperkalemia, hypokalemia, alkalosis, hypernatremia

Contraindications: Hypersensitivity to penicillins; neonates

Precautions: Pregnancy (B), hypersensitivity to cephalosporins

Pharmacokinetics:

PO: 30-60 min, duration 5-6 hr, metabolized in liver, excreted in urine

Interactions/incompatibilities:

• Decreased antimicrobial effectiveness of this drug: tetracyclines, erythromycins

• Increased penicillin concentrations when used with: aspirin, probenicid

NURSING CONSIDERATIONS

Assess:

• I&O ratio; report hematuria, oli-

---

guria since penicillin in high doses is nephrotoxic
• Any patient with compromised renal system, since drug is excreted slowly in poor renal system function; toxicity may occur rapidly
• Liver studies: AST, ALT
• Blood studies: WBC, RBC, H&H, bleeding time
• Renal studies: urinalysis, protein, blood
• Culture, sensitivity before drug therapy; drug may be taken as soon as culture is taken

Administer:
• After C&S completed

Perform/provide:
• Adrenaline, suction, tracheostomy set, endotracheal intubation equipment on unit
• Adequate intake of fluids (2000 ml) during diarrhea episodes
• Scratch test to assess allergy after securing order from physician; usually done when penicillin is only drug of choice
• Storage in dry tight container

Evaluate:
• For therapeutic effectiveness: absence of temperature, draining wounds
• Bowel pattern before, during treatment
• Skin eruptions after administration of penicillin to 1 wk after discontinuing drug
• Respiratory status: rate, character, wheezing, tightness in chest
• Allergies before initiation of treatment; reaction of each medication; place allergies on chart, Kardex in bright red

Teach patient/family:
• Aspects of drug therapy: culture may be taken after completed course of medication
• To report sore throat, fever, fatigue (could indicate superimposed infection)
• To wear or carry a Medic Alert

ID if allergic to penicillins
• To notify nurse of diarrhea stools

Lab test interferences:
False positive: Urine glucose, urine protein
Decrease: Uric acid

Treatment of overdose: Withdraw drug, maintain airway, administer epinephrine, aminophylline, O_2, IV corticosteroids for anaphylaxis

---

bacitracin

(bass-i-tray'sin)
Baci-IM

Func. class.: Antibacterial
Chem. class.: Bacillus subtilis derivative

Action: Inhibits bacterial cell wall synthesis by interfering with osmotic pressure within cell

Uses: Staphylococcal pneumonia, empyema

Dosage and routes:
• *Adults:* IM 10,000-25,000 U q6h, not to exceed 25,000 U/dose
• *Infants >2.5 kg:* IM 1,000 U/kg/day in divided doses q8-12h
• *Infants <2.5 kg:* IM 900 U/kg/day in divided doses q8-12h

Available forms include: Inj IM 10,000, 50,000 U

Side effects/adverse reactions:
INTEG: Rash, urticaria, pruritus, erythema, pain at injection site
SYST: Anaphylaxis
HEMA: Anemia, bone marrow depression, granulocytopenia
GI: Nausea, anorexia, vomiting, diarrhea, rectal itching
GU: Oliguria, albuminuria, anuria, increased BUN, *uremia, tubular, glomerular necrosis*

Contraindications: Hypersensitivity, severe renal disease

Precautions: Myasthenia gravis, multiple sclerosis, pregnancy

Pharmacokinetics: Peak 1-2 hr,

---

italics = common side effects   ***bold italic*** = life threatening reactions

duration >12 hr, metabolized in liver, excreted in feces

Interactions/incompatibilities:

• Increased nephrotoxicity, neurotoxicity: aminoglycosides, polymyxin

• Increased neuromuscular blockage: nondepolarizing skeletal muscle relaxants, anesthetics

NURSING CONSIDERATIONS

Assess:

• I&O ratio; report oliguria, change in urinary output; high doses are nephrotoxic

• Any patient with compromised renal system; drug is excreted slowly in poor renal system function; toxicity may occur rapidly

• Renal studies: urinalysis, protein, blood, BUN, creatinine, urine pH (keep at 6.0)

• C&S before drug therapy; drug may be taken as soon as culture is taken; repeat C&S after treatment

Administer:

• After reconstituting with NS

• IM in deep muscle mass; rotate injection site; do not give IV/SC

Perform/provide:

• Storage in refrigerator; protect from direct sunlight

• Adrenalin, suction, tracheostomy set, endotracheal intubation equipment on unit

• Adequate intake of fluids (2000 ml) during diarrhea episodes

Evaluate:

• Therapeutic response: absence of fever, cough, dyspnea, malaise

• Bowel pattern before, during treatment; if severe diarrhea occurs, drug should be discontinued

• Skin eruptions, itching: rash, urticaria, erythema

• Respiratory status: rate, character, wheezing, tightness in chest, dyspnea on exertion

• Allergies before treatment, reaction of each medication; place allergies on chart, Kardex in bright red letters; notify all people giving drugs

Teach patient/family:

• To report sore throat, fever, fatigue; could indicate superimposed infection

---

bacitracin (ophthalmic)

(bass-i-tray'sin)

Func. class.: Antiinfective

Action: Inhibits bacterial cell wall in organism by preventing amino acids, nucleotides into cell wall

Uses: Infection of eye

Dosage and routes:

• *Adult and child:* Apply to conjunctival sac bid-qid until desired response

Available forms include: Oint 500 U/g

Side effects/adverse reactions:

EENT: Poor corneal wound healing, visual haze (temporary), overgrowth of nonsusceptible organisms

Contraindications: Hypersensitivity

Precautions: Antibiotic hypersensitivity

Interactions/incompatibilities: None known

NURSING CONSIDERATIONS

Administer:

• After washing hands, cleanse crusts or discharge from eye before application

Perform/provide:

• Storage at room temperature

Evaluate:

• Therapeutic response: absence of redness, inflammation, tearing

• Allergy: itching, lacrimation, redness, swelling

Teach patient/family:

• To use drug exactly as prescribed

• Not to use eye makeup, towels, washcloths, eye medication of others; reinfection may occur

• That drug container tip should not be touched to eye
• To report itching, increased redness, burning, stinging, swelling; drug should be discontinued
• That drug may cause blurred vision when ointment is applied

bacitracin (topical)

(bass-i-tray′sin)
Baciguent, Bacitin*
Func. class.: Local antiinfective
Chem. class.: Antibacterial

Action: Interferes with bacterial cell wall function by inhibiting protein synthesis
Uses: Topical staphylococci, streptococci
Dosage and routes:
• *Adult and child:* TOP bid-qid or more often if needed
Available forms include: Oint 500 U/g
Side effects/adverse reactions:
INTEG: Rash, urticaria, stinging, burning
Contraindications: Hypersensitivity
Precautions: Pregnancy, lactation
Interactions/incompatibilities: None known
NURSING CONSIDERATIONS
Administer:
• Enough medication to completely cover lesions
• After cleansing with soap, water before each application, dry well (as ordered)
Perform/provide:
• Storage at room temperature in dry place
Evaluate:
• Allergic reaction: burning, stinging, swelling, redness
• Therapeutic response: decrease in size, number of lesions

Teach patient/family:
• To apply with glove to prevent further infection
• To avoid use of OTC creams, ointments, lotions unless directed by physician
• To use medical asepsis (hand washing) before, after each application to prevent further infection

baclofen

(bak′loe-fen)
Lioresal, Lioresal DS
Func. class.: Skeletal muscle relaxant, central acting
Chem. class.: GABA chlorophenyl derivative

Action: Inhibits synaptic responses in CNS by decreasing GABA, which decreases neurotransmitter function; decreases frequency, severity of muscle spasms
Uses: Spinal cord injury, spasticity in multiple sclerosis
Dosage and routes:
• *Adult:* PO 5 mg tid × 3 days, then 10 mg tid × 3 days, then 15 mg tid × 3 days, then 20 mg tid × 3 days, then titrated to response, not to exceed 80 mg/day
Available forms include: Tabs 10, 20 mg
Side effects/adverse reactions:
CNS: Dizziness, weakness, fatigue, drowsiness, headache, disorientation insomnia, paresthesias, tremors
EENT: Nasal congestion, blurred vision, mydriasis
CV: Hypotension, chest pain, palpitations
GI: Nausea, constipation, vomiting, increased AST, alk phosphatase, abdominal pain, dry mouth, anorexia
GU: Urinary frequency
INTEG: Rash, pruritus

---

italics = common side effects   ***bold italic*** = life threatening reactions

Contraindications: Hypersensitivity

Precautions: Peptic ulcer disease, renal disease, hepatic disease, stroke, seizure disorder, diabetes mellitus, pregnancy

Pharmacokinetics:

PO: Peak 2-3 hr, duration >8 hr, half-life 2½-4 hr, partially metabolized in liver, excreted in urine (unchanged)

Interactions/incompatibilities:

• Increased CNS depression: alcohol, tricylic antidepressants, narcotics, barbiturates, sedatives, hypnotics

NURSING CONSIDERATIONS

Assess:

• For increased seizure activity in epilepsy patient; this drug decreases seizure threshold

• I&O ratio; check for urinary retention, frequency, hesitancy

• ECG in epileptic patients; poor seizure control has occurred in patients taking this drug

Administer:

• With meals for GI symptoms

• Gum, frequent sips of water for dry mouth

Perform/provide:

• Storage in tight container at room temperature

• Assistance with ambulation if dizziness or drowsiness occurs

Evaluate:

• Therapeutic response: decreased pain, spasticity

• Allergic reactions: rash, fever, respiratory distress

• Severe weakness, numbness in extremities

• Psychologic dependency: increased need for medication, more frequent requests for medication, increased pain

• CNS depression: dizziness, drowsiness, psychiatric symptoms

Teach patient/family:

• Not to discontinue medication

quickly; hallucinations, spasticity, tachycardia will occur; drug should be tapered off over 1-2 wk

• Not to take with alcohol, other CNS depressants

• To avoid altering activities while taking this drug

• To avoid hazardous activities if drowsiness or dizziness occurs

• To avoid using OTC medication: cough preparations, antihistamines, unless directed by physician

Lab test interferences:

Increase: AST, alk phosphatase, blood glucose

Treatment of overdose: Induce emesis of conscious patient, lavage, dialysis

---

beclomethasone dipropionate

(be-kloe-meth′a-sone)

Beclovent, Vancenase, Vanceril, Beconase

Func. class.: Corticosteroid, synthetic

Chem. class.: Mineralocorticoid

Action: Prevents inflammation by depression of migration of polymorphonuclear leukocytes, fibroblasts, reversal of increased capillary permeability and lysosomal stabilization; does not suppress hypothalamus and pituitary function

Uses: Steroid-dependent asthma, rhinitis

Dosage and routes:

• *Adult:* INH 2-4 puffs tid-qid, not to exceed 20 inhalations/day

• *Child:* 6-12 yr: INH 1-2 puffs tid-qid, not to exceed 10 inhalations/day

Available forms include: Aerosol 42 µg/actuation

Side effects/adverse reactions:

RESP: Bronchospasm

GI: Dry mouth

EENT: Hoarseness, candidal infections of oral cavity, sore throat

Contraindications: Hypersensitivity, status asthmaticus (primary treatment), nonasthmatic bronchial disease, bacterial, fungal, or viral infections of mouth, throat, or lungs

Precautions: Nasal disease/surgery

Pharmacokinetics:

INH: Onset 10 min, excreted in feces (metabolites), half-life 3-15 hr, crosses placenta, metabolized in lungs, liver, GI system

Interactions/incompatibilities: None significant

NURSING CONSIDERATIONS

Assess:

• Adrenal function periodically for HPA axis suppression

Administer:

• INH with water to decrease possibility of fungal infections

• Titrated dose, use lowest effective dose

Perform/provide:

• Gum, rinsing of mouth for dry mouth

Evaluate:

• Therapeutic response: decreased dyspnea, wheezing, dry rales on auscultation

Teach patient/family:

• That ID as steroid user should be carried

• To notify physician if therapeutic response decreases; dosage adjustment may be needed

• Proper administration technique

• Wash inhaler with warm water and dry after each use

• Teach patient all aspects of drug usage including Cushingoid symptoms

• Symptoms of adrenal insufficiency: nausea, anorexia, fatigue, dizziness, dyspnea, weakness, joint pain, depression

• To keep out of children's reach

beclomethasone dipropionate (nasal)

(be-kloe-meth′a-sone)

Beconase Nasal Inhaler, Vancenase Nasal Inhaler, Beclovent, Vanceril

Func. class.: Synthetic corticosteroid

Chem. class.: Beclomethasone diester

Action: Antiinflammatory, vasoconstrictive properties in nasal passages

Uses: Seasonal or perennial rhinitis

Dosage and routes:

• *Adult and child >12 yr:* IN-STILL 1-2 sprays in each nostril bid-qid

Available forms include: Aero 42 μg/spray

Side effects/adverse reactions:

EENT: Dryness, nasal irritation, burning, sneezing, secretions with blood, nasal ulcerations, ***perforation of nasal septum,*** candida infection, earache

ENDO: Adrenal suppression

INTEG: Rash, urticaria, pruritus

CNS: Headache, paresthesia

Contraindications: Hypersensitivity, systemic corticosteroid therapy

Precautions: Pregnancy (C), lactation, children <12, nasal ulcers, recurrent epistaxis respiration

Pharmacokinetics:

INSTILL: Readily absorbed; peak, concentration, other data have not been determined

Interactions/incompatibilities: None known

NURSING CONSIDERATIONS

Evaluate:

• Adrenal suppression: 17-KS, plasma cortisol for decreased levels

• Nasal passages during long-term treatment for changes in mucous

Administer:
• After cleaning aerosol top daily with warm water, dry thoroughly

Perform/provide:
• Storage in cool environment, do not puncture or incinerate container

Teach patient/family:
• To clear nasal passages if sneezing attack occurs, repeat dose
• To continue using product even if mild nasal bleeding occurs, is usually transient
• Method of installation after providing written instructions from manufacturer
• To clear nasal passages before administration, use decongestant if needed, shake inhaler, invert, tilt head backward, insert nozzle into nostril, away from septum, hold other nostril closed and depress activator, inhale through nose, exhale through mouth

---

belladonna alkaloids

(bell-a-don'a)
Bellafoline

Func. class.: Gastrointestinal anticholinergic
Chem. class.: Belladonna alkaloid

Action: Inhibits muscarinic actions of acetylcholine at postganglionic parasympathetic neurone effector sites

Uses: Treatment of peptic ulcer disease, irritable bowel syndrome in combination with other drugs; for other GI disorders

Dosage and routes:
• *Adult:* PO 0.25-0.5 mg tid; SC 0.125-0.5 mg qd or bid
• *Child >6 yr:* PO 0.125-0.25 mg tid

Available forms include: Tabs 0.25 mg; inj SC 0.5 mg/ml

Side effects/adverse reactions:
*CNS: Confusion, stimulation in el-*derly, headache, insomnia, dizziness, drowsiness, anxiety, weakness, hallucination
GI: Dry mouth, constipation, paralytic ileus, heartburn, nausea, vomiting, dysphagia, absence of taste
GU: Hesitancy, retention, impotence
CV: Palpitations, tachycardia
EENT: Blurred vision, photophobia, mydriasis, cycloplegia, increased ocular tension
INTEG: Urticaria, rash, pruritus, anhidrosis, fever, allergic reactions

Contraindications: Hypersensitivity to anticholinergics, narrow-angle glaucoma, GI obstruction, myasthenia gravis, paralytic ileus, GI atony, toxic megacolon

Precautions: Hyperthyroidism, coronary artery disease, dysrhythmias, CHF, ulcerative colitis, hypertension, hiatal hernia, hepatic disease, renal disease

Pharmacokinetics:
PO: Duration 4-6 hr; metabolized by liver, excreted in urine, half-life 13-38 hr

Interactions/incompatibilities:
• Increased anticholinergic effect: amantadine, tricyclic antidepressants, MAOIs
• Increased effect of: nitrofurantoin
• Decreased effect of: phenothiazines, levodopa

NURSING CONSIDERATIONS

Assess:
• VS, cardiac status: checking for dysrhythmias, increased rate, palpitations
• I&O ratio; check for urinary retention or hesitancy

Administer:
• ½-1 hr ac for better absorption
• Decreased dose to elderly patients; their metabolism may be slowed
• Gum, hard candy, frequent rins-

ing of mouth for dryness of oral cavity

Perform/provide:

• Storage in tight container protected from light

• Increased fluids, bulk, exercise to patient's lifestyle to decrease constipation

Evaluate:

• Therapeutic response: absence of epigastric pain, bleeding, nausea, vomiting

• GI complaints: pain, bleeding (frank or occult), nausea, vomiting, anorexia

Teach patient/family:

• Avoid driving or other hazardous activities until stabilized on medication

• Avoid alcohol or other CNS depressants; will enhance sedating properties of this drug

• To avoid hot environments, stroke may occur, drug suppresses perspiration

• Use sunglasses when outside to prevent photophobia

---

belladonna leaf

(bell-a-don'a)

Belladonna Tincture

Func. class.: Gastrointestinal anticholinergic

Chem. class.: Belladonna alkaloid

Action: Inhibits muscarinic actions of acetylcholine at postganglionic parasympathetic neuroeffector sites

Uses: Treatment of peptic ulcer disease, irritable bowel syndrome, neurogenic bowel disorder, functional GI disorders in combination with other drugs

Dosage and routes:

• *Adult:* PO 10.8-21.6 mg tid-qid (extract); PO 0.3-1 ml tid-qid (tincture)

Available forms include: Extract-tabs 15 mg; tincture-liq 0.3 mg/ml

Side effects/adverse reactions:

CNS: Confusion, stimulation in elderly, headache, insomnia, dizziness, drowsiness, anxiety, weakness, hallucination

GI: Dry mouth, constipation, paralytic ileus, heartburn, nausea, vomiting, dysphagia, absence of taste

GU: Hesitancy, retention, impotence

CV: Palpitations, tachycardia

EENT: Blurred vision, photophobia, mydriasis, cycloplegia, increased ocular tension

INTEG: Urticaria, rash, pruritus, anhidrosis, fever, allergic reactions

Contraindications: Hypersensitivity to anticholinergics, narrow-angle glaucoma, GI obstruction, myasthenia gravis, paralytic ileus, GI atony, toxic megacolon

Precautions: Hyperthyroidism, coronary artery disease, dysrhythmias, CHF, ulcerative colitis, hypertension, hiatal hernia, hepatic disease, renal disease

Pharmacokinetics:

PO: Onset 1-2 hr, duration 4-6 hr; metabolized by liver, excreted in urine

Interactions/incompatibilities:

• Increased anticholinergic effect: amantadine, tricyclic antidepressants, MAOIs

• Increased effect of: nitrofurantoin

• Decreased effect of: phenothiazines, levodopa

NURSING CONSIDERATIONS

Assess:

• VS, cardiac status: checking for dysrhythmias, increased rate, palpitations

• I&O ratio; check for urinary retention or hesitancy

Administer:

• ½-1 hr ac for better absorption

• Decreased dose to elderly patients; their metabolism may be slowed

---

italics = common side effects   ***bold italic*** = life threatening reactions

• Gum, hard candy, frequent rinsing of mouth for dryness of oral cavity

Perform/provide:

• Storage in tight container protected from light

• Increased fluids, bulk, exercise to patient's lifestyle to decrease constipation

Evaluate:

• Therapeutic response: absence of epigastric pain, bleeding, nausea, vomiting

• GI complaints: pain, bleeding (frank or occult), nausea, vomiting, anorexia

Teach patient/family:

• Avoid driving or other hazardous activities until stabilized on medication

• Avoid alcohol or other CNS depressants; will enhance sedating properties of this drug

• To avoid hot environments, stroke may occur, drug suppresses perspiration

• Use sunglasses when outside to prevent photophobia

---

bendroflumethiazide

(ben-droe-floo-meth-eye′a-zide)

Naturetin

Func. class.: Diuretic

Chem. class.: Thiazide; benzothiazide derivative

Action: Acts on distal tubule by increasing excretion of water, sodium, chloride, potassium

Uses: Edema, hypertension

Dosage and routes:

• *Adult:* PO 5-20 mg qd or in 2 divided doses

• *Child:* PO 0.1-0.4 mg/kg qd or in 2 divided doses; maintenance 0.05-0.1 mg/kg/day

Available forms include: Tab 2.5, 5, 10 mg

Side effects/adverse reactions:

GU: Frequency, polyuria, uremia, glucosuria

CNS: Drowsiness, paresthesia, anxiety, depression, headache, dizziness, fatigue, weakness

GI: Nausea, vomiting, anorexia, constipation, diarrhea, cramps, pancreatitis, GI irritation, *hepatitis*

EENT: Blurred vision

INTEG: Rash, urticaria, purpura, photosensitivity, fever

META: Hyperglycemia, hyperuremia, increased creatinine

HEMA: Aplastic anemia, hemolytic anemia, leukopenia, agranulocytosis, thrombocytopenia

CV: Irregular pulse, orthostatic hypotension

ELECT: Hypokalemia, hypercalcemia, hyponatremia, hypochloremia

Contraindications: Hypersensitivity to thiazides or sulfonamides, anuria, renal decompensation

Precautions: Hypokalemia, renal disease, pregnancy, hepatic disease, gout, COPD, lupus erythematosus, diabetes mellitus, pregnancy

Pharmacokinetics:

PO: Onset 2 hr, peak 4 hr, duration 6-12 hr

IV: Onset 15 min, peak ½ hr, duration 2-4 hr

Excreted unchanged in urine 3-6 hr, crosses placenta, excreted in breast milk

Interactions/incompatibilities:

• Increased toxicity: lithium, nondepolarizing skeletal muscle relaxants, digitalis

• Decreased effects of: antidiabetics

• Decreased absorption of thiazides: cholestyramine, colestipol

• Decreased hypotensive response: indomethacin

• Increased action of: quinidine

NURSING CONSIDERATIONS
Assess:
• Weight, I&O daily to determine fluid loss; effect of drug may be decreased if used qd
• Rate, depth, rhythm of respiration, effect of exertion
• B/P lying, standing; postural hypotension may occur
• Electrolytes: potassium, sodium, chloride; include BUN, blood sugar, CBC, serum creatinine, blood pH, ABGs
• Glucose in urine if patient is diabetic

Administer:
• In AM to avoid interference with sleep if using drug as a diuretic
• Potassium replacement if potassium is less than 3.0
• With food if nausea occurs; absorption may be decreased slightly

Evaluate:
• Improvement in edema of feet, legs, sacral area daily if medication is being used in CHF
• Improvement in CVP q8h
• Signs of metabolic acidosis: drowsiness, restlessness
• Signs of hypokalemia: postural hypotension, malaise, fatigue, tachycardia, leg cramps, weakness
• Rashes, temperature elevation qd
• Confusion especially in elderly; take safety precautions if needed

Teach patient/family:
• To increase fluid intake 2-3 L/day unless contraindicated; to rise slowly from lying or sitting position
• To notify physician of muscle weakness, cramps, nausea, dizziness
• Drug may be taken with food or milk
• That blood sugar may be increased in diabetics
• Take early in day to avoid nocturia

Lab test interferences:
Increase: BSP retention, calcium, amylase
Decrease: PBI, PSP
Treatment of overdose: Lavage if taken orally, monitor electrolytes, administer dextrose in saline

bentiromide
(ben-teer'oh-mide)
Chymex
Func. class.: Digestant
Chem. class.: Synthetic peptide with PABA

Action: A peptide that carries a PABA marker that can be detected
Uses: Pancreatic exocrine insufficiency screening, to assess pancreatic enzyme replacement therapy

Dosage and routes:
• *Adult and child >12 yr:* PO 500 mg with 8 oz water
• *Child <12 yr:* PO 14 mg/kg with 8 oz water
Available forms include: Sol 500 mg/7.5 ml

Side effects/adverse reactions:
CNS: Headache, dizziness, drowsiness, weakness
GI: Nausea, vomiting, *diarrhea,* abdominal pain, flatulence, increased liver enzymes
RESP: Acute respiratory distress, stridor

Contraindications: Hypersensitivity
Precautions: Pregnancy (B), lactation, children

Pharmacokinetics:
Peak 2-3 hr, metabolized in liver, excreted in urine (metabolites)

Interactions/incompatibilities:
• Decreased action of: sulfonamides

NURSING CONSIDERATIONS
Administer:
• After 8 hr NPO

• Whole, not to be crushed or chewed

• With water, give 16 oz of water 2 hr after dose, another 16 oz 4-6 hr after dose

Perform/provide:

• Storage at room temperature

• Collection of urine specimens (10-20 ml) for testing at hours 1-6 after drug administration

Evaluate:

• Bowel pattern before, during treatment: diarrhea may occur

Teach patient/family:

• To drink water 2-3 L daily 24 hr following test to promote elimination of drug

• That if retest is needed 1 wk is necessary after previous test

• To void before taking drug

Lab test interferences:

False increase: PABA drugs, arylamines

---

benzalkonium chloride

(benz-al-koe'nee-um)

Benasept, Benzachlor-50,* Bena-All, Ionax Scrub,* Sabol Shampoo,* Zalkon, Zalkonium Chloride, Zephiran, Mercurochrome II, Benza, Dermo-Sterol

Func. class.: Disinfectant

Chem. class.: Quaternary ammonium cationic surfactant

Action: Inhibits and destroys organisms by enzyme inactivation (bactericidal/bacteriostatic)

Uses: Irrigate eye, vagina, body cavities, disinfection of skin before surgery

Dosage and routes:

• *Adult and child:* TOP 1:750 for minor wounds, disinfection before surgery; 1:3,000-20,000 deep infected wounds; 1:2,000-5,000 vaginal irrigation; 1:5,000-10,000 denuded skin, eye, mucous membrane irrigation; 1:5,000-20,000 bladder, urethral irrigation

Available forms include: Top sol 0.1%, 0.13%, 17%, 17.5%, 50%; tinct 0.13%

Side effects/adverse reactions:

CNS: Confusion, restlessness

INTEG: Irritation, contact dermatitis, hypersensitivity, rash, burning

GI: Nausea, vomiting

RESP: Dyspnea, *respiratory paralysis, coma*

Contraindications: Hypersensitivity, occlusive dressing, casts/traction

Interactions/incompatibilities:

• Decreased action when soap is left on skin

• Not to be used with fluorescein, nitrates, lanolin, potassium permanganate, kaolin, zinc sulfate, zinc oxide, caramel, aluminum, iodine, peroxide, yellow oxide of mercury, citrates, sulfonamides

NURSING CONSIDERATIONS

Administer:

• After diluting with sterile water for injection for irrigating wounds

• To body areas only; do not apply to face, lips, mouth, eyes, mucous membrane, anus, meatus

• To ⅓ of body or less to avoid chilling

Perform/provide:

• Rust tablets for cleaning metal objects, or instrument will rust

• Wet dressings using clear solution only; discontinue if necrosis occurs

Evaluate:

• Area of body involved: irritation, rash, breaks, dryness, scales, discharge

Teach patient/family:

• To store at room temperature no longer than 1 wk

• To use applicator, insert high into vagina, notify physician of itching, discharge, burning

Treatment of ingestion: Admin-

---

ister milk, soap solution, gastric lavage, supportive care

---

benzocaine

(ben'zoe-caine)
Americaine, Anbesol, Benzocol, Cloerex, Dermoplast, Hurricaine, Oracin, Ora-Jel, Rhulicream, Solarcaine, Spec-T Anesthetic, Trocaine

Func. class.: Topical anesthetic
Chem. class.: Ethyl ester of PABA

Action: Inhibits nerve impulses from sensory nerves; produces anesthesia
Uses: Pruritus, sunburn, toothache, sore throat, cold sores, oral pain, rectal pain, irritation
Dosage and routes:
• *Adult and child:* SYR/JEL apply to affected area; LOZ suck as needed; OINT apply to affected area bid-tid
Available forms include: Aerosol 20%; gel 6.3%, 7.5%, 10%, 20%; sol 2.5%, 6.3%, 20%; cream 1%, 5%, 6%; oint 2%, 5%; lotion 0.5%
Side effects/adverse reactions:
*HEMA: **Methemoglobinemia***
INTEG: Rash, irritation, sensitization
Contraindications: Hypersensitivity to PABA or procaine, infants <1 yr, application to large areas
Precautions: Child <6 yr, sepsis, pregnancy, denuded skin
Interactions/incompatibilities: None known
NURSING CONSIDERATIONS
Administer:
• After cleansing, drying of affected area
Evaluate
• For allergic reactions: rash, irritation, reddening, swelling
• For therapeutic response: absence of pain, itching of affected area
• Affected area for infection, if in-

fection is present, do not apply
Teach patient/family:
• To report rash, irritation, redness, swelling
• How to apply spray, ointment, jelly; how to use syrup or lozenges

---

benzocaine

(ben-zoe-kane)
Orabase with Benzocaine, Oracin, Ora-Jel, Spec-T Anesthetic, Trocaine, Tyzomint, Solarcaine, Dermoplast, Chiggerex, Benzocal, Americaine

Func. class.: Topical local anesthetic
Chem. class.: Ester

Action: Inhibits conduction of nerve impulses from sensory nerves
Uses: Oral irritation, sore throat, toothache, cold sore, canker sore, sunburn, minor cuts, insect bites, pain, itching
Dosage and routes:
• *Adult and child >12 yr:* TOP apply to affected area; LOZ suck as needed
Available forms include: Cream 1%, 5%; lotion 0.5%, 8%; oint 2%, 5%, 20%; sol 2.1%, 2.5%, 6.3%, 20%; lozenges 3, 5, 6.25, 10 mg; topical aerosol 20%; gel 6.3%, 7.5%, 10%, 20%
Side effects/adverse reactions:
EENT: Itching, irritation in ear
INTEG: Rash, urticaria
Contraindications: Hypersensitivity
Precautions: Pregnancy
Pharmacokinetics:
TOP: Peak 1 min, duration ½-1 hr
Interactions/incompatibilities: None known
NURSING CONSIDERATIONS
Administer:
• To gums as needed for teething pain

---

italics = common side effects **bold italic** = life threatening reactions

• Lozenges for temporary sore throat pain

Perform/provide:

• Storage in tight, light-resistant container; do not freeze, puncture, or incinerate aerosol container

Evaluate:

• Affected area for redness, swelling, pain

Teach patient/family:

• To avoid contact with eyes

• Not to use for prolonged periods of time <1 wk; if condition remains, physician should be contacted

---

benzocaine

(ben'zoe-caine)

Americaine-Otic, Auralgan, Eardro, Myringacaine, Tympagesic, Otocain

Func. class.: Otic

Chem. class.: Paraminobenzoic acid ethyl ester (PABA)

Action: Inhibits nerve impulse conduction in sensory nerves, decreases ear pain

Uses: Removal of cerumen, otitis media pain

Dosage and routes:

• *Adult and child:* INSTILL in ear canal tid × 2 days

Otitis media pain

• *Adult and child:* INSTILL in ear canal, plug with cotton, repeat q1-2h prn

Available forms include: Sol 1.4%, 5%, 20%

Side effects/adverse reactions:

EENT: Itching, irritation in ear

INTEG: Rash, urticaria

Contraindications: Hypersensitivity, perforated eardrum

Pharmacokinetics:

INSTILL: Peak 1 min, duration ½-1 hr

Interactions/incompatibilities: None known

NURSING CONSIDERATIONS

Administer:

• After removing impacted cerumen by irrigation

• After cleaning stopper with alcohol

• After restraining child if necessary

• Warming solution to body temperature

Evaluate:

• Therapeutic response: decreased ear pain

• For redness, swelling, pain in ear, which indicates superimposed infection

Teach patient/family:

• Method of instillation, using aseptic technique including not touching dropper to ear

• That dizziness may occur after instillation

• Report ear pain >48 hr

---

benzocaine (topical)

(ben'zoe-caine)

Americaine, Anbesol, Benzocol, Cloerex, Dermoplast, Hurricaine, Oracin, Ora-Jel, Rhulicream, Solarcaine, Spec T Anesthetic, Trocaine

Func. class.: Topical anesthetic

Chem. class.: PABA ethyl ester

Action: Inhibits nerve impulses from sensory nerves which produces anesthesia

Uses: Pruritus, sunburn, toothache, sore throat, cold sores, oral pain, rectal pain, irritation

Dosage and routes:

• *Adult and child:* Apply syr/gel to affected area; suck loz as needed; apply oint to affected area bid-tid

Available forms include: Aerosol 20%; gel 6.3%, 7.5%, 10%, 20%; sol 2.5%, 6.3%, 20%

Side effects/adverse reactions:

HEMA: Methemoglobinemia (infants)

INTEG: Rash, irritation, sensitization

Contraindications: Hypersensitivity to PABA or procaine, infants <1 yr, application to large areas

Precautions: Child <6 yr, sepsis, pregnancy, denuded skin

Interactions/incompatibilities: None known

NURSING CONSIDERATIONS

Administer:

• After cleansing and drying of affected area

Evaluate:

• Allergy: rash, irritation, reddening, swelling

• Therapeutic response: absence of pain, itching of affected area

• Infection: if affected area is infected, do not apply

Teach patient/family:

• To report rash, irritation, redness, swelling

• How to apply spray, ointment, jelly, and how to use syrup or lozenges

• Not to get aerosol in eyes or inhale spray

---

benzonatate

(ben-zoe'na-tate)

Tessalon

Func. class.: Antitussive, nonnarcotic

Chem. class.: Tetracine derivative

Action: Inhibits cough reflex by anesthetizing stretch receptors in respiratory system, direct action on cough center in medulla

Uses: Nonproductive cough

Dosage and routes:

• *Adult and child:* PO 100 mg tid, not to exceed 600 mg/day

• *Child <10 yr:* PO 8 mg/kg in 3-6 divided doses

Available forms include: Caps 100 mg

Side effects/adverse reactions:

CNS: Dizziness, drowsiness, headache

GI: Nausea, constipation, upset stomach

EENT: Nasal congestion, burning eyes

CV: Increased B/P, chest tightness, numbness

INTEG: Urticaria, rash, pruritus

Contraindications: Hypersensitivity

Precautions: Pregnancy (C), lactation

Pharmacokinetics:

PO: Onset 15-20 min, duration 3-8 hr, metabolized by liver, excreted in urine

Interactions/incompatibilities: None known

NURSING CONSIDERATIONS

Perform/provide:

• Storage in tight, light-resistant containers

• Increased fluids, bulk, exercise to patient's lifestyle to decrease constipation, liquefy sputum

• Chest percussion to bring up secretion if needed

Evaluate:

• Therapeutic response: absence of cough

• Cough: type, frequency, character including sputum

Teach patient/family:

• Avoid driving, other hazardous activities until patient is stabilized on this medication

• Not to chew or break capsules; will anesthetize mouth

• To avoid smoking, smoke-filled rooms, perfumes, dust, environmental pollutants, cleaners

---

benzoyl peroxide

(ben'zoe-ill per-ox'ide)
Benoxyl, Benzac, Benzagel, Desquam-X,* Oxy-5, Oxy-10, Persadox, Persa-Gel, Xerac BP, Pan Oxyl, Propa P.H. Acne

Func. class.: Antiacne medication

Action: Antibacterial activity especially against predominant bacteria causing acne
Uses: Mild-moderate acne
Dosage and routes:
• *Adult and child:* TOP apply to affected area qd or bid
Available forms include: Topical cleansers, lotions, creams, sticks, pads, gels, bars
Side effects/adverse reactions:
INTEG: Local skin irritation, stinging, warmth (dryness), scaling, erythema, edema, allergic, contact dermatitis
Contraindications: Hypersensitivity to benzoic acid derivatives
Precautions: Pregnancy (C), lactation, children <12 yr
Pharmacokinetics:
TOP: 50% absorbed through skin, metabolized to benzoic acid, excreted in urine
Interactions/incompatibilities:
None known
NURSING CONSIDERATIONS
Administer:
• Then wash hands immediately to avoid irritation
Perform/provide:
• Storage at room temperature
Evaluate:
• Therapeutic response: decreased amount of acne on body
• Area of body involved, including time involved, what helps or aggravates condition
• Allergic reaction: rash, irritation, scaling, dermatitis; discontinue use

Teach patient/family:
• To avoid application on normal skin or getting cream in eyes, nose, or other mucous membranes
• To discontinue use if rash or irritation develops
• May cause transitory warmth or stinging over area treated
• Expect dryness, peeling of area treated
• Avoid contact with hair or clothing; they may stain
• Cosmetics may be used over drug
• That dryness and peeling can be expected

benzphetamine HCl

(benz-fet'a-neen)
Didrex

Func. class.: Cerebral stimulant
Chem. class.: Amphetamine

Controlled Substance Schedule III

Action: Increases release of norepinephrine and dopamine in cerebral cortex to reticular activating system.
Uses: Exogenous obesity
Dosage and routes:
• *Adult:* PO 25-50 mg qd-tid
Available forms include: Tabs 25, 50 mg
Side effects/adverse reactions:
CNS: Hyperactivity, insomnia, restlessness, talkativeness, dizziness, headache, chills, stimulation, dysphoria, irritability, aggressiveness
GI: Nausea, vomiting, anorexia, dry mouth, diarrhea, constipation, weight loss, metallic taste, cramps
GU: Impotence, change in libido
CV: Palpitations, tachycardia, hypertension, hypotension
INTEG: Urticaria
Contraindications: Hypersensitivity to sympathomimetic amines, hyperthyroidism, hypertension, glaucoma hypertrophy, severe ar-

teriosclerosis, nephritis, angina pectoris, parkinsonism, drug abuse, cardiovascular disease, anxiety, pregnancy (X)

Precautions: Gilles de la Tourette's disorder, lactation, child <3 yr, diabetes mellitus, elderly

Pharmacokinetics:

PO: Onset 30 min, peak 1-3 hr, duration 4-20 hr; metabolized by liver, excreted by kidneys, crosses placenta, breast milk, half-life 10-30 hr

Interactions/incompatibilities:

• Hypertensive crisis: MAOIs or within 14 days of MAOIs

• Increased effect of this drug: acetazolamide, antacids, sodium bicarbonate, ascorbic acid, ammonium chloride, phenothiazines, haloperidol

• Decreased effects of this drug: barbiturates

• Decreased effects of: guanethidine, other antihypertensives

NURSING CONSIDERATIONS

Assess:

• VS, B/P since this drug may reverse antihypertensives; check patients with cardiac diseases more often

• CBC, urinalysis, in diabetes: blood sugar, urine sugar; insulin changes may need to be made since eating will decrease

• Height, growth rate in children; growth rate may be decreased

Administer:

• At least 6 hr before hs to avoid sleeplessness

• For obesity only if patient is on weight reduction program that includes dietary changes, exercise; patient will develop tolerance and weight loss won't occur without additional methods

• Gum, hard candy, frequent sips of water for dry mouth

If drug is for obesity, 1 hour before meals

Perform/provide:

• Check to see PO medication has been swallowed

Evaluate:

• Mental status: mood, sensorium, affect, stimulation, insomnia, aggressiveness may occur

• Physical dependency; should not be used for extended time; dose should be discontinued gradually

• Withdrawal symptoms: headache, nausea, vomiting, muscle pain, weakness

• Drug tolerance will develop after long-term use

• Dosage should not be increased if tolerance develops

Teach patient/family:

• To decrease caffeine consumption (coffee, tea, cola, chocolate); may increase irritability, stimulation

• Avoid OTC preparations unless approved by physician

• To taper off drug over several weeks, or depression, increased sleeping, lethargy may occur

• To avoid alcohol ingestion

• To avoid hazardous activities until patient is stabilized on medication

• To get needed rest; patients will feel more tired at end of day

Treatment of overdose: Administer fluids, hemodialysis, peritoneal dialysis; antihypertensive for increased B/P; ammonium Cl for increased excretion

---

benzquinamide HCl

(benz-kwin'a-mide)

Emete-Con, Quantril

Func. class.: Antiemetic

Chem. class.: Benzoquinolize amide

Action: Acts centrally by blocking chemoreceptor trigger zone, which in turn acts on vomiting center

Uses: To inhibit nausea, vomiting associated with anesthetic, surgery
Dosage and routes:
• *Adult:* IM 50 mg or 0.5-1 mg/kg, may be repeated in 1 hr, then q3-4 hr prn; IV 25 mg or 0.2-0.4 mg/kg as a one-time dose
Available forms include: Inj 50 mg/vial
Side effects/adverse reactions:
CNS: Drowsiness, fatigue, restlessness, tremor, headache, stimulation, dizziness, insomnia, twitching, excitement, nervousness, extrapyramidal symptoms
GI: Nausea, anorexia
*CV: **Premature atrial** or **ventricular contractions, atrial fibrillation,*** hypertension, hypotension
INTEG: Rash, urticaria, fever, chills, flushing, hives, shivering, sweating, temperature
EENT: Dry mouth, blurred vision, hiccups, salivation
Contraindications: Hypersensitivity, hypertension
Precautions: Children, pregnancy, lactation, elderly
Pharmacokinetics:
IM/IV: Onset 15 min, duration 3-4 hr, metabolized by liver, excreted in urine, feces, half-life 40 min
Interactions/incompatibilities:
None known
NURSING CONSIDERATIONS
Assess:
• Vital signs, B/P; check patients with cardiac disease more often; hypotension, hypertension dysrhythmias may occur
Administer:
• After reconstituting with 2.2 ml sterile water for injection; do not use sodium chloride
Perform/provide:
• Storage of injection before, after reconstitution in light-resistant container

Evaluate:
• Therapeutic response: absence of nausea, vomiting
• Observe for drowsiness; instruct patient not to drive, operate machinery
Treatment of overdose:
• Supportive care; atropine may be helpful

---

benzthiazide
(bens-thye′a-zide)
Aquatag, Exna, Hydrex, Proaqua
Func. class.: Diuretic
Chem. class.: Thiazide; sulfonamide derivative

Action: Acts on distal tubule by increasing excretion of water, sodium, chloride, potassium
Uses: Edema, hypertension
Dosage and routes:
• *Adult:* PO 50-200 mg qd or in divided doses, adjusted to desired response
• *Child:* PO 1-4 mg/kg/day in 3 divided doses
Available forms include: Tabs 25, 50 mg
Side effects/adverse reactions:
GU: Frequency, polyuria, uremia, glucosuria
CNS: Drowsiness, paresthesia, anxiety, depression, headache, dizziness, fatigue, weakness
GI: Nausea, vomiting, anorexia, constipation, diarrhea, cramps, pancreatitis, GI irritation, **hepatitis**
EENT: Blurred vision
INTEG: Rash, urticaria, purpura, photosensitivity, fever
META: Hyperglycemia, hyperuremia, increased creatinine
*HEMA: **Aplastic anemia, hemolytic anemia, leukopenia, agranulocytosis, thrombocytopenia***
CV: Irregular pulse, orthostatic hypotension
ELECT: Hypokalemia, hypercalce-

mia, hyponatremia, hypochloremia
Contraindications: Hypersensitivity to thiazides or sulfonamides, anuria, renal decompensation
Precautions: Hypokalemia, renal disease, pregnancy, hepatic disease, gout, COPD, lupus erythematosus, diabetes mellitus
Pharmacokinetics:
PO: Onset 2 hr, peak 4-6 hr, duration 12-18 hr; crosses placenta, enters breast milk
Interactions/incompatibilities:
• Increased toxicity: lithium, nondepolarizing skeletal muscle relaxants, digitalis
• Decreased effects of: antidiabetics
• Decreased absorption of thiazides: cholestyramine, colestipol
• Decreased hypotensive response: indomethacin
• Increased action of: quinidine
NURSING CONSIDERATIONS
Assess:
• Weight, I&O daily to determine fluid loss; effect of drug may be decreased if used qd
• Rate, depth, rhythm of respiration, effect of exertion
• B/P lying, standing; postural hypotension may occur
• Electrolytes: potassium, sodium, chloride; include BUN, blood sugar, CBC, serum creatinine, blood pH, ABGs
• Glucose in urine if patient is diabetic
Administer:
• In AM to avoid interference with sleep if using drug as a diuretic
• Potassium replacement if potassium is less than 3.0
• With food if nausea occurs; absorption may be decreased slightly
Evaluate:
• Improvement in edema of feet, legs, sacral area daily if medication is being used in CHF
• Improvement in CVP q8h

• Signs of metabolic acidosis: drowsiness, restlessness
• Signs of hypokalemia: postural hypotension, malaise, fatigue, tachycardia, leg cramps, weakness
• Rashes, temperature elevation qd
• Confusion especially in elderly; take safety precautions if needed
Teach patient/family:
• To increase fluid intake 2-3 L/day unless contraindicated, to rise slowly from lying or sitting position
• To notify physician of muscle weakness, cramps, nausea, dizziness
• Drug may be taken with food or milk
• That blood sugar may be increased in diabetics
• Take early in day to avoid nocturia
Lab test interferences:
Increase: BSP retention, calcium, amylase
Decrease: PBI, PSP
Treatment of overdose: Lavage if taken orally, monitor electrolytes, administer dextrose in saline

---

benztropine mesylate
(benz′troe-peen)
Cogentin
Func. class.: Cholinergic blocker
Chem. class.: Tertiary amine

Action: Acts on dopamine receptors in CNS, which decrease involuntary movements
Uses: Parkinson symptoms, dystonia associated with neuroleptic drugs
Dosage and routes:
Dystonia
• *Adult:* IM/IV 2 mg; give PO dose as soon as possible; PO 1-2 mg bid
Parkinson symptoms
• *Adult:* PO 0.5-1 mg qd, increased 0.5 mg q5-6 days titrated to patient response

Available forms include: Tabs 0.5, 1, 2 mg; inj IM, IV 1 mg/ml

Side effects/adverse reactions:

CNS: Confusion, anxiety, restlessness, irritability, delusions, hallucinations, headache, sedation, depression, incoherence, dizziness

EENT: Blurred vision, photophobia, dilated pupils, difficulty swallowing

CV: Palpitations, tachycardia

GI: Dryness of mouth, constipation, nausea, vomiting, abdominal distress, paralytic ileus

GU: Hesitancy, retention

Contraindications: Hypersensitivity, narrow-angle glaucoma, myasthenia gravis, GI/GU obstruction, child <3 yr

Precautions: Pregnancy (C), elderly, lactation, tachycardia, prostatic hypertrophy

Pharmacokinetics:

IM/IV: Onset 15 min, duration 6-10 hr

PO: Onset 1 hr, duration 6-10 hr

Interactions/incompatibilities:

• Increased anticholinergic effect: alcohol, narcotics, barbiturates, antihistamines, MAOIs, phenothiazines, procainamide, quinidine, haloperidol, amantadine

NURSING CONSIDERATIONS

Assess:

• I&O ratio; retention commonly causes decreased urinary output

Administer:

• With or after meals to prevent GI upset; may give with fluids other than water

• At hs to avoid daytime drowsiness in patient with parkinsonism

• Parenteral dose slowly; keep in bed for at least 1 hr after dose

Perform/provide:

• Storage at room temperature

• Hard candy, frequent drinks, gum to relieve dry mouth

Evaluate:

• Parkinsonism, extrapyramidal symptoms: shuffling gait, muscle rigidity, involuntary movements

• Urinary hesitancy, retention; palpate bladder if retention occurs

• Constipation; increase fluids, bulk, exercise if this occurs

• For tolerance over long-term therapy; dose may need to be increased or changed

• Mental status: affect, mood, CNS depression, worsening of mental symptoms during early therapy

Teach patient/family:

• Not to discontinue this drug abruptly; to taper off over 1 wk

• To avoid driving or other hazardous activities, drowsiness may occur

• To avoid OTC medication: cough, cold preparations with alcohol, antihistamines unless directed by physician

---

betamethasone/betamethasone sodium phosphate/betamethasone disodium phosphate/betamethasone acetate, betamethasone sodium phosphate

Betnelan, Celestone/Celestone Phosphate*/Betnesol/Celestone Soluspan

Func. class.: Corticosteroid, synthetic

Chem. class.: Glucocorticoid, long-acting

Action: Decreases inflammation by suppression of migration of polymorphonuclear leukocytes, fibroblasts, reversal of increased capillary permeability and lysosomal stabilization

Uses: Immunosupression, severe inflammation, prevention of neonatal respiratory distress syndrome (by administering to mothers)

Dosage and routes:
• *Adult:* PO 0.6-7.2 mg qd; IM/IV 0.6-7.2 qd in joint or soft tissue (sodium phosphate)
• *Pregnant adult:* IM 12 mg 36-48 hr, before premature delivery, then same dose in 24 hr (betamethasone acetate)
Available forms include: Tabs 0.6 mg; syr 0.6 mg/5 ml; inj 3, 4 mg/ml

Side effects/adverse reactions:
INTEG: Acne, poor wound healing, ecchymosis, bruising, petechiae
CNS: Depression, flushing, sweating, headache, ecchymosis, bruising, mood changes
*CV: Hypotension, **circulatory collapse, thrombophlebitis, embolism,** tachycardia, **necrotizing angiitis, CHF***
*HEMA: **Thrombocytopenia***
MS: Fractures, osteoporosis, weakness
*GI: Diarrhea, nausea, abdominal distention, GI hemorrhage, increased appetite, **pancreatitis***
EENT: Fungal infections, increased intraocular pressure, blurred vision
Contraindications: Psychosis, hypersensitivity, idiopathic thrombocytopenia, acute glomerulonephritis, amebiasis, fungal infections, nonasthmatic bronchial disease, child <2 yr
Precautions: Pregnancy, diabetes mellitus, glaucoma, osteoporosis, seizure disorders, ulcerative colitis, CHF, myasthenia gravis

Pharmacokinetics:
PO: Onset 1-2 hr, peak 1 hr, duration 3 days
IM/IV: Onset 10 min, peak 4-8 hr, duration 1-1½ days
Metabolized in liver, excreted in urine as steroids, crosses placenta
Interactions/incompatibilities:
• Decreased action of this drug: cholestyramine, colestipol, barbiturates, rifampin, ephedrine, phe-

nytoin, theophylline
• Decreased effects of: anticoagulants, anticonvulsants, antidiabetics, ambenonium, neostigmine, isoniazid, toxoids, vaccines
• Increased side effects: alcohol, salicylates, indomethacin, amphotericin B, digitalis preparations
• Increased action of this drug: salicylates, estrogens, indomethacin

NURSING CONSIDERATIONS
Assess:
• Potassium, blood sugar, urine glucose while on long-term therapy; hypokalemia and hyperglycemia
• Weight daily, notify physician of weekly gain >5 lb
• B/P q4h, pulse, notify physician if chest pain occurs
• I&O ratio, be alert for decreasing urinary output and increasing edema
• Plasma cortisol levels during long-term therapy (normal level: 138-635 nmol/L SI units when drawn at 8 AM)
Administer:
• After shaking suspension (parenteral)
• Titrated dose, use lowest effective dose
• IM injection deeply in large mass, rotate sites, avoid deltoid, use 19G needle
• In one dose in AM to prevent adrenal suppression, avoid SC administration, damage may be done to tissue
• With food or milk to decrease GI symptoms
Perform/provide:
• Assistance with ambulation in patient with bone tissue disease to prevent fractures
Evaluate:
• Therapeutic response: ease of respirations, decreased inflammation
• Infection: increased temperature, WBC even after withdrawal of

---

italics = common side effects   **bold italic** = life threatening reactions

medication; drug masks infection symptoms

• Potassium depletion: paresthesias, fatigue, nausea, vomiting, depression, polyuria, dysrhythmias, weakness

• Edema, hypotension, cardiac symptoms

• Mental status: affect, mood, behavioral changes, aggression

Teach patient/family:

• That ID as steroid user should be carried

• To notify physician if therapeutic response decreases; dosage adjustment may be needed

• Not to discontinue this medication abruptly or adrenal crisis can result

• To avoid OTC products: salicylates, alcohol in cough products, cold preparations unless directed by physician

• Teach patient all aspects of drug usage including Cushingoid symptoms

• Symptoms of adrenal insufficiency: nausea, anorexia, fatigue, dizziness, dyspnea, weakness, joint pain

Lab test interferences:

Increase: Cholesterol, sodium, blood glucose, uric acid, calcium, urine glucose

Decrease: Calcium, potassium, T_4, T_3, thyroid ^{131}I uptake test, urine 17-OHCS, 17-KS, PBI

False negative: Skin allergy tests

---

betamethasone benzoate

(bay-ta-meth′a-sone)

Beben, Benisone, Uticort

Func. class.: Topical corticosteroid
Chem. class.: Synthetic fluorinated agent, group III potency

Action: Possesses antipruritic, antiinflammatory actions

Uses: Psoriasis, eczema, contact dermatitis, pruritus

Dosage and routes:

• *Adult and child:* Apply to affected area qid

Available forms include: Oint 0.025%; cream 0.025%; lotion 0.025%; gel 0.025%

Side effects/adverse reactions:

INTEG: Burning, dryness, itching, irritation, acne, folliculitis, hypertrichosis, perioral dermatitis, hypopigmentation, atrophy, striae, miliaria, allergic contact dermatitis, secondary infection

Contraindications: Hypersensitivity to corticosteroids, fungal infections

Precautions: Pregnancy (C), lactation, viral infections, bacterial infections

Interactions/incompatibilities:
None known

NURSING CONSIDERATIONS

Assess:

• Temperature; if fever develops, drug should be discontinued

Administer:

• Only to affected areas; do not get in eyes

• Medication, then cover with occlusive dressing (only if prescribed), seal to normal skin, change q12h

• Only to dermatoses; do not use on weeping, denuded, or infected area

Perform/provide:

• Cleansing before application of drug

• Treatment for a few days after area has cleared

• Storage at room temperature

Evaluate:

• Therapeutic response: absence of severe itching, patches on skin, flaking

Teach patient/family:

• To avoid sunlight on affected area; burns may occur

B

betamethasone dipropionate

(bay-ta-meth'a-sone)
Diprolene, Diprosone

Func. class.: Topical corticosteroid
Chem. class.: Synthetic fluorinated agent, group I-II potency

Action: Possesses antipruritic, antiinflammatory actions
Uses: Psoriasis, eczema, contact dermatitis, pruritus
Dosage and routes:
• *Adult and child:* Apply to affected area bid
Available forms include: Oint 0.05%; cream 0.05%; lotion 0.05%; aerosol 0.05%
Side effects/adverse reactions:
INTEG: Burning, dryness, itching, irritation, acne, folliculitis, hypertrichosis, perioral dermatitis, hypopigmentation, atrophy, striae, miliaria, allergic contact dermatitis, secondary infection
Contraindications: Hypersensitivity to corticosteroids, fungal infections, child <12 yr
Precautions: Pregnancy (C), lactation, viral infections, bacterial infections
Interactions/incompatibilities: None known
NURSING CONSIDERATIONS
Assess:
• Temperature; if fever develops, drug should be discontinued
Administer:
• Only to affected areas; do not get in eyes
• Leave uncovered or use light dressing; do not cover with occlusive dressing
• Only to dermatoses; do not use on weeping, denuded, or infected area

Perform/provide:
• Cleansing before application of drug
• Treatment for a few days after area has cleared
• Storage at room temperature
Evaluate:
• Therapeutic response: absence of severe itching, patches on skin, flaking
Teach patient/family:
• To avoid sunlight on affected area; burns may occur

betamethasone valerate

(bay-ta-meth'a-sone)
Beta-Val, Betatrex, Valnac, Valisone

Func. class.: Topical corticosteroid
Chem. class.: Synthetic fluorinated agent

Action: Possesses antipruritic, antiinflammatory actions
Uses: Psoriasis, eczema, contact dermatitis, pruritus
Dosage and routes:
• *Adult and child:* Apply to affected area qid
Available forms include: Oint 0.1%; cream 0.01%, 0.1%; lotion 0.1%
Side effects/adverse reactions:
INTEG: Burning, dryness, itching, irritation, acne, folliculitis, hypertrichosis, perioral dermatitis, hypopigmentation, atrophy, striae, miliaria, allergic contact dermatitis, secondary infection
Contraindications: Hypersensitivity to corticosteroids, fungal infections
Precautions: Pregnancy (C), lactation, viral infections, bacterial infections
Interactions/incompatibilities: None known

NURSING CONSIDERATIONS
Assess:
• Temperature; if fever develops, drug should be discontinued
Administer:
• Only to affected areas; do not get in eyes
• Medication, then cover with occlusive dressing (only if prescribed), seal to normal skin, change q12h
• Only to dermatoses; do not use on weeping, denuded, or infected area
Perform/provide:
• Cleansing before application of drug
• Treatment for a few days after area has cleared
• Storage at room temperature
Evaluate:
• Therapeutic response: absence of severe itching, patches on skin, flaking
Teach patient/family:
• To avoid sunlight on affected area; burns may occur

---

bethanechol chloride
(be-than'e-kile)
Duvoid, Myotonachol, Urecholine
Func. class.: Cholinergics
Chem. class.: Synthetic choline ester

Action: Stimulates the parasympathetic nervous system directly, which produces contraction to initiate micturition; stimulates gastric motility
Uses: Urinary retention (postoperative, postpartum), neurogenic atony of bladder with retention, abdominal distention, megacolon
Dosage and routes:
• *Adult:* PO/SC 10-30 mg tid-qid
Test dose
• *Adult:* SC 2.5 mg repeated 15-30 min intervals × 4 doses to deter-mine effective dose
Available forms include: Tabs 5, 10, 25, 50 mg; inj SC 5 mg/ml
Side effects/adverse reactions:
INTEG: Rash, urticaria, flushing, increased sweating, hypothermia
CNS: Dizziness, headache, confusion, weakness, *convulsions*
GI: Nausea, bloody diarrhea, vomiting, cramps, fecal incontinence
CV: Hypotension, bradycardia, orthostatic hypotension, reflex tachycardia, *cardiac arrest, circulatory collapse*
GU: Frequency, incontinence
RESP: Acute asthma, dyspnea
EENT: Miosis, increased salivation, lacrimation, blurred vision
Contraindications: Hypersensitivity, severe bradycardia, asthma, severe hypotension, hyperthyroidism, peptic ulcer, parkinsonism, COPD, seizure disorders
Precautions: Hypertension, pregnancy, lactation, child <8 yr
Pharmacokinetics:
PO: Onset 30-90 min, duration 1 hr
SC: Onset 5-15 min, duration 2 hr, excreted by kidneys
Interactions/incompatibilities:
• Increased action of this drug: other cholinergics
• Hypotension: ganglionic blockers
• Decreased action of this drug: procainamide, quinidine

NURSING CONSIDERATIONS
Assess:
• B/P, pulse; observe after parenteral dose for 1 hr
• I&O ratio; check for urinary retention or incontinence
Administer:
• Parenteral dose by SC route; use of IM, IV may result in cardiac arrest
• Only with atropine sulfate available for cholinergic crisis
• Only after all other cholinergics have been discontinued

• Increased doses if tolerance occurs

• With food or milk to decrease GI symptoms (bilateral vagotomy), may decrease action of this drug

• On empty stomach for better absorption

Perform/provide:

• Storage at room temperature

• Bedpan/urinal if given for urinary retention

• Use of rectal tube if ordered to increase passage of gas if used for abdominal distention

Evaluate:

• Therapeutic response: absence of urinary retention, abdominal distention

• Bradycardia, hypotension, bronchospasm, headache, dizziness, convulsions, respiratory depression; drug should be discontinued if toxicity occurs

Teach patient/family:

• To take drug exactly as prescribed

• All aspects of drug: action, side effects, dose, when to notify physician

• To make position changes slowly, orthostatic hypotension may occur

Treatment of overdose: Administer atropine 0.6-1.2 mg IV or IM (adult)

Lab test interferences:

Increase: AST, lipase/amylase, bilirubin, BSP

---

bile salts

Bilron, Biso, Chobile, Ox-Bile, Extract Enseal

Func. class.: Digestant
Chem. class.: Choleretic

Action: Increases bile flow, use of vitamins, cholesterol
Uses: Constipation
Dosage and routes:

• *Adult and child:* PO 300-500 mg

bid-tid pc (tab) or 150-450 mg with or pc (cap)
Available forms include: Tab 324 mg; cap 150, 300 mg
Side effects/adverse reactions:
GI: Diarrhea (increased doses)
Contraindications: Severe liver disease, biliary obstruction
Precautions: Pregnancy
Pharmacokinetics: None known
Interactions/incompatibilities:
None known
NURSING CONSIDERATIONS
Administer:

• During meals for better absorption

• Whole, do not crush or chew tablets

Perform/provide:

• Storage at room temperature
Evaluate:

• Bowel pattern before, after treatment; constipation; nausea, vomiting, abdominal pain, cramps; do not use if these occur

Teach patient/family:

• Not to use often, laxative dependency may occur

---

biperiden HCl, biperiden lactate

(bye-per'i-den)
Akineton, Akineton Lactate

Func. class.: Cholinergic blocker
Chem. class.: Trihexyphenidyl

Action: Acts on dopamine receptors in CNS, which decrease involuntary movements
Uses: Parkinson symptoms, extrapyramidal symptoms
Dosage and routes:
Extrapyramidal symptoms

• *Adult:* PO 2-6 mg bid-tid; IM/IV 2 mg q30 min, if needed, not to exceed 8 mg
Parkinson symptoms

• *Adult:* PO 2 mg tid-qid

Available forms include: Tabs 2 mg; inj IM/IV 5 mg/ml (lactate)

Side effects/adverse reactions:

CNS: Confusion, anxiety, restlessness, irritability, delusions, hallucinations, headache, sedation, depression, incoherence, dizziness

EENT: Blurred vision, photophobia, dilated pupils, difficulty swallowing

CV: Palpitations, tachycardia, postural hypotension

GI: Dryness of mouth, constipation, nausea, vomiting, abdominal distress, paralytic ileus

GU: Hesitancy, retention

Contraindications: Hypersensitivity, narrow-angle glaucoma, myasthenia gravis, GI/GU obstruction, child <3 yr

Precautions: Pregnancy (C), elderly, lactation, tachycardia, prostatic hypertrophy

Pharmacokinetics:

IM/IV: Onset 15 min, duration 6-10 hr

PO: Onset 1 hr, duration 6-10 hr

Interactions/incompatibilities:

• Increased anticholinergic effect: alcohol, narcotics, barbiturates, antihistamines, MAOIs, phenothiazines, amantadine

NURSING CONSIDERATIONS

Assess:

• I&O ratio; retention commonly causes decreased urinary output

Administer:

• Parenteral dose with patient recumbent to prevent postural hypotension

• With or after meals to prevent GI upset; may give with fluids other than water

• At hs to avoid daytime drowsiness in patient with parkinsonism

• Parenteral dose slowly; keep in bed for at least 1 hr after dose

Perform/provide:

• Storage at room temperature

• Hard candy, frequent drinks, gum to relieve dry mouth

Evaluate:

• Parkinsonism, extrapyramidal symptoms: shuffling gait, muscle rigidity, involuntary movements

• Urinary hesitancy, retention; palpate bladder if retention occurs

• Constipation; increase fluids, bulk, exercise if this occurs

• For tolerance over long-term therapy; dose may need to be increased or changed

• Mental status: affect, mood, CNS depression, worsening of mental symptoms during early therapy

Teach patient/family:

• Not to discontinue this drug abruptly, to taper off over 1 wk

• To avoid driving or other hazardous activities, drowsiness may occur

• To avoid OTC medication: cough, cold preparations with alcohol, antihistamines unless directed by physician

---

bisacodyl

(bis-a-koe′dill)

Bisco-Lax, Codylax,* Dulcolax, Rolax,* Theralax, Dacodyl, Deficol

Func. class.: Laxative, stimulant
Chem. class.: Diphenylmethane

Action: Acts directly on intestine by increasing motor activity, thought to irritate colonic intramural plexus

Uses: Short-term treatment of constipation, bowel or rectal preparation for surgery, examination

Dosage and routes:

• *Adult:* PO 10-15 mg in PM or AM, may use up to 30 mg for bowel or rectal preparation; REC 10 mg; ENEMA 1.25 oz

• *Child >3 yr:* PO 5-10 mg

• *Child >2 yr:* REC 10 mg

• *Child <2 yr:* REC 5 mg

• *Child <6 yr:* ENEMA one-half contents of micro enema
Available forms include: Enteric coated tabs 5 mg; rec supp 10 mg
Side effects/adverse reactions:
CNS: Muscle weakness
GI: Nausea, vomiting, anorexia, cramps, diarrhea, rectal burning (suppositories)
META: Protein-losing enteropathy, alkalosis, hypokalemia, *tetany,* electrolyte, fluid imbalances
Contraindications: Hypersensitivity, rectal fissures, abdominal pain, nausea/vomiting, appendicitis, acute surgical abdomen, ulcerated hemorrhoids, acute hepatitis, fecal impaction, intestinal/biliary tract obstruction
Pharmacokinetics:
PO: Onset 6-10 min, acts within 6-12 hr
REC: Onset 15-16 min
Metabolized by liver, excreted in urine, bile, feces, breast milk
Interactions/incompatibilities:
• Gastric irritation: antacids, milk, cimetidine
NURSING CONSIDERATIONS
Assess:
• Blood, urine electrolytes if drug is used often by patient
• I&O ratio to identify fluid loss
Administer:
• Alone for better absorption; do not take within 1 hr of other drugs or within 1 hr of antacids, milk, or cimetidine
• In morning or evening (oral dose)
Evaluate:
• Therapeutic response: decrease in constipation
• Cause of constipation; identify whether fluids, bulk, or exercise is missing from lifestyle
• Cramping, rectal bleeding, nausea, vomiting; if these symptoms occur, drug should be discontinued
Teach patient/family:
• Swallow tabs whole; do not chew

• Not to use laxatives for long-term therapy; bowel tone will be lost
• That normal bowel movements do not always occur daily
• Do not use in presence of abdominal pain, nausea, vomiting
• Notify physician if constipation unrelieved or if symptoms of electrolyte imbalance occur: muscle cramps, pain, weakness, dizziness

bismuth subsalicylate/ bismuth subgallate

(bis-meth)
Pepto-Bismol
Func. class.: Antidiarrheal
Chem. class.: Salicylate

Action: Inhibits prostaglandin synthesis responsible for GI hypermotility
Uses: Diarrhea (cause undetermined), prevention of diarrhea when traveling
Dosage and routes:
• *Adult:* PO 1-2 tabs chewed or swallowed tid (subgallate), or 30 ml or 2 tabs q30-60 min, not to exceed 8 doses for >2 days (subsalicylate)
• *Child 10-14 yr:* PO 20 ml
• *Child 6-10 yr:* PO 10 ml
• *Child 3-6 yr:* PO 5 ml
Available forms include: Chewable tabs 300 mg; susp 262 mg/15 ml
Side effects/adverse reactions:
HEMA: Increased bleeding time
GI: Increased fecal impaction (high doses), dark stools
CNS: Confusion, twitching
EENT: Hearing loss, tinnitus, metallic taste, blue gums
Contraindications: Child <3 yr
Precautions: Salicylate therapy
Pharmacokinetics:
PO: Onset 1 hr, peak 2 hr, duration 4 hr
Interactions/incompatibilities:
• Increased side effects: alcohol,

---

italics = common side effects   ***bold italic*** = life threatening reactions

aminosalicyclic acid, carbonic an-hydrase inhibitors
• Increased action of this drug: ammonium chloride
• Decreased action of this drug: antacids, corticosteroids
• Decreased action of: uricosurics, indomethacin, antidiabetics, sulfonamides

NURSING CONSIDERATIONS
Assess:
• Skin turgor; shift if dehydration is suspected
• Electrolytes (K, Na, Cl) if diarrhea is severe or continues for a long term
Administer:
• For <3 wk
• Increased fluids to rehydrate the patient
Evaluate:
• Therapeutic response: decreased diarrhea or absence of diarrhea when traveling
• Bowel pattern before drug therapy, after treatment
Teach patient/family:
• To chew or dissolve in mouth, do not swallow whole
• To avoid other salicylates unless directed by physician
• Stools may turn gray
Lab test interferences:
Interfere: radiographic studies of GI system

---

bitolterol mesylate

(bye-tole'-ter-ol)
Tornalate
Func. class.: Adrenergic
Chem. class.: Acid ester of colterol

Action: Causes increased contractility and heart rate by acting on β-receptors in heart; also, acts on α-receptors, causing vasoconstriction in blood vessels when larger doses are administered, causing vasodilation in renal, intracerebral, coronary dopaminergic receptors.
Uses: Asthma, bronchospasm
Dosage and routes:
• *Adult and child >12 yr:* INH 2 puffs, wait 1-3 min before 3rd puff if needed, not to exceed 3 INH q6h or 2 INH q4h
Available forms include: Aerosol 0.37 mg/actuation
Side effects/adverse reactions:
CNS: Tremors, anxiety, insomnia, headache, dizziness, stimulation, restlessness, hallucinations
EENT: Dry nose, irritation of nose and throat
CV: Palpitations, tachycardia, hypertension, angina, hypotension
GI: Heartburn, nausea, vomiting
MS: Muscle cramps
RESP: Bronchospasm
Contraindications: Hypersensitivity to sympathomimetics
Precautions: Lactation, pregnancy (C), cardiac disorders, hyperthyroidism, diabetes mellitus
Pharmacokinetics:
INH: Onset 3 min, peak ½-1 hr, duration 8 hr
Interactions/incompatibilities:
• Increased action of: aerosol bronchodilators
• Increased action of this drug: tricyclic antidepressants, MAOIs
• May inhibit action when used with other β-blockers

NURSING CONSIDERATIONS
Assess:
• Respiratory function: vital capacity, forced expiratory volume, ABGs
Administer:
• After shaking, exhale, place mouthpiece in mouth, inhale slowly, hold breath, remove, exhale slowly
• Gum, sips of water for dry mouth
Perform/provide:
• Storage in light-resistant container, do not expose to temperatures over 86° F

Evaluate:
• Therapeutic response: absence of dyspnea, wheezing over 1 hr
Teach patient/family:
• Not to use OTC medications; extra stimulation may occur
• Use of inhaler, review package insert with patient
• To avoid getting aerosol in eyes
• To wash inhaler in warm water and dry qd
• On all aspects of drug; avoid smoking, smoke-filled rooms, persons with respiratory infections
Treatment of overdose: Administer a β-1adrenergic blocker

---

bleomycin sulfate

(blee-oh-mye'sin)
Blenoxane
Func. class.: Antineoplastic, antibiotic
Chem. class.: Glycopeptide

Action: Inhibits synthesis of DNA, RNA, protein; this drug is derived from *Streptomyces verticillus;* replication is decreased by binding to DNA, which causes strand splitting; drug is phase specific in the G_2 and M phases
Uses: Cancer of head, neck, penis, cervix, vulva of squamous cell origin, Hodgkin's disease, lymphosarcoma, reticulum cell sarcoma, testicular carcinoma
Dosage and routes:
• *Adult:* SC/IV/IM 0.25-0.5 U/kg 1-2 × /wk or 10-20 U/m², then 1 U/day or 5 U/wk
Available forms include: Inj IV, SC, IM 5 units
Side effects/adverse reactions:
SYST: Anaphylaxis
HEMA: Thrombocytopenia, leukopenia
GI: Nausea, vomiting, anorexia, stomatitis, weight loss
INTEG: Rash, hyperkeratosis, nail changes, alopecia
RESP: Fibrosis, pneumonitis, wheezing
CNS: Fever, chills
IDIOSYNCRATIC REACTION: Hypotension, confusion, fever, chills, wheezing
Contraindications: Hypersensitivity
Precautions: Renal, hepatic, respiratory disease, pregnancy
Pharmacokinetics: Half-life 2 hr when CrCl of 35 ml/min for lower clearance, half-life is increased, metabolized in liver, 50% excreted in urine (unchanged)
Interactions/incompatibilities:
• Increased toxicity: other antineoplastics or radiation therapy
NURSING CONSIDERATIONS
Assess:
• Pulmonary function tests: chest x-ray before and during therapy; should be obtained q2 wk during treatment
• Monitor temperature q4h; fever may indicate beginning infection
Administer:
• Medications by oral route if possible; avoid IM, SC, IV routes to prevent infections
• Antiemetic 30-60 min before giving drug to prevent vomiting
• Topical or systemic analgesics for pain of stomatitis as ordered
Perform/provide:
• Deep breathing exercises with patient tid-qid; place in semi-Fowler's position
• Liquid diet: carbonated beverage, Jello; dry toast, crackers may be added if patient is not nauseated or vomiting
• Rinsing of mouth tid-qid with water, hydrogen peroxide; brushing of teeth bid-tid with soft brush or cotton-tipped applicators for stomatitis; use unwaxed dental floss
• HOB increased to facilitate breathing

Evaluate:

• Dyspnea, rales, unproductive cough, chest pain, tachypnea, fatigue, increased pulse, pallor, lethargy

• Food preferences; list likes, dislikes

• Effects of alopecia on body image; discuss feelings about body changes

• Buccal cavity q8h for dryness, sores, ulceration, white patches, oral pain, bleeding, dysphagia

• Local irritation, pain, burning, discoloration at injection site

• Symptoms indicating severe allergic reaction: rash, pruritus, urticaria, purpuric skin lesions, itching, flushing

• Storage for 2 wk after reconstituting at room temperature; discard unused portions

Teach patient/family:

• To report any complaints, side effects to nurse or physician

• To report any changes in breathing, coughing

• That hair may be lost during treatment and wig or hairpiece may make patient feel better; tell patient that new hair may be different in color, texture

• To avoid foods with citric acid, hot or rough texture

• To report any bleeding, white spots, ulcerations in mouth; to examine mouth qd and report symptoms

---

boric acid

(bor′ik)

Blinx, Bluboro, Boric acid solution 5%, Borofax, Ting

Func. class.: Disinfectant
Chem. class.: Acid (weak)

Action: Unknown, has fungistatic effect; weak bacteriostatic fungistatic agent

Uses: Athlete's foot, minor conditions of eye, skin, ear, mucous membranes

Dosage and routes:

• *Adult and child:* TOP POWD/SOL apply 1%-4% to affected area; TOP OINT apply 5%, 10% to affected area

Available forms include: Top sol, powd, top oint 5%, 10%

Side effects/adverse reactions:

INTEG: Irritation, rash, alopecia (systemic effect)

GI: Nausea, vomiting, diarrhea, cramps

GU: Renal damage

CNS: Delirium, *convulsions,* restlessness, headache, *coma*

CV: Circulatory collapse, tachycardia

Contraindications: Hypersensitivity, closed wounds, abraded skin, infants, laceration of the eye

Interactions/incompatibilities:

• Do not use with products containing polyvinyl alcohol or tannins

NURSING CONSIDERATIONS

Administer:

• To body areas only; do not apply to face, lips, mouth, eyes, any mucous membrane, anus, meatus

• To small area of body to avoid chilling

Evaluate:

• Area of body involved: irritation, rash, breaks

Teach patient/family:

• Not to share eye solution with others; serious infections may occur

---

boric acid

Ear-Dry, Swim-Ear, Swim'n Clear, Auro-Dri, Aurocaine 2

Func. class.: Otic
Chem. class.: Weak acid

Action: Fungistatic properties used to decrease infection

Uses: Ear infection (external)
Dosage and routes:
• *Adult and child:* INSTILL 3-6 gtts tid-qid
Available forms include: Sol 2.75%
Side effects/adverse reactions:
EENT: Itching, irritation in ear
INTEG: Rash, urticaria
Contraindications: Hypersensitivity, perforated eardrum
Pharmacokinetics: Not known
Interactions/incompatibilities:
• Do not mix with tannins, polyvinyl alcohol
NURSING CONSIDERATIONS
Administer:
• After removing impacted cerumen by irrigation
• After cleaning stopper with alcohol
• After restraining child if necessary
• After warming solution to body temperature
Evaluate:
• Therapeutic response: decreased ear pain
• For redness, swelling, pain in ear, which indicates superimposed infection
Teach patient/family:
• Method of instillation using aseptic technique, including not touching dropper to ear
• That dizziness may occur after instillation

---

bretylium tosylate
(bre-til′ee-um)
Bretylate,* Bretylol
Func. class.: Antidysrhythmic (Class III)
Chem. class.: Quaternary ammonium compound

Action: Inhibits release of norepinephrine in postganglionic nerve endings that control ventricular tachycardia; this drug is able to block norepinephrine release after 2 hr; calms nerve ending excitability
Uses: Serious ventricular tachycardia, cardioversion, ventricular fibrillation; for short-term use only
Dosage and routes:
Severe ventricular fibrillation
• *Adult:* IV BOL 5 mg/kg, increase to 10 mg/kg repeated q15 min; not to exceed 30 mg/kg/day; IV INF 1-2 mg/min after loading dose
Ventricular dysrhythmias
• *Adult:* IV INF 500 mg diluted in 50 ml D₅W or NS, infuse over 8 min at rate of 5-10 mg/kg; may repeat in 1 hr, maintain with 1-2 mg/min or 5-10 mg/kg over 8 min q6h; IM 5-10 mg/kg undiluted; repeat in 1-2 hr if needed; may repeat with 3rd dose q6-8h
Available forms include: Inj IV 50 mg/ml
Side effects/adverse reactions:
CNS: Syncope, dizziness, involuntary movement, confusion, psychosis, anxiety
GI: Nausea, vomiting, diarrhea, abdominal pain, anorexia
CV: Hypotension, postural hypotension, bradycardia, angina, PVCs, substernal pressure
RESP: Respiratory depression
Contraindications: Hypersensitivity, digitalis toxicity, aortic stenosis, pulmonary hypertension, pregnancy, lactation, children
Precautions: Renal disease
Pharmacokinetics:
IV: Onset 5 min
IM: Onset ½-2 hr, peak 6-9 hr, duration 24 hr
Half-life 4-17 hr, excreted unchanged by kidneys (70%-80% in 24 hr), not metabolized
Interactions/incompatibilities:
• Increased or decreased effects of this drug: quinidine, procainamide,

propranolol or other antidys-rhythmics

• Hypotension: antihypertensives

• Toxicity: digitalis

• Incompatible with all medications in solution or syringe

NURSING CONSIDERATIONS

Assess:

• ECG continuously to determine drug effectiveness, PVCs or other dysrhythmias

• IV inf rate to avoid causing nausea, vomiting

• For dehydration or hypovolemia

• B/P continuously for hypotension, hypertension

• I&O ratio

Administer:

• IM inj, rotate sites, inject <5 ml in any one site

• Reduced dosage slowly with ECG monitoring

Perform/provide:

• Place patient in supine position unless otherwise ordered

• Have suction equipment available

Evaluate:

• For rebound hypertension after 1-2 hr

• Cardiac status: rate, rhythm, character, continuously

Lab test interferences:

Decrease: Urinary epinephrine, urinary norepinephrine, urinary VMA epinephrine

Treatment of overdose: O_2, artificial ventilation, ECG, administer dopamine for circulatory depression, administer diazepam or thiopental for convulsions

bromocriptine mesylate

(broe-moe-krip′teen)

Parlodel

Func. class.: Dopamine receptor agonist

Chem. class.: Ergot alkaloid derivative

Action: Stimulates prolactin release by activating postsynaptic dopamine receptors; activation of dopamine receptors could be reason for improvement in Parkinson's disease

Uses: Female infertility, Parkinson's disease, prevention of postpartum lactation, amenorrhea, galactorrhea caused by hyperprolactinemia, acromegaly

Dosage and routes:

Amenorrhea/galactorrhea/postpartum lactation

• *Adult:* PO 2.5 mg bid-tid with meal × 14 days

Parkinson's disease

• *Adult:* PO 1.25 mg bid with meals, may increase q2-4 wk, not to exceed 100 mg qd

Available forms include: Caps 5 mg; tabs 2.5 mg

Side effects/adverse reactions:

EENT: Blurred vision, diplopia, burning eyes

CNS: Headache, depression, restlessness, anxiety, nervousness, confusion, *convulsions,* hallucinations

GU: Frequency, retention, incontinence, diuresis

GI: Nausea, vomiting, anorexia, cramps, constipation, diarrhea, dry mouth, GI hemorrhage

INTEG: Rash on face, arms, alopecia

CV: Orthostatic hypotension, decreased B/P, palpitation, extra systole, *shock,* dysrhythmias

Contraindications: Hypersensitiv-

ity to ergot, severe ischemic disease
Precautions: Pregnancy, lactation, hepatic disease, renal disease
Pharmacokinetics:
PO: Peak 1-3 hr, duration 4-8 hr, 90%-96% protein bound, half-life 3-8 hr, metabolized by liver (inactive metabolites), excreted in urine, feces
Interactions/incompatibilities:
• Decreased action of this drug: phenothiazines, methyldopa, imipramine, haloperidol, droperidol, amitriptyline, oral contraceptives
• Increased action of: antihypertensives, levodopa
NURSING CONSIDERATIONS
Assess:
• B/P; establish baseline, compare with other reading; this drug decreases B/P
Administer:
• With meal to prevent GI symptoms
• HS so dizziness, orthostatic hypotension are not problems
Perform/provide:
• Storage at room temperature in tight container
Evaluate:
• Therapeutic response (Parkinson's disease): decreased dyskinesia, decreased slow movements, drooling
Teach patient/family:
• To change position slowly, to prevent orthostatic hypotension
• To use contraceptives during treatment with this drug; pregnancy may occur; to use methods other than oral contraceptives
• That therapeutic effect may take 2 mo: galactorrhea, amenorrhea
• To avoid hazardous activity if dizziness occurs
Lab test interferences:
Increase: Growth hormone, AST/ALT, CPK, BUN, uric acid, alk phosphatase, GGTP

brompheniramine maleate

(brome-fen-ir′a-meen)
Brombay, Dimetane, Dimetane-Ten, Rolabromophen, Spentane, Veltane, and others
Func. class.: Antihistamine
Chem. class.: Alkylamine, H_1-receptor antagonist

Action: Acts on blood vessels, GI, respiratory system by competing with histamine for H_1-receptor site; decreases allergic response by blocking histamine
Uses: Allergy symptoms, rhinitis
Dosage and routes:
• *Adult:* PO 4-8 mg tid-qid, not to exceed 24 mg/day; TIME REL 8-12 mg bid-tid, not to exceed 24 mg/day; IM/IV/SC 5-20 mg q6-12h, not to exceed 40 mg/day
• *Child >6 yr:* PO 2 mg tid-qid, not to exceed 12 mg/day; IM/IV/SC 0.5 mg/kg/day divided tid or qid
• *Child <6 yr:* Only as directed by physician
Available forms include: Tabs 4 mg; tabs, time rel 8, 12 mg; elix 2 mg/5 ml; inj IM/SC/IV 10, 100 mg/ml
Side effects/adverse reactions:
CNS: Dizziness, drowsiness, poor coordination, fatigue, anxiety, euphoria, confusion, paresthesia, neuritis
CV: Hypotension, palpitations, tachycardia
RESP: Increased thick secretions, wheezing, chest tightness
*HEMA: **Thrombocytopenia, agranulocytosis, hemolytic anemia***
GI: Dry mouth, nausea, vomiting, anorexia, constipation, diarrhea
INTEG: Rash, urticaria, photosensitivity

---

italics = common side effects   ***bold italic*** = life threatening reactions

GU: Retention, dysuria, frequency, impotence

EENT: Blurred vision, dilated pupils, tinnitus, nasal stuffiness, dry nose, throat, mouth

Contraindications: Hypersensitivity to H_1-receptor antagonists, acute asthma attack, lower respiratory tract disease, child <6 yr

Precautions: Increased intraocular pressure, renal disease, cardiac disease, hypertension, bronchial asthma, seizure disorder, stenosed peptic ulcers, hyperthyroidism, prostatic hypertrophy, bladder neck obstruction, pregnancy (C)

Pharmacokinetics:

PO: Peak 2-5 hr, duration to 48 hr; metabolized in liver, excreted by kidneys, excreted in breast milk, half-life 12-34 hr

Interactions/incompatibilities:

• Increased CNS depression: barbiturates, narcotics, hypnotics, tricyclic antidepressants, alcohol

• Decreased effect of: oral anticoagulants, heparin

• Increased drying effect of this drug: MAOIs

NURSING CONSIDERATIONS

Assess:

• I&O ratio; be alert for urinary retention, frequency, dysuria; drug should be discontinued if these occur

• CBC during long-term therapy

Administer:

• Coffee, tea, cola (caffeine) to decrease drowsiness

• With meals if GI symptoms occur; absorption may slightly decrease

Perform/provide:

• Hard candy, gum, frequent rinsing of mouth for dryness

• Storage in tight container at room temperature

Evaluate:

• Therapeutic response: absence of running or congested nose or rashes

• Blood dyscrasias: thrombocytopenia, agranulocytosis (rare)

• Respiratory status: rate, rhythm, increase in bronchial secretions, wheezing, chest tightness

• Cardiac status: palpitations, increased pulse, hypotension

Teach patient/family:

• Not to crush or chew sustained release forms

• All aspects of drug use; to notify physician if confusion, sedation, hypotension occurs

• To avoid driving or other hazardous activities if drowsiness occurs

• To avoid use of alcohol or other CNS depressants while taking drug

Lab test interferences:

False negative: Skin allergy tests

Treatment of overdose: Administer ipecac syrup or lavage, diazepam, vasopressors, barbiturates (short-acting)

---

buclizine HCl

(byoo'kli-zeen)

Bucladin-S, Softran, Equivert, Vibazine

Func. class.: Antiemetic, antihistamine

Chem. class.: H_1-receptor antagonist (piperazine)

Action: Acts centrally by blocking chemoreceptor trigger zone, which in turn acts on vomiting center

Uses: Motion sickness, dizziness, nausea, vomiting

Dosage and routes:

• *Adult:* PO 25-50 mg prn ½ hr before travel; may be repeated q4-6h prn

Available forms include: Tabs 50 mg

Side effects/adverse reactions:

CNS: Drowsiness, dizziness, fatigue, restlessness, headache, insomnia

GI: Nausea, anorexia

EENT: Dry mouth, blurred vision
Contraindications: Hypersensitivity to cyclizines, shock
Precautions: Children, narrow-angle glaucoma, lactation, prostatic hypertrophy, elderly, pregnancy
Pharmacokinetics:
PO: Duration 4-6 hr, other pharmacokinetics not known
Interactions/incompatibilities:
None known
NURSING CONSIDERATIONS
Assess:
• VS, B/P; check patients with cardiac disease more often
Administer:
• Tablets may be swallowed whole, chewed, or allowed to dissolve
Evaluate:
• Signs of toxicity of other drugs or masking of symptoms of disease: brain tumor, intestinal obstruction
• Drowsiness, dizziness
Teach patient/family:
• To avoid hazardous activities or activities requiring alertness; dizziness may occur; instruct patient to request assistance with ambulation
• To avoid alcohol, other depressants

---

bumetanide

(byoo-met′a-nide)
Bumex
Func. class.: Loop diuretic
Chem. class.: Sulfonamide derivative

Action: Acts on ascending loop of Henle by increasing excretion of chloride, sodium
Uses: Edema in CHF, liver disease, renal disease (nephrotic syndrome), pulmonary edema, ascites (nephrotic syndrome)
Dosage and routes:
• *Adult:* PO 0.5-2.0 mg qd, may give 2nd or 3rd dose at 4-5 hr intervals, not to exceed 10 mg/day, may be given on alternate days or intermittently; IV/IM 0.5-1.0 mg/day, may give 2nd or 3rd dose at 2-3 hr intervals, not to exceed 10 mg/day
Available forms include: Tabs 0.5, 1 mg; inj IV, IM
Side effects/adverse reactions:
GU: Polyuria, gynecomastia, ejaculatory problems, *renal failure,* glycosuria
ELECT: Hypokalemia, hypochloremic alkalosis, hypomagnesemia, hyperuricemia, hypocalcemia, hyponatremia
CNS: Headache, fatigue, weakness, vertigo
GI: Nausea, diarrhea, dry mouth, vomiting, anorexia, cramps, upset stomach, abdominal pain, acute pancreatitis, jaundice
EENT: Loss of hearing, ear pain, tinnitus, blurred vision
INTEG: Rash, pruritus, purpura, Stevens-Johnson syndrome, sweating
MS: Cramps, arthritis, stiffness
ENDO: Hyperglycemia
HEMA: Thrombocytopenia, agranulocytosis
CV: Chest pain, hypotension, *circulatory collapse,* ECG changes
Contraindications: Hypersensitivity to sulfonamides, anuria, hypovolemia, children <18 yr, lactation
Precautions: Dehydration, ascites, severe renal disease, pregnancy (C)
Pharmacokinetics:
PO: Onset ½-1 hr, duration 4 hr
IM: Onset 40 min, duration 4 hr
IV: Onset 5 min, duration 2-3 hr, Excreted by kidneys, crosses placenta, excreted by breast milk
Interactions/incompatibilities:
• Increased toxicity: lithium, nondepolarizing skeletal muscle relaxants, digitalis

• Decreased effects of: antidiabetics

• Decreased absorption of thiazides: cholestyramine, colestipol

NURSING CONSIDERATIONS

Assess:

• Weight, I&O daily to determine fluid loss; effect of drug may be decreased if used qd

• Rate, depth, rhythm of respiration, effect of exertion

• B/P lying, standing; postural hypotension may occur

• Electrolytes: potassium, sodium, chloride; include BUN, blood sugar, CBC, serum creatinine, blood pH, ABGs

• Glucose in urine if patient is diabetic

Administer:

• In AM to avoid interference with sleep if using drug as a diuretic

• Potassium replacement if potassium is less than 3.0

• With food if nausea occurs; absorption may be decreased slightly

Evaluate:

• Improvement in edema of feet, legs, sacral area daily if medication is being used in CHF

• Improvement in CVP q8h

• Signs of metabolic acidosis: drowsiness, restlessness

• Signs of hypokalemia: postural hypotension, malaise, fatigue, tachycardia, leg cramps, weakness

• Rashes, temperature elevation qd

• Confusion, especially in elderly; take safety precautions if needed

Teach patient/family:

• To increase fluid intake 2-3 L/day unless contraindicated, to rise slowly from lying or sitting position

• Adverse reactions: muscle cramps, weakness, nausea, dizziness

• Take with food or milk for GI symptoms

• Take early in day to prevent nocturia

Treatment of overdose: Lavage if taken orally, monitor electrolytes, administer dextrose in saline

---

bupivacaine HCl

(byoop-a-va'caine)
Marcaine, Sensorcaine
Func. class.: Local anesthetic
Chem. class.: Amide

Action: Competes with calcium for sites in nerve membrane that control sodium transport across cell membrane; decreases rise of depolarization phase of action potential

Uses: Epidural anesthesia, peripheral nerve block, caudal anesthesia

Dosage and routes:

Varies depending on route of anesthesia

Available forms include: Inj 0.25%, 0.5%, 0.75%; inj with epinephrine 0.25%, 0.5%, 0.75%

Side effects/adverse reactions:

CNS: Anxiety, restlessness, ***convulsions, loss of consciousness,*** drowsiness, disorientation, tremors, shivering

*CV: **Myocardial depression, cardiac arrest, dysrhythmias,*** bradycardia, hypotension, hypertension, fetal bradycardia

GI: Nausea, vomiting

EENT: Blurred vision, tinnitus, pupil constriction

INTEG: Rash, urticaria, allergic reactions, edema, burning, skin discoloration at injection site, tissue necrosis

*RESP: **Status asthmaticus, respiratory arrest, anaphylaxis***

Contraindications: Hypersensitivity, child <12 yr, elderly, severe liver disease

Precautions: Elderly, severe drug allergies, pregnancy (C)

Pharmacokinetics:

Onset 4-17 min, duration 4-8 hr,

excreted in urine (metabolites), metabolized by liver

Interactions/incompatibilities:
• Dysrhythmias: epinephrine, halothane, enflurane
• Hypertension: MAOIs, tricyclic antidepressants, phenothiazines
• Decreased action of this drug: chloroprocaine

NURSING CONSIDERATIONS
Assess:
• B/P, pulse, respiration during treatment
• Fetal heart tones if drug is used during labor

Administer:
• Only with crash cart, resuscitative equipment nearby
• Only drugs without preservatives for epidural or caudal anesthesia

Perform/provide:
• Use of new solution, discard unused portions

Evaluate:
• Therapeutic response: anesthesia necessary for procedure
• Allergic reactions: rash, urticaria, itching
• Cardiac status: ECG for dysrhythmias, pulse, B/P during anesthesia

Treatment of overdose: Airway, O_2, vasopressor, IV fluids, anticonvulsants for seizures

---

buprenorphine HCl
(byoo-preen′or-feen)
Buprenex
Func. class.: Nonnarcotic analgesics
Chem. class.: Nonopiate

Controlled Substance Schedule V
Action: Inhibits ascending pain pathways in limbic system, thalamus, midbrain, hypothalamus
Uses: Moderate to severe pain
Dosage and routes:
• *Adult:* IM/IV 0.3-0.6 mg q6h

prn, reduce dosage in elderly
Available forms include: Inj IM IV 1, 2 mg/ml

Side effects/adverse reactions:
CNS: Drowsiness, dizziness, confusion, headache, sedation, euphoria
GI: Nausea, vomiting, anorexia, constipation, cramps
GU: Increased urinary output, dysuria
INTEG: Rash, urticaria, bruising, flushing, diaphoresis, pruritus
EENT: Tinnitus, blurred vision, miosis, diplopia
CV: Palpitations, bradycardia, change in B/P
*RESP: **Respiratory depression***

Contraindications: Hypersensitivity, addiction (narcotic)
Precautions: Addictive personality, pregnancy (C), lactation, increased intracranial pressure, MI (acute), severe heart disease, respiratory depression, hepatic disease, renal disease

Pharmacokinetics:
IM: Onset 10-30 min, peak ½ hr, duration 3-4 hr
IV: Onset 1 min, peak 5 min, duration 2-5 hr
REC: Onset slow, duration 4-6 hr
Metabolized by liver, excreted by kidneys, crosses placenta, excreted in breast milk, half-life 2½-3½ hr

Interactions/incompatibilities:
• Effects may be increased with other CNS depressants: alcohol, narcotics, sedative/hypnotics, antipsychotics, skeletal muscle relaxants

NURSING CONSIDERATIONS
Assess:
• I&O ratio; check for decreasing output; may indicate urinary retention

Administer:
• With antiemetic if nausea, vomiting occur
• When pain is beginning to return;

---

determine dosage interval by patient response

Perform/provide:

• Assistance with ambulation

• Safety measures: siderails

Evaluate:

• CNS changes, dizziness, drowsiness, hallucinations, euphoria, LOC, pupil reaction

• Allergic reactions: rash, urticaria

• Respiratory dysfunction: respiratory depression, character, rate, rhythm; notify physician if respirations are <12/min

• Need for pain medication, physical dependence

• Therapeutic response: decrease in pain, absence of grimacing

Teach patient/family:

• To report any symptoms of CNS changes, allergic reactions

• That physical dependency may result when used for extended periods of time

Treatment of overdose: Narcan 0.2-0.8 mg IV, O₂, IV fluids, vasopressors

---

busulfan

(byoo-sul'fan)

Myleran

Func. class.: Antineoplastic alkylating agent

Chem. class.: Nitrosurea

Action: Changes essential cellular ions to covalent bonding with resultant alkylation; this interferes with normal biologic function of DNA; activity is not phase specific

Uses: Chronic myelocytic leukemia

Dosage and routes:

• *Adult:* PO 4-12 mg/day initially until WBC levels fall to 10,000/mm³, then drug is stopped until WBC levels raise over 50,000/mm³, then 1-3 mg/day

• *Child:* PO 0.06-0.12 mg/kg or

1.8-4.6 mg/m² day; dose is titrated to maintain WBC levels at 20,000/mm³

Available forms include: Tab 2 mg

Side effects/adverse reactions:

*HEMA: **Thrombocytopenia, leukopenia, pancytopenia***

GI: Nausea, vomiting, diarrhea, weight loss

GU: Impotence, sterility, amenorrhea, gynecomastia, ***renal toxicity,*** hyperuremia

INTEG: Alopecia, dermatitis

*RESP: **Fibrosis,** pneumonitis*

Contraindications: Radiation, chemotherapy, lactation, pregnancy (3rd trimester) (D)

Precautions: Childbearing age men, women

Pharmacokinetics:

Well absorbed orally, excreted in urine, crosses placenta, excreted in breast milk

Interactions/incompatibilities:

Increased toxicity: other antineoplastics or radiation

NURSING CONSIDERATIONS

Assess:

• CBC, differential, platelet count weekly; withhold drug if WBC is <4000 or platelet count is <75,000; notify physician of results

• Pulmonary function tests, chest x-ray films before, during therapy; chest film should be obtained q2wk during treatment

• Renal function studies: BUN, serum uric acid, urine CrCl before, during therapy

• I&O ratio; report fall in urine output of 30 ml/hr

• Monitor temperature q4h (may indicate beginning infection)

Administer:

• Medications by oral route, if possible avoid IM, SC, IV routes to prevent infections

• Antacid before oral agent, give

drug after evening meal, before bedtime

• Antiemetic 30-60 min before giving drug to prevent vomiting

• Allopurinol or sodium bicarbonate to maintain uric acid levels, alkalinization of urine

• Antibiotics for prophylaxis of infection

Perform/provide:

• Strict medical asepsis, protective isolation if WBC levels are low

• Special skin care

• Deep breathing exercises with patient tid-qid; place in semi-Fowler's position

• Liquid diet, including cola, Jello; dry toast or crackers may be added if patient is not nauseated or vomiting

• Increase fluid intake to 2-3 L/day to prevent urate deposits, calculi formation

• Diet low in purines: organ meats (kidney, liver), dried beans, peas to maintain alkaline urine

• Storage in tight container

Evaluate:

• Bleeding: hematuria, guaiac, bruising or petechiae, mucosa or orifices q8h

• Dyspnea, rales, unproductive cough, chest pain, tachypnea

• Food preferences; list likes, dislikes

• Effects of alopecia on body image; discuss feelings about body changes

• Edema in feet, joint, stomach pain, shaking

• Inflammation of mucosa, breaks in skin

Teach patient/family:

• Of protective isolation precautions

• To report any complaints or side effects to nurse or physician

• That impotence or amenorrhea can occur, are reversible after discontinuing treatment

• To report any changes in breathing or coughing

• That hair may be lost during treatment; a wig or hairpiece may make patient feel better; new hair may be different in color, texture

butabarbital/butabarbital sodium

(byoo-ta-bar'bi-tal)

Butisol, Day-Barb,* Medarsed, Neo-Barb/Butalan,* Butatran, Buticaps, Butisol Sodium

Func. class.: Sedative/hypnotic-barbiturate

Chem. class.: Barbitone (intermediate acting)

Controlled Substance Schedule III (USA), Schedule G (Canada)
Action: Depresses activity in brain cells primarily in reticular activating system in brainstem; also selectively depresses neurons in posterior hypothalamus and limbic structures

Uses: Sedation, insomnia, preoperatively

Dosage and routes:
Sedation

• *Adult:* PO 15-30 mg tid or qid

• *Child:* PO 6 mg/kg in divided doses tid, range may vary from 7.5-30 mg tid

Insomnia

• *Adult:* PO 50-100 mg hs

Preoperatively

• *Adult:* PO 50-100 mg 1-2 hr preoperatively

Available forms include: Tabs 15, 30, 50, 100 mg; caps 15, 30 mg; elix 30, 33.3 mg/5 ml, powder

Side effects/adverse reactions:

CNS: Lethargy, drowsiness, hangover, dizziness, stimulation in elderly and children, lightheadedness, physical dependence, CNS depression, mental depression, slurred speech

---

italics = common side effects   ***bold italic*** = life threatening reactions

GI: Nausea, vomiting, diarrhea, constipation

INTEG: Rash, urticaria, pain, abscesses at injection site, angioedema, thrombophlebitis, *Stevens-Johnson syndrome*

CV: Hypotension, bradycardia

RESP: Depression, apnea, *laryngospasm, bronchospasm*

HEMA: Agranulocytosis, thrombocytopenia, megaloblastic anemia (long-term treatment)

Contraindications: Hypersensitivity to barbiturates, respiratory depression, addiction to barbiturates, severe liver impairment, porphyria

Precautions: Anemia, pregnancy, lactation, hepatic disease, renal disease, hypertension, elderly, acute/chronic pain

Pharmacokinetics:

PO: Onset 40-60 min, duration 6-8 hr; metabolized by liver, excreted by kidneys; half-life 32-44 hr

Interactions/incompatibilities:

• Increased CNS depression: alcohol, MAOIs, sedative, narcotics

• Decreased effect of: oral anticoagulants, corticosteroids, griseofulvin, quinidine

• Increased half-life of: doxycycline

NURSING CONSIDERATIONS

Assess:

• Blood studies: Hct, Hgb, RBCs, serum folate (if on long-term therapy); pro-time in patients receiving anticoagulants

• Hepatic studies: AST, ALT, bilirubin; if increased, the drug is usually discontinued

Administer:

• After removal of cigarettes, to prevent fires

• After trying conservative measures for insomnia

• ½-1 hr before hs for sleeplessness

• On empty stomach for best absorption

Perform/provide:

• Assistance with ambulation after receiving dose

• Safety measure: siderails, nightlight, callbell within easy reach

• Checking to see PO medication swallowed

Evaluate:

• Therapeutic response: ability to sleep at night, decreased amount of early morning awakening if taking drug for insomnia

• Mental status: mood, sensorium, affect, memory (long, short)

• Physical dependency: more frequent requests for medication, shakes, anxiety

• Barbiturate toxicity: hypotension; pulmonary constriction; cold, clammy skin; cyanosis of lips; insomnia; nausea; vomiting; hallucinations; delirium; weakness; mild symptoms may occur in 8-12 hr without drug

• Respiratory dysfunction: respiratory depression, character, rate, rhythm; hold drug if respirations are <12 /min or if pupils are dilated

• Blood dyscrasias: fever, sore throat, bruising, rash, jaundice, epistaxis

Teach patient/family:

• That hangover is common

• That drug is indicated only for short-term treatment of insomnia and is probably ineffective after 2 wk

• That physical dependency may result when used for extended periods of time (45-90 days depending on dose)

• To avoid driving or other activities requiring alertness

• To avoid alcohol ingestion or CNS depressants; serious CNS depression may result

• Not to discontinue medication quickly after long-term use; drug should be tapered over 1-2 wk

• To tell all prescribers that a barbiturate is being taken

• That withdrawal insomnia may occur after short-term use; do not start using drug again, insomnia will improve in 1-3 nights

• That effects may take 2 nights for benefits to be noticed

• Alternate measures to improve sleep (reading, exercise several hours before hs, warm bath, warm milk, TV, self-hypnosis, deep breathing)

Lab test interferences:

False increase: Sulfobromophthalein test

Treatment of overdose: Lavage, activated charcoal, warming blanket, vital signs, hemodialysis, alkalinize urine

butoconazole nitrate

(byoo'-toe-kone-a-zole)

Femstat

Func. class.: Local antiinfective

Chem. class.: Antifungal

Action: Interferes with fungal replication; binds sterols in fungal cell membrane, which increases permeability, leaking of cell nutrients

Uses: Vaginal infections caused by candida

Dosage and routes:

• *Adult:* INTRA VAG 1 applicatorful hs × 3 days (nonpregnant), 6 days (2nd/3rd trimester pregnancy)

Available forms include: Vaginal cream 2%

Side effects/adverse reactions:

GU: Rash, stinging, burning, itching

Contraindications: Hypersensitivity

Precautions: Pregnancy (C), lactation

Interactions/incompatibilities: None known

NURSING CONSIDERATIONS

Administer:

• 1 applicatorful every night

Perform/provide:

• Storage at room temperature in dry place

Evaluate:

• Allergic reaction: burning, stinging, itching

• Therapeutic response: decrease in itching, or white discharge

Teach patient/family:

• To apply with applicator only

• To avoid use of any other vaginal product unless directed by physician

• To use medical asepsis (hand washing) before, after each application

• To abstain from sexual intercourse until treatment is completed

butorphanol tartrate

(byoo-tor'fa-nole)

Stadol

Func. class.: Nonnarcotic analgesics

Chem. class.: Nonopiate

Action: Inhibits ascending pain pathways in limbic system, thalamus, midbrain, hypothalamus

Uses: Moderate to severe pain

Dosage and routes:

• *Adult:* IM 1-4 mg q3-4h prn; IV 0.5-2 mg q3-4h prn

Available forms include: Inj IM, IV 1, 2 mg/ml

Side effects/adverse reactions:

CNS: Drowsiness, dizziness, confusion, headache, sedation, euphoria

GI: Nausea, vomiting, anorexia, constipation, cramps

GU: Increased urinary output, dysuria

INTEG: Rash, urticaria, bruising, flushing, diaphoresis, pruritus

---

italics = common side effects   ***bold italic*** = life threatening reactions

EENT: Tinnitus, blurred vision, miosis, diplopia

CV: Palpitations, bradycardia, change in B/P

*RESP: **Respiratory depression***

Contraindications: Hypersensitivity, addiction (narcotic)

Precautions: Addictive personality, pregnancy, lactation, increased intracranial pressure, MI (acute), severe heart disease, respiratory depression, hepatic disease, renal disease, child <18 yr

Pharmacokinetics:

IM: Onset 10-30 min, peak ½ hr, duration 3-4 hr

IV: Onset 1 min, peak 5 min, duration 2-4 hr

REC: Onset slow, duration 4-6 hr, metabolized by liver, excreted by kidneys, crosses placenta, excreted in breast milk, half-life 2½-3½ hr

Interactions/incompatibilities:

• Effects may be increased with other CNS depressants: alcohol, narcotics, sedative/hypnotics, antipsychotics, skeletal muscle relaxants

NURSING CONSIDERATIONS

Assess:

• I&O ratio; check for decreasing output; may indicate urinary retention

Administer:

• With antiemetic if nausea, vomiting occur

• When pain is beginning to return; determine dosage interval by patient response

Perform/provide:

• Storage in light-resistant area at room temperature

• Assistance with ambulation

• Safety measures: siderails, night light, call bell within easy reach

Evaluate:

• Therapeutic response: decrease in pain

• CNS changes: dizziness, drowsiness, hallucinations, euphoria, LOC, pupil reaction

• Allergic reactions: rash, urticaria

• Respiratory dysfunction: respiratory depression, character, rate, rhythm; notify physician if respirations are <12/min

• Need for pain medication, physical dependence

Teach patient/family:

• To report any symptoms of CNS changes, allergic reactions

• That physical dependency may result when used for extended periods of time

• Withdrawal symptoms may occur: nausea, vomiting, cramps, fever, faintness, anorexia

Lab test interferences:

Increase: Amylase

Treatment of overdose: Narcan 0.2-0.8 mg IV, O$_2$, IV fluids, vasopressors

---

caffeine

(kaf-een)

No-Doz, Tirend, Vivarin

Func. class.: Cerebral stimulant

Chem. class.: Xanthine

Action: Increases epinephrine and norepinephrine release from adrenal medulla, which causes CNS stimulation

Uses: Mild CNS stimulation, in combination with analgesics, diuretics for tension and fluid retention associated with menstruation

Dosage and routes:

• *Adult:* PO 100-200 mg q4h prn

Available forms include: Tabs 100, 200 mg; time rel caps 200, 250 mg

Side effects/adverse reactions:

CNS: Hyperactivity, insomnia, restlessness, talkativeness, dizziness, headache, *stimulation,* irritability, aggressiveness, tremors, twitching

GI: Nausea, vomiting, anorexia

GU: Diuresis

CV: Tachycardia

INTEG: Hyperesthesia

Contraindications: Hypersensitivity, gastric or duodenal

Precautions: Dysrhythmias, Gilles de la Tourette's disorder

Pharmacokinetics:

PO: Onset 15 min, peak ½-1 hr, metabolized by liver, excreted by kidneys, crosses placenta, breast milk, half-life 3-10 hr

Interactions/incompatibilities:

• Increased effect of this drug: oral contraceptives, cimetidine

NURSING CONSIDERATIONS

Assess:

• VS, B/P

Perform/provide:

• Check to see PO medication has been swallowed

Evaluate:

• Therapeutic response: increased CNS stimulation, decreased drowsiness

• Mental status: mood, sensorium, affect, stimulation, insomnia, irritability

• Tolerance or dependency: an increased amount may be used to get same effect

• Overdose: pain, fever, dehydration, insomnia, hyperactivity

Teach patient/family:

• To decrease other caffeine consumption (coffee, tea, cola, chocolate), which may increase irritability, stimulation

• To taper off drug over several weeks if used long-term

Lab test interferences:

Increase: Urinary cathecholamines

False positive: Serum urate

Treatment of overdose: Lavage, activated charcoal, monitor electrolytes, VS, administer anticonvulsants if needed

calcifediol

(kal-si-fe-dye'ole)

Calderol

Func. class.: Vitamin D analog

Chem. class.: Sterol

Action: Increases intestinal absorption, provides calcium for bones; increases renal tubular absorption of phosphate

Uses: Metabolic bone disease with chronic renal failure, osteopenia, osteomalacia

Dosage and routes:

• *Adult:* PO 300-350 μg qwk divided into qd or qod doses; may increase q4wk

Available forms include: Caps 20, 50 μg

Side effects/adverse reactions:

EENT: Tinnitus

CNS: Drowsiness, headache, vertigo, fever, lethargy

GI: Nausea, diarrhea, vomiting, jaundice, anorexia, dry mouth, constipation, cramps, metallic taste

MS: Myalgia, arthralgia, decreased bone development

GU: Polyuria, hypercalciuria, hyperphosphatemia, hematuria

Contraindications: Hypersensitivity, renal disease, hyperphosphatemia, hypercalcemia

Precautions: Pregnancy (C), renal calculi, lactation, CV disease

Pharmacokinetics:

PO: Peak 4 hr, duration 15-20 days; half-life 12-22 days

Interactions/incompatibilities:

• Decreased absorption of this drug: cholestyramine, colestipol HCl, mineral oil

• Hypercalcemia: thiazide diuretics

• Cardiac dysrhythmias: cardiac glycosides

• Decreased effect of this drug: corticosteroids

NURSING CONSIDERATIONS
Assess:
• BUN, urinary calcium, AST, ALT, cholesterol, creatinine, uric acid, chloride, magnesium, electrolytes, urine pH, phosphate; may increase, calcium should be kept at 9-10 mg/dl, vitamin D 50-135 IU/dl, phosphate 70 mg/dl
• Alk phosphatase; may be decreased
• For increased blood level since toxic reactions may occur rapidly
Administer:
• PO may be increased q4wk depending on blood level
Perform/provide:
• Storage in tight, light-resistant containers at room temperature
• Restriction of sodium, potassium if required
• Restriction of fluids if required for chronic renal failure
Evaluate:
• For dry mouth, metallic taste, polyuria, bone pain, muscle weakness, headache, fatigue, tinnitus, change in LOC, irregular pulse, dysrhythmias, increased respirations, anorexia, nausea, vomiting, cramps, diarrhea, constipation; may indicate hypercalcemia
• Renal status: decreased urinary output (oliguria, anuria), edema, in extremities, weight gain 5 lb, periorbital edema
• Nutritional status, diet for sources of vitamin D (milk, some seafood), calcium (dairy products, dark green vegetables), phosphates (dairy products)
Teach patient/family:
• The symptoms of hypercalcemia
• Foods rich in calcium
Lab test interferences:
False increase: Cholesterol

calcitonin salmon
(kal-si-toe'nin)
Calcimar

Func. class.: Parathyroid agents (calcium regulator)
Chem. class.: Polypeptide hormone

Action: Decreases bone reabsorption, blood calcium levels; increases deposits of calcium in bones
Uses: Hypercalcemia, postmenopausal osteoporosis, Paget's disease
Dosage and routes:
Osteoporosis/Paget's disease
• *Adult:* SC/IM 100 IU qd, maintenance for Paget's disease 50-100 IU qd or qod
Hypercalcemia
• *Adult:* IM 100-400 IU qd-bid
Available forms include: Inj SC/IM 200 MRC units/ml
Side effects/adverse reactions:
INTEG: Rash
CNS: Headache, flushing, tetany
GU: Diuresis, calcitonin antibody formation
GI: Nausea, diarrhea, vomiting
MS: Swelling, tingling of hands
Contraindications: Hypersensitivity, children, lactation
Precautions: Renal disease, osteoporosis, pernicious anemia, Zollinger-Ellison syndrome, pregnancy (C)
Pharmacokinetics:
IM/SC: Onset 15 min, peak 4 hr, duration 8-24 hr; metabolized by kidneys, excreted as inactive metabolites
Interactions/incompatibilities:
None known
NURSING CONSIDERATIONS
Assess:
• BUN, creatinine, uric acid, chloride, electrolytes, urine pH, urinary

calcium, magnesium, phosphatase, urinalysis, calcitonin antibody formation (calcium should be kept at 9-10 mg/dl, vitamin D 50-135 IU/dl)

• Increased level since toxic reactions may occur rapidly

• Urine for sediment

Administer:

• IM injection in deep muscle mass slowly, rotate sites

Perform/provide:

• Storage in light-resistant area, refrigerate

• Restriction of sodium, potassium if required

Evaluate:

• GI symptoms, polyuria, flushing, head swelling, tingling, headache; may indicate hypercalcemia

• Nutritional status; diet for sources of vitamin D (milk, some seafood), calcium (dairy products, dark green vegetables), phosphates

• Systemic allergic reaction to drug: skin test before 1st dose

Teach patient/family:

• Avoid OTC products

• All aspects of drug: action, side effects, dose, when to notify physician

• To administer drug SC if patient will be responsible for self-medication

---

calcitriol (1,25-Dihydroxycholecalciferol)

(kal-si-tyre′ole)

Rocaltrol

Func. class.: Parathyroid agents (calcium regulator)

Chem. class.: Vitamin D analog

Action: Increases intestinal absorption, provides calcium for bones, increases renal tubular absorption of phosphate

Uses: Hypocalcemia in chronic renal failure, hypoparathyroidism, pseudo-hypoparathyroidism

Dosage and routes:

Hypocalcemia

• *Adult:* PO 0.25 μg qd, may increase by 0.25 μg q4-8wk, maintenance 0.25 μg qod-1.25 μg qd

Hypoparathyroidism/pseudohypoparathyroidism

• *Adult and child >1 yr:* PO 0.25 μg qd, may be increased q4-8wk; maintenance 0.25-2 μg qd

Available forms include: Caps 0.25, 0.5 μg

Side effects/adverse reactions:

EENT: Tinnitus

CNS: Drowsiness, headache, vertigo, fever, lethargy

GI: Nausea, diarrhea, vomiting, jaundice, anorexia, dry mouth, constipation, cramps, metallic taste

MS: Myalgia, arthralgia, decreased bone development

GU: Polyuria, hypercalciuria, hyperphosphatemia, hematuria

Contraindications: Hypersensitivity, hyperphosphatemia, hypercalcemia

Precautions: Pregnancy (C), renal calculi, lactation, CV disease

Pharmacokinetics:

PO: Peak 4 hr, duration 15-20 days, half-life 12-22 days

Interactions/incompatibilities:

• Decreased absorption of this drug: cholestyramine, colestipol, mineral oil

• Hypercalcemia: thiazide diuretics

• Cardiac dysrhythmias: cardiac glycosides

• Decreased effect of this drug: corticosteroids

NURSING CONSIDERATIONS

Assess:

• BUN, urinary calcium, AST, ALT, cholesterol, creatinine, uric acid, chloride, magnesium, electrolytes, urine pH, phosphate; may increase calcium, should be kept at 9-10 mg/dl, vitamin D 50-135 IU/

---

italics = common side effects   ***bold italic*** = life threatening reactions

dl, phosphate 70 mg/dl

• Alk phosphatase; may be decreased

• For increased blood level since toxic reactions may occur rapidly

Administer:

• PO, may be increased q4wk depending on blood level

Perform/provide:

• Storage protected from light, heat, moisture

• Restriction of sodium, potassium if required

• Restriction of fluids if required for chronic renal failure

Evaluate:

• For dry mouth, metallic taste, polyuria, bone pain, muscle weakness, headache, fatigue, tinnitus, change in LOC, irregular pulse, dysrhythmias, increased respirations, anorexia, nausea, vomiting, cramps, diarrhea, constipation; may indicate hypercalcemia

• Renal status: decreased urinary output (oliguria, anuria), edema in extremities, weight gain 75 lb, periorbital edema

• Nutritional status, diet for sources of vitamin D (milk, some seafood), calcium (dairy products, dark green vegetables), phosphates (dairy products) must be avoided

Teach patient/family:

• The symptoms of hypercalcemia

• Foods rich in calcium

• To avoid products with sodium: cured meats, dairy products, cold cuts, olives, beets, pickles, soups, meat tenderizers in chronic renal failure

• To avoid products with potassium: oranges, bananas, dried fruit, peas, dark green leafy vegetables, milk, melons, beans in chronic renal failure

• Avoid OTC products containing calcium, potassium, or sodium in chronic renal failure

• All aspects of drug: action, side effects, dose, when to notify physician

• Avoid all preparations containing vitamin D

Lab test interferences:

False increase: Cholesterol

---

calcium carbonate

Alka-2, Amitone, Biocal Calcilac, Cal-glycine, Dicarbosil, El-Da-Minte, Equilet, Gustalac, Mallamint, P.H. Tablets, Titracid, Titralac, Trialea, Tums, Cal-sup, Caltrate

Func. class.: Antacid, calcium supplement

Chem. class.: Calcium product

Action: Neutralizes gastric acidity

Uses: Antacid

Dosage and routes:

• *Adult:* PO 1 g 4-6 × /day, chewed with water; SUSP 1 g 1 hr pc, hs

Available forms include: Chewable tabs 350, 420, 500, 750 mg; tabs 650 mg; gum 500 mg; susp 1 g/5 ml

Side effects/adverse reactions:

GI: Constipation, anorexia, *obstruction,* nausea, vomiting, flatulence, diarrhea

CV: Hemorrhage, rebound hypertension

META: Hypercalcemia, metabolic alkalosis

GU: Renal dysfunction, renal stones

Contraindications: Hypersensitivity, hypercalcemia, hyperparathyroidism, bone tumors

Precautions: Elderly, fluid restriction, decreased GI motility, GI obstruction, dehydration, renal disease

Pharmacokinetics:

PO: Onset 3 min, excreted in feces

Interactions/incompatibilities:

• Increased plasma levels of: quinidine, amphetamines

• Decreased levels of: salicylates, calcium channel blockers

• Hypercalcemia: thiazide diuretics

NURSING CONSIDERATIONS

Assess:

• Ca⁺ (serum, urine), Ca⁺ should be 8.5-10.5 mg/dl, urine Ca⁺ should be 150 mg/day

Administer:

• Laxatives, or stool softeners if constipation occurs

Evaluate:

• Therapeutic response: absence of pain, decreased acidity

• Milk-alkali syndrome: nausea, vomiting, disorientation, headache

• Constipation; increase bulk in the diet if needed

• Hypercalcemia: headache, nausea, vomiting, confusion

Teach patient/family:

• Increase fluids to 2000 ml unless contraindicated

• Not to switch antacids unless directed by physician

---

calcium chloride/calcium gluceptate/calcium gluconate/calcium lactate

Func. class.: Electrolyte replacements—calcium product

Action: Cation needed for maintenance of nervous, muscular, skeletal, enzyme reactions, normal cardiac contractility, coagulation of blood; affects secretory activity of endocrine, exocrine glands

Uses: Prevention and treatment of hypocalcemia, hypermagnesemia, hypoparathyroidism, neonatal tetany, cardiac toxicity caused by hyperkalemia, lead colic

Dosage and routes:

Calcium chloride

• *Adult:* IV 500 mg-1 g q1-3 days as indicated by serum calcium

levels, give at <1 ml/min; IAV 200-400 mg injected in ventricle of heart

• *Child:* IV 25 mg/kg over several min

Calcium gluceptate

• *Adult:* IV 5-20 ml; IM 2-5 ml

• *Newborn:* 0.5 ml/100 ml of blood transfused

Calcium gluconate

• *Adult:* PO 1-2 g bid-qid; IV 0.5-2 g at 0.5 ml/min (10% solution)

• *Child:* PO/IV 500 mg/kg/day in divided doses

Calcium lactate

• *Adult:* PO 325 mg-1.3 g tid with meals

• *Child:* PO 500 mg/kg/day in divided doses

Available forms include: Many, check product listings

Contraindications: Hypercalcemia, digitalis toxicity, ventricular fibrillation, renal calculi

Precautions: Pregnancy, lactation, children, renal disease, respiratory disease, cor pulmonale, digitalized patient, respiratory failure

Interactions/incompatibilities:

• Increased: digitalis glycosides

• Decreased action: calcium channel blockers

NURSING CONSIDERATIONS

Assess:

• ECG for decreased QT and T wave inversion: hypercalcemia, drug should be reduced or discontinued

• Calcium levels during treatment (8.5-1.5 g/dl is normal level)

Administer:

• Through small-bore needle into large vein, give over several min, if extravasation occurs, necrosis will result (IV)

• In large vein, avoiding scalp

Perform/provide:

• Seizure precautions: padded side rails, decreased stimuli, (noise, light); place airway suction equipment, padded mouth gag if Ca levels are low

• Store at room temperature

Evaluate:

• Cardiac status: rate, rhythm, CVP, (PWP, PAWP if being monitored directly)

• Therapeutic response: decreased twitching, paresthesias, muscle spasms, absence of tremors, convulsions, dysrhythmias, dyspnea, laryngospasm, negative Chvostek's sign, Trousseau's sign

Teach patient/family:

• To remain recumbent ½ hr after IV dose

• To add calcium-rich foods to diet: dairy products, shellfish, dark green leafy vegetables; and decrease oxylate-rich and zinc-rich foods: nuts, legumes, chocolate, spinach, soy

Lab test interferences:

Increase: 11-OCHS

False decrease: Magnesium

Decrease: 17-OHCS

---

calcium polycarbophil

(pol-i-kar'boe-fol)

Mitrolan

Func. class.: Laxative

Chem. class.: Bulk-forming

Action: Attracts water, expands in intestine to increase peristalsis; also absorbs excess water in stool; decreases diarrhea

Uses: Constipation, irritable bowel syndrome (diarrhea), acute, nonspecific diarrhea

Dosage and routes:

• *Adult:* PO 1 g qid prn, not to exceed 6 g/24 hr

• *Child 6-12 yr:* PO 500 mg bid prn, not to exceed 3 g/24 hr

• *Child 3-6 yr:* PO 500 mg bid prn, not to exceed 1.5 g/24 hr

Available forms include: Chew tab 500 mg

Side effects/adverse reactions:

GI: Obstruction, abdominal distention, laxative dependency

Contraindications: Hypersensitivity, GI obstruction

Pharmacokinetics:

PO: Onset 12-24 min, peak 1-3 days

Interactions/incompatibilities:

• Gastric irritation: antacids, milk, cimetidine

NURSING CONSIDERATIONS

Assess:

• Blood, urine electrolytes if drug is used often by patient

• I&O ratio to identify fluid loss

Administer:

• Alone for better absorption; do not take within 1 hr of other drugs or within 1 hr of antacids, milk, or cimetidine

• In morning or evening (oral dose)

Evaluate:

• Therapeutic response: decrease in constipation

• Cause of constipation; identify whether fluids, bulk, or exercise is missing from lifestyle

• Cramping, rectal bleeding, nausea, vomiting; if these symptoms occur, drug should be discontinued

Teach patient/family:

• Swallow tabs whole; do not chew

• Not to use laxatives for long-term therapy; bowel tone will be lost

• That normal bowel movements do not always occur daily

• Do not use in presence of abdominal pain, nausea, vomiting

• Notify physician if constipation unrelieved or if symptoms of electrolyte imbalance occur: muscle cramps, pain, weakness, dizziness

---

*Available in Canada only

capreomycin sulfate

(kap-ree-oh-mye´sin)
Capastat Sulfate

Func. class.: Antitubercular
Chem. class.: S. carpreolus polypeptide antibiotic

Action: Inhibits RNA synthesis, decreases tubercle bacilli replication

Uses: Pulmonary tuberculosis as adjunctive

Dosage and routes:
• *Adult:* IM 15 mg/kg/day × 2-3 mo, then 1 g 2-3 × /wk × 18-24 mo, not to exceed 20 mg/kg/day, must be given with another antitubercular medication

Available forms include: Powder for inj 1 mg/5 ml vial

Side effects/adverse reactions:
INTEG: Pain, irritation, sterile abscess at injection site, photosensitivity, rash, urticaria

CNS: Headache, vertigo, fever

EENT: Tinnitus, *deafness, ototoxicity*

GU: Proteinuria, decreased CrCl, increased BUN, *tubular necrosis,* hypokalemia, alkalosis, *hematuria, albuminuria, nephrotoxicity*

HEMA: Eosinophilia, leukocytosis, leukopenia

Contraindications: Hypersensitivity

Precautions: Renal disease, hearing impairment, allergy history, hepatic disease, myasthenia gravis, parkinsonism

Pharmacokinetics:
IM: Peak 1-2 hr, half-life 4-6 hr; excreted in urine unchanged

Interactions/incompatibilities:
• Increased toxicity: aminoglycosides, polymyxin, colistin, vancomycin
• Increased neuroblocking action: phenothiazine, tubocurarine, neostigmine, ether anesthesia

NURSING CONSIDERATIONS
Assess:
• Liver studies q wk: ALT, AST, bilirubin; potassium
• Renal status: before; q wk: BUN, creatinine, output, sp gr, urinalysis
• Blood levels of drug

Administer:
• After reconstituting with NS or sterile water for injection, wait 2-3 min before giving
• With other antituberculars
• IM in large muscle mass, rotate sites
• After C&S is completed; q mo to detect resistance
• Reduced dosage in renal impairment, if BUN >20 mg/dl, drug should be decreased or discontinued

Evaluate:
• Therapeutic response: decreased dyspnea, fatigue
• Ototoxicity: tinnitus, vertigo, change in hearing; audiometric testing should be done before, during, after treatment
• Hepatic status: decreased appetite, jaundice, dark urine, fatigue

Teach patient/family:
• That compliance with dosage schedule, length is necessary
• Side effects, adverse reactions: hearing loss, change in urine or urinary habits

captopril

(kap´toe-pril)
Capoten

Func. class.: Antihypertensive
Chem. class.: Renin-angiotensin antagonist

Action: Selectively suppresses renin-angiotensin-aldosterone system; inhibits ACE, prevents conversion of angiotensin I to angiotensin II, dilation of arterial, venous vessels

Uses: Hypertension, heart failure not responsive to conventional therapy

Dosage and routes:
Malignant hypertension
• *Adult:* PO 25 mg increasing q2h until desired response, not to exceed 450 mg/day
Hypertension
• *Initial dose:* 25 mg 2-3 × daily; may increase to 50 mg bid-tid at 1-2 wk intervals; usual range: 25-150 mg bid-tid; max 450 mg
CHF
• *Adult:* PO 25 mg tid given with a diuretic, digitalis; may increase to 50 mg tid, after 14 days, may increase to 150 mg tid if needed
Available forms include: Tabs 12.5, 25, 50, 100 mg

Side effects/adverse reactions:
CV: Tachycardia
GU: Impotence, dysuria, nocturia, proteinuria, *nephrotic syndrome, acute reversible renal failure,* polyuria, oliguria, frequency
HEMA: Neutropenia
INT: Rash
RESP: Bronchospasm, dyspnea, cough

Contraindications: Hypersensitivity, pregnancy (C), lactation, heart block, children, K-sparing diuretics

Precautions: Dialysis patients, hypovolemia, leukemia, scleroderma, lupus erythematosis, blood dyscrasias, CHF, diabetes mellitus, renal disease, thyroid disease, COPD, asthma

Pharmacokinetics:
PO: Peak 1 hr; duration 2-6 hr; half-life 6-7 hr, metabolized by liver (metabolites), excreted in urine, crosses placenta, excreted in breast milk

Interactions/incompatibilities:
• Increased hypotension: diuretics,

other antihypertensives, ganglionic blockers, adrenergic blockers
• Do not use with vasodilators, hydralazine, prazosin

NURSING CONSIDERATIONS
Assess:
• Blood studies: neutrophils, decreased platelets
• B/P, pulse q4h; note rate, rhythm, quality during initial therapy
• Apical/radial pulse before administration; notify physician of any significant changes
• Renal studies: protein, BUN, creatinine, watch for increased levels that may indicate nephrotic syndrome
• Baselines in renal, liver function tests before therapy begins
• K levels, although hyperkalemia rarely occurs
• Dip-stick of urine for protein qd in first morning specimen, if protein is increased a 24 hr urinary protein should be collected

Administer:
• IV infusion of 0.9% NaCl (as ordered) to expand fluid volume if severe hypotension occurs

Perform/provide:
• Storage in tight container at 30° C or less
• Supine or Trendelenburg position for severe hypotension

Evaluate:
• Therapeutic response: decrease in B/P in hypertensives, decreased B/P, edema, moist rales (CHF)
• Edema in feet, legs daily
• Allergic reaction: rash, fever, pruritus, urticaria; drug should be discontinued if antihistamines fail to help
• Symptoms of CHF: edema, dyspnea, wet rales, B/P
• Renal symptoms: polyuria, oliguria, frequency

Teach patient/family:
• Administer 1 hr before meals

• Not to discontinue drug abruptly
• Not to use OTC (cough, cold, or allergy) products unless directed by physician
• Tell patient to avoid sunlight or wear sunscreen if in sunlight, photosensitivity may occur
• Stress patient compliance with dosage schedule, even if feeling better
• To rise slowly to sitting or standing position to minimize orthostatic hypotension
• Notify physician of: mouth sores, sore throat, fever, swelling of hands or feet, irregular heartbeat, chest pain, signs of angioedema
• Excessive perspiration, dehydration, vomiting; diarrhea may lead to fall in blood pressure—consult physician if these occur
• May cause dizziness, fainting; light-headedness may occur during 1st few days of therapy
• May cause skin rash or impaired perspiration

Lab test interferences:
False positive: Urine acetone
Treatment of overdose: 0.9% Na Ca IV/INF hemodialysis

---

carbachol
(kar'ba-kole)

Miostat, Carbacel, Isopto Carbachol, Carcholin, Doryl, Lentin, Mistura C, P.V. Carbachol, Murocarb

Func. class.: Miotic, cholinergic

Action: Contracts spinchter muscle of iris, resulting in pupil constriction; causes spasms of ciliary muscle, deepening of anterior chamber; causes vasodilation of intraocular vessels or where intraocular fluids leaves eye
Uses: Ocular surgery, glaucoma (open-angle, narrow-angle)

Dosage and routes:
Ocular surgery
• *Adult:* INSTILL 0.5 ml (intraocular) of 0.01% solution in anterior chamber of eye (done by physician) for miosis during surgery
Glaucoma
• *Adult:* INSTILL 1-2 gtt (topical) of 0.75%-3% solution into eye bid-tid; OINT apply bid
Available forms include: 0.75%, 1.5%, 2.25%, 3.0% sol for topical use; sol, powders for preparing sol for inj, oint

Side effects/adverse reactions:
CV: Marked hypotension, bradycardia, headache
GI: Nausea, vomiting, abdominal discomfort, diarrhea
EENT: Blurred vision, varying degrees of myopia, decreased visual acuity in dim light, slight conjunctival hyperemia, altered distance vision, decreased night vision, eye ache
Contraindications: Hypersensitivity, when miosis is undesirable, corneal abrasions
Precautions: Bradycardia, CAD, hyperthyroidism, asthma, pregnancy, obstruction of GI or urinary tract, peptic ulcer, parkinsonism, epilepsy, peritonitis
Pharmacokinetics:
INSTILL/OINT: Miosis onset 10-20 min, duration 4-8 hr; decreased IOP onset 4 hr duration 8 hr
Interactions/incompatibilities:
None known

NURSING CONSIDERATIONS
Assess:
• Heart, respiratory rate, B/P
Perform/provide:
• Use of reconstituted solution immediately, discard unused potion
Teach patient/family:
• To report change in vision, blurring or loss of sight, trouble breathing, sweating, flushing
• Method of instillation, including

---

italics = common side effects   **bold italic** = life threatening reactions

pressure on lacrimal sac for 1 min, and not to touch dropper to eye
• That long-term therapy may be required in glaucoma
• That blurred vision will decrease with repeated use of drug
• Not to drive during first few days of treatment

---

carbamazepine

(kar-ba-maz′e-peen)
Mazepine,* Tegretol
Func. class.: Anticonvulsant
Chem. class.: Iminostilbene derivative

Action: Inhibits nerve impulses by limiting influx of sodium ions across cell membrane in motor cortex

Uses: Tonic-clonic, complex-partial, mixed seizures; trigeminal neuralgia

Dosage and routes:
Seizures
• *Adult and child >12 yr:* PO 200 mg bid, may be increased by 200 mg/day in divided doses q6-8h; adjustment is needed to minimum dose to control seizures
• *Child <12 yr:* PO 10-20 mg/kg/day in 2-3 divided doses
Trigeminal neuralgia
• *Adult:* PO 100 mg bid, may increase 100 mg q12h until pain subsides, not to exceed 1.2 g/day; maintenance is 200-400 mg bid
Available forms include: Tabs, chewable 100 mg; tabs 200 mg
Side effects/adverse reactions:
*HEMA: **Thrombocytopenia, agranulocytosis, leukocytosis, neutropenia, aplastic anemia, eosinophilia,** increased pro-time*
CNS: Drowsiness, dizziness, confusion, fatigue, paralysis, headache, hallucinations
GI: Nausea, constipation,diarrhea, anorexia, vomiting, abdominal

pain, stomatitis, glossitis, increased liver enzymes, ***hepatitis***
INTEG: Rash, Stevens-Johnson syndrome, urticaria
EENT: Tinnitus, dry mouth, blurred vision, diplopia, nystagmus, conjunctivitis
*CV: **Hypertension, CHF,** hypotension, aggravation of cardiac artery disease*
RESP: Pulmonary hypersensitivity (fever, dyspnea, pneumonitis)
GU: Frequency, retention, albuminuria, glycosuria, increased BUN
Contraindications: Hypersensitivity to carbamazepine or tricyclic antidepressants, bone marrow depression, concomitant use of MAOIs
Precautions: Glaucoma, hepatic disease, renal disease, cardiac disease, psychosis, pregnancy, lactation, child <6 yr
Pharmacokinetics:
PO: Onset slow, peak 4-8 hr, metabolized by liver, excreted in urine, feces, crosses placenta, excreted in breast milk, half-life 14-16 hr
Interactions/incompatibilities:
• Toxicity: troleandomycin, erythromycin, cimetidine, isoniazid, propoxyphene, lithium
• Decreased effects of: phenobarbital, phenytoin, primidone
• Increased effects of: vasopressin, lypressin, desmopressin
NURSING CONSIDERATIONS
Assess:
• Renal studies: urinalysis, BUN, urine creatinine
• Blood studies: RBC, Hct, Hgb, reticulocyte counts q wk for 4 wk then q mo; if myelosupression occurs, drug should be discontinued
• Hepatic studies: ALT, AST, bilirubin, creatinine
• Drug levels during initial treatment; should remain at 6-12 mg/ml

---

Administer:
• With food, milk to decrease GI symptoms
• Chewable tablets; tell patient to chew tablet, not swallow it whole
Perform/provide:
• Storage at room temperature.
• Hard candy, frequent rinsing of mouth, gum for dry mouth
• Assistance with ambulation during early part of treatment; dizziness occurs
Evaluate:
• Therapeutic response: decreased seizure activity, document on patient's chart
• Mental status: mood, sensorium, affect, behavioral changes; if mental status changes notify physician
• Eye problems: need for ophthalmic examinations before, during, after treatment (slit lamp, fundoscopy, tonometry)
• Allergic reaction: purpura, red raised rash, if these occur, drug should be discontinued
• Blood dyscrasias: fever, sore throat, bruising, rash, jaundice
• Toxicity: bone marrow depression, nausea, vomiting, ataxia, diplopia, cardiovascular collapse, Stevens-Johnson syndrome
Teach patient/family:
• To carry ID card or Medic-Alert bracelet stating drugs taken, condition, physician's name, phone number
• To avoid driving, other activities that require alertness
• To avoid alcohol ingestion; convulsions may result
• Not to discontinue medication quickly after long-term use
• Urine may turn pink to brown
• All aspects of drug: action, use, side effects, adverse reactions, when to notify physician
Lab test interferences:
Decrease: Thyroid function tests

Treatment of overdose: Lavage, VS

---

carbamide peroxide

(kar′ba-mide per-ox′ide)
Debrox, Murine Ear Drops
Func. class.: Otic
Chem. class.: Urea compound, hydrogen peroxide

Action: Foaming action facilitates removal of impacted cerumen
Uses: Impacted cerumen, prevention of ceruminosis
Dosage and routes:
• *Adult and child:* INSTILL 5-10 gtts bid × 3-4 days
Available forms include: Sol 6.5%
Side effects/adverse reactions:
EENT: Itching, irritation in ear, redness
Contraindications: Hypersensitivity, otic surgery, perforated eardrum
Pharmacokinetics: Not known
Interactions/incompatibilities: None known
NURSING CONSIDERATIONS
Administer:
• Drug, then irrigate to remove cerumen
• By allowing drops to enter ear canal, do not touch dropper to ear
Evaluate:
• Therapeutic response: loosened cerumen, ability to hear better
Teach patient/family:
• Method of instillation, using aseptic technique

carbamide peroxide (topical)

(kar'ba-mide per-ox'ide)
Cank-aid, Clear drops, Gly-Oxide, Proxigel

Func. class.: Topical anesthetic
Chem. class.: Hydrogen peroxide urea combination

Action: Inhibits nerve impulses from sensory nerves, which produces anesthesia
Uses: Toothache, cold sores, oral pain
Dosage and routes:
• *Adult and child:* Apply to oral mucosa as needed, leave on 5-7 min, expectorate
Available forms include: Gel 11%; sol 10%
Side effects/adverse reactions:
INTEG: Rash, irritation, sensitization
Contraindications: Hypersensitivity, child <3 yr
Precautions: Denuded skin
Interactions/incompatibilities: None known
NURSING CONSIDERATIONS
Administer:
• After cleansing and drying of affected area
Evaluate:
• Allergy: rash, irritation, reddening, swelling
• Therapeutic response: absence of pain, itching of affected area
• Infection: if affected area is infected, do not apply
Teach patient/family:
• To report rash, irritation, redness, swelling
• How to apply ointment, jelly

carbamide peroxide (urea peroxide)

(kar'ba-mide per-ox'ide)
Cank-aid, Clear Drops, Gly-Oxide Liquid, Orajel Brace-Aid Rinse, Proxigel

Func. class.: Topical antiinfective
Chem. class.: Equimolar compound of urea, hydrogen peroxide

Action: Releases oxygen on contact with mouth tissues, this provides cleansing effect; decreases inflammation, pain, mouth odors caused by bacteria
Uses: Oral and lip irritation, sore throat, toothache, cold sore, canker sore, aid to oral hygiene (when dental appliances are worn), cleansing of oral wounds/lesions
Dosage and routes:
• *Adult and child >3 yr:* TOP apply to affected area qid or prn; leave on 1-3 min
Available forms include: Sol 10%; gel 11%
Side effects/adverse reactions:
EENT: Itching, irritation in oral cavity
INTEG: Rash, urticaria
Contraindications: Hypersensitivity, child <3 yr
Interactions/incompatibilities: None known
NURSING CONSIDERATIONS
Administer:
• Gel by placing small amount directly on affected area, massage, do not expectorate or rinse mouth for at least 5 min
• Solution undiluted by placing several drops on affected area, on tongue, mix with saliva, swish 3 min, expectorate
Perform/provide:
• Storage in tight, light-resistant container at room temperature

Evaluate:
• Redness, swelling, pain in mouth or oral cavity
Teach patient/family:
• Not to use over 1 wk; notify physician if increased inflammation, redness, swelling, fever occur; drug should be discontinued
• That foaming will occur on contact with saliva

---

carbarsone

(kar-bar′sone)

Func. class.: Amebicide
Chem. class.: Pentavalent organic arsenic

Action: Organism death occurs in intestinal lumen by inhibition of sulfhydryl enzyme
Uses: Intestinal amebiasis
Dosage and routes:
• *Adult:* PO 250 mg bid-tid × 10 days; REC 2 g/200 ml warm 2% $NaHCO_3$ sol, qod × 5 doses
• *Child:* PO 75 mg/kg/day in 3 divided doses × 10 days
Available forms include: Caps 250 mg; powder
Side effects/adverse reactions:
RESP: Congestion
HEMA: **Agranulocytosis, aplastic anemia**
INTEG: Rash, pruritus, *exfoliative dermatitis*
CNS: Neuritis, **convulsion, hemorrhagic encephalitis, coma**
EENT: Blurred vision, sore throat, retinal edema
GI: Nausea, vomiting, diarrhea, epigastric distress, anorexia, constipation, abdominal cramps, irritation, hepatomegaly, jaundice, **hepatitis,** gastric necrosis, weight decrease
GU: Polyuria, albuminuria, **nephrotoxicity**
CV: Tachycardia, hypotension, edema

Contraindications: Hypersensitivity to this drug or arsenic, renal disease, hepatic disease, contracted visual or color fields
Precautions: Pregnancy
Pharmacokinetics:
PO: Slowly excreted by kidneys, accumulation may occur
Interactions/incompatibilities:
None known
NURSING CONSIDERATIONS
Assess:
• Stools during entire treatment; should be clear at end of therapy, for 1 yr before patient is considered cured
• ECG before, during, after therapy; be aware that inversion of T waves occurs
• Vision by ophthalmologic exam during, after therapy; vision problems occur often
• I&O, stools for number, frequency, character
Administer:
• Dimercaprol for arsenic toxicity as ordered
• PO after meals to avoid GI symptoms
Perform/provide:
• Storage in tight container
Evaluate:
• Allergic reaction: fever, rash, itching, chills; drug should be discontinued if these occur
• Nephrotoxicity: polyuria, albuminuria, hematuria
• Arsenic toxicity: sore throat, edema, pruritus, nausea, vomiting, dizziness, anorexia, epigastric pain, weight decrease, gastritis, hepatitis, visual problems, convulsions, polyuria, agranulocytosis
• Superimposed infection: fever, monilial growth, fatigue, malaise
• Tachycardia, decreasing B/P, GI

symptoms, weakness, neuromuscular symptoms

• Diarrhea for 2-3 days

Teach patient/family:

• To report any side effects

• Proper hygiene after BM: handwashing technique

• Avoid contact of drug with eyes, mouth, nose, other mucous membranes

• Need for compliance with dosage schedule, duration of treatment

Treatment of overdose: Administer dimercaprol, gastric lavage, O_2, IV fluids

---

carbinoxamine maleate

(kar-bi-nox′a-meen)

Clistin

Func. class.: Antihistamine

Chem. class.: Ethanolamine derivative, H_1-receptor antagonist

Action: Acts on blood vessels, GI system, respiratory system, by competing with histamine for H_1-receptor site; decreases allergic response by blocking histamine

Uses: Allergy symptoms, rhinitis

Dosage and routes:

• *Adult:* PO 4-8 mg tid-qid

• *Child >6 yr:* PO 4-6 mg tid-qid

• *Child 3-6 yr:* PO 2-4 mg tid-qid

• *Child 1-3 yr:* 2 mg tid-qid

Available forms include: Tabs 4 mg

Side effects/adverse reactions:

CNS: Dizziness, drowsiness, poor coordination, fatigue, anxiety, euphoria, confusion, paresthesia, neuritis

CV: Hypotension, palpitations, tachycardia

RESP: Increased thick secretions, wheezing, chest tightness

HEMA: Thrombocytopenia, agranulocytosis, hemolytic anemia

GI: Dry mouth, nausea, vomiting, anorexia, constipation, diarrhea

INTEG: Rash, urticaria, photosensitivity

GU: Retention, dysuria, frequency

EENT: Blurred vision, dilated pupils, tinnitus, nasal stuffiness, dry nose, throat, mouth

Contraindications: Hypersensitivity to H_1-receptor antagonists, acute asthma attack, lower respiratory tract disease

Precautions: Increased intraocular pressure, renal disease, cardiac disease, hypertension, bronchial asthma, seizure disorder, stenosed peptic ulcers, hyperthyroidism, prostatic hypertrophy, bladder neck obstruction, pregnancy (C)

Pharmacokinetics:

PO: Onset ½-1 hr, duration 4-6 hr; degraded in liver, excreted by kidneys (inactive)

Interactions/incompatibilities:

• Increased CNS depression: barbiturates, narcotics, hypnotics, tricyclic antidepressants, alcohol

• Decreased effect of: oral anticoagulants, heparin

• Increased effect of: MAOIs

NURSING CONSIDERATIONS

Assess:

• I&O ratio; be alert for urinary retention, frequency, dysuria; drug should be discontinued if these occur

• CBC during long-term therapy

Administer:

• Coffee, tea, cola (caffeine) to decrease drowsiness

• With meals if GI symptoms occur; absorption may slightly decrease

Perform/provide:

• Hard candy, gum, frequent rinsing of mouth for dryness

• Storage in tight container at room temperature

Evaluate:

• Therapeutic response: absence of running or congested nose, rashes

• Blood dyscrasias: thrombocyto-

---

penia, agranulocytosis (rare)
• Respiratory status: rate, rhythm, increase in bronchial secretions, wheezing, chest tightness
• Cardiac status: palpitations, increased pulse, hypotension
Teach patient/family:
• All aspects of drug use; to notify physician if confusion, sedation, hypotension occurs
• To avoid driving or other hazardous activity if drowsiness occurs
• To avoid concurrent use of alcohol, other CNS depressants
Lab test interferences:
False negative: Skin allergy tests
Treatment of overdose: Administer ipecac syrup or lavage, diazepam, vasopressors, barbiturates (short-acting)

---

carboprost trometh-amine

(kar'boe-prost)
Prostin/M15

Func. class.: Oxytocic
Chem. class.: Prostaglandin

Action: Stimulates uterine contractions causing abortion complete in approximately 16 hr
Uses: Abortion between 13-20 wk gestation
Dosage and routes:
• *Adult:* IM 250 μg, then 250 μg q1½-3½ hr, may increase to 500 μg if no response, not to exceed 12 mg total dose
Available forms include: Inj IM 250 μg/ml carboprost, 83 μg/ml tromethamine
Side effects/adverse reactions:
CNS: Fever, chills
GI: Nausea, vomiting, diarrhea
Contraindications: Hypersensitivity, severe hepatic disease, severe renal disease, pelvic inflammatory disease (PID), respiratory disease, cardiac disease

Precautions: Asthma, anemia, jaundice, diabetes mellitus, convulsive disorders, past uterine surgery
Pharmacokinetics: Onset: 15 min peak 2 hr; metabolized in lungs liver, excreted in urine (metabolites)
Interactions/incompatibilities:
None known
NURSING CONSIDERATIONS
Assess:
• B/P, pulse; watch for change that may indicate hemorrhage
• Respiratory rate, rhythm, depth; notify physician of abnormalities
Administer:
• IM in deep muscle mass, rotate injection sites if additional doses are given
• After having crash cart available on unit
Evaluate:
• For length, duration of contraction; notify physician of contractions lasting over 1 min or absence of contractions
Teach patient/family:
• To report increased blood loss, abdominal cramps, increased temperature or foul-smelling lochia

---

carisoprodol

(kar-eye-soe-proe'dole)
Rela, Soma

Func. class.: Skeletal muscle relaxant, central acting
Chem. class.: Meprobamate congener

Action: Depresses CNS by blocking interneuronal activity in descending reticular formation, spinal cord, producing sedation
Uses: Relieving pain in musculoskeletal conditions
Dosage and routes:
• *Adult and child >12 yr:* PO 350 mg tid, hs

---

italics = common side effects   ***bold italic*** = life threatening reactions

Available forms include: Tabs 350 mg

Side effects/adverse reactions:

CNS: Dizziness, weakness, drowsiness, headache, tremor, depression, insomnia

EENT: Diplopia, temporary loss of vision

CV: Postural hypotension, tachycardia

GI: Nausea, vomiting, hiccups

INTEG: Rash, pruritus, fever, facial flushing

Contraindications: Hypersensitivity, child <12 yr, intermittent porphyria

Precautions: Renal disease, hepatic disease, addictive personalities, pregnancy

Pharmacokinetics:

PO: Onset ½ hr, duration 4-6 hr, metabolized by liver, excreted in urine, crosses placenta, excreted in breast milk (large amounts), half-life 8 hr

Interactions/incompatibilities:

• Increased CNS depression: alcohol, tricylic antidepressants, narcotics, barbiturates, sedatives, hypnotics

NURSING CONSIDERATIONS

Assess:

• Blood studies: CBC, WBC, differential; blood dyscrasias may occur

• Liver function studies: AST, ALT, alk phosphatase; hepatitis may occur

• ECG in epileptic patients; poor seizure control has occurred with patients taking this drug

Administer:

• With meals for GI symptoms

Perform/provide:

• Storage in tight container at room temperature

• Assistance with ambulation if dizziness, drowsiness occurs

Evaluate:

• Therapeutic response: decreased pain, spasticity

• Allergic reactions: rash, fever, respiratory distress

• Severe weakness, numbness in extremities

• Psychologic dependency: increased need for medication, more frequent requests for medication, increased pain

• CNS depression: dizziness, drowsiness, psychiatric symptoms

Teach patient/family:

• Not to discontinue the medication quickly; insomnia, nausea, headache, spasticity, tachycardia will occur; drug should be tapered off over 1-2 wk

• Not to take with alcohol, other CNS depressants

• To avoid altering activities while taking this drug

• To avoid hazardous activities if drowsiness, dizziness occurs

• To avoid using OTC medication: cough preparations, antihistamines, unless directed by physician

Treatment of overdose: Induce emesis of conscious patient, lavage, dialysis

---

carmustine (BCNU)

(kar-mus'teen)

BiCNU

Func. class.: Antineoplastic alkylating agent

Chem. class.: Nitrosourea

Action: Alkylates DNA, RNA; is able to inhibit enzymes that allow synthesis of amino acids in proteins

Uses: Brain tumors such as glioblastoma, medulloblastoma, astrocytoma; multiple myeloma, Hodgkin's disease, other lymphomas

Dosage and routes:

• *Adult:* IV 75-100 mg/m^2 over 1-2 hr × 2 days or 200 mg/m^2 × 1

dose q6-8wk; if leukocytes fall below 2000 or platelets below 25,000 only 50% of dose should be given
Available forms include: Inj IV 100 mg; powder
Side effects/adverse reactions:
*HEMA: **Thrombocytopenia, leukopenia, myelosuppression, anemia***
*GI: Nausea, vomiting, anorexia, stomatitis, **hepatotoxicity***
*GU: Azotemia, **renal failure***
INTEG: Burning, hyperpigmentation at injection site
*RESP: **Fibrosis, pulmonary infiltrate***
Contraindications: Hypersensitivity, leukopenia, thrombocytopenia
Precautions: Pregnancy
Pharmacokinetics:
Degraded within 15 min, crosses blood-brain barrier; 70% excreted in urine within 96 hr, 10% excreted as CO_2, fate of 20% is unknown
Interactions/incompatibilities:
• Increased toxicity: other antineoplastics, or radiation
• Enhanced action: Vitamin A or caffeine
• Increased toxicity: cimetidine, other antineoplastics or radiation
NURSING CONSIDERATIONS
Assess:
• CBC, differential, platelet count weekly; withhold drug if WBC is <4000 or platelet count is <75,000; notify physician of results
• Pulmonary function tests, chest x-ray films before, during therapy; chest film should be obtained q2wk during treatment
• Renal function studies: BUN, serum uric acid, urine CrCl before, during therapy
• I&O ratio; report fall in urine output of 30 ml/hr
• Monitor temperature q4h (may indicate beginning infection)
Administer:
• Medications by oral route; if pos-

sible avoid IM, SC, IV routes to prevent infections
• Antiemetic 30-60 min before giving drug to prevent vomiting
• Antibiotics for prophylaxis of infection
Perform/provide:
• Storage in refrigerator
• Strict medical asepsis, protective isolation if WBC levels are low
• Special skin care
• Deep breathing exercises with patient tid-qid; place in semi-Fowler's position
• Liquid diet, including cola, Jello; dry toast or crackers may be added if patient is not nauseated or vomiting
• Increase fluid intake to 2-3 L/day to prevent urate deposits, calculi formation
• Rinsing of mouth tid-qid with water, hydrogen peroxide; brushing of teeth bid-tid with soft brush or cotton tipped applicators for stomatitis; use unwaxed dental floss
• Warm compresses at injection site for inflammation
Evaluate:
• Bleeding: hematuria, guaiac, bruising or petechiae, mucosa or orifices q8h
• Dyspnea, rales, unproductive cough, chest pain, tachypnea
• Food preferences; list likes, dislikes
• Inflammation of mucosa, breaks in skin
Teach patient/family:
• Of protective isolation precautions
• To report any complaints or side effects to nurse or physician
• To report any changes in breathing or coughing
• To avoid foods with citric acid, hot or rough texture
• To report any bleeding, white spots, or ulceration in mouth to

physician; tell patient to examine mouth qd

---

cascara sagrada/cascara sagrada aromatic fluid extract/cascara sagrada fluid extract

(kas-kar'a)

Func. class.: Laxative
Chem. class.: Anthraquinone

Action: Direct chemical irritation in colon; increases propulsion of stool

Uses: Constipation, bowel, or rectal preparation for surgery or examination

Dosage and routes:
• *Adult:* PO 325 mg hs; FLUID 1 ml qd; AROMATIC FLUID 5 ml qd
• *Child 2-12 yr:* PO/FLUID/AROMATIC FLUID ½ adult dose
• *Child <2 yr:* PO/FLUID/AROMATIC FLUID ¼ adult dose

Available forms include: Powder, tabs 325 mg; oral sol

Side effects/adverse reactions:
GI: Nausea, vomiting, anorexia, cramps, diarrhea
META: Hypocalcemia, enteropathy, alkalosis, hypokalemia, tetany

Contraindications: Hypersensitivity, GI bleeding, obstruction, CHF, lactation, abdominal pain, nausea/vomiting, appendicitis, acute surgical abdomen

Pharmacokinetics:
PO: Peak 6-12 hr; metabolized by liver, excreted by kidneys, in feces

Interactions/incompatibilities:
• Decreased absorption: antibiotics, digitalis, nitrofurantoin, salicylates, tetracyclines, oral anticoagulants

NURSING CONSIDERATIONS

Assess:
• Blood, urine electrolytes if drug is used often by patient
• I&O ratio to identify fluid loss

Administer:
• Alone for better absorption; do not take within 1 hr of other drugs or within 1 hr of antacids, milk, or cimetidine
• In morning or evening (oral dose)

Evaluate:
• Therapeutic response: decrease in constipation
• Cause of constipation; identify whether fluids, bulk, or exercise is missing from lifestyle
• Cramping, rectal bleeding, nausea, vomiting; if these symptoms occur, drug should be discontinued

Teach patient/family:
• Swallow tabs whole; do not chew
• Not to use laxatives for long-term therapy; bowel tone will be lost
• That normal bowel movements do not always occur daily
• Do not use in presence of abdominal pain, nausea, vomiting
• Notify physician if constipation unrelieved or if symptoms of electrolyte imbalance occur: muscle cramps, pain, weakness, dizziness

---

castor oil

Alphamul, Neoloid, Purge
Func. class.: Laxative

Action: Directly acts on intestine by increasing motor activity, thought to irritate colonic intramural plexus

Uses: Bowel, rectal preparation for surgery or examination

Dosage and routes:
• *Adult:* PO 1.25-3.7 mg; LIQ 15-60 ml
• *Child >2 yr:* LIQ 5-15 ml
• *Child <2 yr:* LIQ 1.25-7.5 ml
• *Infants:* LIQ 1-4 ml

Available forms include: Liq 36.4%, 60%, 64%, 95%; caps 0.62 ml/cap

Side effects/adverse reactions:
GI: Nausea, vomiting, anorexia, cramps, diarrhea, rebound constipation, colon irritation, flatus
META: Alkalosis, hypokalemia, electrolytes, fluid imbalance

Contraindications: Hypersensitivity, fecal impaction, GI bleeding, pregnancy, lactation, abdominal pain, nausea/vomiting, appendicitis, acute surgical abdomen

Pharmacokinetics:
PO: Peak 2-3 hr; excreted in breast milk

Interactions/incompatibilities:
Unknown

NURSING CONSIDERATIONS
Assess:
• Blood, urine electrolytes if drug is used often by patient
• I&O ratio to identify fluid loss

Administer:
• Alone for better absorption; do not take within 1 hr of other drugs or within 1 hr of antacids, milk, or cimetidine
• In morning or evening (oral dose)

Perform/provide:
• Storage in cool environment, do not freeze

Evaluate:
• Therapeutic response: decrease in constipation
• Cause of constipation; identify whether fluids, bulk, or exercise is missing from lifestyle
• Cramping, rectal bleeding, nausea, vomiting; if these symptoms occur, drug should be discontinued

Teach patient/family:
• Swallow tabs whole; do not chew
• Not to use laxatives for long-term therapy; bowel tone will be lost
• That normal bowel movements do not always occur daily
• Do not use in presence of abdominal pain, nausea, vomiting
• Notify physician if constipation unrelieved or if symptoms of electrolyte imbalance occur: muscle cramps, pain, weakness, dizziness

cefaclor

(sef′a-klor)
Ceclor
Func. class.: Antibiotic, broadspectrum
Chem. class.: Cephalosporin (2nd generation)

Action: Inhibits mucopeptide synthesis in bacterial cell wall synthesis, which renders cell wall osmotically unstable

Uses: Gram-negative bacilli: *H. influenzae, E. coli, P. mirabilis, Klebsiella;* gram-positive organisms: *S. pneumoniae, S. pyogenes, S. aureus;* upper and lower respiratory tract, urinary tract, skin infections, otitis media

Dosage and routes:
• *Adult:* PO 250-500 mg q8h, not to exceed 4 g/day
• *Child >1 mo:* PO 20-40 mg/kg/qd in divided doses q8h, not to exceed 1 g/day

Available forms include: Pulvule 250, 500 mg; oral susp 125, 250 mg/5 ml

Side effects/adverse reactions:
CNS: Headache, dizziness, weakness, paresthesia, fever, chills
GI: Nausea, vomiting, diarrhea, anorexia, pain, glossitis, bleeding, increased AST, ALT, bilirubin, LDH, alk phosphatase, abdominal pain
GU: Proteinuria, vaginitis, pruritus, candidiasis, increased BUN, *nephrotoxicity, renal failure*
HEMA: Leukopenia, *thrombocytopenia, agranulocytosis,* anemia, neutropenia, lymphocytosis, eosin-

ophilia, *pancytopenia, hemolytic anemia*

INTEG: Rash, urticaria, dermatitis, *anaphylaxis*

RESP: Dyspnea

Contraindications: Hypersensitivity to cephalosporins, infants <1 mo

Precautions: Hypersensitivity to penicillins, pregnancy (B), lactation, renal disease

Pharmacokinetics:
Peak ½-1 hr, half-life 36-54 min, 25% bound by plasma proteins, 60%-85% eliminated unchanged in urine in 8 hr, crosses placenta, excreted in breast milk

Interactions/incompatibilities:
• Do not mix with tetracyclines, erythromycins, calcium chloride, magnesium salts in same parenteral fluid
• Decreased effects: tetracyclines, erythromycins
• Increased toxicity: aminoglycosides, furosemides, probenecid, sulfinpyrazone, colistin, ethacrynic acid

NURSING CONSIDERATIONS
Assess:
• Nephrotoxicity: increased BUN, creatinine
• I&O daily
• Blood studies: AST, ALT, CBC, Hct, bilirubin, LDH, alk phosphatase, Coombs' test monthly if patient is on long-term therapy
• Electrolytes: potassium, sodium, chloride monthly if patient is on long-term therapy
• Bowel pattern qd; if severe diarrhea occurs, drug should be discontinued; may indicate pseudomembranous colitis
• IV site for extravasation or phlebitis, change site q72h

Administer:
• For 10-14 days to ensure organism death, prevent superimposed infection

• With food if needed for GI symptoms
• After C&S completed

Evaluate:
• Therapeutic response: decreased fever, malaise, chills
• Urine output; if decreasing, notify physician (may indicate nephrotoxicity)
• Allergic reactions: rash, urticaria, pruritus, chills, fever, joint pain; angioedema may occur a few days after therapy begins
• Bleeding: ecchymosis, bleeding gums, hematuria, stool guaiac daily
• Overgrowth of infection: perineal itching, fever, malaise, redness, pain, swelling, drainage, rash, diarrhea, change in cough, sputum

Teach patient/family:
• To use yogurt or buttermilk to maintain intestinal flora, decrease diarrhea
• Take all medication prescribed for length of time ordered
• To report sore throat, bruising, bleeding, joint pain; may indicate blood dyscrasias (rare)

Lab test interferences:
Increase (false): Creatinine (serum urine), urinary 17-KS
False positive: Urinary protein, direct Coombs', urine glucose
Interference: Cross-matching

Treatment of overdose: Epinephrine, antihistamines, resuscitate if needed (anaphylaxis)

---

cefadroxil monohydrate
(sef-a-drox'ill)
Duricef, Ultracef
Func. class.: Antibiotic, broad-spectrum
Chem. class.: Cephalosporin (1st generation)

Action: Inhibits bacterial cell wall synthesis, rendering cell wall osmotically unstable

Uses: Gram-negative bacilli: *H. influenzae, E. coli, P. mirabilis, Klebsiella;* gram-positive organisms: *S. pneumoniae, S. pyogenes, S. aureus;* upper, lower respiratory tract, urinary tract, skin infections, otitis media; tonsillitis; particularly for urinary tract infections

Dosage and routes:

• *Adult:* PO 1-2 g qd or q12h, give a loading dose of 1 g initially

Available forms include: Caps 500 mg; tabs 1 g; oral susp 125, 250, 500 mg/5 ml

Side effects/adverse reactions:

CNS: Headache, dizziness, weakness, paresthesia, fever, chills

GI: Nausea, vomiting, diarrhea, anorexia, pain, glossitis, bleeding, increased AST, ALT, bilirubin, LDH, alk phosphatase, abdominal pain

GU: Proteinuria, vaginitis, pruritus, candidiasis, increased BUN, ***nephrotoxicity, renal failure***

HEMA: Leukopenia, ***thrombocytopenia, agranulocytosis,*** anemia, neutropenia, lymphocytosis, eosinophilia, ***pancytopenia, hemolytic anemia***

INTEG: Rash, urticaria, dermatitis, ***anaphylaxis***

RESP: Dyspnea

Contraindications: Hypersensitivity to cephalosporins, infants <1 mo

Precautions: Hypersensitivity to penicillins, pregnancy (B), lactation, renal disease

Pharmacokinetics:

Peak 1-1½ hr, half-life 1-2 hr, 20% bound by plasma proteins, crosses placenta, excreted in breast milk

Interactions/incompatibilities:

• Do not mix with tetracyclines, erythromycins, calcium chloride, magnesium salts in same parenteral fluid

• Decreased effects: tetracyclines, erythromycins

• Increased toxicity: aminoglycosides, furosemides, probenecid, sulfinpyrazone, colistin, ethacrynic acid

NURSING CONSIDERATIONS

Assess:

• Nephrotoxicity: increased BUN, creatinine

• I&O daily

• Blood studies: AST, ALT, CBC, Hct, bilirubin, LDH, alk phosphatase, Coombs' test monthly if patient is on long-term therapy

• Electrolytes: potassium, sodium, chloride monthly if patient is on long-term therapy

• Bowel pattern qd; if severe diarrhea occurs drug should be discontinued; may indicate pseudomembranous colitis

• IV site for extravasation or phlebitis, change site q72h

Administer:

• For 10-14 days to ensure organism death, prevent superimposed infection

• With food if needed for GI symptoms

• After C&S completed

Evaluate:

• Therapeutic response: decreased fever, malaise, chills

• Urine output; if decreasing, notify physician; may indicate nephrotoxicity

• Allergic reactions: rash, urticaria, pruritus, chills, fever, joint pain; angioedema; may occur few days after therapy begins

• Bleeding: ecchymosis, bleeding gums, hematuria, stool guaiac daily

• Overgrowth of infection: perineal itching, fever, malaise, redness, pain, swelling, drainage, rash, diarrhea, change in cough, sputum

Teach patient/family:

• To use yogurt or buttermilk to maintain intestinal flora, decrease diarrhea

• Take all medication prescribed

---

italics = common side effects   ***bold italic*** = life threatening reactions

for length of time ordered

• To report sore throat, bruising, bleeding, joint pain; may indicate blood dyscrasias (rare)

Lab test interferences:

Increase (false): Creatinine (serum urine), urinary 17-KS

False positive: Urinary protein, direct Coombs', urine glucose

Interference: Cross-matching

Treatment of overdose: Epinephrine, antihistamines, resuscitate if needed (anaphylaxis)

---

cefamandole nafate

(sef-a-man'dole)

Mandol

Func. class.: Antibiotic, broad spectrum

Chem. class.: Cephalosporin (1st generation)

Action: Inhibits bacterial cell wall synthesis, rendering cell wall osmotically unstable

Uses: Gram-negative bacilli: *H. influenzae, E. coli, P. mirabilis, Klebsiella;* gram-positive organisms: *S. pneumoniae, S. pyogenes, S. aureus;* upper, lower respiratory tract, urinary tract, skin infections, otitis media

Dosage and routes:

• *Adult:* IM/IV 500 mg-1 g q4-8h; may give up to 2 g q4h for severe infections

• *Child >1 mo:* IM/IV 50-100 mg/kg/day in divided doses q4-8h, not to exceed adult dose

Available forms include: Inj IM, IV 500 mg, 1, 2, 10 g; IV 1, 2 g

Side effects/adverse reactions:

CNS: Headache, dizziness, weakness, paresthesia, fever, chills

GI: Nausea, vomiting, diarrhea, anorexia, pain, glossitis, bleeding, increased AST, ALT, bilirubin, LDH, alk phosphatase, abdominal pain

GU: Proteinuria, vaginitis, pruritus, candidiasis, increased BUN, *nephrotoxicity, renal failure*

HEMA: Leukopenia, *thrombocytopenia, agranulocytosis,* anemia, neutropenia, lymphocytosis, eosinophilia, *pancytopenia, hemolytic anemia*

INTEG: Rash, urticaria, dermatitis, *anaphylaxis*

RESP: Dyspnea

Contraindications: Hypersensitivity to cephalosporins, infants <1 mo

Precautions: Hypersensitivity to penicillins, pregnancy, lactation, renal disease

Pharmacokinetics:

Peak 1-1½ hr, half-life 1-2 hr, 25% bound by plasma proteins, crosses placenta, excreted in breast milk

Interactions/incompatibilities:

• Do not mix with tetracyclines, erythromycins, calcium chloride, magnesium salts in same parenteral fluid

• Decreased effects: tetracyclines, erythromycins

• Increased toxicity: aminoglycosides, furosemides, probenecid, sulfinpyrazone, colistin, ethacrynic acid

NURSING CONSIDERATIONS

Assess:

• Nephrotoxicity: increased BUN, creatinine

• I&O daily

• Blood studies: AST, ALT, CBC, Hct, bilirubin, LDH, alk phosphatase, Coombs' test monthly if patient is on long-term therapy

• Electrolytes: potassium, sodium, chloride monthly if patient is on long-term therapy

• Bowel pattern qd, if severe diarrhea occurs drug should be discontinued; may indicate pseudomembranous colitis

• IV site for extravasation or phlebitis, change site q72h

Administer:
• IV, check for irritation, extravasation often
• For 10-14 days to ensure organism death, prevent superimposed infection
• With food if needed for GI symptoms
• After C&S completed

Evaluate:
• Therapeutic response: decreased fever, malaise, chills
• Urine output, if decreasing, notify physician; may indicate nephrotoxicity
• Allergic reactions: rash, urticaria, pruritus, chills, fever, joint pain, angioedema; may occur few days after therapy begins
• Bleeding: ecchymosis, bleeding gums, hematuria, stool guaiac daily
• Overgrowth of infection: perineal itching, fever, malaise, redness, pain, swelling, drainage, rash, diarrhea, change in cough, sputum

Teach patient/family:
• To use yogurt or buttermilk to maintain intestinal flora, decrease diarrhea
• Take all medication prescribed for length of time ordered
• To report sore throat, bruising, bleeding, joint pain; may indicate blood dyscrasias (rare)

Lab test interferences:
Increase (false): Creatinine (serum urine), urinary 17-KS
False positive: Urinary protein, direct Coombs', urine glucose
Interference: Cross-matching
Treatment of overdose: Epinephrine, antihistamines, resuscitate if needed (anaphylaxis)

cefazolin sodium

(sef-a'zoe-lin)
Ancef, Kefzol
Func. class.: Antibiotic, broad-spectrum
Chem. class.: Cephalosporin (2nd generation)

C

Action: Inhibits bacterial cell wall synthesis rendering cell wall osmotically unstable

Uses: Gram-negative bacilli: *H. influenzae, E. coli, P. mirabilis, Klebsiella;* gram-positive organisms: *S. pneumoniae, S. pyogenes, S. aureus;* upper, lower respiratory tract, urinary tract, skin infections, otitis media, peritonitis, septicemia

Dosage and routes:
Life-threatening infections
• *Adult:* IM/IV 1-1.5 g q6h
• *Child >1 mo:* IM/IV 100 mg/kg in 3-4 equal doses
Mild/moderate infections
• *Adult:* IM/IV 250-500 mg q8h
• *Child >1 mo:* IM/IV 25-50 mg/kg in 3-4 equal doses
Available forms include: Inj IM, IV, 250, 500 mg, 1, 5, 10 g

Side effects/adverse reactions:
CNS: Headache, dizziness, weakness, paresthesia, fever, chills
GI: Nausea, vomiting, diarrhea, anorexia, pain, glossitis, bleeding, increased AST, ALT, bilirubin, LDH, alk phosphatase, abdominal pain
GU: Proteinuria, vaginitis, pruritus, candidiasis, increased BUN, *nephrotoxicity, renal failure*
HEMA: Leukopenia, *thrombocytopenia, agranulocytosis,* anemia, neutropenia, lymphocytosis, eosinophilia, *pancytopenia, hemolytic anemia*
INTEG: Rash, urticaria, dermatitis, *anaphylaxis*
RESP: Dyspnea

Contraindications: Hypersensitivity to cephalosporins, infants <1 mo

Precautions: Hypersensitivity to penicillins, pregnancy (B), lactation, renal disease

Pharmacokinetics:

IM: Peak ½-2 hr, half-life 1-2 hr
IV: Peak 10 min, half-life 30 min, eliminated unchanged in urine

Interactions/incompatibilities:

• Do not mix with tetracyclines, erythromycins, calcium chloride, magnesium salts in same parenteral fluid

• Decreased effects: tetracyclines, erythromycins

• Increased toxicity: aminoglycosides, furosemides, probenecid, sulfinpyrazone, colistin, ethacrynic acid

NURSING CONSIDERATIONS

Assess:

• Nephrotoxicity: increased BUN, creatinine   •

• I&O daily

• Blood studies: AST, ALT, CBC, Hct, alk phosphatase, bilirubin, LDH, Coombs' test monthly if patient is on long-term therapy

• Electrolytes: potassium, sodium, chloride monthly if patient is on long-term therapy

• Bowel pattern qd; if severe diarrhea occurs drug should be discontinued; may indicate pseudomembranous colitis

• IV site for extravasation or phlebitis, change site q72h

Administer:

• IV, check for irritation, extravasation often

• For 10-14 days to ensure organism death, prevent superimposed infection

• With food if needed for GI symptoms

• After C&S completed

Evaluate:

• Therapeutic response: decreased fever, malaise, chills

• Urine output, if decreasing, notify physician; may indicate nephrotoxicity

• Allergic reactions: rash, urticaria, pruritus, chills, fever, joint pain, angioedema; may occur few days after therapy begins

• Bleeding: ecchymosis, bleeding gums, hematuria, stool guaiac daily

• Overgrowth of infection: perineal itching, fever, malaise, redness, pain, swelling, drainage, rash, diarrhea, change in cough, sputum

Teach patient/family:

• To use yogurt or buttermilk to maintain intestinal flora, decrease diarrhea

• Take all medication prescribed for length of time ordered

• To report sore throat, bruising, bleeding, joint pain; may indicate blood dyscrasias (rare)

Lab test interferences:

Increase (false): Creatinine (serum urine), urinary 17-KS
False positive: urinary protein, direct Coombs', urine glucose
Interference: Cross-matching

Treatment of overdose: Epinephrine, antihistamines, resuscitate if needed (anaphylaxis)

---

cefonicid sodium

(se-fon′i-sid)
Monocid

Func. class.: Antibiotic, broad-spectrum

Chem. class.: Cephalosporin (1st generation)

Action: Inhibits bacterial cell wall synthesis rendering cell wall osmotically unstable

Uses: Gram-negative bacilli: *H. influenzae, E. coli, P. mirabilis, Klebsiella;* gram-positive organisms: *S. pneumoniae, S. pyogenes, S. aureus;* upper, lower respiratory tract, urinary tract, skin infections, otitis media, peritonitis, septicemia

Dosage and routes:

Life-threatening infections

• *Adult:* IM/IV BOL or INF 1 g/ 24 hr in divided doses

Available forms include: Inj IM, IV, 500 mg, 1, 10 g

Side effects/adverse reactions:

CNS: Headache, dizziness, weakness, paresthesia, fever, chills

GI: Nausea, vomiting, diarrhea, anorexia, pain, glossitis, bleeding, increased AST, ALT, bilirubin, LDH, alk phosphatase, abdominal pain

GU: Proteinuria, vaginitis, pruritus, candidiasis, increased BUN, *nephrotoxicity, renal failure*

HEMA: Leukopenia, *thrombocytopenia, agranulocytosis,* anemia, neutropenia, lymphocytosis, eosinophilia, *pancytopenia, hemolytic anemia*

INTEG: Rash, urticaria, dermatitis, *anaphylaxis*

RESP: Dyspnea

Contraindications: Hypersensitivity to cephalosporins, infants <1 mo

Precautions: Hypersensitivity to penicillins, pregnancy (B), lactation, renal disease

Pharmacokinetics:

IV: Onset 5 min

IM: Peak 1 hr

Half-life 4½ min, excreted in breast milk

Interactions/incompatibilities:

• Do not mix with tetracyclines, erythromycins, calcium chloride, magnesium salts in same parenteral fluid

• Decreased effects: tetracyclines, erythromycins

• Increased toxicity: aminoglycosides, furosemides, probenecid, sulfinpyrazone, colistin, ethacrynic acid

NURSING CONSIDERATIONS

Assess:

• Nephrotoxicity: increased BUN, creatinine

• I&O daily

• Blood studies: AST, ALT, CBC, Hct, bilirubin, LDH, alk phosphatase, Coombs' test monthly if patient is on long-term therapy

• Electrolytes: potassium, sodium, chloride monthly if patient is on long-term therapy

• Bowel pattern qd; if severe diarrhea occurs, drug should be discontinued; may indicate pseudomembranous colitis

Administer:

• IV, check for irritation, extravasation often

• For 10-14 days to ensure organism death, prevent superimposed infection

• With food if needed for GI symptoms

• After C&S completed

Evaluate:

• Therapeutic response: decreased fever, fatigue, malaise

• Urine output; if decreasing, notify physician; may indicate nephrotoxicity

• Allergic reactions: rash, urticaria, pruritus, chills, fever, joint pain, angioedema; may occur few days after therapy begins

• Bleeding: ecchymosis, bleeding gums, hematuria, stool guaiac daily

• Overgrowth of infection: perineal itching, fever, malaise, redness, pain, swelling, drainage, rash, diarrhea, change in cough, sputum

Teach patient/family:

• To use yogurt or buttermilk to maintain intestinal flora, decrease diarrhea

• Take all medication prescribed for length of time ordered

• To report sore throat, bruising, bleeding, joint pain; may indicate blood dyscrasias (rare)

---

italics = common side effects   ***bold italic*** = life threatening reactions

Lab test interferences:
Increase (false): Creatinine (serum urine), urinary 17-KS
False positive: Urinary protein, direct Coombs', urine glucose
Interference: Cross-matching
Treatment of overdose: Epinephrine, antihistamines, resuscitate if needed (anaphylaxis)

---

cefoperazone sodium

(sef-oh-per′a-zone)
Cefobid
Func. class.: Antibiotic, broad-spectrum
Chem. class.: Cephalosporin (3rd generation)

Action: Inhibits bacterial cell wall synthesis rendering cell wall osmotically unstable

Uses: Gram-negative bacilli: *H. influenzae, E. coli, P. mirabilis, Klebsiella, Enterobacter, P. aeruginosa;* upper, lower respiratory tract, urinary tract, skin, bone infections, bacterial septicemia, peritonitis

Dosage and routes:
Mild/moderate infections
• *Adult:* IM/IV 1-2 g q12h
Severe infections
• *Adult:* IM/IV 6-12 g/day divided in 2-4 equal doses
Available forms include: Inj IM, IV, 1, 2 g

Side effects/adverse reactions:
CNS: Headache, dizziness, weakness, paresthesia, fever, chills
GI: (Nausea, vomiting, diarrhea, anorexia), pain, glossitis, bleeding, increased AST, ALT, bilirubin, LDH, alk phosphatase, abdominal pain
GU: Proteinuria, vaginitis, pruritus, candidiasis, increased BUN, *nephrotoxicity, renal failure*
HEMA: Leukopenia, *thrombocytopenia, agranulocytosis,* anemia, neutropenia, lymphocytosis, eosinophilia, *pancytopenia, hemolytic anemia*
INTEG: Rash, urticaria, dermatitis, *anaphylaxis*
RESP: Dyspnea

Contraindications: Hypersensitivity to cephalosporins, infants <1 mo

Precautions: Hypersensitivity to penicillins, pregnancy (B), lactation, renal disease

Pharmacokinetics:
IV: Onset 5 min, peak 5-20 min, duration 6-8 hr
IM: Peak 1-2 hr, duration 6-8 hr
Half-life 2 hr, 70%-75% is eliminated unchanged in bile, 20%-30% unchanged in urine, excreted in breast milk (small amounts)

Interactions/incompatibilities:
• Do not mix with tetracyclines, erythromycins, calcium chloride, magnesium salts in same parenteral fluid
• Decreased effects: tetracyclines, erythromycins
• Increased toxicity: aminoglycosides, furosemides, probenecid, sulfinpyrazone, colistin, ethacrynic acid

NURSING CONSIDERATIONS
Assess:
• Nephrotoxicity: increased BUN, creatinine
• I&O daily
• Blood studies: AST, ALT, CBC, Hct, bilirubin, LDH, alk phosphatase, Coombs' test monthly if patient is on long-term therapy
• Electrolytes: potassium, sodium, chloride monthly if patient is on long-term therapy
• Bowel pattern qd; if severe diarrhea occurs, drug should be discontinued; may indicate pseudomembranous colitis
• IV site for extravasation or phlebitis, change site q72h

Administer:
• For 10-14 days to ensure organism death, prevent superimposed infection
• With food if needed for GI symptoms
• After C&S completed
Evaluate:
• Therapeutic response: decreased fever, malaise, chills
• Urine output, if decreasing, notify physician; may indicate nephrotoxicity
• Allergic reactions: rash, urticaria, pruritus, chills, fever, joint pain, angioedema; may occur few days after therapy begins
• Bleeding: ecchymosis, bleeding gums, hematuria, stool guaiac daily
• Overgrowth of infection: perineal itching, fever, malaise, redness, pain, swelling, drainage, rash, diarrhea, change in cough, sputum
Teach patient/family:
• To use yogurt or buttermilk to maintain intestinal flora, decrease diarrhea
• Take all medication prescribed for length of time ordered
• To report sore throat, bruising, bleeding, joint pain; may indicate blood dyscrasias (rare)
Lab test interferences:
Increase (false): Creatinine (serum urine), urinary 17-KS
False positive: Urinary protein, direct Coombs', urine glucose
Interference: Cross-matching
Treatment of overdose: Epinephrine, antihistamines, resuscitate if needed (anaphylaxis)

ceforanide
(sef-or-aa-nide)
Precef
Func. class.: Antibiotic, broad-spectrum
Chem. class.: Cephalosporin (2nd generation)

Action: Inhibits bacterial cell wall synthesis, rendering cell wall osmotically unstable
Uses: Gram-negative bacilli: *H. influenzae, E. coli, P. mirabilis, Klebsiella;* gram-positive organisms: *S. pneumoniae, S. pyogenes, S. aureus;* upper, lower respiratory tract, urinary tract, skin, bone infections, septicemia, endocarditis
Dosage and routes:
• *Adult:* IM/IV 0.5-1 g q12h
• *Child:* IM/IV 20-40 mg/kg/day in 2 equal doses q12h
Available forms include: Powder for inj IM, IV 500 mg, 1, 10 g
Side effects/adverse reactions:
CNS: Headache, dizziness, weakness, paresthesia, fever, chills
GI: Nausea, vomiting, diarrhea, anorexia, pain, glossitis, bleeding, increased AST, ALT, bilirubin, LDH, alk phosphatase, abdominal pain
GU: Proteinuria, vaginitis, pruritus, increased BUN, *nephrotoxicity, renal failure*
HEMA: Leukopenia, *thrombocytopenia, agranulocytosis,* anemia, neutropenia, lymphocytosis, eosinophilia, *pancytopenia, hemolytic anemia*
INTEG: Rash, urticaria, dermatitis, *anaphylaxis*
RESP: Dyspnea
Contraindications: Hypersensitivity to cephalosporins, infants <1 mo
Precautions: Hypersensitivity to

penicillins, pregnancy (B), lactation, renal disease

Pharmacokinetics:

IV: Peak 2 hr

IM: Peak 1 hr

Half-life 150-210 min, 80% is bound by plasma proteins, 75%-95% is eliminated unchanged in urine in 8 hr; crosses placenta, excreted in breast milk

Interactions/incompatibilities:

• Do not mix with tetracyclines, erythromycins, calcium chloride, magnesium salts in same parenteral fluid

• Decreased effects: tetracyclines, erythromycins

• Increased toxicity: aminoglycosides, furosemides, probenecid, sulfinpyrazone, colistin, ethacrynic acid

NURSING CONSIDERATIONS

Assess:

• Nephrotoxicity: increased BUN, creatinine

• I&O daily

• Blood studies: AST, ALT, CBC, Hct, bilirubin, LDH alk phosphatase, Coombs' test monthly if patient is on long-term therapy

• Electrolytes: potassium, sodium, chloride monthly if patient is on long-term therapy

• Bowel pattern qd; if severe diarrhea occurs, drug should be discontinued; may indicate pseudomembranous colitis

• IV site for extravasation or phlebitis; change site q72h

Administer:

• For 10-14 days to ensure organism death, prevent superimposed infection

• With food if needed for GI symptoms

• After C&S completed

Evaluate:

• Therapeutic response: decreased fever, malaise, chills

• Urine output, if decreasing, notify physician; may indicate nephrotoxicity

• Allergic reactions: rash, urticaria, pruritus, chills, fever, joint pain, angioedema; may occur few days after therapy begins

• Bleeding: ecchymosis, bleeding gums, hematuria, stool guaiac daily

• Overgrowth of infection: perineal itching, fever, malaise, redness, pain, swelling, drainage, rash, diarrhea, change in cough, sputum

Teach patient/family:

• To use yogurt or buttermilk to maintain intestinal flora, decrease diarrhea

• Take all medication prescribed for length of time ordered

• To report sore throat, bruising, bleeding, joint pain; may indicate blood dyscrasias (rare)

Lab test interferences:

Increase (false): Creatinine (serum urine), urinary 17-KS

False positive: Urinary protein, direct Coombs', urine glucose

Interference: Cross-matching

Treatment of overdose: Epinephrine, antihistamines, resuscitate if needed (anaphylaxis)

---

cefotaxime sodium

(sef-oh-taks'eem)

Claforan

Func. class.: Antibiotic, broad-spectrum

Chem. class.: Cephalosporin (3rd generation)

Action: Inhibits bacterial cell wall synthesis, rendering cell wall osmotically unstable

Uses: Gram-negative bacilli: *H. influenzae, E. coli, N. gonorrhea, N. meningitidis, P. mirabilis, Klebsiella;* gram-positive organisms: *S. pneumoniae, S. pyogenes, S. aureus, Enterobacter;* upper, lower serious respiratory tract, urinary tract, skin, bone, gonococcal infections, bacteremia, septicemia

Dosage and routes:
• *Adult:* IM/IV 1 g q12h, not to exceed 12 g/day

Severe infections
• *Adult:* IM/IV 2 g q4h

Available forms include: Powder for inj IM, IV, 1, 2, 10 g, frozen inj/IV 20, 40 mg/ml

Side effects/adverse reactions:
CNS: Headache, dizziness, weakness, paresthesia, fever, chills
GI: Nausea, vomiting, diarrhea, anorexia, pain, glossitis, bleeding, increased AST, ALT, bilirubin, LDH, alk phosphatase, abdominal pain
GU: Proteinuria, vaginitis, pruritus, candidiasis, increased BUN, *nephrotoxicity, renal failure*
HEMA: Leukopenia, *thrombocytopenia, agranulocytosis,* anemia, neutropenia, lymphocytosis, eosinophilia, *pancytopenia, hemolytic anemia*
INTEG: Rash, urticaria, dermatitis, *anaphylaxis*
RESP: Dyspnea

Contraindications: Hypersensitivity to cephalosporins, infants <1 mo

Precautions: Hypersensitivity to penicillins, pregnancy (B), lactation, renal disease

Pharmacokinetics:
IV: Onset 5 min
IM: Onset 30 min
Half-life 1 hr, 35%-65% is bound by plasma proteins, 40%-65% is eliminated unchanged in urine in 24 hr, 25% eliminated (active metabolized), excreted in breast milk (small amounts)

Interactions/incompatibilities:
• Do not mix with tetracyclines, erythromycins, calcium chloride, magnesium salts in same parenteral fluid

• Decreased effects: tetracyclines, erythromycins
• Increased toxicity: aminoglycosides, furosemides, probenecid, sulfinpyrazone, colistin, ethacrynic acid

NURSING CONSIDERATIONS
Assess:
• Nephrotoxicity: increased BUN, creatinine
• I&O daily
• Blood studies: AST, ALT, CBC, Hct, bilirubin, LDH, alk phosphatase, Coombs' test monthly if patient is on long-term therapy
• Electrolytes: potassium, sodium, chloride monthly if the patient is on long-term therapy
• Bowel pattern qd; if severe diarrhea occurs, drug should be discontinued; may indicate pseudomembranous colitis
• IV site for extravasation or phlebitis, change site q72h

Administer:
• For 10-14 days to ensure organism death, prevent superimposed infection
• With food if needed for GI symptoms
• After C&S completed

Evaluate:
• Therapeutic response: decreased fever, malaise, chills
• Urine output; if decreasing, notify physician; may indicate nephrotoxicity
• Allergic reactions: rash, urticaria, pruritis, chills, fever, joint pain, angioedema; may occur few days after therapy begins
• Bleeding: ecchymosis, bleeding gums, hematuria, stool guaiac daily
• Overgrowth of infection: perineal itching, fever, malaise, redness, pain, swelling, drainage, rash, diarrhea, change in cough, sputum

Teach patient/family:
• To use yogurt or buttermilk to

---

maintain intestinal flora, decrease diarrhea

• Take all medication prescribed for length of time ordered

• To report sore throat, bruising, bleeding, joint pain; may indicate blood dyscrasias (rare)

Lab test interferences:

Increase (false): Creatinine (serum urine), urinary 17-KS

False positive: Urinary protein, direct Coombs', urine glucose

Interference: Cross-matching

Treatment of overdose: Epinephrine, antihistamines, resuscitate if needed (anaphylaxis)

---

cefoxitin sodium

(se-fox′i-tin)

Mefoxin

Func. class.: Antibiotic, broad-spectrum

Chem. class.: Cephalosporin (2nd generation)

Action: Inhibits bacterial cell wall synthesis rendering cell wall osmotically unstable

Uses: Gram-negative bacilli: *H. influenzae, E. coli, Proteus, Klebsiella, B. fragilis, N. gonorrhoeae;* gram-positive organisms: *S. pneumoniae, S. pyogenes, S. aureus;* anaerobes including *Clostridium, Fusobacterium;* upper, lower respiratory tract, urinary tract, skin, bone, gonococcal infections, septicemia, peritonitis

Dosage and routes:

• *Adult:* IM/IV 1-2 g q8-12h

Severe infections

• *Adult:* IM/IV 2 g q4h

Available forms include: Powder for inj IM, IV 1, 2, 10 g

Side effects/adverse reactions:

CNS: Headache, dizziness, weakness, paresthesia, fever, chills

GI: Nausea, vomiting, diarrhea, anorexia, pain, glossitis, bleeding,

increased AST, ALT, bilirubin, LDH, alk phosphatase, abdominal pain

GU: Proteinuria, vaginitis, pruritus, candidiasis, increased BUN, *nephrotoxicity, renal failure*

HEMA: Leukopenia, *thrombocytopenia, agranulocytosis,* anemia, neutropenia, lymphocytosis, eosinophilia, *pancytopenia, hemolytic anemia*

INTEG: Rash, urticaria, dermatitis, *anaphylaxis*

RESP: Dyspnea

Contraindications: Hypersensitivity to cephalosporins, infants <1 mo

Precautions: Hypersensitivity to penicillins, pregnancy (B), lactation, renal disease

Pharmacokinetics:

IV: Peak 3 min

IM: Peak 15-60 min

Half-life 1-2 hr, 33%-55% bound by plasma proteins, 90%-100% eliminated unchanged in urine; crosses placenta, blood-brain barrier, eliminated in milk, not metabolized

Interactions/incompatibilities:

• Do not mix with tetracyclines, erythromycins, calcium chloride, magnesium salts in same parenteral fluid

• Decreased effects: tetracyclines, erythromycins

• Increased toxicity: aminoglycosides, furosemides, probenecid, sulfinpyrazone, colistin, ethacrynic acid

NURSING CONSIDERATIONS

Assess:

• Nephrotoxicity: increased BUN, creatinine

• I&O daily

• Blood studies: AST, ALT, CBC, Hct, bilirubin, LDH, alk phosphatase, Coombs' test monthly if patient is on long-term therapy

• Electrolytes: potassium, sodium,

chloride monthly if patient is on long-term therapy
• Bowel pattern qd, if severe diarrhea occurs drug should be discontinued (may indicate pseudomembranous colitis)
• IV site for extravasation or phlebitis, change site q72h

Administer:
• For 10-14 days to ensure organism death, prevent superimposed infection
• With food if needed for GI symptoms
• After C&S completed

Evaluate:
• Therapeutic response: decreased fever, malaise, chills
• Urine output; if decreasing, notify physician; may indicate nephrotoxicity
• Allergic reactions: rash, urticaria, pruritis, chills, fever, joint pain, angioedema; may occur few days after therapy begins
• Bleeding: ecchymosis, bleeding gums, hematuria, stool guaiac daily
• Overgrowth of infection: perineal itching, fever, malaise, redness, pain, swelling, drainage, rash, diarrhea, change in cough, sputum

Teach patient/family:
• To use yogurt or buttermilk to maintain intestinal flora, decrease diarrhea
• Take all medication prescribed for length of time ordered
• To report sore throat, bruising, bleeding, joint pain; may indicate blood dyscrasias (rare)

Lab test interferences:
Increase (false): Creatinine (serum urine), urinary 17-KS
False positive: Urinary protein, direct Coombs', urine glucose
Interference: Cross-matching
Treatment of overdose: Epinephrine, antihistamines, resuscitate if needed (anaphylaxis)

ceftriaxone sodium
Rocephin

Func. class.: Antibiotic, broad-spectrum
Chem. class.: Cephalosporin (3rd generation)

Action: Inhibits bacterial cell wall synthesis, which renders cell wall osmotically unstable

Uses: Gram-negative organisms: *H. influenzae, E. coli, E. aerogenes, P. mirabilis, Klebsiella,* Neisseria, *Morganelli, Enterobacter, Pseudomonas, Serratia;* gram-positive organisms: *S. pneumoniae, S. pyogenes, S. aureus;* upper, lower serious respiratory tract, urinary tract, skin, gonococcal, intraabdominal infections, septicemia meningitis

Dosage and routes:
• *Adult:* IM/IV 1-2 g qd or in two equal doses
• *Child:* IM/IV 50-75 mg/kg/day in equal doses q12h

Meningitis
• *Adult and child:* IM/IV 100 mg/kg/day in equal doses q12h
A vailable forms include: Inj IM, IV 250, 500 mg, 1, 2, 10 g

Side effects/adverse reactions:
CNS: Headache, dizziness, weakness, paresthesia, fever, chills
GI: Nausea, vomiting, diarrhea, anorexia, pain, glossitis, bleeding, increased AST, ALT, bilirubin, LDH, alk phosphatase, abdominal pain
GU: Proteinuria, vaginitis, pruritus, candidiasis, increased BUN, *nephrotoxicity, renal failure*
HEMA: Leukopenia, *thrombocytopenia, agranulocytosis,* anemia, neutropenia, lymphocytosis, eosinophilia, *pancytopenia, hemolytic anemia*

---

italics = common side effects   ***bold italic*** = life threatening reactions

INTEG: Rash, urticaria, dermatitis, ***anaphylaxis***
RESP: Dyspnea
Contraindications: Hypersensitivity to cephalosporins, infants <1 mo
Precautions: Hypersensitivity to penicillins, pregnancy (B), lactation, renal disease
Pharmacokinetics:
IV: Onset 5 min
IM: Peak 1 hr
Half-life 36-54 min, 25% bound by plasma proteins, 60%-85% is eliminated unchanged in urine in 8 hr, crosses placenta, excreted in milk
Interactions/incompatibilities:
• Do not mix with tetracyclines, erythromycins, calcium chloride, magnesium salts in same parenteral fluid
• Decreased effects: tetracyclines, erythromycins
• Increased toxicity: aminoglycosides, furosemides, probenecid, sulfinpyrazone, colistin, ethacrynic acid

NURSING CONSIDERATIONS
Assess:
• Nephrotoxicity: increased BUN, creatinine
• I&O daily
• Blood studies: AST, ALT, CBC, Hct, bilirubin, LDH, alk phosphatase, Coombs' test monthly if patient is on long-term therapy
• Electrolytes: potassium, sodium, chloride monthly if patient is on long-term therapy
• Bowel pattern qd; if severe diarrhea occurs, drug should be discontinued; may indicate pseudomembranous colitis
• IV site for extravasation, phlebitis; change site q72h
Administer:
• For 10-14 days to ensure organism death, prevent superimposed infection

• With food if needed for GI symptoms
• After C&S
Evaluate:
• Therapeutic response: decreased fever, malaise, chills
• Urine output; if decreasing, notify physician; may indicate nephrotoxicity
• Allergic reactions: rash, urticaria, pruritus, chills, fever, joint pain, angioedema; may occur few days after therapy begins
• Bleeding: ecchymosis, bleeding gums, hematuria, stool guaiac daily
• Overgrowth of infection: perineal itching, fever, malaise, redness, pain, swelling, drainage, rash, diarrhea, change in cough, sputum
Teach patient/family:
• To use yogurt or buttermilk to maintain intestinal flora and decrease diarrhea
• To take all medication prescribed for length of time ordered
• To report sore throat, bruising, bleeding, joint pain; may indicate blood dyscrasias (rare)
Lab test interferences:
Increase (false): Creatinine (serum urine); urinary 17-KS
False positive: Urinary protein, direct Coombs', urine glucose
Interference: Cross-matching
Treatment of overdose: Epinephrine, antihistamines, resuscitate if needed (anaphylaxis)

---

cefuroxime sodium

(se-fyoor-ox'eem)
Zinacef
Func. class.: Antibiotic, broadspectrum
Chem. class.: Cephalosporin (2nd generation)

Action: Inhibits bacterial cell wall synthesis, rendering cell wall osmotically unstable

Uses: Gram-negative bacilli: *H. influenzae, E. coli, Neisseria, P. mirabilis, Klebsiella;* gram-positive organisms: *S. pneumoniae, S. pyogenes, S. aureus;* serious lower respiratory tract, urinary tract, skin, gonococcal infections, septicemia, meningitis

Dosage and routes:
• *Adult:* IM/IV 750 mg-1.5 g q8h for 5-10 days

Severe infections
• *Adult:* IM/IV 1.5 g q6h; may give up to 3 g q8h for bacterial meningitis
• *Child >3 mo:* IM/IV 50-100 mg/kg/day; may give up to 200-240 mg/kg/day IV in divided doses for bacterial meningitis

Available forms include: Inj IM, IV 750 mg, 1.5 g, powder, sol

Side effects/adverse reactions:
CNS: Headache, dizziness, weakness, paresthesia, fever, chills
GI: Nausea, vomiting, diarrhea, anorexia, pain, glossitis, bleeding, increased AST, ALT, bilirubin, LDH, alk phosphatase, abdominal pain
GU: Proteinuria, vaginitis, pruritus, candidiasis, increased BUN, *nephrotoxicity, renal failure*
HEMA: Leukopenia, *thrombocytopenia, agranulocytosis,* anemia, neutropenia, lymphocytosis, eosinophilia, *pancytopenia, hemolytic anemia*
INTEG: Rash, urticaria, dermatitis, *anaphylaxis*
RESP: Dyspnea

Contraindications: Hypersensitivity to cephalosporins, infants <1 mo

Precautions: Hypersensitivity to penicillins, pregnancy (B), lactation, renal disease

Pharmacokinetics:
IV: Peak 3 min
IM: Peak 15-60 min
Half-life 1-2 hr, 33%-50% bound

by plasma proteins, 90%-100% eliminated unchanged in urine, crosses placenta, blood-brain barrier, excreted in breast milk, not metabolized

Interactions/incompatibilities:
• Do not mix with tetracyclines, erythromycins, calcium chloride, magnesium salts in the same parenteral fluid
• Decreased effects: tetracyclines, erythromycins
• Increased toxicity: aminoglycosides, furosemides, probenecid, sulfinpyrazone, colistin, ethacrynic acid

NURSING CONSIDERATIONS
Assess:
• Nephrotoxicity: increased BUN, creatinine
• I&O daily
• Blood studies: AST, ALT, CBC, Hct, bilirubin, LDH, alk phosphatase, Coombs' test monthly if patient is on long-term therapy
• Electrolytes: potassium, sodium, chloride monthly if patient is on long-term therapy
• Bowel pattern qd; if severe diarrhea occurs, drug should be discontinued; may indicate pseudomembranous colitis
• IV site for extravasation, phlebitis; change site q72h

Administer:
• For 10-14 days to ensure organism death, prevent superimposed infection
• With food if needed for GI symptoms
• After C&S

Evaluate:
• Therapeutic response: decreased fever, malaise, chills
• Urine output: if decreasing, notify physician; may indicate nephrotoxicity
• Allergic reactions: rash, urticaria, pruritus, chills, fever, joint pain, angioedema; may occur few

---

italics = common side effects   **bold italic** = life threatening reactions

days after therapy begins

• Bleeding: ecchymosis, bleeding gums, hematuria, stool guaiac daily

• Overgrowth of infection: perineal itching, fever, malaise, redness, pain, swelling, drainage, rash, diarrhea, change in cough, sputum

Teach patient/family:

• To use yogurt or buttermilk to maintain intestinal flora, decrease diarrhea

• To take all medication prescribed for length of time ordered

• To report sore throat, bruising, bleeding, joint pain; may indicate blood dyscrasias (rare)

Lab test interferences:

Increase (false): Creatinine (serum urine), urinary 17-KS

False positive: Urinary protein, direct Coombs', urine glucose

Interference: Cross-matching

Treatment of overdose: Epinephrine, antihistamines, resuscitate if needed (anaphylaxis)

---

cephalexin monohydrate

(sef-a-lex′in)

Ceporex,* Keflex, Novolexin*

Func. class.: Antibiotic, broad-spectrum

Chem. class.: Cephalosporin (1st generation)

Action: Inhibits bacterial cell wall synthesis, rendering cell wall osmotically unstable

Uses: Gram-negative bacilli: *H. influenzae, E. coli, P. mirabilis, Klebsiella;* gram-positive organisms: *S. pneumoniae, S. pyogenes, S. aureus;* upper, lower respiratory tract, urinary tract, skin, bone infections, otitis media

Dosage and routes:

• *Adult:* PO 250-500 mg q6h

• *Child:* PO 25-50 mg/kg/day in 4 equal doses

Severe infections

• *Adult:* PO 500 mg-1 g q6h

• *Child:* PO 50-100 mg/kg/day in 4 equal doses

Available forms include: Caps 250, 500 mg; tabs 1000 mg; oral susp 125, 250 mg/5ml; pediatric susp 100 mg/5ml

Side effects/adverse reactions:

CNS: Headache, dizziness, weakness, paresthesia, fever, chills

GI: Nausea, vomiting, diarrhea, anorexia, pain, glossitis, bleeding, increased AST, ALT, bilirubin, LDH, alk phosphatase, abdominal pain

GU: Proteinuria, vaginitis, pruritus, candidiasis, increased BUN, *nephrotoxicity, renal failure*

HEMA: Leukopenia, *thrombocytopenia, agranulocytosis,* anemia, neutropenia, lymphocytosis, eosinophilia, *pancytopenia, hemolytic anemia*

INTEG: Rash, urticaria, dermatitis, *anaphylaxis*

RESP: Dyspnea

Contraindications: Hypersensitivity to cephalosporins, infants <1 mo.

Precautions: Hypersensitivity to penicillins, pregnancy (B), lactation, renal disease

Pharmacokinetics:

PO: Peak 1 hr, duration 6-8 hr, half-life 30-72 min, 5%-15% bound by plasma proteins, 90%-100% eliminated unchanged in urine, crosses placenta, excreted in breast milk

Interactions/incompatibilities:

• Do not mix with tetracyclines, erythromycins, calcium chloride, magnesium salts in same parenteral fluid

• Decreased effects: tetracyclines, erythromycins

• Increased toxicity: aminoglycosides, furosemides, probenecid, sulfinpyrazone, colistin, ethacrynic acid

---

NURSING CONSIDERATIONS
Assess:
• Nephrotoxicity: increased BUN, creatinine
• I&O daily
• Blood studies: AST, ALT, CBC, Hct, bilirubin, LDH, alk phosphatase, Coombs' test monthly if patient is on long-term therapy
• Electrolytes: potassium, sodium, chloride monthly if patient is on long-term therapy
• Bowel pattern qd; if severe diarrhea occurs, drug should be discontinued; may indicate pseudomembranous colitis
• IV site for extravasation, phlebitis; change site q72h
Administer:
• For 10-14 days to ensure organism death, prevent superimposed infection
• With food if needed for GI symptoms
• After C&S
Evaluate:
• Therapeutic response: decreased fever, malaise, chills
• Urine output: if decreasing, notify physician; may indicate nephrotoxicity
• Allergic reactions: rash, urticaria, pruritus, chills, fever, joint pain, angioedema; may occur few days after therapy begins
• Bleeding: ecchymosis, bleeding gums, hematuria, stool guaiac daily
• Overgrowth of infection: perineal itching, fever, malaise, redness, pain, swelling, drainage, rash, diarrhea, change in cough, sputum
Teach patient/family:
• To use yogurt or buttermilk to maintain intestinal flora, decrease diarrhea
• To take all medication prescribed for length of time ordered
• To report sore throat, bruising, bleeding, joint pain; may indicate blood dyscrasias (rare)

Lab test interferences:
Increase (false): Creatinine (serum urine), urinary 17-KS
False positive: Urinary protein, direct Coombs', urine glucose
Interference: Cross-matching
Treatment of overdose: Epinephrine, antihistamines, resuscitate if needed (anaphylaxis)

---

cephalothin sodium

(sef-a'loe-thin)
Ceporacin,* Keflin, Seffin

Func. class.: Antibiotic, broad-spectrum
Chem. class.: Cephalosporin (1st generation)

Action: Inhibits bacterial cell wall synthesis, rendering cell wall osmotically unstable
Uses: Gram-negative bacilli: *H. influenzae, E. coli, P. mirabilis, Klebsiella, Salmonella, Shigella;* gram-positive organisms: *S. pneumoniae, S. pyogenes, S. aureus;* severe respiratory tract, urinary tract, skin, bone infections, septicemia, meningitis, endocarditis, bacterial peritonitis
Dosage and routes:
• *Adult:* IM/IV 500 mg-1 g q4-6h
• *Child:* IM/IV 14-27 mg/kg q4h or 20-40 mg/kg, q6h
Severe infections
• *Adult:* IM/IV 1-2 g q4h
Available forms include: Powder for inj IM, IV 1, 2, 4, 10, 20 g; frozen IV 20, 30, 40 mg/ml
Side effects/adverse reactions:
CNS: Headache, dizziness, weakness, paresthesia, fever, chills
GI: Nausea, vomiting, diarrhea, anorexia, pain, glossitis, bleeding, increased AST, ALT, bilirubin, LDH, alk phosphatase, abdominal pain
GU: Proteinuria, vaginitis, pruritus, candidiasis, increased BUN, ***neph-***

---

italics = common side effects   ***bold italic*** = life threatening reactions

rotoxicity, renal failure

HEMA: Leukopenia, ***thrombocyto-***
penia, agranulocytosis, anemia,
neutropenia, lymphocytosis, eosinophilia, ***pancytopenia, hemolytic***
anemia

INTEG: Rash, urticaria, dermatitis,
anaphylaxis

RESP: Dyspnea

Contraindications: Hypersensitivity to cephalosporins, infants <1 mo

Precautions: Hypersensitivity to
penicillins, pregnancy (B), lactation, renal disease

Pharmacokinetics:

IV: Peak 15 min

IM: Peak 30 min

Half-life ½-1 hr, 25% bound by
plasma proteins, 60%-95% eliminated unchanged in urine in 8 hr,
crosses placenta, excreted in breast
milk, deacetylated in kidneys, liver

Interactions/incompatibilities:

• Do not mix with tetracyclines,
erythromycins, calcium chloride,
magnesium salts in same parenteral
fluid

• Decreased effects: tetracyclines,
erythromycins

• Increased toxicity: aminoglycosides, furosemides, probenecid,
sulfinpyrazone, colistin, ethacrynic acid

NURSING CONSIDERATIONS

Assess:

• Nephrotoxicity: increased BUN,
creatinine

• I&O daily

• Blood studies: AST, ALT, CBC,
Hct, bilirubin, LDH, alk phosphatase, Coombs' test monthly if patient is on long-term therapy

• Electrolytes: potassium, sodium,
chloride monthly if patient is on
long-term therapy

• Bowel pattern qd; if severe diarrhea occurs, drug should be discontinued; may indicate pseudomembranous colitis

• IV site for extravasation, phlebitis; change site q72h

Administer:

• For 10-14 days to ensure organism death, prevent superimposed
infection

• With food if needed for GI
symptoms

• After C&S

Evaluate:

• Therapeutic response: decreased
fever, malaise, chills

• Urine output: if decreasing, notify physician; may indicate nephrotoxicity

• Allergic reactions: rash, urticaria, pruritus, chills, fever, joint
pain, angioedema; may occur few
days after therapy begins

• Bleeding: ecchymosis, bleeding
gums, hematuria, stool guaiac daily

• Overgrowth of infection: perineal
itching, fever, malaise, redness,
pain, swelling, drainage, rash,
diarrhea, change in cough, sputum

Teach patient/family:

• To use yogurt or buttermilk to
maintain intestinal flora, decrease
diarrhea

• To take all medication prescribed
for length of time ordered

• To report sore throat, bruising,
bleeding, joint pain; may indicate
blood dyscrasias (rare)

Lab test interferences:

Increase (false): Creatinine (serum
urine), urinary 17-KS

False positive: Urinary protein, direct Coombs', urine glucose

Interference: Cross-matching

Treatment of overdose: Epinephrine, antihistamines, resuscitate if
needed (anaphylaxis)

cephapirin sodium

(sef-a-pye′rin)
Cefadyl

Func. class.: Antibiotic, broad-spectrum
Chem. class.: Cephalosporin (1st generation)

Action: Inhibits bacterial cell wall synthesis, rendering cell wall osmotically unstable

Uses: Gram-negative bacilli: *H. influenzae, E. coli, P. mirabilis, Klebsiella;* gram-positive organisms: *S. pneumoniae, S. viridans, S. aureus;* serious respiratory tract, urinary tract, skin infections, septicemia, endocarditis

Dosage and routes:
• *Adult:* IM/IV 500 mg-1 g q4-6h
• *Child:* IM/IV 10-20 mg/kg, q6h
Available forms include: Powder for inj IM, IV 1, 2, 20 g; IV only 2, 4 g

Side effects/adverse reactions:
CNS: Headache, dizziness, weakness, paresthesia, fever, chills
GI: Nausea, vomiting, diarrhea, anorexia, pain, glossitis, bleeding, increased AST, ALT, bilirubin, LDH, alk phosphatase, abdominal pain
GU: Proteinuria, vaginitis, pruritus, candidiasis, increased BUN, *nephrotoxicity, renal failure*
HEMA: Leukopenia, thrombocytopenia, agranulocytosis, anemia, neutropenia, lymphocytosis, eosinophilia, *pancytopenia, hemolytic anemia*
INTEG: Rash, urticaria, dermatitis, **anaphylaxis**
RESP: Dyspnea

Contraindications: Hypersensitivity to cephalosporins, infants <1 mo
Precautions: Hypersensitivity to penicillins, pregnancy (B), lactation, renal disease

Pharmacokinetics:
IV: Peak 5 min
IM: Peak 30 min
Half-life 21-47 min, 44%-50% bound by plasma proteins, 70%-95% eliminated unchanged in urine, crosses placenta, excreted in breast milk, metabolized in liver

Interactions/incompatibilities:
• Do not mix with tetracyclines, erythromycins, calcium chloride, magnesium salts in same parenteral fluid
• Decreased effects: tetracyclines, erythromycins
• Increased toxicity: aminoglycosides, furosemides, probenecid, sulfinpyrazone, colistin, ethacrynic acid

NURSING CONSIDERATIONS
Assess:
• Nephrotoxicity: increased BUN, creatinine
• I&O daily
• Blood studies: AST, ALT, CBC, Hct, bilirubin, LDH, alk phosphatase, Coombs' test monthly if patient is on long-term therapy
• Electrolytes: potassium, sodium, chloride monthly if patient is on long-term therapy
• Bowel pattern qd; if severe diarrhea occurs drug should be discontinued; may indicate pseudomembranous colitis
• IV site for extravasation, phlebitis; change site q72h

Administer:
• For 10-14 days to ensure organism death, prevent superimposed infection
• With food if needed for GI symptoms
• After C&S

Evaluate:
• Therapeutic response: decreased fever, malaise, chills
• Urine output: if decreasing, no-

---

italics = common side effects   ***bold italic*** = life threatening reactions

tify physician; may indicate neph-rotoxicity

• Allergic reactions: rash, urti-caria, pruritus, chills, fever, joint pain, angioedema; may occur few days after therapy begins

• Bleeding: ecchymosis, bleeding gums, hematuria, stool guaiac daily

• Overgrowth of infection: perineal itching, fever, malaise, redness, pain, swelling, drainage, rash, diarrhea, change in cough, sputum

Teach patient/family:

• To use yogurt or buttermilk to maintain intestinal flora, decrease diarrhea

• To take all medication prescribed for length of time ordered

• To report sore throat, bruising, bleeding, joint pain; may indicate blood dyscrasias (rare)

Lab test interferences:

Increase (false:) Creatinine (serum urine), urinary 17-KS

False positive: Urinary protein, di-rect Coombs', urine glucose

Interference: Cross-matching

Treatment of overdose: Epineph-rine, antihistamines, resuscitate if needed (anaphylaxis)

---

cephradine

(sef'ra-deen)

Anspor, Velosef

Func. class.: Antibiotic, broad-spectrum

Chem. class.: Cephalosporin (1st generation)

Action: Inhibits bacterial cell wall synthesis, rendering cell wall os-motically unstable

Uses: Gram-negative bacilli: *H. in-fluenzae, E. coli, P. mirabilis, Klebsiella;* gram-positive organ-isms: *S. pneumoniae, S. pyogenes, S. aureus;* serious respiratory tract, urinary tract, skin infections, otitis media

Dosage and routes:

• *Adult:* IM/IV 500 mg-1 g bid-qid, not to exceed 8 g/day; PO 250-500 mg q6h

• *Child >1 yr.:* IM/IV 12-25 mg/kg q6h; PO 6-12 mg/kg q6h

Available forms include: Powder for inj IM, IV 250, 500 mg, 1 g; caps 250, 500 mg; oral susp 125, 250 mg/5 ml

Side effects/adverse reactions:

CNS: Headache, dizziness, weak-ness, paresthesia, fever, chills

GI: Nausea, vomiting, diarrhea, anorexia, pain, glossitis, bleeding, increased AST, ALT, bilirubin, LDH, alk phosphatase, abdominal pain

GU: Proteinuria, vaginitis, pruritus, candidasis, increased BUN, *neph-rotoxicity, renal failure*

HEMA: Leukopenia, *thrombocyto-penia, agranulocytosis,* anemia, neutropenia, lymphocytosis, eosin-ophilia, *pancytopenia, hemolytic anemia*

INTEG: Rash, urticaria, dermatitis, *anaphylaxis*

RESP: Dyspnea

Contraindications: Hypersen-sitivity to cephalosporins, in-fants <1 mo

Precautions: Hypersensitivity to penicillins, pregnancy (B), lacta-tion, renal disease

Pharmacokinetics:

PO: Peak 1 hr

IV: Peak 5 min

IM: Peak 1 hr

Half-life 36-54 min, 20% bound by plasma proteins, 60%-90% elimi-nated unchanged in urine, crosses placenta, excreted in breast milk

Interactions/incompatibilities:

• Do not mix with tetracyclines, erythromycins, calcium chloride, magnesium salts in same parenteral fluid

• Decreased effects: tetracyclines, erythromycins

• Increased toxicity: aminoglycosides, furosemides, probenecid, sulfinpyrazone, colistin, ethacrynic acid

NURSING CONSIDERATIONS
Assess:
• Nephrotoxicity: increased BUN, creatinine
• I&O daily
• Blood studies: AST, ALT, CBC, Hct, bilirubin, LDH, alk phosphatase, Coombs' test monthly if patient is on long-term therapy
• Electrolytes: potassium, sodium, chloride monthly if patient is on long-term therapy
• Bowel pattern qd; if severe diarrhea occurs, drug should be discontinued; may indicate pseudomembranous colitis
• IV site for extravasation, phlebitis; change site q72h

Administer:
• For 10-14 days to ensure organism death, prevent superimposed infection
• With food if needed for GI symptoms
• After C&S

Evaluate:
• Therapeutic response: decreased fever, malaise, chills
• Urine output: if decreasing, notify physician; may indicate nephrotoxicity
• Allergic reactions: rash, urticaria, pruritus, chills, fever, joint pain, angioedema; may occur few days after therapy begins
• Bleeding: ecchymosis, bleeding gums, hematuria, stool guaiac daily
• Overgrowth of infection: perineal itching, fever, malaise, redness, pain, swelling, drainage, rash, diarrhea, change in cough, sputum

Teach patient/family:
• To use yogurt or buttermilk to maintain intestinal flora, decrease diarrhea
• To take all medication prescribed

for length of time ordered
• To report sore throat, bruising, bleeding, joint pain; may indicate blood dyscrasias (rare)

Lab test interferences:
Increase (false): Creatinine (serum urine), urinary 17-KS
False positive: Urinary protein, direct Coombs', urine glucose
Interference: Cross-matching
Treatment of overdose: Epinephrine, antihistamines, resuscitate if needed (anaphylaxis)

---

chenodiol
(kee-noe-dye′ole)
Chenix
Func. class.: Antilithic
Chem. class.: Natural human bile acid

Action: Suppresses synthesis of cholesterol, cholic acid, replacing cholic acid with drug metabolite, which leads to the degradation of gallstones
Uses: Dissolving gallstones instead of surgery

Dosage and routes:
• *Adult:* PO 250 mg bid × 2 wk, then increased by 250 mg/day, not to exceed 16 mg/kg/day × 24 mo
Available forms include: Tabs 250 mg

Side effects/adverse reactions:
*HEMA: **Leukopenia***
GI: Diarrhea, fecal urgency, heartburn, nausea, cramps, increased ALT, AST, LDH, vomiting, dysphagia, absence of taste, ***hepatotoxicity,*** flatulence, dyspepsia
Contraindications: Hypersensitivity, hepatic disease, bile duct obstruction, biliary GI fistula, pregnancy (X)
Precautions: Lactation, children, atherosclerosis
Pharmacokinetics:
Metabolized by liver, excreted in

---

feces (metabolite/unchanged drug), crosses placenta

Interactions/incompatibilities:

• Decreased action of this drug: cholestyramine, colestipol, aluminum antacids, estrogens, clofibrate

NURSING CONSIDERATIONS

Assess:

• Vital signs, cardiac status: checking for dysrhythmias increased rate, palpitations

• I&O ratio; check for urinary retention or hesitancy

• Oral cholecystogram or ultrasonogram q6-9 mo

Administer:

• With meals for better absorption

• Antidiarrheals if diarrhea occurs

Perform/provide:

• Storage at room temperature

• Increased fluids, bulk, exercise to patient's lifestyle to decrease constipation

Evaluate:

• Therapeutic response: absence of pain (epigastric), gallstones on diagnostic testing

• GI complaints: nausea, vomiting, anorexia, diarrhea; if diarrhea is severe drug may need to be decreased

Teach patient/family:

• That stone dissolution may take 6-24 mo, therapy is discontinued in 18 mo if gallstones are still intact

• To notify physician if pregnancy is suspected, birth defects may occur

---

chloral hydrate

(klor-al hye'drate)

Aquachloral Supprettes, Cohidrate, Noctec, Novochlorhydrate*

Func. class.: Sedative-hypnotic
Chem. class.: Chloral derivative

Controlled Substance Schedule IV (USA), Schedule F (Canada)
Action: Reduction product trichloroethanol produces mild cerebral depression, which causes sleep

Uses: Sedation, insomnia

Dosage and routes:

Sedation

• *Adult:* PO/REC 250 mg tid pc

• *Child:* PO 8 mg/kg tid, not to exceed 500 mg tid

Insomnia

• *Adult:* PO/REC 500 mg-1g ½ hr before hs

• *Child:* PO/REC 50 mg/kg in one dose

Available forms include: Caps 250, 500 mg; syr 250, 500 mg/5 ml; supp 325, 500, 650 mg

Side effects/adverse reactions:

*HEMA: **Eosinophilia, leukopenia***
*CNS: **Drowsiness,** dizziness, stimulation, nightmares, ataxia, hangover (rare), lightheadedness, headache, paranoia*
*GI: Nausea, vomiting, flatulence, diarrhea, unpleasant taste, **gastric necrosis***
*INTEG: **Rash,** urticaria, angioedema, fever, purpura, eczema*
CV: Hypotension, dysrhythmias
*RESP: **Depression***

Contraindications: Hypersensitivity to this drug or triclofos, severe renal disease, severe hepatic disease, GI disorders (oral forms), pregnancy, lactation, gastritis

Precautions: Severe cardiac disease, depression, suicidal individuals, asthma, intermittent porphyria

Pharmacokinetics:

PO: Onset 30 min-1 hr, duration 4-8 hr
REC: Onset slow, duration 4-6 hr Metabolized by liver, excreted by kidneys (inactive metabolite) and feces, crosses placenta, excreted in breast milk; half-life 8-11 hr; metabolite is highly protein bound

Interactions/incompatibilities:

• Increased action of: oral anticoagulants

• Increased action of both drugs: alcohol

NURSING CONSIDERATIONS
Assess:

• Blood studies: Hct, Hgb, RBCs serum folate (if on long-term therapy), pro-time in patients receiving anticoagulants

Administer:

• After removal of cigarettes, to prevent fires

• After trying conservative measures for insomnia

• ½-1 hr before hs for sleeplessness

• On empty stomach with full glass of water or juice for best absorption and decrease corrosion (do not chew); after meals to decrease GI symptoms if using for sedation

Perform/provide:

• Assistance with ambulation after receiving dose

• Safety measure: siderails, nightlight, callbell within easy reach

• Checking to see PO medication swallowed

Evaluate:

• Therapeutic response: ability to sleep at night, decreased amount of early morning awakening if taking drug for insomnia

• Mental status: mood, sensorium, affect, memory (long, short)

• Physical dependency: more frequent requests for medication, shakes, anxiety

• Respiratory dysfunction: respiratory depression, character, rate, rhythm; hold drug if respirations are <12/min or if pupils are dilated (rare)

• Blood dyscrasias: fever, sore throat, bruising, rash, jaundice, epistaxis (rare)

• Previous history of substance abuse, cardiac disease, or gastritis

Teach patient/family:

• To avoid driving or other activities requiring alertness

• To avoid alcohol ingestion or CNS depressants; serious CNS depression may result

• Not to discontinue medication quickly after long-term use; drug should be tapered over 1-2 wk

• That effects may take 2 nights for benefits to be noticed

• Alternate measures to improve sleep (reading, exercise several hours before hs, warm bath, warm milk, TV, self-hypnosis, deep breathing)

Lab test interferences:

Interferences: Urine catecholamines, urinary 17-OHCS

False Positive: Urine glucose (copper sulfate test)

Treatment of overdose: Lavage, activated charcoal, monitor electrolytes, vital signs

---

chlorambucil

(klor-am'byoo-sil)

Leukeran

Func. class.: Antineoplastic alkylating agent

Chem. class.: Nitrogen mustard

Action: Alkylates DNA, RNA; inhibits enzymes that allow synthesis of amino acids in proteins

Uses: Chronic lymphocytic leukemia, Hodgkin's disease, other lymphomas

Dosage and routes:

• *Adult:* PO 0.1-0.2 mg/kg/day for 3-6 wk initially, then 2-6 mg/day; maintenance 0.2 mg/kg for 2-4 wk, course may be repeated at 2-4 wk intervals

• *Child:* PO 0.1-0.2 mg/kg/day in divided doses or 4.5 mg/m²/day as 1 dose or in divided doses

Available forms include: Tabs 2 mg

Side effects/adverse reactions:

CNS: Convulsions in children

HEMA: **Thrombocytopenia, leukopenia, pancytopenia**

GI: Nausea, vomiting, diarrhea, weight loss
GU: Hyperuremia
INTEG: Alopecia (rare), dermatitis, rash
RESP: Fibrosis, pneumonitis
Contraindications: Radiation therapy within 1 mo, chemotherapy within 1 mo, thrombocytopenia, smallpox vaccination, pregnancy (1st trimester) (D)
Precautions: Pneumococcus vaccination
Pharmacokinetics:
Well absorbed orally, metabolized in liver, excreted in urine; half-life 2 hr
Interactions/incompatibilities:
• Increased toxicity; other antineoplastics, or radiation
NURSING CONSIDERATIONS
Assess:
• CBC, differential, platelet count weekly; withhold drug if WBC is <4000 or platelet count is <75,000; notify physician of results
• Pulmonary functions test, chest x-ray films before, during therapy; chest film should be obtained q2wk during treatment
• Renal function studies: BUN, serum uric acid, urine CrCl before, during therapy
• I&O ratio; report fall in urine output of 30 ml/hr
• Monitor temperature q4h (may indicate beginning infection)
• Liver function tests before, during therapy (bilirubin, AST, ALT, LDH) as needed or monthly
Administer:
• Medications by oral route; if possible avoid IM, SC, IV routes to prevent infections
• Antacid before oral agent, give drug after evening meal, before bedtime
• Antiemetic 30-60 min before giving drug to prevent vomiting

• Allopurinol or sodium bicarbonate to maintain uric acid levels, alkalinization of urine
• Antibiotics for prophylaxis of infection
Perform/provide:
• Storage in tight container
• Strict medical asepsis, protective isolation if WBC levels are low
• Special skin care
• Liquid diet, including cola, Jello; dry toast or crackers may be added if patient is not nauseated or vomiting
• Increase fluid intake to 2-3 L/day to prevent urate deposits, calculi formation
• Diet low in purines: organ meats (kidney, liver), dried beans, peas to maintain alkaline urine
Evaluate:
• Bleeding: hematuria, guaiac, bruising or petechiae, mucosa or orifices q8h
• Food preferences; list likes, dislikes
• Yellowing of skin, sclera, dark urine, clay-colored stools, itchy skin, abdominal pain, fever, diarrhea
• Dyspnea, rales, unproductive cough, chest pain, tachypnea
• Effects of alopecia on body image; discuss feelings about body changes (rare)
Teach patient/family:
• Of protective isolation precautions
• To report any complaints or side effects to nurse or physician
• To report any changes in breathing or coughing
• That hair may be lost during treatment; a wig or hairpiece may make patient feel better; new hair may be different in color, texture (rare)

chloramphenicol / chlor-amphenicol palmitate / chloramphenicol sodium succinate

Chloromycetin, Mychel, Novo-chlorocap*

Func. class.: Antibacterial / anti-rickettsial

Chem. class.: Dichoroacetic acid derivative

Action: Binds to 50S ribosomal subunit which prevents binding of amino acid to ribosome binding site

Uses: Infections caused by *H. influenzae, S. typhi, Rickettsia, Neisseria,* myoplasma

Dosage and routes:

• *Adult and child:* PO/IV 50-100 mg/kg/day in divided doses q6h, not to exceed 100 mg/kg/day

• *Premature infants and neonates:* IV/PO 25 mg/kg/day in divided doses q6h

Available forms include: Inj (IV) 1 g; caps 250 mg; oral susp 150 mg/ 5 ml

Side effects / adverse reactions:

*HEMA: **Anemia, bone marrow depression, thrombocytopenia, aplastic anemia, granulocytopenia, leukopenia***

EENT: Optic neuritis, blindness

GI: Nausea, vomiting, diarrhea, abdominal pain, xerostomia, glossitis, colitis, pruritis ani

INTEG: Itching, urticaria, contact dermatitis, rash

*CV: **Gray syndrome*** in newborns: failure to feed, pallid, cyanosis, abdominal distention, irregular respiration, vasomotor collapse

Contraindications: Hypersensitivity, severe renal disease, severe hepatic disease, minor infections

Precautions: Hepatic disease, renal disease, infants, children, bone marrow depression (drug-induced), pregnancy, lactation

Pharmacokinetics:

PO/IV: Peak 1-2 hr, duration 8 hr, half-life 1½-4 hr, conjugated in liver, excreted in urine (up to 15% as free drug), breast milk, feces, crosses placenta

Interactions / incompatibilities:

• Increased action of: dicumarol, phenytoin, tolbutamide, chlorpropamide

• Increased prothrombin time: anticoagulants

• Increased action of this drug: phenobarbital, rifampin

• Decreased action of: iron, vitamin B_{12}, folic acid, penicillins, aminoglycosides

• Do not mix with any drug before consulting package inserts; incompatible with many drugs

• Avoid use with myelosuppressive drugs

NURSING CONSIDERATIONS

Assess:

• Any patient with compromised renal system; drug is excreted slowly in poor renal system function; toxicity may occur rapidly

• Liver studies: AST, ALT

• Blood studies: WBC, RBC, Hct, Hgb, platelets, serum iron, reticulocytes; drug should be discontinued if bone marrow depression occurs

• Renal studies: urinalysis, protein, blood, BUN, creatinine

• C&S before drug therapy; may be taken as soon as culture is taken

• Drug level in impaired hepatic, renal systems

Administer:

• IV slowly over at least 1 min

• After reconstituting with 10 ml sterile H_2O/1 g drug; refrigerate

• Oral form on empty stomach with full glass of water

Perform / provide:

• Storage of capsules in tight container at room temperature, reconstituted solution at room temperature for up to 30 days

• Adrenalin, suction, tracheostomy set, endotracheal intubation equipment on unit

• Adequate intake of fluids (2000 ml) during diarrhea episodes

Evaluate:

• Therapeutic response: decreased temperature, negative C&S

• Bowel pattern before, during treatment

• Skin eruptions, itching, dermatitis after administration

• Respiratory status: rate, character, wheezing, tightness in chest

• Allergies before treatment, reaction of each medication; place allergies on chart, Kardex in bright red letters; notify all people giving drugs

• Neonates for beginning gray syndrome: cyanosis, abdominal distention, irregular respiration, failure to feed; drug should be discontinued immediately

Teach patient/family:

• Aspects of drug therapy: need to complete entire course of medication to ensure organism death (10-14 days); culture may be taken after complete course of medication

• To report sore throat, fever, fatigue, unusual bleeding, bruising; could indicate bone marrow depression (may occur weeks or months after termination of drug)

• That drug must be taken in equal intervals around clock to maintain blood levels

• To wear or carry a Medic Alert identification if allergic to this drug

• To notify nurse of diarrhea stools

Treatment of overdose: Withdraw drug, maintain airway, administer epinephrine, aminophylline, O_2, IV corticosteroids

chloramphenicol

Chloromycetin Otic, Sopamycetin*

Func. class.: Otic, broad-spectrum antibiotic

Action: Inhibits protein synthesis in suspectible microorganisms

Uses: Ear infection (external)

Dosage and routes:

• *Adult and child:* INSTILL 2-3 gtts tid

Available forms include: Sol 0.5%

Side effects/adverse reactions:

EENT: Itching, irritation in ear

INTEG: Rash, urticaria, contact dermatitis, burning, angioedema

Contraindications: Hypersensitivity, perforated eardrum

Pharmacokinetics: Not known

Interactions/incompatibilities: None known

NURSING CONSIDERATIONS

Administer:

• After removing impacted cerumen by irrigation

• After cleaning stopper with alcohol

• After restraining child if necessary

• Warming solution to body temperature

Evaluate:

• Therapeutic response: decreased ear pain

• For redness, swelling, pain in ear, which indicates superimposed infection

Teach patient/family:

• Method of instillation, using aseptic technique, including not touching dropper to ear

• That dizziness may occur after instillation

chloramphenicol (ophthalmic)

(klor-am-fen'i-kole)

Antibiopto, Chloromycetin Ophthalmic, Chloroptic, Chloroptic SOP, Econochlor Ophthalmic, Fenicol,* Isopto Fenical,* Ophthoclor Ophthalmic, Pentamycin*

Func. class.: Antiinfective

Action: Inhibits bacterial cell wall in organism by preventing amino acids and nucleotides into cell wall

Uses: Infection of eye

Dosage and routes:

• *Adult and child:* INSTILL 2 gtts in eye qd-qid until desired response; TOP apply oint to conjunctival sac q3-6h as needed or hs if using gtts also

Available forms include: Oint 1%; sol 0.5%, 25 mg

Side effects/adverse reactions:

EENT: Poor corneal wound healing, temporary visual haze, overgrowth of nonsusceptible organisms

Contraindications: Hypersensitivity

Precautions: Antibiotic hypersensitivity

Interactions/incompatibilities: None known

NURSING CONSIDERATIONS

Administer:

• After washing hands, cleanse crusts or discharge from eye before application

• Apply pressure to lacrimal sac for 1 min to prevent systemic absorption

Perform/provide:

• Storage at room temperature, protect from light

Evaluate:

• Therapeutic response: absence of redness, inflammation, tearing

• Allergy: itching, lacrimation, redness, swelling

Teach patient/family:

• To use drug exactly as prescribed

• Not to use eye makeup, towels, washcloths, eye medication of others; reinfection may occur

• That drug container tip should not be touched to eye

• To report itching, increased redness, burning, stinging, swelling; drug should be discontinued

• That drug may cause blurred vision when ointment is applied

chloramphenicol (topical)

(klor-am-fen'i-kole)

Chloromycetin

Func. class.: Local antiinfective

Chem. class.: Antibacterial

Action: Interferes with bacterial ribosome synthesis

Uses: Skin infections (bacterial)

Dosage and routes:

• *Adult and child:* TOP apply to affected area qid-bid

Available forms include: Cream 1%

Side effects/adverse reactions:

INTEG: Rash, urticaria, stinging, burning

Contraindications: Hypersensitivity

Precautions: Pregnancy, lactation

Interactions/incompatibilities: None known

NURSING CONSIDERATIONS

Administer:

• Enough medication to completely cover lesions

• After cleansing with soap, water before each application, dry well

Perform/provide:

• Storage at room temperature in dry place

---

italics = common side effects   ***bold italic*** = life threatening reactions

Evaluate:
• Allergic reaction: burning, stinging, swelling, redness
• Therapeutic response: decrease in size, number of lesions

Teach patient/family:
• To apply with glove to prevent further infection
• To avoid use of OTC creams, ointments, lotions unless directed by physician
• To use medical asepsis (hand washing) before, after each application to prevent further infection

---

chlordiazepoxide HCl

(klor-dye-az-e-pox'ide)
A-poxide,* C-Tran, Libritabs, Librium,* Medilium,* Novopoxide,* Relaxil, Solium,* Lipoxide, SK-Lygen

Func. class.: Antianxiety
Chem. class.: Benzodiazepine

Controlled Substance Schedule IV
Action: Depresses subcortical levels of CNS, including limbic system, reticular formation
Uses: Short-term management of anxiety, acute alcohol withdrawal, preoperatively for relaxation

Dosage and routes:
Mild anxiety
• *Adult:* PO 5-10 mg tid-qid
• *Child >6 yr:* 5 mg bid-qid, not to exceed 10 mg bid-tid
Severe anxiety
• *Adult:* PO 20-25 mg tid-qid
Preoperatively
• *Adult:* PO 5-10 mg tid-qid on day before surgery; IM 50-100 mg 1 hr before surgery
Alcohol withdrawal
• *Adult:* PO/IM/IV 50-100 mg, not to exceed 300 mg/day
Available forms include: Caps 5, 10, 25 mg; tabs 5, 10, 25 mg; powder for IM inj 100 mg

Side effects/adverse reactions:
CNS: Dizziness, drowsiness, confusion, headache, anxiety, tremors, stimulation, fatigue, depression, insomnia, hallucinations
GI: Constipation, dry mouth, nausea, vomiting, anorexia, diarrhea
INTEG: Rash, dermatitis, itching
*CV: Orthostatic hypotension, **ECG changes, tachycardia,*** hypotension
EENT: Blurred vision, tinnitus, mydriasis

Contraindications: Hypersensitivity to benzodiazepines, narrow-angle glaucoma, psychosis, pregnancy (D), child <18 yr
Precautions: Elderly, debilitated, hepatic disease, renal disease
Pharmacokinetics:
PO: Onset 30 min, peak ½ hr, duration 4-6 hr, metabolized by liver, excreted by kidneys, crosses placenta, breast milk, half-life 5-30 hr
Interactions/incompatibilities:
• Decreased effects of this drug: oral contraceptives, rifampin, valproic acid
• Increased effects of this drug: CNS depressants, alcohol, cimetidine, disulfiram, oral contraceptives

NURSING CONSIDERATIONS
Assess:
• B/P (lying, standing), pulse; if systolic B/P drops 20 mm Hg, hold drug, notify physician
• Blood studies: CBC during long-term therapy, blood dyscrasias have occurred rarely
• Hepatic studies: AST, ALT, bilirubin, creatinine, LDH, alk phosphatase
• I&O; may indicate renal dysfunction
Administer:
• By IV 5 ml saline 100 mg/powder, agitate ampule gently; do not use diluent for IM 2 ml/powder
• With food or milk for GI symptoms

---

*Available in Canada only

• Crushed if patient is unable to swallow medication whole
• Sugarless gum, hard candy, frequent sips of water for dry mouth

Perform/provide:
• Assistance with ambulation during beginning therapy, since drowsiness/dizziness occurs
• Safety measure, including siderails
• Check to see PO medication has been swallowed

Evaluate:
• Therapeutic response: decreased anxiety, restlessness, sleeplessness
• Mental status: mood, sensorium, affect, sleeping pattern, drowsiness, dizziness
• Physical dependency, withdrawal symptoms: headache, nausea, vomiting, muscle pain, weakness after long-term use
• Suicidal tendencies

Teach patient/family:
• That drug may be taken with food
• Not to be used for everyday stress or used longer than 4 mo, unless directed by physician
• Avoid OTC preparations unless approved by physician
• To avoid driving, activities that require alertness; drowsiness may occur
• To avoid alcohol ingestion or other psychotropic medications, unless prescribed by physician
• Not to discontinue medication abruptly after long-term use
• To rise slowly or fainting may occur
• That drowsiness might worsen at beginning of treatment

Lab test interferences:
Increase: AST/ALT, serum bilirubin
False increase: 17-OHCS
Decrease: RAIU

Treatment of overdose: Lavage, VS, supportive care

chlorhexidine gluconate

Exidine, Hibistat

Func. class.: Disinfectant
Chem. class.: Polychlorinated phenol derivative

Action: Inhibits growth of gram-positive bacteria

Uses: Surgical scrub, bacteriostatic skin cleanser, gram-positive infection when other treatment has been ineffective

Dosage and routes:
• *Adult and child:* Use prn
Available forms include: Top soap, emulsion

Side effects/adverse reactions:
INTEG: Irritation, dryness, dermatitis, scaling
GI: Nausea, vomiting, diarrhea
CNS: Delirium, convulsions, restlessness, headache, confusion, tremors, dizziness

Contraindications: Hypersensitivity, occlusive dressings, infants, burns

Interactions/incompatibilities:
None known

NURSING CONSIDERATIONS

Administer:
• To body areas only, do not apply to face, lips, mouth, eyes, mucous membrane, anus, meatus
• Only to adults; repeated use may lead to systemic absorption

Evaluate:
• Area of body involved: irritation, rash, breaks, redness, dryness, itching

Teach patient/family:
• To report itching, irritation, dizziness, headache, confusion; discontinue drug immediately

Treatment of ingestion: Gastric lavage, administer vegetable oil, saline laxative, supportive treatment

---

chloroprocaine HCl

(klor'-oh-pro-kane)

Nesacaine, Nesacaine-CE

Func. class.: Local anesthetic
Chem. class.: Ester

Action: Competes with calcium for sites in nerve membrane that control sodium transport across cell membrane; decreases rise of depolarization phase of action potential

Uses: Epidural anesthesia, peripheral nerve block, caudal anesthesia, infiltration block

Dosage and routes:
Varies depending on route of anesthesia

Available forms include: Inj 1%, 2%, 3%

Side effects/adverse reactions:

CNS: Anxiety, restlessness, ***convulsions, loss of consciousness,*** drowsiness, disorientation, tremors, shivering

CV: ***Myocardial depression, cardiac arrest, dysrhythmias,*** bradycardia, hypotension, hypertension, fetal bradycardia

GI: Nausea, vomiting

EENT: Blurred vision, tinnitus, pupil constriction

INTEG: Rash, urticaria, allergic reactions, edema, burning, skin discoloration at injection site, tissue necrosis

RESP: ***Status asthmaticus, respiratory arrest, anaphylaxis***

Contraindications: Hypersensitivity, child <12 yr, elderly, severe liver disease

Precautions: Elderly, severe drug allergies, pregnancy (C)

Pharmacokinetics:
Duration ½-1 hr, metabolized by liver, excreted in urine (metabolites)

Interactions/incompatibilities:
• Dysrhythmias: epinephrine, halothane, enflurane

• Hypertension: MAOIs, tricyclic antidepressants, phenothiazines

NURSING CONSIDERATIONS

Assess:

• B/P, pulse, respiration during treatment

• Fetal heart tones if drug is used during labor

Administer:

• Only with crash cart, resuscitative equipment nearby

• Only drugs without preservatives for epidural or caudal anesthesia

Perform/provide:

• Use of new solution, discard unused portions

Evaluate:

• Therapeutic response: anesthesia necessary for procedure

• Allergic reactions: rash, urticaria, itching

• Cardiac status: ECG for dysrhythmias, pulse, B/P during anesthesia

Treatment of overdose: Airway, O_2, vasopressor, IV fluids, anticonvulsants for seizures

chloroquine HCl/ chloroquine phosphate

(klor'oh-kwin)

Aralen HCl, Aralen Phosphate, Chlorocon, Novochloroquine*

Func. class.: Antimalarial
Chem. class.: Synthetic 4-aminoquinoline derivative

Action: Inhibits parasite replications, transcription of DNA to RNA by forming complexes with DNA of parasite

Uses: Malaria caused by *Plasmodium vivax, P. malariae, P. ovale, P. falciparum* (some strains), rheumatoid arthritis, amebiasis

Dosage and routes:
Malaria suppression
• *Adult and child:* PO 5 mg/kg/wk

on same day of week, not to exceed 300 mg; treatment should begin 2 wk before exposure and for 8 wk after; if treatment begins after exposure, 600 mg for adult and 10 mg/kg for children in 2 divided doses 6 hr apart

Extraintestinal amebiasis

• *Adult:* IM 160-200 mg (HCl) up to 12 days, then 1 g (phosphate) qd × 2 days, then 500 mg qd × 2-3 wk; PO 600 mg qd × 2 days, then 300 mg qd × 2-3 wk

• *Child:* IM/PO 10 mg/kg (HCl) × 2-3 wk, not to exceed 300 mg/ day

Rheumatoid arthritis

• *Adult:* PO 250 mg (phosphate) qd with evening meal

Available forms include: Tabs 250, 500 mg; inj IM 40 mg/ml

Side effects/adverse reactions:

CV: Hypotension, heart block, asystole with syncope, ECG changes

INTEG: Pruritus, pigmentary changes, skin eruptions, lichen planus–like eruptions, eczema, *exfoliative dermatitis,* alopecia

CNS: Headache, stimulation, fatigue, irritability, *convulsion,* bad dreams, dizziness, confusion, psychosis, decreased reflexes

EENT: Blurred vision, corneal changes, retinal changes, difficulty focusing, tinnitus, vertigo, deafness, photophobia, corneal edema

GI: Nausea, vomiting, anorexia, diarrhea, cramps, weight loss, stomatitis

HEMA: Thrombocytopenia, agranulocytosis, hemolytic anemia, leukopenia

Contraindications: Hypersensitivity, retinal field changes, porphyria, children (long-term)

Precautions: Pregnancy, children, blood dyscrasias, severe GI disease, neurologic disease, alcoholism, hepatic disease, G-6-PD deficiency, psoriasis, eczema

Pharmacokinetics:

PO: Peak 1-2 hr, half-life 3-5 days, metabolized in the liver, excreted in urine, feces, breast milk, crosses placenta

Interactions/incompatibilities:

• Decreased action of this drug: magnesium or aluminum compounds

NURSING CONSIDERATIONS

Assess:

• Ophthalmic test if long-term treatment or drug dosage >150 mg/day

• Liver studies q wk: AST, ALT, bilirubin

• Blood studies: CBC, since blood dyscrasias occur

• For decreased reflexes: knee, ankle; watch for depression of T waves, widening of QRS complex

• ECG during therapy

Administer:

• Before or after meals at same time each day to maintain drug level

• IM after aspirating to avoid injection into blood system, which may cause hypotension, asystole, heart block; rotate injection sites

Perform/provide:

• Storage in tight, light-resistant containers at room temperature; injection should be kept in cool environment

Evaluate:

• Allergic reactions: pruritus, rash, urticaria

• Blood dyscrasias: malaise, fever, bruising, bleeding (rare)

• For ototoxicity (tinnitus, vertigo, change in hearing); audiometric testing should be done before, after treatment

• For toxicity: blurring vision, difficulty focusing, headache, dizziness, knee, ankle reflexes; drug should be discontinued immediately

---

italics = common side effects　　　**bold italic** = life threatening reactions

Teach patient/family:
• To use sunglasses in bright sunlight to decrease photophobia
• That urine may turn rust or brown color
• To report hearing, visual problems, fever, fatigue, bruising, bleeding, which may indicate blood dyscrasias
Treatment of overdose: Induce vomiting, gastric lavage, administer barbiturate (ultrashort-acting), vasopressin; tracheostomy may be necessary

---

chlorothiazide

(klor-oh-thye′a-zide)
Diachlor, Diuril, Ro-Chlorozide
Func. class.: Diuretic
Chem. class.: Thiazide; sulfonamide derivative

Action: Acts on distal tubule by increasing excretion of water, sodium, chloride, potassium
Uses: Edema, hypertension, diuresis
Dosage and routes:
Edema, hypertension
• *Adult:* PO/IV 500 mg-2 g qd in 2 divided doses
Diuresis
• *Child >6 mo:* PO/IV 20 mg/kg/day in divided doses
• *Child <6 mo:* PO/IV up to 30 mg/kg/day in 2 divided doses
Available forms include: Tabs 250, 500 mg; oral susp 250 mg/5 ml; inj 500 mg
Side effects/adverse reactions:
GU: Frequency, polyuria, uremia, glucosuria
CNS: Drowsiness, paresthesia, anxiety, depression, headache, dizziness, fatigue, weakness
GI: Nausea, vomiting, anorexia, constipation, diarrhea, cramps, pancreatitis, GI irritation, *hepatitis*
EENT: Blurred vision

INTEG: Rash, urticaria, purpura, photosensitivity, fever
META: Hyperglycemia, hyperuremia, increased creatinine
HEMA: Aplastic anemia, hemolytic anemia, leukopenia, agranulocytosis, thrombocytopenia
CV: Irregular pulse, orthostatic hypotension
ELECT: Hypokalemia, hypercalcemia, hyponatremia, hypochloremia
Contraindications: Hypersensitivity to thiazides or sulfonamides, anuria, renal decompensation
Precautions: Hypokalemia, renal disease, pregnancy, hepatic disease, gout, COPD, lupus erythematosus, diabetes mellitus
Pharmacokinetics:
PO: Onset 2 hr, peak 4 hr, duration 6-12 hr; crosses placenta, excreted in breast milk
Interactions/incompatibilities:
• Increased toxicity: lithium, nondepolarizing skeletal muscle relaxants, digitalis
• Decreased effects of: antidiabetics
• Decreased absorption of thiazides: cholestyramine, colestipol
• Decreased hypotensive response: indomethacin
• Increased action of: quinidine
NURSING CONSIDERATIONS
Assess:
• Weight, I&O daily to determine fluid loss; effect of drug may be decreased if used qd
• Rate, depth, rhythm of respiration, effect of exertion
• B/P lying, standing; postural hypotension may occur
• Electrolytes: potassium, sodium, chloride; include BUN, blood sugar, CBC, serum creatinine, blood pH, ABGs

• Glucose in urine if patient is diabetic

Administer:
• In AM to avoid interference with sleep if using drug as a diuretic
• Potassium replacement if potassium is less than 3.0
• With food if nausea occurs; absorption may be decreased slightly

Evaluate:
• Improvement in edema of feet, legs, sacral area daily if medication is being used in CHF
• Improvement in CVP q8h
• Signs of metabolic acidosis: drowsiness, restlessness
• Signs of hypokalemia: postural hypotension, malaise, fatigue, tachycardia, leg cramps, weakness
• Rashes, temperature elevation qd
• Confusion, especially in elderly; take safety precautions if needed

Teach patient/family:
• To increase fluid intake 2-3 L/day unless contraindicated, to rise slowly from lying or sitting position
• To notify physician of muscle weakness, cramps, nausea, dizziness
• Drug may be taken with food or milk
• That blood sugar may be increased in diabetics
• Take early in day to avoid nocturia

Lab test interferences:
Increase: BSP retention, calcium, amylase
Decrease: PBI, PSP

Treatment of overdose: Lavage if taken orally, monitor electrolytes, administer dextrose in saline

chlorotrianisene
(klor-oh-trye-an′i-seen)
Tace

Func. class.: Estrogen
Chem. class.: Nonsteroidal synthetic estrogen

Action: Needed for adequate functioning of female reproductive system, it affects release of pituitary gonadotropins, inhibits ovulation, adequate calcium use in bone structures

Uses: Breast engorgement, prostatic cancer, menopause, female hypogonadism, atrophic vaginitis, kraurosis vulvae

Dosage and routes:
Breast engorgement
• *Adult:* PO 72 mg bid × 2 days, or 50 mg q6h × 6 doses, or 12 mg qid × 1 wk, begin dose 8 hr after delivery

Prostatic cancer
• *Adult:* PO 12-25 mg qd

Menopause
• *Adult:* PO 12-25 mg qd × 30 days or 3 wk on 1 wk off

Female hypogonadism
• *Adult:* PO 12-25 mg × 21 days, then progesterone 100 mg IM or 5 days of progesterone PO given with last 5 days of medroxyprogesterone 5-10 mg

Vaginitis
• *Adult:* PO 12-25 mg qd × 30-60 days

Available forms include: Caps 12, 25, 72 mg

Side effects/adverse reactions:
CNS: Dizziness, headache, migraines, depression
CV: Hypotension, ***thrombophlebitis,*** edema, ***thromboembolism, stroke, pulmonary embolism, myocardial infarction***
GI: Nausea, vomiting, diarrhea, anorexia, pancreatitis, cramps, con-

stipation, increased appetite, increased weight, cholestatic jaundice

EENT: Contact lens intolerance, increased myopia, astigmatism

GU: Amenorrhea, cervical erosion, breakthrough bleeding, dysmenorrhea, vaginal candidiasis, breast changes, *gynecomastia, testicular atrophy, impotence*

INTEG: Rash, urticaria, acne, hirsutism, alopecia, oily skin, seborrhea, purpura, melasma

META: Folic acid deficiency, hypercalcemia, hyperglycemia

Contraindications: Breast cancer, thromboembolic disorders, reproductive cancer, genital bleeding (abnormal, undiagnosed), pregnancy (X)

Precautions: Hypertension, asthma, blood dyscrasias, gallbladder disease, CHF, diabetes mellitus, bone disease, depression, migraine headache, convulsive disorders, hepatic disease, renal disease, family history of cancer of the breast or reproductive tract

Pharmacokinetics:

PO: Degraded in liver, excreted in urine, crosses placenta, excreted in breast milk

Interactions/incompatibilities:

• Decreased action of: anticoagulants, oral hypoglycemics

• Toxicity: tricyclic antidepressants

• Decreased action of this drug: anticonvulsants, barbiturates, phenylbutazone, rifampin

• Increased action of: corticosteroids

NURSING CONSIDERATIONS

Assess:

• Urine glucose in patient with diabetes, increased urine glucose may occur

• Weight daily, notify physician if weekly weight gain is >5 lb, if increase, diurectic may be ordered

• B/P q4h, watch for increase

caused by water and sodium retention

• I&O ratio, be alert for decreasing urinary output and increasing edema

• Liver function studies, including AST, ALT, bilirubin, alk phosphatase

Administer:

• Titrated dose, use lowest effective dose

• In one dose in AM, for prostatic cancer, vaginitis, hypogonadism

• With food or milk to decrease GI symptoms

Evaluate:

• Therapeutic response: absence of breast engorgement, reversal of menopause or decrease in tumor size in prostatic cancer

• Edema, hypertension, cardiac symptoms, jaundice

• Mental status: affect, mood, behavioral changes, aggression

• Hypercalcemia

Teach patient/family:

• To weigh weekly, report gain >5 lb

• To report breast lumps, vaginal bleeding, edema, jaundice, dark urine, clay colored stools, dyspnea, headache, blurred vision, abdominal pain, numbness or stiffness in legs, chest pain; male to report impotence or gynecomastia

• To avoid sunlight or wear sunscreen, burns may occur

Lab test interferences:

Increase: BSP retention test, PBI, T_4, serum sodium, platelet aggressability, thyroxine-binding globulin (TBG), prothrombin, factors VII, VIII, IX, X, triglycerides

Decrease: Serum folate, serum triglyceride, T_3 resin uptake test, glucose tolerance test, antithrombin III, pregnanediol, metyrapone test

False positive: LE prep, antinuclear antibodies

chlorphenesin carbamate

(klor-fen′e-sin)
Maolate
Func. class.: Skeletal muscle relaxant, central acting
Chem. class.: Carbamate

Action: Unknown; may be related to sedative properties; does not directly relax muscle or depress nerve conduction

Uses: Relieving pain in musculoskeletal conditions

Dosage and routes:
• *Adult:* PO 800 mg tid, maintenance 400 mg qid, not to exceed 8 wk

Available forms include: Tabs 400 mg

Side effects/adverse reactions:
CNS: Dizziness, weakness, drowsiness, headache, tremor, depression, insomnia
EENT: Diplopia, temporary loss of vision
CV: Postural hypotension, tachycardia
GI: Nausea, vomiting, hiccups
INTEG: Rash, pruritus, fever, facial flushing

Contraindications: Hypersensitivity, child <12 yr, intermittent porphyria

Precautions: Renal disease, hepatic disease, addictive personalities

Pharmacokinetics:
PO: Onset ½ hr, duration 4-6 hr, metabolized by liver, excreted in urine, crosses placenta, excreted in breast milk (large amounts), half-life 8 hr

Interactions/incompatibilities:
• Increased CNS depression: alcohol, tricylic antidepressants, narcotics, barbiturates, sedatives, hypnotics

NURSING CONSIDERATIONS
Assess:
• Blood studies: CBC, WBC, differential; blood dyscrasias may occur
• Liver function studies: AST, ALT, alk phosphatase; hepatitis may occur
• ECG in epileptic patients; poor seizure control has occurred with patients taking this drug

Administer:
• With meals for GI symptoms

Perform/provide:
• Storage in tight container at room temperature
• Assistance with ambulation if dizziness, drowsiness occurs

Evaluate:
• Therapeutic response: decreased pain, spasticity
• Allergic reactions: rash, fever, respiratory distress
• Severe weakness, numbness in extremities
• Psychologic dependency: increased need for medication, more frequent requests for medication, increased pain
• CNS depression: dizziness, drowsiness, psychiatric symptoms

Teach patient/family:
• Not to discontinue medication quickly, insomnia, nausea, headache, spasticity, tachycardia will occur; drug should be tapered off over 1-2 wk
• Not to take with alcohol, other CNS depressants
• To avoid altering activities while taking this drug
• To avoid hazardous activities if drowsiness, dizziness occurs
• To avoid using OTC medication: cough preparations, antihistamines, unless directed by physician

Treatment of overdose: Give physostigmine IV; monitor cardiac function

---

italics = common side effects   ***bold italic*** = life threatening reactions

chlorpheniramine maleate

(klor-fen-eer'a-meen)

Alleroid-OD, AL-R, Chlormene, Chlortab, Chlor-Trimeton, Chlor-Tripolon,* Histaspan, Novopheniram,* Pyranistan, Teldrin

Func. class.: Antihistamine
Chem. class.: Alkylamine, H_1-receptor antagonist

Action: Acts on blood vessels, GI system, respiratory system, by competing with histamine for H_1-receptor site; decreases allergic response by blocking histamine

Uses: Allergy symptoms, rhinitis

Dosage and routes:

• *Adult:* PO 2-4 mg tid-qid, not to exceed 24 mg/day; TIME-REL 8-12 mg bid-tid, not to exceed 24 mg/day; IM/IV/SC 5-40 mg/day

• *Child 6-12 yr:* PO 2 mg q4-6h, not to exceed 12 mg/day; SUS REL 8 mg hs or qd, SUS REL not recommended for child <6 yr

• *Child 2-5 yr:* PO 1 mg q4-6h, not to exceed 4 mg/day

Available forms include: Tabs, chewable 2 mg; tabs 4 mg; tabs, time-rel 8, 12 mg, caps, time-rel 8, 12 mg; syr 2 mg/5 ml; inj IM, SC, IV 10, 100 mg/ml

Side effects/adverse reactions:

CNS: Dizziness, drowsiness, poor coordination, fatigue, anxiety, euphoria, confusion, paresthesia, neuritis

CV: Hypotension, palpitations, tachycardia

RESP: Increased thick secretions, wheezing, chest tightness

HEMA: Thrombocytopenia, agranulocytosis, hemolytic anemia

GI: Dry mouth, nausea, vomiting, anorexia, constipation, diarrhea

INTEG: Rash, urticaria, photosensitivity

GU: Retention, dysuria, frequency

EENT: Blurred vision, dilated pupils, tinnitus, nasal stuffiness, dry nose, throat, mouth

Contraindications: Hypersensitivity to H_1-receptor antagonists, acute asthma attack, lower respiratory tract disease

Precautions: Increased intraocular pressure, renal disease, cardiac disease, hypertension, bronchial asthma, seizure disorder, stenosed peptic ulcers, hyperthyroidism, prostatic hypertrophy, bladder neck obstruction, pregnancy

Pharmacokinetics:

PO: Onset 20-60 min, duration 8-12 hr; detoxified in liver, excreted by kidneys, (metabolites/free drug), half-life 20-24 hr

Interactions/incompatibilities:

• Increased CNS depression: barbiturates, narcotics, hypnotics, tricyclic antidepressants, alcohol

• Decreased effect of: oral anticoagulants, heparin

• Increased effect of this drug: MAOIs

NURSING CONSIDERATIONS

Assess:

• I&O ratio; be alert for urinary retention, frequency, dysuria; drug should be discontinued if these occur

• CBC during long-term therapy

Administer:

• Coffee, tea, cola (caffeine) to decrease drowsiness

• With meals if GI symptoms occur; absorption may slightly decrease

Perform/provide:

• Hard candy, gum, frequent rinsing of mouth for dryness

• Storage in tight container at room temperature

Evaluate:

• Therapeutic response: absence of running or congested nose or rashes

• Blood dyscrasias: thrombocyto-

---

* Available in Canada only

penia, agranulocytosis (rare)
• Respiratory status: rate, rhythm, increase in bronchial secretions, wheezing, chest tightness
• Cardiac status: palpitations, increased pulse, hypotension
Teach patient/family:
• Not to chew or crush sustained release forms
• All aspects of drug use; to notify physician if confusion, sedation, hypotension occurs
• To avoid driving or other hazardous activity if drowsiness occurs
• To avoid concurrent use of alcohol or other CNS depressants
Lab test interferences:
False negative: Skin allergy tests
Treatment of overdose: Administer ipecac syrup or lavage, diazepam, vasopressors, barbiturates (short-acting)

---

chlorpromazine HCl

(klor-proe′ma-zeen)

Chlor-Promanyl,* Clorazine, Klorazine, Largactil,* Ormazine, Promapar, Promaz, Thorazine, Thor-Prom

Func. class.: Antipsychotic/neuroleptic
Chem. class.: Phenothiazine-aliphatic

Action: Depresses cerebral cortex, hypothalamus, limbic system, which control activity aggression; blocks neurotransmission produced by dopamine at synapse; exhibits a strong α-adrenergic, anticholinergic blocking action; mechanism for antipsychotic effects is unclear
Uses: Psychotic disorders, mania, schizophrenia, intractable hiccups, nausea, vomiting, preoperatively for relaxation
Dosage and routes:
Psychiatry
• *Adult:* PO 10-50 mg q1-4h ini-

tially, then increase up to 200 mg if necessary
• *Adult:* IM 10-50 mg q1-4h
• *Child:* PO 0.25 mg/lb q4-6h or 0.5 mg/kg
• *Child:* IM 0.25 mg/lb q6h or 0.5 mg/kg
• *Child:* REC 0.5 mg/lb q6h or 1 mg/kg
Nausea and vomiting
• *Adult:* PO 10-25 mg q4-6h prn; IM 25-50 mg q3h prn; REC 50-100 mg q6-8h prn
• *Child:* PO 0.25 mg/lb q4-6h prn, not to exceed 40 mg/day; (<5 yr) or 75 mg/day (5-12 yr); IM 0.25 mg/lb q6-8h prn; REC 0.5 mg/lb q6-8h prn
• *Adult:* IV 25-5 mg qd-qid
• *Child:* IV 0.55 mg/kg q6-8h
Intractable hiccups
• *Adult:* PO 25-50 mg tid-qid; IM 25-50 mg (used only if PO dose does not work); IV 25 mg (only for severe hiccups)
Available forms include: Tabs 10, 25, 50, 100, 200 mg; time-release caps 30, 75, 150, 200, 300 mg; syr 10 mg/5ml; conc 30, 100 mg/ml; supp 25, 100 mg; inj IM, IV 25 mg/ml
Side effects/adverse reactions:
*RESP: **Laryngospasm,** dyspnea, **respiratory depression***
CNS: Extrapyramidal symptoms: pseudoparkinsonism, akathisia, dystonia, tardive dyskinesia, seizures, headache
HEMA: Anemia, leukopenia, leukocytosis, ***agranulocytosis***
INTEG: Rash, photosensitivity, dermatitis
EENT: Blurred vision, glaucoma
GI: Dry mouth, nausea, vomiting, anorexia, constipation, diarrhea, jaundice, weight gain
GU: Urinary retention, urinary frequency, enuresis, impotence, amenorrhea, gynecomastia
CV: Orthostatic hypotension, hy-

pertension, *cardiac arrest,* ECG changes, *tachycardia*

Contraindications: Hypersensitivity, circulatory collapse, liver damage, cerebral arteriosclerosis, coronary disease, severe hypertension/hypotension, blood dyscrasias, coma, child <2 years, brain damage, bone marrow depression, alcohol and barbiturate withdrawal states

Precautions: Pregnancy, lactation, seizure disorders, hypertension, hepatic disease, cardiac disease

Pharmacokinetics:

PO: Onset erratic, peak 2-4 hr, duration may be detected for up to 6 mo after last dose

IM: Onset 15-30 min, peak 15-20 min, duration may be detected for up to 6 mo after last dose

IV: Onset 5 min, peak 10 min, duration may be detected for up to 6 mo after last dose

REC: Onset erratic, peak 3 hr

Metabolized by liver, excreted in urine (metabolites), crosses placenta, enters breast milk; 95% bound to plasma proteins; elimination half-life 10-20 hr

Interactions/incompatibilities:

• Oversedation: other CNS depressants, alcohol, barbiturate anesthetics

• Toxicity: epinephrine

• Decreased absorption: aluminum hydroxide or magnesium hydroxide antacids

• Decreased effects of: lithium, levodopa

• Increased effects of both drugs: β-adrenergic blockers, alcohol

• Increased anticholinergic effects: anticholinergics

NURSING CONSIDERATIONS

Assess:

• Swallowing of PO medication; check for hoarding or giving of medication to other patients

• I&O ratio; palpate bladder if low

urinary output occurs

• Bilirubin, CBC, liver function studies monthly

• Urinalysis is recommended before, during prolonged therapy

Administer:

• Antiparkinsonian agent, to be used if EPS occur

• Drug in elixir form mixed in glass of juice or cola, if hoarding is suspected

Perform/provide:

• Decreased noise input by dimming lights, avoiding loud noises

• Supervised ambulation until stabilized on medication; do not involve in strenuous exercise program because fainting is possible; patient should not stand still for long periods of time

• Increased fluids to prevent constipation

• Sips of water, candy, gum for dry mouth

• Storage in tight, light-resistant container, oral solutions in amber bottles

Evaluate:

• Therapeutic response: decrease in emotional excitement, hallucinations, delusions, paranoia, reorganization of patterns of thought, speech

• Affect, orientation, LOC, reflexes, gait, coordination, sleep pattern disturbances

• B/P standing and lying; take pulse and respirations q4h during initial treatment; establish baseline before starting treatment; report drops of 30 mm Hg

• Dizziness, faintness, palpitations, tachycardia on rising

• EPS including akathisia (inability to sit still, no pattern to movements), tardive dyskinesia (bizarre movements of the jaw, mouth, tongue, extremities), pseudoparkinsonism (rigidity, tremors, pill rolling, shuffling gait)

• Skin turgor daily

• Constipation, urinary retention daily; if these occur, increase bulk, water in diet

Teach patient/family:

• That orthostatic hypotension occurs often, and to rise from sitting or lying position gradually

• To remain lying down after IM injection for at least 30 min

• To avoid hot tubs, hot showers, or tub baths since hypotension may occur

• To avoid abrupt withdrawal of this drug or EPS may result; drug should be withdrawn slowly

• To avoid OTC preparations (cough, hayfever, cold) unless approved by physician since serious drug interactions may occur; avoid use with alcohol or CNS depressants; increased drowsiness may occur

• To use a sunscreen during sun exposure to prevent burns

• Regarding compliance with drug regimen

• About EPS and necessity for meticulous oral hygiene since oral candidiasis may occur

• To report sore throat, malaise, fever, bleeding, mouth sores; if these occur, CBC should be drawn and drug discontinued

• In hot weather, heat stroke may occur; take extra precautions to stay cool

Lab test interferences:

Increase: Liver function tests, cardiac enzymes, cholesterol, blood glucose, prolactin, bilirubin, PBI, cholinesterase, ^{131}I

Decrease: Hormones (blood and urine)

False positive: Pregnancy tests, PKU

False negative: Urinary steroids, 17-OHCS

Treatment of overdose: Lavage, if orally ingested, provide an air-way; *do not induce vomiting*

chlorpropamide

(klor-proe'pa-mide)

Chloronase,* Diabinese, Novo-propamide,* Stabinol*

Func. class.: Antidiabetic

Chem. class.: Sulfonylurea (1st generation)

Action: Causes functioning β-cells in pancreas to synthesize, release insulin, leading to drop in blood glucose levels; stimulation of insulin results in increased insulin binding; not effective if patient lacks functioning β-cells

Uses: Stable adult-onset diabetes mellitus (type II)

Dosage and routes:

• *Adult:* PO 100-250 mg qd, initially, then 100-500 mg maintenance according to response; not to exceed 750 mg/day

Available forms include: Tabs 100, 250 mg

Side effects/adverse reactions:

CNS: Headache, weakness, dizziness, drowsiness

*GI: **Hepatotoxicity, cholestatic jaundice,** nausea, vomiting, diarrhea, constipation, anorexia*

*HEMA: **Leukopenia, thrombocytopenia, agranulocytosis, aplastic anemia, pancytopenia, hemolytic anemia***

INTEG: Rash, allergic reactions, pruritus, urticaria, eczema, photosensitivity, erythema

*ENDO: **Hypoglycemia***

Contraindications: Hypersensitivity to sulfonylureas, juvenile or brittle diabetes, renal disease, hepatic disease

Precautions: Pregnancy, elderly, cardiac disease, thyroid disease, severe hypoglycemic reactions

Pharmacokinetics:

PO: Completely absorbed by GI

C

italics = common side effects   ***bold italic*** = life threatening reactions

route, onset 1 hr, peak 3-6 hr, duration 24 hr, half-life 36 hr, metabolized in liver, excreted in urine (metabolites and unchanged drug), breast milk, 90%-95% is plasma protein bound

Interactions/incompatibilities:
• Adverse effects: oral anticoagulants, hydantoins, salicylates, sulfonamides, nonsteroidal antiinflammatories
• Increased effects of this drug: insulin, MAOIs
• Decreased action of this drug: calcium channel blockers, corticosteroids, oral contraceptives, thiazide diuretics, thyroid preparations, estrogens

NURSING CONSIDERATIONS

Administer:
• Drug 30 min before meals

Perform/provide:
• Storage in tight container in cool environment

Evaluate:
• Therapeutic response: decrease in polyuria, polydipsia, polyphagia, clear sensorium, absence of dizziness, stable gait
• Hypoglycemic/hyperglycemic reaction that can occur soon after meals

Teach patient/family:
• To check for symptoms of cholestatic jaundice: dark urine, pruritus, yellow sclera; if these occur, physician should be notified
• To use capillary blood glucose test while on this drug
• To test urine glucose levels with Chemstrip approximately 2 hr after each meal
• Symptoms of hypo/hyperglycemia, what to do about each
• That this drug must be continued on daily basis; explain consequence of discontinuing drug abruptly
• To take drug in morning to prevent hypoglycemic reactions at night

• To avoid OTC medications unless prescribed by physician
• That diabetes is life-long illness, drug will not cure disease
• That all food included in diet plan must be eaten in order to prevent hypoglycemia
• To carry Medic-Alert ID for emergency purposes

Treatment of overdose: 10%-50% glucose solution

---

chlorprothixene

(klor-proe-thix'een)
Taractan, Tarasan*
Func. class.: Antipsychotic/neuroleptic
Chem. class.: Thioxanthene

Action: Depresses cerebral cortex, hypothalamus, limbic system, which control activity, aggression; blocks neurotransmission produced by dopamine at synapse; exhibits strong α-adrenergic, anticholinergic blocking action; mechanism for antipsychotic effects is unclear

Uses: Psychotic disorders, schizophrenia, neurosis

Dosage and routes:
• *Adult:* PO 25-50 mg tid or qid, increased to desired response, max dosage 500 mg/qd; IM 25-50 mg tid or qid
• *Child >6 yr:* PO 10-25 mg tid or qid

Available forms include: Tabs 10, 25, 50, 100 mg; conc 100 mg/5 ml; inj IM 12 mg/ml

Side effects/adverse reactions:
RESP: **Laryngospasm,** dyspnea, *respiratory depression*
CNS: Extrapyramidal symptoms: pseudoparkinsonism, akathisia, dystonia, tardive dyskinesia, drowsiness, headache, seizures
HEMA: Anemia, leukopenia, leukocytosis, **agranulocytosis**

INTEG: Rash, photosensitivity, dermatitis

EENT: Blurred vision, glaucoma

GI: Dry mouth, nausea, vomiting, anorexia, constipation, diarrhea, jaundice, weight gain

GU: Urinary retention, urinary frequency, enuresis, impotence, amenorrhea, gynecomastia

CV: Orthostatic hypotension, hypertension, *cardiac arrest,* ECG changes, *tachycardia*

Contraindications: Hypersensitivity, circulatory collapse, liver damage, cerebral arteriosclerosis, coronary disease, severe hypertension/hypotension, blood dyscrasias, coma, child <6 yr (PO), <12 yr (IM), brain damage, bone marrow depression, alcohol and barbiturate withdrawal states

Precautions: Pregnancy, lactation, seizure disorders, hypertension, hepatic disease, cardiac disease

Pharmacokinetics:

PO: Onset erratic, peak 2-4 hr; duration may be detected for up to 6 mo after last dose

IM: Onset 10-30 min, duration may be detected for up to 6 mo after last dose

Metabolized by liver, excreted in urine (metabolites), crosses placenta, enters breast milk

Interactions/incompatibilities:

• Oversedation: other CNS depressants, alcohol, barbiturate anesthetics

• Toxicity: epinephrine

• Decreased effects of: levodopa, lithium

• Increased effects of both drugs: β-adrenergic blockers, alcohol

• Increased anticholinergic effects: anticholinergics

NURSING CONSIDERATIONS

Assess:

• Swallowing of PO medication; check for hoarding or giving of medication to other patients

• I&O ratio; palpate bladder if low urinary output occurs

• Bilirubin, CBC, liver function studies monthly

• Urinalysis is recommended before and during prolonged therapy

Administer:

• Antiparkinsonian agent, to be used if EPS occur

• Drug in concentrate form mixed in milk, water, fruit juice, coffee, tea, carbonated beverage, or undiluted

• IM injection into large muscle mass; to minimize postural hypotension give injection with patient seated or recumbent

Perform/provide:

• Decreased noise input by dimming lights, avoiding loud noises

• Supervised ambulation until stabilized on medication; do not involve in strenuous exercise program because fainting is possible; patient should not stand still for long periods of time

• Increased fluids to prevent constipation

• Sips of water, candy, or gum for dry mouth

• Storage in tight, light-resistant container in cool environment

Evaluate:

• Therapeutic response: decrease in emotional excitement, hallucinations, delusions, paranoia, reorganization of patterns of thought, speech

• Affect, orientation, LOC, reflexes, gait, coordination, sleep pattern disturbances

• B/P standing and lying; take pulse and respirations q4h during initial treatment; establish baseline before starting treatment; report drops of 30 mm Hg

• Dizziness, faintness, palpitations, tachycardia on rising

• EPS including akathisia (inability to sit still, no pattern to movements), tardive dyskinesia (bizarre movements of the jaw, mouth, tongue, extremities), pseudoparkinsonism (rigidity, tremors, pill rolling, shuffling gait)

• Skin turgor daily

• Constipation, urinary retention daily, if these occur, increase bulk, water in diet

Teach patient/family:

• That orthostatic hypotension occurs often, and to rise from sitting or lying position gradually

• To avoid hot tubs, hot showers, or tub baths since hypotension may occur

• To avoid abrupt withdrawal of this drug or EPS may result; drug should be withdrawn slowly

• To avoid OTC preparations (cough, hayfever, cold) unless approved by physician since serious drug interactions may occur; avoid use with alcohol or CNS depressants; increased drowsiness may occur

• To use a sunscreen during sun exposure to prevent burns

• Regarding compliance with drug regimen

• About EPS and necessity for meticulous oral hygiene since oral candidiasis may occur

• To report sore throat, malaise, fever, bleeding, mouth sores; if these occur, CBC should be drawn and drug discontinued

• In hot weather, heat stroke may occur; take extra precautions to stay cool

Lab test interferences:

Increase: Liver function tests, cardiac enzymes, cholesterol, blood glucose, prolactin, bilirubin, PBI, cholinesterase, ^{131}I

Decrease: Hormones (blood and urine)

False positive: Pregnancy tests, PKU

False negative: Urinary steroids, 17-OHCS

Treatment of overdose: Lavage, if orally ingested, provide an airway; *do not induce vomiting*

---

chlortetracycline HCl (topical)

(klor-te-tra-sye'kleen)

Aureomycin

Func. class.: Local antiinfective
Chem. class.: Antibacterial

Action: Interferes with bacterial cell synthesis

Uses: Pyogenic skin infections

Dosage and routes:

• *Adult and child:* TOP rub into affected area qid-bid

Available forms include: Oint 3%

Side effects/adverse reactions:

INTEG: Rash, urticaria, stinging, burning

Contraindications: Hypersensitivity

Precautions: Pregnancy (C), lactation

Interactions/incompatibilities: None known

NURSING CONSIDERATIONS

Administer:

• Enough medication to completely cover lesions

• After cleansing with soap, water before each application, dry well

Perform/provide:

• Storage at room temperature in dry place

Evaluate:

• Allergic reaction: burning, stinging, swelling, redness

• Therapeutic response: decrease in size, number of lesions

Teach patient/family:

• To apply with glove to prevent further infection

• To avoid use of OTC creams, ointments, lotions unless directed by physician

---

• To use medical asepsis (hand washing) before, after each application

• To avoid squeezing or poking-lesions or spreading may occur

---

chlorthalidone

(klor-thal'i-done)

Hygroton, Hylidone, Novothalidone,* Thalitone, Uridon*

Func. class.: Diuretic

Chem. class.: Thiazide-like; phthalimidine derivative

Action: Acts on distal tubule by increasing excretion of water, sodium, chloride, potassium

Uses: Edema, hypertension

Dosage and routes:

• *Adult:* PO 25-100 mg/day or 100 mg 3 × /wk

• *Child:* PO 2 mg/kg 3 × /wk

Available forms include: Tabs 25, 50, 100 mg

Side effects/adverse reactions:

GU: Frequency, polyuria, uremia, glucosuria

CNS: Drowsiness, paresthesia, anxiety, depression, headache, dizziness, fatigue, weakness

GI: Nausea, vomiting, anorexia, constipation, diarrhea, cramps, pancreatitis, GI irritation, *hepatitis*

EENT: Blurred vision

INTEG: Rash, urticaria, purpura, photosensitivity, fever

META: Hyperglycemia, hyperuremia, increased creatinine

HEMA: Aplastic anemia, hemolytic anemia, leukopenia, agranulocytosis, thrombocytopenia

CV: Irregular pulse, orthostatic hypotension

ELECT: Hypokalemia, hypercalcemia, hyponatremia, hypochloremia

Contraindications: Hypersensitivity to thiazides or sulfonamides, anuria, renal decompensation

Precautions: Hypokalemia, renal

disease, pregnancy (C), hepatic disease, gout, COPD, lupus erythematosus, diabetes mellitus

Pharmacokinetics:

PO: Onset 2 hr, peak 6 hr, duration 24-72 hr; excreted unchanged by kidneys, crosses placenta, enters breast milk, half-life 35-55 hr

Interactions/incompatibilities:

• Increased toxicity: lithium, nondepolarizing skeletal muscle relaxants, digitalis

• Decreased effects of: antidiabetics

• Decreased absorption of thiazides: cholestyramine, colestipol

• Decreased hypotensive response: indomethacin

• Increased action of: quinidine

NURSING CONSIDERATIONS

Assess:

• Weight, I&O daily to determine fluid loss; effect of drug may be decreased if used qd

• Rate, depth, rhythm of respiration, effect of exertion

• B/P lying, standing; postural hypotension may occur

• Electrolytes: potassium, sodium, chloride; include BUN, blood sugar, CBC, serum creatinine, blood pH, ABGs

• Glucose in urine if patient is diabetic

Administer:

• In AM to avoid interference with sleep if using drug as a diuretic

• Potassium replacement if potassium is less than 3.0

• With food if nausea occurs; absorption may be decreased slightly

Evaluate:

• Improvement in edema of feet, legs, sacral area daily if medication is being used in CHF

• Improvement in CVP q8h

• Signs of metabolic acidosis: drowsiness, restlessness

• Signs of hypokalemia: postural hypotension, malaise, fatigue,

---

tachycardia, leg cramps, weakness
• Rashes, temperature elevation qd
• Confusion, especially in elderly; take safety precautions if needed
Teach patient/family:
• To increase fluid intake 2-3 L/day unless contraindicated, to rise slowly from lying or sitting position
• To notify physician of muscle weakness, cramps, nausea, dizziness
• Drug may be taken with food or milk
• That blood sugar may be increased in diabetics
• Take early in day to avoid nocturia
Lab test interferences:
Increase: BSP retention, calcium, cholesterol, triglycerides, amylase
Decrease: PBI, PSP
Treatment of overdose: Lavage if taken orally, monitor electrolytes, administer dextrose in saline

---

chlorzoxazone

(klor-zox'a-zone)
Paraflex, and others
Func. class.: Skeletal muscle relaxant
Chem. class.: Benzoxazole derivative

Action: Inhibits multisynaptic reflex arcs
Uses: Relieving pain in musculoskeletal conditions
Dosage and routes:
• *Adult:* PO 250-750 mg tid-qid
• *Child:* PO 20 mg/kg/day in divided doses bid-tid
Available forms include: Tabs 250 mg
Side effects/adverse reactions:
HEMA: Granulocytopenia, anemia
CNS: Dizziness, drowsiness, headache, insomnia, stimulation
GI: Nausea, vomiting, anorexia,

diarrhea, constipation, *hepatotoxicity, jaundice*
INTEG: Rash, pruritus, petechiae, ecchymoses, angioedema
SYST: Anaphylaxis
Contraindications: Hypersensitivity
Precautions: Pregnancy, lactation, hepatic disease
Pharmacokinetics:
PO: Onset 1 hr, peak 3-4 hr, duration 6 hr, half-life 1 hr, metabolized in liver, excreted in urine (metabolites)
Interactions/incompatibilities:
• Increased CNS depression: alcohol, tricylic antidepressants, narcotics, barbiturates, sedatives, hypnotics

NURSING CONSIDERATIONS
Assess:
• Blood studies: CBC, WBC, differential; blood dyscrasias may occur
• Liver function studies: AST, ALT, alk phosphatase; hepatitis may occur
• ECG in epileptic patients; poor seizure control has occurred with patients taking this drug
Administer:
• With meals for GI symptoms
Perform/provide:
• Storage in tight container at room temperature
• Assistance with ambulation if dizziness or drowsiness occurs
Evaluate:
• Therapeutic response: decreased pain, spasticity
• Allergic reactions: rash, fever, respiratory distress
• Severe weakness, numbness in extremities
• Psychologic dependency: increased need for medication, more frequent requests for medication, increased pain

---

• CNS depression: dizziness, drowsiness, psychiatric symptoms
Teach patient/family:
• Not to discontinue the medication quickly; insomnia, nausea, headache, spasticity, tachycardia will occur; drug should be tapered off over 1-2 wk
• Not to take with alcohol, other CNS depressants
• To avoid altering activities while taking this drug
• To avoid hazardous activities if drowsiness, dizziness occurs
• To avoid using OTC medication: cough preparations, antihistamines, unless directed by physician
Treatment of overdose: Gastric lavage or induce emesis, then administer activated charcoal; use other supportive treatment as necessary; monitor cardiac function

---

cholestyramine

(koe-less-tir′a-meen)
Questran
Func. class.: Antilipemic
Chem. class.: Bile acid sequestrant

Action: Absorbs, combines with bile acids to form insoluble complex that is excreted through feces; loss of bile acids lowers cholesterol levels
Uses: Primary hyperlipidemia, pruritus, diarrhea caused by excess bile acid, digitalis toxicity
Dosage and routes:
• *Adult:* PO 4 g ac, and hs, not to exceed 32 g/day
• *Child:* PO 240 mg/kg/day in 3 divided doses; administer with food or drink
Available forms include: Powd
Side effects/adverse reactions:
GI: Constipation, abdominal pain, nausea, fecal impaction, hemorrhoids, flatulence, vomiting, steatorrhea

INTEG: Rash, irritation of perianal area, tongue, skin
HEMA: Decreased vitamin A, D, K, ***hyperchloremic acidosis***
Contraindications: Hypersensitivity, biliary obstruction
Precautions: Pregnancy (C), lactation, children
Pharmacokinetics:
PO: Excreted in feces, maximum effect in 2 wk
Interactions/incompatibilities:
• Decreased absorption of phenylbutazone, warfarin, thiazides, digitalis, penicillin G, tetracyclines, phenobarbital, folic acid, corticosteroids, iron, thyroid, clindamycin, trimethoprim, chendiol

NURSING CONSIDERATIONS
Assess:
• Cardiac glycoside level, if both drugs are being administered
• For signs of vitamin A, D, K deficiency
• Serum cholesterol, triglyceride levels, electrolytes if on extended therapy
Administer:
• Drug ac, hs; give all other medications 1 hr before cholestyramine or 4 hr after cholestyramine to avoid poor absorption
• Drug sprinkled on food or stirred into beverage; let stand for 2 min
• Supplemental doses of vitamins A, D, K, if levels are low
Evaluate:
• Bowel pattern daily; increase bulk, water in diet if constipation develops
• Therapeutic response: decreased triglyceride, cholesterol level (hyperlipidemia); diarrhea, pruritus (excess bile area)
Teach patient/family:
• Symptoms of hypothrombinemia: bleeding mucous membranes, dark tarry stools, petechiae; report immediately
• Stress patient compliance since

---

italics = common side effects   ***bold italic*** = life threatening reactions

toxicity may result if doses are missed

• That risk factors should be decreased: high fat diet, smoking, alcohol consumption, absence of exercise

• That OTC preparations should be avoided unless directed by physician

Lab test interferences:
Increase: Liver function studies, chloride, PO$_4$
Decrease: Electrolytes (+)

---

choline
(koe′leen)

Func. class.: Miscellaneous GI agent

Action: Acts as a precursor to acetylcholine, a neurotransmitter; a phospholipid
Uses: Hepatic disease, poor fat metabolism
Dosage and routes:
• *Adult and child:* PO 650-750 mg qd
Available forms include: Tabs 250, 500 mg; powder
Side effects/adverse reactions:
CNS: Dizziness, vertigo
GI: GI irritation
META: Ketosis
INTEG: Foul body odor, halitosis
Contraindications: Hypersensitivity
Pharmacokinetics: Not known
Interactions/incompatibilities: Not known
NURSING CONSIDERATIONS
Administer:
• PO, usually in AM
Perform/provide:
• Storage at room temperature
Evaluate:
• Nutritional status: egg yolk, dairy products, beans, peas, beef, liver (high in choline)

Teach patient/family:
• Food high in choline, that diet should contain 500-900 mg/day

---

choline magnesium trisalicylate
(koe′leen)
Trilisate

Func. class.: Nonnarcotic analgesic
Chem. class.: Salicylate

Action: Blocks pain impulses in CNS that occur in response to inhibition of prostaglandin synthesis; antipyretic action results from inhibition of hypothalamic heat-regulating center
Uses: Mild to moderate pain or fever including arthritis, juvenile rheumatoid arthritis
Dosage and routes:
Arthritis
• *Adult:* PO 1-3 tsp or tabs bid
• *Child 12-37 kg:* PO 50 mg/kg/day in divided doses
• *Child > 37 kg:* PO 2250 mg in divided doses
Pain/fever
• *Adult:* PO 2-3 g/day in divided doses
• *Child 12-37 kg:* PO 50 mg/kg/day in divided doses
Available forms include: Liq 870 mg/5 ml
Side effects/adverse reactions:
*HEMA: **Thrombocytopenia, agranulocytosis, leukopenia, neutropenia, hemolytic anemia,*** increased pro-time
CNS: Stimulation, drowsiness, dizziness, confusion, convulsion, headache, flushing, hallucinations, coma
GI: Nausea, vomiting, GI bleeding, diarrhea, heartburn, anorexia, ***hepatitis***
INTEG: Rash, urticaria, bruising
EENT: Tinnitus, hearing loss

CV: Rapid pulse, pulmonary edema
RESP: Wheezing, hyperpnea
ENDO: Hypoglycemia, hyponatremia, hypokalemia

Contraindications: Hypersensitivity to salicylates, GI bleeding, bleeding disorders, children < 3 yr, pregnancy, lactation, vitamin K deficiency

Precautions: Anemia, hepatic disease, renal disease, Hodgkin's disease

Pharmacokinetics:
PO: Onset 15-30 min, peak 1-2 hr, duration 4-6 hr, metabolized by liver, excreted by kidneys, crosses placenta, excreted in breast milk, half-life 1-3½ hr

Interactions/incompatibilities:
• Decreased effects of this drug: antacids, steroids, urinary alkalizers
• Increased blood loss: alcohol, heparin
• Increased effects of: anticoagulants, insulin, methotrexate
• Decreased effects of: probenecid, spironolactone, sulfinpyrazone, sulfonylamides
• Toxic effects: PABA
• Decreased blood sugar levels: salicylates

NURSING CONSIDERATIONS
Assess:
• Liver function studies: AST, ALT, bilirubin, creatinine if patient is on long-term therapy
• Renal function studies: BUN, urine creatinine if patient is on long-term therapy
• Blood studies: CBC, Hct, Hgb, pro-time if patient is on long-term therapy
• I&O ratio; decreasing output may indicate renal failure (long-term therapy)

Administer:
• To patient crushed or whole; chewable tablets may be chewed
• With food or milk to decrease gastric symptoms; give 30 min before or 2 hr after meals

Perform/provide:
• Repositioning to decrease pain
• Cool cloth for fever

Evaluate:
• Hepatotoxicity: dark urine, clay-colored stools, yellowing of skin, sclera, itching, abdominal pain, fever, diarrhea if patient is on long-term therapy
• Allergic reactions: rash, urticaria; if these occur, drug may need to be discontinued
• Renal dysfunction: decreased urine output
• Ototoxicity: tinnitus, ringing, roaring in ears; audiometric testing is needed before, after long-term therapy
• Visual changes: blurring, halos, corneal, retinal damage
• Edema in feet, ankles, legs
• Prior drug history; there are many drug interactions

Teach patient/family:
• To report any symptoms of hepatotoxicity, renal toxicity, visual changes, ototoxicity, allergic reactions (long-term therapy)
• Not to exceed recommended dosage; acute poisoning may result
• To read label on other OTC drugs; many contain aspirin
• That therapeutic response takes 2 wk (arthritis)
• To avoid alcohol ingestion; GI bleeding may occur

Lab test interferences:
Increase: Coagulation studies, liver function studies, serum uric acid, amylase, CO_2, urinary protein
Decrease: Serum potassium, PBI, cholesterol
Interfere: Urine catecholamines, pregnancy test

Treatment of overdose: Lavage, activated charcoal, monitor electrolytes, VS

---

italics = common side effects   ***bold italic*** = life threatening reactions

choline salicylate

(koe′leen)

Arthropan

Func. class.: Nonnarcotic analgesic

Chem. class.: Salicylate

Action: Blocks pain impulses in CNS that occur in response to inhibition of prostaglandin synthesis; antipyretic action results from inhibition of hypothalamic heat-regulating center to produce vasodilation to allow heat dissipation

Uses: Mild to moderate pain or fever including arthritis, juvenile rheumatoid arthritis

Dosage and routes:

Arthritis

• *Adult:* PO 870-1740 mg qid

Pain/fever

• *Adult:* PO 870 mg q3-4h prn

• *Child 3-6 yr:* PO 105-210 mg q4h prn

Available forms include: Liq 870 mg/5 ml

Side effects/adverse reactions:

*HEMA: **Thrombocytopenia, agranulocytosis, leukopenia, neutropenia, hemolytic anemia,** increased pro-time*

CNS: Stimulation, drowsiness, dizziness, confusion, convulsion, headache, flushing, hallucinations, coma

*GI: Nausea, vomiting, GI bleeding, diarrhea, heartburn, anorexia, **hepatitis***

INTEG: Rash, urticaria, bruising

EENT: Tinnitus, hearing loss

CV: Rapid pulse, pulmonary edema

RESP: Wheezing, hyperpnea

ENDO: Hypoglycemia, hyponatremia, hypokalemia

Contraindications: Hypersensitivity to salicylates, GI bleeding, bleeding disorders, children < 3 yr,

pregnancy, lactation, vitamin K deficiency

Precautions: Anemia, hepatic disease, renal disease, Hodgkin's disease

Pharmacokinetics:

PO: Onset 15-30 min, metabolized by liver, excreted by kidneys, crosses placenta, excreted in breast milk

Interactions/incompatibilities:

• Decreased effects of this drug: antacids, steroids, urinary alkalizers

• Increased blood loss: alcohol, heparin

• Increased effects of: anticoagulants, insulin, methotrexate

• Decreased effects of: probenecid, spironolactone, sulfinpyrazone, sulfonylamides

• Toxic effects: PABA

• Decreased blood sugar levels: salicylates

NURSING CONSIDERATIONS

Assess:

• Liver function studies: AST, ALT, bilirubin, creatinine if patient is on long-term therapy

• Renal function studies: BUN, urine creatinine if patient is on long-term therapy

• Blood studies: CBC, Hct, Hgb, pro-time if patient is on long-term therapy

• I&O ratio; decreasing output may indicate renal failure (long-term therapy)

Administer:

• To patient crushed or whole; chewable tablets may be chewed

• With food or milk to decrease gastric symptoms; give 30 min before or 2 hr after meals

Perform/provide:

• Repositioning to decrease pain

• Cool cloth for fever

Evaluate:

• Hepatotoxicity: dark urine, clay-colored stools, yellowing of skin,

sclera, itching, abdominal pain, fever, diarrhea if patient is on long-term therapy
• Allergic reactions: rash, urticaria; if these occur, drug may need to be discontinued
• Renal dysfunction: decreased urine output
• Ototoxicity: tinnitus, ringing, roaring in ears; audiometric testing needed before, after long-term therapy
• Visual changes: blurring, halos, corneal, retinal damage
• Edema in feet, ankles, legs
• Prior drug history; there are many drug interactions

Teach patient/family:
• To report any symptoms of hepatotoxicity, renal toxicity, visual changes, ototoxicity, allergic reactions (long-term therapy)
• Not to exceed recommended dosage; acute poisoning may result
• To read label on other OTC drugs; many contain aspirin
• That therapeutic response takes 2 wk (arthritis)
• To avoid alcohol ingestion; GI bleeding may occur

Lab test interferences:
Increase: Coagulation studies, liver function studies, serum uric acid, amylase, CO_2, urinary protein
Decrease: Serum potassium, PBI, cholesterol
Interfere: Urine catecholamines, pregnancy test

Treatment of overdose: Lavage, activated charcoal, monitor electrolytes, VS

chorionic gonadotropin, human

(go-nad'oh-troe-pin)
Android HCG, APL, Chorex, Follutein, Glukor, Gonic, Libigen, Pregnyl, Profasi HP, Stemutrolin

Func. class.: Human chorionic gonadotropin
Chem. class.: Polypeptide hormone

Action: Stimulates production of gonadal steroids, androgens; stimulates corpus luteum to produce progesterone
Uses: Infertility, anovulation, hypogonadism, nonobstructive cryptorchidism

Dosage and routes:
Infertility/anovulation
• *Adult:* IM 10,000 U 1 day after last dose of menotropins
Hypogonadism
• *Adult:* IM 500-1000 U 3 × wk × 3 wk, then 2 × wk × 3 wk, or 4000 U 3 × wk × 6-9 mo, then 2000 U 3 × wk × 3 mo
Cryptorchidism
• *Child (boy 4-9 yr):* IM 5000 U qod × 4 doses
Available forms include: Powder for inj 200, 1000, 2000 U/ml

Side effects/adverse reactions:
CNS: Headache, depression, fatigue, anxiety, irritability
GU: Gynecomastia, early puberty, edema, ectopic pregnancy
INTEG: Pain at injection site
Contraindications: Hypersensitivity, pituitary hypertrophy/tumor, early puberty, prostatic CA
Precautions: Asthma, migraine headache, convulsive disorders, cardiac disease, renal disease
Pharmacokinetics:
IM: Peak 6 hr, half-life 11-24 hr, excreted by kidneys

Interactions/incompatibilities:
None known
NURSING CONSIDERATIONS
Assess:
• Weight weekly; notify physician if weekly weight gain is >5 lb
• B/P before, during treatment
• Be alert for decreasing urinary output, increasing edema
Administer:
• Only after clomiphene citrate has been tried on anovulatory client
• After reconstitution with diluent enclosed in package
Perform/provide:
• Refrigeration for up to 2 mo
Evaluate:
• Edema, hypertension
Teach patient/family:
• All aspects of drug usage
• To report facial, axillary, pubic hair, change in voice, penile enlargement, acne in male, abdominal pain, distention, vaginal bleeding in women
• To report symptoms of ectopic pregnancy: dizziness, pain on one side, shoulder, pallor, weak thready pulse, hemorrhage, shock; may proceed rapidly

---

chymopapain
(kye'moe-pa-pane)
Chymodiactin, Discase
Func. class.: Enzyme
Chem. class.: Proteolytic

Action: Hydrolyzes noncollagenous polypeptides that maintain structure of chondromucoprotein; this activity decreases pressure on disk
Uses: Herniated lumbar intervertebral disk
Dosage and routes:
• *Adult:* INJ 2000-4000 U/disk injected intradiskally, not to exceed 10,000 U in a multiple herniation

Available forms include: Powder for inj 4000, 10,000 U/vial
Side effects/adverse reactions:
*CNS: **Paraplegia, cerebral hemorrhage,** headache, dizziness, paresthesia, numbness of extremities
INTEG: Rash, urticaria, itching
GI: Nausea, paralytic ileus
MS: Back pain, stiffness, spasm, acute transverse myelitis, weakness
*SYSTEM: **Anaphylaxis***
GU: Urinary retention
Contraindications: Hypersensitivity to this drug, papaya, meat tenderizer; severe spondylolisthesis; severe progressing paralysis; spinal cord tumor; cauda equina lesion
Precautions: Pregnancy, children
Pharmacokinetics:
Onset 30 min, duration 24 hr
Interactions/incompatibilities:
• Dysrhythmias: halothane anesthetics plus epinephrine
NURSING CONSIDERATIONS
Assess:
• RBCs, ESR before treatment
• Respiratory rate, rhythm, depth; notify physician of abnormalities
• Anaphylaxis for several days after injection
Administer:
• Only with epinephrine available for anaphylaxis
• Only in lumbar spine by physician
• After diluting with sterile water for injection
• After completing allergy test (ChymoFAST)
Evaluate:
• Therapeutic response: absence of back pain, increased mobility
• For allergies: iodine, papaya, meat tenderizer; if allergies are identified, drug should not be used
Teach patient/family
• To report allergic reactions that have occurred up to 2 wk after injection

chymotrypsin and mixtures

(kye'moe-trip-sen)
Avazyme, Chymoral, Orenzyme
Func. class.: Enzyme
Chem. class.: Proteolytic

Action: Unknown; may increase tissue permeability in inflamed areas, restores body fluids, frees blood flow in inflamed area
Uses: Episiotomy pain
Dosage and routes:
• *Adult:* PO 20,000-40,000 U (USP) qid
Available forms include: Tabs 20,000, 40,000 USP Units, 50,000, 100,000 Armour Units; 50,000, 100,000 USP Units
Side effects/adverse reactions:
HEMA: Bleeding
CNS: Chills, fever, dizziness
GU: Hematuria, albuminuria
GI: Nausea, diarrhea, vomiting, anorexia
INTEG: Rash, itching, urticaria
*SYSTEM: **Anaphylaxis***
Contraindications: Hypersensitivity to this drug, trypsin; septicemia; acute infection; hemophilia
Precautions: Severe renal disease, severe hepatic disease
Pharmacokinetics: Unknown
Interactions/incompatibilities:
• Increased effect of: anticoagulants

NURSING CONSIDERATIONS
Evaluate:
• Therapeutic response: decreased episiotomy pain
Teach patient/family
• To notify physician if bleeding occurs
• That allergic reactions, nausea, vomiting, diarrhea may occur

ciclopirox olamine (topical)

(sye-kloe-peer'ox)
Loprox
Func. class.: Local antiinfective
Chem. class.: Antifungal

Action: Interferes with fungal DNA replication; binds sterols in fungal cell membrane, which increases permeability, leaking of cell nutrients
Uses: Tinea cruris, tinea corporis, cutaneous candidiasis
Dosage and routes:
• *Adult and child >10 yr:* TOP rub into affected area bid
Available forms include: Cream 1%
Side effects/adverse reactions:
INTEG: Rash, urticaria, stinging, burning, pruritus
Contraindications: Hypersensitivity
Precautions: Pregnancy (B), lactation, child <10 yr
Interactions/incompatibilities: None known
NURSING CONSIDERATIONS
Administer:
• Enough medication to completely cover lesions
• After cleansing with soap, water before each application, dry well
Perform/provide:
• Storage at room temperature in dry place
Evaluate:
• Allergic reaction: burning, stinging, swelling, redness
• Therapeutic response: decrease in size, number of lesions
Teach patient/family:
• To apply with glove to prevent further infection
• To avoid use of OTC creams, ointments, lotions unless directed by physician

---

italics = common side effects   ***bold italic*** = life threatening reactions

• To use medical asepsis (hand washing) before, after each application
• Not to cover with occlusive dressing

---

cimetidine

(sye-met'i-deen)
Tagamet
Func. class.: Antihistamine—H_2 receptor
Chem. class.: Imidazole derivative

Action: Inhibits histamine at H_2 receptor site in parietal cells, which inhibits gastric acid secretion
Uses: Short-term treatment of duodenal ulcers and maintenance
Dosage and routes:
• *Adult and child: PO* 300 mg qid with meals, hs × 8 wk or 400 mg bid, after 8 wk give hs dose only; IV BOL 300 mg/20 ml 0.9% NaCl over 1-2 min q6h; IV INF 300 mg/50 ml D_5W over 15-20 min; IM 300 mg q6h, not to exceed 2400 mg
Prophylaxis of duodenal ulcer
• *Adult and child >16 yr:* 400 mg hs
Available forms include: Tabs 200, 300, 400, 800 mg; liq 300 mg/15 ml; inj 300 mg/2 ml, 300 mg/50 ml 0.9% NaCl
Side effects/adverse reactions:
CNS: Confusion, headache, depression, dizziness, anxiety, weakness, psychosis, tremors, *convulsions*
GI: Diarrhea, abdominal cramps, paralytic ileus, *jaundice*
GU: Gynecomastia, galactorrhea, impotence, increase in BUN, creatinine
CV: Bradycardia, tachycardia
HEMA: Agranulocytosis, thrombocytopenia, neutropenia, aplastic anemia, increase in pro-time
INTEG: Urticaria, rash, alopecia, sweating, flushing, *exfoliative dermatitis*

Contraindications: Hypersensitivity
Precautions: Pregnancy, lactation, child <16 yr, OBS, hepatic disease, renal disease
Pharmacokinetics:
PO: Peak 1-1½ hr, half-life 1½ hr; metabolized by liver, excreted in urine (unchanged), crosses placenta, enters breast milk
Interactions/incompatibilities:
• Increased toxicity: benzodiazepines, metoprolol, propranolol, phenytoins, quinidine, theophyllines, tricyclic antidepressants, carmustine, lidocaine, procainamide
• Decreased action of this drug: antacids
NURSING CONSIDERATIONS
Assess:
• Gastric pH (>5 should be maintained)
• I&O ratio, BUN, creatinine
Administer:
• With meals for prolonged drug effect
• Antacids 1 hr before or 1 hr after cimetidine
• IV slowly, bradycardia may occur, give over 30 min
Perform/provide:
• Storage at room temperature
Teach patient/family:
• That gynecomastia, impotence may occur, but is reversible
• Avoid driving or other hazardous activities until patient is stabilized on this medication
• To avoid black pepper, caffeine, alcohol, harsh spices, extremes in temperature of food
• To avoid OTC preparations: aspirin, cough, cold preparations
Lab test interferences:
Increase: Alk phosphatase, AST, creatinine
False positive: Gastric bleeding test

---

cinoxacin

(sin-ox′a-sin)
Cinobac

Func. class.: Urinary tract antiseptic

Action: Interferes with conversion of intermediate DNA fragments into high-molecular-weight DNA in bacteria

Uses: Urinary tract infections caused by *E. coli, Klebsiella, Enterobacter, P. mirabilis, P. vulgaris, P. morgani, Serratia, Citrobacter*

Dosage and routes:
• *Adult and child >12 yr:* PO 1 g/day in 2-4 divided doses × 1-2 wk
Available forms include: Caps 250, 500 mg

Side effects/adverse reactions:
INTEG: Pruritus, rash, urticaria, photosensitivity, edema
CNS: Dizziness, headache, agitation, insomnia, confusion
GI: Nausea, vomiting, anorexia, abdominal cramps, diarrhea
EENT: Sensitivity to light, visual disturbances, blurred vision, tinnitus

Contraindications: Hypersensitivity to this drug, anuria, CNS damage

Precautions: Renal disease, hepatic disease, pregnancy, nursing mothers

Pharmacokinetics:
PO: Duration 6-8 hr, half-life 1½ hr, excreted in urine (unchanged/inactive metabolites)

Interactions/incompatibilities:
• May increase action of this drug: probenecid

NURSING CONSIDERATIONS
Assess:
• Kidney, liver function studies: BUN, creatinine, AST, ALT
• I&O ratio, urine pH; <5.5 is ideal

Administer:
• After clean-catch urine is obtained for C&S
• Two daily doses if urine output is high or if patient has diabetes

Perform/provide:
• Limited intake of alkaline foods, drugs: milk, dairy products, peanuts, vegetables, alkaline antacids, sodium bicarbonate

Evaluate:
• Therapeutic response: decreased pain, frequency, urgency, C&S absence of infection
• CNS symptoms: insomnia, vertigo, headache, agitation, confusion
• Allergic reactions: fever, flushing, rash, urticaria, pruritus

Teach patient/family:
• That photosensitivity occurs; that patient should avoid sunlight or use sunscreen to prevent burns
• Fluids must be increased to 3 L/day to avoid crystallization in kidneys
• If dizziness occurs, ambulate/activities with assistance
• Complete full course of drug therapy
• Contact physician if adverse reactions occur
• Take with food/milk to decrease GI irritation

Lab test interferences:
Increase: AST/ALT, BUN, creatinine, alk phosphatase

cisplatin

(sis′pla-tin)
Platinol

Func. class.: Antineoplastic alkylating agent
Chem. class.: Inorganic heavy metal

Action: Alkylates DNA, RNA; inhibits enzymes that allow synthesis of amino acids in proteins

---

italics = common side effects   ***bold italic*** = life threatening reactions

Uses: Advanced bladder cancer, adjunctive in metastatic testicular cancer, adjunctive in metastatic ovarian cancer

Dosage and routes:

Testicular cancer

• *Adult:* IV 20 mg/m^2 qd × 5 days, repeat q3wk for 3 cycles or more, depending on response

Bladder cancer

• *Adult:* IV 50-70 mg/m^2 q3-4wk

Ovarian cancer

• *Adult:* IV 100 mg/m^2 q4wk or 50 mg/m^2 q3wk with doxorubicin therapy; mix with 2 L of NaCl and 37.5 g mannitol over 6 hr

Available forms include: Inj IV 10, 50 mg

Side effects/adverse reactions:

EENT: Tinnitus, hearing loss, vestibular toxicity

*HEMA: **Thrombocytopenia, leukopenia, pancytopenia***

CV: Cardiac abnormalities

GI: Nausea, vomiting, diarrhea, weight loss

*GU: **Renal tubular damage,** renal insufficiency, impotence, sterility, amenorrhea, gynecomastia, hyperuremia*

INTEG: Alopecia, dermatitis

*CNS: **Convulsions***

*RESP: **Fibrosis***

META: Hypomagnesemia, hypocalcemia, hypokalemia, hypophosphatemia

Contraindications: Radiation therapy within 1 mo, chemotherapy within 1 mo, thrombocytopenia, smallpox vaccination

Precautions: Pneumococcus vaccination, pregnancy (1st trimester)

Pharmacokinetics:

Well absorbed orally, metabolized in liver, excreted in urine; half-life 2 hr

Interactions/incompatibilities:

• Increased toxicity: aminoglycosides

• Decreased effects of: phenytoin

NURSING CONSIDERATIONS

Assess:

• CBC, differential, platelet count weekly; withhold drug if WBC is <4000 or platelet count is <75,000; notify physician of results

• Renal function studies: BUN, serum uric acid, urine CrCl before, during therapy

• I&O ratio; report fall in urine output of 30 ml/hr

• Monitor temperature q4h (may indicate beginning infection)

• Liver function tests before, during therapy (bilirubin, AST, ALT, LDH) as needed or monthly

Administer:

• Medications by oral route; if possible avoid IM, SC, IV routes to prevent infections

• Antacid before oral agent, give drug after evening meal, before bedtime

• Antiemetic 30-60 min before giving drug to prevent vomiting

• Allopurinol or sodium bicarbonate to maintain uric acid levels, alkalinization of urine

• Antibiotics for prophylaxis of infection

Perform/provide:

• Strict medical asepsis, protective isolation if WBC levels are low

• Storage protected from light at room temperature for 20 hr

• Special skin care

• Deep breathing exercises with patient tid-qid; place in semi-Fowler's position

• Liquid diet, including cola, Jello; dry toast or crackers may be added if patient is not nauseated or vomiting

• Increase fluid intake to 2-3 L/day to prevent urate deposits, calculi formation

• Diet low in purines: organ meats (kidney, liver), dried beans, peas to maintain alkaline urine

---

* Available in Canada only

Evaluate:
• Bleeding: hematuria, guaiac, bruising or petechiae, mucosa or orifices q8h
• Dyspnea, rales, unproductive cough, chest pain, tachypnea
• Food preferences; list likes, dislikes
• Effects of alopecia on body image, discuss feelings about body changes
• Yellowing of skin, sclera, dark urine, clay-colored stools, itchy skin, abdominal pain, fever, diarrhea
• Edema in feet, joint pain, stomach pain, shaking
• Inflammation of mucosa, breaks in skin

Teach patient/family:
• Of protective isolation precautions
• To report any complaints or side effects to nurse or physician
• That impotence or amenorrhea can occur, reversible after discontinuing treatment
• To report any changes in breathing or coughing
• That hair may be lost during treatment; a wig or hairpiece may make patient feel better; new hair may be different in color, texture

---

clemastine fumarate

(klem'as-teen)
Tavist, Tavist-1
Func. class.: Antihistamine
Chem. class.: Ethanolamine derivative, H_1-receptor antagonist

Action: Acts on blood vessels, GI, respiratory system by competing with histamine for H_1-receptor site; decreases allergic response by blocking histamine
Uses: Allergy symptoms, rhinitis, angioedema, urticaria

Dosage and routes:
• *Adult and child >12 yr:* PO 1.34-2.68 mg bid-tid, not to exceed 8.04 mg/day
Available forms include: Tabs 1.34, 2.68 mg; syr 0.67 mg/ml
Side effects/adverse reactions:
CNS: Dizziness, drowsiness, poor coordination, fatigue, anxiety, euphoria, confusion, paresthesia, neuritis
CV: Hypotension, palpitations, tachycardia
RESP: Increased thick secretions, wheezing, chest tightness
*HEMA: **Thrombocytopenia, agranulocytosis, hemolytic anemia***
GI: Dry mouth, nausea, vomiting, anorexia, constipation, diarrhea
INTEG: Rash, urticaria, photosensitivity
GU: Retention, dysuria, frequency
EENT: Blurred vision, dilated pupils, tinnitus, nasal stuffiness, dry nose, throat, mouth
Contraindications: Hypersensitivity to H_1-receptor antagonists, acute asthma attack, lower respiratory tract disease
Precautions: Increased intraocular pressure, renal disease, cardiac disease, hypertension, bronchial asthma, seizure disorder, stenosed peptic ulcers, hyperthyroidism, prostatic hypertrophy, bladder neck obstruction, pregnancy (B)
Pharmacokinetics:
PO: Peak 5-7 hr, duration 10-12 hr or more; metabolized in liver, excreted by kidneys
Interactions/incompatibilities:
• Increased CNS depression: barbiturates, narcotics, hypnotics, tricyclic antidepressants, alcohol
• Decreased effect of: oral anticoagulants, heparin
• Increased effect of this drug: MAOIs

NURSING CONSIDERATIONS
Assess:
• I&O ratio; be alert for urinary retention, frequency, dysuria; drug should be discontinued if these occur
• CBC during long-term therapy
Administer:
• Coffee, tea, cola (caffeine) to decrease drowsiness
• With meals if GI symptoms occur; absorption may slightly decrease
Perform/provide:
• Hard candy, gum, frequent rinsing of mouth for dryness
• Storage in tight container at room temperature
Evaluate:
• Therapeutic response: absence of running or congested nose or rashes
• Blood dyscrasias: thrombocytopenia, agranulocytosis (rare)
• Respiratory status: rate, rhythm, increase in bronchial secretions, wheezing, chest tightness
• Cardiac status: palpitations, increased pulse, hypotension
Teach patient/family:
• All aspects of drug use; to notify physician if confusion, sedation, hypotension occurs
• To avoid driving or other hazardous activity if drowsiness occurs
• To avoid concurrent use of alcohol or other CNS depressants
• To change position slowly, as drug may cause dizziness, hypotension (elderly)
Lab test interferences:
False negative: Skin allergy tests
Treatment of overdose: Administer ipecac syrup or lavage, diazepam, vasopressors, barbiturates (short-acting)

clidinium bromide
(kli'di-nee-um)
Quarzan

Func. class.: Gastrointestinal anticholinergic
Chem. class.: Synthetic quaternary ammonium antimuscarinic

Action: Inhibits muscarinic actions of acetylcholine at postganglionic parasympathetic neuroeffector sites
Uses: Treatment of peptic ulcer disease in combination with other drugs
Dosage and routes:
• *Adult:* PO 2.5-5 mg tid-qid ac, hs
• *Elderly:* PO 2.5 mg tid ac
Available forms include: Caps 2.5, 5 mg
Side effects/adverse reactions:
CNS: Confusion, stimulation in elderly, headache, insomnia, dizziness, drowsiness, anxiety, weakness, hallucination
GI: Dry mouth, constipation, paralytic ileus, heartburn, nausea, vomiting, dysphagia, absence of taste
GU: Hesitancy, retention, impotence
CV: Palpitations, tachycardia
EENT: Blurred vision, photophobia, mydriasis, cycloplegia, increased ocular tension
INTEG: Urticaria, rash, pruritus, anhidrosis, fever, allergic reactions
Contraindications: Hypersensitivity to anticholinergics, narrow-angle glaucoma, GI obstruction, myasthenia gravis, paralytic ileus, GI atony, toxic megacolon
Precautions: Hyperthyroidism, coronary artery disease, dysrhythmias, CHF, ulcerative colitis, hypertension, hiatal hernia, hepatic disease, renal disease

---

Pharmacokinetics:

PO: Onset 1 hr, duration 3 hr; ionized, excreted in urine

Interactions/incompatibilities:

• Increased anticholinergic effect: amantadine, tricyclic antidepressants, MAOIs

• Increased effect of: nitrofurantoin

• Decreased effect of: phenothiazines, levodopa

NURSING CONSIDERATIONS

Assess:

• VS, cardiac status: checking for dysrhythmias, increased rate, palpitations

• I&O ratio; check for urinary retention or hesitancy

Administer:

• ½-1 hr ac for better absorption

• Decreased dose to elderly patients since their metabolism may be slowed

• Gum, hard candy, frequent rinsing of mouth for dryness of oral cavity

Perform/provide:

• Storage in tight container protected from light

• Increased fluids, bulk, exercise to patient's lifestyle to decrease constipation

Evaluate:

• Therapeutic response: absence of epigastric pain, bleeding, nausea, vomiting

• GI complaints: pain, bleeding (frank or occult), nausea, vomiting, anorexia

Teach patient/family:

• Avoid driving or other hazardous activities until stabilized on medication

• Avoid alcohol or other CNS depressants; will enhance sedating properties of this drug

• To avoid hot environments, stroke may occur, drug suppresses perspiration

• Use sunglasses when outside to prevent photophobia

clindamycin HCl/clindamycin palmitate HCl/clindamycin phosphate

(klin-da-mye′sin)

Cleocin, Dalacin C*

Func. class.: Antibacterial macrolide

Chem. class.: Lincomycin derivative

Action: Binds to 50S subunit of bacterial ribosomes, suppresses protein synthesis

Uses: Infections caused by staphylococci, streptococci, pneumococci, *Rickettsia, Fusobacterium, Actinomyces, Peptococcus, Clostridium*

Dosage and routes:

• *Adults:* PO 150-450 mg q6h; IM/IV 300 mg q6-12h, not to exceed 2700 mg/day

• *Child >1 mo:* PO 8-25 mg/kg/day in divided doses q6-8h; IM/IV 15-40 mg/kg/day in divided doses q6h

Available forms include: Inj 150 mg/ml; caps 50, 75 mg; oral sol 75 mg/ml

Side effects/adverse reactions:

HEMA: **Leukopenia, eosinophilia, agranulocytosis, thrombocytopenia**

GI: Nausea, vomiting, abdominal pain, diarrhea, **Pseudomembranous colitis**

GU: Increased AST, ALT, bilirubin, alk phosphatase, jaundice, *vaginitis,* urinary frequency

EENT: Rash, urticaria, pruritus, erythema, pain, abscess at injection site

Contraindications: Hypersensitivity to this drug or lincomycin, ulcerative colitis/enteritis, infants <1 mo

Precautions: Renal disease, liver

---

disease, GI disease, elderly, pregnancy, lactation

Pharmacokinetics:
PO: Peak 45 min, duration 6 hr
IM: Peak 3 hr, duration 8-12 hr
Half-life 2½ hr, metabolized in liver, excreted in urine, bile, feces as active/inactive metabolites, crosses placenta, excreted in breast milk

Interactions/incompatibilities:
• Increased neuromuscular blockage: nondepolarizing muscle relaxants
• Decreased action of: chloramphenicol, erythromycin
• Decreased rate of absorption of: opiates, diphenoxylate

NURSING CONSIDERATIONS
Assess:
• Any patient with compromised renal system; drug is excreted slowly in poor renal system function; toxicity may occur rapidly
• Liver studies: AST, ALT
• Blood studies: WBC, RBC, Hct, Hgb, platelets, serum iron, reticulocytes; drug should be discontinued if bone marrow depression occurs
• Renal studies: urinalysis, protein, blood, BUN, creatinine
• C&S before drug therapy; drug may be taken as soon as culture is taken
• Drug level in impaired hepatic, renal systems
• B/P, pulse in patient receiving drug parenterally

Administer:
• IV by infusion only; do not administer bolus dose
• IM deep injection; rotate sites
• Orally with at least 8 oz water

Perform/provide:
• Storage at room temperature (capsules) and up to 2 wk (reconstituted solution)
• Adrenalin, suction, tracheostomy set, endotracheal intubation equipment on unit
• Adequate intake of fluids (2000 ml) during diarrhea episodes

Evaluate:
• Therapeutic response: decreased temperature, negative C&S
• Bowel pattern before, during treatment
• Skin eruptions, itching, dermatitis after administration
• Respiratory status: rate, character, wheezing, tightness in chest
• Allergies before treatment, reaction of each medication; place allergies on chart, Kardex in bright red letters; notify all people giving drugs

Teach patient/family:
• To take oral drug with full glass of water; may give with food if GI symptoms occur
• Aspects of drug therapy: need to complete entire course of medication to ensure organism death (10-14 days); culture may be taken after completed medication course
• To report sore throat, fever, fatigue; could indicate superimposed infection
• That drug must be taken in equal intervals around clock to maintain blood levels
• To wear or carry Medic Alert ID if allergic to this drug
• To notify nurse of diarrhea stools

Lab test interferences:
Increase: Alk phosphatase, bilirubin, CPK, AST, ALT

Treatment of overdose: Withdraw drug, maintain airway, administer epinephrine, aminophylline, O_2, IV corticosteroids

---

clobetasol propionate

(klo-bet′-a-sol)
Temovate

Func. class.: Topical corticosteroid
Chem. class.: Synthetic fluorinated
agent, group I potency

Action: Possesses antipruritic, antiinflammatory actions
Uses: Psoriasis, eczema, contact
dermatitis, pruritus; usually re-
served for severe dermatoses that
have not responded to less potent
formulation
Dosage and routes:
• *Adult and child:* Apply to affected area bid
Available forms include: Oint
0.05%; cream 0.05%
Side effects/adverse reactions:
INTEG: Burning, dryness, itching,
irritation, acne, folliculitis, hypertrichosis, perioral dermatitis, hypopigmentation, atrophy, striae,
miliaria, allergic contact dermatitis, secondary infection
Contraindications: Hypersensitivity to corticosteroids, fungal infections
Precautions: Pregnancy (C), lactation, viral infections, bacterial infections
Interactions/incompatibilities:
None known
NURSING CONSIDERATIONS
Assess:
• Temperature, if fever develops,
drug should be discontinued
Administer:
• Only to affected areas; do not get
in eyes
• Leaving uncovered or lightly
covered, occlusive dressing is not
recommended
• Only to dermatoses; do not use on
weeping, denuded, or infected area

Perform/provide:
• Cleansing before application of
drug
• Treatment for a few days after
area has cleared
• Storage at room temperature
Evaluate:
• Therapeutic response: absence of
severe itching, patches on skin,
flaking
Teach patient/family:
• To avoid sunlight on affected
area; burns may occur
• To limit treatment to 14 days us-
ing <50 g/wk

clocortolone pivalate

(klo-kort′-oo-lone)
Cloderm

Func. class.: Topical corticosteroid
Chem. class.: Synthetic fluorinated
agent, group IV potency

Action: Possesses antipruritic, antiinflammatory actions
Uses: Psoriasis, eczema, contact
dermatitis, pruritus
Dosage and routes:
• *Adult and child:* Apply to affected area tid
Available forms include: Cream
0.1%
Side effects/adverse reactions:
INTEG: Burning, dryness, itching,
irritation, acne, folliculitis, hypertrichosis, perioral dermatitis, hypopigmentation, atrophy, striae,
miliaria, allergic contact dermatitis, secondary infection
Contraindications: Hypersensitivity to corticosteroids, fungal infections
Precautions: Pregnancy (C), lactation, viral infections, bacterial infections
Interactions/incompatibilities:
None known

NURSING CONSIDERATIONS
Assess:
• Temperature; if fever develops, drug should be discontinued
Administer:
• Only to affected areas; do not get in eyes
• Medication, then cover with occlusive dressing (only if prescribed), seal to normal skin, change q12h
• Only to dermatoses; do not use on weeping, denuded, or infected area
Perform/provide:
• Cleansing before application of drug
• Treatment for a few days after area has cleared
• Storage at room temperature
Evaluate:
• Therapeutic response: absence of severe itching, patches on skin, flaking
Teach patient/family:
• To avoid sunlight on affected area; burns may occur

---

clofibrate
(kloe-fye'brate)
Atromide-S, Claripex*
Func. class.: Antilipemic
Chem. class.: Aryloxyisobutyric acid derivative

Action: Inhibits biosynthesis of VLDL, LDL, which are responsible for cholesterol development, mobilizes cholesterol from tissue, increases excretion of neutrol
Uses: Hyperlipidemia, xanthoma tuberosum, type III hyperlipidemia, (type III, IV, V hyperlipoproteinemia)
Dosage and routes:
• *Adult:* PO 2 g/day in 4 divided doses
Available forms include: Caps 500 mg

Side effects/adverse reactions:
GI: Nausea, vomiting, dyspepsia, increased liver enzymes, stomatitis, flatulence, hepatomegaly, gastritis, increased cholelithiasis
INTEG: Rash, urticaria, pruritus, dry hair and skin, alopecia
HEMA: Leukopenia, anemia, eosinophilia
CNS: Fatigue, weakness, headache
GU: Decreased libido, impotence, dysuria, proteinuria, oliguria
MS: Myalgias, arthralgias
CV: Angina, dysrhythmias, thrombophlebitis, *pulmonary emboli*
Contraindications: Severe hepatic disease, severe renal disease, primary biliary cirrhosis, pregnancy, lactation
Precautions: Peptic ulcer
Pharmacokinetics:
PO: Peak 2-6 hr, plasma protein binding >90%; half-life 6-25 hr, excreted in urine, metabolized in liver
Interactions/incompatibilities:
• Increased effects of: sulfonylureas
• Increased toxicity of: probenecid
• Increased anticoagulant effects of: oral anticoagulants
• Decreased effects of: rifampin
NURSING CONSIDERATIONS
Assess:
• Renal and hepatic levels if patient is on long-term therapy
• For signs of vitamin A, D, K deficiency
Administer:
• Drug with meals if GI symptoms occur
Evaluate:
• Therapeutic response: decreased triglycerides, cholesterol level (hyperlipidemia); diarrhea, pruritus (excess bile area)
• Bowel pattern daily; increase bulk, water in diet if constipation develops

---

Teach patient/family:
• Symptoms of hypothrombinemia: bleeding mucous membranes, dark tarry stools, petechiae; report immediately
• That patient compliance is needed since toxicity may result if doses are missed
• That risk factors should be decreased: high fat diet, smoking, alcohol consumption, absence of exercise
• That OTC preparations should be avoided unless directed by physician
• Birth control should be practiced while on this drug
• To report GU symptoms: decreased libido, impotence, dysuria, proteinuria, oliguria

Lab test interferences:
Increase: Liver function studies, CPK, BSP, thymol turbidity

---

clomiphene citrate

(kloe'mi-feen)
Clomid, Serophene
Func. class.: Ovulation stimulant
Chem. class.: Nonsteroidal antiestrogenic

Action: Increases LH, FSH, which increase maturation of ovarian follicle, ovulation, development of corpus luteum
Uses: Female infertility
Dosage and routes:
• *Adult:* PO 50-100 mg qd × 5 days or 50-100 mg qd beginning on day 5 of cycle; may be repeated until conception occurs or 3 cycles of therapy have been completed
Available forms include: Tabs 50 mg
Side effects/adverse reactions:
EENT: Blurred vision, diplopia, photophobia
*HEMA: **Hemolytic anemia***
CNS: Headache, depression, restlessness, anxiety, nervousness, fatigue, insomnia
GI: Nausea, vomiting, constipation, increased appetite, abdominal pain
INTEG: Rash, dermatitis, urticaria, alopecia
GU: Polyuria, frequency, birth defects, spontaneous abortions, multiple ovulation, breast pain, oliguria
CV: Phlebitis, deep vein thrombosis
Contraindications: Hypersensitivity, pregnancy, fibroidphlebitis, thrombophlebitis, hepatic disease, undiagnosed vaginal bleeding
Precautions: Hypertension, depression, convulsions, diabetes mellitus
Pharmacokinetics: Detoxified in liver, excreted in feces, stored in fat
Interactions/incompatibilities:
None known
NURSING CONSIDERATIONS
Administer:
• At same time qd to maintain drug level
Teach patient/family:
• Multiple births are common after drug is taken
• To notify physician if low abdominal pain occurs; may indicate ovarian cyst, cyst rupture
• Method for taking, recording basal body temperature to determine whether ovulation has occurred
• If ovulation can be determined (there is a slight decrease then a sharp increase for ovulation) to attempt coitus 3 days before and qod until after ovulation
• If pregnancy is suspected, physician must be notified immediately
Lab test interferences:
Increase: FSH/LH, BSP, thyroxine, TBG

---

clonazepam

(kloe-na'zi-pam)
Klonopin, Rivotril

Func. class.: Anticonvulsant
Chem. class.: Benzodiazapine derivative

Controlled Substance Schedule IV

Action: Inhibits spike, wave formation in absence seizures (petit mal), decreases amplitude, frequency, duration, spread of discharge in minor motor seizures

Uses: Absence, atypical absence, akinetic, myoclonic seizures

Dosage and routes:
• *Adult:* PO Not to exceed 1.5 mg/day in 3 divided doses; may be increased 0.5-1 mg q3 days until desired response, not to exceed 20 mg/day
• *Child <10 yr or 30 kg:* PO 0.01-0.03 mg/kg/day in divided doses q8h, not to exceed 0.05 mg/kg/day; may be increased 0.25-0.5 mg q3 days until desired response, not to exceed 0.1-0.2 mg/kg/day

Available forms include: Tabs 0.5, 1, 2 mg

Side effects/adverse reactions:
HEMA: Thrombocytopenia, leukocytosis, eosinophilia
CNS: Drowsiness, dizziness, confusion, behavioral changes, tremors, insomnia, headache, suicidal tendencies
GI: Nausea, constipation, polyphagia, anorexia, xerostomia, diarrhea
INTEG: Rash, alopecia, hirsutism
EENT: Increased salivation, nystagmus, diplopia, abnormal eye movements, sore gums
RESP: Respiratory depression, dyspnea, congestion
CV: Palpitations, bradycardia
Contraindications: Hypersensitivity to benzodiazepines, acute narrow-angle glaucoma

Precautions: Open-angle glaucoma, chronic respiratory disease

Pharmacokinetics:
PO: Peak 1-2 hr, metabolized by liver, excreted in urine, half-life 18-50 hr

Interactions/incompatibilities:
• Increased CNS depression: alcohol, barbiturates, narcotics, antidepressants, other anticonvulsants
• Decreased effect of: carbamazepine
• Seizures: valproic acid

NURSING CONSIDERATIONS
Assess:
• Renal studies: urinalysis, BUN, urine creatinine
• Blood studies: RBC, Hct, Hgb, reticulocyte counts q wk for 4 wk then q mo
• Hepatic studies: ALT, AST, bilirubin, creatinine
• Drug levels during initial treatment

Administer:
• With food, milk to decrease GI symptoms

Perform/provide:
• Storage at room temperature
• Hard candy, frequent rinsing of mouth, gum for dry mouth
• Assistance with ambulation during early part of treatment; dizziness occurs

Evaluate:
• Therapeutic response: decreased seizure activity, document on patient's chart
• Mental status: mood, sensorium, affect, behavioral changes; if mental status changes, notify physician
• Eye problems: need for ophthalmic examinations before, during, after treatment (slit lamp, fundoscopy, tonometry)
• Allergic reaction: red raised rash; if this occurs, drug should be discontinued

---

* Available in Canada only

• Blood dyscrasias: fever, sore throat, bruising, rash, jaundice
• Toxicity: bone marrow depression, nausea, vomiting, ataxia, diplopia, cardiovascular collapse

Teach patient/family:
• To carry ID card to Medic-Alert bracelet stating drugs taken, condition, physician's name, phone number
• To avoid driving, other activities that require alertness
• To avoid alcohol ingestion or CNS depressants, increased sedation may occur
• Not to discontinue medication quickly after long-term use; taper off over several weeks
• All aspects of the drug: action, use, side effects, adverse reactions, when to notify physician

Lab test interferences:
Increase: AST, alk phosphatase

Treatment of overdose: Lavage, activated charcoal, monitor electrolytes, VS, administer vasopressors

---

clonidine HCl

(kloe′ni-deen)
Catapres, Dixarit*
Func. class.: Antihypertensive
Chem. class.: Central α-adrenergic agonist

Action: Inhibits sympathetic vasomotor center in CNS, which reduces impulses in sympathetic nervous system; blood pressure decreases, pulse rate, cardiac output decreases

Uses: Hypertension

Dosage and routes:
Hypertension
• *Adult:* PO/TRANS 0.1 mg bid, then increase by 0.1 mg/day or 0.2 mg/day until desired response; range 0.2-0.8 mg/day in divided doses

Available forms include: Tabs 0.1,

0.2, 0.3 mg; trans sys 0.1, 0.2, 0.3 mg/24 hr

Side effects/adverse reactions:
CV: Hypotension, orthostatic palpitations
CNS: Drowsiness, sedation, headache, fatigue, nightmares, insomnia, mental changes, anxiety, depression, hallucinations, delirium
GI: Nausea, vomiting, malaise, constipation, dry mouth
INTEG: Rash, alopecia, facial pallor, pruritus, hives, edema, burning papules, excoriation (transdermal patches)
EENT: Taste change, parotid pain
ENDO: Hyperglycemia
MS: Muscle/joint pain, leg cramps
GU: Impotence, dysuria, *nocturia,* gynecomastia

Contraindications: Hypersensitivity

Precautions: MI (recent), diabetes mellitus, chronic renal failure, Raynaud's disease, thyroid disease, depression, COPD, child <12 (patches), asthma, pregnancy, lactation

Pharmacokinetics:
PO: Peak 3-5 hr; half-life 6-20 hr, metabolized by liver (metabolites), excreted in urine (unchanged, inactive metabolites, feces), crosses blood-brain barrier, excreted in breast milk

Interactions/incompatibilities:
• Increased CNS depression: narcotics, sedatives, alcohol, anesthetics
• Decreased hypotension effects: tricyclic antidepressants, MAOIs
• Increased hypotensive effects: diuretics
• Increased bradycardia: β-blockers, cardiac glycosides

NURSING CONSIDERATIONS
Assess:
• Blood studies: neutrophils, decreased platelets

• Renal studies: protein, BUN, creatinine; watch for increased levels that may indicate nephrotic syndrome
• Baselines in renal, liver function tests before therapy begins
• K levels, although hyperkalemia rarely occurs
• Dip-stick of urine for protein qd in first morning specimen, if protein is increased, a 24 hr urinary protein should be collected

Administer:
• IV infusion of 0.9% NaCl (as ordered) to expand fluid volume if severe hypotension occurs

Perform/provide:
• Storage of patches in cool environment, tablets in tight containers

Evaluate:
• Therapeutic response: decrease in B/P in hypertension
• Edema in feet, legs daily
• Allergic reaction: rash, fever, pruritus, urticaria; drug should be discontinued if antihistamines fail to help
• Allergic reaction from patches: rash, urticaria, angioedema; should not continue to use
• Symptoms of CHF: edema, dyspnea, wet rales, B/P
• Renal symptoms: polyuria, oliguria, frequency

Teach patient/family:
• To avoid hazardous activities
• Administer 1 hr before meals
• Not to discontinue drug abruptly or withdrawal symptoms may occur: anxiety, increased B/P, headache, insomnia, increased pulse, tremors, nausea, sweating
• Not to use OTC (cough, cold, or allergy) products unless directed by physician
• Tell patient to avoid sunlight or wear sunscreen if in sunlight, photosensitivity may occur
• Stress patient compliance with dosage schedule even if feeling better
• To rise slowly to sitting or standing position to minimize orthostatic hypotension
• Notify physician of: mouth sores, sore throat, fever, swelling of hands or feet, irregular heartbeat, chest pain, signs of angioedema
• Excessive perspiration, dehydration, vomiting; diarrhea may lead to fall in blood pressure—consult physician if these occur
• May cause dizziness, fainting; light-headedness may occur during 1st few days of therapy
• That compliance is necessary, not to skip or stop drug unless directed by physician
• May cause skin rash or impaired perspiration

Lab test interferences:
Increase: Blood glucose
Decrease: VMA, catecholamines, aldosterone

Treatment of overdose: Supportive treatment, administer Prescoline for severe overdose

---

clorazepate dipotassium

(klor-az′e-pate)
Tranxene

Func. class.: Antianxiety
Chem. class.: Benzodiazepine

Controlled Substance Schedule IV

Action: Depresses subcortical levels of CNS, including limbic system, reticular formation

Uses: Anxiety, acute alcohol withdrawal, adjunct in seizure disorders

Dosage and routes:
Anxiety
• *Adult:* PO 15-60 mg/day
Alcohol withdrawal
• *Adult:* PO 30 mg then 30-60 mg in divided doses; day 2, 45-90 mg in divided doses; day 3, 22.5-45 mg

in divided doses; day 4, 15-30 mg in divided doses; then reduce daily dose to 7.5-15 mg

Seizure disorders

• *Adult and child >12 yr:* PO 7.5 mg tid, may increase by 7.5 mg/wk or less, not to exceed 90 mg/day

• *Child 9-12 yr:* PO 7.5 mg bid, may increase by 7.5 mg/wk or less, not to exceed 60 mg/day

Available forms include: Caps 3.75, 7.5, 15 mg; tabs 3.75, 7.5, 15 mg, single dose tab 11.25, 22.5 mg

Side effects/adverse reactions:

CNS: Dizziness, drowsiness, confusion, headache, anxiety, tremors, stimulation, fatigue, depression, insomnia, hallucinations

GI: Constipation, dry mouth, nausea, vomiting, anorexia, diarrhea

INTEG: Rash, dermatitis, itching

*CV: Orthostatic hypotension, **ECG changes, tachycardia,*** hypotension

EENT: Blurred vision, tinnitus, mydriasis

Contraindications: Hypersensitivity to benzodiazepines, narrow-angle glaucoma, psychosis, pregnancy (D), child <18 yr

Precautions: Elderly, debilitated, hepatic disease, renal disease

Pharmacokinetics:

PO: Onset 15 min, peak 1-2 hr, duration 4-6 hr, metabolized by liver, excreted by kidneys, crosses placenta, breast milk, half-life 30-100 hr

Interactions/incompatibilities:

• Decreased effects of this drug: oral contraceptives, rifampin, valproic acid

• Increased effects of this drug: CNS depressants, alcohol, cimetidine, disulfiram, oral contraceptives

NURSING CONSIDERATIONS

Assess:

• B/P (lying, standing), pulse; if systolic B/P drops 20 mm Hg, hold drug, notify physician

• Blood studies: CBC during long-term therapy, blood dyscrasias have occurred rarely

• Hepatic studies: AST, ALT, bilirubin, creatinine, LDH, alk phosphatase

• I&O; may indicate renal dysfunction

Administer:

• With food or milk for GI symptoms

• Crushed if patient is unable to swallow medication whole

• Sugarless gum, hard candy, frequent sips of water for dry mouth

Perform/provide:

• Assistance with ambulation during beginning therapy, since drowsiness/dizziness occurs

• Safety measures, including siderails

• Check to see PO medication has been swallowed

Evaluate:

• Therapeutic response: decreased anxiety, restlessness, insomnia

• Mental status: mood, sensorium, affect, sleeping pattern, drowsiness, dizziness

• Physical dependency, withdrawal symptoms: headache, nausea, vomiting, muscle pain, weakness after long-term use

• Suicidal tendencies

Teach patient/family:

• That drug may be taken with food

• Not to be used for everyday stress or used longer than 4 mo, unless directed by physician

• Avoid OTC preparations unless approved by physician

• To avoid driving, activities that require alertness; drowsiness may occur

• To avoid alcohol ingestion or other psychotropic medications, unless prescribed by physician

• Not to discontinue medication abruptly after long-term use

italics = common side effects   ***bold italic*** = life threatening reactions

• To rise slowly or fainting may occur
• That drowsiness might worsen at beginning of treatment
Lab test interferences:
Increase: AST/ALT, serum bilirubin
Decrease: RAIU
False increase: 17-OHCS
Treatment of overdose: Lavage, VS, supportive care

clotrimazole (topical)

(kloe-trim′a-zole)

Canesten,* Gyne-Lotrimin, Mycelex, Mycelex-G

Func. class.: Local antiinfective
Chem. class.: Imidazole derivative

Action: Interferes with fungal DNA replication; binds sterols in fungal cell membrane, which increases permeability, leaking of cell nutrients
Uses: Tinea pedis, tinea cruris, tinea corporis, tinea versicolor, candida albican infection of the vagina, vulva, throat, mouth
Dosage and routes:
• *Adult and child:* TOP rub into affected area bid × 1-8 wk; LOZ dissolve in mouth 5×/day × 2 wk; INTRA VAG 1 applicator/1 tab × 1-2 wk hs
Available forms include: Cream, sol, lotion 1%; vag tabs 100, 500 mg; vag cream 1%
Side effects/adverse reactions:
INTEG: Rash, urticaria, stinging, burning
Contraindications: Hypersensitivity
Precautions: Pregnancy, lactation
Interactions/incompatibilities: None known
NURSING CONSIDERATIONS
Administer:
• 1 applicator or 1 tablet intravaginally each night

• Enough medication to completely cover lesions
• After cleansing with soap, water before each application, dry well
Perform/provide:
• Storage at room temperature in dry place
Evaluate:
• Allergic reaction: burning, stinging, swelling, redness
• Therapeutic response: decrease in size, number of lesions, decrease in itching or white patches around vulva
Teach patient/family:
• To apply with glove to prevent further infection
• To avoid use of OTC creams, ointments, lotions unless directed by physician
• To use medical asepsis (hand washing) before, after each application
• To abstain from sexual intercourse during vaginal/vulvular treatment

cloxacillin sodium

(klox-a-sill′in)

Apo Cloxi,* Bactopen,* Cloxapen, Novocloxin,* Orbenin,* Tegopen

Func. class.: Broad spectrum antibiotic
Chem. class.: Penicillinase-resistant penicillin

Action: Interferes with cell wall replication of susceptible organisms; the cell wall, rendered osmotically unstable, swells, bursts from osmotic pressure
Uses: Effective for gram-positive cocci *(S. aureus, S. pyogenes, E. pyogenes, S. pneumoniae)*
Dosage and routes:
• *Adult:* PO 1-4 g/day in divided doses q6h
• *Child:* PO 50-100 mg/kg in divided doses q6h

Available forms include: Caps 250, 500 mg; powder for oral susp 125 mg/ml

Side effects/adverse reactions:
HEMA: Anemia, increased bleeding time, ***bone marrow depression, granulocytopenia***
GI: Nausea, vomiting, diarrhea, increased AST, ALT, abdominal pain, glossitis, colitis
GU: Oliguria, proteinuria, hematuria, *vaginitis, moniliasis,* ***glomerulonephritis***
CNS: Lethargy, hallucinations, anxiety, depression, twitching, ***coma, convulsions***
META: Hyperkalemia, hypokalemia, alkalosis, hypernatremia
Contraindications: Hypersensitivity to penicillins; neonates
Precautions: Pregnancy, hypersensitivity to cephalosporins
Pharmacokinetics:
PO: Peak 1 hr, duration 6 hr; half-life 30-60 min, metabolized in liver, excreted in urine, bile, breast milk, crosses placenta
Interactions/incompatibilities:
• Decreased antimicrobial effectiveness of this drug: tetracyclines, erythromycins
• Increased penicillin concentrations when used with: aspirin, probenicid

NURSING CONSIDERATIONS
Assess:
• I&O ratio; report hematuria, oliguria since penicillin in high doses is nephrotoxic
• Any patient with compromised renal system, since drug is excreted slowly in poor renal system function; toxicity may occur rapidly
• Liver studies: AST, ALT
• Blood studies: WBC, RBC, H&H, bleeding time
• Renal studies: urinalysis, protein, blood
• Culture, sensitivity before drug therapy; drug may be taken as soon as culture is taken
Administer:
• After C&S completed
Perform/provide:
• Adrenaline, suction, tracheostomy set, endotracheal intubation equipment on unit
• Adequate intake of fluids (2000 ml) during diarrhea episodes
• Scratch test to assess allergy after securing order from physician; usually done when penicillin is only drug of choice
• Storage in tight container; after reconstituting, store in refrigerator
Evaluate:
• Therapeutic effectiveness: absence of temperature, draining wounds
• Bowel pattern before, during treatment
• Skin eruptions after administration of penicillin to 1 wk after discontinuing drug
• Respiratory status: rate, character, wheezing, tightness in chest
• Allergies before initiation of treatment; reaction of each medication; place allergies on chart, Kardex in bright red
Teach patient/family:
• Aspects of drug therapy including need to complete entire course of medication to ensure organism death (10-14 days); culture may be taken after completed course of medication
• To report sore throat, fever, fatigue (could indicate superimposed infection)
• To wear or carry a Medic Alert ID if allergic to penicillins
• To notify nurse of diarrhea stools
Lab test interferences:
False positive: Urine glucose, urine protein
Decrease: Uric acid
Treatment of overdose: Withdraw drug, maintain airway, administer

epinephrine, aminophylline, O_2, IV corticosteroids for anaphylaxis

---

codeine sulfate/codeine phosphate
(koe'deen)

Func. class.: Narcotic analgesics
Chem. class.: Opiate, phenathrene derivative

Controlled Substance Schedule II
Action: Inhibits ascending pain pathways in CNS, increases pain threshold, alters pain perception
Uses: Moderate to severe pain, nonproductive cough
Dosage and routes:
Pain
• *Adult:* PO 15-60 mg q4h prn; IM/SC 15-60 mg q4h prn
• *Child:* PO 3 mg/kg/day in divided doses q4h prn
Cough
• *Adult:* PO 8-20 mg q4-6h, not to exceed 120 mg/day
• *Child:* PO 1-1.5 mg/kg/day in 4 divided doses, not to exceed 60 mg/day
Available forms include: Inj IM, SC 15, 30, 60 mg/ml; tabs 15, 30, 60 mg
Side effects/adverse reactions:
CNS: Drowsiness, sedation, dizziness, agitation, dependency, lethargy, restlessness
GI: Nausea, vomiting, anorexia, constipation
RESP: Respiratory depression, respiratory paralysis
CV: Bradycardia, palpitations, orthostatic hypotension, tachycardia
GU: Urinary retention
INTEG: Flushing, rash, urticaria
Contraindications: Hypersensitivity to opiates, respiratory depression, increased intracranial pressure, seizure disorders, severe respiratory disorders

Precautions: Elderly, cardiac dysrhythmias
Pharmacokinetics: Onset 15-30 min, peak 1-2 hr, duration 4-6 hr; metabolized by liver, excreted by kidneys, crosses placenta, excreted in breast milk, half-life 2½-4 hr
Interactions/incompatibilities:
• Effects may be increased with other CNS depressants: alcohol, narcotics, sedative/hypnotics, antipsychotics, skeletal muscle relaxants

NURSING CONSIDERATIONS
Assess:
• I&O ratio; check for decreasing output; may indicate urinary retention
Administer:
• With antiemetic if nausea, vomiting occur
• With milk or food for GI symptoms
• When pain is beginning to return; determine dosage interval by patient response
Perform/provide:
• Storage in light-resistant container at room temperature
• Assistance with ambulation
• Safety measures: siderails, night light, call bell
Evaluate:
• Therapeutic response: decrease in pain, absence of grimacing or decreased cough
• Cough: type, duration, ability to raise secretion
• CNS changes, dizziness, drowsiness, hallucinations, euphoria, LOC, pupil reaction
• Allergic reactions: rash, urticaria
• Respiratory dysfunction: respiratory depression, character, rate rhythm; notify physician if respirations are <12/min
• Need for pain medication, physical dependence
Teach patient/family:
• To report any symptoms of CNS

---

changes, allergic reactions
• That physical dependency may result when used for extended periods of time
• To change position slowly, orthostatic hypotension may occur
• To avoid hazardous activities if drowsiness or dizziness occurs
• To avoid alcohol unless directed by physician

co-trimoxazole (sulfamethoxazole and trimethoprim)

(koe-trye-mox′a-zole)
Apo-Sulfatrim,* Bactrim, Cotrim, Septra, Sulfatrim, Bethaprim

Func. class.: Antibiotic
Chem. class.: Miscellaneous sulfonamide

Action: Sulfamethoxazole interferes with bacterial biosynthesis of proteins by competitive antagonism of PABA when adequate levels are maintained; trimethoprim blocks synthesis of tetrahydrofolic acid; this combination blocks 2 consecutive steps in bacterial synthesis of essential nucleic acids, protein
Uses: Urinary tract infections, otitis media, chronic prostatitis, shigellosis, *Pneumocystis carinii* pneumonitis, chronic bronchitis

Dosage and routes:
Urinary tract infections
• *Adult:* PO 160 mg TMP/800 mg SMZ q12h × 10-14 days
• *Child:* PO 8 mg/kg TMP/40 mg/kg SMZ qd in 2 divided doses q12h × 10 days; IV 8-10 kg/day (based on TMP component) in 2-4 divided doses for up to 14 days
Otitis media
• *Child:* PO 8 mg/kg TMP/40 mg/kg SMZ qd in 2 divided doses q12h × 10 days
Chronic bronchitis
• *Adult:* PO 100 mg TMP/800

mg SMZ q12h × 14 days
Pneumocystis carinii pneumonitis
• *Adult and child:* PO 20 mg/kg TMP/100 mg/kg SMZ qd in 2 divided doses q6h × 14 days; IV 15-20 mg/kg/day (based on TMP) in 3-4 divided doses for up to 14 days
Available forms include: Tabs 80 mg trimethoprim/400 mg sulfamethoxazole, 160 mg trimethoprim/800 mg sulfamethoxazole; susp 40 mg/200 mg/5 ml; IV inj 16 mg/80 mg/ml

Side effects/adverse reactions:
*SYST: **Anaphylaxis***
GI: Nausea, vomiting, abdominal pain, stomatitis, ***hepatitis,*** glossitis, pancreatitis, diarrhea, ***enterocolitis***
CNS: Headache, confusion, insomnia, hallucinations, depression, vertigo, fatigue, anxiety, convulsions, drug fever, chills
*HEMA: **Leukopenia, neutropenia, thrombocytopenia, agranulocytosis, hemolytic anemia***
INTEG: Rash, dermatitis, urticaria, ***Stevens-Johnson syndrome,*** erythema, photosensitivity, pain, inflammation at injection site
*GU: **Renal failure, toxic nephrosis,*** increased BUN, creatinine, crystalluria
*CV: **Allergic myocarditis***
Contraindications: Hypersensitivity to trimethoprim or sulfonamides, pregnancy at term, megaloblastic anemia, infants <2 mo, CrCl <15 ml/min
Precautions: Pregnancy (C), lactation, renal disease, elderly, G-6-PD deficiency, impaired hepatic function, possible folate deficiency, severe allergy, bronchial asthma
Pharmacokinetics:
PO: Rapidly absorbed, peak 1-4 hr; half-life 8-13 hr, excreted in urine (metabolites and unchanged), breast milk, crosses placenta,

highly bound to plasma proteins
Interactions/incompatibilities:
• Increased hypoglycemic response: sulfonylurea agents
• Do not mix with silver preparations
• Increased anticoagulant effects: oral anticoagulants
• Decreased renal excretion of: methotrexate
• Decreased hepatic clearance of: phenytoin

NURSING CONSIDERATIONS
Assess:
• I&O ratio; note color, character, pH of urine if drug administered for urinary tract infections; output should be 800 ml less than intake; if urine is highly acidic, alkalization may be needed
• Kidney function studies: BUN, creatinine, urinalysis if on long-term therapy
• Drug level (therapeutic range 5-15 mg/dl)
Administer:
• With full glass of water to maintain adequate hydration; increase fluids to 2000 ml/day to decrease crystallization in kidneys
• Medication after C&S; repeat C&S after full course of medication completed
• After dilution with D_5W infuse over 1-1½ hr; use immediately after reconstituting
• With resuscitative equipment available; severe allergic reactions may occur
Perform/provide:
• Storage in tight, light-resistant containers at room temperature
Evaluate:
• Therapeutic response: absence of pain, fever, C&S negative
• Blood dyscrasias: skin rash, fever, sore throat, bruising, bleeding, fatigue, joint pain
• Allergic reaction: rash, dermatitis, urticaria, pruritus, dyspnea, bronchospasm
Teach patient/family:
• To take each oral dose with full glass of water to prevent crystalluria
• To complete full course of treatment to prevent superimposed infection
• To avoid sunlight or use sunscreen to prevent burns
• To avoid OTC medications (aspirin, vitamin C) unless directed by physician
• To use alternative contraceptive measures; decreased effectiveness of oral contraceptives may result
• To notify physician if skin rash, sore throat, fever, mouth sores, unusual bruising, bleeding occur
Lab test interferences:
Increase: Alk phosphatase, creatinine, bilirubin
False positive: Urinary glucose test

---

colchicine
(kol'chi-seen)
Colsalide, Novocolchine
Func. class.: Antigout agent
Chem. class.: Colchicum autumnale alkaloid

Action: Inhibits microtubule formation in leukocytes, which decreases phagocytosis in joints
Uses: Gout, gouty arthritis (prevention, treatment), hepatic cirrhosis
Dosage and routes:
Prevention
• *Adult:* PO 0.5-1.8 mg qd depending on severity
Treatment
• *Adult:* PO 1-1.2 mg, then 0.5-0.6 mg q1h, or 1-1.2 mg q2h until pain decreases or side effects occur; IV 2 mg, then 2 mg after 12 hr, not to exceed 4 mg/24 hr
Available forms include: Tabs 0.5,

0.6 mg; inj IV 1 mg/2 ml

Side effects/adverse reactions:

*HEMA: **Agranulocytosis, thrombocytopenia, aplastic anemia, pancytopenia***

CNS: Headache, drowsiness, neuritis, dizziness

GI: Nausea, vomiting, anorexia, malaise, metallic taste, cramps, peptic ulcer

EENT: Retinopathy, cataracts

INTEG: Stomatitis, fever, chills, dermatitis, pruritus, purpura, erythema

Contraindications: Hypersensitivity, cardiac dyscrasias

Precautions: Severe renal disease, blood dyscrasias

Pharmacokinetics:

PO: Peak ½-2 hr, half-life 20 min, deacetylates in liver, excreted in feces (metabolites/active drug)

Interactions/incompatibilities:

• Increased action of this drug: acidifiers, alkalinizers, alcohol

• Decreased action of: CNS depressants, vitamin B$_{12}$

NURSING CONSIDERATIONS

Assess:

• I&O ratio; observe for decrease in urinary output

• CBC, platelets, reticulocytes before, during therapy (q3 mo)

• Coombs' test to determine Coombs' negative hemolytic anemia

Administer:

• On empty stomach only, to facilitate absorption

Evaluate:

• Therapeutic response: decreased stone formation on x-ray, decreased pain in kidney region, absence of hematuria

Teach patient/family:

• To avoid alcohol, OTC preparations that contain alcohol; skin rashes have occurred

• To report any pain, redness, or hard area usually in legs

• Stress patient compliance with medical regimen; bone marrow depression may occur

Lab test interferences:

Increase: Alk phosphatase, AST/ALT

False positive: RBC, Hgb

colestipol HCl

(koe-les'ti-pole)

Colestid

Func. class.: Antilipemic

Chem. class.: Bile sequestrant, resin exchange agent

Action: Absorbs, combines with bile acids to form insoluble complex that is excreted through feces; loss of bile acids lowers cholesterol levels

Uses: Primary hypercholesterolemia, xanthomas, digitalis toxicity, pruritus

Dosage and routes:

• *Adult:* PO 15-30 g/day in 2-4 divided doses

Available forms include: Susp

Side effects/adverse reactions:

GI: Constipation, abdominal pain, nausea, fecal impaction, hemorrhoids, flatulence, vomiting, steatorrhea

INTEG: Rash, irritation of perianal area, tongue, skin

*HEMA: Decreased vitamins A, D, K, **hyperchloremic acidosis***

Contraindications: Hypersensitivity, biliary obstruction

Precautions: Pregnancy (B), lactation, children, bleeding disorders

Pharmacokinetics:

PO: Excreted in feces

Interactions/incompatibilities:

• May reduce action of: thiazide, digitalis

• May reduce action of this drug: oral hypoglycemic agents

• Decreased action of: thiazide diuretics, digitalis

• Decreased action of this drug: oral hypoglycemics

NURSING CONSIDERATIONS

Assess:

• Cardiac glycoside levels, if both drugs are being administered

• For signs of vitamins A, D, K deficiency

• Serum cholesterol, triglyceride levels, electrolytes if on extended therapy

Administer:

• Drug ac, hs; give all other medications 1 hr before cholestyramine or 4 hr after cholestyramine to avoid poor absorption

• Drug sprinkled on food or stirred into beverage; let stand for 2 min

• Supplemental doses of vitamins A, D, K if levels are low

Evaluate:

• Therapeutic response: decreased triglycerides, cholesterol level (hyperlipidemia); diarrhea, pruritus (excess bile area)

• Bowel pattern daily; increase bulk, water in diet if constipation develops

Teach patient/family:

• Symptoms of hypothrombinemia: bleeding mucous membranes, dark tarry stools, petechiae; report immediately

• That patient compliance is needed since toxicity may result if doses are missed

• That risk factors should be decreased: high fat diet, smoking, alcohol consumption, absence of exercise

• That OTC preparations should be avoided unless directed by physician

Lab test interferences:

Increase: Liver function studies, chloride, PO$_4$

Decrease: Electrolytes ($^+$)

---

colistimethate sodium/ colistin sulfate

(koe-lis′ti-meth-ate)
Coly-Mycin M / Coly-Mycin S
Func. class.: Antibacterial
Chem. class.: Polymixin

Action: Interacts with phospholipids, penetrates cell wall; changes occur immediately in bacterial cytoplasmic membrane causing leakage of essential intracellular metabolites

Uses: Infections caused by *Pseudomonas, Enterobacter, E. coli, Klebsiella, Shigella, Brucella, Haemophilus, Salmonella,* some strains of *Proteus, Serratia, Bordetella, Vibrio, N. gonorrhoeae, N. meningitidis*

Dosage and routes:

• *Adult and child:* IM/IV 2.5-5 mg/kg/day in divided doses q6-12h, not to exceed 5 mg/kg/day in normal renal function

Shigella/E. coli

• *Infant and child:* PO 5-15 mg/kg/day in divided doses q6-8h

• *Child >1 month:* PO 8-25 mg/kg/day in divided doses q6-8h; IM/IV 15-40 mg/kg/day in divided doses q6h

Available forms include: Inj IM, IV 150 mg; oral powder for susp 25 mg/ml

Side effects/adverse reactions:

INTEG: Pruritus, urticaria, rash, pain at injection site

*HEMA: **Leukopenia, agranulocytosis***

GI: Nausea, vomiting, diarrhea, increased ALT, AST, abdominal pain, glossitis, colitis, *hepatotoxicity*

*RESP: **Arrest,** dyspnea*

*GU: **Oliguria, proteinuria, hematuria,** vaginitis, moniliasis, **glo-***

---

merulonephritis, acute tubular necrosis

CNS: Paresthesia, dizziness, ataxia, slurred speech, psychosis, *coma,* drug fever, confusion

EENT: Blurred vision

Contraindications: Hypersensitivity, severe renal disease

Precautions: Elderly, pregnancy

Pharmacokinetics:

IM: Peak 2 hr, duration <12 hr

IV: Peak 2 hr, duration <12 hr

Half-life 1½-8 hr IM, IV; 2-3 days PO, excreted in urine (active drug, metabolites)

Interactions/incompatibilities:

• Increased neurotoxicity, nephrotoxicity: cephalothin, aminoglycosides, amphotericin B, polymixin, vancomycin, capreomycin, methoxyflurane

• Increased neuromuscular blockade: tubocurarine, decamethonium, succinylcholine, gallamine

NURSING CONSIDERATIONS

Assess:

• Any patient with compromised renal system; drug is excreted slowly in poor renal system function; toxicity may occur rapidly

• Liver studies: AST, ALT

• Blood studies: WBC, RBC, Hct, Hgb, platelets, serum iron, reticulocytes; drug should be discontinued if bone marrow depression occurs

• Renal studies: urinalysis, protein, blood, BUN, creatinine

• C&S before drug therapy; drug may be taken as soon as culture is taken

• Drug level in impaired hepatic, renal systems

• B/P, pulse in patient receiving drug parenterally

Administer:

• IV by infusion only; do not administer bolus dose

• IM deep injection; rotate sites

• Orally with at least 8 oz water

Perform/provide:

• Storage of colistimethate sodium in refrigerator after reconstitution, use within 1 wk; colistin oral solution stored in refrigerator for up to 2 wk, protect from light

• Adrenalin, suction, tracheostomy set, endotracheal intubation equipment on unit; respiratory arrest has occurred following IM dose

• Adequate intake of fluids (2000 ml) during diarrhea episodes

Evaluate:

• Therapeutic response: decreased temperature, negative C&S

• Bowel pattern before, during treatment

• Skin eruptions, itching, dermatitis

• Respiratory status: rate, character, wheezing, tightness in chest

• Allergies before treatment, reaction of each medication; place allergies on chart, Kardex in bright red letters; notify all people giving drugs

Teach patient/family:

• To take oral drug with full glass of water; may give with food if GI symptoms occur

• Aspects of drug therapy: need to complete entire course of medication to ensure organism death (10-14 days); culture may be taken after completed course of medication

• To report sore throat, fever, fatigue; could indicate superimposed infection

• That drug must be taken in equal intervals around clock to maintain blood levels

• To wear or carry a Medic Alert ID if allergic to this drug

• To notify nurse of diarrhea stools

Treatment of overdose: Withdraw drug, maintain airway, administer epinephrine, aminophylline, O_2, IV corticosteroids

---

collagenase

(kol'la-je-nase)
Biozyme-C, Santyl
Func. class.: Topical enzyme preparation

Action: Effective in removing debris on skin by digesting collagen deposits
Uses: Debriding dermal ulcers, severely burned areas
Dosage and routes:
• *Adult and child:* TOP apply to lesion qd or qod
Available forms include: Top oint 250 U/g
Side effects/adverse reactions:
INTEG: Pain, burning, redness, irritation, hypersensitivity reactions
Contraindications: Hypersensitivity, elderly
Precautions: Pregnancy
Interactions/incompatibilities:
• Inhibited enzymatic activity of collagenase: benzalkonium chloride, hexachlorophene, nitrofurazone, iodine, heavy metal drugs
NURSING CONSIDERATIONS
Administer:
• After removing debris using hydrogen peroxide solution or modified Dakin solution; use sterile gauze to cover area
• As often as needed if area becomes soiled
• With tongue depressor or wooden spatula to deep wounds, use gauze for superficial wounds
• After covering healthy skin with a protectant such as petrolatum or zinc oxide paste
Perform/provide:
• Removal of gauze bandage, cream by applying mineral oil before cleaning area, make sure all cream is removed
Evaluate:
• Therapeutic response: separation of burn eschar; clean, pink ulcer area
• Area of body involved, including time involved, what helps or aggravates condition
Teach patient/family:
• To avoid application on normal skin or getting ointment in eyes
• To discontinue use if rash or irritation occur
• That healing may take 1-2 wk; use only until necrotic tissue is gone, healthy tissue is present

compound benzoin tincture

(ben'zoin)
Benzoin Spray
Func. class.: Emollient/protectant

Action: Decreases irritation, soothes skin
Uses: Cracked nipples, decubitus ulcers, fissures of lips, anus, croup, bronchitis
Dosage and routes:
• *Adult:* TOP apply qd-bid
• *Adult and child:* INH 1 tsp/pt boiling water, inhale vapors
Side effects/adverse reactions:
INTEG: Contact dermatitis
Interactions/incompatibilities:
None known
NURSING CONSIDERATIONS
Administer:
• After mixing with magnesium-aluminum hydroxide for decubitus ulcers
Perform/provide:
• Skin cleansing at least qd or more often if needed
Evaluate:
• Therapeutic response: smooth, moist skin, absence of fissures, ulcers
• For infection (increased temperature, redness), often bacteria are trapped underneath

Teach patient/family:
• To avoid inhaling vapors directly, may be added to boiling water for inhalation in croup, bronchitis

---

corn oil
Lipamul
Func. class.: Caloric

Action: Provides fat, calories needed for energy
Uses: Increased intake of calories
Dosage and routes:
• *Adult:* PO 45 ml bid-qid
• *Child:* PO 30 ml qd-qid
Available forms include: Oil 10 g/15 ml
Side effects/adverse reactions:
GI: Nausea, vomiting, diarrhea, anorexia
Precautions: Gall bladder disease, diabetes mellitus
Interactions/incompatibilities:
None known
NURSING CONSIDERATIONS
Assess:
• Urine, blood glucose levels if used for diabetic patient
Administer:
• With food or milk to decrease GI symptoms
Evaluate:
• Therapeutic response: increased weight
• Nutritional status: calorie count by dietician
Teach patient/family
• This treatment is short-term, not intended to replace normal nutritional intake

---

corticotropin (ACTH)
(kor-ti-koe-troe'pin)
ACTHAR, Cortigel-80, Cortrophin Gel, Cortrophin Zinc, Duracton,* H.P. Acthar Gel
Func. class.: Pituitary hormone
Chem. class.: Adrenocorticotropic hormone

Action: Stimulates adrenal cortex to produce, secrete corticosterone, cortisol
Uses: Testing adrenocortical function, treatment of adrenal insufficiency caused by administration of corticosteroids (long term), myasthenia gravis, multiple sclerosis
Dosage and routes:
Testing of adrenocortical function
• *Adult:* IM/SC up to 80 units in divided doses; IV 10-25 units in 500 ml D₅W given over 8 hr
Inflammation
• *Adult:* SC/IM 40 units in 4 divided doses (aqueous) or 40 units q12-24h (gel/repository form)
Available forms include: Inj IM, IV, SC 25, 40 U/vial
Side effects/adverse reactions:
INTEG: Impaired wound healing, rash, urticaria, hirsutism, petechiae, ecchymoses, sweating, acne, hyperpigmentation
CNS: Convulsions, dizziness, euphoria, insomnia, headache, mood swings, behavioral changes, depression, psychosis
HEMA: Agranulocytosis, leukopenia, thrombocytopenia
GI: Nausea, vomiting, peptic ulcer perforation, pancreatitis, distention, ulcerative esophagitis
MS: Myalgia, arthralgia
GU: Water, sodium retention, hypokalemia, menstrual irregularities
EENT: Cataracts, glaucoma
MS: Weakness, osteoporosis, compression fractures, muscle

---

atrophy, growth retardation in children, steroid myopathy

ENDO: Cushingoid symptoms, diabetes mellitus, antibody formation

Contraindications: Hypersensitivity, idiopathic thrombocytopenia, purpura, acute glomerulonephritis, scleroderma, osteoporosis, CHF, peptic ulcer disease, hypertension, systemic infections, small pox vaccination, recent surgery, ocular herpes simplex, primary adrenocortical insufficiency/hyperfunction

Precautions: Pregnancy, lactation, latent TB, hepatic disease, hypothyroiditis, child bearing-age women, psychiatric diagnosis, myasthenia gravis, acute gouty arthritis

Pharmacokinetics:

IV/IM/SC: Onset <6 hr, duration 2-4 hr, half life <20 min, excreted in urine

Interactions/incompatibilities:

• Possible ulceration: salicylates, alcohol, corticosteroids

• Hypokalemia: diuretics (K-depleting), amphotericin B

• Decreased anticoagulant's effect: when used with oral anticoagulants

NURSING CONSIDERATIONS

Assess:

• Baseline ECG, B/P, chest x-ray, GTT

• Pulse, B/P

• I&O ratio; weight q wk, report gain over 5 lb/wk

• 2 hr postprandial, chest x-ray, serum potassium, 17 KS, 17-OHCS, cortisol, during long-term treatment

Administer:

• Test for hypersensitivity for individuals allergic to pork products

• Decreased sodium, increase potassium for dependent edema

• Increase protein diet for nitrogen loss

• Gel at room temperature, give

deep IM using 21G needle

• May be used to treat edema

• IV for diagnostic purpose only

Perform/provide:

• Storage in refrigerator of unused portion; use within 24 hr

Evaluate:

• Therapeutic response: absence of inflammation, pain, increased muscle strength in myasthenia gravis

• Dependent edema, moon face, pulmonary edema, cerebral edema

• Infection; drug may mask infections

• Increased stress in patient's life that may require increased corticosteroids

• Mental status: affect, mood, increased aggressiveness, irritability; a change in mental status may require decreased steroids

• Growth rate of child

• Hypoadrenalism in neonates if drug was given during pregnancy

• Allergic reaction: rash, urticaria, fever, nausea, vomiting, dyspnea; drug should be discontinued immediately, administer epinephrine 1:1000

Teach patient/family:

• To avoid vaccinations during drug treatment

• To maintain adequate hydration up to 2000 ml/day unless contraindicated

• Avoid OTC products: salicylates, products with alcohol

• All aspects of drug: action, side effects, dose, when to notify physician

• Not to discontinue medication abruptly, thyroid crisis may occur; drug should be tapered off over several wk

• To wear Medic Alert ID specifying steroid therapy

• That drug does not cure condition, only decreases symptoms

• To notify physician of infection:

increased temperature, sore throat, muscular pain

• To tell patient to notify anyone involved in medical or dental care that this drug is being taken

---

cortisone acetate

(kor′-ti-sone)
Cortistan, Cortone

Func. class.: Corticosteroid, synthetic

Chem. class.: Glucocorticoid, short-acting

Action: Decreases inflammation by suppression of migration of polymorphonuclear leukocytes, fibroblasts, reversal of increased capillary permeability and lysosomal stabilization

Uses: Inflammation, severe allergy, adrenal insufficiency

Dosage and routes:

• *Adult:* PO/IM 25-300 mg qd or q2 days, titrated to patient response

Available forms include: Tabs 5, 10, 25 mg; inj IM 25, 50 mg/ml

Side effects/adverse reactions:

INTEG: Acne, poor wound healing, ecchymosis, bruising, petechiae

CNS: Depression, flushing, sweating, headache, mood changes

*CV: Hypotension, **circulatory collapse, thrombophlebitis, embolism,** tachycardia, **necrotizing angiitis, CHF***

*HEMA: **Thrombocytopenia***

MS: Fractures, osteoporosis, weakness

*GI: Diarrhea, nausea, abdominal distention, GI hemorrhage, increased appetite, **pancreatitis***

EENT: Fungal infections, increased intraocular pressure, blurred vision

Contraindications: Psychosis, hypersensitivity, idiopathic thrombocytopenia, acute glomerulonephritis, amebiasis, fungal infections, nonasthmatic bronchial disease, child <2 yr

Precautions: Pregnancy, diabetes mellitus, glaucoma, osteoporosis, seizure disorders, ulcerative colitis, CHF, myasthenia gravis

Pharmacokinetics:

PO: Peak 2 hr, duration 1½ days

IM: Peak 20-48 hr, duration 1½ days

Interactions/incompatibilities:

• Decreased action of this drug: cholestyramine, colestipol, barbiturates, rifampin, ephedrine, phenytoin, theophylline

• Decreased effects of: anticoagulants, anticonvulsants, antidiabetics, ambenonium, neostigmine, isoniazid, toxoids, vaccines

• Increased side effects: alcohol, salicylates, indomethacin, amphotericin B, digitalis preparations

• Increased action of this drug: salicylates, estrogens, indomethacin

NURSING CONSIDERATIONS

Assess:

• Potassium, blood sugar, urine glucose while on long-term therapy; hypokalemia and hyperglycemia

• Weight daily, notify physician of weekly gain >5 lb

• B/P q4h, pulse, notify physician if chest pain occurs

• I&O ratio, be alert for decreasing urinary output and increasing edema

• Plasma cortisol levels during long-term therapy (normal level: 138-635 nmol/L SI units if drawn at 8 AM)

Administer:

• After shaking suspension (parenteral)

• Titrated dose, use lowest effective dose

• IM inj deeply in large mass, rotate sites, avoid deltoid, use a 19G needle

• In one dose in AM to prevent ad-

---

renal suppression, avoid SC administration, damage may be done to tissue
• With food or milk to decrease GI symptoms
Perform/provide:
• Assistance with ambulation in patient with bone tissue disease to prevent fractures
Evaluate:
• Therapeutic response: ease of respirations, decreased inflammation
• Infection: increased temperature, WBC even after withdrawal of medication; drug masks symptoms of infection
• Potassium depletion: paresthesias, fatigue, nausea, vomiting, depression, polyuria, dysrhythmias, weakness
• Edema, hypotension, cardiac symptoms
• Mental status: affect, mood, behavioral changes, aggression
Teach patient/family:
• That ID as steroid user should be carried at all times
• To notify physician if therapeutic response decreases; dosage adjustment may be needed
• Not to discontinue this medication abruptly or adrenal crisis can result
• To avoid OTC products: salicylates, alcohol in cough products, cold preparations unless directed by physician
• Teach patient all aspects of drug usage, including Cushingoid symptoms
• Symptoms of adrenal insufficiency: nausea, anorexia, fatigue, dizziness, dyspnea, weakness, joint pain
Lab test interferences:
Increase: Cholesterol, sodium, blood glucose, uric acid, calcium, urine glucose
Decrease: Calcium, potassium, T_4, T_3, thyroid ^{131}I uptake test, urine

17-OHCS, 17-KS, PBI
False negative: Skin allergy tests

---

cosyntropin

(koe-sin-troe'pin)
Cortrosyn, Synacthen Depot*
Func. class.: Pituitary hormone
Chem. class.: Synthetic polypeptide

Action: Stimulates adrenal cortex to produce, secrete corticosterone, cortisol
Uses: Testing adrenocortical function
Dosage and routes:
• *Adult and child >2 yr:* IM/IV 0.25-1 mg between blood sampling
• *Child <2 yr:* IM/IV 0.125 mg
Available forms include: Inj IM, IV 0.25 mg/vial
Side effects/adverse reactions:
INTEG: Rash urticaria, pruritus, flushing
Contraindications: Hypersensitivity
Pharmacokinetics:
IV/IM: Onset 5 min, peak 1 hr, duration 2-4 hr
Interactions/incompatibilities:
None known
NURSING CONSIDERATIONS
Assess:
• Plasma cortisol levels at ½-1 hr after drug administered (>5 µg/dl is normal), at end of 1 hr, levels should have doubled
Administer:
• After reconstitution with 1 ml 0.9% NaCl/0.25 mg
Perform/provide:
• Storage at room temperature for 24 hr or refrigerated for 3 wk

cromolyn sodium

(kroe'moe-lin)
Opticrom
Func. class.: Ophthalmic
Chem. class.: Mast cell stabilizer

Action: Inhibits degranulation of mast cells after contact with antigens, which decreases release of histamine and SRS-A from mast cell
Uses: Vernal keratoconjunctivitis, conjunctivitis, vernal keratitis, allergic keratoconjunctivitis
Dosage and routes:
• *Adult:* INSTILL 1-2 gtts in both eyes q4-6h
Available forms include: Sol 40 mg/ml
Side effects/adverse reactions:
EENT: Stinging, burning, itching, lacrimation, puffiness
Contraindications: Hypersensitivity
Interactions/incompatibilities: None known
NURSING CONSIDERATIONS
Perform/provide:
• Storage at room temperature
Teach patient/family:
• To report stinging, burning, itching, lacrimation, puffiness
• Method of instillation, including pressure on lacrimal sac for 1 min, and not to touch dropper to eye
• Not to wear soft contact lens, use may be reinstituted 4-6 hr after therapy is discontinued

cromolyn sodium (disodium cromoglycate)

(kroe'moe-lin)
Intal, Intal p,* Nasalcrom, Rynacrom*

Func. class.: Antiasthmatic
Chem. class.: Mast cell stabilizer

Action: Inhibits histamine, slow-reacting substance of anaphylaxis from mast cells in respiratory tract; this decreases allergic response
Uses: Allergic rhinitis, severe perennial bronchial asthma, exercise-induced bronchospasm (prevention, treatment)
Dosage and routes:
Allergic rhinitis
• *Adult and child >5 yr:* INH 1 spray in each nostril tid-qid, not to exceed 6 doses/day
Bronchospasm
• *Adult and child >5 yr:* INH 20 mg <1 hr before exercise
Bronchial asthma
• *Adult and child >5 yr:* INH 20 mg qid; NEB 20 mg qid by nebulization
Available forms include: Sol 40 mg/ml; inh, caps for inh, 20 mg
Side effects/adverse reactions:
EENT: Throat irritation, cough, nasal congestion, burning eyes
CNS: Headache, dizziness, neuritis
GU: Frequency, dysuria
GI: Nausea, vomiting, anorexia, dry mouth, bitter taste
INTEG: Rash, urticaria, angioedema
MS: Joint pain/swelling
Contraindications: Hypersensitivity to this drug or lactose, child <5 yr, status asthmaticus
Precautions: Pregnancy, lactation, renal disease, hepatic disease
Pharmacokinetics:
INH: Peak 15 min, duration 4-6 hr,

---

italics = common side effects   **bold italic** = life threatening reactions

excreted unchanged in feces, half-life 80 min

Interactions/incompatibilities:
None known

NURSING CONSIDERATIONS
Assess:
• Eosinophil count during treatment

Administer:
• By inhalation/nebulizer only; not to be given PO
• Gargle, sip of water to decrease irritation in throat

Evaluate:
• Respiratory status: respiratory rate, rhythm, characteristics, cough, wheezing, dyspnea

Teach patient/family:
• To clear mucous before using
• Proper inhalation technique: exhale, using inhaler, inhale deeply, remove, hold breath, exhale, repeat until all of drug is inhaled
• That therapeutic effect may take up to 4 wk
• Not to swallow capsule

---

crotamiton
(kroe-tam′i-tonn)
Eurax
Func. class.: Scabicide
Chem. class.: Synthetic chloroformate salt

Action: Unknown, toxic to *Sarcoptes scabiei*
Uses: Scabies, pruritus
Dosage and routes:
• *Adult and child:* CREAM wash area with soap, water; remove visible crusts, apply cream, apply another coat in 24 hr, remove with soap, water in 48 hr; for pruritus, massage into affected area, repeat as necessary
Available forms include: Cream 10%; lotion 10%
Side effects/adverse reactions:
INTEG: Itching, rash, irritation,

contact dermatitis
Contraindications: Hypersensitivity, inflammation of skin, abrasions, or breaks in skin, mucous membranes

Precautions: Children, pregnancy
Pharmacokinetics: Not available
Interactions/incompatibilities:
None known

NURSING CONSIDERATIONS
Administer:
• After patient bathes with soap, water; remove all crusts
• To body areas, scalp only, do not apply to face, lips, mouth, eyes, any mucous membrane, anus, or meatus
• Topical corticosteroids as ordered to decrease contact dermatitis
• Lotions of menthol or phenol to control itching
• Topical antibiotics for infection

Perform/provide:
• Storage in tight, light-resistant container
• Isolation until areas on skin, scalp have cleared; treatment is completed

Evaluate:
• Area of body involved, including crusts, brownish trails on skin, itching papules in skin folds

Teach patient/family:
• Shake well before using
• To wash all inhabitants' clothing, using hot water, dryed in hot dryers for >20 min; preventative treatment may be required of all persons living in same house using lotion or shampoo to decrease spread of infection
• That itching may continue for 4-6 wk
• That drug must be reapplied if accidently washed off or treatment will be ineffective
• To avoid contact with eyes, face, meatus or mucous membranes or irritation may occur

cyanocobalamin (vitamin B₁₂)/hydroxocobalamin (vitamin B₁₂a)

(sye-an-oh-koe-bal'a-min)
Anacobin,* Bedoce, Bedoz,* Berubigen, Betalin-12, Crystimin, Cyanabin,* Kaybovit, Pernavite, Poyamin, Rubesol, Rubion,* Rubramin, Sigamine/Alpha Rediso, Alpha-Ruvite, Codroxomin, Droxomin, Neo-Betalin 12, Rubesol-LA

Func. class.: Vitamin B₁₂, fat-soluble vitamin

Action: Needed for adequate nerve functioning, protein and carbohydrate metabolism, normal growth, RBC development and cell reproduction

Uses: Vitamin B₁₂ deficiency, pernicious anemia, vitamin B₁₂ malabsorption syndrome, Schilling test, increased requirements with pregnancy thyrotoxicosis, hemolytic anemia, hemorrhage, renal and hepatic disease

Dosage and routes:
• *Adult:* PO 25 μg qd × 5-10 days, maintenance 100-200 mg IM q mo; IM/SC 30-100 μg qd × 5-10 days, maintenance 100-200 mg IM q mo
• *Child:* PO 1 μg qd × 5-10 days, maintenance 60 μg IM q mo or more; IM/SC 1-30 μg qd × 5-10 days, maintenance 60 μg IM q mo or more

Pernicious anemia/malabsorption syndrome
• *Adult:* IM 100-1000 μg qd × 2 wk, then 100-1000 μg IM q mo
• *Child:* IM 1000-5000 μg over 2 wk or more given in 100-500 μg doses, then 60 μg IM/SC monthly

Schilling test
• *Adult and child:* IM 1000 μg in one dose

Available forms include: Tabs 25, 50, 100, 250, 500, 1000 μg; inj IM 100, 120, 1000 μg/ml

Side effects/adverse reactions:
CNS: Flushing, optic nerve atrophy
GI: Diarrhea
CV: **CHF,** peripheral vascular thrombosis, pulmonary edema
INTEG: Itching, rash
META: Hypokalemia

Contraindications: Hypersensitivity, optic nerve atrophy

Precautions: Pregnancy, lactation, children

Pharmacokinetics: Stored in liver, kidneys, stomach; 50%-90% excreted in urine; crosses placenta, breast milk

Interactions/incompatibilities:
• Decreased absorption: aminoglycosides, anticonvulsants, colchicine, chloramphenicol, aminosalicylic acid, potassium preparation
• Increased absorption: prednisone

NURSING CONSIDERATIONS
Assess:
• GI function: diarrhea, constipation
• Potassium levels during beginning treatment
• CBC for increase in reticulocyte count during 1st week of therapy, then increase in RBC and hemoglobin

Administer:
• With fruit juice to disguise taste
• With meals if possible for better absorption
• By IM injection for pernicious anemia unless contraindicated

Evaluate:
• Therapeutic response: decreased anorexia, dyspnea on excretion palpitations, paresthesias, psychosis, visual disturbances
• Nutritional status: egg yolks, fish, organ meats, dairy products, clams, oysters, which are good sources for vitamin B₁₂
• For pulmonary edema, or worsening of CHF in cardiac patients

C

Teach patient/family
• That treatment must continue for life if diagnosed as having pernicious anemia
• Well balanced diet
• Avoid contact with persons with infection

Lab test interferences:
False positive: Intrinsic factor
Treatment of overdose: Discontinue drug

---

cyclacillin
(sye-kla-sill'in)
Cyclapen-W
Func. class.: Broad-spectrum antibiotic
Chem. class.: Aminopenicillin

Action: Interferes with cell wall replication of susceptible organisms; osmotically unstable cell wall swells, bursts from osmotic pressure

Uses: Otitis media and skin, soft tissue, urinary tract, respiratory tract infections by gram-positive cocci *(S. aureus, S. pneumoniae)*, gram-negative cocci, gram-negative bacilli *(E. coli, H. influenzae, P. mirabilis)*

Dosage and routes:
• *Adult:* PO 250-500 mg q6h
• *Child:* PO 50-100 mg/kg/day q6h in equally divided doses
Available forms include: Tabs 250, 500 mg; powder for oral susp 125, 250 mg/5 ml

Side effects/adverse reactions:
HEMA: Anemia, increased bleeding time, *bone marrow depression, granulocytopenia*
GI: Nausea, vomiting, diarrhea, increased AST, ALT, abdominal pain, glossitis, colitis
GU: Oliguria, proteinuria, hematuria, *vaginitis, moniliasis, glomerulonephritis*
CNS: Lethargy, hallucinations, anxiety, depression, twitching, *coma, convulsions*
META: Hyperkalemia, hypokalemia, alkalosis, hypernatremia
Contraindications: Hypersensitivity to penicillins
Precautions: Hypersensitivity to cephalosporins, child <2 mo

Pharmacokinetics:
PO: peak 40-60 min, half-life 30-40 min, metabolized in liver, excreted in urine (unchanged)

Interactions/incompatibilities:
• Decreased antimicrobial effectiveness of this drug: tetracyclines, erythromycins
• Increased penicillin concentrations when used with: aspirin, probenecid

NURSING CONSIDERATIONS
Assess:
• I&O ratio; report hematuria, oliguria since penicillin in high doses is nephrotoxic
• Any patient with compromised renal system since drug is excreted slowly in poor renal system function; toxicity may occur rapidly
• Liver studies: AST, ALT
• Blood studies: WBC, RBC, H&H, bleeding time
• Renal studies: urinalysis, protein, blood
• C&S before drug therapy; drug may be taken as soon as culture is taken

Administer:
• Drug after C&S has been completed

Perform/provide:
• Adrenalin, suction, tracheostomy set, endotracheal intubation equipment
• Adequate fluid intake (2000 ml) during diarrhea episodes
• Scratch test to assess allergy, after securing order from physician; usually done when penicillin is only drug of choice

• Storage in tight container; after reconstituting, store in refrigerator
Evaluate:
• Therapeutic effectiveness: absence of fever, draining wounds
• Bowel pattern before, during treatment
• Skin eruptions after administration of penicillin to 1 wk after discontinuing drug
• Respiratory status: rate, character, wheezing, tightness in chest
• Allergies before initiation of treatment, reaction of each medication; highlight allergies on chart, Kardex
Teach patient/family:
• Aspects of drug therapy, including need to complete course of medication to ensure organism death (10-14 days); culture may be taken after completed course
• To report sore throat, fever, fatigue; could indicate superimposed infection
• To wear or carry Medic Alert ID if allergic to penicillins
• To notify nurse of diarrhea stools
Lab test interferences:
Decrease: Uric acid
False positive: Urine glucose, urine protein
Treatment of overdose: Withdraw drug, maintain airway, administer epinephrine, aminophylline, O_2, IV corticosteroids for anaphylaxis

---

cyclandelate
(sye-klan'da-late)
Cyclospasmol
Func. class.: Peripheral vasodilator
Chem. class.: Nonnitrate

Action: Relaxes vascular smooth muscle, dilates peripheral vascular smooth muscle by direct action
Uses: Angina, intermittent claudication, arteriosclerosis, thrombophlebitis, Raynaud's phenomenon, ischemic cerebrovascular disease
Dosage and routes:
• *Adult:* PO 200 mg qid, not to exceed 400 mg qid; maintenance dose is 400-800 mg/day in 2-4 divided doses
Available forms include: Tabs 100, 200 mg; caps 200, 400 mg
Side effects/adverse reactions:
HEMA: Increased bleeding time (rare)
*CV: **Tachycardia***
CNS: Headache, paresthesias, dizziness, weakness
GI: Heartburn, eructation, nausea, pyrosis
INTEG: Sweating, flushing
Contraindications: Hypersensitivity, severe obliterative coronary artery or cerebrovascular disease
Precautions: Glaucoma, pregnancy/lactation, recent MI, hypertension
Pharmacokinetics:
PO: Onset 15 min, peak 1½ hr, duration 4 hr
Interactions/incompatibilities:
None known

NURSING CONSIDERATIONS
Assess:
• Bleeding time in individuals with bleeding disorders
Administer:
• With meals to reduce GI symptoms
Perform/provide:
• Storage in tight container at room temperature
Evaluate:
• Therapeutic response: ability to walk without pain, increased temperature in extremities, increased pulse volume
• Cardiac status: B/P, pulse, rate, rhythm, character; watch for increasing pulse
Teach patient/family:
• That medication is not cure, may need to be taken continuously

---

italics = common side effects   ***bold italic*** = life threatening reactions

• That it is necessary to quit smoking to prevent excessive vasoconstriction
• That improvement may be sudden, but usually occurs gradually over several weeks
• To report headache, weakness, increased pulse, as drug may need to be decreased or discontinued
• To avoid hazardous activities until stabilized on medication; dizziness may occur

---

cyclizine HCl, cyclizine lactate

(sye'kli-zeen)

Marezine, Marzine, Meclizine

Func. class.: Antiemetic, antihistamine

Chem. class.: H_2-receptor antagonist, piperazine derivative

Action: Acts centrally by blocking chemoreceptor trigger zone, which in turn acts on vomiting center
Uses: Motion sickness, prevention of postoperative vomiting
Dosage and routes:
Vomiting
• *Adult:* IM 50 mg ½ hr before termination of surgery, then q4-6h prn (lactate)
• *Child:* IM 3 mg/kg divided in 3 equal doses
Motion sickness
• *Adult:* PO 50 mg then q4-6h prn, not to exceed 200 mg/day (HCl)
• *Child:* PO 25 mg q4-6h prn
Available forms include: Tabs 50 mg; inj 50 mg/ml
Side effects/adverse reactions:
CNS: Drowsiness, dizziness, fatigue, restlessness, headache, insomnia
GI: Nausea, anorexia
EENT: Dry mouth, blurred vision
Contraindications: Hypersensitivity to cyclizines, shock, lactation, pregnancy

Precautions: Children, narrow-angle glaucoma, urinary retention, lactation, prostatic hypertrophy, elderly, pregnancy
Pharmacokinetics:
PO: Duration 4-6 hr, other pharmacokinetics not known
Interactions/incompatibilities:
• May increase effect of: alcohol, tranquilizers, narcotics
NURSING CONSIDERATIONS
Assess:
• VS, B/P; check patients with cardiac disease more often
Administer:
• IM injection in large muscle mass, aspirate to avoid IV administration
• Tablets may be swallowed whole, chewed, or allowed to dissolve
Evaluate:
• Signs of toxicity of other drugs or masking of symptoms of disease: brain tumor, intestinal obstruction
• Observe for drowsiness, dizziness
Teach patient/family:
• That a false negative result may occur with skin testing; skin testing procedures should not be scheduled for 4 days after discontinuing use
• To avoid hazardous activities or activities requiring alertness; dizziness may occur; instruct patient to request assistance with ambulation
• Avoid alcohol, other depressants
Lab test interferences:
False negative: Allergy skin testing

---

cyclobenzaprine

(sye-kloe-ben'za-preen)

Flexeril

Func. class.: Skeletal muscle relaxant, central acting
Chem. class.: Tricyclic amine salt

Action: Unknown; may be related to antidepressant effects

Uses: Relieving pain in musculo-skeletal conditions

Dosage and routes:

• *Adult:* PO 10 mg tid × 1 wk, not to exceed 60 mg/day × 3 wk

Side effects/adverse reactions:

CNS: Dizziness, weakness, drowsiness, headache, tremor, depression, insomnia

EENT: Diplopia, temporary loss of vision

CV: Postural hypotension, tachycardia

GI: Nausea, vomiting, hiccups, dry mouth

INTEG: Rash, pruritus, fever, facial flushing

Contraindications: Hypersensitivity, child <12 yr, intermittent porphyria, thyroid disease

Precautions: Renal disease, hepatic disease, addictive personalities

Pharmacokinetics:

PO: Onset 1 hr, peak 3-8 hr, duration 12-24 hr, half-life 1-3 days, metabolized by liver, excreted in urine, crosses placenta, excreted in breast milk

Interactions/incompatibilities:

• Increased CNS depression: alcohol, tricylic antidepressants, narcotics, barbiturates, sedatives, hypnotics

NURSING CONSIDERATIONS

Assess:

• Blood studies: CBC, WBC, differential; blood dyscrasias may occur

• Liver function studies: AST, ALT, alk phosphatase; hepatitis may occur

• ECG in epileptic patients; poor seizure control has occurred in patients taking this drug

Administer:

• With meals for GI symptoms

Perform/provide:

• Storage in tight container at room temperature

• Assistance with ambulation if dizziness, drowsiness occurs

Evaluate:

• Therapeutic response: decreased pain, spasticity

• Allergic reactions: rash, fever, respiratory distress

• Severe weakness, numbness in extremities

• Psychologic dependency: increased need for medication, more frequent requests for medication, increased pain

• CNS depression: dizziness, drowsiness, psychiatric symptoms

Teach patient/family:

• Not to discontinue medication quickly; insomnia, nausea, headache, spasticity, tachycardia will occur; drug should be tapered off over 1-2 wk

• Not to take with alcohol, other CNS depressants

• To avoid altering activities while taking this drug

• To avoid hazardous activities if drowsiness, dizziness occurs

• To avoid using OTC medication: cough preparations, antihistamines, unless directed by physician

Treatment of overdose: Empty stomach with emesis, gastric lavage, then administer activated charcoal; use anticonvulsants if indicated; monitor cardiac function

---

cyclopentolate HCl (optic)

(sye-kloe-pen'toe-late)

AK-Pentolate, Cyclogyl, Mydplegic*

Func. class.: Mydriatic, cycloplegic, anticholinergic

Action: Blocks response of iris sphincter muscle, muscle of accommodation of ciliary body to cholinergic stimulation, resulting

---

in dilation, paralysis of accommodation

Uses: Cycloplegic refraction, mydriasis

Dosage and routes:

• *Adult:* INSTILL SOL 1 gtt of a 1% sol, then 1 gtt in 5 min

• *Child >6 yr:* INSTILL SOL 1 gtt of a 0.5%-2% sol, then 1 gtt in 5 min of a 0.5%-1% sol

Available forms include: Sol 0.5%, 1%, 2%

Side effects/adverse reactions:

SYST: Tachycardia, confusion, fever, flushing, dry skin, dry mouth, abdominal discomfort (infants: bladder distention, irregular pulse, *respiratory depression)*

EENT: Blurred vision, temporary burning sensation on instillation, eye dryness, photophobia, conjunctivitism, increased intraocular pressure

CNS: Psychotic reaction, behavior disturbances, ataxia, restlessness, hallucinations, somnolence, disorientation, failure to recognize people, *grand mal seizures*

GI: Abdominal distention, vomiting

Contraindications: Hypersensitivity, infants <3 mo, local or systemic glaucoma, conjunctivitis

Pharmacokinetics:

INSTILL: Peak 30-60 min (mydriasis), 25-74 min (cyclopegia), duration ¼-1 day

Interactions/incompatibilities:
None known

NURSING CONSIDERATIONS
Administer:

• After shaking vial to mix drug to clear solution, push stopper to mix sterile water with powder

• After cleaning stopper with alcohol (rubbing)

• Immediately after reconstituting, discard unused portion

Teach patient/family:

• To report change in vision, blur-

ring, or loss of sight, trouble breathing, sweating, flushing

• Method of instillation: pressure on lacrimal sac for 1 min, do not touch dropper to eye

• That blurred vision will decrease with repeated use of drug

• That drug will burn when instilled

• Wear dark sunglasses for photophobia

• Not to do hazardous duties until able to see

---

cyclophosphamide

(sye-kloe-foss'fa-mide)
Cytoxan, Neosar, Procytox*

Func. class.: Antineoplastic alkylating agent

Chem. class.: Nitrogen mustard

Action: Alkylates DNA, RNA; inhibits enzymes that allow synthesis of amino acids in proteins; is also responsible for cross linking DNA strands

Uses: Hodgkin's disease, lymphomas, leukemia, cancer of female reproductive tract

Dosage and routes:

• *Adult:* PO initially 1-5 mg/kg over 2-5 days, maintenance is 1-5 mg/kg; IV initially 40-50 mg/kg in divided doses over 2-5 days, maintenance 10-15 mg/kg q7-10d, or 3-5 mg/kg q3d

• *Child:* PO/IV 2-8 mg/kg or 60-250 mg/m^2 in divided doses for 6 or more days; maintenance 10-15 mg/kg q7-10d or 30 mg/kg q3-4w; dose should be reduced by half when bone marrow depression occurs

Available forms include: Powder for inj IV 100, 200, 500 mg, 1, 2 g; tabs 25, 50 mg

Side effects/adverse reactions:

CV: Cardiotoxicity (high doses)

HEMA: Thrombocytopenia, leuko-

penia, pancytopenia
GI: Nausea, vomiting, diarrhea, weight loss, colitis, ***hepatotoxicity***
GU: Hemorrhagic cystitis, hematuria, neoplasms, amenorrhea, azoospermia, impotence, sterility, ovarian fibrosis
INTEG: Alopecia, dermatitis
*RESP: **Fibrosis***
CNS: Headache, dizziness
Contraindications: Lactation
Precautions: Radiation therapy, pregnancy (1st trimester)
Pharmacokinetics:
Metabolized by liver, excreted in urine; half-life 4-6½ hr; 50% bound to plasma proteins
Interactions/incompatibilities:
• Increased toxicity: aminoglycosides
• Increased metabolism of this drug: phenobarbital
• Potentiation of this drug: succinylcholine
• Increased bone marrow depression: allopurinol
NURSING CONSIDERATIONS
Assess:
• CBC, differential, platelet count weekly; withhold drug if WBC is <4000 or platelet count is <75,000; notify physician of results
• Pulmonary function tests, chest x-ray films before, during therapy; chest film should be obtained q2wk during treatment
• Renal function studies: BUN, serum uric acid, urine CrCl before, during therapy
• I&O ratio; report fall in urine output of 30 ml/hr
• Monitor temperature q4h (may indicate beginning infection)
• Liver function tests before, during therapy (bilirubin, AST, ALT, LDH) as needed or monthly
Administer:
• Medications by oral route; if possible avoid IM, SC, IV routes to

prevent infections
• Antacid before oral agent, give drug after evening meal, before bedtime
• Antiemetic 30-60 min before giving drug to prevent vomiting
• Allopurinol or sodium bicarbonate to maintain uric acid levels, alkalinization of urine
• Antibiotics for prophylaxis of infection
• Slow IV infusion using 21-, 23-, 25-gauge needle
• Topical or systemic analgesics for pain
• Local or systemic drugs for infection
Perform/provide:
• Storage in tight container at room temperature
• Strict medical asepsis, protective isolation if WBC levels are low
• Special skin care
• Deep breathing exercises with patient tid-qid; place in semi-Fowler's position
• Liquid diet, including cola, Jello; dry toast or crackers may be added if patient is not nauseated or vomiting
• Increase fluid intake to 2-3 L/day to prevent urate deposits, calculi formation
• Diet low in purines: organ meats (kidney, liver), dried beans, peas to maintain alkaline urine
• Rinsing of mouth tid-qid with water, hydrogen peroxide; brushing of teeth bid-tid with soft brush or cotton-tipped applicators for stomatitis; use unwaxed dental floss
• Warm compresses at injection site for inflammation
Evaluate:
• Bleeding: hematuria, guaiac, bruising or petechiae, mucosa or orifices q8h
• Dyspnea, rales, unproductive cough, chest pain, tachypnea

• Food preferences; list likes, dislikes

• Effects of alopecia on body image, discuss feelings about body changes

• Yellowing of skin, sclera, dark urine, clay-colored stools, itchy skin, abdominal pain, fever, diarrhea

• Edema in feet, joint pain, stomach pain, shaking

• Inflammation of mucosa, breaks in skin

• Buccal cavity q8h for dryness, sores or ulceration, white patches, oral pain, bleeding, dysphagia

• Symptoms indicating severe allergic reaction: rash, pruritus, urticaria, purpuric skin lesions, itching, flushing

• Tachypnea, ECG changes, dyspnea, edema, fatigue

Teach patient/family:

• Of protective isolation precautions

• To report any complaints or side effects to nurse or physician

• That impotence or amenorrhea can occur, reversible after discontinuing treatment

• To report any changes in breathing or coughing

• That hair may be lost during treatment; a wig or hairpiece may make patient feel better; new hair may be different in color, texture

• To avoid foods with citric acid, hot or rough texture

• To report any bleeding, white spots or ulcerations in mouth to physician; tell patient to examine mouth qd

cycloserine

(sye-kloe-ser'een)
Seromycin Pulvules

Func. class.: Antitubercular
Chem. class.: S. oichidaceus, antibiotic

Action: Inhibits RNA synthesis, decreases tubercle bacilli replication

Uses: Pulmonary tuberculosis, extrapulmonary as adjunctive

Dosage and routes:

• *Adult:* PO 250 mg q12h × 14 days, then 250 mg q8h × 2 wk if there are no signs of toxicity, then 250 mg q6h if there are no signs of toxicity, not to exceed 1 g/day

Available forms include: Caps 250 mg

Side effects/adverse reactions:

INTEG: Dermatitis, photosensitivity

*CV: **CHF, dysrhythmias***

CNS: Headache, anxiety, drowsiness, tremors, *convulsions,* lethargy, depression, confusion, psychosis, aggression

EENT: Blurred vision, optic neuritis, photophobia, leukocytosis, tubular necrosis, hypokalemia, alkalosis

*HEMA: **Megaloblastic anemia,*** vitamin B_{12}, folic acid deficiency

Contraindications: Hypersensitivity, seizure disorders, renal disease, alcoholism (chronic)

Precautions: Pregnancy, children

Pharmacokinetics:

PO: Peak 3-4 hr; excreted unchanged in urine, crosses placenta, excreted in breast milk

Interactions/incompatibilities:

• Seizures: alcohol

• May increase toxicity: ethionamide, isoniazid, phenytoin

C

NURSING CONSIDERATIONS
Assess:
• Liver studies q wk: ALT, AST, bilirubin
• Renal status: before; q mo: BUN, creatinine, output, sp gr, urinalysis
• Blood levels of drug; keep at <30 $\mu m/ml$ or toxicity may occur
Administer:
• With meals to decrease GI symptoms
• Antiemetic if vomiting occurs
• After C&S is completed, q mo to detect resistance
• Pyridoxine if ordered to prevent neurotoxicity
Perform/provide:
• Storage in tight container at room temperature
Evaluate:
• Mental status often: affect, mood, behavioral changes, psychosis may occur
• Hepatic status: decreased appetite, jaundice, dark urine, fatigue
Teach patient/family:
• Avoid alcohol while taking drug
• That compliance with dosage schedule, length is necessary
• To report neurotoxicity: confusion, headache, drowsiness, tremors, paresthesias, mental changes
• To avoid hazardous activities if drowsiness or dizziness occurs
Lab test interferences:
Increase: AST/ALT
Treatment of overdose: Administer vitamin B_6, anticonvulsants, lavage, O_2, assisted respiration

---

cyclosporine
(sye′kloe-spor-een)
Sandimmune

Func. class.: Immunosuppressant
Chem. class.: Fungus-derived peptide

Action: Produces immunosuppression by inhibiting lymphocytes (T)

Uses: Organ transplants to prevent rejection
Dosage and routes:
• *Adult and child:* PO 15 mg/kg several hours before surgery, daily for 2 wk, reduce dosage by 2.5 mg/kg/wk to 5-10 mg/kg/day; IV 4-5 mg/kg several hours before surgery, daily, switch to PO form as soon as possible
Available forms include: Oral sol 100 mg/ml; inj IV 50 mg/ml
Side effects/adverse reactions:
GI: Nausea, vomiting, diarrhea, oral *Candida, gum hyperplasia, hepatotoxicity*
INTEG: Rash, acne, *hirsutism*
CNS: Tremors, headache
GU: Albuminuria, hematuria, proteinuria, renal failure
Contraindications: Hypersensitivity
Precautions: Severe renal disease, severe hepatic disease
Pharmacokinetics: Peak 4 hr, highly protein bound, half-life (biphasic) 1.2 hr, 25 hr; metabolized in liver, excreted in feces, crosses placenta, excreted in breast milk
Interactions/incompatibilities:
• Increased action of this drug: amphotericin B, cimetidine, ketoconazole
• Decreased action of this drug: phenytoin, rifampin
NURSING CONSIDERATIONS
Assess:
• Renal studies: BUN, creatinine at least monthly during treatment, 3 mo after treatment
• Liver function studies: alk phosphatase, AST, ALT, bilirubin
• Drug blood levels during treatment
Administer:
• For several days before transplant surgery
• With corticosteroids
• With meals for GI upset

• With oral nystatin for *Candida* infections

Evaluate:

• Hepatotoxicity: dark urine, jaundice, itching, light-colored stools; drug should be discontinued

Teach patient/family:

• To report fever, chills, sore throat, fatigue since serious infections may occur

• To use contraceptive measures during treatment, for 12 wk after ending therapy

---

cyclothiazide

(cye-kloe-thye′a-zide)

Anhydron, Fluidil

Func. class.: Diuretic

Chem. class.: Thiazide; sulfonamide derivative

Action: Acts on distal tubule by increasing excretion of water, sodium, chloride, potassium

Uses: Edema, hypertension, diuresis

Dosage and routes:

• *Adult:* PO 1-2 mg/day up to 4-6 mg/day

• *Child:* PO 0.02-0.04 mg/kg/day

Available forms include: Tabs 2 mg

Side effects/adverse reactions:

GU: Frequency, polyuria, uremia, glucosuria

CNS: Drowsiness, paresthesia, anxiety, depression, headache, dizziness, fatigue, weakness

GI: Nausea, vomiting, anorexia, constipation, diarrhea, cramps, pancreatitis, GI irritation, *hepatitis*

EENT: Blurred vision

INTEG: Rash, urticaria, purpura, photosensitivity, fever

META: Hyperglycemia, hyperuremia, increased creatinine

HEMA: Aplastic anemia, hemolytic anemia, leukopenia, agranulocytosis, thrombocytopenia

CV: Irregular pulse, orthostatic hypotension

ELECT: Hypokalemia, hypercalcemia, hyponatremia, hypochloremia

Contraindications: Hypersensitivity to thiazides or sulfonamides, anuria, renal decompensation

Precautions: Hypokalemia, renal disease, pregnancy, hepatic disease, gout, COPD, lupus erythematosus, diabetes mellitus

Pharmacokinetics:

PO: Onset 6 hr, peak 7-12 hr, duration 18-24 hr; excreted by kidneys, crosses placenta, enters breast milk

Interactions/incompatibilities:

• Increased toxicity: lithium, nondepolarizing skeletal muscle relaxants, digitalis

• Decreased effects of: antidiabetics

• Decreased absorption of thiazides: cholestyramine, colestipol

• Decreased hypotensive response: indomethacin

• Increased action of: quinidine

NURSING CONSIDERATIONS

Assess:

• Weight, I&O daily to determine fluid loss; effect of drug may be decreased if used qd

• Rate, depth, rhythm of respiration, effect of exertion

• B/P lying, standing; postural hypotension may occur

• Electrolytes: potassium, sodium, chloride; include BUN, blood sugar, CBC, serum creatinine, blood pH, ABGs

• Glucose in urine if patient is diabetic

Administer:

• In AM to avoid interference with sleep if using drug as a diuretic

• Potassium replacement if potassium is less than 3.0

• With food, if nausea occurs, absorption may be decreased slightly

---

Evaluate:
• Improvement in edema of feet, legs, sacral area daily if medication is being used in CHF
• Improvement in CVP q8h
• Signs of metabolic acidosis: drowsiness, restlessness
• Signs of hypokalemia: postural hypotension, malaise, fatigue, tachycardia, leg cramps, weakness
• Rashes, temperature elevation qd
• Confusion, especially in elderly; take safety precautions if needed

Teach patient/family:
• To increase fluid intake 2-3 L/day unless contraindicated, to rise slowly from lying or sitting position
• To notify physician of muscle weakness, cramps, nausea, dizziness
• Drug may be taken with food or milk
• That blood sugar may be increased in diabetics
• Take early in day to avoid nocturia

Lab test interferences:
Increase: BSP retention, calcium, amylase
Decrease: PBI, PSP

Treatment of overdose: Lavage if taken orally, monitor electrolytes, administer dextrose in saline

---

cyproheptadine HCI

(si-proe-hep'-ta-deen)
Periactin, Vimicon*
Func. class.: Antihistamine, H_1 receptor antagonist
Chem. class.: Piperidine

Action: Acts on blood vessels, GI, respiratory system by competing with histamine for H_1-receptor site; decreases allergic response by blocking histamine
Uses: Allergy symptoms, rhinitis, pruritus

Dosage and routes:
• *Adult:* PO 4 mg tid-qid, not to exceed 0.5 mg/kg/day
• *Child 7-14 yr:* PO 4 mg bid-tid, not to exceed 16 mg/day
• *Child 2-6 yr:* PO 2 mg bid-tid, not to exceed 12 mg/day
Available forms include: Tabs 4 mg; syr 2 mg/5 ml

Side effects/adverse reactions:
CNS: Dizziness, drowsiness, poor coordination, fatigue, anxiety, euphoria, confusion, paresthesia, neuritis
CV: Hypotension, palpitations, tachycardia
RESP: Increased thick secretions, wheezing, chest tightness
GI: Dry mouth, nausea, vomiting, anorexia, constipation, diarrhea
INTEG: Rash, urticaria, photosensitivity
GU: Retention, dysuria, frequency, increased appetite
EENT: Blurred vision, dilated pupils, tinnitus, nasal stuffiness, dry nose, throat, mouth

Contraindications: Hypersensitivity to H_1-receptor antagonist, acute asthma attack, lower respiratory tract disease

Precautions: Increased intraocular pressure, renal disease, cardiac disease, hypertension, bronchial asthma, seizure disorder, stenosed peptic ulcers, hyperthyroidism, prostatic hypertrophy, bladder neck obstruction, pregnancy (B)

Pharmacokinetics:
PO: Duration 4-6 hr, metabolized in liver, excreted by kidneys, excreted in breast milk

Interactions/incompatibilities:
• Increased CNS depression: barbiturates, narcotics, hypnotics, tricyclic antidepressants, alcohol
• Decreased effect of: oral anticoagulants, heparin
• Increased effect of this drug: MAOIs

---

italics = common side effects   ***bold italic*** = life threatening reactions

NURSING CONSIDERATIONS
Assess:
• I&O ratio; be alert for urinary retention, frequency, dysuria; drug should be discontinued if these occur
• CBC during long-term therapy
Administer:
• Coffee, tea, cola (caffeine) to decrease drowsiness
• With meals if GI symptoms occur; absorption may slightly decrease
Perform/provide:
• Hard candy, gum, frequent rinsing of mouth for dryness
• Storage in tight container at room temperature
Evaluate:
• Therapeutic response: absence of running or congested nose or rashes
• Respiratory status: rate, rhythm, increase in bronchial secretions, wheezing, chest tightness
• Cardiac status: palpitations, increased pulse, hypotension
Teach patient/family:
• All aspects of drug use; to notify physician if confusion, sedation, hypotension occurs
• To avoid driving or other hazardous activity if drowsiness occurs
• To avoid concurrent use of alcohol or other CNS depressants
Lab test interferences:
False negative: Skin allergy tests
Treatment of overdose: Administer ipecac syrup or lavage, diazepam, vasopressors, barbiturates (short-acting)

---

cytarabine (ARA-C, cytosine arabinoside)
(sye-tare′a-been)
Cytosar-U
Func. class.: Antineoplastic, antimetabolite
Chem. class.: Pyrimidine nucleoside

Action: Competes with physiologic substrate that inhibits DNA synthesis; interferes with cell replication at S phase, directly before mitosis
Uses: Acute myelocytic leukemia, acute lymphocytic leukemia, chronic myelocytic leukemia, and in combination for non-Hodgkin's lymphomas in children
Dosage and routes:
Acute myelocytic leukemia
• *Adult:* IV INF 200 mg/m^2/day × 5 days; INTRATHECAL 5-50 mg/m^2/day × 3 days/wk or 30 mg/m^2/day q4 days
In combination
• *Child:* IV INF 100 mg/m^2/day × 5-10 days
Available forms include: Inj IV, intrathecal 100, 500 mg
Side effects/adverse reactions:
*HEMA: Thrombophlebitis, bleeding, **thrombocytopenia, leukopenia, myelosuppression, anemia***
*GI: Nausea, vomiting, anorexia, diarrhea, stomatitis, **hepatotoxicity,** abdominal pain, hematemesis, GI hemorrhage*
EENT: Sore throat, conjunctivitis
GU: Urinary retention, ***renal failure, hyperuricemia***
INTEG: Rash, fever, freckling, cellulitis
*RESP: **Pneumonia,** dyspnea*
CV: Chest pain, ***cardiopathy***
CNS: Neuritis, dizziness, headache, personality changes, ***coma***
CYTARABINE SYNDROME: Fever, myalgia, bone pain, chest pain,

rash, conjunctivitis, malaise (6-12 hr after administration)

Contraindications: Hypersensitivity, infants, pregnancy (1st trimester)

Precautions: Renal disease, hepatic disease, pregnancy (C)

Pharmacokinetics:

INTRATHECAL: Half-life 2 hr, metabolized in liver, excreted in urine (primarily inactive metabolite), crosses blood-brain barrier, placenta

IV: Distribution half-life 10 min, elimination half-life 1-3 hr

Interactions/incompatibilities:

• Increased toxicity: radiation or other antineoplastics

• Decreased effects of: oral digoxin

NURSING CONSIDERATIONS

Assess:

• CBC (RBC, Hct, Hgb), differential, platelet count weekly; withhold drug if WBC is <4000/mm,³ platelet count is <75,000/mm,³ or RBC, Hct, Hgb are low; notify physician of these results

• Renal function studies: BUN, serum uric acid, urine creatinine clearance, electrolytes before and during therapy

• I&O ratio; report fall in urine output to <30 ml/hr

• Monitor temperature q4h; fever may indicate beginning infection

• Liver function tests before and during therapy: bilirubin, ALT, AST, alk phosphatase, as needed or monthly

• Blood uric acid levels during therapy

Administer:

• Medications by oral route if possible; avoid IM, SC, IV routes to prevent infections

• Antiemetic 30-60 min before giving drug to prevent vomiting

• Allopurinol or sodium bicarbonate to maintain uric acid levels and alkalinization of the urine

• Antibiotics for prophylaxis of infection

• Slow IV infusion using 21-, 23-, 25-gauge needle

• Topical or systemic analgesics for pain

• Transfusion for anemia

• Antispasmodic for GI symptoms

Perform/provide:

• Strict medical asepsis and protective isolation if WBC levels are low

• Liquid diet: carbonated beverage, Jello; dry toast, crackers may be added when patient is not nauseated or vomiting

• Increase fluid intake to 2-3 L/day to prevent urate deposits and calculi formation, unless contraindicated

• Diet low in purines: absence of organ meats (kidney, liver), dried beans, peas to prevent increased urate deposits

• Rinsing of mouth tid-qid with water, hydrogen peroxide; brushing of teeth bid-tid with soft brush or cotton-tipped applicators for stomatitis; use unwaxed dental floss

• Warm compresses qid at injection site for inflammation, pain

• HOB increased to facilitate breathing if dyspnea or pneumonia occurs

Evaluate:

• Cytarabine syndrome: fever, myalgia, bone pain, chest pain, rash, conjunctivitis, malaise; corticosteroids may be ordered

• Bleeding: hematuria, guaiac, bruising or petechiae, mucosa or orifices q8h

• Dyspnea, rales, unproductive cough, chest pain, tachypnea, fatigue, increased pulse, pallor, lethargy, personality changes, with high doses

• Food preferences; list likes, dislikes

• Edema in feet, joint pain, stomach pain, shaking

• Inflammation of mucosa, breaks in skin

• Yellowing of skin, sclera, dark urine, clay-colored stools, itchy skin, abdominal pain, fever, diarrhea

• Buccal cavity q8h for dryness, sores or ulceration, white patches, oral pain, bleeding, dysphagia

• Local irritation, pain, burning, discoloration at injection site

• GI symptoms: frequency of stools, cramping

• Acidosis, signs of dehydration: rapid respirations, poor skin turgor, decreased urine output, dry skin, restlessness, weakness

Teach patient/family:

• Why protective isolation precautions are necessary

• To report any coughing, chest pain, or changes in breathing, which may indicate beginning pneumonia

• To avoid foods with citric acid, hot or rough texture if stomatitis is present

• To report stomatitis: any bleeding, white spots, ulcerations in mouth; tell patient to examine mouth qd, report any symptoms

---

dacarbazine (DTIC)

(da-kar′ba-zeen)
DTIC-Dome

Func. class.: Antineoplastic alkylating agent
Chem. class.: Cytotoxic triazine

Action: Alkylates DNA, RNA; inhibits enzymes that allow synthesis of amino acids in proteins; also responsible for cross-linking DNA strands

Uses: Hodgkin's disease, sarcomas, neuroblastoma, malignant melanoma

Dosage and routes:

• *Adult:* IV 2-4.5 mg/kg or 70-160 mg/m^2 qd × 10 days, repeat q4wk depending on response or 250 mg/m^2 qd × 5 days, repeat q3wk

Available forms include: Inj IV 100, 200 mg

Side effects/adverse reactions:

*HEMA: **Thrombocytopenia, leukopenia,** anemia*

*GI: Nausea, anorexia, vomiting, **hepatotoxicity***

CNS: Facial paresthesia, flushing, fever, malaise

INTEG: Alopecia, dermatitis, pain at injection site

Contraindications: Lactation

Precautions: Radiation therapy, pregnancy (1st trimester) (C)

Pharmacokinetics:

Metabolized by liver, excreted in urine; half-life 35 min, terminal 5 hr, 5% protein bound

Interactions/incompatibilities:

Decreased effectiveness of this drug: phenytoin, phenobarbital

NURSING CONSIDERATIONS

Assess:

• CBC, differential, platelet count weekly; withhold drug if WBC is <4000 or platelet count is <75,000; notify physician of results

• Monitor temperature q4h (may indicate beginning infection)

• Liver function tests before, during therapy (bilirubin, AST, ALT, LDH) as needed or monthly

Administer:

• Medications by oral route if possible; avoid IM, SC, IV routes to prevent infections

• Antiemetic 30-60 min before giving drug to prevent vomiting

• Antibiotics for prophylaxis of infection

• Slow IV infusion using 21-, 23-, 25-gauge needle

Perform/provide:

• Storage in light-resistant container, dry area

• Strict medical asepsis, protective

isolation if WBC levels are low
• Special skin care
• Liquid diet, including cola, Jello; dry toast or crackers may be added if patient is not nauseated or vomiting
• Increase fluid intake to 2-3 L/day to prevent urate deposits, calculi formation
• Warm compresses at injection site for inflammation

Evaluate:
• Bleeding: hematuria, guaiac, bruising or petechiae, mucosa or orifices q8h
• Food preferences; list likes, dislikes
• Effects of alopecia on body image, discuss feelings about body changes
• Yellowing of skin, sclera, dark urine, clay-colored stools, itchy skin, abdominal pain, fever, diarrhea
• Inflammation of mucosa, breaks in skin

Teach patient/family:
• Of protective isolation precautions
• To report any complaints or side effects to nurse or physician

---

dactinomycin (actinomycin D)

(dak-ti-noe-mye'sin)
Cosmegen
Func. class.: Antineoplastic, antibiotic

Action: Inhibits DNA, RNA, protein synthesis; derived from *Streptomyces parrullus;* replication is decreased by binding to DNA, which causes strand splitting; cell cycle nonspecific
Uses: Sarcomas, melanomas, trophoblastic tumors in women, testicular cancer, Wilms' tumor, rhabdomyosarcoma

Dosage and routes:
• *Adult:* IV 500 µg/m²/day × 5 days; stop drug for 2-4 wk; then repeat cycle
• *Child:* IV 15 µg/kg/day × 5 days, not to exceed 500 µg/day; stop drug until bone marrow recovery, then repeat cycle
Available forms include: Inj IV 500 µg

Side effects/adverse reactions:
*HEMA: **Thrombocytopenia, leukopenia, myelosuppression, aplastic anemia***
*GI: Nausea, vomiting, anorexia, stomatitis, **hepatotoxicity,** abdominal pain, diarrhea*
INTEG: Rash, alopecia, pain at injection site, folliculitis, acne
EENT: Chelitis, dysphagia, esophagitis
CNS: Malaise, fatigue, lethargy, fever
MS: Myalgia

Contraindications: Hypersensitivity, herpes infections, child <6 months
Precautions: Renal disease, hepatic disease, pregnancy (C), lactation, bone marrow depression
Pharmacokinetics: Half-life 36 hr; IV: onset 2-5 min, concentrates in kidneys, liver, spleen; does not cross blood-brain barrier, excreted in bile and urine
Interactions/incompatibilities:
• Increased toxicity: other antineoplastics or radiation

NURSING CONSIDERATIONS

Assess:
• CBC, differential, platelet count weekly; withhold drug if WBC is <4000/mm³ or platelet count is <75,000/mm³; notify physician of these results
• Renal function studies: BUN, serum uric acid, urine CrCl, electrolytes before, during therapy
• I&O ratio; report fall in urine output to <30 ml/hr

---

italics = common side effects   ***bold italic*** = life threatening reactions

• Monitor temperature q4h; fever may indicate beginning infection
• Liver function tests before, during therapy: bilirubin, AST, ALT, alk phosphatase, as needed or monthly

Administer:
• Medications by oral route if possible; avoid IM, SC, IV routes to prevent infections
• Antiemetic 30-60 min before giving drug to prevent vomiting
• Antibiotics as ordered for prophylaxis of infection
• Slow IV infusion using 21-, 23-, 25-gauge needle
• Topical or systemic analgesics for pain
• Local or systemic drugs for infection
• Transfusion for anemia
• Antispasmodic for GI symptoms

Evaluate:
• Bleeding: hematuria, guaiac, bruising, petechiae, mucosa or orifices q8h
• Food preferences; list likes, dislikes
• Effects of alopecia on body image; discuss feelings about body changes
• Edema in feet; joint, stomach pain; shaking
• Inflammation of mucosa, breaks in skin
• Yellowing of skin, sclera, dark urine, clay-colored stools, itchy skin, abdominal pain, fever, diarrhea
• Buccal cavity q8h for dryness, sores, ulceration, white patches, oral pain, bleeding, dysphagia
• Local irritation, pain, burning at injection site
• Symptoms indicating severe allergic reaction: rash, pruritus, urticaria, purpuric skin lesions, itching, flushing
• GI symptoms: frequency of stools, cramping

• Acidosis, signs of dehydration: rapid respirations, poor skin turgor, decreased urine output, dry skin, restlessness, weakness

Perform/provide:
• Strict medical asepsis, protective isolation if WBC levels are low
• Liquid diet: carbonated beverages, Jello; dry toast, crackers may be added if patient is not nauseated or vomiting
• Rinsing of mouth tid-qid with water, hydrogen peroxide; brushing of teeth bid-qid with soft brush or cotton-tipped applicators for stomatitis; use unwaxed dental floss
• Warm compresses at injection site for inflammation; check for extravasation
• Storage in darkness in cool environment

Teach patient/family:
• Why protective isolation precautions are necessary
• To report any complaints, side effects to nurse or physician
• That hair may be lost during treatment and wig or hairpiece may make patient feel better; tell patient that new hair may be different in color, texture
• To avoid foods with citric acid, hot or rough texture
• To report any bleeding, white spots, ulcerations in mouth to physician; tell patient to examine mouth qd

Lab test interferences:
Increase: Uric acid

---

danazol

(da′na-zole)
Cyclomen,* Danocrine

Func. class.: Androgen
Chem. class.: α-Ethinyl testosterone derivative

Action: Decreases FSH, LH, which are controlled by pituitary;

this leads to amenorrhea/anovulation, atrophy of endometrial tissue

Uses: Endometriosis, prevention of hereditary angioedema, fibrocystic breast disease

Dosage and routes:

Endometriosis

• *Adult:* PO initial dose 500 mg bid then decreased to 400 mg bid × 3-9 mo

Fibrocystic breast disease

• *Adult:* PO 100-400 mg qd in 2 divided doses × 2-6 mo

Hereditary angioedema

• *Adult:* PO 200 mg bid-tid until desired response, then decrease dose to 100 mg at 1-3 mo intervals

Available forms include: Caps 50, 100, 200 mg

Side effects/adverse reactions:

INTEG: Rash, acneiform lesions, oily hair, skin, flushing, sweating, acne vulgaris, alopecia, hirsutism

CNS: Dizziness, headache, fatigue, tremors, paresthesias, flushing, sweating, anxiety, lability, insomnia

MS: Cramps, spasms

CV: Increased B/P

GU: Hematuria, amenorrhea, vaginitis, decreased libido, decreased breast size, clitoral hypertrophy, testicular atrophy

GI: Nausea, vomiting, constipation, weight gain, *cholestatic jaundice*

EENT: Carpal tunnel syndrome, conjunctional edema, nasal congestion

ENDO: Abnormal GTT

Contraindications: Severe renal disease, severe cardiac disease, severe hepatic disease, hypersensitivity, pregnancy, lactation, genital bleeding (abnormal)

Precautions: Migraine headaches, seizure disorders

Pharmacokinetics:

Data unavailable

Interactions/incompatibilities:

• Increased effects of: oral antidiabetics, oxyphenbutazone

• Increased prothrombin time: anticoagulants

• Edema: ACTH, adrenal steroids

• Decreased effects of: insulin

NURSING CONSIDERATIONS

Assess:

• Semen q3-4 mo for count, viscosity, volume—especially adolescent

• Potassium, blood sugar, urine glucose while on long-term therapy

• Weight daily; notify physician if weekly weight gain is >5 lb

• I&O ratio; be alert for decreasing urinary output, increasing edema

• Growth rate in children since growth rate may be decreased when used for extended periods of time

• Liver function studies: AST, ALT, alk phosphatase

Administer:

• With food or milk to decrease GI symptoms

Perform/provide:

• Storage in tight container at room temperature

• ROM exercise for patients who are immobile

Evaluate:

• Therapeutic response: decreased pain in endometriosis, decreased size, pain in fibrocystic breast disease

• Edema, hypertension, cardiac symptoms, jaundice

• Mental status: affect, mood, behavioral changes, aggression, sleep disorders, depression

• Signs of virilization: deepening of voice, decreased libido, facial hair (may not be reversible)

• Hypercalcemia: GI symptoms, polydipsia, polyuria, increased calcium levels, decrease in muscle tone

Teach patient/family:

• To notify physician if therapeutic

D

---

response decreases
• Not to discontinue medication abruptly but to taper over several weeks
• Teach patient all aspects of drug usage
• Women to report menstrual irregularities, that amenorrhea usually occurs but menstruation resumes 2-3 mo after termination of therapy
• Routine breast self-exam, report any increase in nodule size
• Drug should induce anovulation; reversible within 60-90 days after drug is discontinued

Lab test interferences:
Increase: Cholesterol
Decrease: Cholesterol, T_4, T_3, thyroid ^{131}I uptake test, 17-KS, PBI
Interferes: GTT

---

dantrolene sodium

(dan'troe-leen)
Dantrium, Dantrium IV

Func. class.: Skeletal muscle relaxant, direct acting
Chem. class.: Hydantoin

Action: Contracts skeletal muscle directly by decreasing release of calcium in muscle
Uses: Spasticity in multiple sclerosis, stroke, spinal cord injury, cerebral palsy, malignant hyperthermia

Dosage and routes:
Spasticity
• *Adult:* PO 25 mg/day; may increase by 25-100 mg bid-qid, not to exceed 400 mg/day × 1 wk
• *Child:* PO 1 mg/kg/day given in divided doses bid-tid; may increase gradually, not to exceed 100 mg qid
Malignant hyperthermia
• *Adult and child:* IV 1 mg/kg, may repeat to total dose of 10 mg/kg; PO 4-8 mg/kg/day in 4 divided doses × 3 days to prevent further hyperthermia

Available forms include: Caps 25, 50, 100 mg; powder for inj IV 20 mg/vial
Side effects/adverse reactions:
CNS: Dizziness, weakness, fatigue, drowsiness, headache, disorientation, insomnia, paresthesias, tremors
EENT: Nasal congestion, blurred vision, mydriasis
CV: Hypotension, chest pain, palpitations
GI: Nausea, constipation, vomiting, increased AST, alk phosphatase, abdominal pain, dry mouth, anorexia
GU: Urinary frequency
INTEG: Rash, pruritus
Contraindications: Hypersensitivity
Precautions: Peptic ulcer disease, renal disease, hepatic disease, stroke, seizure disorder, diabetes mellitus
Pharmacokinetics:
PO: Peak 5 hr, highly protein bound, half-life 8 hr, metabolized in liver, excreted in urine (metabolites)
Interactions/incompatibilities:
• Increased CNS depression: alcohol, tricylic antidepressants, narcotics, barbiturates, sedatives, hypnotics
NURSING CONSIDERATIONS
Assess:
• For increased seizure activity in epilepsy patient; this drug decreases seizure threshold
• I&O ratio; check for urinary retention, frequency, hesitancy
• ECG in epileptic patients; poor seizure control has occurred with patients taking this drug
• Hepatic function by frequent determination of AST, ALT
Administer:
• With meals for GI symptoms

• Gum, frequent sips of water for dry mouth

Perform/provide:
• Storage in tight container at room temperature
• Assistance with ambulation if dizziness, drowsiness occurs

Evaluate:
• Therapeutic response: decreased pain, spasticity
• Allergic reactions: rash, fever, respiratory distress
• Severe weakness, numbness in extremities
• Psychologic dependency: increased need for medication, more frequent requests for medication, increased pain
• CNS depression: dizziness, drowsiness, psychiatric symptoms

Teach patient/family:
• Not to discontinue medication quickly; hallucinations, spasticity, tachycardia will occur; drug should be tapered off over 1-2 wk
• Not to take with alcohol, other CNS depressants
• To avoid altering activities while taking this drug
• To avoid hazardous activities if drowsiness, dizziness occurs
• To avoid using OTC medication: cough preparations, antihistamines, unless directed by physician

Treatment of overdose: Induce emesis of conscious patient, lavage, dialysis

---

dapsone (DDS)

(dap′sone)
Avlosulfon*
Func. class.: Leprostatic
Chem. class.: Sulfone

Action: Competitive inhibition of bacterial replication of folic acid from PABA

Uses: Leprosy

Dosage and routes:
• *Adult:* PO 100 mg qd with rifampin 600 mg qd × 6 mo

Available forms include: Tabs 25, 100 mg

Side effects/adverse reactions:
INTEG: Dermatitis, photosensitivity
CV: **CHF, dysrhythmias**
CNS: Headache, anxiety, drowsiness, tremors, **convulsions,** lethargy, depression, confusion, psychosis, aggression
EENT: Blurred vision, optic neuritis, photophobia, leukocytosis, tubular necrosis, hypokalemia, alkalosis
HEMA: **Megaloblastic anemia,** vitamin B_{12}, folic acid deficiency

Contraindications: Hypersensitivity to sulfones, renal amyloidosis, severe anemia

Precautions: Renal disease, hepatic disease, G-6-PD deficiency

Pharmacokinetics:
Rapid complete absorption 25-31 hr; highly bound to plasma protein

Interactions/incompatibilities:
• Increased action of this drug: probenecid, PABA, folic acid antagonists, rifampin

NURSING CONSIDERATIONS

Assess:
• Temperature, if <101° F, drug should be reduced
• Liver studies q wk: ALT, AST, bilirubin
• Renal status: BUN, creatinine, output, sp gr, urinalysis before; q mo
• Blood levels of drug

Administer:
• With meals to decrease GI symptoms
• Antiemetic if vomiting occurs
• After C&S is completed; q mo to detect resistance

Perform/provide:
• Infants to be kept with mothers infected with leprosy, breastfeed-

---

italics = common side effects   ***bold italic*** = life threatening reactions

ing during drug therapy is encouraged

Evaluate:

• Mental status often: affect, mood, behavioral changes; psychosis may occur

• Hepatic status: decreased appetite, jaundice, dark urine, fatigue

Teach patient/family:

• That therapeutic effects may occur after 3-6 mo of drug therapy

• That compliance with dosage schedule, length is necessary

• That scheduled appointments must be kept or relapse may occur

---

daunorubicin HCl

(daw-noe-roo'bi-sin)

Cerubidine

Func. class.: Antineoplastic, antibiotic

Chem. class.: Anthracycline glycoside

Action: Inhibits DNA synthesis, primarily; derived from *Streptomyces verticillus;* replication is decreased by binding to DNA, which causes strand splitting; cell cycle specific (S phase)

Uses: Myelogenous, monocytic leukemia, acute nonlymphocytic leukemia

Dosage and routes:

Single agent

• *Adult:* IV 60 mg/m^2/day × 3-5 day q4 wk

In combination

• *Adult:* IV 45 mg/m^2/day × 3 days, then 2 days of subsequent courses with cytosine arabinoside

Available forms include: Inj IV 20 mg

Side effects/adverse reactions:

HEMA: Thrombocytopenia, leukopenia, myelosuppression, anemia

GI: Nausea, vomiting, anorexia, mucositis, hepatotoxicity

GU: Impotence, sterility, amenor-

rhea, gynecomastia, hyperuricemia

INTEG: Rash, necrosis at injection site, dermatitis, reversible alopecia, cellulitis, thrombophlebitis at injection site

CV: CHF, cardiopathy

CNS: Fever, chills

Contraindications: Hypersensitivity, pregnancy (1st trimester), lactation, systemic infections

Precautions: Renal, hepatic, cardiac disease, gout, bone marrow depression

Pharmacokinetics: Half-life 18½ hr, metabolized by liver, crosses placenta, appears in breast milk, excreted in urine, bile

Interactions/incompatibilities:

• Increased toxicity: other antineoplastics or radiation

• Do not mix with other drugs in solution or syringe

NURSING CONSIDERATIONS

Assess:

• CBC, differential, platelet count weekly; withhold drug if WBC is <4000/mm^3 or platelet count is <75,000/mm^3; notify physician of these results

• Blood, urine uric acid levels

• Renal function studies: BUN, serum uric acid, urine CrCl, electrolytes before, during therapy

• I&O ratio; report fall in urine output to <30 ml/hr

• Monitor temperature q4h; fever may indicate beginning infection

• Liver function tests before, during therapy: bilirubin, AST, ALT, alk phosphatase as needed or monthly

• ECG; watch for ST-T wave changes, low QRS and T, possible dysrhythmias (sinus tachycardia, heart block, PVCs)

Administer:

• Medications by oral route if possible; avoid IM, SC, IV routes to prevent infections

• Antiemetic 30-60 min before giv-

ing drug to prevent vomiting
• Antibiotics for prophylaxis of infection
• Allopurinol or sodium bicarbonate to maintain uric acid levels, alkalinization of urine
• Slow IV infusion using 21-, 23-, 25-gauge needle; check for extravasation
• Topical or systemic analgesics for pain
• Transfusion for anemia
• Antispasmodic for GI symptoms
Evaluate:
• Bleeding: hematuria, guaiac, bruising or petechiae, mucosa or orifices q8h
• Food preferences; list likes, dislikes
• Effects of alopecia on body image; discuss feelings about body changes
• Edema in feet, joint, stomach pain, shaking
• Inflammation of mucosa, breaks in skin
• Yellowing of skin, sclera, dark urine, clay-colored stools, itchy skin, abdominal pain, fever, diarrhea
• Buccal cavity q8h for dryness, sores or ulceration, white patches, oral pain, bleeding, dysphagia
• Local irritation, pain, burning at injection site
• GI symptoms: frequency of stools, cramping
• Acidosis, signs of dehydration: rapid respirations, poor skin turgor, decreased urine output, dry skin, restlessness, weakness
• Cardiac status: B/P, pulse, character, rhythm, rate
Perform/provide:
• Strict medical asepsis and protective isolation if WBC levels are low
• Liquid diet: carbonated beverages, Jello; dry toast, crackers may be added if patient is not nauseated or vomiting

• Increased fluid intake to 2-3 L/day to prevent urate and calculi formation
• Diet low in purines: absence of organ meats (kidney, liver), dried beans, peas to maintain alkaline urine
• Rinsing of mouth tid-qid with water, hydrogen peroxide; brushing of teeth bid-qid with soft brush or cotton-tipped applicators for stomatitis; use unwaxed dental floss
• Warm compresses at injection site for inflammation; check for extravasation
• Storage at room temperature for 24 hr after reconstituting or 48 hr refrigerated
Teach patient/family:
• Why protective isolation precautions are necessary
• To report any complaints, side effects to nurse or physician
• That hair may be lost during treatment and wig or hairpiece may make patient feel better; tell patient that new hair may be different in color, texture
• To avoid foods with citric acid, hot or rough texture
• To report any bleeding, white spots, ulcerations in mouth; tell patient to examine mouth qd
• That urine may be red-orange for 48 hr
Lab test interferences:
Increase: Uric acid

---

deferoxamine mesylate

(de-fer-ox′a-meen)
Desferal
Func. class.: Heavy metal antagonist
Chem. class.: Chelating agent

Action: Binds iron ions (ferric ions) to form water-soluble complex that is removed by kidneys

Uses: Acute, chronic iron intoxication

Dosage and routes:

Acute

• *Adult and child:* IM/IV 1 g, then 500 mg q4h × 2 doses, then 500 mg q4-12h × 2 doses, not to exceed 15 mg/kg/hr or 6 g/24 hr

Chronic

• *Adult and child:* IM 500 mg-1 g/day plus IV INF 2 g given by separate line with each blood transfusion, not to exceed 15 mg/kg/hr or 6 gm/24 hr; SC 1-2 g over 8-24 hr by SC infusion pump

Available forms include: Powder for inj IV, IM, SC 500 mg/vial

Side effects/adverse reactions:

INTEG: Urticaria, erythema, pruritus, pain at injection site, fever

CV: Hypotension, tachycardia

GI: Diarrhea, abdominal cramps

EENT: Blurred vision, cataracts

MS: Leg cramps

GU: Dysuria, pyelonephritis

SYST: Anaphylaxis

Contraindications: Hypersensitivity, anuria, severe renal disease, child <3 yr

Precautions: Pregnancy, lactation

Pharmacokinetics:

Metabolized by plasma enzymes, excreted by kidneys as complex, unchanged drug

Interactions/incompatibilities:

None known

NURSING CONSIDERATIONS

Assess:

• VS

• I&O, kidney function studies: BUN, creatinine, CrCl

Administer:

• IV (used for shock) after diluting in D$_5$W or LR or NS; run at <15 mg/kg/hr; to be used only for short time; IM is preferred route

• IM after diluting with 2 ml sterile water for injection per 500 mg of drug; rotate injection sites

• Only when epinephrine 1:1000 is on unit for anaphylaxis

Evaluate:

• Allergic reactions: rash, urticaria; if these occur, drug should be discontinued

---

dehydrocholic acid

(dee-hye-droe-koe′lik)

Atrocholin, Cholan-DH, Decholin, Dycholium,* Hepahydrin

Func. class.: Laxative-stimulant
Chem. class.: Unconjugated oxidized acid

Action: Facilitates drainage from gallbladder by increasing volume, water content, flow of low-viscosity diluted bile

Uses: Constipation, biliary tract conditions

Dosage and routes:

• *Adult:* PO 250-500 mg bid-tid pc not to exceed 1.5 g/24 hr

Available forms include: Tabs 130, 250 mg; powder

Side effects/adverse reactions:

None known

Contraindications: Hypersensitivity, cholelithiasis, hepatic disease, obstruction in hepatic system, abdominal pain, nausea, vomiting

Precautions: Asthma, prostatic hypertrophy, hepatitis, child <12 yr, elderly, pregnancy

Pharmacokinetics:

PO: Concentrated in liver, excreted in bile

Interactions/incompatibilities:

None known

NURSING CONSIDERATIONS

Administer:

• During meals for better absorption

• Whole, not to be crushed or chewed

Perform/provide:
• Storage at room temperature
Evaluate:
• Bowel pattern before, after treatment, constipation; nausea, vomiting, abdominal pain, cramps; do not use if these occur
Teach patient/family:
• Not to use often, laxative dependency may occur
Lab test interference:
Interfere: BSP

---

demecarium bromide
(dem-e-kare′ee-um)
Humorsol, Tosmilen, Tonilen, Visumiotic
Func. class.: Miotic
Chem. class.: Cholinesterase inhibitor

Action: Produces intense miosis by constricting iris sphincter, also increases accommodation by contracting ciliary muscles; causing widening of trabecular network, resulting in decrease in intraocular pressure by facilitating aqueous humor outflow
Uses: Postiridectomy, glaucoma (open-angle), accommodative esotropia; also used following iridectomy, in management of esotropia
Dosage and routes:
• *Adult:* INSTILL 1-2 gtt of 0.125% or 0.25% sol up to bid
• *Child:* INSTILL 1 gtt of 0.125% sol in both eyes qd × 3-4 wk, then 1 gtt 2 ×/wk for up to 4 mo
Available forms include: Ophthalmic sol 0.125%, 0.25%
Side effects/adverse reactions:
GU: Frequency
CV: Hypotension, bradycardia, *cardiac arrest*
INTEG: Sweating, pallor, cyanosis
RESP: Bronchospasm
GI: Nausea, vomiting, abdominal cramps, diarrhea

EENT: Blurred vision, stinging, burning, lacrimation, lid muscle twitching, conjunctival, ciliary redness, browache, headache, induced myopia, iris cysts, hyperemia, hyphema
Contraindications: Hypersensitivity, retinal detachment, hypotension, CHF, bradycardia, recent MI, epilepsy, parkinsonism
Interactions/incompatibilities:
• Decreased effect of this drug: pilocarpine
• Increased effect of both drugs: ambenonium, edrophonium, neostigmine, physostigmine, pyridostigmine
• Increased effects of: general anesthetics
NURSING CONSIDERATIONS
Administer:
• Immediately after reconstituting, discard unused portion
• Gently remove (wipe away) any excess solution after administration to minimize/prevent any possible systemic absorption
Perform/provide:
• Storage in airtight containers
• Protect from light
• Always have atropine sulfate available for systemic toxicity
Teach patient/family:
• To avoid systemic absorption, press finger to lacrimal sac during, for 1-2 min after instillation
• Always wash hands before, after procedure
• To report change in vision, blurring or loss of sight, trouble breathing, sweating, flushing
• Method of instillation, including pressure on lacrimal sac for 1 min, not to touch dropper to eye
• That long-term therapy may be required
• That blurred vision will decrease with repeated use of drug
• That drug may be taken at night to minimize resulting visual effects

---

• To adhere to prescribed drug concentration to avoid systemic effects
• To avoid having skin come in contact with drug
• To avoid driving, to use caution during night vision

---

demeclocycline HCl

(dem-e-kloe-sye'kleen)
Declomycin, DMCT, Ledermycin

Func. class.: Broad-spectrum antibiotic/antiinfective
Chem. class.: Tetracycline

Action: Inhibits protein synthesis, phosphorylation in microorganisms by binding to 30S ribosomal subunits, reversibly binding to 50S ribosomal subunits

Uses: Gram-positive/gram-negative bacteria, protozoa, rickettsia, mycoplasma, diuretic, inappropriate ADH syndrome

Dosage and routes:
• *Adult:* PO 150 mg q6h or 300 mg q12h
• *Child >8 yr:* PO 6-12 mg/kg/day in divided doses q6-12h
Gonorrhea
• *Adult:* PO 600 mg, then 300 mg q12h × 4 days, total 3 g
Chlamydia trachomatis
• *Adult:* PO 300 mg qid × 7 days
Inappropriate ADH syndrome
• *Adult:* PO 600-1200 mg/day in divided doses
Available forms include: Tabs 150, 300 mg; caps 150 mg

Side effects/adverse reactions:
CNS: Fever, headache, paresthesia
HEMA: Eosinophilia, neutropenia, thrombocytopenia, leukocytosis, hemolytic anemia
EENT: Dysphagia, glossitis, decreased calcification of deciduous teeth, abdominal pain, oral candidiasis
GI: Nausea, vomiting, diarrhea, anorexia, enterocolitis, ***hepato-***

toxicity, flatulence, abdominal cramps, epigastric burning, stomatitis, ***psuedomembranous colitis***
CV: Pericarditis
GU: Increased BUN, polyuria, polydipsia, renal failure, nephrotoxicity
*INTEG: Rash, urticaria, photosenitivity, increased pigmentation, **exfoliative dermatitis,*** pruritus, angioedema

Contraindications: Hypersensitivity to tetracyclines, children <8 yr, pregnancy

Precautions: Renal disease, hepatic disease, lactation

Pharmacokinetics:
PO: Peak 3-6 hr, duration 48-72 hr, half-life 10-17 hr, excreted in urine, crosses placenta, excreted in breast milk, 36%-91% bound to serum protein

Interactions/incompatibilities:
• Decreased effect of this drug: antacids, $NaHCO_3$, dairy, alkali products
• Increased effect: anticoagulants
• Decreased effect: penicillins
• Nephrotoxicity: methoxyflurane

NURSING CONSIDERATIONS
Assess:
• I&O ratio
• Blood studies: PT, CBC, AST, ALT, BUN, creatinine
Administer:
• On empty stomach 1 hr ac or 2 hr pc with 8 oz of water
• After C&S obtained
• 2 hr before or after laxative or ferrous products; 3 hr after antacid
Perform/provide:
• Storage in tight, light-resistant container at room temperature
Evaluate:
• Therapeutic response: decreased temperature, absence of lesions, negative C&S
• Allergic reactions: rash, itching, pruritus, angioedema

• Nausea, vomiting, diarrhea; administer antiemetic, antacids as ordered
• Overgrowth of infection: increased temperature, malaise, redness, pain, swelling, drainage, perineal itching, diarrhea, changes in cough, sputum

Teach patient/family:
• To avoid sun exposure since burns may occur; sunscreen does not seem to decrease photosensitivity
• Of diabetic to avoid use of Clinistix, Diastix, or Tes-Tape for urine glucose testing
• That all prescribed medication must be taken to prevent superimposed infection
• To avoid milk products

Lab test interferences:
False positive: Urine glucose with Clinistix or Tes-Tape
False increase: Urinary catecholamines

---

deserpidine

(de-ser'pi-deen)
Harmonyl

Func. class.: Antihypertensive
Chem. class.: Antiadrenergic agent, rauwolfia alkaloid

Action: Inhibits norepinephrine release, depleting norepinephrine stores in adrenergic nerve endings
Uses: Hypertension, relief of symptoms in agitated psychotic states (e.g., schizophrenia) in patient unable to tolerate phenothiazines or who require antihypertensive medication

Dosage and routes:
Hypertension
• *Adult:* PO 0.25 mg tid, qid for up to 2 wk, then 0.25 mg qd maintenance; psychiatric dose: initial 0.5 mg/day (range 0.1-1 mg); do

not adjust dosage more frequently than 10-14 days
Available forms include: Tabs 0.1, 0.25 mg

Side effects/adverse reactions:
CV: Bradycardia, chest pain, dysrhythmias
CNS: Drowsiness, fatigue, lethargy, dizziness, depression, anxiety, headache, increased dreaming, nightmares, convulsions, Parkinson's, EPS (high doses)
GI: Nausea, vomiting, cramps, peptic ulcer, dry mouth, increased appetite, anorexia
HEMA: Prolonged bleeding time, *thrombocytopenia,* purpura
INTEG: Rash, purpura, alopecia, flushing, warm feeling, pruritus, ecchymosis
EENT: Lacrimation, miosis, blurred vision, ptosis, dry mouth, epistaxis, *glaucoma*
GU: Impotence, dysuria, nocturia, sodium, water retention, edema, breast engorgement, galactorrhea, gynecomastia
RESP: Bronchospasm, dyspnea, cough, rales

Contraindications: Hypersensitivity, depression/suicidal patients, active peptic ulcer disease, ulcerative colitis
Precautions: Pregnancy, lactation, seizure disorders
Pharmacokinetics:
PO: Onset is slow because several days are required to develop norepinephrine stores; half-life 50-100 hr, extensive metabolism by liver, crosses blood-brain barrier

Interactions/incompatibilities:
• Increased hypotension: diuretics, hypotension, beta blockers, methotrimeprazine
• Dysrhythmias: cardiac glycosides
• Increased cardiac depression: quinidine, procainamide
• Excitation, hypertension: MAOIs

• Increased CNS depression: barbiturates, alcohol, narcotics
• Decreased pressor effect: epinephrine, isoproterenol, norepinephrine
• Ephedrine, amphetamine

NURSING CONSIDERATIONS
Assess:
• Renal function studies in renal impairment (BUN, creatinine)
• Bleeding time, check for ecchymosis, thrombocytopenia, purpura
• I&O in renal disease patient

Evaluate:
• Cardiac status: B/P, pulse, watch for hypotension
• Edema in feet, legs daily; take weight daily
• Skin turgor, dryness of mucous membranes for hydration status
• Symptoms of CHF: edema, dyspnea, wet rales

Teach patient/family:
• To avoid driving, hazardous activities if drowsiness occurs
• Not to discontinue drug abruptly
• Not to use OTC products unless directed by physician: cough, cold preparations
• To report bradycardia, dizziness, confusion, depression, fever or sore throat
• That impotence, gynecomastia may occur but is reversible
• That therapeutic effects may take 2-4 wk

Lab test interferences:
Increase: VMA excretion, 5-HIAA excretion
Interferences: 17-OHCS, 17-KS
Treatment of overdose: Lavage, IV atropine for bradycardia, supportive therapy

desipramine HCl

(dess-ip'ra-meen)
Norpramin, Pertofrane
Func. class.: Antidepressant, tricyclic
Chem. class.: Dibenzazepine, secondary amine

Action: Blocks reuptake of norepinephrine, serotonin into nerve endings, increasing action of norepinephrine, serotonin in nerve cells
Uses: Depression
Dosage and routes:
• *Adult:* PO 75-150 mg/day in divided doses, may increase to 300 mg/day or may give daily dose hs
• *Adolescent/geriatric:* PO 25-50 mg/day, may increase to 100 mg/day
Available forms include: Tabs 10, 25, 50, 75, 100, 150 mg; caps 25, 50 mg
Side effects/adverse reactions:
*HEMA: **Agranulocytosis, thrombocytopenia, eosinophilia, leukopenia***
CNS: Dizziness, drowsiness, confusion, headache, anxiety, tremors, stimulation, weakness, insomnia, nightmares, EPS (elderly), increased psychiatric symptoms, paresthesia
GI: Diarrhea, dry mouth, nausea, vomiting, ***paralytic ileus,*** increased appetite, cramps, epigastric distress, jaundice, ***hepatitis,*** stomatitis
*GU: Retention, **acute renal failure***
INTEG: Rash, urticaria, sweating, pruritus, photosensitivity
*CV: Orthostatic hypotension, ECG changes, tachycardia, **hypertension,** palpitations*
EENT: Blurred vision, tinnitus, mydriasis, ophthalmoplegia
Contraindications: Hypersensitiv-

ity to tricyclic antidepressants, recovery phase of myocardial infarction, narrow-angle glaucoma, convulsive disorders, prostatic hypertrophy, child <12 yr

Precautions: Suicidal patients, severe depression, increased intraocular pressure, narrow-angle glaucoma, elderly, pregnancy (C)

Pharmacokinetics:

PO: Steady state 2-11 days; metabolized by liver, excreted by kidneys, crosses placenta, half-life 14-62 hr

Interactions/incompatibilities:

• Decreased effects of: guanethidine, clonidine, indirect acting sympathomimetics (ephedrine)

• Increased effects of: direct acting sympathomimetics (epinephrine) alcohol, barbiturates, benzodiazepines, CNS depressants

• Hyperpyretic crisis, convulsions, hypertensive episode: MAOI (pargyline [Eutonyl])

NURSING CONSIDERATIONS
Assess:

• B/P (lying, standing), pulse q4h; if systolic B/P drops 20 mm Hg hold drug, notify physician; take vital signs q4h in patients with cardiovascular disease

• Blood studies: CBC, leukocytes, differential, cardiac enzymes if patient is receiving long-term therapy

• Hepatic studies: AST, ALT, bilirubin, creatinine

• Weight qwk, appetite may increase with drug

• ECG for flattening of T wave, bundle branch block, AV block, dysrhythmias in cardiac patients

Administer:

• Increased fluids, bulk in diet if constipation, urinary retention occur

• With food or milk for GI symptoms

• Crushed if patient is unable to swallow medication whole

• Dosage hs if over-sedation occurs during day; may take entire dose hs; elderly may not tolerate once/day dosing

• Gum, hard candy, or frequent sips of water for dry mouth

Perform/provide:

• Storage at room temperature

• Assistance with ambulation during beginning therapy since drowsiness/dizziness occurs

• Safety measures including siderails primarily in elderly

• Checking to see PO medication swallowed

Evaluate:

• EPS primarily in elderly: rigidity, dystonia, akathisia

• Mental status: mood, sensorium, affect, suicidal tendencies, an increase in psychiatric symptoms: depression, panic

• Urinary retention, constipation; constipation is more likely to occur in children

• Withdrawal symptoms: headache, nausea, vomiting, muscle pain, weakness; do not usually occur unless drug was discontinued abruptly

• Alcohol consumption; if alcohol is consumed, hold dose until morning

Teach patient/family:

• That therapeutic effects may take 2-3 wk

• Use caution in driving or other activities requiring alertness because of drowsiness, dizziness, blurred vision

• To avoid alcohol ingestion, other CNS depressants

• Not to discontinue medication quickly after long-term use, may cause nausea, headache, malaise

• To wear sunscreen or large hat since photosensitivity occurs

Lab test interferences:

Increase: Serum bilirubin, blood

---

glucose, alk phosphatase
False increase: Urinary catecholamines
Decrease: VMA, 5-HIAA
Treatment of overdose: ECG monitoring, induce emesis, lavage, activated charcoal, administer anticonvulsant

---

desmopressin acetate

(des-moe-press'in)
DDAVP, Stimate
Func. class.: Pituitary hormone
Chem. class.: Synthetic antidiuretic hormone

Action: Promotes reabsorption of water by action on renal tubular epithelium, smooth muscles, causing constriction with a vasopressor effect
Uses: Hemophilia A, von Willebrand's disease, nonnephrogenic diabetes insipidus, symptoms of polyuria/polydipsia caused by pituitary dysfunction
Dosage and routes:
Diabetes insipidus
• *Adult:* INTRANASAL 0.1-0.4 ml qd in divided doses: IV/IM 0.5-1 ml qd in divided doses
• *Child 3 mo to 12 yr:* INTRANASAL 0.05-0.3 ml qd in divided doses
Hemophilia/von Willebrand's disease
• *Adult and child:* IV 0.3 μg/kg in NaCl over 15-30 min; may repeat if needed
Available forms include: INTRANASAL 0.1 ml; inj IV, IM 4 μg/ml
Side effects/adverse reactions:
EENT: Nasal irritation, congestion, rhinitis
CNS: Drowsiness, headache, lethargy, flushing
GU: Vulval pain
GI: Nausea, heartburn, cramps

CV: Increased B/P
Contraindications: Hypersensitivity, nephrogenic diabetes insipidus
Precautions: Pregnancy (B), CAD, lactation, hypertension
Pharmacokinetics:
NASAL: Onset 1 hr, peak 1-5 hr, duration 8-20 hr, half-life 8 min, 76 min (terminal), excreted in breast milk
Interactions/incompatibilities:
• Decreased response: anticoagulants, alcohol, lithium
• Increased response: carbamazepine, chlorpropamide, clofibrate, fludrocortisone
NURSING CONSIDERATIONS
Assess:
• Pulse, B/P when giving drug IV or IM
• I&O ratio; weight daily, check for edema in extremities; if water retention is severe, diuretic may be prescribed
Perform/provide:
• Storage in refrigerator or cool environment
Evaluate:
• Therapeutic response: absence of severe thirst, decreased urine output, osmolality
• Water intoxication: lethargy, behavioral changes, disorientation, neuromuscular excitability
• Intranasal use: nausea, congestion, cramps, headache, usually decreased with decreased dose
Teach patient/family:
• Technique for nasal instillation: to insert tube into nasal cavity to instill drug
• Avoid OTC products: cough, hayfever products since these preparations may contain epinephrine, decrease drug response; do not use with alcohol
• All aspects of drug: action, side effects, dose, when to notify physician

---

* Available in Canada only

• To wear Medic Alert ID specifying therapy

---

desonide

(dess'oh-nide)

Des Owen, Tridesilon

Func. class.: Topical corticosteroid
Chem. class.: Synthetic nonfluorinated agent, group IV potency

---

Action: Possesses antipruritic, antiinflammatory actions
Uses: Psoriasis, eczema, contact dermatitis, pruritus
Dosage and routes:
• *Adult and child:* Apply to affected area bid-tid
Available forms include: Cream 0.05%; oint 0.05%
Side effects/adverse reactions:
INTEG: Burning, dryness, itching, irritation, acne, folliculitis, hypertrichosis, perioral dermatitis, hypopigmentation, atrophy, striae, miliaria, allergic contact dermatitis, secondary infection
Contraindications: Hypersensitivity to corticosteroids, fungal infections
Precautions: Pregnancy (C), lactation, viral infections, bacterial infections
Interactions/incompatibilities: None known
NURSING CONSIDERATIONS
Assess:
• Temperature; if fever develops, drug should be discontinued
Administer:
• Only to affected areas; do not get in eyes
• Medication, then cover with occlusive dressing (only if prescribed), seal to normal skin, change q12h
• Only to dermatoses; do not use on weeping, denuded, or infected area

Perform/provide:
• Cleansing before application of drug
• Treatment for a few days after area has cleared
• Storage at room temperature
Evaluate:
• Therapeutic response: absence of severe itching, patches on skin, flaking
Teach patient/family:
• To avoid sunlight on affected area; burns may occur

---

desoximetasone

(des-ox-i-met'a-sone)

Topicort, Topicort LP

Func. class.: Topical corticosteroid
Chem. class.: Synthetic fluorinated agent, group II potency (0.25%), group III potency (0.05%)

Action: Possesses antipruritic, antiinflammatory actions
Uses: Psoriasis, eczema, contact dermatitis, pruritus
Dosage and routes:
• *Adult and child:* Apply to affected area bid-tid
Available forms include: Cream 0.05% (LP), 0.25%; oint 0.25%; gel 0.05%
Side effects/adverse reactions:
INTEG: Burning, dryness, itching, irritation, acne, folliculitis, hypertrichosis, perioral dermatitis, hypopigmentation, atrophy, striae, miliaria, allergic contact dermatitis, secondary infection
Contraindications: Hypersensitivity to corticosteroids, fungal infections
Precautions: Pregnancy (C), lactation, viral infections, bacterial infections
Interactions/incompatibilities: None known

---

italics = common side effects   ***bold italic*** = life threatening reactions

NURSING CONSIDERATIONS
Assess:
• Temperature; if fever develops, drug should be discontinued
Administer:
• Only to affected areas; do not get in eyes
• Medication, then cover with occlusive dressing (only if prescribed), seal to normal skin, change q12h; use occlusive dressing with extreme caution (group II potency)
• Only to dermatoses; do not use on weeping, denuded, or infected area
Perform/provide:
• Cleansing before application of drug
• Treatment for a few days after area has cleared
• Storage at room temperature
Evaluate:
• Therapeutic response: absence of severe itching, patches on skin, flaking
Teach patient/family:
• To avoid sunlight on affected area; burns may occur

---

desoxycorticosterone acetate/desoxycorticosterone pivalate
(des-ox-i-kor-ti-koe-ster'one)
Doca Acetate, Percorten Acetate/ Percorten Pivalate

Func. class.: Corticosteroid
Chem. class.: Mineralocorticoid

Action: Promotes increased reabsorption of sodium and loss of potassium from the renal tubules
Uses: Adrenal insufficiency, salt-losing adrenogenital syndrome
Dosage and routes:
• *Adult:* IM 2-5 mg qd (acetate); IM 25-100 mg q4wk (pivalate);

PELLET 1 pellet/0.5 mg of injected dose
Available forms include: Pellet 125 mg; inj IM 5 mg/ml
Side effects/adverse reactions:
INTEG: Acne, poor wound healing, petechiae, ecchymosis
CNS: Depression, flushing, sweating, headache, mood changes
*CV: Hypotension, **circulatory collapse, thrombophlebitis, embolism,*** tachycardia
*HEMA: **Thrombocytopenia***
MS: Fractures, osteoporosis, weakness
*GI: Diarrhea, nausea, abdominal distention, GI hemorrhage, increased appetite, **pancreatitis***
EENT: Fungal infections, increased intraocular pressure, blurred vision
Contraindications: Psychosis, hypersensitivity, idiopathic thrombocytopenia, acute glomerulonephritis, amebiasis, fungal infections, nonasthmatic bronchial disease, child <2 yr
Precautions: Pregnancy (C), diabetes mellitus, glaucoma, osteoporosis, seizure disorders, ulcerative colitis, CHF, myasthenia gravis
Pharmacokinetics:
IM: Duration 24-48 hr
Pellet: Duration 8-12 mo
Interactions/incompatibilities:
• Decreased action of this drug: cholestyramine, colestipol, barbiturates, rifampin, ephedrine, phenytoin, theophylline
• Decreased effects of: anticoagulants, anticonvulsants, antidiabetics, ambenonium, neostigmine, isoniazid, toxoids, vaccines
• Increased side effects: alcohol, salicylates, indomethacin, amphotericin B, digitalis preparations
• Increased action of this drug: salicylates, estrogens, indomethacin

D

NURSING CONSIDERATIONS
Assess:
• Potassium, blood sugar, urine glucose while on long-term therapy; hypokalemia and hyperglycemia
• Weight daily, notify physician of weekly gain >5 lb
• B/P q4h, pulse, notify physician if chest pain occurs
• I&O ratio, be alert for decreasing urinary output and increasing edema
• Plasma cortisol levels during long-term therapy (normal level: 138-635 nmol/L SI units when drawn at 8 AM)

Administer:
• Titrated dose, use lowest effective dose
• IM inj deeply in large mass, rotate sites, avoid deltoid, use 19G needle
• In one dose in AM to prevent adrenal suppression, avoid SC administration, damage may be done to tissue
• With food or milk to decrease GI symptoms

Perform/provide:
• Assistance with ambulation in patient with bone tissue disease to prevent fractures

Evaluate:
• Therapeutic response: ease of respirations, decreased inflammation
• Infection: increased temperature, WBC even after withdrawal of medication; drug masks symptoms of infection
• Potassium depletion: paresthesias, fatigue, nausea, vomiting, depression, polyuria, dysrhythmias, weakness
• Edema, hypotension, cardiac symptoms
• Mental status: affect, mood, behavioral changes, aggression

Teach patient/family:
• That ID as steroid user should be carried
• To notify physician if therapeutic response decreases; dosage adjustment may be needed
• Not to discontinue this medication abruptly or adrenal crisis can result
• To avoid OTC products: salicylates, alcohol in cough products, cold preparations unless directed by physician
• Teach patient all aspects of drug usage, including Cushingoid symptoms
• Symptoms of adrenal insufficiency: nausea, anorexia, fatigue, dizziness, dyspnea, weakness, joint pain

Lab test interferences:
Increase: Cholesterol, sodium, blood glucose, uric acid, calcium, urine glucose
Decrease: Calcium, potassium, T_4, T_3, thyroid ^{131}I uptake test, urine 17-OHCS, 17-KS, PBI
False negative: Skin allergy tests

---

dexamethasone
(dex-a-meth'a-sone)
Aeroseb-Dex, Decaderm, Deca-spray

Func. class.: Topical corticosteroid
Chem. class.: Synthetic fluorinated agent

Action: Possesses antipruritic, antiinflammatory actions
Uses: Corticosteroid-responsive dermatoses
Dosage and routes:
• *Adult and child:* TOP apply to affected area bid-qid
Available forms include: Gel 0.1%; aerosol 0.01%, 0.04%
Side effects/adverse reactions:
INTEG: Burning, dryness, itching, irritation, acne, folliculitis, hyper-

---

trichosis, perioral dermatitis, hypopigmentation, atrophy, striae, miliaria, allergic contact dermatitis, secondary infection

Contraindications: Hypersensitivity to corticosteroids, fungal infections, viral infections

Precautions: Pregnancy (C), lactation, viral infections, bacterial infections

Pharmacokinetics: Not known

Interactions/incompatibilities: None known

NURSING CONSIDERATIONS
Assess:
• Temperature, if fever develops drug should be discontinued

Administer:
• Only to affected areas, do not get in eyes
• Then cover with occlusive dressing if ordered, seal to normal skin, change q12h
• Only to dermatoses, do not use on weeping, denuded or infected area

Perform/provide:
• Cleansing before application of drug
• Treatment for a few days after area has cleared
• Storage at room temperature

Evaluate:
• Systemic absorption: fever, infection, irritation
• Therapeutic response: absence of severe itching, patches on skin, flaking

Teach patient/family:
• To avoid sunlight on affected area, burns may occur

dexamethasone
(dex-a-meth′a-sone)
Aeroseb-Dex, Decaderm, Decaspray

Func. class.: Topical corticosteroid
Chem. class.: Synthetic fluorinated agent, group V or VI potency

Action: Possesses antipruritic, antiinflammatory actions

Uses: Psoriasis, eczema, contact dermatitis, pruritus

Dosage and routes:
• *Adult and child:* Apply to affected area bid-qid

Available forms include: Gel 0.01%; aerosol 0.01%, 0.04%

Side effects/adverse reactions:
INTEG: Burning, dryness, itching, irritation, acne, folliculitis, hypertrichosis, perioral dermatitis, hypopigmentation, atrophy, striae, miliaria, allergic contact dermatitis, secondary infection

Contraindications: Hypersensitivity to corticosteroids, fungal infections

Precautions: Pregnancy (C), lactation, viral infections, bacterial infections

Interactions/incompatibilities: None known

NURSING CONSIDERATIONS
Assess:
• Temperature; if fever develops, drug should be discontinued

Administer:
• Only to affected areas; do not get in eyes
• Medication, then cover with occlusive dressing (only if prescribed), seal to normal skin, change q12h
• Only to dermatoses; do not use on weeping, denuded, or infected area

Perform/provide:
• Cleansing before application of drug
• Treatment for a few days after area has cleared
• Storage at room temperature
Evaluate:
• Therapeutic response: absence of severe itching, patches on skin, flaking
Teach patient/family:
• To avoid sunlight on affected area; burns may occur

---

dexamethasone/dexamethasone acetate/ dexamethasone sodium phosphate

(dex-a-meth'a-sone)
Decadron, Dexamethasone Intensol, Dexasone,* Dexone, Hexadrol/Dalalone-LA, Decadron-LA, Decaject-LA, Decameth-LA, Dexcen-LA, Dexasone-LA, Dexone-LA/Decadron Phosphate, Decaject, Decameth, Dexacen-4, Dexasone, Dexone, Dezone, Hexadrol Phosphate, Savacort-D

Func. class.: Corticosteroid
Chem. class.: Glucocorticoid, long-acting

Action: Decreases inflammation by suppression of migration of polymorphonuclear leukocytes, fibroblasts, reversal of increase capillary permeability and lysosomal stabilization
Uses: Inflammation, allergies, neoplasms, cerebral edema, shock
Dosage and routes:
Inflammation
• *Adult:* PO 0.25-4 mg bid-qid IM 4-16 mg q1-3 wk (acetate)
Shock
• *Adult:* IV 1-6 mg/kg or 40 mg q2-6h (phosphate)
Cerebral edema
• *Adult:* IV 10 mg, then 4-6 mg IM q6h × 2-4 days, then taper over 1 wk
• *Child:* PO 0.2 mg/kg/day in divided doses
Available forms include: Tabs 0.25, 0.5, 0.75, 1, 1.5, 3, 4, 6 mg; inj IM acetate 8, 16 mg/ml; inj IV phosphate 4, 10 mg/ml; elix 0.5 mg/5 ml; oral sol 0.5 mg/5 ml, 0.5 mg/0.5 ml
Side effects/adverse reactions:
INTEG: Acne, poor wound healing, ecchymosis, petechiae
CNS: Depression, flushing, sweating, headache, mood changes
*CV: Hypotension, **circulatory collapse, thrombophlebitis, embolism,** tachycardia
*HEMA: **Thrombocytopenia***
MS: Fractures, osteoporosis, weakness
*GI: Diarrhea, nausea, abdominal distention, GI hemorrhage, increased appetite, **pancreatitis***
EENT: Fungal infections, increased intraocular pressure, blurred vision
Contraindications: Psychosis, hypersensitivity, idiopathic thrombocytopenia, acute glomerulonephritis, amebiasis, fungal infections, nonasthmatic bronchial disease, child <2 yr
Precautions: Pregnancy, diabetes mellitus, glaucoma, osteoporosis, seizure disorders, ulcerative colitis, CHF, myasthenia gravis
Pharmacokinetics:
PO: Peak 1-2 h, duration 2⅓
IM: Peak 8 h, duration 6 days
Half-life 3-4½ h
Interactions/incompatibilities:
• Decreased action of this drug: cholestyramine, colestipol, barbiturates, rifampin, ephedrine, phenytoin, theophylline
• Decreased effects of: anticoagulants, anticonvulsants, antidiabetics, ambenonium, neostigmine, isoniazid, toxoids, vaccines

---

italics = common side effects   ***bold italic*** = life threatening reactions

• Increased side effects: alcohol, salicylates, indomethacin, amphotericin B, digitalis preparations

• Increased action of this drug: salicylates, estrogens, indomethacin

NURSING CONSIDERATIONS

Assess:

• Potassium, blood sugar, urine glucose while on long-term therapy; hypokalemia and hyperglycemia

• Weight daily, notify physician of weekly gain >5 lb

• B/P q4h, pulse, notify physician if chest pain occurs

• I&O ratio, be alert for decreasing urinary output and increasing edema

• Plasma cortisol levels during long-term therapy (normal level: 138-635 nmol/L SI units when drawn at 8 AM)

Administer:

• After shaking suspension (parenteral)

• Titrated dose, use lowest effective dose

• IM inj deeply in large mass, rotate sites, avoid deltoid, use 19G needle

• In one dose in AM to prevent adrenal suppression, avoid SC administration, damage may be done to tissue

• With food or milk to decrease GI symptoms

Perform/provide:

• Assistance with ambulation in patient with bone tissue disease to prevent fractures

Evaluate:

• Therapeutic response: ease of respirations, decreased inflammation

• Infection: increased temperature, WBC even after withdrawal of medication; drug masks symptoms of infection

• Potassium depletion: paresthesias, fatigue, nausea, vomiting, depression, polyuria, dysrhythmias, weakness

• Edema, hypotension, cardiac symptoms

• Mental status: affect, mood, behavioral changes, aggression

Teach patient/family:

• That ID as steroid user should be carried

• To notify physician if therapeutic response decreases; dosage adjustment may be needed

• Not to discontinue this medication abruptly or adrenal crisis can result

• To avoid OTC products: salicylates, alcohol in cough products, cold preparations unless directed by physician

• Teach patient all aspects of drug usage, including Cushingoid symptoms

• Symptoms of adrenal insufficiency: nausea, anorexia, fatigue, dizziness, dyspnea, weakness, joint pain

Lab test interferences:

Increase: Cholesterol, sodium, blood glucose, uric acid, calcium, urine glucose

Decrease: Calcium, potassium, T_4, T_3, thyroid ^{131}I uptake test, urine 17-OHCS, 17-KS, PBI

False negative: Skin allergy tests

---

dexamethasone/dexamethasone sodium phosphate

(dex-a-meth′a-sone)

Ophthalmic Suspension/Decadron Phosphate Ophthalmics, Maxidex Ophthalmic

Func. class.: Ophthalmic antiinflammatory

Action: Results in decreased inflammation, resulting in decreased pain, photophobia, hyperemia, cellular infiltration

Uses: Inflammation of eye, lids, conjunctiva, cornea, uveitis, iridocyclitis, allergic condition, burns, foreign bodies

Dosage and routes:
• *Adult and child:* Instill 1-2 gtts into conjunctival sac q1-4h depending on condition

Available forms include: Oint 0.05%; ophthalmic sol 0.1%

Side effects/adverse reactions:
*EENT: **Increased intraocular pressure,** poor corneal wound healing, increased possibility of corneal infection, glaucoma exacerbation, **optic nerve damage,** decreased acuity, visual field, cataracts*

Contraindications: Hypersensitivity, acute superficial herpes simplex, fungal/viral diseases of the eye or conjunctiva, active diabetes mellitus, ocular TB, infections of the eye

Precautions: Corneal abrasions, glaucoma

Interactions/incompatibilities: None known

NURSING CONSIDERATIONS
Evaluate:
• Allergic reactions: redness, itching, swelling, lacrimation
• Therapeutic response: absence of swelling, redness, exudate

Teach patient/family:
• Instillation method: pressure on lacrimal sac for 1 min
• Not to share eye medications with others

dexamethasone sodium phosphate
(dex-a-meth′a-sone)
Decadron Phosphate

Func. class.: Topical corticosteroid
Chem. class.: Synthetic fluorinated agent, group VI potency

Action: Possesses antipruritic, antiinflammatory actions

Uses: Psoriasis, eczema, contact dermatitis, pruritus

Dosage and routes:
• *Adult and child:* Apply to affected area tid-qid

Available forms include: Cream 0.1%

Side effects/adverse reactions:
INTEG: Burning, dryness, itching, irritation, acne, folliculitis, hypertrichosis, perioral dermatitis, hypopigmentation, atrophy, striae, miliaria, allergic contact dermatitis, secondary infection

Contraindications: Hypersensitivity to corticosteroids, fungal infections

Precautions: Pregnancy (C), lactation, viral infections, bacterial infections

Interactions/incompatibilities: None known

NURSING CONSIDERATIONS
Assess:
• Temperature; if fever develops, drug should be discontinued

Administer:
• Only to affected areas; do not get in eyes
• Medication, then cover with occlusive dressing (only if prescribed), seal to normal skin, change q12h
• Only to dermatoses; do not use on weeping, denuded, or infected area

Perform/provide:
• Cleansing before application of drug
• Treatment for a few days after area has cleared
• Storage at room temperature

Evaluate:
• Therapeutic response: absence of severe itching, patches on skin, flaking

Teach patient/family:
• To avoid sunlight on affected area; burns may occur

---

dexamethasone sodium phosphate (nasal)

(dex-a-meth'a-sone)
Decadron Phosphate Turbinaire
Func. class.: Steroid, intranasal
Chem. class.: Glucocorticoid

Action: Long-acting synthetic adrenocorticoid with antiinflammatory activity, minimal mineralocorticoid properties

Uses: Inflammation (not within sinuses), nasal polyps, allergic conditions of nose

Dosage and routes:
• *Adult:* AERO 1-2 sprays bid-tid, not to exceed 12/day
• *Child 6-12 yr:* AERO 1-2 sprays bid, not to exceed 8/day

Available forms include: Aero 100 μg dexamethasone/spray

Side effects/adverse reactions:
EENT: Nasal irritation, dryness, rebound congestion, epistaxis, sneezing

INTEG: Urticaria
CNS: Headache, dizziness
SYSTEMIC: CHF, convulsions, increased sodium, hypertension

Contraindications: Hypersensitivity, child <12 yr, localized infection of nose

Precautions: Lactation, nasal trauma

Interactions/incompatibilities:
None known

NURSING CONSIDERATIONS
Administer:
• After cleaning daily with warm water, dry thoroughly

Perform/provide:
• Storage in cool environment, do not puncture or incinerate container

Evaluate:
• Adrenal suppression: 17-KS, plasma cortisol for decreased levels
• Nasal passages during long-term treatment for changes in mucus
• For edema, increased B/P, increase in K^+ during treatment, which indicates systemic absorption

Teach patient/family:
• To clear nasal passages if sneezing attack occurs, repeat dose
• To continue using product even if mild nasal bleeding occurs, is usually transient
• Method of instillation after providing written instructions from manufacturer
• To clear nasal passages before administration, use decongestant if needed, shake inhaler, invert, tilt head backward, insert nozzle into nostril, away from septum, hold other nostril closed, depress activator, inhale through nose, exhale through mouth
• To decrease gradually if drug has been used consistently
• That only 1 person should use a single-container drug
• If irritation, dryness, epistaxis occur, drug may need to be discontinued
• Benefit requires regular use, will not occur after several days

dexamethasone sodium phosphate
(dex-a-meth'a-sone)
Decadron Phosphate

Func. class.: Topical corticosteroid
Chem. class.: Synthetic fluorinated agent

Action: Possesses antipruritic, antiinflammatory actions
Uses: Corticosteroid-responsive dermatoses
Dosage and routes:
• *Adult and child:* TOP apply to affected area bid-tid
Available forms include: Cream 0.1%
Side effects/adverse reactions:
INTEG: Burning, dryness, itching, irritation, acne, folliculitis, hypertrichosis, perioral dermatitis, hypopigmentation, atrophy, striae, miliaria, allergic contact dermatitis, secondary infection
Contraindications: Hypersensitivity to corticosteroids, fungal infections, viral infections
Precautions: Pregnancy (C), lactation, viral infections, bacterial infections
Pharmacokinetics: Not known
Interactions/incompatibilities: None known
NURSING CONSIDERATIONS
Assess:
• Temperature, if fever develops drug should be discontinued
Administer:
• Only to affected areas, do not get in eyes
• Then cover with occlusive dressing if ordered, seal to normal skin, change q12h
• Only to dermatoses, do not use on weeping, denuded or infected area

Perform/provide:
• Cleansing before application of drug
• Treatment for a few days after area has cleared
• Storage at room temperature
Evaluate:
• For systemic absorption: fever, infection, irritation
• Therapeutic response: absence of severe itching, patches on skin, flaking
Teach patient/family:
• To avoid sunlight on affected area, burns may occur

dexchlorpheniramine maleate
(dex-klor-fen-eer'a-meen)
Polaramine

Func. class.: Antihistamine
Chem. class.: Alkylamine derivative, H_1-receptor antagonist

Action: Acts on blood vessels, GI, respiratory system by competing with histamine for H_1-receptor site; decreases allergic response by blocking histamine
Uses: Allergy symptoms, rhinitis, pruritus, contact dermatitis
Dosage and routes:
• *Adult:* PO 1-2 mg tid-qid; REPEAT ACTION 4-6 mg bid-tid
• *Child 6-11 yr:* PO 1 mg q4-6h, or TIME REL 4 mg hs
• *Child 2-5 yr:* PO 0.5 mg q4-6h; do not use repeat action form
Available forms include: Tabs 2 mg; repeat-action tab 4, 6 mg; syr 2 mg/5 ml
Side effects/adverse reactions:
CNS: Dizziness, drowsiness, poor coordination, fatigue, anxiety, euphoria, confusion, paresthesia, neuritis
CV: Hypotension, palpitations, tachycardia
RESP: Increased thick secretions,

wheezing, chest tightness

GI: Dry mouth, nausea, vomiting, anorexia, constipation, diarrhea

INTEG: Rash, urticaria, photosensitivity

GU: Retention, dysuria, frequency

EENT: Blurred vision, dilated pupils, tinnitus, nasal stuffiness, dry nose, throat, mouth

Contraindications: Hypersensitivity to H_1-receptor antagonist; acute asthma attack, lower respiratory tract disease

Precautions: Increased intraocular pressure, renal disease, cardiac disease, hypertension, bronchial asthma, seizure disorder, stenosed peptic ulcers, hyperthyroidism, prostatic hypertrophy, bladder neck obstruction, pregnancy (B)

Pharmacokinetics:

PO: Onset 15 min, peak 3 hr, duration 3-6 hr, metabolized in liver, excreted by kidneys (inactive metabolites), excreted in breast milk (small amounts)

Interactions/incompatibilities:

• Increased CNS depression: barbiturates, narcotics, hypnotics, tricyclic antidepressants, alcohol

• Decreased effect of: oral anticoagulants, heparin

• Increased effect of this drug: MAOIs

NURSING CONSIDERATIONS
Assess:

• I&O ratio; be alert for urinary retention, frequency, dysuria; drug should be discontinued if these occur

• CBC during long-term therapy

Administer:

• Coffee, tea, cola (caffeine) to decrease drowsiness

• With meals if GI symptoms occur, absorption may slightly decrease

Perform/provide:

• Hard candy, gum, frequent rinsing of mouth for dryness

• Storage in tight container at room temperature

Evaluate:

• Therapeutic response: absence of running or congested nose or rashes

• Respiratory status: rate, rhythm, increase in bronchial secretions, wheezing, chest tightness

• Cardiac status: palpitations, increased pulse, hypotension

Teach patient/family:

• All aspects of drug use; to notify physician if confusion, sedation, hypotension occurs

• To avoid driving or other hazardous activity if drowsiness occurs

• To avoid concurrent use of alcohol or other CNS depressants

Lab test interferences:

False negative: Skin allergy tests

Treatment of overdose: Administer ipecac syrup or lavage, diazepam, vasopressors, barbiturates (short-acting)

---

dexpanthenol
(dex-pan'the-nole)
Panthoderm

Func. class.: Emollient/protectant
Chem. class.: Pantothenic acid derivative

Action: Prevents irritation of surgical areas by preventing evaporation of moisture

Uses: Diaper rash, decubitus ulcers, itching, eczema, insect bites

Dosage and routes:

• *Adult:* TOP apply qd bid

Available forms include: Cream, lotion 2%

Side effects/adverse reactions: None known

Contraindications: Hemophilia patients, wounds

Interactions/incompatibilities: None known

NURSING CONSIDERATIONS
Administer:
• Only to intact skin, never apply to raw, denuded, blistered, or oozing wounds
Perform/provide:
• Skin cleansing at least qd or more often if needed
Evaluate:
• For infection (increased temperature, redness), often bacteria are trapped underneath
Teach patient/family:
• To report color change on skin, redness, increased temperature

---

dexpanthenol
(dex-pan'the-nole)
Ilopan, Intrapan, Tonestat
Func. class.: Cholinergic
Chem. class.: Pantothenic acid analog

Action: Action is unknown, but this drug is precursor of pantothenic acid, which is needed for acetylcholine production, which maintains normal intestinal functioning
Uses: Prevention of paralytic ileus, postoperative abdominal distention
Dosage and routes:
Distention
• *Adult and child:* IM 250-500 mg, may repeat in 2 hr, 6 hr; IV INF 500 mg in D_5, or LR slowly
Paralytic ileus
• *Adult and child >16 yr:* IM 500 mg, may repeat in 2 hr, then q4-6h
Available forms include: Inj IM, IV 250 mg/ml
Side effects/adverse reactions:
HEMA: Increased bleeding time
GI: Diarrhea, hyperperistalsis, flatulence
INTEG: Urticaria, rash, pruritus, allergic reactions
Contraindications: Hypersensitivity, hemophilia, GI obstruction

Precautions: Pregnancy, children, lactation
Pharmacokinetics: Excreted in urine (pantothenic acid)
Interactions/incompatibilities:
None known

NURSING CONSIDERATIONS
Assess:
• Bleeding time, drug should be discontinued if bleeding time is increased
• I&O ratio; check for urinary retention or hesitancy
Administer:
• This drug at least 12 hr after parasympathomimetics
• Increased doses in hypokalemia patient
• IV after dilution
Perform/provide:
• Storage at room temperature
• Insertion of rectal tube if ordered
Evaluate:
• Allergic reaction: rash, urticaria; drug should be discontinued
• Therapeutic response: flatulence, bowel sounds present, abdomen soft, absence of pain
Teach patient/family:
• To report flatulence, decreased pain in abdomen

---

dextran 40
Gentran 40, Rheomacrodex
Func. class.: Plasma volume expander
Chem. class.: Low molecular weight polysaccharide

Action: Similar to human albumin which expands plasma volume
Uses: Expand plasma volume, prophylaxis of embolism, thrombosis
Dosage and routes:
Shock
• *Adult:* IV INF 500 ml over 15-30 min, then subsequent doses given slowly, if given >4 days, not to exceed 10 ml/kg/day

---

Thrombosis/embolism

• *Adult:* IV INF 500-1000 ml, then 500 ml/day × 3 days, then 500 ml q2-3 days × 2 wk if needed

Available forms include: 10% dextran 40/5% dextrose, 10% dextran 40/0.9% sodium chloride

Side effects/adverse reactions:

HEMA: Decreased hematocrit, increased bleeding/coagulation times

INTEG: Rash, urticaria, pruritus, angioedema, chills, fever, flushing

RESP: Wheezing, dyspnea, ***bronchospasm, pulmonary edema***

CV: Hypotension, ***cardiac arrest***

*GU: **Osmotic nephrosis, renal failure, stasis, blocking***

GI: Nausea, vomiting, increased AST, ALT

*SYST: **Anaphylaxis***

Contraindications: Hypersensitivity, renal failure, CHF (severe), extreme dehydration

Precautions: Active hemorrhage, pregnancy

Pharmacokinetics:

IV: Expands blood volume 1-2 × amount infused, excreted in urine and feces

Interactions/incompatibilities: None known

NURSING CONSIDERATIONS
Assess:

• VS q5 min × 30 min

• CVP during infusion (5-10 sm H₂—normal range)

• Urine output q1h; watch for increase in urinary output, which is common; if output does not increase, infusion should be decreased or discontinued

• I&O ratio and specific gravity, urine osmolarity; if specific gravity is very low, renal clearance is low, drug should be discontinued

Administer:

• After crossmatch is drawn, if blood is to be given also

• Dextran 1 (Promit) to prevent anaphylaxis if ordered

Perform/provide:

• Storage at constant temperature 25° C (77° F); discard unused portions

Evaluate:

• Allergy: rash, urticaria, pruritus, wheezing, dyspnea, bronchospasm, drug should be discontinued immediately

• Circulatory overload: increased pulse, respirations, SOB, wheezing, chest tightness, chest pain

• Dehydration after infusion: decreased output, increased temperature, poor skin turgor, increased specific gravity, dry skin

Lab test interferences:

False increase: Blood glucose, urinary protein, bilirubin, total protein

Interference: Rh test, blood typing/crossmatching

---

dextran 70/75
Gentran 75, Macrodex

Func. class.: Plasma volume expander

Chem. class.: Low molecular weight polysaccharide

Action: Similar to human albumin, which expands plasma volume

Uses: Expand plasma volume, prophylaxis of embolism, thrombosis

Dosage and routes:

• *Adult:* IV INF 500 ml not to exceed 20 ml/kg/24 hr, not to exceed 10 ml/kg/24 hr if therapy >24 hr

Side effects/adverse reactions:

HEMA: Decreased hematocrit, increased bleeding/coagulation times

INTEG: Rash, urticaria, pruritus, angioedema, chills, fever, flushing

RESP: Wheezing, dyspnea, ***bronchospasm, pulmonary edema***

CV: Hypotension, ***cardiac arrest***

*GU: **Osmotic nephrosis, renal fail-***

ure, stasis, blocking

GI: Nausea, vomiting, increase AST, ALT

*SYST: **Anaphylaxis***

Contraindications: Hypersensitivity, renal failure, CHF (severe), extreme dehydration

Precautions: Active hemorrhage, pregnancy

Pharmacokinetics:

IV: Expands blood volume 1-2 × amount infused, excreted in urine and feces

Interactions/incompatibilities: None known

NURSING CONSIDERATIONS

Assess:

• VS q5 min × 30 min

• CVP during infusion (5-10 sm H_2—normal range)

• Urine output q1h, watch for increase in urinary output which is common; if output does not increase, infusion should be decreased or discontinued

• I&O ratio and specific gravity, urine osmolarity; if specific gravity is very low, renal clearance is low, drug should be discontinued

Administer:

• After crossmatch is drawn, if blood is to be given also

• Dextran 1 (Promit) to prevent anaphylaxis

Perform/provide:

• Storage at constant temperature 25° C (77° F); discard unused portions

Evaluate:

• Allergy: rash, urticaria, pruritus, wheezing, dyspnea, bronchospasm, drug should be discontinued immediately

• Circulatory overload: increased pulse, respirations, SOB, wheezing, chest tightness, chest pain

• Dehydration after infusion: decreased output, increased temperature, poor skin turgor, increased

specific gravity, dry skin

Lab test interferences:

False increase: Blood glucose, urinary protein, bilirubin, total protein

Interferes: Rh test, blood typing/crossmatching

dextranomer

(dex-tran'oh-mer)

Debrisan

Func. class.: Miscellaneous topical drug

Chem. class.: Hydrophilic dextran polymer

Action: Absorbs exudate, particles from wound surface reducing inflammation, edema

Uses: Cleaning of wet ulcers: decubitus ulcers, surgical wounds, venous stasis ulcers

Dosage and routes:

• *Adult and child:* TOP apply ¼-inch thick on affected area bid, prn, cover with gauze dressing

Available forms include: Topical beads, topical paste

Side effects/adverse reactions:

INTEG: Erythema, pain, irritation, blistering, bleeding when dressings are changed

Contraindications: Hypersensitivity, deep fistulas, sinus tracts

Precautions: Pregnancy

Interactions/incompatibilities: None known

NURSING CONSIDERATIONS

Administer:

• After cleaning wound, do not dry

• Cover with dressing, do not pack wound tightly

• After mixing beads with glycerin, not to be mixed with other substances; do not reuse left-over mixture

Perform/provide:

• Storage in tight, closed container in dry place at room temperature

---

italics = common side effects   ***bold italic*** = life threatening reactions

Evaluate:

• Therapeutic response: drying of area, with eventual closure of wound

• Area of body involved, including time involved, what helps or aggravates condition

Teach patient/family:

• That treatment may take 1-2 wk

• To notify physician if condition lasts longer than 2 wk

---

dextroamphetamine sulfate

(dex-troe-am-fet′a-meen)

Dexampex, Dexedrine, Ferndex, Robese, Spancap #1

Func. class.: Cerebral stimulant

Chem. class.: Amphetamine

Controlled Substance Schedule II

Action: Increases release of norepinephrine, dopamine in cerebral cortex to reticular activating system

Uses: Narcolepsy, exogenous obesity, attention deficit disorder with hyperactivity

Dosage and routes:

Narcolepsy

• *Adult:* PO 5-60 mg qd in divided doses

• *Child >12 yr:* PO 10 mg qd increasing by 10 mg/wk

• *Child 6-12 yr:* PO 5 mg qd increasing by 5 mg/wk

Attention deficit disorder

• *Child >6 yr:* PO 5 mg qd-bid increasing by 5 mg/wk

• *Child 3-6 yr:* PO 2.5 mg qd increasing by 2.5 mg/wk

Obesity

• *Adult:* PO 5-30 mg qd in divided doses 30 min before meals

Available forms include: Tabs 5, 10 mg; caps 15 mg; caps susp rel 5, 10, 15 mg; elix 5 mg/5 ml

Side effects/adverse reactions:

CNS: Hyperactivity, insomnia, rest-lessness, talkativeness, dizziness, headache, chills, stimulation, dysphoria, irritability, aggressiveness

GI: Nausea, vomiting, anorexia, dry mouth, diarrhea, constipation, weight loss, metallic taste, cramps

GU: Impotence, change in libido

CV: Palpitations, tachycardia, hypertension, hypotension

INTEG: Urticaria

Contraindications: Hypersensitivity to sympathomimetic amines, hyperthyroidism, hypertension, glaucoma hypertrophy, severe arteriosclerosis, nephritis, angina pectoris, parkinsonism, drug abuse, cardiovascular disease, anxiety

Precautions: Gilles de la Tourette's disorder, pregnancy (C), lactation, child <3 yr, diabetes mellitus, elderly

Pharmacokinetics:

PO: Onset 30 min, peak 1-3 hr, duration 4-20 hr, metabolized by liver, excreted by kidneys, crosses placenta, breast milk, half-life 10-30 hr

Interactions/incompatibilities:

• Hypertensive crisis: MAOIs or within 14 days of MAOIs

• Increased effect of this drug: acetazolamide, antacids, sodium bicarbonate, ascorbic acid, ammonium chloride, phenothiazines, haloperidol

• Decreased effects of this drug: barbiturates

• Decreased effects of: guanethidine, other antihypertensives

NURSING CONSIDERATIONS

Assess:

• VS, B/P since this drug may reverse antihypertensives check patients with cardiac disease more often

• CBC, urinalysis; in diabetes: blood sugar, urine sugar; insulin changes may need to be made since eating will decrease

• Height, growth rate in children; growth rate may be decreased

Administer:

• At least 6 hr before hs to avoid sleeplessness

• For obesity only if the patient is on a weight reduction program including dietary changes and exercise; patient will develop tolerance and weight loss won't occur without additional methods.

• Gum, hard candy, frequent sips of water for dry mouth

• If drug is being given for obesity 1 hour before meals

Perform/provide:

• Check to see PO medication has been swallowed

Evaluate:

• Therapeutic response: increased CNS stimulation, decreased drowsiness

• Mental status: mood, sensorium, affect, stimulation, insomnia, irritability

• Tolerance or dependency: an increased amount may be used to get same effect

• Overdose: pain, fever, dehydration, insomnia, hyperactivity

• Drug tolerance; will develop after long-term use

• Dosage not to increase; instead discontinue

Teach patient/family:

• To decrease caffeine consumption (coffee, tea, cola, chocolate) which may increase irritability, stimulation

• Avoid OTC preparations unless approved by the physician

• To taper off drug over several weeks or depression, increased sleeping, lethargy

• To avoid alcohol ingestion

• To avoid hazardous activities until patient is stabilized on medication

• To get needed rest, patients will

feel more tired at end of day

Treatment of overdose: Administer fluids, hemodialysis or peritoneal dialysis; antihypertensive for increased B/P, ammonium Cl for increased excretion

---

D

dextromethorphan hydrobromide

(dex-troe-meth-or'fan)

Creamcoat, Pertussin 8-hour, Mediquell, Sucrets, Hold

Func. class.: Antitussive, nonnarcotic

Chem. class.: Levorphanol derivative

Action: Depresses cough center in medulla

Uses: Nonproductive cough

Dosage and routes:

• *Adult:* PO 10-20 mg q4h, or 30 mg q6-8h, not to exceed 120 mg/day; CON-REL LIQ 60 mg bid, not to exceed 120 mg/day

• *Child 6-12 yr:* PO 5-10 mg q4h; CON-REL LIQ 30 mg bid, not to exceed 60 mg/day

• *Child 2-6 yr:* PO 2.5-5 mg q4h, or 7.5 mg q6-8h, not to exceed 30 mg/day

Available forms include: Loz 5 mg; sol 5, 7.5, 10, 15 mg/5 ml

Side effects/adverse reactions:

CNS: Dizziness

GI: Nausea

Contraindications: Hypersensitivity, asthma/emphysema, productive cough

Precautions: Nausea/vomiting, increased temperature, persistent headache

Pharmacokinetics:

PO: Onset 15-30 min, duration 3-6 hr

Interactions/incompatibilities:

• Do not give with MAOIs, penicillins, salicylates, tetracyclines, phenobarbital, iodines (high doses)

---

italics = common side effects   ***bold italic*** = life threatening reactions

NURSING CONSIDERATIONS
Administer:
• Decreased dose to elderly patients; their metabolism may be slowed
Perform/provide:
• Increased fluids to liquefy secretions
• Humidification of patient's room
Evaluate:
• Therapeutic response: absence of cough
• Cough: type, frequency, character including sputum
Teach patient/family:
• Avoid driving or other hazardous activities until patient is stabilized on this medication
• Avoid smoking, smoke-filled rooms, perfumes, dust, environmental pollutants, cleaners that increase cough

---

dextrose (*D*-glucose)
Func. class.: Caloric

Action: Needed for adequate utilization of amino acids, decreases protein, nitrogen loss, prevents ketosis
Uses: Increases intake of calories, increases fluids in patients unable to take adequate fluids, calories orally
Dosage and routes:
• *Adult and child:* IV depends on individual requirements
Available forms include: Inj IV
Side effects/adverse reactions:
CNS: Confusion, loss of consciousness, dizziness
CV: Hypertension, *CHF, pulmonary edema*
GU: Glycosuria, osmotic diuresis
ENDO: Hyperglycemia, rebound hypoglycemia, hyperosmolar syndrome, hyperosmolar hyperglycemic nonketotic syndrome
INTEG: Chills, flushing, warm feeling, rash, urticaria, extravasation necrosis
Contraindications: Hyperglycemia, delirum tremens, hemorrhage (cranial/spinal), CHF
Precautions: Renal, liver, cardiac disease
Interactions/incompatibilities: None known

NURSING CONSIDERATIONS
Assess:
• Electrolytes (K, Na, Ca, Cl, Mg), blood glucose, ammonia, phosphate
• Renal, liver function studies: BUN, creatinine, ALT, AST, bilirubin
• Injection site for extravasation: redness along vein, edema at site, necrosis, pain, hard tender area; site should be changed immediately
• Monitor respiratory function q4h: auscultate lung fields bilaterally for rales, respirations, quality, rate, rhythm
• Monitor temperature q4h for increased fever, indicating infection; if infection suspected, infusion is discontinued, tubing, bottle cultured
• Urine glucose q6h using Tes-Tape, Clinistix, Keto-Diastix, which are not affected by infusion substances
Administer:
• After changing IV catheter, dressing q24h with aseptic technique
Evaluate for:
• Therapeutic response: increased weight
• Nutritional status: calorie count by dietician
Teach patient/family
• Reason for dextrose infusion

---

dextrothyroxine sodium

(dex-troe-thye-rox'een)
Choloxin

Func. class.: Antilipemic
Chem. class.: Hormone isomer

Action: Stimulates hepatic catabolism, excretion of cholesterol; increases bile products into feces

Uses: Hyperlipidemia in euthyroid patients with no evidence of organic heart disease

Dosage and routes:
• *Adult:* PO 1-2 mg/day, may increase 1-2 mg/day q mo, not to exceed 8 mg/day
• *Child:* PO 0.05 mg/kg/day, may increase 0.5 mg/kg/day q mo, not to exceed 4 mg/day

Available forms include: Tabs 1, 2, 4, 6 mg

Side effects/adverse reactions:
GI: Nausea, vomiting, diarrhea, constipation, anorexia, weight loss, jaundice
INTEG: Flushing, alopecia, sweating, hyperthermia
CV: Palpitations, dysrhythmias, *myocardial infarction, ischemic myocardial changes*
EENT: Visual disturbances, ptosis, retinopathy, lid lag
GU: Menstrual irregularities, change in libido
CNS: Insomnia, tremors, headache, dizziness, paresthesia, decreased sensorium

Contraindications: Severe hepatic disease, severe renal disease, organic heart disease, Hx of myocardial infarction, cardiac dysrhythmias, rheumatic heart disease, CHF, hypertension, iodism, pregnancy, lactation

Precautions: Obesity, hepatic disease, renal disease

Pharmacokinetics: Not known

Interactions/incompatibilities:
• Decreased effects of this drug: cholestyramine, colestipol
• Increased effects of: digitalis, oral anticoagulants
• Increase stimulation: tricyclic antidepressants
• Increases blood sugar levels in patients with diabetes
• Decreased effects of: beta blockers

NURSING CONSIDERATIONS

Assess:
• Renal and hepatic levels, if patient is on long-term therapy
• For signs of vitamin A, D, K deficiency

Administer:
• Drug before meals, at bedtime

Evaluate:
• Therapeutic response: decreased triglyceride, cholesterol levels, (hyperlipidemia); diarrhea, pruritus (excess bile area)
• Bowel pattern daily; increase bulk, water in diet if constipation develops

Teach patient/family:
• Symptoms of hypothrombinemia: bleeding mucous membranes, dark tarry stools, petechiae; report immediately
• That compliance is needed since toxicity may result if doses are missed
• That risk factors should be decreased: high fat diet, smoking, alcohol consumption, absence of exercise
• That OTC preparations should be avoided unless directed by physician
• Birth control should be practiced while on this drug

---

italics = common side effects   ***bold italic*** = life threatening reactions

diazepam

(dye-az'-e-pam)
D-Tran,* E-Pam,* Meval,* Novo-
dipam,* Stress-Pam,* Valium, Val-
release, Vivol*

Func. class.: Antianxiety
Chem. class.: Benzodiazepine

Controlled Substance Schedule IV

Action: Depresses subcortical
levels of CNS, including limbic
system, reticular formation

Uses: Anxiety, acute alcohol withdrawal, adjunct in seizure disorders

Dosage and routes:

Anxiety/convulsive disorders

• *Adult:* PO 2-10 mg tid-qid; EXT
REL 15-30 mg qd

• *Child >6 mo:* PO 1-2.5 mg tid-
qid

Tetanic muscle spams

• *Child >5 yr:* IM/IV 5-10 mg q3-
4 hr prn

• *Infants >30 days:* IM/IV 1-2 mg
q 3-4 hr prn

Status epilepticus

• *Adult:* IV BOLUS 5-20 mg, 2
mg/min, may repeat q5-10 min,
not to exceed 60 mg, may repeat in
30 min if seizures reappear

• *Child:* IV BOLUS 0.1-0.3 mg/
kg (1 mg/min over 3 min), may
repeat q15 min × 2 doses

Available forms include: Tabs 2,
5, 10 mg; caps sust rel 15 mg, IM/
IV inj

Side effects/adverse reactions:

CNS: Dizziness, drowsiness, confusion, headache, anxiety, tremors,
stimulation, fatigue, depression,
insomnia, hallucinations

GI: Constipation, dry mouth, nausea, vomiting, anorexia, diarrhea

INTEG: Rash, dermatitis, itching

*CV: Orthostatic hypotension, ECG
changes, tachycardia,* hypotension

EENT: Blurred vision, tinnitus, mydriasis

Contraindications: Hypersensitivity to benzodiazepines, narrow-
angle glaucoma, psychosis, pregnancy (D), child <18 yr

Precautions: Elderly, debilitated,
hepatic disease, renal disease

Pharmacokinetics:

PO: Onset ½, duration 2-3 hr

IM: Onset 15-30 min, duration 1-
1½ hr

IV: Onset 1-5 min, duration 15 min
Metabolized by liver, excreted by
kidneys, crosses placenta, breast
milk, half-life 20-50 hr

Interactions/incompatibilities:

• Decreased effects of this drug:
oral contraceptives, rifampin, valproic acid

• Increased effects of this drug:
CNS depressants, alcohol, cimetidine, disulfiram, oral contraceptives

• Incompatible with all drugs in solution or syringe

NURSING CONSIDERATIONS

Assess:

• B/P (lying, standing), pulse; if
systolic B/P drops 20 mm Hg, hold
drug, notify physician; respirations
q5-15 min if given IV

• Blood studies: CBC during long-
term therapy, blood dyscrasias have
occurred rarely

• Hepatic studies: AST, ALT, bilirubin, creatinine, LDH, alk phosphatase

Administer:

• IV into large vein to decrease
chance of extravasation

• With food or milk for GI symptoms

• Crushed if patient is unable to
swallow medication whole

• Sugarless gum, hard candy, frequent sips of water for dry mouth

Perform/provide:

• Assistance with ambulation during beginning therapy, since drows-

iness/dizziness occurs
• Safety measures, including side-rails
• Check to see PO medication has been swallowed

Evaluate:
• Therapeutic response: decreased anxiety, restlessness, insomnia
• Mental status: mood, sensorium, affect, sleeping pattern, drowsiness, dizziness
• Physical dependency, withdrawal symptoms: headache, nausea, vomiting, muscle pain, weakness after long-term use
• Suicidal tendencies

Teach patient/family:
• That drug may be taken with food
• Not to be used for everyday stress or used longer than 4 mo, unless directed by physician
• Avoid OTC preparations unless approved by physician
• To avoid driving, activities that require alertness; drowsiness may occur
• To avoid alcohol ingestion or other psychotropic medications, unless prescribed by physician
• Not to discontinue medication abruptly after long-term use
• To rise slowly or fainting may occur
• That drowsiness might worsen at beginning of treatment

Lab test interferences:
Increase: AST/ALT, serum bilirubin
False increase: 17-OHCS
Decrease: RAIU

Treatment of overdose: Lavage, VS, supportive care

diazoxide

(dye-az-ox´ide)
Hyperstat
Func. class.: Antihypertensive
Chem. class.: Vasodilator

Action: Vasodilates arteriolar smooth muscle by direct relaxation; a reduction in blood pressure with concomitant increases in heart rate, cardiac output

Uses: Hypertensive crisis when urgent decrease of diastolic pressure required

Dosage and routes:
• *Adult:* IV BOL 1-3 mg/kg rapidly up to a max of 150 mg in a single injection, dose may be repeated at 5-15 min intervals until desired response is achieved; give IV in 30 sec or less
• *Child:* IV BOL 1-2 mg/kg rapidly; administration same as adult, not to exceed 150 mg

Available forms include: Inj IV 15 mg/ml

Side effects/adverse reactions:
CV: **Hypotension,** T wave changes, angina pectoris, palpitations, *supraventricular tachycardia, edema,* rebound hypertension
CNS: Headache, sleepiness, euphoria, anxiety, extrapyramidal symptoms, confusion, tinnitus, blurred vision, dizziness, weakness
GI: Nausea, vomiting, dry mouth
INTEG: Rash
HEMA: Decreased hemoglobulin, hematocrit, *thrombocytopenia*
GU: Breast tenderness, increased BUN, fluid, electrolyte imbalances, sodium, water retention
ENDO: Hyperglycemia in diabetics, transient hyperglycemia in nondiabetics

Contraindications: Hypersensitivity to thiazides, sulfonamides, hypertension associated with aortic coarctation or AV shunt, pheochromocytoma, dissecting aortic aneurysm

Precautions: Tachycardia, fluid, electrolyte imbalances, pregnancy (B), lactation, impaired cerebral or cardiac circulation, children

Pharmacokinetics:

PO: Onset 1 hr, duration 6-8 hr

IV: Onset 1-2 min, peak 5 min, duration 3-12 hr

Half-life 20-36 hr, excreted slowly in urine, crosses blood-brain barrier, placenta

Interactions/incompatibilities:

• Effects: thiazide diuretics, antihypertensives, coumadin, guanethidine

• Do not mix with any drug in syringe or solution

• Increased effects of: warfarin, other coumarins

• Hyperglycemia/hyperuricemia: thiazides, diuretics

• Decreased pharmacologic effects of both: sulfonylureas

NURSING CONSIDERATIONS

Assess:

• B/P q5 min × 2 hr, then q1h × 2 hr, then q4h

• Pulse, jugular venous distention q4h

• Electrolytes, blood studies: potassium, sodium, chloride, CO_2, CBC, serum glucose

• Weight daily, I&O

Administer:

• To patient in recumbent position, keep in that position for 1 hr after administration

Perform/provide:

• Protection from light

Evaluate:

• Therapeutic response: decreased B/P, primarily diastolic pressure

• Edema in feet, legs daily

• Skin turgor, dryness of mucous membranes for hydration status

• Rales, dyspnea, orthopnea

• IV site for extravasation, rate

• Signs of CHF: dyspnea, edema, wet rales

• Postural hypotension, take B/P sitting, standing

Teach patient/family:

• That hirsutism is reversible after drug is discontinued

Treatment of overdose: Administer levarterenol, dopamine, or norepinephrine for hypotension, dialysis

---

diazoxide (oral)

(dye-az-ox'ide)

Proglycem

Func. class.: Hyperglycemic

Chem. class.: Benzothiadiazine

Action: Decreases release of insulin from β-cells in pancreas, decreases use of glucose in body

Uses: Hypoglycemia caused by hyperinsulinism

Dosage and routes:

• *Adult and child:* PO 3-8 mg/kg/day in 3 divided doses q8h

• *Infants and neonates:* PO 8-15 mg/kg/day in 2-3 divided doses q8-12h

Available forms include: Caps 50 mg; oral susp 50 mg/ml

Side effects/adverse reactions:

EENT: Diplopia

HEMA: **Thrombocytopenia, leukopenia**

INTEG: Increased hair growth

GI: Nausea, vomiting, anorexia

CV: Dysrhythmias

META: Hyperuricemia, sodium/fluid retention, ketoacidosis

Contraindications: Hypersensitivity to this drug or thiazides, CV disease

Precautions: Pregnancy, lactation, renal disease, diabetes mellitus

Pharmacokinetics:

PO: Onset 1 hr, duration 8 hr, half-life 20-36 min, excreted unchanged

---

by kidneys, crosses blood-brain barrier, placenta

Interactions/incompatibilities:
• Increased effects of: antihypertensives, oral anticoagulants
• Decreased effects of this drug: α-adrenergic blockers

NURSING CONSIDERATIONS
Assess:
• I&O ratio, weight weekly
• Electrolytes (K, Na, Cl), glucose, Hct, Hgb, platelets, differential
• Urine for glucose, ketones qd

Administer:
• Shake before using

Perform/provide:
• Storage protected from light

Evaluate:
• Therapeutic response: adequate blood, urine glucose, absence of ketones in urine

Teach patient/family:
• That if drug is not effective within 2-3 wk, drug is discontinued
• That if hirsutism occurs, it is reversible after discontinuing treatment

Lab test interferences:
Increase: Bilirubin, uric acid, blood glucose
Decrease: Creatinine, Hgb, Hct, plasma-free fatty acids

---

dibucaine

(dye′byoo-kane)
D-Caine, Nupercainal
Func. class.: Topical anesthetic
Chem. class.: Amide. long acting

Action: Inhibits nerve impulses from sensory nerves; produces anesthesia
Uses: Pruritus, sunburn, toothache, sore throat, cold sores, oral pain, rectal pain, irritation
Dosage and routes:
• *Adult and child:* TOP apply qid prn; REC insert tid, after each BM

Available forms include: Cream 0.5%, oint 1%, rec supp 2.5 mg
Side effects/adverse reactions:
INTEG: Rash, irritation, sensitization
Contraindications: Hypersensitivity
Precautions: Child <6 yr, pregnancy
Interactions/incompatibilities: None known

NURSING CONSIDERATIONS
Administer:
• After moistening suppository before insertion

Perform/provide:
• Storage of suppositories in cool environment

Evaluate:
• For allergic reactions: rash, irritation, reddening, swelling
• For therapeutic response: absence of pain of affected area
• Affected area for infection, if infection present, do not apply

Teach patient/family:
• To report rash, irritation, redness, swelling
• How to apply ointment, cream, rectal suppositories

---

dibucaine HCl (topical)

(dye′byoo-kane)
D-Caine, Nupercainal
Func. class.: Topical anesthetic
Chem. class.: Amide

Action: Inhibits nerve impulses from sensory nerves, which produces anesthesia
Uses: Pruritus, sunburn, toothache, sore throat, cold sores, oral pain, rectal pain and irritation
Dosage and routes:
• *Adult and child:* TOP apply qid as needed; REC insert tid and after each BM
Available forms include: Cream 0.5%; rec or top oint 1%

Side effects/adverse reactions:
INTEG: Rash, irritation, sensitization
Contraindications: Hypersensitivity, infants <1 yr, application to large areas
Precautions: Child <6 yr, sepsis, pregnancy, denuded skin
Interactions/incompatibilities: None known
NURSING CONSIDERATIONS
Administer:
• After cleansing and drying of affected area
Evaluate:
• Allergy: rash, irritation, reddening, swelling
• Therapeutic response: absence of pain, itching of affected area
• Infection: if affected area is infected, do not apply
Teach patient/family:
• To report rash, irritation, redness, swelling
• How to apply cream, ointment

---

dichlorphenamide

(dye-klor-fen'a-mide)
Daranide, Oratrol

Func. class.: Diuretic; carbonic anhydrase inhibitor
Chem. class.: Sulfonamide derivative

Action: Decreases production of aqueous humor in eye, which lowers intraocular pressure
Uses: Adjunct in glaucoma (used with miotics), preoperatively in narrow-angle glaucoma when surgery is delayed
Dosage and routes:
• *Adult:* PO 100-200 mg, then 100 mg q12h until desired response occurs; maintenance 25-50 mg bid or tid given with miotics
Available forms include: Tabs 50 mg

Side effects/adverse reactions:
GU: Frequency, hypokalemia, polyuria uremia, glucosuria, hematuria, decreased libido, impotence
CNS: Drowsiness, paresthesia, anxiety, depression, headache, dizziness, confusion, stimulation, fatigue, *convulsions*
GI: Nausea, vomiting, anorexia, constipation, diarrhea, melena, weight loss, hepatic insufficiency
EENT: Myopia, tinnitus
INTEG:Rash, pruritus, urticaria, fever, photosensitivity
ENDO: Hypoglycemia
HEMA: Hyperchloremia, *aplastic anemia, hemolytic anemia, leukopenia, agranulocytosis, thrombocytopenia, purpura, pancytopenia*
Contraindications: Hypersensitivity to sulfonamides, severe renal disease, severe hepatic disease, electrolyte imbalances (hyponatremia, hypokalemia), hypochloremic acidosis, Addison's disease
Precautions: Hypercalciuria, pregnancy, COPD
Pharmacokinetics:
PO: Onset ½-1 hr, peak 2-4 hr, duration 6-12 hr, 65% absorbed if fasting (oral), 75% absorbed if given with food; half-life 2½-5½ hr, excreted unchanged by kidneys (80% within 24 hr), crosses placenta
Interactions/incompatibilities:
• Increased action of: amphetamines, procainamide, quinidine, tricyclics, digitalis
• Decreased effects of: salicylates, lithium, barbiturates, methotrexate, chlorpropamide
• Hypokalemia: with other diuretics, corticosteroids, amphotericin B
NURSING CONSIDERATIONS
Assess:
• Weight, I&O daily to determine

---

fluid loss; effect of drug may be decreased if used qd
• Rate, depth, rhythm of respiration, effect of exertion
• B/P lying, standing; postural hypotension may occur
• Electrolytes: potassium, sodium, chloride; include BUN, blood sugar, CBC, serum creatinine, blood pH, ABGs

Administer:
• In AM to avoid interference with sleep if using drug as a diuretic
• Potassium replacement if potassium is less than 3.0
• With food, if nausea occurs, absorption may be decreased slightly

Evaluate:
• Therapeutic response: improvement in edema of feet, legs, sacral area daily if medication is being used in CHF; or decrease in aqueous humor if medication is being used in glaucoma
• Improvement in CVP q8h
• Signs of metabolic acidosis: drowsiness, restlessness
• Signs of hypokalemia: postural hypotension, malaise, fatigue, tachycardia, leg cramps, weakness
• Rashes, temperature elevation qd
• Confusion, especially in elderly; take safety precautions if needed

Teach patient/family:
• To increase fluid intake 2-3 L/day unless contraindicated; to rise slowly from lying or sitting position
• To notify physician if sore throat, unusual bleeding, bruising, paresthesias, tremors, flank pain, or skin rash occurs
• To avoid hazardous activities if drowsiness occurs

Lab test interferences:
False Positive: Urinary protein

Treatment of overdose: Lavage if taken orally, monitor electrolytes, administer dextrose in saline

dicloxacillin sodium

(dye-klox-a-sill′-in)
Dycill, Dynapen, Pathocil
Func. class.: Broad-spectrum antibiotic
Chem. class.: Penicillinase-resistant penicillin

D

Action: Interferes with cell wall replication of susceptible organisms; osmotically unstable cell wall swells, bursts from osmotic pressure

Uses: Effective for gram-positive cocci *(S. aureus, S. pyogenes, S. viridans, S. faecalis, S. bovis, S. pneumoniae)*, infections caused by penicillinase-producing *Staphylococcus*

Dosage and routes:
• *Adult:* PO 1-2 g/day in divided doses q6h
• *Child:* PO 12.5-25 mg/kg in divided doses q6h

Available forms include: Caps 125, 250, 500 mg; powder for oral susp 62.5 mg/5 ml

Side effects/adverse reactions:
HEMA: Anemia, increased bleeding time, ***bone marrow depression, granulocytopenia***
GI: Nausea, vomiting, diarrhea, increased AST, ALT, abdominal pain, glossitis, colitis
GU: Oliguria, proteinuria, hematuria, *vaginitis, moniliasis,* ***glomerulonephritis***
CNS: Lethargy, hallucinations, anxiety, depression, twitching, ***coma, convulsions***
META: Hyperkalemia, hypokalemia, alkalosis, hypernatremia

Contraindications: Hypersensitivity to penicillins; neonates

Precautions: Hypersensitivity to cephalosporins

Pharmacokinetics:
PO: Peak 1 hr, duration 4-6 hr, half-

life 30-60 min, metabolized in liver, excreted in urine, bile, breast milk, crosses placenta

Interactions/incompatibilities:

• Decreased antimicrobial effectiveness of this drug: tetracyclines, erythromycins

• Increased penicillin concentrations when used with: aspirin, probenecid

NURSING CONSIDERATIONS

Assess:

• I&O ratio; report hematuria, oliguria since penicillin in high doses is nephrotoxic

• Any patient with compromised renal system since drug is excreted slowly in poor renal system function; toxicity may occur rapidly

• Liver studies: AST, ALT

• Blood studies: WBC, RBC, H&H, bleeding time

• Renal studies: urinalysis, protein, blood

• C&S before drug therapy; drug may be taken as soon as culture is taken

Administer:

• Drug after C&S has been completed

Perform/provide:

• Adrenalin, suction, tracheostomy set, endotracheal intubation equipment

• Adequate fluid intake (2000 ml) during diarrhea episodes

• Scratch test to assess allergy, after securing order from physician; usually done when penicillin is only drug of choice

• Storage in tight container; after reconstituting, store in refrigerator

Evaluate:

• Therapeutic effectiveness: absence of fever, draining wounds

• Bowel pattern before, during treatment

• Skin eruptions after administration of penicillin to 1 wk after discontinuing drug

• Respiratory status: rate, character, wheezing, tightness in chest

• Allergies before initiation of treatment, reaction of each medication; highlight allergies on chart, Kardex

Teach patient/family:

• Aspects of drug therapy, including need to complete course of medication to ensure organism death (10-14 days); culture may be taken after completed course

• To report sore throat, fever, fatigue; could indicate superimposed infection

• To wear or carry Medic Alert ID if allergic to penicillins

• To notify nurse of diarrhea stools

Lab test interferences:

Decrease: Uric acid

False positive: Urine glucose, urine protein

Treatment of overdose: Withdraw drug, maintain airway, administer epinephrine, aminophylline, O_2, IV corticosteroids for anaphylaxis

---

dicumarol

(dye-koo'ma-role)

Dicumarol, Bishydroxycoumarin

Func. class.: Anticoagulant

Chem. class.: Coumarin

Action: Indirectly interferes with blood clotting; depresses hepatic synthesis of vitamin K-dependent coagulation factors (II, VII, IX, X)

Uses: Deep vein thrombosis, pulmonary emboli, rheumatic heart disease, myocardial infarction, atrial dysrhythmias, transient cerebral, ischemic attacks

Dosage and routes:

• *Adult:* PO 200-300 mg, then 25-200 mg qd depending on PT

Available forms include: Tabs 25, 50, 100 mg

Side effects/adverse reactions:

GI: Diarrhea, nausea, vomiting,

anorexia, stomatitis, abdominal cramps, *hepatitis*
GU: Hematuria
INTEG: Rash, dermatitis, urticaria, alopecia, pruritus
CNS: Fever
*HEMA: **Hemorrhage, agranulocytosis, leukopenia***
Contraindications: Hypersensitivity, hemophilia, leukemia with bleeding, peptic ulcer disease, thrombocytopenic purpura, hepatic disease (severe), renal disease (severe), severe hypertension, subacute bacterial endocarditis, blood dyscrasias, acute nephritis, pregnancy
Precautions: Alcoholism, elderly
Pharmacokinetics:
PO: Onset 2-12 hr, peak ½-3 days, duration 2-5 days; half-life ½-3 days, metabolized by liver, excreted in urine, feces, crosses placenta, excreted in breast milk
Interactions/incompatibilities:
• Increased action: allopurinol, chloramphenicol, clofibrate, amiodarone, diflunisal, heparin, steroids, cimetidine, disulfiram, thyroid, glucagon, metronidazole, quinidine, sulindac, sulfinpyrazone, sulfonamides, tricyclic antidepressants, inhalation anesthetics, salicylates, ethacrynic acid, indomethacin, mefenamic acid, oxyphenbutazones, phenylbutazone
• Decreased action: barbiturates, griseofulvin, haloperidol, ethchlorvynol, carbamazepine, rifampin, cholestyramine
• Increased or decreased action: chloral hydrate, glutethimide, sulfinpyrazone, triclofos sodium, alcohol
NURSING CONSIDERATIONS
Assess:
• Blood studies (Hct, platelets, occult blood in stools) q3 mo
• Prothrombin time, which should be 1½-2 × control, PT; often done qd
• B/P, watch for increasing signs of hypertension
Administer:
• At same time each day to maintain steady blood levels
• Alone, do not give with food
• Avoiding all IM injections that may cause bleeding
Perform/provide:
• Storage in tight container
Evaluate:
• Therapeutic response: decrease of deep vein thrombosis
• Bleeding gums, petechiae, ecchymosis, black tarry stools, hematuria
• Fever, skin rash, urticaria
• Needed dosage change q 1-2 wk
Teach patient/family:
• To avoid OTC preparations (aspirin or aspirin-containing products) that may cause serious drug interactions unless directed by physician
• That urine may turn orange/red
• Drug may be held during active bleeding (menstruation)
• To use soft-bristle toothbrush to avoid bleeding gums
• To carry a Medic-Alert ID identifying drug taken
• Stress patient compliance
• On all aspects of adjustments: dosage, route, action, side effects, when to notify physician
• To report any signs of bleeding: gums, under skin, urine, stools
• To avoid hazardous activities (football, hockey, skiing) or dangerous work
Lab test interferences:
Increase: T$_3$ uptake
Decrease: Uric acid
Treatment of overdose: Administer vitamin K

---

italics = common side effects   ***bold italic*** = life threatening reactions

dicyclomine HCl

(dye-sye′kloe-meen)

Antispas, Bentyl, Bentylol, Dibent, Formulex,* Neoquess, Nospaz, Rocyclo, Stannitol, Viserol*

Func. class.: Gastrointestinal anticholinergic

Chem. class.: Synthetic tertiary amine

Action: Inhibits muscarinic actions of acetylcholine at postganglionic parasympathetic neuroeffector sites

Uses: Treatment of peptic ulcer disease in combination with other drugs; infant colic

Dosage and routes:

• *Adult:* PO 10-20 mg tid-qid; IM 20 mg q4-6h

• *Child:* PO 10 mg tid-qid

• *Infant:* PO 5 mg tid-qid

Available forms include: Caps 10, 20 mg; tabs 20 mg; syr 10 mg/5 ml; inj IM 10 mg/ml

Side effects/adverse reactions:

CNS: Confusion, stimulation in elderly, headache, insomnia, dizziness, drowsiness, anxiety, weakness, hallucination

GI: Dry mouth, constipation, paralytic ileus, heartburn, nausea, vomiting, dysphagia, absence of taste

GU: Hesitancy, rentention, impotence

CV: Palpitations, tachycardia

EENT: Blurred vision, photophobia, mydriasis, cycloplegia, increased ocular tension

INTEG: Urticaria, rash, pruritus, anhidrosis, fever, allergic reactions

Contraindications: Hypersensitivity to anticholinergics, narrow-angle glaucoma, GI obstruction, myasthenia gravis, paralytic ileus, GI atony, toxic megacolon

Precautions: Hyperthyroidism, coronary artery disease, dysrhyth-mias, CHF, ulcerative colitis, hypertension, hiatal hernia, hepatic disease, renal disease

Pharmacokinetics:

PO: Onset 1-2 hr, duration 3-4 hr; metabolized by liver, excreted in urine

Interactions/incompatibilities:

• Increased anticholinergic effect: amantadine, tricylic antidepressants, MAOIs

• Increased effect of: nitrofurantoin

• Decreased effect of: phenothiazines, levodopa

NURSING CONSIDERATIONS

Assess:

• VS, cardiac status: checking for dysrhythmias, increased rate, palpitations

• I&O ratio; check for urinary retention or hesitancy

Administer:

• ½-1 hr ac for better absorption

• Decreased dose to elderly patients; their metabolism may be slowed

• Gum, hard candy, frequent rinsing of mouth for dryness of oral cavity

Perform/provide:

• Storage in tight container protected from light

• Increased fluids, bulk, exercise to patient's lifestyle to decrease constipation

Evaluate:

• Therapeutic response: absence of epigastric pain, bleeding, nausea, vomiting

• GI complaints: pain, bleeding (frank or occult), nausea, vomiting, anorexia

Teach patient/family:

• Avoid driving or other hazardous activities until stabilized on medication

• Avoid alcohol or other CNS depressants; will enhance sedating properties of this drug

• To avoid hot environments,

stroke may occur, drug suppresses perspiration
• Use sunglasses when outside to prevent photophobia

dienestrol

(dye-en-ess'trole)
DV, Estraguard, Ortho Dienestrol
Func. class.: Estrogen
Chem. class.: Nonsteroidal synthetic estrogen

Action: Needed for adequate functioning of female reproductive system, it affects release of pituitary gonadotropins, inhibits ovulation, adequate calcium use in bone structures

Uses: Atrophic vaginitis, kraurosis vulvae

Dosage and routes:
• *Adult:* VAG CREAM 1-2 applications qd × 2 wk, then $\frac{1}{2}$ dose × 2 wk, then 1 applicator
Available forms include: Vag cream 0.01%

Side effects/adverse reactions:
CNS: Dizziness, headache, migraines, depression
CV: Hypotension, thrombophlebitis, edema, *thromboembolism, stroke, pulmonary embolism, myocardial infarction*
GI: Nausea, vomiting, diarrhea, anorexia, pancreatitis, cramps, constipation, increased appetite, increased weight, cholestatic jaundice
EENT: Contact lens intolerance, increased myopia, astigmatism
GU: Amenorrhea, cervical erosion, breakthrough bleeding, dysmenorrhea, vaginal candidiasis, breast changes, *gynecomastia, testicular atrophy, impotence*
INTEG: Rash, urticaria, acne, hirsutism, alopecia, oily skin, seborrhea, purpura, melasma
META: Folic acid deficiency, hy-

percalcemia, hyperglycemia
Contraindications: Breast cancer, thromboembolic disorders, reproductive cancer, genital bleeding (abnormal, undiagnosed), pregnancy (X)
Precautions: Hypertension, asthma, blood dyscrasias, gallbladder disease, CHF, diabetes mellitus, bone disease, depression, migraine headache, convulsive disorders, hepatic disease, renal disease, family history of cancer of the breast or reproductive tract
Pharmacokinetics:
TOP: Degraded in liver, excreted in urine, crosses placenta, excreted in breast milk
Interactions/incompatibilities:
• Decreased action of: anticoagulants, oral hypoglycemics
• Toxicity: tricyclic antidepressants
• Decreased action of this drug: anticonvulsants, barbiturates, phenylbutazone, rifampin
• Increased action of: corticosteroids
NURSING CONSIDERATIONS
Assess:
• Weight daily; notify physician of weekly weight gain >5 lb
• B/P q4h
• I&O ratio, be alert for decreasing urinary output and increasing edema
• Liver function studies including ALT, AST, bilirubin
Administer:
• At hs for better absorption
• Titrated dose, use lowest effective dose, to prevent adverse reactions
• Dosage reduction should continue at 3-6 month intervals
Perform/provide:
• Storage in tight, light-resistant container in refrigerator
Evaluate:
• Edema, hypertension, cardiac

symptoms, jaundice
• Mental status: affect, mood, behavioral changes, aggression
• Hypercalcemia
Teach patient/family:
• How to fill applicator and insert cream
• To report breast lumps, vaginal bleeding, edema, jaundice, dark urine, clay colored stools, dyspnea, headache, blurred vision, abdominal pain, numbness or stiffness in legs, chest pain

---

diethylpropion HCl

Nobesine, Nu-Dispoz, Regibon, Ro-Diet, Tenuate, Tepanil

Func. class.: Cerebral stimulant
Chem. class.: Amphetamine derivative

Controlled Substance Schedule IV

Action: Increases release of norepinephrine and dopamine in cerebral cortex to reticular activating system
Uses: Exogenous obesity
Dosage and routes:
• *Adult:* PO 25 mg ac, or 75 mg controlled release qd midmorning
Available forms include: Tabs 25 mg, tabs susp rel 75 mg
Side effects/adverse reactions:
CNS: Hyperactivity, restlessness
GI: Nausea, vomiting, anorexia, dry mouth, diarrhea, constipation
GU: Impotence, change in libido, menstrual irregularities
CV: Palpitations, tachycardia hypertension
INTEG: Urticaria
Contraindications: Hypersensitivity, hyperthyroidism, hypertension, glaucoma, angina pectoris, drug abuse, cardiovascular disease
Precautions: Convulsive disorders, diabetes mellitus, anxiety

Pharmacokinetics:
PO: Duration 4 hr
CONT REL: Duration 10-14 hr; metabolized by liver, excreted by kidneys, crosses placenta, breast milk, half-life 1-3½ hr
Interactions/incompatibilities:
• Hypertensive crisis: MAOIs or within 14 days of MAOIs
• Increased effect of this drug: acetazolamide, antacids, sodium bicarbonate, ascorbic acid, ammonium chloride, phenothiazines, haloperidol
• Decreased effects of this drug: barbiturates
• Decreased effects of: guanethidine, other antihypertensives
NURSING CONSIDERATIONS
Assess:
• VS, B/P since this drug may reverse antihypertensives; check patients with cardiac disease more often
• CBC, urinalysis, in diabetes: blood sugar, urine sugar; insulin changes may need to be made since eating will decrease
• Height, growth rate in children; growth rate may be decreased
Administer:
• At least 6 hr before hs to avoid sleeplessness
• For obesity only if patient is on weight reduction program, including dietary changes, exercise; patient will develop tolerance, and weight loss won't occur without additional methods
• Gum, hard candy, frequent sips of water for dry mouth
• If the drug is being given for obesity, 1 hour before meals
Perform/provide:
• Check to see PO medication has been swallowed
Evaluate:
• Mental status: mood, sensorium, affect, stimulation, insomnia, aggressiveness

• Physical dependency: should not be used for extended time; dose should be discontinued gradually
• Withdrawal symptoms: headache, nausea, vomiting, muscle pain, weakness
• Drug tolerance after long-term use
• Dosage should not be increased if tolerance develops

Teach patient/family:
• To decrease caffeine consumption (coffee, tea, cola, chocolate); may increase irritability, stimulation
• Avoid OTC preparations unless approved by physician
• To taper off drug over several weeks, or depression, increased sleeping, lethargy will occur
• To avoid alcohol ingestion
• To avoid hazardous activities until patient is stabilized on medication
• To get needed rest, patients will feel more tired at end of day

Treatment of overdose: Administer fluids, hemodialysis for peritoneal dialysis; antihypertensive for increased B/P; ammonium Cl for increased excretion

---

diethylstilbestrol/diethylstilbestrol diphosphate

(dye-eth-il-stil-bess'trole)
DES, Stilboestrol*/Honvol,* Stilphostrol

Func. class.: Estrogen
Chem. class.: Nonsteroidal synthetic estrogen

Action: Needed for adequate functioning of female reproductive system, it affects release of pituitary gonadotropins, inhibits ovulation, adequate calcium use in bone structures

Uses: Atrophic vaginitis, kraurosis vulvae, menopause, postcoital contraception hypogonadism, castration, primary ovarian failure, breast engorgement, breast cancer, prostatic cancer

Dosage and routes:
Atrophic vaginitis/kraurosis vulvae
• *Adult:* VAG SUPP 0.1-1 mg qd × 10-14 days with oral therapy or up to 5 mg q wk
Menopause
• *Adult:* PO 0.1-2 mg qd 3 wk on, 1 wk off
Contraception
• *Adult:* PO 25 mg bid × 5 days, within 72 hr of intercourse
Hypogonadism/castration/ovarian failure
• *Adult:* PO 0.2-0.5 mg qd
Breast engorgement
• *Adult:* PO 5 mg qd-tid, not to exceed 30 mg
Prostatic cancer
• *Adult:* PO 1-3 mg qd, then 1 mg qd; PO 50-200 mg tid (diphosphate); IM 5 mg 2×/wk, then 4 mg 2×/wk; IV 0.25-1 g qd × 5 days, then 1-2×/wk
Breast cancer
• *Adult:* PO 15 mg qd
Available forms include: Tabs 1, 5 mg; tabs enteric coated 0.1, 0.25, 0.5, 1, 5 mg; vag supp 0.1, 0.5 mg

Side effects/adverse reactions:
CNS: Dizziness, headache, migraines, depression
CV: Hypotension, thrombophlebitis, edema, ***thromboembolism, stroke, pulmonary embolism, myocardial infarction***
GI: Nausea, vomiting, diarrhea, anorexia, pancreatitis, cramps, constipation, increased appetite, increased weight, cholestatic jaundice
EENT: Contact lens intolerance, increased myopia, astigmatism
GU: Amenorrhea, cervical erosion, breakthrough bleeding, dysmenorrhea, vaginal candidiasis, breast

---

changes, *gynecomastia, testicular atrophy, impotence*

INTEG: Rash, urticaria, acne, hirsutism, alopecia, oily skin, seborrhea, purpura, melasma

META: Folic acid deficiency, hypercalcemia, hyperglycemia

Contraindications: Breast cancer, thromboembolic disorders, reproductive cancer, genital bleeding (abnormal, undiagnosed), pregnancy (X)

Precautions: Hypertension, asthma, blood dyscrasias, gallbladder disease, CHF, diabetes mellitus, bone disease blocking agents

Interactions/incompatibilities:
• Decreased action of: anticoagulants, oral hypoglycemics
• Toxicity: tricyclic antidepressants
• Decreased action of this drug: anticonvulsants, barbiturates, phenylbutazone, rifampin
• Increased action of: corticosteroids

NURSING CONSIDERATIONS

Assess:
• Urine glucose in patient with diabetes; increased urine glucose may occur
• Weight daily, notify physician of weekly weight gain >5 lb; if increase, diuretic may be ordered
• B/P q4h, watch for increase caused by water and sodium retention
• I&O ratio, be alert for decreasing urinary output and increasing edema
• Liver function studies, including AST, ALT, bilirubin, alk phosphatase

Administer:
• Titrated dose, use lowest effective dose
• IM injection deeply in large muscular mass
• In one dose in AM for prostatic cancer, vaginitis, hypogonadism
• With food or milk to decrease GI symptoms

Evaluate:
• Therapeutic response: absence of breast engorgement, reversal of menopause or decrease in tumor size in prostatic cancer
• Edema, hypertension, cardiac symptoms, jaundice
• Mental status: affect, mood, behavioral changes, aggression
• Hypercalcemia

Teach patient/family:
• To weigh weekly, report gain >5 lb
• To report breast lumps, vaginal bleeding, edema, jaundice, dark urine, clay colored stools, dyspnea, headache, blurred vision, abdominal pain, numbness or stiffness in legs, chest pain; male to report impotence or gynecomastia
• To avoid sunlight or wear sunscreen; burns may occur

Lab test interferences:
Increase: BSP retention test, PBI, T_4, serum sodium, platelet aggressability, thyroxine-binding globulin (TBG), prothrombin, factors VII, VIII, IX, X, triglycerides
Decrease: Serum folate, serum triglyceride, T_3 resin uptake test, glucose tolerance test, antithrombin III, pregnanediol, metyraponetest
False positive: LE prep, antinuclear antibodies

---

diflorasone diacetate

(die-floor'-a-sone)
Maxifloor

Func. class.: Topical corticosteroid
Chem. class.: Synthetic fluorinated agent, group II potency

Action: Possesses antipruritic, antiinflammatory actions
Uses: Psoriasis, eczema, contact dermatitis, pruritus

Dosage and routes:
• *Adult and child:* Apply to affected area qd-tid
Available forms include: Cream 0.05%; oint 0.05%
Side effects/adverse reactions:
INTEG: Burning, dryness, itching, irritation, acne, folliculitis, hypertrichosis, perioral dermatitis, hypopigmentation, atrophy, striae, miliaria, allergic contact dermatitis, secondary infection
Contraindications: Hypersensitivity to corticosteroids, fungal infections
Precautions: Pregnancy (C), lactation, viral infections, bacterial infections
Interactions/incompatibilities: None known
NURSING CONSIDERATIONS
Assess:
• Temperature; if fever develops, drug should be discontinued
Administer:
• Only to affected areas; do not get in eyes
• Medication, then cover with occlusive dressing (only if prescribed), seal to normal skin, change q12h; use occlusive dressing with extreme caution
• Only to dermatoses; do not use on weeping, denuded, or infected area
Perform/provide:
• Cleansing before application of drug
• Treatment for a few days after area has cleared
• Storage at room temperature
Evaluate:
• Therapeutic response: absence of severe itching, patches on skin, flaking
Teach patient/family:
• To avoid sunlight on affected area; burns may occur

diflunisal
(dye-floo′ni-sal)
Dolobid
Func. class.: Nonnarcotic analgesic
Chem. class.: Salicylate

D

Action: Blocks pain impulses in CNS that occur in response to inhibition of prostaglandin synthesis; antipyretic action results from inhibition of hypothalamic heat-regulating center to produce vasodilation to allow heat dissipation
Uses: Mild to moderate pain or fever including arthritis, juvenile rheumatoid arthritis
Dosage and routes:
Pain/fever
• *Adult:* PO 500-1000 mg/day in 2 divided doses, q12h, not to exceed 1500 mg/day
Available forms include: Tabs 250, 500 mg
Side effects/adverse reactions:
*HEMA: **Thrombocytopenia, agranulocytosis, leukopenia, neutropenia, hemolytic anemia,*** increased pro-time
CNS: Stimulation, drowsiness, dizziness, confusion, convulsion, headache, flushing, hallucinations, coma
GI: Nausea, vomiting, GI bleeding, diarrhea, heartburn, anorexia, ***hepatitis***
INTEG: Rash, urticaria, bruising
EENT: Tinnitus, hearing loss
CV: Rapid pulse, pulmonary edema
RESP: Wheezing, hyperpnea
ENDO: Hypoglycemia, hyponatremia, hypokalemia
Contraindications: Hypersensitivity to salicylates, GI bleeding, bleeding disorders, children <3 yr, pregnancy, lactation, vitamin K deficiency
Precautions: Anemia, hepatic dis-

ease, renal disease, Hodgkin's disease

Pharmacokinetics:

PO: Onset 15-30 min, peak 2-3 hr, metabolized by liver, excreted by kidneys, crosses placenta, 99% protein bound, excreted in breast milk

Interactions/incompatibilities:

• Decreased effects of this drug: antacids, steroids, urinary alkalizers

• Increased blood loss: alcohol, heparin

• Increased effects of: anticoagulants, insulin, methotrexate

• Decreased effects of: probenecid, spironolactone, sulfinpyrazone, sulfonylmides

• Toxic effects: PABA

• Decreased blood sugar levels: salicylates

NURSING CONSIDERATIONS

Assess:

• Liver function studies: AST, ALT, bilirubin, creatinine if patient is on long-term therapy

• Renal function studies: BUN, urine creatinine if patient is on long-term therapy

• Blood studies: CBC, Hct, Hgb, pro-time if patient is on long-term therapy

• I&O ratio; decreasing output may indicate renal failure (long-term therapy)

Administer:

• To patient crushed or whole; chewable tablets may be chewed

• With food or milk to decrease gastric symptoms; give 30 min before or 2 hr after meals

Perform/provide:

• Repositioning to decrease pain

• Cool cloth for fever

Evaluate:

• Hepatotoxicity: dark urine, clay-colored stools, yellowing of skin, sclera, itching, abdominal pain, fever, diarrhea if patient is on long-term therapy

• Allergic reactions: rash, urticaria; if these occur, drug may need to be discontinued

• Renal dysfunction: decreased urine output

• Ototoxicity: tinnitus, ringing, roaring in ears; audiometric testing is needed before, after long-term therapy

• Visual changes: blurring, halos, corneal, retinal damage

• Edema in feet, ankles, legs

• Prior drug history; there are many drug interactions

Teach patient/family:

• To report any symptoms of hepatotoxicity, renal toxicity, visual changes, ototoxicity, allergic reactions (long-term therapy)

• Not to exceed recommended dosage; acute poisoning may result

• To read label on other OTC drugs; many contain aspirin

• That therapeutic response takes 2 wk (arthritis)

• To avoid alcohol ingestion; GI bleeding may occur

Lab test interferences:

Increase: Coagulation studies, liver function studies, serum uric acid, amylase, CO_2, urinary protein

Decrease: Serum potassium, PBI, cholesterol

Interfere: Urine catecholamines, pregnancy test

Treatment of overdose: Lavage, activated charcoal, monitor electrolytes, VS

---

digitoxin

(di-ji-tox'in)

Crystodigin, Purodigin

Func. class.: Antidysrhythmic, cardiac glycoside cardiotonic

Chem. class.: Digitalis preparation

Action: Acts by influx of calcium

ions from extracellular to intracellular cytoplasm, increasing force of contraction and cardiac output

Uses: Congestive heart failure, atrial fibrillation, atrial flutter, atrial tachycardia, rapid digitalization in these disorders

Dosage and routes:

• *Adult:* PO 0.6 mg then 0.4 mg and 0.2 mg at intervals 4-6 hr divided doses over 24 hr, maintenance is 0.05-0.3 mg/day

• *Child 2-12 yr:* IM/IV/PO .03 mg/kg or 0.075 mg/m^2 in divided doses over 24 hr, maintenance .003 mg/kg or 0.75 mg/m^2 qd

• *Child 1-2 yr:* IM/IV/PO 0.04 mg/kg in divided doses over 24 hr maintenance 0.004 mg/kg qd

• *Child 2 wk-1 yr:* IM/IV/PO 0.045 mg/kg in divided doses over 24 hr, maintenance 0.0045 mg/kg qd

• *Neonates:* IM/IV/PO 0.022 mg/kg in divided doses over 24 hrs., maintenance 0.0022 mg/kg qd

• *Avoid IM route; causes painful local reaction*

Available forms include: Tabs IV 0.05, 0.1, 0.15 g, 0.2 mg

Side effects/adverse reactions:

CNS: Headache, drowsiness, apathy, confusion, disorientation, fatigue, depression, hallucinations

CV: Dysrhythmias, hypotension, bradycardia, AV block

GI: Nausea, vomiting, anorexia, abdominal pain, diarrhea

EENT: Blurred vision, yellow-green halos, photophobia, diplopia

MS: Muscular weakness

Contraindications: Hypersensitivity to digitalis, ventricular fibrillation, ventricular tachycardia, carotid sinus syndrome

Precautions: Renal disease, hepatic disease, acute MI, AV block, severe respiratory disease, hypothyroidism, elderly

Pharmacokinetics:

IV: Onset 30-125 min, peak 4-12 hr, duration variable, half-life 5-7 days metabolized in liver, excreted in urine

Interactions/incompatibilities:

• Hypokalemia: diuretics, amphotericin B, carbenicillin, ticarcillin, corticosteroids

• Blood levels increased: propantheline bromide, spironolactone

• Decreased effects: antihistamines, anticonvulsants, hypoglycemic agents, phenylbutazone, barbiturates, cholestyramine, colestipol, penicillamine

• Toxicity: adrenergics, amphotericin, corticosteroids, diuretics, glucose, insulin, reserpine, succinylcholine, thyroid agents, quinidine, thioamines

• Incompatible with all medications in syringe or solution

NURSING CONSIDERATIONS

Assess:

• Apical pulse for 1 min before giving drug; if pulse <60, take again in 1 hr; if <60, call physician

• Electrolytes: potassium, sodium, chloride, calcium; renal function studies: BUN, creatinine; blood studies: ALT, AST, bilirubin

• Monitor drug levels (therapeutic level 25-35ng/ml)

Administer:

• Potassium supplements if ordered for potassium levels <3.0

Evaluate:

• Cardiac status: apical pulse, character, rate, rhythm

• Therapeutic response: decreased weight, edema, pulse, respiration and increased urine output

Teach patient/family:

• Not to stop drug abruptly; teach all aspects of drug

• To avoid OTC medications, since many adverse drug interactions may occur

---

italics = common side effects   ***bold italic*** = life threatening reactions

Lab test interferences:
Increase: CPK
Treatment of overdose: Discontinue drug, administer potassium, monitor EKG

---

digoxin
(di-jox'in)
Lanoxicaps, Lanoxin

Func. class.: Antidysrhythmic, cardic glycoside
Chem. class.: Digitalis preparation

Action: Acts by influx of calcium ions from extracellular to intracellular cytoplasm; increases cardiac contractility and cardiac output
Uses: Congestive heart failure, atrial fibrillation, atrial flutter, atrial tachycardia, rapid digitalization in these disorders
Dosage and routes:
• *Adult:* IV 0.5 mg in divided doses over 24 hr; PO 0.125-0.5 mg qd, may require loading dose of 1 mg; IV 8-12 μg/kg
• *Elderly:* PO 0.125 qd maintenance
• *Child >2 yr:* PO 0.02-0.04 mg/kg divided q8h over 24 hr, maintenance 0.012 mg/kg qd in divided doses q12hr; IV loading dose 0.015-0.035 mg/kg
• *Child 1 mo-2 yr:* IV 0.03-0.05 mg/kg, change to PO as soon as possible; PO 0.035-0.060 mg/kg divided in 3 doses over 24 hr, maintenance 0.01-0.02 mg/kg in divided doses q12h
• *Neonates:* IV loading dose 0.02-0.03 mg/kg, change to PO as soon as possible; PO loading dose 0.035 mg/kg divided q8h, over 24h, maintenance 0.01 mg/kg in divided doses q12h
• *Premature infants:* IV 0.015-0.025 mg/kg divided in 3 doses over 24 hr, maintenance 0.01 mg/kg in divided doses q12hr

Available forms include: Caps 50, 100, 200 μg; elix 50 μg/ml; tabs 125, 250, 500 μg; inj 100, 250 μg/ml
Side effects/adverse reactions:
CNS: Headache, drowsiness, apathy, confusion, disorientation, fatigue, depression, hallucinations
CV: Dysrhythmias, hypotension, bradycardia, *AV block*
GI: Nausea, vomiting, anorexia, abdominal pain, diarrhea
EENT: Blurred vision, yellow-green halos, photophobia, diplopia
MS: Muscular weakness
Contraindications: Hypersensitivity to digitalis, ventricular fibrillation, ventricular tachycardia, carotid sinus syndrome
Precautions: Renal disease, hepatic disease, acute MI, AV block, severe respiratory disease, hypothyroidism, elderly
Pharmacokinetics:
IV: Onset 5-30 min, peak 1-5 hr, duration variable, half-life 1.5 days excreted in urine
Interactions/incompatibilities:
• Hypokalemia: diuretics, amphotericin B, carbenicillin, ticarcillin, corticosteroids
• Increased blood levels: propantheline bromide, spironolactone quinidine, verapamil, aminoglycosides PO, amiodarone, anticholinergics, quinine
• Toxicity: adrenergics, amphotericin, corticosteroids, diuretics, glucose, insulin, reserpine, succinylcholine, thyroid agents, quinidine, thioamines
• Incompatible with all medications in syringe or solution
NURSING CONSIDERATIONS
Assess:
• Apical pulse for 1 min before giving drug; if pulse <60, take again in 1 hr; if <60, call physician
• Electrolytes: potassium, sodium, chloride, calcium; renal function

---

studies: BUN, creatinine; blood studies: ALT, AST, bilirubin

• I&O ratio, daily weights

• Monitor drug levels (therapeutic level 0.5-2 mg/ml)

Administer:

• Potassium supplements if ordered for potassium levels <3.0

Evaluate:

• Cardiac status: apical pulse, character, rate, rhythm

• Therapeutic response: decreased weight, edema, pulse, respiration and increased urine output

Teach patient/family:

• Not to stop drug abruptly; teach all aspects of drug

• To avoid OTC medications, since many adverse drug interactions may occur; do not take antacid at same time

Lab test interferences:

Increase: CPK

Treatment of overdose: Discontinue drug, administer potassium, monitor EKG, administer an adrenergic blocking agent

---

dihydroergotamine mesylate

(dye-hye-droe-er-got′a-meen)

D.H.E. 45

Func. class.: Adrenergic blocker

Chem. class.: Ergot alkaloid (dihydrogenated)

Action: Constricts smooth muscle in periphery, cranial blood vessels

Uses: Vascular headache (migraine or histamine)

Dosage and routes:

• *Adult:* IM/IV 1 mg, may repeat q1-2 hr if needed, not to exceed 3 mg/day or 6 mg/wk

Available forms include: Inj 1 mg/ml

Side effects/adverse reactions:

CNS: Numbness in fingers, toes

CV: Transient tachycardia, chest pain, bradycardia, increase or decrease in B/P

GI: Nausea, vomiting

MS: Muscle pain

Contraindications: Hypersensitivity to ergot preparations, occlusion (peripheral, vascular), CAD, hepatic disease, pregnancy, renal disease, peptic ulcer, hypertension

Precautions: Pregnancy, lactation, children

Pharmacokinetics:

IM: Onset 15-30 min, peak 45 min, duration 3-4 hr

IV: Onset 5 min, peak 45 min, duration 3-4 hr

Half-life 1.3-4 hr

Interactions/incompatibilities:

• Increased effects: troleandomycin

• Increased vasoconstriction: beta blockers

NURSING CONSIDERATIONS

Assess:

• Weight daily, check for peripheral edema in feet, legs

Administer:

• IM dose, which takes 20 min for effect, or use IV for immediate effect

• At beginning of headache, dose must be titrated to patient response

• Give with meals or after meals to avoid GI symptoms

• Only to women who are not pregnant, harm to fetus may occur

Perform/provide:

• Storage in dark area, do not use discolored solutions

• Quiet, calm environment with decreased stimulation for noise, or bright light or excessive talking

Evaluate:

• Therapeutic response: decrease in frequency, severity of headache

• For stress level, activity, recreation, coping mechanisms of patient

• Neurological status: LOC, blurring vision, nausea, vomiting, tin-

---

italics = common side effects   ***bold italic*** = life threatening reactions

gling in extremities that occur preceding the headache

• Ingestion of tyramine foods (pickled products, beer, wine, aged cheese), food additives, preservatives, colorings, artificial sweeteners, chocolate, caffeine, which may precipitate these types of headaches

Teach patient/family:

• Not to use OTC medications, serious drug interactions may occur

• To maintain dose at approved level, not to increase even if drug does not relieve headache

• To report side effects: increased vasoconstriction starting with cold extremities, then paresthesia, weakness

• That an increase in headaches may occur when this drug is discontinued after long-term use

• Keep drug out of reach of children, death may occur

---

dihydrotachysterol

(dye-hye-droe-tak-iss′ter-ole)
DHT Intensol, DHT Oral Solution, Hytakerol

Func. class.: Parathyroid agent (calcium regulator)
Chem. class.: Vitamin D analog

Action: Increases intestinal absorption, provides calcium for bones, increases renal tubular absorption of phosphate

Uses: Renal osteodystrophy, hypoparathyroidism, pseudo hypoparathyroidism, familial hypophosphatemia

Dosage and routes:
Hypophosphatemia

• *Adult and child:* PO 0.5-2 mg qd, maintenance 0.3-1.5 mg qd

Hypoparathyroidism/pseudohypoparathyroidism

• *Adult:* PO 0.8-2.4 mg qd × 1 wk, maintenance 0.2-2 mg qd reg-

ulated by serum Ca levels

• *Child:* PO 1-5 mg qd × 1 wk, maintenance 0.2-1 mg qd regulated by serum Ca levels

Renal osteodystrophy

• *Adult:* PO 0.1-0.6 mg qd

Available forms include: Tabs 0.125, 0.2, 0.4 mg; caps 0.125 mg; oral sol 0.2, 0.25 mg/5 ml

Side effects/adverse reactions:

EENT: Tinnitus

CNS: Drowsiness, headache, vertigo, fever, lethargy

GI: Nausea, diarrhea, vomiting, jaundice, anorexia, dry mouth, constipation, cramps, metallic taste

MS: Myalgia, arthralgia, decreased bone development

GU: Polyuria, hypercalciuria, hyperphosphatemia, hematuria

Contraindications: Hypersensitivity, renal disease, hyperphosphatemia, hypercalcemia

Precautions: Pregnancy (C), renal calculi, lactation, CV disease

Pharmacokinetics:

PO: Onset 2 wk; metabolized by liver, excreted in feces (active/inactive)

Interactions/incompatibilities:

• Decreased absorption of this drug: cholestyramine, colestipol, HCl, mineral oil

• Hypercalcemia: thiazide diuretics

• Cardiac dysrhythmias: cardiac glycosides

• Decreased effect of this drug: corticosteroids

NURSING CONSIDERATIONS
Assess:

• BUN, urinary calcium, AST, ALT, cholesterol, creatinine, uric acid, chloride, magnesium, electrolytes, urine pH, phosphate; may increase calcium, should be kept at 9-10 mg/dl, vitamin D 50-135 IU/dl, phosphate 70 mg/dl

• Alk phosphatase; may be decreased

• For increased blood level since

toxic reactions may occur rapidly
Administer:
• PO, may be increased q4wk depending on blood level
Perform/provide:
• Storage in tight, light-resistant containers at room temperature
• Restriction of sodium, potassium if required
• Restriction of fluids if required for chronic renal failure
Evaluate:
• For dry mouth, metallic taste, polyuria, bone pain, muscle weakness, headache, fatigue, tinnitus, change in LOC, irregular pulse, dysrhythmias, increased respirations, anorexia, nausea, vomiting, cramps, diarrhea, constipation; may indicate hypercalcemia
• Renal status: decreased urinary output (oliguria, anuria), edema in extremities, weight gain 5 lb, periorbital edema
• Nutritional status, diet for sources of vitamin D (milk, some seafood), calcium (dairy products, dark green vegetables), phosphates (dairy products) must be avoided
Teach patient/family:
• The symptoms of hypercalcemia
• Foods rich in calcium
Lab test interferences:
False increase: Cholesterol

---

dihydroxyaluminum sodium carbonate

(dye-hye-drox'-ee-a-loom-aa-nim)
Rolaids
Func. class.: Antacid
Chem. class.: Aluminum product

Action: Neutralizes gastric acidity, reduces pepsin
Uses: Antacid
Dosage and routes:
• *Adult:* PO 1-2 as needed
Available forms include: Chewable tab 334 mg

Side effects/adverse reactions:
GI: Constipation, **obstruction**
Contraindications: Hypersensitivity to aluminum products
Precautions: Elderly, sodium/fluid restriction, decreased GI motility, GI obstruction, dehydration, severe renal disease, CHF
Pharmacokinetics:
PO: Onset 20-40 min, excreted in feces
Interactions/incompatibilities:
• Decreased effectiveness of: tetracyclines
NURSING CONSIDERATIONS
Administer:
• Laxatives or stool softeners if constipation occurs
Evaluate:
• Therapeutic response: absence of pain, decreased acidity
• Constipation; increase bulk in the diet if needed
Teach patient/family:
• Increase fluids to 2000 ml/day unless contraindicated

---

diltiazem HCl

(dil-tye'a-zem)
Cardizem
Func. class.: Calcium channel blocker
Chem. class.: Benzothiazepine

Action: Inhibits calcium ion influx across cell membrane during cardiac depolarization; produces relaxation of coronary vascular smooth muscle, dilates coronary arteries
Uses: Chronic stable angina pectoris, vasospastic angina, coronary artery spasm, dysrhythmias
Dosage and routes:
• *Adult:* PO 30 mg qid, increasing dose gradually to 240 mg/day in divided doses
Available forms include: Tabs 30, 60 mg

Side effects/adverse reactions:

CV: Dysrhythmia, edema, CHF, bradycardia, hypotension, palpitations

GI: Nausea, vomiting, diarrhea, gastric upset, constipation, increased liver function studies

GU: Nocturia, polyuria, *acute renal failure*

INTEG: Rash, pruritus, flushing, photosensitivity

CNS: Headache, fatigue, drowsiness, dizziness, anxiety, depression, weakness, insomnia, confusion

Contraindications: Sick sinus syndrome, 2nd or 3rd degree heart block, hypotension less than 90 mm Hg systolic

Precautions: CHF, hypotension, hepatic injury, pregnancy, lactation, children, renal disease

Pharmacokinetics: Onset 30-60 min, peak 2-3 hr, half-life 3½-9 hr; metabolized by liver, excreted in urine (96% as metabolites)

Interactions/incompatibilities:

• Increased effects: β-blockers, digitalis

NURSING CONSIDERATIONS
Assess:

• Blood levels (therapeutic levels: 0.025-0.1 μg/ml)

Administer:

• Before meals, hs

Perform/provide:

• Storage in tight container at room temperature

Evaluate:

• Therapeutic response: decreased anginal pain

• Cardiac status: B/P, pulse, respiration, ECG

Teach patient/family:

• How to take pulse before taking drug; record or graph should be kept

• To avoid hazardous activities until stabilized on drug; dizziness is no longer a problem

• To limit caffeine consumption

• To avoid OTC drugs unless directed by a physician

• Stress patient compliance to all areas of medical regimen: diet, exercise, stress reduction, drug therapy

Treatment of overdose: Defibrillation, atropine for AV block, vasopressor for hypotension

---

dimenhydrinate

(dye-men-hye′dri-nate)

Dimen, Dimentabs, Dipendrate, Dramamine, Dymenate, Gravol,* Hydrate, Nauseal,* Nauseatol,* Novodimenate,* Reidamine, Travamine,* Vertiban

Func. class.: Antiemetic, antihistamine

Chem. class.: H₁-receptor antagonist, ethanolamine derivative

Action: Acts centrally by blocking chemoreceptor trigger zone, which in turn acts on vomiting center

Uses: Motion sickness, nausea, vomiting

Dosage and routes:

• *Adult:* PO 50-100 mg q4h; REC 100 mg qd or bid; IM/IV 50 mg as needed

• *Child:* IM/PO 5 mg/kg divided in 4 equal doses

Available forms include: Tabs 50 mg; inj 500 mg/ml; liq 12.5/4 ml; supp 50, 100 mg

Side effects/adverse reactions:

CNS: Drowsiness, restlessness, headache, dizziness, insomnia, confusion, nervousness, tingling, vertigo

GI: Nausea, anorexia, diarrhea, vomiting, constipation

CV: Hypertension, hypotension, palpitation

INTEG: Rash, urticaria, fever, chills, flushing

EENT: Dry mouth, blurred vision,

diplopia, nasal congestion, photosensitivity

Contraindications: Hypersensitivity to narcotics, shock

Precautions: Children, cardiac dysrhythmias, elderly, asthma, pregnancy, prostatic hypertrophy, bladder-neck obstruction, narrow-angle glaucoma, stenosing peptic ulcer, pyloroduodenal obstruction

Pharmacokinetics:

IM/PO: Duration 4-6 hr

Interactions/incompatibilities:

• Increased effect: alcohol, other CNS depressants

• May mask ototoxic symptoms associated with antibiotics

NURSING CONSIDERATIONS
Assess:

• VS, B/P; check patients with cardiac disease more often

Administer:

• IM injection in large muscle mass; aspirate to avoid IV administration

• Tablets may be swallowed whole, chewed, or allowed to dissolve

Evaluate:

• Signs of toxicity of other drugs or masking of symptoms of disease: brain tumor, intestinal obstruction

• Observe for drowsiness, dizziness

Teach patient/family:

• That a false negative result may occur with skin testing; these procedures should not be scheduled for 4 days after discontinuing use

• Avoid hazardous activities, activities requiring alertness; dizziness may occur; instruct patient to request assistance with ambulation

• Avoid alcohol, other depressants

Lab test interferences:

False negative: Allergy skin testing

dimercaprol

(dye-mer-kap'role)
BAL in Oil

Func. class.: Heavy metal antagonist

Chem. class.: Chelating agent (dithiol compound)

D

Action: Binds ions from arsenic, gold, mercury, lead, copper to form water-soluble complex removed by kidneys

Uses: Arsenic, gold, mercury, lead poisoning

Dosage and routes:

Severe gold/arsenic poisoning

• *Adult:* IM 3 mg/kg q4h × 2 days, then qid × 1 day, then bid × 10 days

Mild gold/arsenic poisoning

• *Adult:* IM 2.5 mg/kg qid × 2 days, then bid × 1 day, then qd × 10 days

Acute lead poisoning

• *Adult:* IM 4 mg/kg, then q4h with edetate calcium disodium 12.5 mg/kg IM, not to exceed 5 mg/kg/dose

Mercury poisoning

• *Adult:* IM 5 mg/kg, then 2.5 mg/kg/day or bid × 10 days

Available forms include: Inj IM 100 mg/ml

Side effects/adverse reactions:

CNS: Headache, paresthesia, anxiety, tremors, ***convulsions, shock***

INTEG: Urticaria, erythema, pruritus, pain at injection site, fever

CV: Hypertension, tachycardia

GI: Nausea, vomiting

*SYST: **Anaphylaxis,*** metabolic acidosis

Contraindications: Hypersensitivity, anuria, hepatic insufficiency, poisoning of other metals, severe renal disease, child <3 yr

Precautions: Hypertension, pregnancy, lactation

Pharmacokinetics:
Metabolized by plasma enzymes, excreted by kidneys as complex, unchanged drug

Interactions/incompatibilities:
• Increased toxicity: iron, selenium, uranium, cadmium

NURSING CONSIDERATIONS

Assess:
• B/P, increasing B/P or tachycardia
• Monitor I&O, kidney function studies: BUN, creatinine, CrCl; report decreases in output
• Urine: pH, albumin, casts, blood
• Metal levels daily

Administer:
• IM in deep muscle mass; rotate injection sites
• Only when epinephrine 1 : 1000 is on unit for anaphylaxis
• Being careful not to allow drug to touch skin, contact dermatitis can occur
• Acetazolamide or sodium citrate to decrease pH of urine, which decreases renal damage

Evaluate:
• Allergic reactions (rash, urticaria); if these occur, drug should be discontinued

Teach patient/family:
• That breath may be odorous

Lab test interferences:
Decrease: RAIU test

---

dinoprost tromethamine

(dye'noe-prost)
PGF$_2$a, Prostin F$_2$ Alpha
Func. class.: Oxytocic
Chem. class.: Prostaglandin F$_2$ alpha

Action: Stimulates uterine contractions causing abortion, complete in approximately 16 hr
Uses: Abortion during 2nd trimester

Dosage and routes:
• *Adult:* INJ 40 mg injection into amniotic sac after determining that there is absence of blood in transabdominal intraamniotic tap, wait 24 hr, give 10-40 mg if abortion is incomplete

Available forms include: Inj 5 mg/ml

Side effects/adverse reactions:
CNS: Headache, dizziness, fainting
CV: Hypotension
GI: Nausea, vomiting, diarrhea, cramps, epigastric pain
INTEG: Flushing, hot flashes
RESP: Wheezing, ***bronchospasm***

Contraindications: Hypersensitivity, uterine fibrosis, cervical stenosis, pelvic surgery, pelvic inflammatory disease (PID), respiratory disease

Precautions: Hepatic disease, renal disease, cardiac disease, asthma, anemia, convulsive disorders, hypertension, glaucoma

Pharmacokinetics:
ONSET: 15 min, peak 2 hr; metabolized in lungs, liver, excreted in urine (metabolites)

Interactions/incompatibilities:
None known

NURSING CONSIDERATIONS

Assess:
• B/P, pulse; watch for change that may indicate hemorrhage
• Respiratory rate, rhythm, depth; notify physician of abnormalities

Administer:
• IM in deep muscle mass, rotate injection sites if additional doses are given
• After having crash cart available on unit

Evaluate:
• For length, duration of contraction; notify physician of contractions lasting over 1 min or absence of contractions

Teach patient/family:
• To report increased blood loss,

abdominal cramps, increased temperature or foul-smelling lochia

---

dinoprostone

(dye-noe-prost'one)

PGE$_2$, Prostin E$_2$

Func. class.: Oxytocic

Chem. class.: Prostaglandin E$_2$

Action: Stimulates uterine contractions causing abortion; acts within 30 hr for complete abortion

Uses: Abortion during 2nd trimester, benign hydatidiform mole, expulsion of uterine contents in fetal deaths to 28 wk, missed abortion

Dosage and routes:

• *Adult:* VAG SUPP 20 mg, repeat q3-5h until abortion occurs

Available forms include: Vag supp 20 mg

Side effects/adverse reactions:

CNS: Headache, dizziness

CV: Hypotension

GI: Nausea, vomiting, diarrhea

GU: Vaginitis, vaginal pain, vulvitis, vaginismus

INTEG: Rash, skin color changes

MS: Leg cramps, joint swelling, weakness

EENT: Blurred vision, decreased tinnitus

Contraindications: Hypersensitivity, uterine fibrosis, cervical stenosis, pelvic surgery, pelvic inflammatory disease (PID), respiratory disease

Precautions: Hepatic disease, renal disease, cardiac disease, asthma, anemia, jaundice, diabetes mellitus, convulsive disorders, hypertension, hypotension

Pharmacokinetics:

SUPP: Onset 10 min, duration 2-3 hr; metabolized in spleen, kidney, lungs, excreted in urine

Interactions/incompatibilities: None known

NURSING CONSIDERATIONS

Assess:

• Respiratory rate, rhythm, depth; notify physician of abnormalities

• Vaginal discharge: check for itching, irritation; indicates vaginal infection

Administer:

• Antiemetic/antidiarrheal before administration of this drug

• High in vagina

• After warming suppository by running warm water over package

Evaluate:

• For length, duration of contraction; notify physician of contractions lasting over 1 min or absence of contractions

• For fever, chills: increase fluids, or give tepid sponge bath or blanket

Teach patient/family:

• To remain supine for 10-15 min after insertion

---

diphenhydramine HCl

(dye-fen-hye'dra-meen)

Allerdryl, Baramine, Bax, Benachlor, Benadryl, Benahist, Bendylate, Bentract, Compoz, Diphenacen, Fenylhist, Nordryl, Rohydra, Span-Lanin, Valdrene, Wehdryl

Func. class.: Antihistamine

Chem. class.: Ethanolamine derivative, H$_1$-receptor antagonist

Action: Acts on blood vessels, GI, respiratory system by competing with histamine for H$_1$-receptor site; decreases allergic response by blocking histamine

Uses: Allergy symptoms, rhinitis, motion sickness, antiparkinsonism, nighttime sedation, infant colic, nonproductive cough

Dosage and routes:

• *Adult:* PO 25-50 mg q4-6h, not to exceed 400 mg/day; IM/IV 10-50 mg, not to exceed 400 mg/day

• *Child >12 kg:* PO/IM/IV 5 mg/

---

kg/day in 4 divided doses, not to exceed 300 mg/day

Available forms include: Caps 25, 50 mg; tabs 50 mg; elix 12.5 mg/ml; syr 12.5 mg/5ml; inj IM, IV 10, 50 mg/ml

Side effects/adverse reactions:

CNS: Dizziness, drowsiness, poor coordination, fatigue, anxiety, euphoria, confusion, paresthesia, neuritis

CV: Hypotension, palpitations, tachycardia

RESP: Increased thick secretions, wheezing, chest tightness

HEMA: Thrombocytopenia, agranulocytosis, hemolytic anemia

GI: Dry mouth, nausea, vomiting, anorexia, constipation, diarrhea

INTEG: Rash, urticaria, photosensitivity

GU: Retention, dysuria, frequency

EENT: Blurred vision, dilated pupils, tinnitus, nasal stuffiness, dry nose, throat, mouth

Contraindications: Hypersensitivity to H_1-receptor antagonist, acute asthma attack, lower respiratory tract disease

Precautions: Increased intraocular pressure, renal disease, cardiac disease, hypertension, bronchial asthma, seizure disorder, stenosed peptic ulcers, hyperthyroidism, prostatic hypertrophy, bladder neck obstruction, pregnancy

Pharmacokinetics:

PO: Peak 1-3 hr, duration 4-7 hr, metabolized in liver, excreted by kidneys, crosses placenta, excreted in breast milk, half-life 2-7 hr

Interactions/incompatibilities:

• Increased CNS depression: barbiturates, narcotics, hypnotics, tricyclic antidepressants, alcohol

• Decreased effect of: oral anticoagulants, heparin

• Increased effect of this drug: MAOIs

NURSING CONSIDERATIONS
Assess:

• I&O ratio; be alert for urinary retention, frequency, dysuria; drug should be discontinued if these occur

• CBC during long-term therapy

Administer:

• Coffee, tea, cola (caffeine) to decrease drowsiness

• With meals if GI symptoms occur, absorption may slightly decrease

• Deep IM in large muscle; rotate site

Perform/provide:

• Hard candy, gum, frequent rinsing of mouth for dryness

• Storage in tight container at room temperature

Evaluate:

• Therapeutic response: absence of running or congested nose or rashes

• Respiratory status: rate, rhythm, increase in bronchial secretions, wheezing, chest tightness

• Cardiac status: palpitations, increased pulse, hypotension

Teach patient/family:

• All aspects of drug use; to notify physician if confusion, sedation, hypotension occurs

• To avoid driving or other hazardous activity if drowsiness occurs

• To avoid concurrent use of alcohol or other CNS depressants

Lab test interferences:

False negative: Skin allergy tests

Treatment of overdose: Administer ipecac syrup or lavage, diazepam, vasopressors, barbiturates (short-acting)

diphenidol

(dye-fen′-i-dole)
Vontrol

Func. class.: Antiemetic
Chem. class.: Trihexyphenidyl derivative

Action: May act as dopamine antagonist at chemoreceptor trigger zone to inhibit vomiting
Uses: Nausea, vomiting, peripheral dizziness
Dosage and routes:
• *Adult:* PO 25-50 mg q4h
• *Children >23 kg:* PO 25 mg q4h prn; do not exceed 5.5 mg/kg/24 hr
Available forms include: Tabs 25 mg
Side effects/adverse reactions:
CNS: Drowsiness, fatigue, restlessness, tremor, headache, stimulation, dizziness, insomnia, twitching, disorientation, confusion, sleep disturbance, auditory, visual hallucination, depression
GI: Nausea, indigestion
CV: Hypotension
INTEG: Rash
EENT: Dry mouth, blurred vision
Contraindications: Hypersensitivity, psychosis, anuria
Precautions: Children, prostatic hypertrophy, glaucoma, pyloric and duodenal stenosis, elderly
Pharmacokinetics:
PO: Onset 30-45 min, duration 3-6 hr, metabolized by liver, excreted by kidneys
Interactions/incompatibilities:
None known
NURSING CONSIDERATIONS
Assess:
• VS, B/P; check patients with cardiac disease more often
• Observe for CNS adverse effects: confusion, hallucination

• Monitor I&O (90% excreted in urine)
Administer:
• Tabs may be swallowed whole, chewed, or allowed to dissolve
Evaluate:
• Signs of toxicity of other drugs or masking of symptoms of disease: brain tumor, intestinal obstruction
• Drowsiness, dizziness
Teach patient/family:
• To avoid alcohol, other depressants
• That drug should be used only under close supervision

diphenoxylate HCl with atropine sulfate

(dye-fen-ox′i-late)
Colonaid, Lofene, Loflo, Lomo-Plus, Lomotil, Lo-Trol

Func. class.: Antidiarrheal
Chem. class.: Phenylipeperidine derivative, opiate agonist

Controlled Substance Schedule V
Action: Inhibits gastric motility by acting on mucosal receptors responsible for peristalsis
Uses: Diarrhea (cause undetermined)
Dosage and routes:
• *Adult:* PO 5 mg qid, titrated to patient response
• *Child 2-12 yr:* PO 0.3-0.4 mg/kg/day in divided doses
Available forms include: Tabs 2.5 mg
Side effects/adverse reactions:
CNS: Drowsiness, headache, sedation, depression, weakness, lethargy
GI: Nausea, vomiting, abdominal pain, glossitis, colitis, paralytic ileus, toxic megacolon
EENT: Blurred vision, nystagmus, mydriasis
INTEG: Rash, urticaria, pruritus, angioneurotic edema

Contraindications: Hypersensitivity, severe liver disease, pseudomembranous enterocolitis, glaucoma, child <2 yr, electrolyte imbalances

Precautions: Hepatic disease, renal disease, ulcerative colitis

Pharmacokinetics:

PO: Onset 45-60 min, peak 2 hr, duration 3-4 hr, half-life 2½ hr; metabolized in liver to active, inactive metabolites; excreted in urine, feces, breast milk

Interactions/incompatibilities:

• Do not use with MAOIs; hypertensive crisis may occur

• Increased action of: alcohol, narcotics, barbiturates, other CNS depressants

NURSING CONSIDERATIONS

Assess:

• Electrolytes (K, Na, Cl) if on long-term therapy

Administer:

• For 48 hr only

Evaluate:

• Therapeutic response: decreased diarrhea

• Bowel pattern before; for rebound constipation after termination of medication

• Response after 48 hr; if no response, drug should be discontinued

• Dehydration in children

• Abdominal distention, toxic megacolon, which may occur in ulcerative colitis

Teach patient/family:

• To avoid OTC products unless directed by physician; may contain alcohol

• Not to exceed recommended dose

diphtheria and tetanus toxoids and pertussis vaccine (DPT)

Tri-Immunol

Func. class.: Vaccine/toxoid

Action: Provide immunity to diphtheria, tetanus, pertussis by stimulating antibody/antitoxin production

Uses: Prevention of diphtheria, tetanus, pertussis

Dosage and routes:

• *Child >6 wk-6 yr:* IM 0.5 ml at 2, 4, 6 mos, 1½ yr; booster needed 0.5 ml at age 6

Available forms include: Inj IM diphtheria 12.5 LfU, tetanus 5 LfU, pertussis 4 U/0.5 ml

Side effects/adverse reactions:

GI: Nausea, vomiting, anorexia

INTEG: Skin abscess, urticaria, itching, swelling, erythema, edema at site

CV: Tachycardia, hypotension

SYST: Lymphadenitis, *anaphylaxis,* fever, chills, malaise

CNS: Crying, fretfulness, fever, drowsiness

MS: Osteomyelitis

Contraindications: Hypersensitivity, active infection, poliomyelitis outbreak, immunosuppression

Precautions: Pregnancy

Interactions/incompatibilities:

• Decreased response to toxoid: immunosuppressive agents: antineoplastics, corticosteroids, radiation therapy

NURSING CONSIDERATIONS

Assess:

• For skin reactions: swelling, rash, urticaria

Administer:

• At least 4 wk apart × 3 doses

• Only with epinephrine 1:1000 on unit to treat laryngospasm

• IM only; not to be given SC (vas-

tus lateralis in infants, deltoid in adults)
Evaluate:
• For history of allergies, skin conditions (eczema, psoriasis, dermatitis), reactions to vaccinations
• For anaphylaxis: inability to breathe, bronchospasm
Teach patient/family:
• That doses are given at least 4 wk apart × 3 doses, booster needed at 10 yr intervals

---

dipivefrin HCl

(dye-pi've-frin)
Propine

Func. class.: Adrenergic agonist
Chem. class.: Diesterified epinephrine

Action: Converted to epinephrine, which decreases aqueous production and increases outflow
Uses: Open-angle glaucoma
Dosage and routes:
• *Adult:* INSTILL 1 gtt q12h
Available forms include: Sol 0.1%
Side effects/adverse reactions:
CV: Hypertension, tachycardia
EENT: Burning, stinging, mydriasis, photophobia
Contraindications: Hypersensitivity, narrow-angle glaucoma
Precautions: Pregnancy (B), lactation, children, aphakia
Pharmacokinetics:
INSTILL: Onset 30 min, duration 1 hr
Interactions/incompatibilities: None known
NURSING CONSIDERATIONS
Perform/provide:
• Storage at room temperature
Teach patient/family:
• To report stinging, burning, itching, lacrimation, puffiness
• Method of instillation, including pressure on lacrimal sac for 1 min and not to touch dropper to eye

dipyridamole

(dye-peer-id'a-mole)
Persantine, Pyridamole

Func. class.: Coronary vasodilator, antiplatelet
Chem. class.: Nonnitrate

Action: Increases oxygen saturation in coronary tissues, coronary blood flow; acts on small resistance vessels with little effect on vascular resistance; may increase development of collateral circulation
Uses: Angina, prevention of transient ischemic attacks, inhibition of platelet adhesion to prevent myocardial reinfarction, thromboembolism, with warfarin in prosthetic heart valves, prevention of coronary bypass graft occlusion with aspirin
Dosage and routes:
Angina/TIA
• *Adult:* PO 50 mg tid, 1 hr ac, not to exceed 400 mg qd
Inhibition of platelet adhesion
• *Adult:* PO 100-400 mg qd
Available forms include: Tabs 25, 50, 75 mg
Side effects/adverse reactions:
CV: Postural hypotension, increased anginal attacks, ***myocardial ischemia***
CNS: Headache, dizziness, weakness, fainting, syncope
GI: Nausea, vomiting, anorexia, diarrhea
INTEG: Rash, flushing
Contraindications: Hypersensitivity, hypotension
Precautions: Pregnancy
Pharmacokinetics:
PO: Onset 30 sec, peak 2-2½ min, duration 3-5 min
Therapeutic response may take several months, metabolized in liver, excreted in bile, undergoes enterohepatic recirculation

---

italics = common side effects   ***bold italic*** = life threatening reactions

Interactions/incompatibilities:

• Increased hypotension: alcohol, beta blockers, antihypertensives, narcotics, tricyclics, anticoagulants

• Decreased effects: sympathomimetics

NURSING CONSIDERATIONS

Assess:

• B/P, pulse during treatment until stable; take B/P lying, standing; orthostatic hypotension is common

Administer:

• On an empty stomach: 1 hr before meals or 2 hr after

Perform/provide:

• Storage at room temperature

Evaluate:

• Therapeutic response: decreased chest pain (angina), decreased platelet count

• Cardiac status: chest pain, what aggravates or ameliorates condition

Teach patient/family:

• That medication is not cure, may need to be taken continuously; therapeutic response may not be evident for 2-3 mo

• That it is necessary to quit smoking to prevent excessive vasoconstriction

• To avoid hazardous activities until stabilized on medication; dizziness may occur

Treatment of overdose: Administer IV phenylephrine, ergotamine tartrate

---

disopyramide

(dye-soe-peer'a-mide)

Rythmodan, Norpace, DSP, Narpamide (Major), Norpaceor

Func. class.: Antidysrhythmic (Class A)

Chem. class.: Nonnitrate

Action: Shortens sinus node recovery time, increases atrial/ventricular refractory time, suppresses ectopic focal activity, reduces duration of action potential between normal, infracted myocardium

Uses: PVCs, ventricular tachycardia

Dosage and routes:

• *Adult:* PO 150-200 mg q6h, in renal dysfunction 100 mg q6h; SUS REL CAPS 1 q12h

• *Child 12-18 yr:* PO 6-15 mg/kg/day, in divided doses q6h

• *Child 4-12 yr:* PO 10-15 mg/kg/day, in divided doses q6h

• *Child 1-4 yr:* PO 10-20 mg/kg/day, in divided doses q6h

• *Child <1 yr:* PO 10-30 mg/kg/day, in divided doses q6h

Available forms include: Caps 100 mg (as phosphate)

Side effects/adverse reactions:

GU: Retention, hesitancy

CNS: Headache, dizziness, psychosis, fatigue, depression, paresthesias

GI: Dry mouth, constipation, nausea, anorexia, flatulence

CV: Hypotension, bradycardia, angina, PVCs, tachycardia, increases QRS, QT segments, *cardiac arrest,* edema, weight gain, AV block

META: Hypoglycemia

INTEG: Rash, pruritus, urticaria, photosensitivity

MS: Weakness, pain in extremities

EENT: Blurred vision, dry nose, throat, eyes, narrow-angle glaucoma

HEMA: Thrombocytopenia, agranulocytosis, anemia (rare)

Contraindications: Hypersensitivity, 2nd/3rd degree block, cardiogenic shock, CHF (uncompensated), hypokalemia

Precautions: Pregnancy, lactation, diabetes mellitus, renal disease, children, hepatic disease, myasthenia gravis, narrow-angle glaucoma, sick sinus syndrome, cardiomyopathy

Pharmacokinetics:

IV: Onset 30 min-3½ hr, peak 1-2

hr, duration 1½-8½ hr

IM: Onset 30 min, peak 60-90 min, duration 6-8 hr

Half-life 4-10 hr, metabolized in liver, excreted in feces, urine, breast milk, crosses placenta

Interactions/incompatibilities:

• Increased effects of this drug: quinidine, procainamide, propranolol, lidocaine, atenolol

• Increased effects of: oral anticoagulants

• Increased side effects of this drug: anticholinergics

• Decreased effects: phenytoin, rifampin

NURSING CONSIDERATIONS

Assess:

• Apical pulse for 1 min, if less than 60 check again in 1 hr; if still less than 60, notify physician

• ECG, check for increased QT, widening QRS; drug should be discontinued

• Blood level during treatment (therapeutic level 2-4 mEq/ml)

• Weight daily, a rapid weight gain should be reported

• For dehydration or hypovolemia, I&O ratio, electrolytes (Na, K, Cl)

• Liver, kidney function studies (AST, ALT, bilirubin, BUN, creatinine) during treatment

• Diabetics for signs of hypoglycemia

• B/P continuously for hypotension, hypertension

Administer:

• Sugar-free gum, frequent sips of water for dry mouth

• Reduced dosage slowly with ECG monitoring

Evaluate:

• Increase in QRS, QT; drug should be discontinued

• For rebound hypertension after 1-2 hr

• Constipation, increase bulk in diet, water, stool softeners or laxatives needed

• Cardiac rate, respiration: rate, rhythm, character

• Urinary hesitancy, frequency or a change in I&O ratio; check for edema daily; check for toxicity

Teach patient/family:

• To take drug exactly as prescribed

• To avoid alcohol or severe hypotension may occur; to avoid OTC drugs or serious drug interactions may occur

• To make position change slowly during early therapy to prevent fainting

• To avoid sun exposure or use sunscreen to prevent burns

• To avoid hazardous activities if dizziness or blurred vision occurs

• Stress patient compliance with drug regimen; tell patient that this drug does not cure condition

Treatment of overdose: O_2, artificial ventilation, ECG, administer dopamine for circulatory depression, administer diazepam or thiopental for convulsions

Lab test interferences:

Increase: Blood glucose, liver enzymes, lipids, BUN, creatinine

Decrease: Hgb/Hct

---

disulfiram

(dye-sul'fi-ram)

Antabuse, Cronetal, Ro-Sulfiram

Func. class.: Alcohol deterrent

Chem. class.: Aldehyde dehydrogenase inhibitor

Action: Blocks oxidation of alcohol at acetaldehyde stage

Uses: Chronic alcoholism (as adjunct)

Dosage and routes:

• *Adult:* PO 250-500 mg qam × 1-2 wk, then 125-500 mg qd until desired response

Available forms include: Tabs 250, 500 mg

Side effects/adverse reactions:

CNS: Headache, drowsiness, restlessness, dizziness, fatigue, tremors, psychosis, neuritis, sweating, *convulsions, death*

GI: Nausea, vomiting, anorexia, *hepatotoxicity*

INTEG: Rash, dermatitis, urticaria

GU: Severe thirst

RESP: Respiratory depression, hyperventilation

CV: Tachycardia, chest pain, hypotension, *dysrhythmias*

Contraindications: Hypersensitivity, alcohol intoxication, psychoses, CV disease

Precautions: Hypothyroidism, hepatic disease, diabetes mellitus, seizure disorders, nephritis

Pharmacokinetics:

PO: Onset 12 hr, oxidized by liver, excreted unchanged in feces

Interactions/incompatibilities:

• Increased effects of: tricyclic antidepressants, diazepam, oral anticoagulants, paraldehyde, phenytoin, diazepam, chloriazepoxide, isoniazid

• Disulfiram reaction: alcohol

• Psychosis: metronidazole

NURSING CONSIDERATIONS

Assess:

• Liver function studies q2 wk during therapy: AST, ALT

• CBC, SMA q3-6 mo to detect any abnormality including increased cholesterol

Administer:

• Vitamin B_6 to decrease cholesterol levels, which often increase with this drug

• Once per day in the AM or hs if drowsiness occurs

• Only after patient has not been drinking for >12 hr

Evaluate:

• Mental status: affect, mood, drug history, ability to follow treatment, abstain from alcohol

Teach patient/family:

• Effect of this drug if alcohol is taken; written consent for disulfiram therapy should be obtained

• That shaving lotions, creams, lotin, cough preparations, skin products must be checked for alcohol content; even in small amount, alcohol can produce a reaction

• That tolerance will not develop if treatment is prolonged

• That reaction may occur for 2 wk after last dose

• That tablets can be crushed, mixed with beverage

• To carry ID listing disulfiram therapy

• To avoid driving or hazardous tasks if drowsiness occurs

• That disulfiram reaction can be fatal, occurs 15 min after drinking

Lab test interferences:

Increase: Cholesterol

Decrease: ^{131}I uptake, PBI, VMA

Treatment of overdose: IV vitamin C, ephedrine sulfate, antihistamines, O_2

---

dobutamine HCl

(doe-byoo'ta-meen)

Dubutrex

Func. class.: Adrenergic direct-acting β-blocker

Chem. class.: Catecholamine

Action: Causes increased contractility and heart rate by acting on β-1 receptors in heart

Uses: Cardiac surgery, refractory heart failure

Dosage and routes:

• *Adult:* IV INF 2.5-10 μg/kg/min, may increase to 40 μg/kg/min if needed

Available forms include: Inj 250 mg vial IV

Side effects/adverse reactions:

CNS: Anxiety, headache, dizziness

CV: Palpitations, tachycardia, hy-

pertension, PVCs, angina
GI: Heartburn, nausea, vomiting
MS: Muscle cramps (leg)
Contraindications: Hypersensitivity, idiopathic hypertropic subaortic stenosis
Precautions: Pregnancy, lactation, children, hypertension
Pharmacokinetics:
IV: Onset 1-5 min, peak 10 min, half-life 2 min, metabolized in liver (inactive metabolites), excreted in urine
Interactions/incompatibilities:
• Dysrhythmias: general anesthetics
• Decreased action of this drug: other β-blockers
• Increased B/P: oxytocics
• Increased pressor effect: tricyclic antidepressant, MAOIs
• Incompatible with alkaline solutions: Na, HCO$_3$

NURSING CONSIDERATIONS
Assess:
• Therapeutic level (40-190 mg/ml)
• I&O ratio
• ECG during administration continuously; if B/P increases, drug is decreased
• B/P and pulse q5min after parenteral route
• CVP or PWP during infusion if possible
Administer:
• Plasma expanders for hypovolemia
• Parenteral (IV) dose slowly, after reconstituting, then diluting with at least 50 ml of D$_5$, 0.9% NS, or Na lactate
Perform/provide:
• Storage of reconstituted solution if refrigerated for no longer than 24 hr
Evaluate:
• Therapeutic response: increased B/P with stabilization

Teach patient/family:
• Reason for drug administration
Treatment of overdose: Administer a β-1 adrenergic blocker

---

docusate calcium/docusate potassium/docusate sodium
D

(dok'yoo-sate)
Surfak/Kasof/Bu-lax, Colace, Doxinate, D.S.S., Laxinate, Regutol, Roctate

Func. class.: Laxative, emollient
Chem. class.: Anionic surface

Action: Increases water, fat penetration in intestine; allows for easier passage of stool
Uses: To soften stools
Dosage and routes:
• *Adult:* PO 50-300 mg qd (sodium) or 240 mg (calcium or potassium) prn; ENEMA 5 ml (potassium)
• *Child >12 yr:* ENEMA 2 ml (potassium)
• *Child 6-12 yr:* PO 40-120 mg qd (sodium)
• *Child 3-6 yr:* PO 20-60 mg qd (sodium)
• *Child <3 yr:* PO 10-40 mg qd (sodium)
Available forms include: Caps 50, 100, 240, 250, 300 mg; tabs 50, 100 mg; oral sol 10, 50 mg/ml, 16.7, 20 mg/5 ml
Side effects/adverse reactions:
GI: Nausea, anorexia, cramps
INTEG: Rash
EENT: Bitter taste, throat irritation
Contraindications: Hypersensitivity, obstruction, fecal impaction, nausea/vomiting
Pharmacokinetics:
Not known
Interactions/incompatibilities:
None known

NURSING CONSIDERATIONS
Assess:
• Blood, urine electrolytes if drug is used often by patient
• I&O ratio to identify fluid loss
Administer:
• Alone for better absorption; do not take within 1 hr of other drugs or within 1 hr of antacids, milk, or cimetidine
• In morning or evening (oral dose)
Perform/provide:
• Storage in cool environment, do not freeze
Evaluate:
• Therapeutic response: decrease in constipation
• Cause of constipation; identify whether fluids, bulk, or exercise is missing from lifestyle
• Cramping, rectal bleeding, nausea, vomiting; if these symptoms occur, drug should be discontinued
Teach patient/family:
• Swallow tabs whole; do not chew
• That normal bowel movements do not always occur daily
• Do not use in presence of abdominal pain, nausea, vomiting
• Notify physician if constipation unrelieved or if symptoms of electrolyte imbalance occur: muscle cramps, pain, weakness, dizziness

---

dopamine HCl
(doe′pa-meen)
Dopastat, Intropin, Revimine*
Func. class.: Adrenergic β-blocker
Chem. class.: Catecholamine

Action: Causes increased contractility and heart rate by acting on β-receptors in heart; also, acts on α-receptors, causing vasoconstriction in blood vessels; when larger doses are administered, causes vasodilation in renal, intracerebral, coronary dopaminergic receptors

Uses: Shock, increase perfusion, hypotension
Dosage and routes:
• *Adult:* IV INF 2-5 μg/kg/min, not to exceed 50 μg/kg/min, titrate to patient's response
Available forms include: Inj 0.8, 1.6, 40, 80, 160 mg/ml
Side effects/adverse reactions:
CNS: Headache
CV: Palpitations, tachycardia, hypertension, ectopic beats, angina
GI: Nausea, vomiting
INTEG: Necrosis, tissue sloughing with extravasation, ***gangrene***
Contraindications: Hypersensitivity, ventricular fibrillation, tachydysrhythmias, pheochromocytoma
Precautions: Pregnancy, lactation, arterial embolism, peripheral vascular disease
Pharmacokinetics:
IV: Onset 5 min, duration <10 min, metabolized in liver, excreted in urine (metabolites)
Interactions/incompatibilities:
• Do not use within 2 wk of MAOIs, or hypertensive crisis may result
• Dysrhythmias: general anesthetics
• Decreased action of this drug: other β-blockers
• Increased B/P: oxytocics
• Increased pressor effect: tricyclic antidepressant, MAOIs
• Incompatible with alkaline solutions: Na, HCO_3

NURSING CONSIDERATIONS
Assess:
• Therapeutic level (40-190 ng/ml)
• I&O ratio
• ECG during administration continuously; if B/P increases, drug is decreased
• B/P and pulse q5min after parenteral route
• CVP or PWP during infusion if possible

Administer:
• Plasma expanders for hypovolemia
• Parenteral IV dose slowly, after reconstituting

Perform/provide:
• Storage of reconstituted solution if refrigerated for no longer than 24 hr
• Do not use discolored solutions

Evaluate:
• Paresthesias and coldness of extremities, perpiperal blood flow may decrease
• Injection site: tissue sloughing if this occurs, administer phentolamine mixed with NS
• Therapeutic response: increased B/P with stabilization

Teach patient/family:
• Reason for drug administration
Treatment of overdose: Administer a β-1 adrenergic blocker

---

doxapram HCl

(dox'a-pram)
Dopram
Func. class.: Cerebral stimulants

Action: Respiratory stimulation through stimulation of respiratory center in medulla

Uses: Chronic obstructive pulmonary disease (COPD), postanesthesia respiratory stimulation, acute hypercapnia, drug-induced CNS depression

Dosage and routes:
• *Adult:* IV INJ 0.5-1 mg/kg, not to exceed 4 mg/kg or 3 g/day; IV INF 0.5-1 mg/kg, not to exceed 4 mg/kg or 3 g/day, run at 1-3 mg/min

COPD
• *Adult:* IV INF 1-2 mg/min, not to exceed 3 mg/min for no longer than 24 hr
• *Child 3-6 yr:* PO 2.5 mg qd increasing by 2.5 mg/wk

Available forms include: Inj IV 20 mg/ml

Side effects/adverse reactions:
CNS: Convulsions, headache, restlessness, dizziness, confusion, paresthesias, flushing, sweating, bilateral Babinski's sign, rigidity (clonus/generalized), depression
GI: Nausea, vomiting, anorexia, diarrhea, hiccups
GU: Retention, incontinence
CV: Chest pain, hypotension, change in heart rate, lowered T waves, tachycardia
INTEG: Pruritus, irritation at injection site
EENT: Pupil dilation, sneezing
RESP: Laryngospasm, bronchospasm, rebound hypoventilation, dyspnea

Contraindications: Hypersensitivity, seizure disorders, severe hypertension, severe bronchial asthma, severe dyspnea, severe cardiac disorders, pneumothorax, pulmonary embolism, severe respiratory disease

Precautions: Bronchial asthma, hyperthyroidism, pheochromocytoma, severe tachycardia, dysrhythmias, cerebral edema, increase cerebrospinal fluid

Pharmacokinetics:
IV: Onset 20-40 sec, peak 1-2 hr, duration 5-10 hr; metabolized by liver, excreted by kidneys (metabolites)

Interactions/incompatibilities:
• Synergistic pressor effect: MAOIs, sympathomimetics
• Cardiac dysrhythmias: halothane, cyclopropane, enflurane
• Do not mix in alkaline solution including thiopental sodium

NURSING CONSIDERATIONS

Assess:
• BP, HR, deep tendon reflexes, ABGs before administration, q30min

---

italics = common side effects   ***bold italic*** = life threatening reactions

• PO$_2$, Pco$_2$, O$_2$ saturation during treatment

Administer:

• IV at 1-3 mg/min, adjust for desired respiratory response

• Only after adequate airway is established

• After O$_2$, IV barbiturates, resuscitative equipment is available

• Using infusion pump IV

Perform/provide:

• Placing patient in Sims' position to prevent aspiration of vomitus

• Discontinue infusion if side effects occur

Evaluate:

• Hypertension, dysrhythmias, tachycardia, dyspnea, skeletal muscle hyperactivity; may indicate overdosage; discontinue if these occur

• Respiratory stimulation: increased respiratory rate, abnormal rhythm

• Extravasation, change IV site q48h

Treatment of overdose: Lavage, activated charcoal, monitor electrolytes, vital signs

---

doxepin HCl

(dox'e-pin)

Adapin, Sinequan

Func. class.: Antidepressant, tricyclic

Chem. class.: Dibenzoxepin, tertiary amine

Action: Blocks reuptake of norepinephrine, serotonin into nerve endings, increasing action of norepinephrine, serotonin in nerve cells

Uses: Endogenous depression, anxiety

Dosage and routes:

• *Adult:* PO 50-75 mg/day in divided doses, may increase to 300 mg/day or may give daily dose hs

Available forms include: Caps 10, 25, 50, 75, 100, 150 mg; oral conc 10 mg/ml

Side effects/adverse reactions:

*HEMA: **Agranulocytosis, thrombocytopenia, eosinophilia, leukopenia***

CNS: Dizziness, drowsiness, confusion, headache, anxiety, tremors, stimulation, weakness, insomnia, nightmares, EPS (elderly), increased psychiatric symptoms, paresthesia

GI: Diarrhea, dry mouth, nausea, vomiting, ***paralytic ileus,*** increased appetite, cramps, epigastric distress, jaundice, ***hepatitis,*** stomatitis

*GU: Retention, **acute renal failure***

INTEG: Rash, urticaria, sweating, pruritus, photosensitivity

*CV: Orthostatic hypotension, ECG changes, tachycardia, **hypertension,*** palpitations

EENT: Blurred vision, tinnitus, mydriasis, ophthalmoplegia, glossitis

Contraindications: Hypersensitivity to tricyclic antidepressants, urinary retention, narrow-angle glaucoma, prostatic hypertrophy

Precautions: Suicidal patients, elderly, pregnancy (C)

Pharmacokinetics:

PO: Steady state 2-8 days; metabolized by liver, excreted by kidneys, crosses placenta, excreted in breast milk, half-life 8-24 hr

Interactions/incompatibilities:

• Decreased effects of: guanethidine, clonidine, indirect acting sympathomimetics (ephedrine)

• Increased effects of: direct acting sympathomimetics (epinephrine), alcohol, barbiturates, benzodiazepines, CNS depressants

• Hyperpyretic crisis, convulsions, hypertensive episode: MAOI (pargyline [Eutonyl])

NURSING CONSIDERATIONS
Assess:
• B/P (lying, standing), pulse q4h; if systolic B/P drops 20 mm Hg hold drug, notify physician; take vital signs q4h in patients with cardiovascular disease
• Blood studies: CBC, leukocytes, differential, cardiac enzymes if patient is receiving long-term therapy
• Hepatic studies: AST, ALT, bilirubin, creatinine
• Weight qwk, appetite may increase with drug
• ECG for flattening of T wave, bundle branch block, AV block, dysrhythmias in cardiac patients

Administer:
• Increased fluids, bulk in diet if constipation, urinary retention occur
• With food or milk for GI symptoms
• Dosage hs if over-sedation occurs during day; may take entire dose hs; elderly may not tolerate once/day dosing
• Gum, hard candy, or frequent sips of water for dry mouth
• Concentrate with fruit juice, water, or milk to disguise taste

Perform/provide:
• Storage protected from direct sunlight, in tight container
• Assistance with ambulation during beginning therapy since drowsiness/dizziness occurs
• Safety measures including siderails primarily in elderly
• Checking to see PO medication swallowed

Evaluate:
• EPS primarily in elderly: rigidity, dystonia, akathisia
• Mental status: mood, sensorium, affect, suicidal tendencies, an increase in psychiatric symptoms: depression, panic
• Urinary retention, constipation; constipation is more likely to occur in children
• Withdrawal symptoms: headache, nausea, vomiting, muscle pain, weakness; do not usually occur unless drug was discontinued abruptly
• Alcohol consumption; if alcohol is consumed, hold dose until morning

Teach patient/family:
• That therapeutic effects may take 2-3 wk
• Use caution in driving or other activities requiring alertness because of drowsiness, dizziness, blurred vision
• To avoid alcohol ingestion, other CNS depressants
• Not to discontinue medication quickly after long-term use, may cause nausea, headache, malaise
• To wear sunscreen or large hat since photosensitivity occurs

Lab test interferences:
Increase: Serum bilirubin, blood glucose, alk phosphatase
False increase: Urinary catecholamines
Decrease: VMA, 5-HIAA

Treatment of overdose: ECG monitoring, induce emesis, lavage, activated charcoal, administer anticonvulsant

---

doxorubicin HCl
(dox-oh-roo′bi-sin)
Adriamycin
Func. class.: Antineoplastic, antibiotic
Chem. class.: Anthracycline glycoside

Action: Inhibits DNA synthesis, primarily; derived from *Streptomyces peucetius;* replication is decreased by binding to DNA, which causes strand splitting; active throughout entire cell cycle

---

Uses: Myeloblastic leukemia, Wilms' tumor, bladder, breast, cervical, head, neck, liver, lung, ovarian, prostatic, stomach, testicular, thyroid cancer, Hodgkin's disease, acute lymphoblastic leukemia, neuroblastomas, lymphomas, sarcomas

Dosage and routes:
• *Adult:* 60-75 mg/m² q3 wk, or 30 mg/m² on days 1-3 of 4-wk cycle, not to exceed 550 mg/m² cumulative dose

Available forms include: Inj IV 10, 20, 50 mg

Side effects/adverse reactions:
HEMA: Thrombocytopenia, leukopenia, myelosuppression, anemia
GI: Nausea, vomiting, anorexia, mucositis, *hepatotoxicity*
GU: Impotence, sterility, amenorrhea, gynecomastia, hyperuricemia
INTEG: Rash, necrosis at injection site, dermatitis, reversible alopecia, cellulitis, thrombophlebitis at injection site
CV: CHF, cardiopathy
CNS: Fever, chills

Contraindications: Hypersensitivity, pregnancy (1st trimester), lactation, systemic infections

Precautions: Renal, hepatic, cardiac disease, gout, bone marrow depression (severe)

Pharmacokinetics: Triphasic pattern of elimination; half-life 12 min, 3⅓ hr, 29⅔ hr, metabolized by liver, crosses placenta, appears in breast milk, excreted in urine, bile

Interactions/incompatibilities:
• Increased toxicity: other antineoplastics or radiation
• Do not mix with other drugs in solution or syringe

NURSING CONSIDERATIONS

Assess:
• CBC, differential, platelet count weekly; withhold drug if WBC is <4000/mm³ or platelet count is <75,000/mm³; notify physician of these results
• Blood, urine uric acid levels
• Renal function studies: BUN, serum uric acid, urine CrCl, electrolytes before, during therapy
• I&O ratio; report fall in urine output to <30 ml/hr
• Monitor temperature q4h; fever may indicate beginning infection
• Liver function tests before, during therapy: bilirubin, AST, ALT, alk phosphatase as needed or monthly
• ECG; watch for ST-T wave changes, low QRS and T, possible dysrhythmias (sinus tachycardia, heart block, PVCs)

Administer:
• Medications by oral route if possible; avoid IM, SC, IV routes to prevent infections
• Antiemetic 30-60 min before giving drug to prevent vomiting
• Antibiotics for prophylaxis of infection
• Allopurinol or sodium bicarbonate to maintain uric acid levels, alkalinization of urine
• Slow IV infusion using 21-, 23-, 25-gauge needle; check for extravasation
• Topical or systemic analgesics for pain
• Transfusion for anemia
• Antispasmodic for GI symptoms

Perform/provide:
• Strict medical asepsis and protective isolation if WBC levels are low
• Liquid diet: carbonated beverages, Jello; dry toast, crackers may be added if patient is not nauseated or vomiting
• Increased fluid intake to 2-3 L/day to prevent urate, calculi formation
• Diet low in purines: absence of organ meats (kidney, liver), dried beans, peas to maintain alkaline urine

• Rinsing of mouth tid-qid with water, hydrogen peroxide; brushing of teeth bid-tid with soft brush or cotton-tipped applicators for stomatitis; use unwaxed dental floss

• Warm compresses at injection site for inflammation; check for extravasation

• Storage at room temperature for 24 hr after reconstituting or 48 hr refrigerated

Evaluate:

• Bleeding: hematuria, guaiac, bruising or petechiae, mucosa or orifices q8h

• Food preferences; list likes, dislikes

• Effects of alopecia on body image; discuss feelings about body changes

• Edema in feet, joint, stomach pain, shaking

• Inflammation of mucosa, breaks in skin

• Yellowing of skin, sclera, dark urine, clay-colored stools, itchy skin, abdominal pain, fever, diarrhea

• Buccal cavity q8h for dryness, sores, ulceration, white patches, oral pain, bleeding, dysphagia

• Local irritation, pain, burning at injection site

• GI symptoms: frequency of stools, cramping

• Acidosis, signs of dehydration: rapid respirations, poor skin turgor, decreased urine output, dry skin, restlessness, weakness

• Cardiac status: B/P, pulse, character, rhythm, rate

Teach patient/family:

• Why protective isolation precautions are necessary

• To report any complaints, side effects to nurse or physician

• That hair may be lost during treatment and wig or hairpiece may make the patient feel better; tell patient that new hair may be different in color, texture

• To avoid foods with citric acid, hot or rough texture

• To report any bleeding, white spots, ulcerations in mouth to physician; tell patient to examine mouth qd

• That urine may be red-orange for 48 hr

Lab test interferences:

Increase: Uric acid

---

doxycycline hyclate

(dox-i-sye′kleen)
Doxy-Caps, Doxychel, Doxy-Tabs, Vibramycin, Vibra-Tabs, Vivox

Func. class.: Broad spectrum antibiotic/antiinfective
Chem. class.: Tetracycline

Action: Inhibits protein synthesis, prosphorylation in microorganisms by binding to 30S ribosomal subunits, reversibly binding to 50S ribosomal subunits

Uses: Syphilis, chlamydia trachomatis, gonorrhea, lymphogranuloma venereum

Dosage and routes:

• *Adult:* PO 100 mg q12h on day 1, then 100 mg/day; IV 200 mg in 1-2 inf on day 1, then 100-200 mg/day

• *Child >8 yr:* PO/IV 4.4 mg/kg/day in divided doses q12h on day 1, then 2.2-4.4 mg/kg/day

Gonorrhea

• *Adult:* PO 200 mg, then 100 mg hs and 100 mg bid × 3 days or 300 mg, then 300 mg in 1 hr

Chlamydia trachomatis

• *Adult:* PO 100 mg bid × 7 days

Syphilis

• *Adult:* PO 300 mg/day in divided doses × 10 days

Available forms include: Tabs 100 mg; caps 50, 100 mg; syr 50 mg/ml; powder for inj IV 100, 200 mg

Side effects/adverse reactions:
CNS: Fever, headache, paresthesia
HEMA: **Eosinophilia, neutropenia, thrombocytopenia, leukocytosis, hemolytic anemia**
EENT: Dysphagia, glossitis, decreased calcification of deciduous teeth, abdominal pain, oral candidiasis
GI: Nausea, vomiting, diarrhea, anorexia, enterocolitis, **hepatotoxicity,** flatulence, abdominal cramps, gastric burning, stomatitis, pseudomembranous colitis
CV: Pericarditis
GU: Increased BUN, polyuria, polydipsia, renal failure, nephrotoxicity
INTEG: Rash, urticaria, photosensitivity, increased pigmentation, **exfoliative dermatitis,** pruritus, angioedema
Contraindications: Hypersensitivity to tetracyclines, children <8 yr, pregnancy
Precautions: Renal disease, hepatic disease, lactation
Pharmacokinetics:
PO: Peak 1½-4 hr, half-life 15-22 hr; excreted in bile, 25%-93% protein bound
Interactions/incompatibilities:
• Decreased effects of this drug: antacids, NaHCO₃, dairy products, alkali products
• Increased effect: anticoagulants
• Decreased effects: penicillins
• Nephrotoxicity: methoxyflurane
NURSING CONSIDERATIONS
Assess:
• I&O ratio
• Blood studies: PT, CBC, AST, ALT, BUN, creatinine
Administer:
• On empty stomach 1 hr ac or 2 hr pc with 8 oz of water
• After C&S obtained
• 2 hr before or after laxative or ferrous products; 3 hr after antacid

Perform/provide:
• Storage in tight, light-resistant container at room temperature
Evaluate:
• Therapeutic response: decreased temperature, absence of lesions, negative C&S
• Allergic reactions: rash, itching, pruritus, angioedema
• Nausea, vomiting, diarrhea; administer antiemetic, antacids as ordered
• Overgrowth of infection: increased temperature, malaise, redness, pain, swelling, drainage, perineal itching, diarrhea, changes in cough or sputum
Teach patient/family:
• To avoid sun exposure since burns may occur; sunscreen does not seem to decrease photosensitivity
• Of diabetic to avoid use of Clinistix, Diastix, or Tes-Tape for urine glucose testing
• That all prescribed medication must be taken to prevent superimposed infection
• To avoid milk products
Lab test interferences:
False positive: Urine glucose with Clinistix or Tes-Tape
False increase: Urinary catecholamines

D-penicillamine

(pen-i-sill'a-meen)
Cuprimine, Depen

Func. class.: Heavy metal antagonist
Chem. class.: Chelating agent (thiol compound)

Action: Binds with ions of lead, mercury, copper, iron, zinc to form a water-soluble complex excreted by kidneys
Uses: Wilson's disease, rheumatoid arthritis, cystinuria

Dosage and routes:
Cystinuria
• *Adult:* PO 250 mg qid ac, not to exceed 5 g/day
• *Child:* PO 30 mg/kg/day in divided doses qid ac
Wilson's disease
• *Adult:* PO 250 mg qid ac
• *Child:* PO 20 mg/kg/day in divided doses ac
Rheumatoid arthritis
• *Adult:* PO 250 mg/day, then increased 250 mg q2-3 mo if needed, not to exceed 1 g/day
Available forms include: Caps 125, 250 mg; tabs 250 mg
Side effects/adverse reactions:
*HEMA: **Thrombocytopenia, granulocytopenia, leukopenia, eosinophilia,** Lupus-syndrome,* increased sedimentation rate
INTEG: Urticaria, erythema, pruritus, fever, ecchymosis
CV: Hypotension, tachycardia
*GI: Diarrhea, abdominal cramping, nausea, vomiting, **hepatotoxicity***
EENT: Tinnitus, optic neuritis
MS: Arthralgia
*GU: **Proteinuria, nephrotic syndrome, glomerulonephritis***
*SYST: **Anaphylaxis***
RESP: Pneumonitis
Contraindications: Hypersensitivity, anuria, agranulocytosis, severe renal disease
Precautions: Pregnancy
Pharmacokinetics:
PO: Peak 1 hr, metabolized in liver, excreted in urine
Interactions/incompatibilities:
• Increased side effects: oxyphenbutazone, phenylbutazone, gold salts, antimalarials, cytotoxics
NURSING CONSIDERATIONS
Assess:
• Monitor hepatic, renal studies: AST/ALT, alk phosphatase, BUN, creatinine
• Monitor I&O

• Monitor platelet, neutropenia, WBC, H&H; if WBC <3500/mm^3 or if platelets <100,000/mm^3, drug should be discontinued
Administer:
• On an empty stomach, ½-1 hr before meals or at least 2 hr after meals
• Vitamin B$_6$ daily, depleted when this drug is used
• Only when epinephrine 1:1000 is on unit for anaphylaxis
• Fluids to 3 L/day to prevent renal failure
Evaluate:
• Therapeutic response: absence of pain, rigidity in joints (rheumatoid arthritis), specific gravity L 1.010 (cystinuria)
• Allergic reactions (rash, urticaria); if these occur, drug should be discontinued
Teach patient/family:
• That urine may be red in color
• That therapeutic effect may take 1-3 mo
• To report sore throat, easy bruising, bleeding from mucous membranes; may indicate bone marrow depression

---

dromostanolone propionate

(droe-moe-stan'oh-lone)
Drolban

Func. class.: Antineoplastic
Chem. class.: Hormone: androgen

Action: Acts as synthetic steroid, similar to testosterone
Uses: Metastatic breast cancer in postmenopausal women
Dosage and routes:
• *Adult:* IM 100 mg 3 × /wk; treatment should be continued for 8-12 wk before evaluation of effectiveness is completed
Available forms include: Inj IM 50 mg/ml

Side effects/adverse reactions:
GU: Clitoral enlargement
INTEG: Acne, *facial hair*
EENT: Deepening voice
Contraindications: Hypersensitivity, premenopausal women, carcinoma of male breast
Precautions: Edema, hepatic disease, nephritis, pregnancy, cardiac disease, prostate cancer
Pharmacokinetics: Not known
Interactions/incompatibilities:
• Increased effects of: oral anticoagulants

NURSING CONSIDERATIONS
Assess:
• I&O ratio
• Liver function tests before, during therapy (bilirubin, AST, ALT, LDH) as needed or monthly
• Weight daily for increase
Administer:
• Diuretics for increased edema
Perform/provide:
• Storage protected from light at room temperature; *do not refrigerate*
• Warm compresses at injection site for inflammation
• Limitation of calcium intake (dairy products)
Evaluate:
• Edema in feet, hands, ankles, oliguria
• Yellowing of skin, sclera, dark urine, clay-colored stools, itchy skin, abdominal pain, fever, diarrhea
• Local irritation, pain, burning, discoloration at injection site
• Mood swings, nervousness, aggression, depression
• Voice change, hair growth on face, acne, oily skin
• Anorexia, nausea, vomiting, constipation, weakness, loss of muscles: may indicate hypercalcemia
Teach patient/family:
• To report any complaints, side effects to nurse or physician
• That facial hair can occur, is reversible after discontinuing treatment

---

droperidol

(droe-per′i-dole)
Inapsine

Func. class.: Antianxiety agent
Chem. class.: Butyrophenone derivative

Action: Acts on CNS at subcortical levels, produces tranquilization, sleep
Uses: Premedication for surgery, induction, maintenance in general anesthesia
Dosage and routes:
Induction
• *Adult:* IV 2.5 mg/20-25 lb given with analgesic or general anesthetic
• *Child 2-12 yr:* IV 1-1.5 mg/20-25 lb, titrated to response needed
Premedication
• *Adult:* IM 2.5-10 mg ½-1 hr before surgery
• *Child 2-12 yr:* IM 1-1.5 mg/20-25 lb
Maintaining general anesthesia
• *Adult:* IV 1.25-2.5 mg
Available forms include: Inj IM, IV 2.5 mg/ml
Side effects/adverse reactions:
RESP: **Laryngospasm, bronchospasm**
CNS: Dystonia, akathisia, flexion of arms, fine tremors, dizziness, anxiety, drowsiness, restlessness, hallucination, depression
CV: Tachycardia, hypotension
EENT: Upward rotation of eyes, oculogyric crisis
INTEG: Chills, facial sweating, shivering
Contraindications: Hypersensitivity, child <2 yr, pregnancy (C)
Precautions: Elderly, cardiovascular disease (hypotension, brady-

dysrhythmias), renal disease, liver disease, Parkinson's disease

Pharmacokinetics:

IM/IV: Onset 3-10 min, peak ½ hr, duration 3-6 hr; metabolized in liver, excreted in urine as metabolites, crosses placenta

Interactions/incompatibilities:

• Increased CNS depression: alcohol, narcotics, barbiturates, antipsychotics or other CNS depressants

• Decreased effects of: amphetamines, anticonvulsants, anticoagulants, when given with this drug

• Increased intraocular pressure: anticholinergics, antiparkinson drugs

• Increased side effects of: lithium

• Do not mix with barbiturates in solution

NURSING CONSIDERATIONS

Assess:

• VS q10 min during IV administration, q30 min after IM dose

Administer:

• Anticholinergics (benztropine, diphenhydramine) for extrapyramidal reaction

• Only with crash cart, resuscitative equipment nearby

• IV slowly only

Perform/provide:

• Slow movement of patient to avoid orthostatic hypotension

Evaluate:

• Therapeutic response: decreased anxiety, absence of vomiting during surgery

• Extrapyramidal reactions: dystonia, akathisia

• For increasing heart rate or decreasing B/P, notify physician at once; do not place patient in Trendelenburg position or sympathetic blockade may occur causing respiratory arrest

dyclonine HCl

(dye-kloe'neen)
Dyclone
Func. class.: Topical anesthetic
Chem. class.: Ketone

D

Action: Inhibits nerve impulses from sensory nerves; produces anesthesia

Uses: Pruritus ani, insect bites, sunburn

Dosage and routes:

• *Adult and child:* TOP apply tidqid; sol instill 10 ml into urethra after cystourethroscopy

Available forms include: Sol 0.5%, 1%

Side effects/adverse reactions:

INTEG: Rash, irritation, sensitization, edema

Contraindications: Hypersensitivity

Precautions: Child <6 yr, pregnancy

Interactions/incompatibilities: None known

NURSING CONSIDERATIONS

Administer:

• After cleansing, drying of affected area

Evaluate:

• For allergic reactions: rash, irritation, reddening, swelling

• For therapeutic response: absence of pain, itching of affected area

• Affected area for infection, if infection present, do not apply

Teach patient/family:

• To report rash, irritation, redness, swelling

• How to apply solution

---

italics = common side effects   ***bold italic*** = life threatening reactions

dyclonine HCl (topical)

(dye-kloe-neen)
Dyclone
Func. class.: Topical anesthetic
Chem. class.: Organic ketone

Action: Inhibits nerve impulses from sensory nerves, which produces anesthesia

Uses: Topical anesthesia prior to diagnostic examination, suppress gag reflex, itching of pruritus ani or vulvae

Dosage and routes:
• *Adult and child:* TOP apply tid-qid; INSTILL 10 ml sol into urethra after cysturethroscopy

Available forms include: Sol 0.5%, 1%

Side effects/adverse reactions:
INTEG: Rash, irritation, sensitization, edema, urticaria, burning

Contraindications: Hypersensitivity, infants, application to large areas

Precautions: Children, sepsis, pregnancy, denuded skin

Interactions/incompatibilities: None known

NURSING CONSIDERATIONS

Administer:
• After cleansing and drying of affected area

Evaluate:
• Allergy: rash, irritation, reddening, swelling
• Therapeutic response: anesthesia of area, absence of gag reflex

Teach patient/family:
• To report rash, irritation, redness, swelling

dyphylline

(dye'fi-lin)
Air-Tabs, Brophylline, Dilin, Dilor, Dyflex, Dylline, Emfabid, Lufyllin, Protophylline*

Func. class.: Spasmolytic
Chem. class.: Xanthine, ethylene-diamine

Action: Relaxes smooth muscle of respiratory system by blocking phosphodiesterase, which increases cyclic AMP

Uses: Bronchial asthma, bronchospasm in chronic bronchitis, COPD

Dosage and routes:
• *Adult:* PO 200-800 mg q6h; IM 250-500 mg q6h injected slowly
• *Child >6 yr:* PO 4-7 mg/kg/day in 4 divided doses

Available forms include: Tabs 200, 400 mg; elix 100, 160 mg/15 ml; inj IM 250 mg/ml

Side effects/adverse reactions:
CNS: Anxiety, restlessness, insomnia, dizziness, convulsions, headache, light-headedness
CV: Palpitations, sinus tachycardia, hypotension
GI: Nausea, vomiting, anorexia, dyspepsia
INTEG: Flushing, urticaria

Contraindications: Hypersensitivity to xanthines, tachydysrhythmias

Precautions: Elderly, CHF, cor pulmonale, hepatic disease, active peptic ulcer disease, diabetes mellitus, hyperthyroidism, hypertension, children, renal disease

Pharmacokinetics:
Peak 1 hr, half-life 2 hr, excreted in urine unchanged

Interactions/incompatibilities:
• Do not mix in syringe with other drugs
• Increased action of this drug: cimetidine, propranolol, erythromycin, troleandomycin

---

• May increase effects of: anticoagulants

• Cardiotoxicity: β-blockade

NURSING CONSIDERATIONS
Assess:

• Dyphylline blood levels; toxicity may occur with small increase above 20 μg/ml

• Monitor I&O; diuresis occurs, dehydration may result in elderly or children

• Whether theophylline was given recently

Administer:

• PO after meals to decrease GI symptoms; absorption may be affected

• Avoid IM injection; pain occurs

Evaluate:

• Therapeutic response: decreased dyspnea, respiratory rate, rhythm

• Auscultate lung fields bilaterally; notify physician of abnormalities

• Allergic reactions: rash, urticaria; if these occur, drug should be discontinued

Teach patient/family

• To check OTC medications, current prescription medications for ephedrine; will increase stimulation

• To avoid hazardous activities; dizziness, drowsiness, blurred vision may occur

• On all aspects of drug therapy: dosage, routes, side effects, when to notify the physician

• If GI upset occurs, to take drug with 8 oz of water; avoid food, since absorption may be decreased

---

echothiophate iodide

(ek-oh-thye′oh-fate)

Phospholine Iodide, Echodide

Func. class.: Miotic

Chem. class.: Cholinesterase inhibitor, irreversible

Action: Prevents breakdown of neurotransmitter acetylcholine, which then accumulates, causing enhancement, prolongation of its physiologic effects

Uses: Glaucoma (open-angle), accommodative esotropia, treatment of obstructed aqueous outflow; extremely effective in control of chronic wide-angle glaucoma, aphakic glaucoma, congenital glaucoma

Dosage and routes:

• *Adult and child:* INSTILL 1 gtt of 0.03%, or 0.125% sol qd in conjunctival sac, not to exceed 1 gtt bid

Available forms include: Powder for reconstitution, 1.5 mg (0.03%), 3 mg (0.06%), 6.25 mg (0.125%), 12.5 mg (0.25%) in 5 ml diluent

Side effects/adverse reactions:

GU: Frequency

CV: Hypotension, bradycardia, ***cardiac arrest***

INTEG: Sweating, pallor, cyanosis

RESP: ***Bronchospasm***

GI: Nausea, vomiting, abdominal cramps, diarrhea

EENT: Blurred vision, stinging, burning, lacrimation, lid muscle twitching, conjunctival, ciliary redness, browache, headache, induced myopia, iris cysts, hyperemia, hyphema

Contraindications: Hypersensitivity

Precautions: Asthma, bradycardia, parkinsonism, peptic ulcer

Interactions/incompatibilities:

• Decreased effect of this drug: pilocarpine

• Increased effect of both drugs: ambenonium, edrophonium, neostigmine, physostigmine, pyridostigmine

• Increased effects of: general anesthetics

NURSING CONSIDERATIONS
Administer:

• After checking vial for concentration

• Immediately after reconstituting; discard unused portion

Evaluate:

• Specific condition being treated

• History of client's previous/current conditions (e.g., asthma, cardiac), possible sensitivity, contraindications, drug interactions

Teach patient/family:

• Instruct as to why client is receiving medication; client, family should have a clear regimen as well as name of medication

• To report change in vision, blurring or loss of sight, trouble breathing, sweating, flushing

• Method of instillation, including pressure on lacrimal sac for 1 min, not to touch dropper to eye

• That long-term therapy may be required

• That blurred vision will decrease with repeated use of drug

• That they may experience stinging sensation, dull ache or tearing which should subside in a few minutes; if it persists, contact physician

• Client may experience decreased visual ability at night; instruct not to drive

• To use drops at night to eliminate hazardous, transient blurring

---

econazole nitrate (topical)

(e-kone′a-zole)

Ecostatin, Spectazole

Func. class.: Local antiinfective
Chem. class.: Imidazole derivative, antifungal

Action: Interferes with fungal DNA replication; binds sterols in fungal cell membrane, which increases permeability, leaking of cell nutrients

Uses: Tinea pedis, tinea cruris, tinea corporis, tinea versicolor, cutaneous candidiasis

Dosage and routes:

• *Adult and child:* TOP apply to affected area qid-bid depending on condition

Available forms include: Cream 1%

Side effects/adverse reactions:

INTEG: Rash, urticaria, stinging, burning, pruritus

Contraindications: Hypersensitivity

Precautions: Pregnancy, lactation

Interactions/incompatibilities: None known

NURSING CONSIDERATIONS

Administer:

• Enough medication to completely cover lesions

• After cleansing with soap, water before each application, dry well

Perform/provide:

• Storage at room temperature in dry place

Evaluate:

• Allergic reaction: burning, stinging, swelling, redness

• Therapeutic response: decrease in size, number of lesions

Teach patient/family:

• To apply with glove to prevent further infection

• To avoid use of OTC creams, ointments, lotions unless directed by physician

• To use medical asepsis (hand washing) before, after each application

• Not to cover with occlusive dressing

edetate calcium disodium

(ed'e-tate)

Calcium Disodium Versenate, Calcium EDTA

Func. class.: Heavy metal antagonist

Chem. class.: Chelating agent

Action: Binds ions from lead to form a water-soluble complex is removed by kidneys

Uses: Lead poisoning, acute lead encephalopathy

Dosage and routes:

Acute lead encephalopathy

• *Adult and child:* 1.5 g/m^2/day × 3-5 days, with dimercaprol, may be given again after 4 days off drug

Lead poisoning

• *Adult:* IV 1 g/250-500 ml D$_5$W or 0.9% NaCl over 1-2 hr or q12h × 3-5 days, may repeat after 2 days, not to exceed 50 mg/kg/day

• *Child:* IM 35 mg/kg/day in divided doses q8-12 hr, not to exceed 50 mg/kg/day

Available forms include: Inj IM, IV 200 mg/ml

Side effects/adverse reactions:

CNS: Headache, paresthesia

INTEG: Urticaria, erythema, pruritus, pain at injection site, fever, cheilosis

CV: Hypotension, dysrhythmias

GI: Vomiting, *diarrhea, abdominal cramps, anorexia*

EENT: Nasal congestion, sneezing

MS: Leg cramps, myalgia, arthralgia, weakness

GU: Hematuria, renal tubular necrosis, proteinuria

Contraindications: Hypersensitivity, anuria, hepatic insufficiency, poisoning of other metals, severe renal disease, child <3 yr

Precautions: Hypertension, pregnancy, lactation

Pharmacokinetics:

Not metabolized, excreted in urine, half-life: 20-60 min (IV), 90 min (IM)

Interactions/incompatibilities:

None known

NURSING CONSIDERATIONS   **E**

Assess:

• VS, B/P, pulse, respirations

• Monitor I&O, kidney function studies: BUN, creatinine, CrCl; watch for decreasing urine output

• Urine: pH, albumin, casts, blood, coproporphyrins, calcium

Administer:

• EDTA, BAL separately

• IV slowly, IM is preferred route

• IM in large muscle mass; rotate injection sites

• Only when epinephrine 1:1000 is on unit for anaphylaxis

• IV fluids to ensure adequate hydration before administration of drug

Evaluate:

• Cardiac abnormalities: dysrhythmias, hypotension, tachycardia

• Allergic reactions (rash, urticaria); if these occur drug should be discontinued

Teach patient/family:

• That compliance to dosage schedule must be followed

Lab test interferences:

Decrease: Cholesterol/triglycerides, potassium

edetate disodium

(ed'e-tate)

Disodium EDTA, Disotate, Endrate

Func. class.: Metal antagonist

Chem. class.: Chelating agent

Action: Binds with ions of calcium, zinc, magnesium to form a water-soluble complex excreted from kidneys

Uses: Hypercalcemic crisis

Dosage and routes:

• *Adult and child:* IV INF 15-50 mg/kg/500 ml of D₅W or 0.9% NaCl, given over 3-4 hr, not to exceed 3 g/day (adult) or 70 mg/kg/day (child)

Available forms include: Inj conc 150 mg/ml

Side effects/adverse reactions:

*CNS: Headache, paresthesia, **convulsions***

INTEG: Urticaria, erythema, pain at injection site

CV: Hypotension, thrombophlebitis

GI: Nausea, vomiting, anorexia, diarrhea, abdominal cramps

GU: Dysuria, pyelonephritis, ***nephrotoxicity,*** hyperuricemia, hypomagnesemia, polyuria, ***proteinuria, renal tubular necrosis***

Contraindications: Hypersensitivity, anuria, hepatic insufficiency, poisoning of other metals, severe renal disease, child <3 yr

Precautions: Hypertension, pregnancy, lactation

Pharmacokinetics:

Excreted in urine as calcium chelate

Interactions/incompatibilities:

None known

NURSING CONSIDERATIONS

Assess:

• VS, B/P, pulse; if hypotension occurs, drug should be discontinued

• Monitor I&O, kidney function studies: BUN, creatinine, CrCl

Administer:

• Only when IV calcium preparation is on unit for emergency use

• EDTA, BAL separately

• IV slowly, use infusion pump

• IV fluids to ensure adequate hydration before administration of drug

Perform/provide:

• Assistance with ambulation

Evaluate:

• Hypocalcemia: numbness of feet, hands, tongue, lips; positive Chvostek's, Trousseau's signs; convulsions; stupor

• Cardiac abnormalities: dysrhythmias, hypotension, tachycardia

• Allergic reactions (rash, urticaria); if these occur, drug should be discontinued

Teach patient/family:

• To remain recumbent for ½ hr to prevent postural hypotension

• To make position changes slowly to prevent fainting

• That compliance to dosage schedule must be followed

• That breath may be odorous

Lab test interferences:

False decrease: Calcium

Decrease: Magnesium, alk phosphatase

---

edrophonium chloride

(ed-roe-foe′nee-um)

Tensilon

Func. class.: Cholinergics, anticholinesterase

Chem. class.: Quaternary ammonium compound

Action: Inhibits destruction of acetylcholine, which increases concentration at sites where acetylcholine is released; this facilitates transmission of impulses across myoneural junction

Uses: To diagnose myasthenia gravis, curare antagonist, differentiation of myasthenic crisis from cholinergic crisis, paroxysmal supraventricular tachycardia

Dosage and routes:

Tensilon test

• *Adult:* IV 1-2 mg, then 8 mg if no response

• *Child >34 kg:* IV 2 mg, if no

response in 45 sec then 1 mg q45 sec, not to exceed 10 mg
• *Child <34 kg:* IV 1 mg, if no response in 45 sec, then 1 mg q45 sec, not to exceed 5 mg
• *Infant:* IV 0.5 mg
Curare antagonist
• *Adult:* IV 10 mg over 30-45 sec, may repeat, not to exceed 40 mg
Differentiation of myasthenic crisis from cholinergic crisis
• *Adult:* IV 1 mg, if no response in 1 min, may repeat
Paroxysmal supraventricular tachycardia
• *Adult:* IV 10 mg over 1 min
Available forms include: Inj IV 10 mg/ml
Side effects/adverse reactions:
INTEG: Rash, urticaria
CNS: Dizziness, headache, sweating, confusion, weakness, convulsions, incoordination, paralysis
GI: Nausea, diarrhea, vomiting, cramps
CV: Tachycardia
GU: Frequency, incontinence
RESP: Respiratory depression, bronchospasm, constriction
EENT: Miosis, blurred vision, lacrimation
Contraindications: Bradycardia, hypotension, obstruction of intestine, renal system
Precautions: Seizure disorders, bronchial asthma, coronary occlusion, hyperthyroidism, dysrhythmias, peptic ulcer, megacolon, poor GI motility
Pharmacokinetics:
IV: Onset 30-60 sec, duration 6-24 min
IM: Onset 2-10 min, duration 12-45 min
Interactions/incompatibilities:
• Decreased action of this drug: procainamide, quinidine
• Bradycardia: digitalis

NURSING CONSIDERATIONS:
Assess:
• VS, respiration during test
Administer:
• Only with atropine sulfate available for cholinergic crisis
• Only after all other cholinergics have been discontinued
Perform/provide:
• Storage at room temperature
Evaluate:
• Therapeutic response: increased muscle strength, hand grasp, improved gait, absence of labored breathing (if severe)
Teach patient/family:
• To wear Medic Alert ID specifying myasthenia gravis, drugs taken

---

emetine HCl
(em'e-teen)

Func. class.: Amebicide
Chem. class.: Ipecac alkaloid

Action: Inhibits protein synthesis in developing trophozoites
Uses: Amebic dysentery (acute fulminating), amebic hepatitis, amebic abscess
Dosage and routes:
Amebic dysentery
• *Adult:* SC/IM 1 mg/kg/day, not to exceed 60 mg/day × 3-5 days simultaneously with another amebicide
• *Child:* IM 1 mg/kg/day in 2 divided doses × 5 days, not to exceed 60 mg/day
Amebic hepatitis/abscess
• *Adult:* SC/IM 60 mg/day × 10 days
• *Child:* IM 1 mg/kg in 2 doses × 5 days, not to exceed 60 mg/day (use only if other amebicides have failed)
Available forms include: Inj SC, IM 65 mg/ml

Side effects/adverse reactions:

CV: Hypotension, tachycardia, dysrhythmia, pericarditis, ECG abnormalities, *CHF,* chest pain, gallop rhythm, palpitations, hypotension, myocarditis, *cardiac arrest,* T wave inversion, increased QT, widening QRS

HEMA: Thrombocytopenia

INTEG: Rash, pruritus, necrosis, abscesses

GI: Nausea, vomiting, diarrhea, epigastric distress, anorexia

CNS: Weakness, tremors, aching, fatigue, depression, paresthesia, *paralysis,* encephalitis

Contraindications: Hypersensitivity, renal disease, hepatic disease, pregnancy

Precautions: Elderly, lactation, surgery patients, hypotension, children

Pharmacokinetics:

SC/IM: Metabolized in liver, excreted in urine slowly over 40-60 days

Interactions/incompatibilities:
None known

NURSING CONSIDERATIONS
Assess:

• Stools during entire treatment; should be clear at end of therapy, for 1 yr before patient is considered cured

• ECG q2-3 days before, after 5th dose, after therapy, 1 wk after; be aware that inversion of T waves occurs

• Vision by ophthalmalogic exam during, after therapy; vision problems occur often

• Injection site for irritation, absence of necrosis q8h

• I&O, stools for number, frequency, character

• B/P, pulse q4h; watch for decrease in B/P; discontinue

Administer:

• Being careful not to get drug in eyes; causes mucous membrane irritation

• Cleansing enema if ordered before beginning treatment

• SC or IM, never IV; rotate injection sites

• PO after meals to avoid GI symptoms

Perform/provide:

• Storage in tight, light-resistant container

Evaluate:

• Allergic reaction: fever, rash, itching, chills; drug should be discontinued if these occur

• Superimposed infection: fever, monilial growth, fatigue, malaise

• Tachycardia, decreasing B/P, GI symptoms, weakness, neuromuscular symptoms

• Diarrhea for 2-3 days

Teach patient/family:

• Proper hygiene after BM: handwashing technique

• Avoid contact of drug with eyes, mouth, nose, other mucous membranes

• Need for compliance with dosage schedule, duration of treatment

---

enalapril maleate

(en-al-a′prel)
Vasotec

Func. class.: Antihypertensive
Chem. class.: Renin-angiotensin antagonist

Action: Selectively suppresses renin-angiotensin-aldosterone system; inhibits ACE, prevents conversion of angiotensin I to angiotensin II

Uses: Hypertension not responsive to other hypertensive medications

Dosage and routes:

• *Adult:* PO 5 mg/day, may increase or decrease to desired response

Available forms include: Tabs 5, 10, 20 mg

Side effects/adverse reactions:

CV: Hypotension, chest pain, tachycardia, dysrhythmias

CNS: Insomnia, dizziness, paresthesias, headache, fatigue, anxiety

GI: Nausea, vomiting, colitis, cramps, diarrhea, constipation flatulence, dry mouth

INTEG: Rash, purpura, alopecia

HEMA: Agranulocytosis

EENT: Tinnitus, visual changes, sore throat, double vision, dry burning eyes

GU: Proteinuria, renal failure, increased frequency of polyurea or oliguria

RESP: Dyspnea, cough, rales

Contraindications: Pregnancy (C), lactation

Precautions: Renal disease, hyperkalemia

Pharmacokinetics:

PO: Peak 4-6 hr; half-life 1½ hr; metabolized by liver to active metabolite, excreted in urine

Interactions/incompatibilities:

• Severe hypotension: diuretics, other antihypertensives

• Decreased effects when used with: aspirin

• Increased potassium levels: salt substitutes, potassium-sparing diuretics, potassium supplements

• May increase effects of: ergots, neuromuscular blocking agents, antihypertensives, hypoglycemics, barbiturates, reserpine, levodopa

• Effects may be increased by phenothiazines, diuretics, phenytoin, quinidine

NURSING CONSIDERATIONS

Assess:

• B/P, pulse q4h; note rate, rhythm, quality

• Electrolytes: K, Na, Cl

• Apical/radial pulse before administration; notify physician of any significant changes

• Baselines in renal, liver function tests before therapy begins

Evaluate:

• Edema in feet, legs daily

• Skin turgor, dryness of mucous membranes for hydration status

• Symptoms of CHF: edema, dyspnea, wet rales

Teach patient/family:

• Not to discontinue drug abruptly

• Not to use OTC products unless directed by physician

• To rise slowly to sitting or standing position to minimize orthostatic hypotension

Lab test interferences:

Interference: Glucose/insulin tolerance tests

Treatment of overdose: Lavage, IV atropine for bradycardia, IV theophylline for bronchospasm, digitalis, O_2, diuretic for cardiac failure, hemodialysis

---

ephedrine sulfate

(e-fed'rin)

Vatronol Nose Drops, Efedron Nasal

Func. class.: Nasal decongestant

Chem. class.: Indirect/direct sympathomimetic amine

Action: Relaxes bronchial smooth muscle, increases diameter of nasal passage by action on β-2 adrenergic receptors

Uses: Nasal congestion associated with colds, hayfever, sinusitis, other allergic conditions, adjunct in middle ear infections

Dosage and routes:

• *Adult and child:* INSTILL 3-4 gtts, q4h or small amount of gel in each nostril

Available forms include: Sol 0.5% sulfate, gel 0.6% HCl

Side effects/adverse reactions:

GI: Nausea, vomiting, anorexia

EENT: Irritation, burning, sneezing, stinging, dryness, rebound congestion

INTEG: Contact dermatitis

CNS: Anxiety, restlessness, tremors, weakness, insomnia, dizziness, fever, headache

Contraindications: Hypersensitivity to sympathomimetic amines

Precautions: Child <6 yr, elderly, diabetes, cardiovascular disease, hypertension, hyperthyroidism, increase ICP, prostatic hypertrophy

Interactions/incompatibilities:

• Hypertension: MAOIs, β-adrenergic blockers

• Hypotension: methyldopa, mecamylamine, reserpine

NURSING CONSIDERATIONS
Administer:

• No more than q4h

• For <4 consecutive days

Perform/provide:

• Environmental humidification to decrease nasal congestion, dryness

• Storage in light-resistant containers; do not expose to high temperatures

Evaluate:

• Redness, swelling, pain in nasal passages

Teach patient/family:

• Stinging may occur for a few applications; drying of mucosa may be decreased by environmental humidification

• To notify physician if irregular pulse, insomnia, dizziness, or tremors occur

• Proper administration to avoid systemic absorption

ephedrine sulfate
(e-fed′rin)

Efedrin, Vatronol

Func. class.: Adrenergic, indirect acting

Chem. class.: Phenylisopropylamine

Action: Causes increased contractility and heart rate by acting on β-receptors in the heart; also, acts on α-receptors, causing vasoconstriction in blood vessels; when larger doses are administered, causes vasodilation in renal, intracerebral, coronary dopaminergic receptors; dilates bronchi, produces mydriasis when used in eye

Uses: Shock, increase perfusion, hypotension, bronchodilation

Dosage and routes:

• *Adult:* IM/SC 25-50 mg, not to exceed 150 mg/24 hr

IV 10-25 mg, not to exceed 150 mg/24 hr

• *Child:* SC/IV 3 mg/kg/day in divided doses q4-6h

Bronchodilator

• *Adult:* PO 12.5-50 mg bid-qid, not to exceed 400 mg/day

• *Child:* PO 2-3 mg/kg/day in 4-6 divided doses

Available forms include: Inj 25, 50 mg/ml, IM, SC, IV; caps 25, 50 mg; syr 11, 20 mg/5 ml

Side effects/adverse reactions:

CNS: Tremors, anxiety, insomnia, headache, dizziness, confusion, hallucinations, *convulsions, CNS depression*

EENT: Dry nose, irritation of nose and throat

CV: Palpitations, tachycardia, hypertension, chest pain, *dysrhythmias*

GI: Anorexia, nausea, vomiting

RESP: Depression

Contraindications: Hypersensitiv-

ity to sympathomimetics, narrow-angle glaucoma

Precautions: Pregnancy, cardiac disorders, hyperthyroidism, diabetes mellitus, prostatic hypertrophy

Pharmacokinetics:

PO: Onset 15-60 min, duration 2-4 hr

IV: Onset 5 min, duration 2 hr

Metabolized in liver, excreted in urine (unchanged), crosses blood-brain barrier, placenta, breast milk

Interactions/incompatibilities:

• Do not use with MAOIs or tricyclic antidepressants; hypertensive crisis may occur

• Decreased effect of this drug: methyldopa, urinary acidifiers, rauwolfia alkaloids

• Increased effect of this drug: urinary alkalizers

NURSING CONSIDERATIONS

Assess:

• I&O ratio

• ECG during administration continuously, if B/P increases, drug is decreased

• B/P and pulse q5 min after parenteral route

• CVP or PWP during infusion if possible

Administer:

• Plasma expanders for hypovolemia

Perform/provide:

• Storage of reconstituted solution if refrigerated for no longer than 24 hr

• Do not use discolored solutions

Evaluate:

• For paresthesias and coldness of extremities, peripheral blood flow may decrease

• Injection site: tissue sloughing if this occurs administer phentolamine mixed with NS

• Therapeutic response: increased B/P with stabilization

Teach patient/family:

• Reason for drug administration

Treatment of overdose: Administer an α-blocker, then norepinephrine for severe hypotension

---

epinephrine/ epinephrine bitartrate/ epinephrine HCl

(ep-i-nef'rin)

Bronkaid Mist, Primatene Mist/ AsthmaHaler, Medihaler-Epi/ Adrenalin, Sus-Phrine

Func. class.: Adrenergic
Chem. class.: Catecholamine

Action: Causes increased contractility and heart rate by acting on β-receptors in heart; also, acts on α-receptors, causing vasoconstriction in blood vessels; when larger doses are administered, causes vasodilation in renal, intracerebral, coronary dopaminergic receptors

Uses: Acute asthmatic attacks, hemostasis, bronchospasm, anaphylaxis, allergic reactions, cardiac arrest

Dosage and routes:

• *Adult:* IM/SC 0.1-0.5 ml of 1:1000 sol, may repeat q10-15 min IV 0.1-0.25 ml of 1:1000 sol

• *Child:* SC 0.01 ml of 1:1000/kg, may repeat q20 min to 4 hr; INH 0.005 ml/kg of 1:200 solution, may repeat q8-12h

Asthma

• *Adult and child:* INH 1-2 puffs of 1:100 or 2.25% racemic q1-5 min

Hemostasis

• *Adult:* TOP 1:50,000-1:1000 applied as needed to stop bleeding

Cardiac arrest

• *Adult:* IC 0.5-1 mg followed by IV INF at 1-4 μg/min

• *Child:* IC 10 μg/kg or 5-10 μg/kg

Available forms include: Aerosol 0.16 mg/spray, 0.2 mg/spray,

E

0.25 mg/spray, inj 1:1000 (1 mg/ml), 1:200 (5 mg/ml) IM, IV, SC; sol for nebulization 1:100, 1.25% 2.25% (base)

Side effects/adverse reactions:

CNS: Tremors, anxiety, insomnia, headache, dizziness, confusion, hallucinations, *convulsions, CNS depression*

EENT: Dry nose, irritation of nose and throat

CV: Palpitations, tachycardia, hypertension, chest pain, *dysrhythmias*

GI: Anorexia, nausea, vomiting

RESP: Depression

Contraindications: Hypersensitivity to sympathomimetics, narrow-angle glaucoma

Precautions: Pregnancy, cardiac disorders, hyperthyroidism, diabetes mellitus, prostatic hypertrophy

Pharmacokinetics:

SC: Onset 3-5 min, duration 20 min
PO, INH: Onset 1 min

Interactions/incompatibilities:

• Do not use with MAOIs or tricyclic antidepressants; hypertensive crisis may occur

• Decreased effect of this drug: methyldopa, urinary acidifiers, rauwolfia alkaloids

• Increased effect of this drug: urinary alkalizers

NURSING CONSIDERATIONS
Assess:

• I&O ratio

• ECG during administration continuously; if B/P increases, drug is decreased

• B/P and pulse q5 min after parenteral route

• CVP or PWP during infusion if possible

Administer:

• Plasma expanders for hypovolemia

• Parenteral IV dose slowly, after reconstituting with D_5W, 0.9% NS

Perform/provide:

• Storage of reconstituted sol if refrigerated for no longer than 24 hr

• Do not use discolored solutions

Evaluate:

• Paresthesias and coldness of extremities, peripheral blood flow may decrease

• Injection site: tissue sloughing; if this occurs administer phentolamine mixed with NS

• Therapeutic response: increased B/P with stabilization

Teach patient/family:

• Reason for drug administration

Treatment of overdose: Administer an α-blocker, then norepinephrine for severe hypotension

---

epinephrine bitartrate/ epinephrine HCl/ epinephryl borate (optic)

(ep-i-nef'rin)

Epitrate, Mytrate/Epifrin, Glaucon/Epinal, Eppy*

Func. class.: Mydriatic
Chem. class.: Sympathomimetic amine

Action: Blocks response of iris sphincter muscle, muscle of accommodation of ciliary body to cholinergic stimulation, resulting in dilation, paralysis of accommodation

Uses: During ocular surgery, open-angle glaucoma

Dosage and routes:

• *Adult and child:* INTRAOCULAR INJ 0.1-0.2 ml of a 0.01 or 0.1% sol (HCl); INSTILL SOL 1-2 gtts of a 1%-2% sol, determined by tonometric reading (Bitartrate); 1 gtt of a 0.5%-2% sol (HCl) or 0.5%-1% (Borate)

During surgery

• *Adult and child:* INSTILL SOL

1 or more gtts of a 0.1% sol (HCl) up to 3 × / day
Available forms include: Sol 0.1% (HCl)
Side effects/adverse reactions:
CV: Palpitations, tachycardia
*RESP: **Bronchospasm***
EENT: Blurred vision
Contraindications: Hypersensitivity to sympathomimetic amines, narrow-angle glaucoma, dysrhythmias, cardiogenic shock, cerebral arteriosclerosis
Precautions: Elderly, prostatic hypertension, diabetes mellitus, hyperthymus, TB, Parkinson's disease, pregnancy (C)
Pharmacokinetics:
INSTILL: Onset 1 hr, peak 4-8 hr, duration 12-24 hr
Interactions/incompatibilities:
• Dysrhythmias: cyclopropane, halogenated hydrocarbons
• Increased pressor effects: tricyclic antidepressants, antihistamines

NURSING CONSIDERATIONS
Assess:
• Tonometer readings during long-term treatment
• B/P, pulse, respirations
Evaluate:
• Allergic reaction: itching, edema of eyelids, eye discharge; drug should be discontinued
Teach patient/family:
• To report change in vision, blurring or loss of sight, trouble breathing, sweating, flushing
• Method of instillation: pressure on lacrimal sac for 1 min, do not touch dropper to eye
• That long-term therapy may be required if using for glaucoma

epinephrine HCl
(ep-i-nef′rin)
Adrenalin Chloride

Func. class.: Nasal decongestant
Chem. class.: Sympathomimetic amine

Action: Relaxes bronchial smooth muscle, increases diameter of nasal passage by action on β-2 adrenergics
Uses: Nasal congestion, superficial bleeding
Dosage and routes:
• *Adult and child:* TOP apply to affected area with sterile swab
Available forms include: Sol 0.1%
Side effects/adverse reactions:
GI: Nausea, vomiting, anorexia
EENT: Irritation, burning, sneezing, stinging, dryness, rebound congestion
INTEG: Contact dermatitis
CNS: Anxiety, restlessness, tremors, weakness, insomnia, dizziness, fever, headache
Contraindications: Hypersensitivity to sympathomimetic amines
Precautions: Child <6 yr, elderly, diabetes, cardiovascular disease, hypertension, hyperthyroidism, increased ICP, prostatic hypertrophy
Interactions/incompatibilities:
• Hypertension: MAOIs, β-adrenergic blockers
• Hypotension: methyldopa, mecamylamine, reserpine

NURSING CONSIDERATIONS
Administer:
• No more than q4h
• For <4 consecutive days
Perform/provide:
• Environmental humidification to decrease nasal congestion, dryness
• Storage in light-resistant containers; do not expose to high temperatures

---

Evaluate:
• Redness, swelling, pain in nasal passages

Teach patient/family:
• Stinging may occur for several applications; drying of mucosa may be decreased by environmental humidification
• To notify physician if irregular pulse, insomnia, dizziness, or tremors occur
• Proper administration to avoid systemic absorption

---

epinephrine HCl (nasal)

(ep-i-nef'rin)
Adrenalin Chloride
Func. class.: Nasal decongestant
Chem. class.: Sympathomimetic amine

Action: Relaxes bronchial smooth muscle, increases diameter of nasal passage by action on β-adrenergics
Uses: Nasal congestion, superficial bleeding

Dosage and routes:
• *Adult and child >6 yr old:* TOP apply to affected area with sterile swab
Available forms include: Sol 0.1%
Side effects/adverse reactions:
GI: Nausea, vomiting, anorexia
EENT: Irritation, burning, sneezing, stinging, dryness, rebound congestion
INTEG: Contact dermatitis
CNS: Anxiety, restlessness, tremors, weakness, insomnia, dizziness, fever, headache
Contraindications: Hypersensitivity to sympathomimetic amines
Precautions: Child <6 yr, elderly, diabetes, cardiovascular disease, hypertension, hyperthyroidism, increased ICP, prostatic hypertrophy
Interactions/incompatibilities:
• Hypertension: MAOIs, β-adrenergic blockers

• Hypotension: methyldopa, mecamylamine, reserpine

NURSING CONSIDERATIONS
Administer:
• No more than q4h
• For <4 consecutive days
Perform/provide:
• Environmental humidification to decrease nasal congestion, dryness
• Storage in light-resistant containers; do not expose to high temperatures
Evaluate:
• For redness, swelling, pain in nasal passages
Teach patient/family:
• Stinging may occur for a few applications; drying of mucosa may be decreased by environmental humidification
• To notify physician if irregular pulse, insomnia, dizziness, or tremors occur
• Proper administration to avoid systemic absorption

---

ergonovine maleate

(er-goe-noe'veen)
Ergotrate Maleate
Func. class.: Oxytocic
Chem. class.: Ergot alkaloid

Action: Stimulates uterine contractions, decreases bleeding
Uses: Treatment of hemorrhage associated with postpartum or post-abortion

Dosage and routes:
• *Adult:* IM 0.2 mg q2-4h, not to exceed 5 doses; IV 0.2 mg given over 1 min; PO 0.2-0.4 mg q6-12h × 2-7 days after initial IM or IV dose
Available forms include: Inj IM, IV 0.2 mg/ml; tabs 0.2 mg
Side effects/adverse reactions:
CNS: Headache, dizziness, fainting
CV: Hypertension, chest pain
GI: Nausea, vomiting

INTEG: Sweating
RESP: Dyspnea
EENT: Tinnitus
GU: Cramping

Contraindications: Hypersensitivity to ergot medication, augmentation of labor, before delivery of placenta, spontaneous abortion (threatened), pelvic inflammatory disease (PID)

Precautions: Hepatic disease, renal disease, cardiac disease, asthma, anemia, convulsive disorders, hypertension, glaucoma

Pharmacokinetics:
PO: Onset 5-25 min, duration 3 hr
IM: Onset 2-5 min, duration 3 hr
IV: Onset immediate, duration 45 min
Metabolized in liver, excreted in urine

Interactions/incompatibilities: None known

NURSING CONSIDERATIONS
Assess:
• B/P, pulse; watch for change that may indicate hemorrhage
• Respiratory rate, rhythm, depth; notify physician of abnormalities

Administer:
• IM in deep muscle mass, rotate injection sites if additional doses are given
• After having crash cart available on unit

Evaluate:
• For length, duration of contraction; notify physician of contractions lasting over 1 min or absence of contractions

Teach patient/family:
• To report increased blood loss, abdominal cramps, increased temperature or foul-smelling lochia

ergotamine tartrate
(er-got'a-meen)
Ergomar, Ergostat, Gynergen, Medihaler-Ergotamine, Wigrettes
Func. class.: Adrenergic blocker
Chem. class.: Ergot alkaloid-amino acid

Action: Constricts smooth muscle in periphery, cranial blood vessels
Uses: Vascular headache (migraine or histamine)

Dosage and routes:
• *Adult:* 2 mg, then 1-2 mg qh or q½ hr for SL, not to exceed 6 mg/day or 10 mg/wk; INH 1 puff, may repeat in 5 min, not to exceed 6/24 hr

Available forms include: SL tabs 2 mg; tabs 1 mg; oral inh 360 μg/dose

Side effects/adverse reactions:
CNS: Numbness in fingers, toes, headache
CV: Transient tachycardia, chest pain, bradycardia
GI: Increase or decrease in B/P, nausea, vomiting
MS: Muscle pain

Contraindications: Hypersensitivity to ergot preparations, occlusion (peripheral, vascular), CAD, hepatic disease, renal disease, peptic ulcer, hypertension

Precautions: Pregnancy, lactation, children

Pharmacokinetics:
PO: Peak 30 min-3 hr; metabolized in liver, excreted as metabolites in feces, crosses blood-brain barrier, excreted in breast milk

Interactions/incompatibilities:
• Increased effects: troleandomycin
• Increased vasoconstriction: β-blockers

NURSING CONSIDERATIONS
Assess:
• Weight daily, check for peripheral edema in feet, legs
Administer:
• IM dose, which takes 20 min for effect, or use IV for immediate effect
• At beginning of headache, dose must be titrated to patient response
• By SL route if possible for better, faster absorption
• With meals or after meals to avoid GI symptoms
• Only to women who are not pregnant, harm to fetus may occur
Perform/provide:
• Storage in dark area, do not use discolored solutions
• Quiet, calm environment with decreased stimulation for noise, or bright light or excessive talking
Evaluate:
• Therapeutic response: decrease in frequency, severity of headache
• For stress level, activity, recreation, coping mechanisms of patient
• Neurological status: LOC, blurring vision, nausea, vomiting, tingling in extremities that occur preceding the headache
• Ingestion of tyramine foods (pickled products, beer, wine, aged cheese), food additives, preservatives, colorings, artificial sweeteners, chocolate, caffeine, which may precipitate these types of headaches
Teach patient/family:
• Not to use OTC medications, serious drug interactions may occur
• To maintain dose at approved level, not to increase even if drug does not relieve headache
• To report side effects including increased vasoconstriction starting with cold extremities, then paresthesia, weakness
• That an increase in headaches

may occur when this drug is discontinued after long-term use
• Keep drug out of reach of children, death may occur

---

erythrityl tetranitrate
(e-ri'thri-till)
Cardilate
Func. class.: Vasodilator, coronary
Chem. class.: Nitrate

Action: Decreases preload, afterload, which is responsible for decreasing left ventricular end diastolic pressure, systemic vascular resistance
Uses: Chronic stable angina pectoris, prophylaxis of angina pain
Dosage and routes:
• *Adult:* PO 10-30 mg tid; SL 5-15 mg before stress
Available forms include: Chew tabs 10 mg; tabs PO, SL 5, 10 mg
Side effects/adverse reactions:
CV: Postural hypotension, tachycardia, collapse
GI: Nausea, vomiting
INTEG: Pallor, sweating
CNS: Headache, flushing, dizziness
Contraindications: Hypersensitivity to this drug or nitrites, anemia, increased intracranial pressure, cerebral hemorrhage, acute MI, pregnancy, lactation
Precautions: Postural hypotension, glaucoma
Pharmacokinetics:
PO: Onset 30 min, peak 1-1½ hr, duration 2-4 hr
SL: Onset 5-10 min, peak 30-45 min, duration 2 hr
Metabolized by liver, excreted in urine
Interactions/incompatibilities:
• Increased effects: β-blockers, narcotics, tricyclics, diuretics, antihypertensives
• Decreased effects: sympathomimetics

NURSING CONSIDERATIONS
Assess:
• B/P, pulse, respirations during beginning therapy
Administer:
• With 8 oz of water on empty stomach (oral tablet)
Evaluate:
• Pain: duration, time started, activity being performed, character
• Tolerance if taken over long period of time
• Headache, lightheadedness, decreased B/P; may indicate a need for decreased dosage
Teach patient/family:
• That drug may be taken before stressful activity: exercise, sexual activity
• That SL may sting when drug comes in contact with mucous membranes
• To avoid hazardous activities if dizziness occurs
• Stress patient compliance with complete medical regimen
• To make position changes slowly to prevent fainting

erythromycin (ophthalmic)
(er-ith-roe-mye'sin)
Ilotycin Ophthalmic
Func. class.: Antiinfective

Action: Inhibits bacterial cell wall in organism by preventing amino acids, nucleotides into cell wall
Uses: Infection of eye
Dosage and routes:
• *Adult and child:* Apply oint qd-qid as needed
Ophthalmia neonatorum
• *Neonates:* Apply oint to conjunctival sacs immediately after delivery
Available forms include: Oint 0.5%

Side effects/adverse reactions:
EENT: Poor corneal wound healing, temporary visual haze, overgrowth of nonsusceptible organisms
Contraindications: Hypersensitivity
Precautions: Antibiotic hypersensitivity
Interactions/incompatibilities: None known
NURSING CONSIDERATIONS
Administer:
• After washing hands, cleanse crusts or discharge from eye before application
Perform/provide:
• Storage at room temperature, in tight container
Evaluate:
• Therapeutic response: absence of redness, inflammation, tearing
• Allergy: itching, lacrimation, redness, swelling
Teach patient/family:
• To use drug exactly as prescribed
• Not to use eye makeup, towels, washcloths, eye medication of others; reinfection may occur
• That drug container tip should not be touched to eye
• To report itching, increased redness, burning, stinging, swelling; drug should be discontinued
• That drug may cause blurred vision when ointment is applied

erythromycin (topical)
(er-ith-roe-mye'sin)
A/T/S, Eryderm, Staticin
Func. class.: Local antiinfective
Chem. class.: Macrolide antibacterial

Action: Interferes with bacterial DNA replication
Uses: Pyoderma, acne vulgaris
Dosage and routes:
• Adult and child: TOP apply to affected area tid-qid

Available forms include: Top sol 2%

Side effects/adverse reactions:
INTEG: Rash, urticaria, stinging, burning, pruritus, dry or oily skin
Contraindications: Hypersensitivity

Precautions: Pregnancy (C), lactation

Interactions/incompatibilities:
Avoid use with clindamycin

NURSING CONSIDERATIONS
Administer:
• Enough medication to completely cover lesions
• After cleansing with soap, water before each application, dry well
Perform/provide:
• Storage at room temperature in dry place
Evaluate:
• Allergic reaction: burning, stinging, swelling, redness
• Therapeutic response: decrease in size, number of lesions
Teach patient/family:
• To apply with glove to prevent further infection
• To avoid use of OTC creams, ointments, lotions unless directed by physician
• To use medical asepsis (hand washing) before, after each application

---

erythromycin base, erythromycin estolate, erythromycin ethylsuccinate, erythromycin glucceptate, erythromycin lactobionate, erythromycin stearate

(er-ith-roe-mye'sin)

E-Mycin, ERYC, Ery-Tab, Erythromid,* Ethril, Ilotycin, Novorythro,* Robimycin, Staticin, Ilosone, E.E.S., Erythrocin, Pediamycin, Wyamycin Liquid, E-Biotic, Erypar, Wintrocin, Wyamycin

Func. class.: Antibacterial
Chem. class.: Macrolide antibiotic

Action: Interacts with phospholipids, penetrates cell wall; changes occur immediately in membrane
Uses: Infections caused by *N. gonorrhoeae,* mild to moderate respiratory tract, skin, soft tissue infections caused by *D. pneumoniae, M. pneumoniae, C. diphtheriae, B. pertussis, L. monocytogenes,* syphilis, Legionnaire's disease, *C. trachomatis*
Dosage and routes:
Soft tissue infections
• *Adult:* PO 250-500 mg q6h (base, estolate, stearate); PO 400-800 mg q6h (ethylsuccinate); IV INF 15-20 mg/kg/day (ethylsuccinate)
• *Child:* PO 30-50 mg/kg/day in divided doses q6h (salts); IV 15-20 mg/kg/day in divided doses q4-6h (salts)

N. gonorrhoeae/PID
• *Adult:* IV 500 mg q6h × 3 days (glucceptate, lactobionate), then PO 250 mg (base, estolate, stearate) or 400 mg (ethylsuccinate) q6h × 1 wk

Syphilis
• *Adult:* PO 500 mg q6h × 15 days (base, estolate, stearate)

Chlamydia

• *Adult:* PO 500 mg q6h × 1 wk or 250 mg qid × 2 wk

• *Infant:* PO 50 mg/kg/day in 4 divided doses × 3 wk or more

• *Newborn:* PO 50 mg/kg/day in 4 divided doses × 2 wk or more

Intestinal amebiasis

• *Adult:* PO 250 mg q6h × 10-14 days (base, estolate, stearate)

• *Child:* PO 30-50 mg/kg/day in divided doses q6h × 10-14 days (base, estolate, stearate)

Available forms include: Base: tabs, enteric-coated 250, 333, 500 mg; tabs film-coated 250, 500 mg; caps, enteric-coated 125, 250 mg; estolate: tabs chewable 125, 250 mg; tabs 500 mg; caps 125, 250 mg; drops 100 mg/ml; susp 125, 250 mg/5ml; stearate: tabs, film-coated 250, 500 mg; ethylsuccinate: tabs, chewable 200 mg; tabs, film-coated 400 mg/2.5 ml, 200, 400 mg/5 ml; susp 200, 400 mg

Side effects/adverse reactions:

INTEG: Rash, urticaria, pruritus

GI: Nausea, vomiting, diarrhea, *hepatotoxicity,* abdominal pain, stomatitis, heartburn, anorexia, pruritus ani

GU: Vaginitis, moniliasis

EENT: Hearing loss, tinnitus

Contraindications: Hypersensitivity

Precautions: Pregnancy, hepatic disease

Pharmacokinetics: Peak 4 hr, duration 6 hr, half-life 1-3 hr, metabolized in liver, excreted in bile, feces

Interactions/incompatabilities:

• Increased action of: oral anticoagulants, digitalis, theophylline, methylprednisolone, cyclospurine

• Decreased action of: clindamycin, penicillins

NURSING CONSIDERATIONS

Assess:

• I&O ratio; report hematuria, oliguria in renal disease

• Liver studies: AST, ALT

• Renal studies: urinalysis, protein, blood

• C&S before drug therapy; drug may be taken as soon as culture is taken; C&S may be repeated after treatment

Administer:

• IM deep injection; rotate sites

• Enteric-coated tablets may be given with food

Perform/provide:

• Storage at room temperature

• Adequate intake of fluids (2000 ml) during diarrhea episodes

Evaluate:

• Bowel pattern before, during treatment

• Skin eruptions, itching

• Respiratory status: rate, character, wheezing, tightness in chest; discontinue drug if these occur

• Allergies before treatment, reaction of each medication; place allergies on chart, Kardex in bright red letters; notify all people giving drugs

Teach patient/family:

• To take oral drug with full glass of water; may give with food if GI symptoms occur

• Do not take with fruit juice

• To report sore throat, fever, fatigue; could indicate superimposed infection

• To notify nurse of diarrhea stools

• To take at evenly spaced intervals; complete dosage regimen

Lab test interferences:

False increase: 17-OHCS/17-KS, AST/ALT

Decrease: Folate assay

Treatment of overdose: Withdraw drug, maintain airway, administer epinephrine, aminophylline, O_2, IV corticosteroids

E

---

italics = common side effects   ***bold italic*** = life threatening reactions

essential crystalline amino acid solution

Aminosyn-RF, Nephramine, Ren-Amine 6.5

Func. class.: Caloric

Action: Needed for anabolism to maintain structure, decrease catabolism, promote healing

Uses: Renal decompensation

Dosage and routes:
• *Adult:* CENT IV 0.3-0.5 g/kg, 250 ml of amino acid/500 ml D70, given at rate of 20-30 ml/hr, increased by 10 ml/hr q24h, not to exceed 100 ml/hr
• *Child:* CENT IV 1 g/kg/day or less, depending on patient's needs

Available forms include: Inj central line only, many types

Side effects/adverse reactions:
CNS: Dizziness, headache, confusion, loss of consciousness
CV: Hypertension, *CHF, pulmonary edema*
GI: Nausea, vomiting, liver fat deposits, abdominal pain
GU: Glycosuria, osmotic diuresis
ENDO: Hyperglycemia, rebound hypoglycemia, electrolyte imbalances, hyperosmolar syndrome, hyperosmolar hyperglycemic non-ketotic syndrome, alkalosis, acidosis, hypophosphatemia, hyperammonemia, dehydration, hypocalcemia
INTEG: Chills, flushing, warm feeling, rash, urticaria, extravasation necrosis, phlebitis at injection site

Contraindications: Hypersensitivity, severe electrolyte imbalances, anuria, severe liver damage, maple syrup urine disease

Precautions: Renal disease, pregnancy, children, diabetes mellitus, CHF

Interactions/incompatibilities:
None known

NURSING CONSIDERATIONS

Assess:
• Electrolytes (K, Na, Ca, Cl, Mg), blood glucose, ammonia, phosphate
• Renal, liver function studies: BUN, creatinine, ALT, AST, bilirubin
• Injection site for extravasation: redness along vein, edema at site, necrosis, pain, hard tender area, site should be changed immediately
• Monitor respiratory function q4h: auscultate lung fields bilaterally for rales, respirations, quality, rate, rhythm
• Monitor temperature q4h for increased fever, indicating infection; if infection suspected, infusion is discontinued, tubing, bottle cultured
• Urine glucose q6h using Tes-Tape, Clinistix, Keto-Diastix, which are not affected by infusion substances

Administer:
• TPN must be used only mixed with dextrose to promote protein synthesis
• Immediately after mixing in pharmacy under strict aseptic technique using laminar flowhood; use infusion pump, in-line filter
• Using careful monitoring technique; do not speed up infusion; pulmonary edema, glucose overload will result

Perform/provide
• Storage depends on type of solution, consult manufacturer
• Changing dressing on IV site to prevent infection q24-48h

Evaluate:
• Hyperammonemia: nausea, vomiting, malaise, tremors, anorexia, convulsions
• Therapeutic response: weight gain, decreased jaundice in liver disorders

Teach patient/family
• Reason for use of TPN
• If chills, sweating are experienced, they should be reported at once

---

esterified estrogens

Climestrone,* Estabs, Estratab, Menest, Ms-Med, Neo-Estrone*

Func. class.: Estrogen
Chem. class.: Nonsteroidal synthetic estrogen

Action: Needed for adequate functioning of female reproductive system; affects release of pituitary gonadotropins, inhibits ovulation, adequate calcium use in bone structures
Uses: Menopause, breast cancer, prostatic cancer hypogonadism, castration, primary ovarian failure
Dosage and routes:
Menopause
• *Adult:* PO 0.3-3.75 mg qd 3 wk on, 1 wk off
Hypogonadism/castration/ovarian failure
• *Adult:* PO 2.5 mg qd-tid 3 wk on, 1 wk off
Prostatic cancer
• *Adult:* PO 1.25-2.5 mg tid
Breast cancer
• *Adult:* PO 10 mg tid × 3 months or longer
Available forms include: Tabs 0.3, 0.625, 1.25, 2.5 mg
Side effects/adverse reactions:
CNS: Dizziness, headache, migraines, depression
CV: Hypotension, thrombophlebitis, edema, *thromboembolism, stroke, pulmonary embolism, myocardial infarction*
GI: Nausea, vomiting, diarrhea, anorexia, pancreatitis, cramps, constipation, increased appetite, increased weight, cholestatic jaundice

EENT: Contact lens intolerance, increased myopia, astigmatism
GU: Amenorrhea, cervical erosion, breakthrough bleeding, dysmenorrhea, vaginal candidiasis, breast changes, *gynecomastia, testicular atrophy, impotence*
INTEG: Rash, urticaria, acne, hirsutism, alopecia, oily skin, seborrhea, purpura, melasma
META: Folic acid deficiency, hypercalcemia, hyperglycemia
Contraindications: Breast cancer, thromboembolic disorders, reproductive cancer, genital bleeding (abnormal, undiagnosed), pregnancy (X)
Precautions: Hypertension, asthma, blood dyscrasias, gallbladder disease, CHF, diabetes mellitus, bone disease, depression, migraine headache, convulsive disorders, hepatic disease, renal disease, family history of cancer of breast or reproductive tract
Pharmacokinetics:
PO: Degraded in liver, excreted in urine, crosses placenta, excreted in breast milk
Interactions/incompatibilities:
• Decreased action of: anticoagulants, oral hypoglycemics
• Toxicity: tricyclic antidepressants
• Decreased action of this drug: anticonvulsants barbiturates, phenylbutazone, rifampin
• Increased action of: corticosteroids
NURSING CONSIDERATIONS
Assess:
• Urine glucose in patient with diabetes, increased urine glucose may occur
• Weight daily, notify physician of weekly weight gain >5 lb; if increase, diuretic may be ordered
• B/P q4h, watch for increase caused by water and sodium retention

---

E

• I&O ratio, be alert for decreasing urinary output and increasing edema
• Liver function studies, including AST, ALT, bilirubin, alk phosphatase

Administer:
• Titrated dose, use lowest effective dose
• With food or milk to decrease GI symptoms

Evaluate:
• Therapeutic response: absence of breast engorgement, reversal of menopause or decrease in tumor size in prostatic cancer
• Edema, hypertension, cardiac symptoms, jaundice
• Mental status: affect, mood, behavioral changes, aggression
• Hypercalcemia

Teach patient/family:
• To weigh weekly, report gain >5 lb
• To report breast lumps, vaginal bleeding, edema, jaundice, dark urine, clay colored stools, dyspnea, headache, blurred vision, abdominal pain, numbness or stiffness in legs, chest pain, male to report impotence or gynecomastia
• To avoid sunlight or wear sunscreen, burns may occur

estradiol/estradiol cypionate/estradiol valerate

(ess-tra-dye'ole)

Estrace/Depo-Estradiol Cypionate, Depogen, Dura Estrin, E-Ionate PA, Estro-Cyp, Estroject-LA/Delestrogen,* Dioval Duragen, Estradiol LA, Estraval, Retestrin, Valergen, Hormogen Depot, Deladiol

Func. class.: Estrogen
Chem. class.: Nonsteroidal synthetic estrogen

Action: Needed for adequate functioning of female reproductive system; affects release of pituitary gonadotropins, inhibits ovulation, adequate calcium use in bone structures

Uses: Menopause, breast cancer, prostatic cancer, atrophic vaginitis, kraurosis vulvae, hypogonadism, castration, primary ovarian failure

Dosage and routes:
Menopause/hypogonadism/castration/ovarian failure
• *Adult:* PO 1-2 mg qd 3 wk on, 1 wk off or 5 days on, 2 days off; IM 0.2-1 mg q wk

Prostatic cancer
• *Adult:* IM 30 mg q 1-2 wk (valerate); PO 1-2 mg tid (oral estradiol)

Breast cancer
• *Adult:* PO 10 mg tid × 3 mo or longer

Atropic vaginitis
• *Adult:* VAG CREAM 2-4 g qd × 1-2 wk, then 1 g 1-3 ×/wk

Kraurosis valvae
• *Adult:* IM 1-1.5 mg 1-2 ×/wk

Available forms include: Estradiol-tabs 1, 2 mg; cypionate-injection IM 1, 5 mg/ml; valerate-injection IM 10, 20, 40 mg/ml

Side effects/adverse reactions:
CNS: Dizziness, headache, migraines, depression
CV: Hypotension, thrombophlebitis, edema, *thromboembolism, stroke, pulmonary embolism, myocardial infarction*
GI:Nausea, vomiting, diarrhea, anorexia, pancreatitis, cramps, constipation, increased appetite, increased weight, cholestatic jaundice
EENT: Contact lens intolerance, increased myopia, astigmatism
GU: Amenorrhea, cervical erosion, breakthrough bleeding, dysmenorrhea, vaginal candidiasis, breast changes, *gynecomastia, testicular atrophy, impotence*
INTEG: Rash, urticaria, acne, hirsutism, alopecia, oily skin, seborrhea, purpura, melasma
META: Folic acid deficiency, hypercalcemia, hyperglycemia
Contraindications: Breast cancer, thromboembolic disorders, reproductive cancer, genital bleeding (abnormal, undiagnosed), pregnancy (X)
Precautions: Hypertension, asthma, blood dyscrasias, gallbladder disease, CHF, diabetes mellitus, bone disease, depression, migraine headache, convulsive disorders, hepatic disease, renal disease, family history of cancer of breast or reproductive tract
Pharmacokinetics:
PO/IH/TOP: Degraded in liver, excreted in urine, crosses placenta, excreted in breast milk
Interactions/incompatibilities:
• Decreased action of: anticoagulants, oral hypoglycemics
• Toxicity: tricyclic antidepressants
• Decreased action of this drug: anticonvulsants, barbiturates, phenylbutazone, rifampin

• Increased action of: corticosteroids
NURSING CONSIDERATIONS
Assess:
• Urine glucose in patient with diabetes, increased urine glucose may occur
• Weight daily, notify physician of weekly weight gain >5 lb; if increase, diuretic may be ordered
• B/P q4h, watch for increase caused by water and sodium retention
• I&O ratio, be alert for decreasing urinary output and increasing edema
• Liver function studies, including AST, ALT, bilirubin, alk phosphatase
Administer:
• Titrated dose, use lowest effective dose
• IM injection deeply in large muscle mass
• With food or milk to decrease GI symptoms (oral)
Evaluate:
• Therapeutic response: absence of breast engorgement, reversal of menopause or decrease in tumor size in prostatic cancer
• Edema, hypertension, cardiac symptoms, jaundice, hypercalcemia
• Mental status: affect, mood, behavioral changes, aggression
Teach patient/family:
• To weigh weekly, report gain >5 lb
• To report breast lumps, vaginal bleeding, edema, jaundice, dark urine, clay-colored stools, dyspnea, headache, blurred vision, abdominal pain, numbness or stiffness in legs, chest pain; male to report impotence or gynecomastia
• To avoid sunlight or wear sunscreen; burns may occur
Lab test interferences:
Increase: BSP retention test, PBI,

E

T_4, serum sodium, platelet aggregation, thyroxine-binding globulin (TBG), prothrombin, factors VII, VIII, IX, X, triglycerides
Decrease: Serum folate, serum triglyceride, T_3 resin uptake test, glucose tolerance test, antithrombin III, pregnanediol, metyraponetest
False positive: LE prep, antinuclear antibodies

estramustine phosphate sodium

(ess-tra-muss'teen)
Emcyt

Func. class.: Antineoplastic
Chem. class.: Hormone: estrogen

Action: Precise actions unknown
Uses: Metastatic prostate cancer
Dosage and routes:
• *Adult:* PO 10-16 mg/kg in 3-4 divided doses; treatment may continue for 3 mo or more
Available forms include: Caps 140 mg (12.5 mg sodium/cap)
Side effects/adverse reactions:
*HEMA: **Thrombocytopenia, leukopenia***
*GI: Nausea, vomiting, anorexia, **hepatotoxicity***
*GU: **Renal failure,** impotence, gynecomastia*
INTEG: Rash, urticaria, pruritus, flushing
RESP: Dyspnea, emboli, hoarseness
*CV: **Myocardial infarction,** hypertension, **CHF, CVA***
CNS: Headache, anxiety, seizures, insomnia, mood swings
Contraindications: Hypersensitivity to estradiol, thromboembolic disorders
Precautions: Edema, hepatic disease, CVA, MI, seizures, hypertension, diabetes mellitus, pregnancy
Pharmacokinetics:
PO: Peak 1-2 hr, metabolized in liver, excreted in bile, half-life 20 hr (terminal)
Interactions/incompatibilities: None known
NURSING CONSIDERATIONS
Assess:
• CBC, differential, platelet count weekly; withhold drug if WBC is <4000 or platelet count is <75,000; notify physician of these results
• Pulmonary function tests, chest film before, during therapy; chest x-ray should be obtained q2 wk during treatment
• Renal function studies: BUN, serum uric acid, urine CrCl, electrolytes before, during therapy
• I&O ratio; report fall in urine output of 30 ml/hr
• Liver function tests before, during therapy (bilirubin, AST, ALT, LDH) as needed or monthly
• Monitor VS q4h, ECG before, during treatment
Administer:
• Medications by oral route if possible; avoid IM, SC, IV routes to prevent infections
• Antacid before oral agent; give drug after evening meal before bedtime
• Antiemetic 30-60 min before giving drug to prevent vomiting
Perform/provide:
• Strict medical asepsis, protective isolation if WBC levels are low
• Special skin care
• Deep breathing exercises with patient 3-4 times/day; place in semi-Fowler's position
• Liquid diet, including cola, Jello; dry toast or crackers may be added if patient is not nauseated or vomiting
Evaluate:
• Bleeding: hematuria, guaiac, bruising, petechiae, mucosa or orifices q8h
• Dyspnea, rales, unproductive

cough, chest pain, tachypnea, fatigue, increased pulse, pallor, lethargy
• Food preferences; list likes, dislikes
• Edema in feet, joint, stomach pain, shaking
• Inflammation of mucosa, breaks in skin
• Yellowing of skin and sclera, dark urine, clay-colored stools, itchy skin, abdominal pain, fever, diarrhea
• Symptoms indicating severe allergic reaction: rash, pruritus, urticaria, purpuric skin lesions, itching, flushing
• Tachycardia, ECG changes, dyspnea, edema, fatigue, leg cramps; may indicate cardiac toxicity

Teach patient/family:
• Protective isolation precautions
• To report any complaints, side effects to nurse or physician
• That gynecomastia, impotence can occur and are reversible after discontinuing treatment
• To report any changes in breathing, coughing

---

estrogenic substances, conjugated

Estrocon, Premarin, Progens
Func. class.: Estrogen
Chem. class.: Nonsteroidal synthetic estrogen

Action: Needed for adequate functioning of female reproductive system; it affects release of pituitary gonadotropins, inhibits ovulation, adequate calcium use in bone structures

Uses: Menopause, breast cancer, prostatic cancer, abnormal uterine bleeding, hypogonadism, castration, primary ovarian failure, osteoporosis

Dosage and routes:
Menopause
• *Adult:* PO 0.3-1.25 mg qd 3 wk on, 1 wk off
Prostatic cancer
• *Adult:* PO 1.25-2.5 mg tid
Breast cancer
• *Adult:* PO 10 mg tid × 3 mo or longer
Abnormal uterine bleeding
• *Adult:* IV/IM 25 mg, repeat in 6-12 hr
Castration/primary ovarian failure/osteoporosis
• *Adult:* PO 1.25 mg qd 3 wk on, 1 wk off
Hypogonadism
• *Adult:* PO 2.5 mg bid-tid × 20 days/mo
Available forms include: Tabs 0.3, 0.625, 0.9, 1.25, 2.5 mg

Side effects/adverse reactions:
CNS: Dizziness, headache, migraine, depression
CV: Hypotension, thrombophlebitis, edema, *thromboembolism, stroke, pulmonary embolism, myocardial infarction*
GI: Nausea, vomiting, diarrhea, anorexia, pancreatitis, cramps, constipation, increased appetite, increased weight, cholestatic jaundice
EENT: Contact lens intolerance, increased myopia, astigmatism
GU: Amenorrhea, cervical erosion, breakthrough bleeding, dysmenorrhea, vaginal candidiasis, breast changes, *gynecomastia, testicular atrophy, impotence*
INTEG: Rash, urticaria, acne, hirsutism, alopecia, oily skin, seborrhea, purpura, melasma
META: Folic acid deficiency, hypercalcemia, hyperglycemia

Contraindications: Breast cancer, thromboembolic disorders, reproductive cancer, genital bleeding (abnormal, undiagnosed), pregnancy (X)

Precautions: Hypertension, asthma, blood dyscrasias, gallbladder disease, CHF, diabetes mellitus, bone disease, depression, migraine headache, convulsive disorders, hepatic disease, renal disease, family history of cancer of breast or reproductive tract

Pharmacokinetics:

PO/IV/IM: Degraded in liver, excreted in urine, crosses placenta, excreted in breast milk

Interactions/incompatibilities:

• Decreased action of: anticoagulants, oral hypoglycemics

• Toxicity: tricyclic antidepressants

• Decreased action of this drug: anticonvulsants, barbiturates, phenylbutazone, rifampin

• Increased action of: corticosteroids

NURSING CONSIDERATIONS

Assess:

• Urine glucose in patient with diabetes; increased urine glucose may occur

• Weight daily, notify physician of weekly weight gain >5 lb; if increase, diurectic may be ordered

• B/P q4h; watch for increase caused by water and sodium retention

• I&O ratio, be alert for decreasing urinary output and increasing edema

• Liver function studies, including AST, ALT, bilirubin, alk phosphatase

Administer:

• Titrated dose, use lowest effective dose

• IM injection deeply in large muscle mass

• With food or milk to decrease GI symptoms PO

Evaluate:

• Therapeutic response: absence of breast engorgement, reversal of menopause, or decrease in tumor size in prostatic cancer

• Edema, hypertension, cardiac symptoms, jaundice, hypercalcemia

• Mental status: affect, mood, behavioral changes, aggression

Teach patient/family:

• To weigh weekly, report gain >5 lb

• To report breast lumps, vaginal bleeding, edema, jaundice, dark urine, clay-colored stools, dyspnea, headache, blurred vision, abdominal pain, numbness or stiffness in legs, chest pain; male to report impotence or gynecomastia

• To avoid sunlight or wear sunscreen; burns may occur

---

estrone

(ess'trone)

Bestrone, Kestrone-5, Theelin Aqeous, Esmone A

Func. class.: Estrogen
Chem. class.: Nonsteroidal synthetic estrogen

Action: Needed for adequate functioning of female reproductive system; affects release of pituitary gonadotropins, inhibits ovulation, promotes adequate calcium use in bone structures

Uses: Menopause, prostatic cancer, atrophic vaginitis, hypogonadism, primary ovarian failure

Dosage and routes:

Menopause/atrophic vaginitis

• *Adult:* IM 0.1-0.5 mg 2-3 × /wk

Prostatic cancer

• *Adult:* IM 2-4 mg 2-3 × /wk

Female hypogonadism/primary ovarian failure

• *Adult:* IM 0.1-1 mg q wk in one dose or divided doses

Available forms include: Inj IM 2, 5 mg/ml

Side effects/adverse reactions:

CNS: Dizziness, headache, migraine, depression

CV: Hypotension, thrombophlebitis, edema, *thromboembolism, stroke, pulmonary embolism, myocardial infarction*

GI:Nausea, vomiting, diarrhea, anorexia, pancreatitis, cramps, constipation, increased appetite, increased weight, cholestatic jaundice

EENT: Contact lens intolerance, increased myopia, astigmatism

GU: Amenorrhea, cervical erosion, breakthrough bleeding, dysmenorrhea, vaginal candidiasis, breast changes, *gynecomastia, testicular atrophy, impotence*

INTEG: Rash, urticaria, acne, hirsutism, alopecia, oily skin, seborrhea, purpura, melasma

META: Folic acid deficiency, hypercalcemia, hyperglycemia

Contraindications: Breast cancer, thromboembolic disorders, reproductive cancer, genital bleeding (abnormal, undiagnosed), pregnancy (X)

Precautions: Hypertension, asthma, blood dyscrasias, gallbladder disease, CHF, diabetes mellitus, bone disease, depression, migraine headache, convulsive disorders, hepatic disease, renal disease, family history of cancer of the breast or reproductive tract

Pharmacokinetics:

IM: Degraded in liver, excreted in urine, crosses placenta, excreted in breast milk

Interactions/incompatibilities:

• Decreased action of: anticoagulants, oral hypoglycemics

• Toxicity: tricyclic antidepressants

• Decreased action of this drug: anticonvulsants, barbiturates, phenylbutazone, rifampin

• Increased action of: corticosteroids

NURSING CONSIDERATIONS
Assess:

• Urine glucose in patient with diabetes; increased urine glucose may occur

• Weight daily, notify physician of weekly weight gain >5 lb; if increase, diurectic may be ordered

• B/P q4h, watch for increase caused by water and sodium retention

• I&O ratio, be alert for decreasing urinary output and increasing edema

• Liver function studies, including AST, ALT, bilirubin, alk phosphatase

Administer:

• Titrated dose, use lowest effective dose

• IM injection deeply in large muscle mass

Evaluate:

• Therapeutic response: absence of breast engorgement, reversal of menopause, or decrease in tumor size in prostatic cancer

• Edema, hypertension, cardiac symptoms, jaundice, hypercalcemia

• Mental status: affect, mood, behavioral changes, aggression

Teach patient/family:

• To weigh weekly, report gain >5 lb

• To report breast lumps, vaginal bleeding, edema, jaundice, dark urine, clay-colored stools, dyspnea, headache, blurred vision, abdominal pain, numbness or stiffness in legs, chest pain; male to report impotence or gynecomastia

• To avoid sunlight or wear sunscreen, burns may occur

E

---

italics = common side effects   ***bold italic*** = life threatening reactions

ethacrynate sodium/ ethacrynic acid

(eth-a-kri′nate)

Sodium Edecrin

Func. class.: Loop diuretic
Chem. class.: Ketone derivative

Action: Acts on loop of Henle by increasing excretion of chloride, sodium

Uses: Pulmonary edema, edema in CHF, liver disease, renal disease

Dosage and routes:

• *Adult:* PO 50-200 mg/day may give up to 200 mg bid

• *Child:* PO 25 mg, increased by 25 mg/day until desired effect occurs

Pulmonary edema

• *Adult:* IV 50 mg given over several minutes or 0.5-1 ml/kg

Available forms include: Tabs 25, 50 mg; powder for inj 50 mg

Side effects/adverse reactions:

GU: Polyuria, gynecomastia, ejaculatory problems, *renal failure,* glycosuria

ELECT: Hypokalemia, hypochloremic alkalosis, hypomagnesemia, hyperuricemia, hypocalcemia, hyponatremia

CNS: Headache, fatigue, weakness, vertigo

GI: Nausea, diarrhea, dry mouth, vomiting, anorexia, cramps, upset stomach, abdominal pain, acute pancreatitis, jaundice, *GI bleeding*

EENT: Loss of hearing, ear pain, tinnitus, blurred vision

INTEG: Rash, pruritus, purpura, Stevens-Johnson syndrome, sweating

MS: Cramps, arthritis, stiffness

ENDO: Hyperglycemia

HEMA: Thrombocytopenia, agranulocytosis, leukopenia, neutropenia

CV: Chest pain, hypotension, *cir-*

culatory collapse, ECG changes

Contraindications: Hypersensitivity to sulfonamides, anuria, hypovolemia, children <18 yr, lactation, electrolyte depletion

Precautions: Dehydration, ascites, severe renal disease, pregnancy (B)

Pharmacokinetics:

PO: Onset ½ hr, peak 2 hr, duration 6-8 hr

IV: Onset 5 min, peak 15-30 min, duration 2 hr

Excreted by kidneys, crosses placenta, half-life 30-70 min

Interactions/incompatibilities:

• Increased toxicity: lithium, nondepolarizing skeletal muscle relaxants, digitalis

• Decreased absorption of thiazides: cholestyramine, colestipol

• Increased anticoagulant activity: anticoagulants

NURSING CONSIDERATIONS

Assess:

• Weight, I&O daily to determine fluid loss; effect of drug may be decreased if used qd

• Rate, depth, rhythm of respiration, effect of exertion

• B/P lying, standing; postural hypotension may occur

• Electrolytes: potassium, sodium, chloride; include BUN, blood sugar, CBC, serum creatinine, blood pH, ABGs

• Glucose in urine if patient is diabetic

Administer:

• In AM to avoid interference with sleep if using drug as a diuretic

• Potassium replacement if potassium is less than 3.0

• With food, if nausea occurs, absorption may be decreased slightly

Evaluate:

• Improvement in edema of feet, legs, sacral area daily if medication is being used in CHF

• Improvement in CVP q8h

• Signs of metabolic acidosis:

drowsiness, restlessness

• Signs of hypokalemia: postural hypotension, malaise, fatigue, tachycardia, leg cramps, weakness

• Rashes, temperature elevation qd

• Confusion, especially in elderly, take safety precautions if needed

Teach patient/family:

• To increase fluid intake 2-3 L/day unless contraindicated; to rise slowly from lying or sitting position

• Adverse reactions: muscle cramps, weakness, nausea, dizziness

• Take with food or milk for GI symptoms

• Take early in day to prevent nocturia

Treatment of overdose: Lavage if taken orally, monitor electrolytes, administer dextrose in saline

---

ethambutol HCl

(e-tham′byoo-tole)
Etibi,* Myambutol
Func. class.: Antitubercular
Chem. class.: Diisopropylethylene diamide derivative

Action: Inhibits RNA synthesis, decreases tubercle bacilli replication

Uses: Pulmonary tuberculosis as an adjunctive

Dosage and routes:

• *Adult and child >13 yr:* PO 15 mg/kg/day as a single dose

Retreatment

• *Adult and child >13 yr:* PO 25 mg/kg/day as single dose × 2 mo with at least 1 other drug, then decrease to 15 mg/kg/day as single dose

Available forms include: Tabs 100, 400 mg

Side effects/adverse reactions:

INTEG: Dermatitis, photosensitivity

CV: CHF, dysrhythmias

CNS: Headache, anxiety, drowsiness, tremors, *convulsions,* lethargy, depression, confusion, psychosis, aggression

EENT: Blurred vision, optic neuritis, photophobia

HEMA: Megaloblastic anemia, vitamin B_{12}, folic acid deficiency

Contraindications: Hypersensitivity, optic neuritis, child <13 yr

Precautions: Pregnancy, renal disease, diabetic retinopathy, cataracts, ocular defects

Pharmacokinetics:

PO: Peak 2-4 hr, half-life 3 hr; metabolized in liver, excreted in urine (unchanged drug/inactive metabolites, feces)

Interactions/incompatibilities:

• Increased toxicity: aminoglycosides, cisplatin, aluminum salts

NURSING CONSIDERATIONS

Assess:

• Temperature, if <101° F, drug should be reduced

• Liver studies q wk: ALT, AST, bilirubin

• Renal status: before, q mo: BUN, creatinine, output, sp gr, urinalysis

• Blood level of drug

Administer:

• With meals to decrease GI symptoms

• Antiemetic if vomiting occurs

• After C&S is completed; q mo to detect resistance

Evaluate:

• Ototoxicity: tinnitus, vertigo, change in hearing

• Mental status often: affect, mood, behavioral changes; psychosis may occur

• Hepatic status: decreased appetite, jaundice, dark urine, fatigue

Teach patient/family:

• That compliance with dosage schedule, length is necessary

• That scheduled appointments must be kept or relapse may occur

---

ethaverine HCl

(eth'a-ver-een)

Circubid, Etalent, Ethaquin, Etha-tabe, Ethavex, Isovex, Pavaspan, Spasodil

Func. class.: Peripheral vasodilator

Chem. class.: Isoquinoline derivative

Action: Relaxes all smooth muscles, dilates coronary blood vessels; vasodilation occurs by cyclic nucleotide phosphodiesterase and increased levels of intracellular AMP

Uses: Peripheral, vascular insufficiency associated with arterial spasm, spastic condition of GI, GU tracts

Dosage and routes:
• *Adult:* PO 100-200 mg tid; SUS REL 150 mg q12h; may be increased to 300 mg q12h

Available forms include: Tabs 100 mg, caps 100 mg, time-release caps 150 mg

Side effects/adverse reactions:
CV: Hypotension, **cardiac depression, cardiac dysrhythmias**
RESP: Respiratory depression
CNS: Headache, dizziness, drowsiness
GI: Nausea, vomiting, anorexia, abdominal pain, dry throat, jaundice, constipation, diarrhea, **hepatic hypersensitivity**
INTEG: Flushing, sweating, rash

Contraindications: Hypersensitivity, arterioventricular dissociation
Precautions: Glaucoma, pregnancy, lactation
Pharmacokinetics:
INH: Onset 30 sec, duration 3-5 min
Interactions/incompatibilities:
• Increased hypotension: alcohol, beta blockers, antihypertensives, narcotics, tricyclics, anticoagulants

• Decreased effects: sympathomimetics

NURSING CONSIDERATIONS
Assess:
• GI symptoms: jaundice, increased liver enzymes, which may indicate hepatic hypersensitivity; notify physician
• B/P, pulse during treatment until stable; take B/P lying, standing; orthostatic hypotension is common
Administer:
• An ordered analgesic if headache develops
• With meals to reduce GI upset
Perform/provide:
• Storage at room temperature
Evaluate:
• Therapeutic response: decreased chest pain (angina), decreased platelet count
• Respiratory status: rate, rhythm; watch for respiratory depression
• Cardiac status: chest pain, what aggravates or ameliorates condition
Teach patient/family:
• That medication is not cure, may need to be taken continuously; therapeutic response may not be evident for 2-3 mo
• That it is necessary to quit smoking to prevent excessive vasoconstriction
• To avoid hazardous activities until stabilized on medication; dizziness may occur
• Not to crush or chew sustained-release tabs

ethchlorvynol

(eth-klor-vi'nole)

Placidyl

Func. class.: Sedative-hypnotic
Chem. class.: Tertiary acetylenic alcohol

Controlled Substance Schedule IV (USA), Schedule F (Canada)
Action: Produces cerebral depres-

sion, exact action is unknown

Uses: Sedation, insomnia

Dosage and routes:

Sedation

• *Adult:* PO 100-250 mg bid or tid

Insomnia

• *Adult:* PO 500 mg-1g ½ hr before hs, may repeat 100-200 mg if needed

Medication for EEG

• *Child:* PO 25 mg/kg in one dose not to exceed 1 g

Available forms include: Caps 200, 500, 750 mg

Side effects/adverse reactions:

HEMA: Thrombocytopenia

CNS: Fatigue, drowsiness, dizziness, sedation, ataxia, nightmares, hangover, giddiness, weakness, hysteria

GI: Nausea, vomiting

INTEG: Rash, urticaria

EENT: Blurred vision, bitter aftertaste

CV: Hypotension

Contraindications: Hypersensitivity to this drug, severe pain, porphyria, pregnancy (1st and 2nd trimester)

Precautions: Depression, hepatic disease, renal disease, suicidal individual, pregnancy (3rd trimester) (C), elderly

Pharmacokinetics:

PO: Onset 15-30 min, peak 1-1½ hr, duration 5 hr; metabolized by liver, excreted by kidneys; half-life 10-20 hr, 21-100 hr terminal

Interactions/incompatibilities:

• Decreased hypoprothrombinemic effect: dicumarol, warfarin

NURSING CONSIDERATIONS

Assess:

• Blood studies: Hct, Hgb, RBCs before and after treatment if blood dyscrasias are suspected

• Hepatic studies: AST, ALT, bilirubin if hepatic disease is present

Administer:

• After removal of cigarettes, to prevent fires

• After trying conservative measures for insomnia

• ½-1 hr before hs for sleeplessness

• With food or meals to decrease dizziness, giddiness

• For only 1 wk, not intended for long-term treatment

Perform/provide:

• Assistance with ambulation after receiving dose

• Safety measures: siderails, nightlight, callbell within easy reach

• Checking to see PO medication swallowed

• Storage in tight container in cool environment

Evaluate:

• Therapeutic response: ability to sleep at night, decreased amount of early morning awakenings if taking drug for insomnia

• Mental status: mood, sensorium, affect, memory (long, short)

• Physical dependency: more frequent requests for medication, shakes, anxiety

• Toxicity: hypotension, hypothermia, weakness, poor muscle coordination, visual problems; drug should be discontinued

• Respiratory dysfunction: respiratory depression, character, rate, rhythm; hold drug if respirations are <12/min or if pupils are dilated (rare)

• Blood dyscrasias: fever, sore throat, bruising, rash, jaundice, epistaxis (rare)

• Allergy to tartrazine: this drug contains tartrazine and should not be used in patients allergic to this dye

Teach patient/family:

• To avoid driving or other activities requiring alertness

• To avoid alcohol ingestion or

E

CNS depressants; serious CNS depression may result

• That effects may take 2 nights for benefits to be noticed

• Alternate measures to improve sleep: reading, exercise several hours before hs, warm bath, warm milk, TV, self-hypnosis, deep breathing

Treatment of overdose: Lavage, activated charcoal, monitor electrolytes, vital signs

---

ethinamate

(e-thin′a-mate)
Valmid

Func. class.: Sedative-hypnotic
Chem. class.: Carbamic acid derivative

Controlled Substance Schedule IV (USA), Schedule F (Canada)
Action: Acts at level of thalamus to produce CNS mood alterations by interfering with nerve impulse transmission in sensory cortex
Uses: Insomnia, preanesthetic
Dosage and routes:
Insomnia
• *Adult:* PO 500 mg-1 g ½ hr before hs
• *Elderly:* PO 250 mg ½ hr before hs
Preanesthetic
• *Adult:* PO 500 mg-1 g 2½ hr before surgery
Available forms include: Caps 500 mg
Side effects/adverse reactions:
*HEMA: **Thrombocytopenia***
CNS: Stimulation
GI: Nausea
INTEG: Rash, purpura, fever
Contraindications: Hypersensitivity, severe pain
Precautions: Depression, suicidal individual, elderly, drug abuse, pregnancy (C)

Pharmacokinetics:
PO: Onset 20 min, duration 3-5 hr
Metabolized by liver, excreted by kidneys; half-life 2½ hr
Interactions/incompatibilities:
• Increased CNS depression: barbiturates, alcohol, narcotics
NURSING CONSIDERATIONS
Assess:
• Blood studies: Hct, Hgb, RBCs (if on long-term therapy)
• Hepatic studies: AST, ALT, bilirubin
Administer:
• After removal of cigarettes, to prevent fires
• After trying conservative measures for insomnia
• ½-1 hr before hs for sleeplessness
• With food or meals to decrease dizziness, giddiness
Perform/provide:
• Assistance with ambulation after receiving dose
• Safety measures: siderails, nightlight, callbell within easy reach
• Checking to see PO medication swallowed
• Storage in tight container in cool environment
Evaluate:
• Therapeutic response: ability to sleep at night, decreased amount of early morning awakening if taking drug for insomnia
• Mental status: mood, sensorium, affect, memory (long, short)
• Physical dependency: more frequent requests for medication, shakes, anxiety
• Withdrawal: confusion, tremors, insomnia, seizures, hallucinations, hyperreflexia
• Respiratory dysfunction: respiratory depression, character, rate, rhythm; hold drug if respirations are <12/min or if pupils are dilated (rare)
• Blood dyscrasias: fever, sore

---

throat, bruising, rash, jaundice, epistaxis (rare)

Teach patient/family:
• To avoid driving or other activities requiring alertness
• To avoid alcohol ingestion or CNS depressants; serious CNS depression may result
• That effects may take 2 nights for benefits to be noticed
• Alternate measures to improve sleep: reading, exercise several hours before hs, warm bath, warm milk, TV, self-hypnosis, deep breathing

Lab test interferences:
False Increase: Urinary 17-KS

Treatment of overdose: Lavage, activated charcoal, monitor electrolytes, vital signs

---

ethinyl estradiol

(eth'in-il ess-tra-dye'ole)
Estinyl, Feminone
Func. class.: Estrogen
Chem. class.: Nonsteroidal synthetic estrogen

Action: Needed for adequate functioning of female reproductive system; affects release of pituitary gonadotropins, inhibits ovulation, promotes adequate calcium use in bone structures

Uses: Menopause, prostatic cancer, breast cancer, breast engorgement, hypogonadism

Dosage and routes:
Menopause
• *Adult:* PO 0.02-0.5 mg qd 3 wk on, 1 wk off
Prostatic cancer
• *Adult:* PO 0.15-2 mg qd
Hypogonadism
• *Adult:* PO 0.05 mg qd-tid × 2 wk/mo, then 2 wk progesterone, then 3-6 mo cycles, then 2 mo off
Breast cancer
• *Adult:* PO 1 mg tid

Breast engorgement
• *Adult:* PO 0.5-1 mg qd × 3 days, then tapered off over 7 days
Available forms include: Tabs 0.02, 0.05, 0.5 mg

Side effects/adverse reactions:
CNS: Dizziness, headache, migraine, depression
CV: Hypotension, thrombophlebitis, edema, *thromboembolism, stroke, pulmonary embolism, myocardial infarction*
GI:Nausea, vomiting, diarrhea, anorexia, pancreatitis, cramps, constipation, increased appetite, increased weight, cholestatic jaundice
EENT: Contact lens intolerance, increased myopia, astigmatism
GU: Amenorrhea, cervical erosion, breakthrough bleeding, dysmenorrhea, vaginal candidiasis, breast changes, *gynecomastia, testicular atrophy, impotence*
INTEG: Rash, urticaria, acne, hirsutism, alopecia, oily skin, seborrhea, purpura, melasma
META: Folic acid deficiency, hypercalcemia, hyperglycemia

Contraindications: Breast cancer, thromboembolic disorders, reproductive cancer, genital bleeding (abnormal, undiagnosed), pregnancy (X)

Precautions: Hypertension, asthma, blood dyscrasias, gallbladder disease, CHF, diabetes mellitus, bone disease, depression, migraine headache, convulsive disorders, hepatic disease, renal disease, family history of cancer of breast or reproductive tract

Pharmacokinetics:
PO: Degraded in liver, excreted in urine, crosses placenta, excreted in breast milk

Interactions/incompatibilities:
• Decreased action of: anticoagulants, oral hypoglycemics

E

---

italics = common side effects   ***bold italic*** = life threatening reactions

• Toxicity: tricyclic antidepressants
• Decreased action of this drug: anticonvulsants, barbiturates, phenylbutazone, rifampin
• Increased action of: corticosteroids

NURSING CONSIDERATIONS
Assess:
• Urine glucose in patient with diabetes; increased urine glucose may occur
• Weight daily, notify physician of weekly weight gain >5 lb; if increase, diuretic may be ordered
• B/P q4h, watch for increase caused by water and sodium retention
• I&O ratio, be alert for decreasing urinary output and increasing edema
• Liver function studies: AST, ALT, bilirubin, alk phosphatase
Administer:
• Titrated dose, use lowest effective dose
• IM injection deeply in large muscle mass
• With food or milk to decrease GI symptoms
Evaluate:
• Therapeutic response: absence of breast engorgement, reversal of menopause, or decrease in tumor size in prostatic cancer
• Edema, hypertension, cardiac symptoms, jaundice, hypercalcemia
• Mental status: affect, mood, behavioral changes, aggression
Teach patient/family:
• To weigh weekly, report gain >5 lb
• To report breast lumps, vaginal bleeding, edema, jaundice, dark urine, clay-colored stools, dyspnea, headache, blurred vision, abdominal pain, numbness or stiffness in legs, chest pain; male to report impotence or gynecomastia

• To avoid sunlight or wear sunscreen; burns may occur

---

ethionamide
(e-thye-on-am-ide)
Trecator SC
Func. class.: Antitubercular
Chem. class.: Thiomine derivative

Action: Inhibits RNA synthesis, decreases tubercle bacilli replication

Uses: Pulmonary, extrapulmonary tuberculosis when other antitubercular drugs are not feasible

Dosage and routes:
• *Adult:* PO 500 mg-1 g qd in divided doses, with another antitubercular drug and pyridoxine
• *Child:* PO 12-15 mg/kg/day in 3-4 doses, not to exceed 750 mg
Available forms include: Tabs 250 mg

Side effects/adverse reactions:
INTEG: Dermatitis, photosensitivity
*CV: **CHF, dysrhythmias***
CNS: Headache, anxiety, drowsiness, tremors, ***convulsions***, lethargy, depression, confusion, psychosis, aggression
*GI: **Anorexia, nausia, vomiting,*** diarrhea, metallic taste
EENT: Blurred vision, optic neuritis, photophobia
*HEMA: **Megaloblastic anemia,*** vitamin B_{12}, folid acid deficiency

Contraindications: Hypersensitivity, optic neuritis

Precautions: Pregnancy, renal disease, diabetic retinopathy, cataracts, ocular defects, child <13 yr

Pharmacokinetics:
PO: Peak 3 hr, duration 9 hr, half-life 3 hr; metabolized in liver, excreted in urine (unchanged drug/inactive), crosses placenta

Interactions/incompatibilities:
• Increased neurotoxicity: cycloserine, ethyl alcohol

• Increased adverse reactions: TB test agents, anti-TB drugs

NURSING CONSIDERATIONS
Assess:
• Temperature, if <101° F, drug should be reduced
• Liver studies q wk: ALT, AST, bilirubin
• Renal status: before, q mo: BUN, creatinine, output, sp gr, urinalysis
Administer:
• With meals to decrease GI symptoms
• Antiemetic if vomiting occurs
• After C&S is completed, q mo to detect resistance
Evaluate:
• Ototoxicity: tinnitus, vertigo, change in hearing
• Mental status often: affect, mood, behavioral changes; psychosis may occur
• Hepatic status: decreased appetite, jaundice, dark urine, fatigue
Teach patient/family:
• That compliance with dosage schedule, length is necessary
• That scheduled appointments must be kept or relapse may occur
• Avoid alcohol while taking this drug

---

ethosuximide

(eth-oh-sux′i-mide)
Zarontin
Func. class.: Anticonvulsant
Chem. class.: Succinimide

Action: Inhibits spike, wave formation in absence seizures (petit mal), decreases amplitude, frequency, duration, spread of discharge in minor motor seizures
Uses: Absence seizures, partial seizures, tonic-clonic seizures.
Dosage and routes:
• *Adult and child >6 yr:* PO 250 mg bid initially; may increase by 250 mg q4-7 days, not to exceed 1.5 g/day
• *Child 3-6 yr:* PO 250 mg/day or 125 mg bid; may increase by 250 mg q4-7 days, not to exceed 1.5 g/day
Available forms include: Caps 250 mg, syr 250 mg/5 ml
Side effects/adverse reactions:
*HEMA: **Agranulocytosis, aplastic anemia, thrombocytopenia, leukocytosis, eosinophilia, pancytopenia***
CNS: Drowsiness, dizziness, fatigue, euphoria, lethargy, anxiety, aggressiveness, irritability, depression, insomnia
GI: Nausea, vomiting, heartburn, anorexia, diarrhea, abdominal pain, cramps, constipation
*GU: Vaginal bleeding, **hematuria, renal damage***
*INTEG: Urticaria, pruritic erythema, hirsutism, **Stevens-Johnson syndrome***
EENT: Myopia, gum hypertrophy, tongue swelling, blurred vision
Contraindications: Hypersensitivity to succinimide derivatives
Precautions: Lactation, pregnancy, hepatic disease, renal disease
Pharmacokinetics:
PO: Peak 1-7 hr, steady state 4-7 days, metabolized by liver, excreted in urine, bile, feces, half-life 24-60 hr
Interactions/incompatibilities:
• Antagonist effect: tricyclic antidepressants (imipramine, doxepin)
• Decreased effects of: estrogens, oral contraceptives
NURSING CONSIDERATIONS
Assess:
• Renal studies: urinalysis, BUN, urine creatinine
• Blood studies: CBC, Hct, Hgb, reticulocyte counts q wk for 4 wk, then q mo

E

• Hepatic studies: AST, ALT, bilirubin, creatinine
• Drug levels during initial treatment, therapeutic range (40-80 μg/ml

Administer:
• With food, milk to decrease GI symptoms

Perform/provide:
• Hard candy, frequent rinsing of mouth, gum for dry mouth
• Assistance with ambulation during early part of treatment; dizziness occurs

Evaluate:
• Therapeutic response: decreased seizure activity, document on patient's chart
• Mental status: mood, sensorium, affect, behavioral changes; if mental status changes, notify physician
• Eye problems: need for ophthalmic examinations before, during, after treatment (slit lamp, fundoscopy, tonometry)
• Allergic reaction: red raised rash, exfoliative dermatitis; if these occur, drug should be discontinued
• Blood dyscrasias: fever, sore throat, bruising, rash, jaundice
• Toxicity: bone marrow depression, nausea, vomiting, ataxia, diplopia, cardiovascular collapse, Stevens-Johnson syndrome

Teach patient/family:
• To carry ID card or Medic-Alert bracelet stating drugs taken, condition, physician's name, phone number
• To avoid driving, other activities that require alertness
• To avoid alcohol ingestion, CNS depressants; increased sedation may occur
• Not to discontinue medication quickly after long-term use
• All aspects of drug: action, use, side effects, adverse reactions, when to notify physician

Lab test interferences:
Increase: Coombs' test
Treatment of overdose: Lavage, activated charcoal, monitor electrolytes, VS

---

ethotoin

(eth'oh-toyin)
Peganone
Func. class.: Anticonvulsant
Chem. class.: Hydantoin derivative

Action: Inhibits nerve in impulses in the motor cortex by decreasing sodium ion influx, limiting tetanic stimulation

Uses: Generalized tonic-clonic or complex-partial seizures

Dosage and routes:
• *Adult:* PO 250 mg qid initially; may increase over several days to 3 g/day in divided doses
• *Child:* PO 250 mg bid; may increase by 250 mg qid

Available forms include: Tabs 250, 500 mg

Side effects/adverse reactions:
HEMA: Agranulocytosis, thrombocytopenia, leukopenia, pancytopenia, megaloblastic anemia, lymphadenopathy
CNS: Fatigue, insomnia, numbness, fever, headache
GI: Nausea, vomiting, diarrhea, gingival hypertrophy
INTEG: Rash
EENT: Nystagmus, diplopia

Contraindications: Hypersensitivity to hydantoins, blood dyscrasias, hematologic disease, hepatic disease

Pharmacokinetics: Metabolized by liver, excreted in urine, half-life 3-9 hr

Interactions/incompatibilities:
• Decreased effects of: rifampin, chronic alcohol, barbiturates, antihistamines, antacids, other anticonvulsants antineoplastics, calcium

products, folic acid, oxacillin
• Increased effects of: benzodiaze-pines, cimetidine, salicylates, sul-fonamide, pyrazolones, phenothi-azines, estrogens, disulfiram, chloramphenicol, anticoagulants
• Seizures: valproic acid
• Myocardial depressions: lido-caine, propranolol, sympathomi-metics

NURSING CONSIDERATIONS
Assess:
• Renal studies: urinalysis, BUN, urine creatinine
• Blood studies: RBC, Hct, Hgb, reticulocyte counts q wk for 4 wk then q mo
• Hepatic studies: AST, ALT, bili-rubin, creatinine
• Drug levels during initial treat-ment, therapeutic level (15-50 μg/ml)
Administer:
• With food, milk to decrease GI symptoms
• After meals
Perform/provide:
• Hard candy, frequent rinsing of mouth, gum for dry mouth
• Assistance with ambulation dur-ing early part of treatment; dizzi-ness occurs
Evaluate:
• Therapeutic response: decreased seizure activity, document on pa-tient's chart
• Mental status: mood, sensorium, affect, behavioral changes; if men-tal status changes, notify physician
• Eye problems: need for ophthal-mic examinations before, during, after treatment (slit lamp, fundos-copy, tonometry)
• Allergic reaction: red raised rash; if this occurs, drug should be dis-continued
• Blood dyscrasias: fever, sore throat, bruising, rash, jaundice
• Toxicity: bone marrow depres-sion, nausea, vomiting, ataxia, dip-

lopia, cardiovascular collapse, Ste-vens-Johnson syndrome
Teach patient/family:
• To carry ID card or Medic-Alert bracelet stating drugs taken, con-dition, physician's name, phone number
• To avoid driving, other activities that require alertness
• To avoid alcohol ingestion, CNS depressants; increased sedation may occur
• Not to discontinue medication quickly after long-term use, taper off over several weeks
• All aspects of drug: action, use, side effects, adverse reactions, when to notify physician
Lab test interferences:
Increase: Serum glucose, BSP, alk phosphatase
Decrease: Urinary steroids, PBI, dexamethasone/metyrapone tests
Treatment of overdose: Lavage, activated charcoal, monitor electro-lytes, VS

---

ethyl chloride (topical)
(eth-il)
Func. class.: Topical anesthetic

Action: Inhibits nerve impulses from sensory nerves, which pro-duces anesthesia
Uses: Pruritus, sunburn, toothache, sore throat, cold sores, oral pain, rectal pain and irritation
Dosage and routes:
• *Adult and child:* TOP apply spray to affected area holding 1 ft away
Available forms include: Aerosol
Side effects/adverse reactions:
INTEG: Rash, irritation, sensitiza-tion
Contraindications: Hypersensitiv-ity, infants <1 yr, application to large areas
Precautions: Child <6 yr, sepsis, pregnancy, denuded skin

Interactions/incompatibilities: None known

NURSING CONSIDERATIONS

Administer:
• After cleansing and drying of affected area

Evaluate:
• Allergy: rash, irritation, reddening, swelling
• Therapeutic response: absence of pain, itching in affected area
• Infection: if affected area is infected, do not apply

Teach patient/family:
• To report rash, irritation, redness, swelling
• How to apply spray

---

ethylestrenol

(eth-il-ess'tre-nole)

Maxibolin

Func. class.: Androgenic anabolic steroid

Chem. class.: Hydantoin derivative

Action: Increases weight by building body tissue, increases potassium, phosphorus, chloride, and nitrogen levels, increases bone development

Uses: To increase weight, combat tissue depletion, osteoporosis, immobility, refractory anemias, catabolic effects of corticosteroid therapy

Dosage and routes:
• *Adult:* PO 4-8 mg qd, decreased at beginning clinical response
• *Child:* PO 1-3 mg qd, not to exceed treatment of 6 wk

Available forms include: Tabs 2 mg; elix 2 mg/5 ml

Side effects/adverse reactions:
INTEG: Rash, acneiform lesions, oily hair, skin, flushing, sweating, acne vulgaris, alopecia, hirsutism
CNS: Dizziness, headache, fatigue, tremors, paresthesias, flushing, sweating, anxiety, lability, insomnia
MS: Cramps, spasms
CV: Increased B/P
GU: Hematuria, amenorrhea, vaginitis, decreased libido, decreased breast size, clitoral hypertrophy, testicular atrophy
GI: Nausea, vomiting, constipation, weight gain, *cholestatic jaundice*
EENT: Carpal tunnel syndrome, conjunctional edema, nasal congestion
ENDO: Abnormal GTT

Contraindications: Severe renal disease, severe cardiac disease, severe hepatic disease, hypersensitivity, pregnancy (C), lactation, genital bleeding (abnormal)

Precautions: Migraine headaches, seizure disorders

Pharmacokinetics:
PO: Metabolized in liver, excreted in urine, crosses placenta, excreted in breast milk

Interactions/incompatibilities:
• May increase effects of: oral anticoagulants, antidiabetics, oxyphenbutazone, phenylbutazone
• May decrease effect of this drug: barbiturates

NURSING CONSIDERATIONS

Assess:
• Weight daily, notify physician if weekly weight gain is >5 lb
• B/P q4h
• I&O ratio; be alert for decreasing urinary output, increasing edema
• Growth rate in children since growth rate may be uneven (linear/bone growth) used for extended periods of time; periodic x-rays are done to assure changes in bone growth
• Electrolytes: K, Na, Cl; cholesterol
• Liver function studies; ALT, AST, bilirubin

• Blood sugar in diabetes (may become hypoglycemic)
Administer:
• Titrated dose, use lowest effective dose
• With food or milk to decrease GI symptoms
Perform/provide:
• Diet with increased calories, protein; decrease sodium if edema occurs
Evaluate:
• Therapeutic response: increased appetite, increased stamina
• Edema, hypertension, cardiac symptoms, jaundice
• Mental status: affect, mood, behavioral changes, aggression
• Signs of masculinization in female: increased libido, deepening of voice, breast tissue, enlarged clitoris, menstrual irregularities; male: gynecomastia, impotence, testicular atrophy
• Hypercalcemia: lethargy, polyuria, polydipsia, nausea, vomiting, constipation, drug may need to be decreased
• Hypoglycemia in diabetics, since oral anticoagulant action is decreased
Teach patient/family:
• Drug needs to be combined with complete health plan: diet, rest, exercise
• To notify physician if therapeutic response decreases
• Not to discontinue medication abruptly
• Teach patient all aspects of drug usage, including change in sex characteristics
Lab test interferences:
Increase: Cholesterol
Decrease: Cholesterol, T_4, T_3, thyroid ^{131}I uptake test, 17-KS, PBI
Interferes: GTT

ethylnorepinephrine HCl

(eth-il-nor-ep-i-nef'rin)
Bronkephrine
Func. class.: Adrenergic
Chem. class.: Catecholamine

Action: Causes increased contractility and heart rate by acting on β-receptors in heart; also, acts on α-receptors causing vasoconstriction in blood vessels; when larger doses are administered, causes vasodilation in renal, intracerebral, coronary dopaminergic receptors
Uses: Bronchospasm
Dosage and routes:
• *Adult:* IM/SC 0.5-1 ml
• *Child:* IM/SC 0.1-0.5 ml
Available forms include: Inj 2 mg/ml IM, SC
Side effects/adverse reactions:
CNS: Tremors, anxiety, insomnia, headache, dizziness, confusion, hallucinations, ***convulsions, CNS depression***
EENT: Dry nose, irritation of nose and throat
CV: Palpitations, tachycardia, hypertension, chest pain, ***dysrhythmias***
GI: Anorexia, nausea, vomiting
RESP: Depression
Contraindications: Hypersensitivity to sympathomimetics, narrow-angle glaucoma
Precautions: Pregnancy, cardiac disorders, hyperthyroidism, diabetes mellitus, prostatic hypertrophy
Pharmacokinetics:
IM/SC: Onset 6-12 min, duration 1-2 hr
Interactions/incompatibilities:
• Do not use with MAOIs or tricyclic antidepressants; hypertensive crisis may occur
• May decrease effect of this drug when used with methyldopa, uri-

nary acidifiers, rauwolfia alkaloids
• May increase effect of this drug when used with urinary alkalizers

NURSING CONSIDERATIONS

Assess:

• I&O ratio

• ECG during administration continuously; if B/P increases, drug is decreased

• B/P and pulse q5 min after parenteral route

• CVP or PWP during infusion if possible

Administer:

• Plasma expanders for hypovolemia

• Parenteral IV dose slowly, after reconstituting with D_5W, 0.9% NS

Perform/provide:

• Storage of reconstituted solution if refrigerated for no longer than 24 hr

• Do not use discolored solutions

Evaluate:

• Paresthesias and coldness of extremities, peripheral blood flow may decrease

• Injection site: tissue sloughing; if this occurs, administer phentolamine mixed with NS

• Therapeutic response: increased B/P with stabilization

Teach patient/family:

• The reason for drug administration

Treatment of overdose: Administer an α-blocker, then norepinephrine for severe hypotension

---

etidocaine HCl

(et-ee′-doe-kane)
Duranest

Func. class.: Local anesthetic
Chem. class.: Amide

Action: Competes with calcium for sites in nerve membrane that control sodium transport across cell membrane; decreases rise of de-

polarization phase of action potential

Uses: Peripheral nerve block, caudal anesthesia, central neural block, vaginal block

Dosage and routes:

Varies depending on route of anesthesia

Available forms include: Inj 1%, 1.5%

Side effects/adverse reactions:

CNS: Anxiety, restlessness, ***convulsions, loss of consciousness,*** drowsiness, disorientation, tremors, shivering

*CV: **Myocardial depression, cardiac arrest, dysrhythmias,*** bradycardia, hypotension, hypertension, fetal bradycardia

GI: Nausea, vomiting

EENT: Blurred vision, tinnitus, pupil constriction

INTEG: Rash, urticaria, allergic reactions, edema, burning, skin discoloration at injection site, tissue necrosis

*RESP: **Status asthmaticus, respiratory arrest, anaphylaxis***

Contraindications: Hypersensitivity, child <12 yr, elderly, severe liver disease

Precautions: Elderly, severe drug allergies, pregnancy (B)

Pharmacokinetics:

Onset 2-8 min, duration 3-6 hr; metabolized by liver, excreted in urine (metabolites)

Interactions/incompatibilities:

• Dysrhythmias: epinephrine, halothane, enflurane

• Hypertension: MAOIs, tricyclic antidepressants, phenothiazines

• Decreased action of this drug: chloroprocaine

NURSING CONSIDERATIONS

Assess:

• B/P, pulse, respiration during treatment

• Fetal heart tones if drug is used during labor

Administer:
• Only with crash cart, resuscitative equipment nearby
• Only drugs without preservatives for epidural or caudal anesthesia

Perform/provide:
• Use of new solution, discard unused portions

Evaluate:
• Therapeutic response: anesthesia necessary for procedure
• Allergic reactions: rash, urticaria, itching
• Cardiac status: ECG for dysrhythmias, pulse, B/P during anesthesia

Treatment of overdose: Airway, O_2, vasopressor, IV fluids, anticonvulsants for seizures

---

etidronate disodium

(e-ti-droe′nate)
Didronel

Func. class.: Parathyroid agents (calcium regulator)
Chem. class.: Diphosphate

Action: Increases bone resorption, new bone development

Uses: Paget's disease, heterotropic ossification

Dosage and routes:
Paget's disease
• *Adult:* PO 5 mg/kg/day 2 hr ac with water, not to exceed 20 mg/kg/day, max 6 mo

Heterotropic ossification
• *Adult:* PO 20 mg/kg qd × 2 wk, then 10 mg/kg/day for 10 wk, total 12 wk

Available forms include: Tabs 200 mg

Side effects/adverse reactions:
GI: Nausea, diarrhea
MS: Bone pain, hypocalcemia, decreased mineralization of noneffected bones

Contraindications: Pathologic fractures, children, colitis

Precautions: Pregnancy (B), renal disease, lactation, restricted vitamin D/calcium

Pharmacokinetics: Not metabolized, excreted in urine/feces, therapeutic response: 1-3 mo

Interactions/incompatibilities:
None known

NURSING CONSIDERATIONS

Assess:
• I&O ratio, check for decreased output in renal patients
• BUN, creatinine, uric acid, chloride, electrolytes, pH, urine calcium, magnesium, alk phosphatase, urinalysis, calcium should be kept at 9-10 mg/dl, vitamin D 50-135 IU/dl
• Increased level since toxic reactions may occur rapidly

Administer:
• On empty stomach with water 2 hr ac
• Drug should not last longer than 6 mo

Evaluate:
• Muscle spasm, laryngospasm, paresthesias, facial twitching, colic; may indicate hypocalcemia
• Nutritional status, diet for sources of vitamin D (milk, some seafood), calcium (dairy products, dark green vegetables), phosphates—adequate intake is necessary
• Persistent nausea or diarrhea

Teach patient/family:
• Avoid OTC products
• All aspects of drug: action, side effects, dose, when to notify physician
• Therapeutic response may take 1-3 mo, effects persist for months after drug is discontinued
• Adequate intake of Ca^+, vitamin D is necessary

---

italics = common side effects   ***bold italic*** = life threatening reactions

etomidate

(e-tom′i-date)

Amidate, Hypnomidate

Func. class.: General anesthetic

Chem. class.: Nonbarbiturate hypnotic

Action: Acts at level of reticular-activating system to produce anesthesia

Uses: Induction of general anesthesia

Dosage and routes:

• *Adult and child >10 yr:* IV 0.2-0.6 mg/kg over ½-1 min

Available forms include: Inj IV 2 mg/ml

Side effects/adverse reactions:

GI: Nausea, vomiting (postoperatively)

CNS: Tonic movements, myoclonic movements, averting movements

CV: Tachycardia, hypotension, hypertension, bradycardia

ENDO: Decreases steroid production

RESP: Laryngospasm

Contraindications: Hypersensitivity, labor/delivery

Precautions: Pregnancy, child <10 yr, lactation

Pharmacokinetics:

IV: Onset 20 sec, peak 1 min, duration 3-5 min; half-life 75 min, metabolized in liver, excreted in urine

Interactions/incompatibilities:

None known

NURSING CONSIDERATIONS

Assess:

• I&O ratio for increasing urine output

• VS q10 min during IV administration, q30 min after IM dose

• Plasma cortisol levels if administered over several hours (5-20 μg/100 ml normal level of cortisol)

Administer:

• Corticosteroids for severe hypotension

• Only with crash cart, resuscitative equipment nearby

• IV slowly only, muscular twitching is reduced with fentanyl before anesthesia induction

Evaluate:

• Increasing or decreasing heart rate or dysrhythmias shown on ECG

etoposide (VP-16)

(e-toe-poe′side)

VePesid

Func. class.: Antineoplastic

Chem. class.: Semisynthetic podophyllotoxin

Action: Inhibits mitotic activity through metaphase to mitosis; also inhibits cells from entering mitosis, depresses DNA, RNA synthesis

Uses: Leukemias, lung, testicular cancer, lymphomas, neuroblastoma

Dosage and routes:

• *Adult:* IV 45-75 mg/m^2/day × 3-5 days given q3-5 wk or 200-250 mg/m^2/wk, or 125-140 mg/m^2/day 3 × wk, q5 wk

Available forms include: Inj IV 20 mg/ml

Side effects/adverse reactions:

HEMA: Thrombocytopenia, leukopenia, myelosuppression, anemia

GI: Nausea, vomiting, anorexia, hepatotoxicity

INTEG: Rash, alopecia, phlebitis

RESP: Bronchospasm

CV: Hypotension

CNS: Headache, fever

Contraindications: Hypersensitivity, bone marrow depression, severe hepatic disease, severe renal disease, bacterial infection

Precautions: Renal disease, hepatic disease, lactation, pregnancy, children, gout

Pharmacokinetics: Half-life 3 hr, terminal 15 hr, metabolized in liver, excreted in urine, crosses placental barrier

Interactions/incompatibilities:

• Do not use with radiation

• Do not use with dextrose solution

NURSING CONSIDERATIONS

Assess:

• CBC, differential, platelet count weekly; withhold drug if WBC is <4000 or platelet count is <75,000; notify physician of results

• Pulmonary function tests, chest X-ray studies before, during therapy; chest X-ray film should be obtained q2 wk during treatment

• Renal function studies: BUN, serum uric acid, urine CrCl, electrolytes before, during therapy

• I&O ratio, report fall in urine output of 30 ml/hr

• Monitor temperature q4h; may indicate beginning infection

• Liver function tests before, during therapy (bilirubin, AST, ALT, LDH) as needed or monthly

• RBC, Hct, Hgb since these may be decreased

Administer:

• Medications by oral route if possible; avoid IM, SC, IV routes to prevent infections

• Antiemetic 30-60 min before giving drug to prevent vomiting

• Allopurinol or sodium bicarbonate to maintain uric acid levels, alkalinization of urine

• Antibiotics for prophylaxis of infection

• IV infusion using 21-, 23-, 25-gauge needle; administer by slow IV infusion over 30 min

• Topical or systemic analgesics for pain

• Local or systemic drugs for infection

• Transfusion for anemia

• Antispasmodic

Perform/provide:

• Strict medical asepsis, protective isolation if WBC levels are low

• Special skin care

• Deep-breathing exercises with patient 3-4 × day; place in semi-Fowler's position

• Liquid diet: cola, Jell-O; dry toast or crackers may be added if patient is not nauseated or vomiting

• Increase fluid intake to 2-3 L/day to prevent urate deposits, calculi formation

• Diet low in purines: organ meats (kidney, liver), dried beans, peas to maintain alkaline urine

• Warm compresses at injection site for inflammation

• Nutritious diet with iron, vitamin supplements

• HOB increased to facilitate breathing

Evaluate:

• Bleeding: *hematuria, guaiac, bruising or petechiae, mucosa or orifices* q8h

• Dyspnea, rales, unproductive cough, chest pain, tachypnea, fatigue, increased pulse, pallor, lethargy

• Food preferences; list likes, dislikes

• Effects of alopecia on body image; discuss feelings about body changes

• Edema in feet, joint pain, stomach pain, shaking

• Inflammation of mucosa, breaks in skin

• Yellowing of skin and sclera, dark urine, clay-colored stools, itchy skin, abdominal pain, fever, diarrhea

• Buccal cavity q8h for dryness, sores or ulceration, white patches, oral pain, bleeding, dysphagia

• Local irritation, pain, burning, discoloration at injection site

E

---

italics = common side effects   ***bold italic*** = life threatening reactions

• Symptoms indicating severe allergic reaction: rash, pruritus, urticaria, purpuric skin lesions, itching, flushing

• Frequency of stools, characteristics: cramping, acidosis; signs of dehydration: rapid respirations, poor skin turgor, decreased urine output, dry skin, restlessness, weakness

Teach patient/family:

• Of protective isolation precautions

• To report any complaints or side effects to nurse or physician

• To report any changes in breathing or coughing

• That hair may be lost during treatment, a wig or hairpiece may make patient feel better; tell patient that new hair may be different in color, texture

---

factor IX complex (human)

Konyne HT, Profilnine, Proplex T, Proplex SX-T

Func. class.: Hemostatic
Chem. class.: Factors II, VII, IX, X

Action: Directly replaces deficient clotting factors II, VII, IX, X

Uses: Hemophilia B (Christmas disease), anticoagulant reversal, control bleeding in hemophilia A

Dosage and routes:

• *Adult and child:* IV 1 U/kg × desired % increase

Available forms include: Inj IV (number of units noted on label)

Side effects/adverse reactions:

GI: Nausea, vomiting, abdominal cramps, jaundice, *viral hepatitis*
INTEG: Rash, flushing, *urticaria*
CNS: Headache, dizziness, malaise, paresthesia, *lethargy, chills, fever, flushing*

HEMA: **Thrombosis, hemolysis, AIDS**
CV: Hypotension, tachycardia
RESP: **Bronchospasm**
EENT: Visual disturbances

Contraindications: Hypersensitivity, hepatic disease, DIC, elective surgery, mild factor IX deficiency

Precautions: Neonates/infants

Pharmacokinetics:

IV: Half-life 4-6 hr, terminal half-life 22.5 hr

Interactions/incompatibilities:
None known

NURSING CONSIDERATIONS

Assess:

• I&O for decreasing urinary output

• Blood studies (coagulation factors assays by % normal: 5% prevents spontaneous hemorrhage, 30%-50% for surgery, 80%-100% for severe hemorrhage)

• Increased B/P, pulse

Administer:

• IV slowly, with plastic syringe only

• After dilution with provide diluent

• After crossmatch is completed if patient has blood type A, B, AB, to determine incompatibility with factor

Perform/provide:

• Storage of reconstituted solution for 12 hr at room temp or up to 2 yr refrigeration (powder); check expiration date

Evaluate:

• Allergic or pyrogenic reaction: fever, chills, rash, itching, slow infusion rate if not severe

• DIC: bleeding, ecchymosis, hypersensitivity, changes in coagulation tests

Teach patient/family:

• To report any signs of bleeding: gums, under skin, urine, stools, emesis

• Risk of viral hepatitis

---

italics = common side effects   ***bold italic*** = life threatening reactions

- That immunization for hepatitis B may be given first

---

famotidine

(fam-oo'-te-dine)

Pepcid

Func. class.: H_2 histamine antagonist

Action: Competitively inhibits histamine at histamine H_2 receptor site, decreasing gastric secretion while pepsin remains at stable level
Uses: Short-term treatment of active duodenal ulcer, maintenance therapy for duodenal ulcer, Zollinger-Ellison syndrome, multiple endocrine adenomas

Dosage and routes:
Duodenal ulcer
- *Adult:* PO 40 mg qd hs $\times$ 4-8 wk, then 20 mg qd hs (maintenance); IV 20 mg q12h if unable to take PO

Hypersecretory conditions
- *Adult:* PO 20 mg q6h, may give 160 mg q6h if needed; IV 20 mg q12h if unable to take PO
Available forms include: Tabs 20, 40 mg; powder for oral susp 40 mg/5 ml; inj IV 10 mg/ml

Side effects/adverse reactions:
HEMA: Thrombocytopenia

CNS: Headache, dizziness, paresthesia, seizure, depression, anxiety, somnolence, insomnia, fever
GI: Constipation, nausea, vomiting, anorexia, cramps, abnormal liver enzymes

RESP: Bronchospasm
EENT: Taste change, tinnitus, orbital edema
INTEG: Rash
MS: Myalgia, arthralgia
GU: Decreased libido

Contraindications: Hypersensitivity
Precautions: Pregnancy (C), lactation, children, severe renal disease, severe hepatic function, elderly

Pharmacokinetics:
PO: Peak 1-3 hr, plasma protein-binding 15%-20%; metabolized in liver (active metabolites), excreted by kidneys, half-life 2.5-3.5 hr

Interactions/incompatibilities:
None known

NURSING CONSIDERATIONS
Assess:
- Blood counts during therapy, watch for decreasing platelets, if low, therapy may need to be discontinued and restarted after hematologic recovery

Administer:
- IV after diluting with water for injection, NS, D_5, D_{10}, LR, or NaHCO3 injection
- IV after diluting 2 ml of drug in IV solution to total volume of 5-10 ml, inject over >2 min
- IV infusion after diluting 2 ml of drug in 100 ml of IV solution and run over 15-30 min

Perform/provide:
- Storage in cool environment (oral), IV solution is stable for 48 hr at room temperature

Evaluate:
- Blood dyscrasias (thrombocytopenia): bruising, fatigue, bleeding, poor healing

Teach patient/family:
- That drug must be continued for prescribed time to be effective
- To report bleeding, bruising, fatigue, malaise since blood dyscrasias do occur
- Discuss possibility of decreased libido, reversible after discontinuing therapy

---

italics = common side effects   ***bold italic*** = life threatening reactions

fat emulsions

Intralipid 10%, 20%; Liposysn 10%, 20%; Soyacal 10%, 20%; Trava-mulsion 10%

Func. class.: Caloric
Chem. class.: Fatty acid, long chain

Action: Needed for energy, heat production; consist of neutral tri-glycerides, primarily unsaturated fatty acids
Uses: Increase calorie intake, fatty acid deficiency, prevention
Dosage and routes:
Deficiency
• *Adult and child:* IV 8%-10% of required calorie intake (intralipid)
Adjunct to TPN
• *Adult:* IV 1 ml/min over 15-30 min (10%) or 0.5 ml/min over 15-30 min (20%); may increase to 500 ml over 4-8 hr if no adverse reactions occur, not to exceed 2.5 gm/kg
• *Child:* IV 0.1 ml/min over 10-15 min (10%) or 0.05 ml/min over 10-15 min (20%); may increase to 1 g/kg over 4 hr if no adverse reactions occur, not to exceed 4 gm/kg
Prevention of deficiency
• *Adult:* IV 500 ml twice a wk (10%), given 1 ml/min for 30 min, not to exceed 500 ml over 6 hr
• *Child:* IV 5-10 ml/kg/day (10%), given 0.1 ml/min for 30 min, not to exceed 100 ml/hr
Available forms include: Inj IV many types
Side effects/adverse reactions:
CNS: Dizziness, headache, drowsiness, focal seizures
CV: Shock
GI: Nausea, vomiting, *hepatomegaly*
RESP: Dyspnea, *fat in lung tissue*
HEMA: Hyperlipemia, hypercoagulation, thrombocytopenia, leukopenia, leukocytosis
Contraindications: Hypersensitivity, hyperlipemia, lipid necrosis, acute pancreatitis accompanied by hyperlipemia
Precautions: Severe liver disease, diabetes mellitus, thrombocytopenia, gastric ulcers, premature, term newborns
Interactions/incompatibilities:
• Do not mix with any drug, electrolytes, solutions, vitamin
NURSING CONSIDERATIONS
Assess:
• Triglycerides, free fatty acid levels, platelet counts daily to prevent fat overload, thrombocytopenia
• Liver function studies: AST, ALT
Administer:
• After changing IV tubing at each infusion: infection may occur with old tubing
• With infusion pump: do not use in-line filter; clogging will occur
Perform/provide:
• Use of mixed solutions that are not separated or oily looking
Evaluate:
• Therapeutic response: increased weight
• Nutritional status: calorie count by dietician
Teach patient/family
• Reason for use of lipids

fenfluramine HCl

(fen-fluer'a-meen)
Ponderal, Pondimin

Func. class.: Cerebral stimulant
Chem. class.: Amphetamine derivative

Controlled Substance Schedule IV
Action: Increases release of nor-epinephrine, dopamine in cerebral cortex to reticular activating system
Uses: Exogenous obesity

Dosage and routes:
• *Adult:* PO 20 mg ac, not to exceed 40 mg tid
Available forms include: Tabs 20 mg
Side effects/adverse reactions:
CNS: Insomnia, talkativeness, dizziness, drowsiness, headache, irritability
GI: Nausea, vomiting, anorexia, *dry mouth, diarrhea,* constipation, abdominal pain
GU: Impotence, change in libido, dysuria, urinary frequency
CV: Palpitations, tachycardia, hypertension, hypotension
INTEG: Urticaria, rash, burning, sweating, chills, fever
Contraindications: Hypersensitivity to sympathomimetic amine, glaucoma, drug abuse, cardiovascular disease, alcoholism
Precautions: Diabetes mellitus, hypertension, depression, pregnancy (C)
Pharmacokinetics:
PO: Onset 1-2 min, duration 4-6 hr, metabolized by liver, excreted by kidneys
Interactions/incompatibilities:
• Hypertensive crisis: MAOIs or within 14 days of MAOIs
• Increased effect of this drug: acetazolamide, antacids, sodium bicarbonate, ascorbic acid, ammonium chloride, phenothiazines, haloperidol
• Decreased effects of this drug: barbiturates
• Decrease effects of: guanethidine, other antihypertensives
NURSING CONSIDERATIONS
Assess:
• VS, B/P since this drug may reverse antihypertensives; check patients with cardiac disease more often
• CBC, urinalysis, in diabetes: blood sugar, urine sugar; insulin changes may need to be made since

eating will decrease
• Height, growth rate in children; growth rate may be decreased
Administer:
• At least 6 hr before hs to avoid sleeplessness
• For obesity only if patient is on weight reduction program, including dietary changes, exercise; patient will develop tolerance and weight loss won't occur without additional methods
• Gum, hard candy, frequent sips of water for dry mouth
• If drug is being given for obesity, 1 hr before meals
Perform/provide:
• Check to see PO medication has been swallowed
Evaluate:
• Mental status: mood, sensorium, affect, stimulation, insomnia, aggressiveness may occur
• Physical dependency: should not be used for extended time; dose should be discontinued gradually
• Withdrawal symptoms: headache, nausea, vomiting, muscle pain, weakness
• Drug tolerance will develop after long-term use
• Dosage should not be increased if tolerance develops
Teach patient/family:
• To decrease caffeine consumption (coffee, tea, cola, chocolate); may increase irritability, stimulation
• Avoid OTC preparations unless approved by physician
• To taper off drug over several weeks, or depression, increased sleeping, lethargy may ensue
• To avoid alcohol ingestion
• To avoid hazardous activities until patient is stabilized on medication
• To get needed rest; patients will feel more tired at end of day
Treatment of overdose: Admin-

ister fluids, hemodialysis or peritoneal dialysis; antihypertensive for increased B/P; ammonium Cl for increased excretion

---

fenoprofen calcium

(fen-oh-proe'fen)
Nalfon
Func. class.: Nonsteroidal
Chem. class.: Propionic acid derivative

Action: Inhibits prostaglandin synthesis by decreasing enzyme needed for biosynthesis; possesses analgesic, antiinflammatory, antipyretic properties
Uses: Mild to moderate pain, osteoarthritis, rheumatoid arthritis, acute gout, arthritis, ankylosing spondylitis
Dosage and routes:
Pain
• *Adult:* PO 200 mg q4-6h as needed
Arthritis
• *Adult:* PO 300-600 mg qid, not to exceed 3.2 g/day
Available forms include: Caps 200, 300 mg; tabs 600 mg
Side effects/adverse reactions:
GI: Nausea, anorexia, vomiting, diarrhea, jaundice, ***cholestatic hepatitis,*** constipation, flatulence, cramps, dry mouth, peptic ulcer
CNS: Dizziness, drowsiness, fatigue, tremors, confusion, insomnia, anxiety, depression
CV: Tachycardia, peripheral edema, palpitations, dysrhythmias
INTEG: Purpura, rash, pruritus, sweating
GU: ***Nephrotoxicity:*** dysuria, hematuria, oliguria, azotemia
HEMA: ***Blood dyscrasias***
EENT: Tinnitus, hearing loss, blurred vision
Contraindications: Hypersensitivity, asthma, severe renal disease,
severe hepatic disease
Precautions: Pregnancy, lactation, children, bleeding disorders, GI disorders, cardiac disorders, hypersensitivity to other antiinflammatory agents
Pharmacokinetics:
PO: Peak 2 hr, half-life 3-3½ hr, metabolized in liver, excreted in urine (metabolites), breast milk
Interactions/incompatibilities:
• May increase the action of coumarin, phenytoin, sulfonamides when with this drug
NURSING CONSIDERATIONS
Assess:
• Renal, liver, blood studies: BUN, creatinine, AST, ALT, Hgb, before treatment, periodically thereafter
• Audiometric, ophthalmic exam before, during, after treatment
Administer:
• With food to decrease GI symptoms; however, best to take on empty stomach to facilitate absorption
Perform/provide:
• Storage at room temperature
Evaluate:
• Therapeutic response: decreased pain, stiffness in joints, decreased swelling in joints, ability to move more easily
• For eye, ear problems: blurred vision, tinnitus; may indicate toxicity
Teach patient/family:
• To report blurred vision, ringing, roaring in ears; may indicate toxicity
• To avoid driving, other hazardous activities if dizziness, drowsiness occurs
• To report change in urine pattern, increased weight, edema, increased pain in joints, fever, blood in urine; indicates nephrotoxicity
• That therapeutic effects may take up to 1 mo

---

fentanyl citrate

(fen'ta-nill)
Sublimaze

Func. class.: Narcotic analgesics
Chem. class.: Opiate, synthetic
phenylpiperdine derivative

Controlled Substance Schedule II
Action: Inhibits ascending pain
pathways in CNS, increases pain
threshold, alters pain perception
Uses: Preoperatively, postopera-
tively; adjunct to general anesthetic
Dosage and routes:
Anesthetic
• *Adult:* IV 0.05-0.1 mg q2-3min
prn
Preoperatively
• *Adult:* IM 0.05-0.1 mg q30-
60 min before surgery
Postoperatively
• *Adult:* IM 0.05-0.1 mg ql-2h prn
• *Child:* IM 0.02-0.03 mg/9 kg
Available forms include: Inj IM,
IV 0.05 mg/ml
Side effects/adverse reactions:
CNS: Dizziness, delirium, euphoria
GI: Nausea, vomiting
MS: Muscle rigidity
EENT: Blurred vision, miosis
CV: **Bradycardia, arrest,** hypoten-
sion
RESP: **Respiratory depression, ar-
rest, laryngospasm**
Contraindications: Hypersensitiv-
ity to opiates, myasthenia gravis
Precautions: Elderly, respiratory
depression, increased intracranial
pressure, seizure disorders, severe
respiratory disorders, cardiac dys-
rhythmias, pregnancy (C)
Pharmacokinetics:
IM: Onset 7-15 min, peak 30 min,
duration 1-2 hr
IV: Onset immediate, peak 3-5 min,
duration ½-1 hr
Metabolized by liver, excreted by
kidneys, crosses placenta, excreted
in breast milk, half-life 2½-4 hr
Interactions/incompatibilities:
• Effects may be increased with
other CNS depressants: alcohol,
narcotics, sedative/hypnotic, antipsychotics, skeletal muscle relaxants

NURSING CONSIDERATIONS
Assess:
• VS after parenteral route, note
muscle rigidity
Administer:
• By injection (IM, IV), give
slowly to prevent rigidity
• With milk or food for GI symp-
toms
• Only with resuscitative equip-
ment available
Perform/provide:
• Storage in light-resistant area at
room temperature
• Coughing, turning, deep breath-
ing for postoperative patients
• Safety measures: siderails, night
light, call bell after returning to
room
Evaluate:
• CNS changes: dizziness, drows-
iness, hallucinations, euphoria,
LOC, pupil reaction
• Allergic reactions: rash, urticaria
• Respiratory dysfunction: respi-
ratory depression, character, rate,
rhythm; notify physician if respirations are <12/min
Teach patient/family:
• To report any symptoms of CNS
changes, allergic reactions
• That physical dependency may
result when used for extended periods of time

F

fentanyl citrate/droperidol combination

(fen'ta-nil) (droe-per'i-dole)
Innovar

Func. class.: General anesthetic/narcotic analgesic
Chem. class.: Phenylpiperone derivative

Controlled Substance Schedule II
Action: Action at subcortical levels to reduce motor activity, produces analgesia

Uses: Premedication, adjunct to general anesthesia, maintenance of anesthesia

Dosage and routes:
Induction
• *Adult:* IV 1 ml/20-25 lb
• *Child:* IV 0.5 ml/20 lb
Premedication
• *Adult:* IM 0.5-2 ml 45-60 min before surgery or procedure
• *Child:* IM 0.25 ml/20 lb 45-60 min before surgery or procedure
Available forms include: Inj IM, IV 0.05 mg fentanyl, 2.5 mg droperidol/ml

Side effects/adverse reactions:
RESP: Laryngospasm, bronchospasm, respiratory arrest
CNS: Dystonia, akathisia, flexion of arms, fine tremors, dizziness, anxiety, drowsiness, restlessness, hallucination, depression
CV: Tachycardia, hypotension, circulatory depression
EENT: Upward rotation of eyes, oculogyric crisis, blurred vision
INTEG: Chills, facial sweating, shivering, diaphoresis
GI: Nausea, vomiting

Contraindications: Hypersensitivity, child < 2 yr, myasthenia gravis
Precautions: Elderly, increased intracranial pressure, cardiovascular disease (bradydysrhythmias), renal disease, liver disease, Parkinson's disease, COPD

Pharmacokinetics:
IV: Onset 20 sec, peak 2-5 min, duration ½-2 hr
IM: Onset 7 min, duration 1-2 hr, metabolized in liver, excreted in urine metabolites (90%)

Interactions/incompatibilities:
• Increased CNS depression: alcohol, narcotics, barbiturates, antipsychotics or other CNS depressants
• Decreased effects of: amphetamines, anticonvulsants, anticoagulants
• Increased intraocular pressure: anticholinergics, antiparkinson drugs
• Increased side effects of: lithium
• Do not mix with barbiturates in solution

NURSING CONSIDERATIONS
Assess:
• VS q10 min during IV administration, q30 min after IM dose
Administer:
• Anticholinergics (benztropine, diphenhydramine) for extrapyramidal reaction
• Only with crash cart, resuscitative equipment nearby
• IV slowly only
Perform/provide:
• Slow movement of patient to avoid orthostatic hypotension
Evaluate:
• Therapeutic response: decreased anxiety, absence of vomiting, maintenance of anesthesia
• Rigidity of skeletal muscles
• Extrapyramidal reactions: dystonia, akathisia
• Increasing heart rate or decreasing B/P, notify physician at once; do not place patient in Trendelenburg position or sympathetic blockade may occur causing respiratory arrest

Teach patient/family:
• To use deep breathing, turning, coughing after surgery to prevent increased secretions in lungs

---

ferrous fumarate

Eldofe, Farbegen, Fecot, Femiron, Feostat, Ferranol,* Fersamal, Fumasorb, Fumerin, Hemocyte, Ircon, Laud-Iron, Maniron, Neofer, Novofumar,* Palafer,* Palmiron

Func. class.: Hematinic
Chem. class.: Iron preparation

Action: Replaces iron stores needed for red blood cell development, energy and O_2 transport, utilization; drug contains 33% iron.
Uses: Iron deficiency anemia
Dosage and routes:
• *Adult:* PO 200 mg tid-qid
• *Child:* PO 100-300 mg qd divided in 3-4 doses
Available forms include: Tabs 60, 195, 200, 300, 324, 325 mg; tabs chewable 100 mg; tabs extended-release 300 mg; oral susp 100 mg/ 5 ml, 45 mg/0.6 ml
Side effects/adverse reactions:
GI: Nausea, constipation, epigastric pain, black and red tarry stools, vomiting, diarrhea
INTEG: Temporarily discolored tooth enamel and eyes
Contraindications: Hypersensitivity, ulcerative colitis/regional enteritis, hemosiderosis/hemochromatosis, peptic ulcer disease, hemolytic anemia, cirrhosis
Precautions: Anemia (long-term)
Pharmacokinetics:
PO: Excreted in feces, urine, skin, breast milk
Interactions/incompatibilities:
• Decreased absorption of both drugs: tetracycline
• Decreased absorption of iron preparations: chloramphenicol, antacids, penicillamine
• Increased absorption of iron preparation: ascorbic acid
NURSING CONSIDERATIONS
Assess:
• Blood studies: Hct, Hgb, reticulocytes, bilirubin before treatment, at least monthly
Administer:
• Only with vitamin E supplements to infants or hemolytic anemia may occur
• Between meals for best absorption, may give with juice; do not give with antacids or milk, delay at least 1 hr; if GI symptoms occur, give PC if absorption is decreased
• Through plastic straw to avoid discoloration of tooth enamel; dilute thoroughly
• At least 1 hr before hs since corrosion may occur in stomach
• For <6 months for anemia
Perform/provide:
• Storage in tight, light-resistant container
Evaluate:
• Toxicity: nausea, vomiting, diarrhea (green then tarry stools), hematemesis, pallor, cyanosis, shock, coma
• Elimination; if constipation occurs, increase water, bulk, activity
• Nutrition: amount of iron in diet (meat, dark green leafy vegetables, dried beans, dried fruits, eggs)
• Cause of iron loss or anemia, including salicylates, sulfonamides, antimalarials, quinidine
• Therapeutic response: improvement in Hct, Hgb, reticulocytes, decreased fatigue, weakness
Teach patient/family:
• That iron will change stools black or dark green
• That iron poisoning may occur if increased beyond recommended level

F

---

italics = common side effects   ***bold italic*** = life threatening reactions

• Not to crush; swallow tablet whole
• Keep out of reach of children
• Do not substitute one iron salt for another; elemental iron content differs (e.g., 300 mg ferrous fumarate contains about 100 mg elemental iron whereas 300 mg ferrous gluconate contains only about 30 mg elemental iron)
• Avoid reclining position for 15-30 min after taking drug to avoid esophageal corrosion

Lab test interferences:
False-positive: Occult blood
Treatment of overdose: Induce vomiting; give eggs, milk until lavage can be done

ferrous gluconate

Fergon, Ferralet, Fertinic,* Novo-ferrogluc*

Func. class.: Hematinic
Chem. class.: Iron preparation

Action: Replaces iron stores needed for red blood cell development; drug contains 11.6% iron
Uses: Iron deficiency anemia
Dosage and routes:
• *Adult:* PO 200-600 mg tid
• *Child 6-12 yr:* 300-900 mg qd
• *Child <6 yr:* 100-300 mg qd
Available forms include: Tabs 300, 320, 325 mg; caps 325, 435 mg; tabs film-coated 300 mg; elix 300 mg/5 ml

Side effects/adverse reactions:
GI: Nausea, constipation, epigastric pain, black and red tarry stools, vomiting, diarrhea
INTEG: Temporarily discolored tooth enamel, eyes

Contraindications: Hypersensitivity, ulcerative colitis/regional enteritis, hemosiderosis/hemochromatosis, peptic ulcer disease, hemolytic anemia, cirrhosis
Precautions: Anemia (long-term)

Pharmacokinetics:
PO: Excreted in feces, urine, through skin, breast milk
Interactions/incompatibilities:
• Decreased absorption of both drugs: tetracycline
• Decreased absorption of iron preparations: chloramphenicol, antacids, penicillamine
• Increased absorption of iron preparation: ascorbic acid

NURSING CONSIDERATIONS
Assess:
• Blood studies: Hct, Hgb, reticulocytes, bilirubin before treatment, at least monthly
Administer:
• Only with vitamin E supplements to infants or hemolytic anemia may occur.
• Between meals for best absorption, may give with juice; do not give with antacids, eggs, milk, delay at least 1 hr; if GI symptoms occur, give PC if absorption is decreased
• Through plastic straw to avoid discoloration of tooth enamel; dilute thoroughly
• At least 1 hr before hs since corrosion may occur in stomach
• For <6 months for anemia
Perform/provide:
• Storage in tight, light-resistant container
Evaluate:
• Toxicity: nausea, vomiting, diarrhea (green then tarry stools), hematemesis, pallor, cyanosis, shock, coma
• Elimination: if constipation occurs, increase water, bulk, activity
• Nutrition: amount of iron in diet (meat, dark green leafy vegetables, dried beans, dried fruits, eggs)
• Cause of iron loss or anemia including salicylates, sulfonamides, antimalarials, quinidine
• Therapeutic reponse: improve-

ment in Hct, Hgb, reticulocytes, decreased fatigue, weakness

Teach patient/family:

• That iron will change stools black or dark green

• That iron poisoning may occur if increased beyond recommended level

• Not to crush; swallow tablet whole

• Keep out of reach of children

• Do not substitute one iron salt for another; elemental iron content differs (e.g., 300 mg ferrous fumarate contains about 100 mg elemental iron whereas 300 mg ferrous gluconate contains only about 30 mg elemental iron)

• Avoid reclining position for 15-30 min after taking drug to avoid esophageal corrosion

Lab test interferences:

False positive: Occult blood

Treatment of overdose: Induce vomiting; give eggs, milk until lavage can be done

---

ferrous sulfate

Fer-in-Sol, Fero-Grad,* Fero-Gradumet, Ferolix, Ferospace, Fesofor,* Irospan, Mol-Iron, Novoferrosulfa,* Slow-Fe, Telefon

Func. class.: Hematinic
Chem. class.: Iron preparation

Action: Replaces iron stores needed for red blood cell development. Drug contains 20% iron.

Uses: Iron deficiency anemia, prophylaxis for iron deficiency in pregnancy

Dosage and routes:

• *Adult:* PO 0.750-1.5 g in divided doses tid; SUS REL 225, 525, 900 mg

• *Child 6-12 yr:* 600 mg in divided doses

Pregnancy

• *Adult:* PO 300-600 mg in divided doses

Available forms include: Powder, tabs, 195, 300, 325 mg; tabs enteric-coated 325 mg; tabs extended-release 525 mg; caps timed-release 150, 225, 250, 390, 525 mg; tabs film-coated 300 mg; caps 150, 225, 250, 390 mg; sol 90 mg/5 ml, 125 mg/ml, 220 mg/5 ml, 75 mg/0.6 ml; caps dried 190, caps extended 150, 159, 167 mg, tabs dried 200 mg, tabs ext-release dried 160 mg

Side effects/adverse reactions:

GI: Nausea, constipation, epigastric pain, black and red tarry stools, vomiting, diarrhea

INTEG: Temporarily discolored tooth enamel, eyes

Contraindications: Hypersensitivity, ulcerative colitis/regional enteritis, hemosiderosis/hemochromatosis, peptic ulcer disease, hemolytic anemia, cirrhosis

Precautions: Anemia (long-term)

Pharmacokinetics:

PO: Excreted in feces, urine, through skin, breast milk

Interactions/incompatibilities:

• Decreased absorption of both drugs: tetracycline

• Decreased absorption of iron preparations: chloramphenicol, antacids, penicillamine

• Increased absorption of iron preparation: ascorbic acid

NURSING CONSIDERATIONS

Assess:

• Blood studies: Hct, Hgb, reticulocytes, bilirubin before treatment, at least monthly

Administer:

• Only with vitamin E supplements to infants or hemolytic anemia may occur

• Between meals for best absorption, may give with juice; do not give with antacids, eggs, milk, delay at least 1 hr; if GI symptoms occur, give PC if absorption is decreased

• Through plastic straw to avoid discoloration of tooth enamel; dilute thoroughly

• At least 1 hr before hs since corrosion may occur in stomach

• For <6 months for anemia

Perform/provide:

• Storage in tight, light-resistant container

Evaluate:

• Toxicity: nausea, vomiting, diarrhea (green then tarry stools), hematemesis, pallor, cyanosis, shock, coma

• Elimination: if constipation occurs, increase water, bulk, activity

• Nutrition: amount of iron in diet (meat, dark green leafy vegetables, dried beans, dried fruits, eggs)

• Cause of iron loss or anemia, including salicylates, sulfonamides, antimalarials, quinidine

• Therapeutic response: Improvement in Hct, Hgb, reticulocytes, decreased fatigue, weakness

Teach patient/family:

• That iron will change stools black or dark green

• That iron poisoning may occur if increased beyond recommended level

• Not to crush; swallow tablet whole

• Keep out of reach of children

• Do not substitute one iron salt for another; elemental iron content differs (e.g., 300 mg ferrous fumarate contains about 100 mg elemental iron whereas 300 mg ferrous gluconate contains about 30 mg elemental iron)

• Avoid reclining position for 15-30 min after taking drug to avoid esophageal corrosion

Lab test interferences:

False-positive: Occult blood

Treatment of overdose: Induce

vomiting, give eggs, milk until lavage can be done

---

fibrinolysin/desoxyribonuclease

(fye-bri-noe-lye′sin)
Elase

Func. class.: Enzyme
Chem. class.: Proteolytic-bovine

Action: Dissolves fibrin in clots, attacks DNA in areas of disintegrating cells

Uses: Debridement of wounds, intravaginally; irrigating wounds, topically

Dosage and routes:

Debridement/intravaginally

• *Adult:* OINT 5 g

Irrigating

• *Adult:* IRIG dilution depends on type of wound

Available forms include: Fibrinolysin with desoxyribonuclease 666.6 U/g; top sol fibrinolysin 25 U/desoxyribonuclease 15,000 U

Side effects/adverse reactions:

INTEG: Hyperemia

Contraindications: Hypersensitivity to bovine or mercury products, hematoma

Interactions/incompatibilities:
None known

NURSING CONSIDERATIONS

Administer:

• After reconstituting with 10 ml sterile Nacl solution

• After removing necrotic debris, dry eschar

• Wet dressing by mixing 1 vial elase/10-50 ml saline solution, saturate gauze with solution, pack area, remove in 6-8 hr, repeat tid-qid

Perform/provide:

• Cleaning of wound, cover with drug, cover, change at least qd

Evaluate:

• Therapeutic response: decrease in

wound scarring, tissue necrosis
• Wound: drainage, color, odor

---

flavoxate HCl

(fla-vox′ate)
Urispas
Func. class.: Spasmolytic
Chem. class.: Flavone derivative

Action: Relaxes smooth muscles in urinary tract
Uses: Relief of nocturia, incontinence, suprapubic pain, dysuria, frequency associated with urologic conditions (symptomatic only)
Dosage and routes:
• *Adult and child >12 yr:* PO 100-200 mg tid-qid
Available forms include: Tabs 100 mg
Side effects/adverse reactions:
HEMA: Leukopenia, eosinophilia
CNS: Anxiety, restlessness, dizziness, convulsions, headache, drowsiness, confusion
CV: Palpitations, sinus tachycardia, hypotension
GI: Nausea, vomiting, anorexia, abdominal pain, constipation
GU: Dysuria
INTEG: Urticaria, dermatitis
EENT: Blurred vision, increased intraocular tension, dry mouth, throat
Contraindications: Hypersensitivity, GI obstruction, GI hemorrhage, GU obstruction
Precautions: Pregnancy (B), lactation, suspected glaucoma, children <12 yr
Pharmacokinetics: Excreted in urine
Interactions/incompatibilities:
None known
NURSING CONSIDERATIONS
Evaluate:
• Urinary status: dysuria, frequency, nocturia, incontinence
• Allergic reactions: rash, urticaria;

if these occur, drug should be discontinued
Teach patient/family
• To avoid hazardous activities; dizziness may occur
• On all aspects of drug therapy: dosage, routes, side effects, when to notify physician

---

flecainide acetate

(fle-kay′nide)
Tambocor
Func. class.: Antidysrhythmic (Class IC)
Chem. class.: Lidocaine analog

Action: Increases electrical stimulation threshold of ventrical, HIS-Purkinge system, which stabilizes cardiac membrane
Uses: Ventricular tachycardia, ventricular dysrhythmias during cardiac surgery, myocardial infarction
Dosage and routes:
• *Adult:* PO 100 mg q12h, may increase q4 days by 50 mg bid to desired response, not to exceed 400 mg/day
Available forms include: Tabs 100 mg
Side effects/adverse reactions:
CNS: Headache, dizziness, involuntary movement, confusion, psychosis, restlessness, irritability, paresthesias
EENT: Tinnitus, *blurred vision,* hearing loss
GI: Nausea, vomiting, anorexia
CV: Hypotension, bradycardia, angina, PVCs, *heart block, cardiovascular collapse, arrest, dysrhythmias*
RESP: Dyspnea, *respiratory depression*
INTEG: Rash, urticaria, edema, swelling
Contraindications: Hypersensitivity, severe heart block, cardiogenic shock

---

Precautions: Pregnancy, lactation, children, renal disease, liver disease, CHF, respiratory depression, myasthenia gravis

Pharmacokinetics:

PO: Peak 1 hr; half-life 7-20 hr; metabolized by liver, excreted unchanged by kidneys (10%), excreted in breast milk

Interactions/incompatibilities:

• May increase effects when used with cimetidine, phenytoin, propranolol, quinidine

NURSING CONSIDERATIONS

Assess:

• ECG continuously to determine increased PR or QRS segments; if these develop, discontinue

• IV infusion rate using infusion pump, run at less than 4 mg/min

• Blood levels

• B/P continuously for fluctuations

Administer:

• IM injection in deltoid; aspirate to avoid intravascular administration

Evaluate:

• Malignant hyperthermia: tachypnea, tachycardia, changes in B/P, increased temperature

• Cardiac rate, respiration: rate, rhythm, character, continuously

• Respiratory status: rate, rhythm, lung fields for rales

• CNS effects: dizziness, confusion, psychosis, paresthesias, convulsions; drug should be discontinued

• Lung fields, bilateral rales may occur in CHF patient

• Increased respiration, increased pulse; drug should be discontinued

Lab test interferences:

Increase: CPK

Treatment of overdose: O₂, artificial ventilation, ECG, administer dopamine for circulatory depression, administer diazepam or thiopental for convulsions

---

floxuridine

(flox-yoor′i-deen)

FUDR

Func. class.: Antineoplastic, antimetabolite

Chem. class.: Pyrimidine antagonist

Action: Inhibits DNA synthesis; interferes with cell replication by competitively inhibiting thymidylate synthesis

Uses: Cancer of breast, head, neck, liver, brain, gallbladder, bile duct; GI adenocarcinoma metastatic to liver

Dosage and routes:

• *Adult:* INTRAARTERIAL: 0.1-0.6 mg/kg/day × 1-6 wk; HEPATIC ARTERY INJ: 0.4-0.6 mg/kg/day × 1-6 wk

Available forms include: Powder for inj (intraarterial, hepatic artery) 500 mg/5 ml vial

Side effects/adverse reactions:

*HEMA: **Thrombocytopenia, leukopenia, myelosuppression, anemia***

GI: Anorexia, stomatitis, diarrhea, nausea, vomiting, ***hemorrhage***

*GU: **Renal failure***

EENT: Epistaxis

INTEG: Rash, alopecia, fever

CNS: Lethargy, malaise, weakness

Contraindications: Hypersensitivity, myelosuppression, pregnancy, poor nutritional states, serious infections

Precautions: Renal disease, hepatic disease, bone marrow depression

Pharmacokinetics: Half-life 10-20 min, 20 hr terminal, metabolized in liver, excreted in urine (active metabolite), crosses blood-brain barrier

Interactions/incompatibilities:

• Increased toxicity: radiation or other antineoplastics

NURSING CONSIDERATIONS
Assess:
• CBC, differential, platelet count weekly; withhold drug if WBC is $<3500/mm^3$ or platelet count is $<100,000/mm^3$; notify physician of these results; drug should be discontinued

• Renal function studies: BUN, serum uric acid, urine CrCl, electrolytes before, during therapy

• I&O ratio: report fall in urine output to <30 ml/hr

• Monitor temperature q4h; fever may indicate beginning infection

• Liver function tests before, during therapy: bilirubin, alk phosphatase, AST, ALT, LDH; as needed or monthly

Administer:
• Medications by oral route if possible; avoid IM, SC, IV routes to prevent infections

• Antiemetic 30-60 min before giving drug to prevent vomiting

• Antibiotics for prophylaxis of infection

• Topical or systemic analgesics for pain

• Transfusion for anemia

• Antispasmodic for diarrhea

Perform/provide:
• Strict medical asepsis and protective isolation if WBC levels are low

• Liquid diet: carbonated beverage, Jello; dry toast, crackers may be added when patient is not nauseated or vomiting

• Increased fluid intake to 2-3 L/day to prevent dehydration unless contraindicated

• Rinsing of mouth tid-qid with water, hydrogen peroxide; brushing of teeth bid-tid with soft brush or cotton-tipped applicators for stomatitis; use unwaxed dental floss

• Nutritious diet with iron, vitamin supplements as ordered

Evaluate:
• Bleeding: hematuria, guaiac, bruising or petechiae, mucosa or orifices q8h

• Food preferences; list likes, dislikes

• Effects of alopecia on body image; discuss feelings about body changes

• Inflammation of mucosa, breaks in skin

• Buccal cavity q8h for dryness, sores or ulceration, white patches, oral pain, bleeding, dysphagia

• Symptoms indicating severe allergic reaction: rash, urticaria, itching, flushing

• GI symptoms: frequency of stools, cramping

• Acidosis, signs of dehydration: rapid respirations, poor skin turgor, decreased urine output, dry skin, restlessness, weakness

Teach patient/family:
• Why protective isolation precautions are necessary

• To report any complaints, side effects to nurse or physician

• That hair may be lost during treatment, and wig or hairpiece may make the patient feel better; tell patient that new hair may be different in color, texture

• To avoid foods with citric acid, hot or rough texture if stomatitis is present

• To report stomatitis: any bleeding, white spots, ulcerations in mouth; tell patient to examine mouth qd, report symptoms

Lab test interferences:
Increase: Liver function studies

---

flucytosine

(floo-sye'toe-seen)
Ancobon, Ancotil*

Func. class.: Antifungal
Chem. class.: Pyrimidine (fluorinated)

Action: Converts drug to fluoruracil after entering fungi, which destroys organism's DNA

Uses: *Candida* infections (septicemia, endocarditis, pulmonary, urinary tract infections), *Cryptococcus* (meningitis, pulmonary, urinary tract infections)

Dosage and routes:
• *Adult and child >50 kg:* PO 50-150 mg/kg/day q6h
• *Adult and child <50 kg:* PO 1.5-4.5 g/m²/day in 4 divided doses
Available forms include: Caps 250, 500 mg

Side effects/adverse reactions:
INTEG: Rash

CNS: Headache, confusion, dizziness, sedation

GI: Nausea, vomiting, anorexia, diarrhea, cramps, enterocolitis, increased AST, ALT, alk phosphatase, *bowel perforation* (rare)

HEMA: Thrombocytopenia, agranulocytosis, anemia, leukopenia, pancytopenia

GU: Increased BUN, creatinine

Contraindications: Hypersensitivity

Precautions: Renal disease, bone marrow depression, blood dyscrasias, radiation/chemotherapy

Pharmacokinetics:
PO: Peak 2½-6 hr, half-life 3-6 hr, excreted in urine (unchanged), well-distributed to CSF, aqueous humor, joints

Interactions/incompatibilities:
• Synergisim: Amphotericin B

NURSING CONSIDERATIONS
Assess:
• VS q15-30 min during first infusion, note changes in pulse and B/P
• Blood studies: CBC, including platelets
• Drug level during treatment (therapeutic level 25-100 μg/ml); if renal impairment is present dose usually kept <100 μg/ml

Administer:
• Drug only after C&S confirms organism, drug needed to treat condition
• Few caps at a time to decrease nausea, vomiting over 15 min

Perform/provide:
• Symptomatic treatment as ordered for adverse reactions: aspirin, antihistamines, antiemetics, antispasmodics
• Storage in tight, light-resistant containers at room temperature

Evaluate:
• Therapeutic response: decreased fever, malaise, rash, negative C&S for infecting organism
• For renal toxicity: increasing BUN, serum creatinine; if serum creatinine >1.7 mg/100 dl, dosage may be reduced
• For hepatotoxicity: increasing AST, ALT, alk phosphatase
• For allergic reaction: dermatitis, rash; drug should be discontinued, antihistamines (mild reaction) or epinephrine (severe reaction) administered
• For blood dyscrasias, fatigue, bruising, malaise, dark urine

Teach patient/family:
• That long-term therapy may be needed to clear infection (1-2 mo depending on type of infection)
• To report symptoms of blood dyscrasias: fatigue, bruising, malaise, dark urine

Lab test interferences:
False-increase: Creatinine

fludrocortisone acetate

(floo-droe-kor'ti-sone)
Florinef Acetate

Func. class.: Corticosteroid
Chem. class.: Mineralocorticoid

Action: Promotes increased reabsorption of sodium and loss of potassium from the renal tubules

Uses: Adrenal insufficiency, salt-losing adrenogenital syndrome

Dosage and routes:
• *Adult:* PO 0.1-0.2 mg qd

Available forms include: Tabs 0.1 mg

Side effects/adverse reactions:
INTEG: Acne, poor wound healing, ecchymosis, petechiae
CNS: Depression, flushing, sweating, headache, mood changes
CV: Hypotension, **circulatory collapse, thrombophlebitis, embolism,** tachycardia
*HEMA: **Thrombocytopenia***
MS: Fractures, osteoporosis, weakness
GI: Diarrhea, nausea, abdominal distention, GI hemorrhage, increased appetite, ***pancreatitis***
EENT: Fungal infections, increased intraocular pressure, blurred vision

Contraindications: Psychosis, hypersensitivity, idiopathic thrombocytopenia, acute glomerulonephritis, amebiasis, fungal infections, nonasthmatic bronchial disease

Precautions: Pregnancy, diabetes mellitus, glaucoma, osteoporosis, seizure disorders, ulcerative colitis, CHF, myasthenia gravis

Pharmacokinetics:
PO: Half-life 30 min, metabolized by liver, excreted in urine

Interactions/incompatibilities:
• Decreased action of this drug: cholestyramine, colestipol, barbiturates, rifampin, ephedrine, phenytoin, theophylline

• Decreased effects of: anticoagulants, anticonvulsants, antidiabetics, ambenonium, neostigmine, isoniazid, toxoids, vaccines
• Increased side effects: alcohol, salicylates, indomethacin, amphotericin B, digitalis preparations
• Increased action of this drug: salicylates, estrogens, indomethacin

NURSING CONSIDERATIONS

Assess:
• Potassium, blood sugar, urine glucose while on long-term therapy; hypokalemia and hyperglycemia
• Weight daily, notify physician of weekly gain >5 lb
• B/P q4h, pulse, notify physician if chest pain occurs
• I&O ratio, be alert for decreasing urinary output and increasing edema
• Plasma cortisol levels during long-term therapy (normal level: 138-635 nmol/L SI units when drawn at 8 AM)

Administer:
• Titrated dose, use lowest effective dose
• With food or milk to decrease GI symptoms

Perform/provide:
• Assistance with ambulation in patient with bone tissue disease to prevent fractures

Evaluate:
• Therapeutic response: ease of respirations, decreased inflammation
• Infection: increased temperature, WBC, even after withdrawal of medication; drug masks symptoms of infection
• Potassium depletion: paresthesias, fatigue, nausea, vomiting, depression, polyuria, dysrhythmias, weakness
• Edema, hypotension, cardiac symptoms
• Mental status: affect, mood, behavioral changes, aggression

---

italics = common side effects   ***bold italic*** = life threatening reactions

Teach patient/family:

• That ID as steroid user should be carried

• To notify physician if therapeutic response decreases; dosage adjustment may be needed

• Not to discontinue this medication abruptly or adrenal crisis can result

• To avoid OTC products: salicylates, alcohol in cough products, cold preparations unless directed by physician

• Teach patient all aspects of drug use, including Cushingoid symptoms

• Symptoms of adrenal insufficiency: nausea, anorexia, fatigue, dizziness, dyspnea, weakness, joint pain

Lab test interferences:

Increase: Cholesterol, sodium, blood glucose, uric acid, calcium, urine glucose

Decrease: Calcium, potassium, T_4, T_3, thyroid ^{131}I uptake test, urine 17-OHCS, 17-KS, PBI

False negative: Skin allergy tests

---

flunisolide

(floo-niss'oh-lide)

Nasalide Nasal Solution

Func. class.: Steroid, intranasal
Chem. class.: Glucocorticoid

Action: Long-acting synthetic adrenocorticoid with antiinflammatory activity, minimal mineralocorticoid properties

Uses: Rhinitis (seasonal or perennial)

Dosage and routes:

• *Adult:* INSTILL 2 sprays in each nostril bid, then increase to tid if needed, not to exceed 8 sprays in each nostril/day

• *Child 6-14 yr:* INSTILL 1 spray in each nostril tid or 2 sprays bid, not to exceed 4 sprays in each nostril/day

Available forms include: Aerosol $25\mu g$/spray

Side effects/adverse reactions:

EENT: Nasal irritation, dryness, rebound congestion, epistaxis, sneezing

INTEG: Urticaria

CNS: Headache, dizziness

*SYST: **Congestive heart failure, convulsions,** increased sodium, hypertension*

Contraindications: Hypersensitivity, child <12 yr, localized infection of nose

Precautions: Lactation

Pharmacokinetics:

AERO: Half-life 6 min, terminal half-life 1.8 hr, metabolized in liver, excreted in urine

Interactions/incompatibilities:
None known

NURSING CONSIDERATIONS

Administer:

• No more than q4h

• For <4 consecutive days

Perform/provide:

• Storage in light-resistant container; discard open container after 3 mo

Evaluate:

• Redness, swelling, pain in nasal passages

Teach patient/family:

• Stinging may occur for several applications; drying of mucosa may be decreased by environmental humidification

• To notify physician if irregular pulse, insomnia, dizziness, or tremors occur

• Proper administration to avoid systemic absorption

---

flunisolide

(floo-niss'oh-lide)
Aerobid, Nasalide

Func. class.: Corticosteroid
Chem. class.: Glucocorticoid

Action: Decreases inflammation by suppression of migration of polymorphonuclear leukocytes, fibroblasts, reversal of increased capillary permeability and lysosomal stabilization; does not depress hypothalamus

Uses: Rhinitis, allergies, nasal polyps

Dosage and routes:
• *Adult and child >6 yr:* INH 2 puffs bid, not to exceed 4 puffs bid
Available forms include: Nasal sol 250 µg/ml

Side effects/adverse reactions:
CNS: Headache
EENT: Bloody mucus, nosebleeds, sore throat, stuffy nose, sneezing
GI: Nausea, vomiting

Contraindications: Hypersensitivity, child <6 yr

Precautions: Nasal ulcers, respiratory TB, untreated fungal, bacterial, or viral infections, pregnancy (C), glaucoma

Pharmacokinetics:
INH: Duration 1 hr

Interactions/incompatibilities:
None known

NURSING CONSIDERATIONS

Administer:
• Titrated dose, use lowest effective dose

Evaluate:
• Therapeutic response: ease of respirations, decreased inflammation
• Infection: increased temperature, WBC, even after withdrawal of medication; drug masks symptoms of infection

Teach patient/family:
• That ID as steroid user should be carried
• To notify physician if therapeutic response decreases; dosage adjustment may be needed
• Proper administration technique
• Compliance to therapy
• To check with physician before using any other nasal medications
• Teach patient all aspects of drug use, including Cushingoid symptoms
• Symptoms of adrenal insufficiency: nausea, anorexia, fatigue, dizziness, dyspnea, weakness, joint pain

fluocinonide

(floo-oh-sin'oh-nide)
Lidex, Lidex-E

Func. class.: Topical corticosteroid
Chem. class.: Synthetic fluorinated agent, group II potency

Action: Possesses antipruritic, antiinflammatory actions

Uses: Psoriasis, eczema, contact dermatitis, pruritus

Dosage and routes:
• *Adult and child:* Apply to affected area tid-qid

Available forms include: Oint 0.05%; cream 0.5%; sol 0.05%; gel 0.05%

Side effects/adverse reactions:
INTEG: Burning, dryness, itching, irritation, acne, folliculitis, hypertrichosis, perioral dermatitis, hypopigmentation, atrophy, striae, miliaria, allergic contact dermatitis, secondary infection

Contraindications: Hypersensitivity to corticosteroids, fungal infections

Precautions: Pregnancy (C), lactation, viral infections, bacterial infections

---

italics = common side effects   ***bold italic*** = life threatening reactions

Interactions/incompatibilities:
None known
NURSING CONSIDERATIONS
Assess:
• Temperature; if fever develops, drug should be discontinued
Administer:
• Only to affected areas; do not get in eyes
• Medication, then cover with occlusive dressing (only if prescribed), seal to normal skin, change q12h; use occlusive dressings with extreme caution
• Only to dermatoses; do not use on weeping, denuded, or infected area
Perform/provide:
• Cleansing before application of drug
• Treatment for a few days after area has cleared
• Storage at room temperature
Evaluate:
• Therapeutic response: absence of severe itching, patches on skin, flaking
Teach patient/family:
• To avoid sunlight on affected area; burns may occur

---

fluorescein sodium
(flure'e-seen)
Fluorescite, Fluor-I-Strip, Ful-Glo, Funduscein Injections
Func. class.: Diagnostic agent, optic
Chem. class.: Fluorescent dye

Action: Allows breaks in the corneal tissue to absorb dye and show up as bright green under cobalt blue light
Uses: Diagnostic aid in identifying foreign bodies, fitting hard contact lenses, fundus photography, tonometry, identifying corneal abrasions, retinal angiography

Dosage and routes:
• *Adult:* INSTILL 1 gtt of 2% sol, irrigated or wet strip with sterile water and touch conjunctiva or fornix, flush eye with irrigating sol
Retinal angiography
• *Adult:* IV 5 ml 10% sol or 3 ml 25% sol injected in antecubital vein
• *Child:* IV 0.077 ml 10% sol or 0.044 ml 25% sol injected in antecubital vein
Available forms include: Inj IV 10%, 25%; sol 2%; strips 0.6, 9 mg, 1 g
Side effects/adverse reactions:
CNS: Headache, dizziness, paresthesia, *convulsions*
CV: Bradycardia, *shock, cardiac arrest*
RESP: Dyspnea, acute pulmonary edema
GI: Nausea, vomiting
EENT: Stinging, burning, conjunctival redness
Contraindications: Hypersensitivity
Precautions: Bronchial asthma
Interactions/incompatibilities:
None known
NURSING CONSIDERATIONS
Administer:
• Solution, have patient close eyelids for 1 min
• Only with resuscitative equipment nearby
Perform/provide:
• Storage at room temperature
Evaluate:
• Eye color after application: defects are green under normal light or bright yellow under cobalt blue light
• For allergic reaction: rash, urticaria, pruritus, angioedema
Teach patient/family:
• To report stinging, burning, itching, lacrimation, puffiness

---

fluorometholone

(flure-oh-meth'oh-lone)

FML Liquifilm Ophthalmic

Func. class.: Ophthalmic antiinflammatory

Action: Decreases inflammation, resulting in decreased pain, photophobia, hyperemia, cellular infiltration

Uses: Inflammation of eye, lids, conjunctiva, cornea, uveitis, iridocyclitis, allergic condition, burns, foreign bodies

Dosage and routes:
• *Adult and child:* Instill 1-2 gtts into conjunctival sac 1hr × 2 days if needed then bid-qid

Available forms include: Oint 0.1%; ophthalmic susp 0.1%

Side effects/adverse reactions:
EENT: ***Increased intraocular pressure,*** poor corneal wound healing, increased possibility of corneal infections, glaucoma exacerbation, ***optic nerve damage,*** decreased activity, visual field

Contraindications: Hypersensitivity, acute superficial herpes simplex, fungal/viral diseases of the eye or conjunctiva, active diabetes mellitus, ocular TB, infections of the eye

Precautions: Corneal abrasions, glaucoma

Interactions/incompatibilities: None known

NURSING CONSIDERATIONS
Evaluate:
• Allergic reactions: redness, itching, swelling, lacrimation
• Therapeutic response: absence of swelling, redness, exudate

Administer:
• After shaking

Perform/provide:
• Storage in tight, light-resistant container

Teach patient/family:
• Instillation method: pressure on lacrimal sac for 1 min
• Not to share eye medications with others

fluorouracil

(flure-oh-yoor'a-sil)

Efudex, Fluoroplex

Func. class.: Topical antineoplastic

Chem. class.: Antimetabolite

Action: Inhibits synthesis of DNA, RNA in susceptible cells

Uses: Keratosis (multiple/actinic), basal cell carcinoma

Dosage and routes:
• *Adult and child:* TOP apply to affected area bid

Available forms include: Sol 1%, 2%, 5%; cream 1%, 5%

Side effects/adverse reactions:
INTEG: Rash, irritation, pain, burning, contact dermatitis, scaling, swelling, soreness, hyperpigmentation, pruritus

Contraindications: Hypersensitivity

Precautions: Pregnancy

Interactions/incompatibilities: None known

NURSING CONSIDERATIONS
Assess:
• WBC, platelets at least monthly

Administer:
• Only 5% sol/cream for basal cell carcinoma
• Using gloves or applicator

Perform/provide:
• Covering of lesion with porous gauze dressing only
• Washing of hands after application if gloves or applicator are not used
• Storage at room temperature

Evaluate:
• Therapeutic response: decreased size of lesion

• Area of body involved for redness, swelling
• Check oral cavity qd for stomatitis; if present discontinue drug
Teach patient/family:
• To avoid application on normal skin or getting cream in eyes
• To discontinue use if rash or irritation occurs
• To avoid sunlight or use sunscreen, photosensitivity may occur
• To wash hands after application
• Not to change application and use exactly as prescribed
• Lesion will disappear in 1-2 mo

---

fluorouracil (5-fluorouracil)

(flure-oh-yoor'a-sil)
Adrucil, 5-FU

Func. class.: Antineoplastic, antimetabolite
Chem. class.: Pyrimidine antagonist

Action: Inhibits DNA synthesis; interferes with cell replication by competitively inhibiting thymidylate synthesis
Uses: Cancer of breast, colon, rectum, stomach, pancreas
Dosage and routes:
• *Adult:* IV 12 mg/kg/day × 4 days, not to exceed 800 mg/day; may repeat with 6 mg/kg on day 6, 8, 10, 12; maintenance is 10-15 mg/kg/wk as a single dose, not to exceed 1 g/wk
Available forms include: Inj IV 50 mg/ml
Side effects/adverse reactions:
*HEMA: **Thrombocytopenia, leukopenia, myelosuppression, anemia***
GI: Anorexia, stomatitis, diarrhea, nausea, vomiting, **hemorrhage**
*GU: **Renal failure***
EENT: Epistaxsis
INTEG: Rash, alopecia, fever
CNS: Lethargy, malaise, weakness

Contraindications: Hypersensitivity, myelosuppression, pregnancy, poor nutritional states, serious infections
Precautions: Renal disease, hepatic disease, bone marrow depression
Pharmacokinetics: Half-life 10-20 min, 20 hr terminal, metabolized in the liver, excreted in the urine, crosses blood-brain barrier
Interactions/incompatibilities:
• Increased toxicity: radiation or other antineoplastics

NURSING CONSIDERATIONS
Assess:
• CBC, differential, platelet count weekly; withhold drug if WBC is <3500/mm³ or platelet count is <100,000/mm³; notify physician of these results; drug should be discontinued
• Renal function studies: BUN, serum uric acid, urine CrCl, electrolytes before, during therapy
• I&O ratio: report fall in urine output to <30 ml/hr
• Monitor temperature q4h; fever may indicate beginning infection
• Liver function tests before, during therapy: bilirubin, alk phosphatase, AST, ALT, LDH; as needed or monthly
Administer:
• Medications by oral route if possible; avoid IM, SC, IV routes to prevent infections
• Antiemetic 30-60 min before giving drug to prevent vomiting
• Antibiotics for prophylaxis of infection
• Topical or systemic analgesics for pain
• Transfusion for anemia
• Antispasmodic for diarrhea
Perform/provide:
• Strict medical asepsis, protective isolation if WBC levels are low
• Liquid diet: carbonated beverage, Jello; dry toast, crackers may be

added when patient is not nauseated or vomiting

• Increase fluid intake to 2-3 L/day to prevent dehydration, unless contraindicated

• Rinsing of mouth tid-qid with water, hydrogen peroxide; brushing of teeth bid-tid with soft brush or cotton-tipped applicators for stomatitis; use unwaxed dental floss.

• Nutritious diet with iron, vitamin supplements as ordered

Evaluate:

• Bleeding: hematuria, guaiac, bruising or petechiae, mucosa or orifices q8h

• Food preferences; list likes, dislikes

• Effects of alopecia on body image; discuss feelings about body changes

• Inflammation of mucosa, breaks in skin

• Buccal cavity q8h for dryness, sores or ulceration, white patches, oral pain, bleeding, dysphagia

• Symptoms indicating severe allergic reaction: rash, urticaria, itching, flushing

• GI symptoms: frequency of stools, cramping

• Acidosis, signs of dehydration: rapid respirations, poor skin turgor, decreased urine output, dry skin, restlessness, weakness

Teach patient/family:

• Why protective isolation precautions are necessary

• To report any complaints, side effects to the nurse or physician

• That hair may be lost during treatment and wig or hairpiece may make patient feel better; tell patient that new hair may be different in color, texture

• To avoid foods with citric acid, hot or rough texture if stomatitis is present

• To report stomatitis: any bleeding, white spots, ulcerations in mouth; tell patient to examine mouth qd, report symptoms

Lab test interferences:

Increase: Liver function studies

---

fluoxymesterone

(floo-ox-ee-mess'te-rone)

Android-F, Halotestin, Ora-Testryl

Func. class.: Androgenic anabolic steroid

Chem. class.: Halogenated testosterone derivative

Action: Increases weight by building body tissue, increases potassium, phosphorus, chloride, nitrogen levels, increases bone development

Uses: Impotence from testicular deficiency, hypogonadism, breast engorgement, palliative treatment of female breast cancer

Dosage and routes:

Hypogonadism/impotence

• *Adult:* PO 2-10 mg qd

Breast engorgement

• *Adult:* PO 2.5 mg qd, then 5-10 mg qd × 5 days

Breast cancer

• *Adult:* PO 15-30 mg qd in divided doses until therapeutic effect occurs, then dosage should be reduced

Available forms include: Tabs 2, 5, 10 mg

Side effects/adverse reactions:

INTEG: Rash, acneiform lesions, oily hair, skin, flushing, sweating, acne vulgaris, alopecia, hirsutism

CNS: Dizziness, headache, fatigue, tremors, paresthesias, flushing, sweating, anxiety, lability, insomnia

MS: Cramps, spasms

CV: Increased B/P

GU: Hematuria, amenorrhea, vaginitis, decreased libido, decreased

---

breast size, clitoral hypertrophy, testicular atrophy

GI: Nausea, vomiting, constipation, weight gain, ***cholestatic jaundice***

EENT: Carpal tunnel syndrome, conjunctival edema, nasal congestion

ENDO: Abnormal GTT

Contraindications: Severe renal disease, severe cardiac disease, severe hepatic disease, hypersensitivity, pregnancy (X), lactation, genital bleeding (abnormal)

Precautions: Diabetes mellitus, CV disease, MI

Pharmacokinetics:

PO: Metaboblized in liver, excreted in urine, crosses placenta, excreted in breast milk

Interactions/incompatibilities:
- Increased effects of: oral antidiabetics, oxyphenbutazone
- Increased PT with anticoagulants
- Edema: ACTH, adrenal steroids
- Decreased effects of: insulin

NURSING CONSIDERATIONS

Assess:
- Weight daily, notify physician if weekly weight gain is >5 lb
- B/P q4h
- I&O ratio; be alert for decreasing urinary output, increasing edema
- Growth rate in children since growth rate may be uneven (linear/bone growth) if used for extended periods of time
- Electrolytes: K, Na, Cl, cholesterol
- Liver function studies: ALT, AST, bilirubin

Administer:
- Titrated dose, use lowest effective dose
- With food or milk to decrease GI symptoms

Perform/provide:
- Diet with increased calories, protein; decrease sodium, if edema occurs

Evaluate:
- Therapeutic response: increased appetite, stamina
- Edema, hypertension, cardiac symptoms, jaundice
- Mental status: affect, mood, behavioral changes, aggression
- Signs of masculinization in female: increased libido, deepening of voice, breast tissue, enlarged clitoris, menstrual irregularities; male: gynecomastia, impotence, testicular atrophy
- Hypercalcemia: lethargy, polyuria, polydipsia, nausea, vomiting, constipation, drug may need to be decreased
- Hypoglycemia in diabetics, since oral anticoagulant action is decreased

Teach patient/family:
- Drug needs to be combined with complete health plan: diet, rest, exercise
- To notify physician if therapeutic response decreases
- Not to discontinue medication abruptly
- Teach patient all aspects of drug usage, including change in sex characteristics
- Females to report menstrual irregularities
- 1-3 mo course is necessary for response in breast cancer

Lab test interferences:

Increase: Serum cholesterol, blood glucose, urine glucose

Decrease: Serum calcium, serum potassium, T_4, T_3, thyroid ^{131}I uptake test, urine 17-OHCS, 17-KS, PBI, BSP

fluphenazine decanoate/fluphenazine enanthate/fluphenazine HCl

(floo-fen'-a-zeen)

Modecate Decanoate,* Prolixin Decanoate/Moditen Enanthate, Prolixin Enanthate/Moditen HCl,* Permitil HCl,* Prolixin HCl

Func. class.: Antipsychotic/neuroleptic
Chem. class.: Phenothiazine, piperazine

Action: Depresses cerebral cortex, hypothalamus, limbic system, which control activity and aggression; blocks neurotransmission produced by dopamine at synapse; exhibits strong α-adrenergic and anticholinergic blocking action; mechanism for antipsychotic effects is unclear

Uses: Psychotic disorders, schizophrenia

Dosage and routes:
Enanthate, decanoate
• *Adult and child >12 yr:* SC 12.5-25 mg ql-3wk
HCl
• *Adult:* PO 0.5-10 mg, in divided doses q6-8h, not to exceed 20 mg qd; IM 1.25-2.5 mg q6-8h, daily dose may range from 2.5-10 mg in divided doses q6-8h

Available forms include: HCl Tabs 2.5, 5, 10 mg; elix 2.5 mg/5 ml; conc 5 mg/ml; inj IM, enanthate, decanoate, inj SC, IM 2.5 mg/ml

Side effects/adverse reactions:
RESP: Laryngospasm, dyspnea, *respiratory depression*
CNS: Extrapyramidal symptoms: pseudoparkinsonism, akathisia, dystonia, tardive dyskinesia, drowsiness, headache, seizures
HEMA: Anemia, leukopenia, leukocytosis, *agranulocytosis*
INTEG: Rash, photosensitivity, dermatitis
EENT: Blurred vision, glaucoma
GI: Dry mouth, nausea, vomiting, anorexia, constipation, diarrhea, jaundice, weight gain
GU: Urinary retention, urinary frequency, enuresis, impotence, amenorrhea, gynecomastia
CV: Orthostatic hypotension, hypertension, *cardiac arrest,* ECG changes, *tachycardia*

Contraindications: Hypersensitivity, circulatory collapse, liver damage, cerebral arteriosclerosis, coronary disease, severe hypertension/hypotension, blood dyscrasias, coma, child <6 yr, brain damage, bone marrow depression, alcohol and barbiturate withdrawal states
Precautions: Pregnancy, lactation, seizure disorders, hypertension, hepatic disease, cardiac disease
Pharmacokinetics:
PO/IM (HCl): Onset 1 hr, peak 2-4 hr, duration 6-8 hr
SC (enanthate): Onset 1-2 days, peak 2-3 days, duration 1-3 wk, half-life 3.5-4 days; decanoate: onset 1-3 days, peak 1-2 days, duration over 4 wk, half-life (single dose) 6.8-9.6 days, (multiple dose) 14.3 days Metabolized by liver, excreted in urine (metabolites), crosses placenta, enters breast milk
Interactions/incompatibilities:
• Oversedation: other CNS depressants, alcohol, barbiturate anesthetics
• Toxicity: epinephrine
• Decreased effects of: levodopa, lithium
• Increased effects of both drugs: β-adrenergic blockers, alcohol
• Increased anticholinergic effects: anticholinergics
NURSING CONSIDERATIONS
Assess:
• Swallowing of PO medication;

check for hoarding or giving of medication to other patients

• I&O ratio; palpate bladder if low urinary output occurs

• Bilirubin, CBC, liver function studies monthly

• Urinalysis is recommended before and during prolonged therapy

Administer:

• Antiparkinsonian agent, to be used if EPS occurs

• IM injection into large muscle mass, to minimize postural hypotension give injection with patient seated or recumbent

Perform/provide:

• Decreased noise input by dimming lights, avoiding loud noises

• Supervised ambulation until stabilized on medication; do not involve in strenuous exercise program because fainting is possible; patient should not stand still for long periods of time

• Increased fluids to prevent constipation

• Sips of water, candy, gum for dry mouth

• Storage in tight, light-resistant container in cool environment

Evaluate:

• Therapeutic response: decrease in emotional excitement, hallucinations, delusions, paranoia, reorganization of patterns of thought, speech

• Affect, orientation, LOC, reflexes, gait, coordination, sleep pattern disturbances

• B/P standing and lying; take pulse and respirations q4h during initial treatment; establish baseline before starting treatment; report drops of 30 mm Hg

• Dizziness, faintness, palpitations, tachycardia on rising

• EPS including akathisia (inability to sit still, no pattern to movements), tardive dyskinesia (bizarre movements of jaw, mouth, tongue, extremities), pseudoparkinsonism (rigidity, tremors, pill rolling, shuffling gait)

• Skin turgor daily

• Constipation, urinary retention daily; if these occur, increase bulk, water in diet

Teach patient/family:

• That orthostatic hypotension occurs often, to rise from sitting or lying position gradually

• To avoid hot tubs, hot showers, or tub baths since hypotension may occur

• To avoid abrupt withdrawal of this drug or EPS may result; drug should be withdrawn slowly

• To avoid OTC preparations (cough, hayfever, cold) unless approved by physician since serious drug interactions may occur; avoid use with alcohol or CNS depressants; increased drowsiness may occur

• To use a sunscreen during sun exposure to prevent burns

• Regarding compliance with drug regimen

• About EPS and necessity for meticulous oral hygiene since oral candidiasis may occur

• To report sore throat, malaise, fever, bleeding, mouth sores; if these occur, CBC should be drawn and drug discontinued

• In hot weather heat stroke may occur; take extra precautions to stay cool

Lab test interferences:

Increase: Liver function tests, cardiac enzymes, cholesterol, blood glucose, prolactin, bilirubin, PBI, cholinesterase, [131]I

Decrease: Hormones (blood and urine)

False positive: Pregnancy tests, PKU

False negative: Urinary steroids, 17-OHCS

Treatment of overdose: Lavage,

if orally injested, provide an airway; *do not induce vomiting*

---

flurandrenolide

(flure-an-dren'oh-lide)

Cordran, Drenison 1/4, Drenison Tape

Func. class.: Topical corticosteroid
Chem. class.: Synthetic fluorinated agent

Action: Possesses antipruritic, antiinflammatory actions
Uses: Corticosteroid-responsive dermatoses, pruritus
Dosage and routes:
• *Adult and child:* TOP apply to affected area tid-qid
Available forms include: Oint 0.025%, 0.05%; cream 0.025%, 0.05%; lotion 0.05%; tape 4 μg/cm²
Side effects/adverse reactions:
INTEG: Burning, dryness, itching, irritation, acne, folliculitis, hypertrichosis, perioral dermatitis, hypopigmentation, atrophy, striae, miliaria, allergic contact dermatitis, secondary infection
Contraindications: Hypersensitivity to corticosteroids, fungal infections, viral infections
Precautions: Pregnancy (C), lactation, viral infections, bacterial infections
Pharmacokinetics: Not known
Interactions/incompatibilities:
None known
NURSING CONSIDERATIONS
Assess:
• Temperature, if fever develops drug should be discontinued
Administer:
• Only to affected areas, do not get in eyes
• Then cover with occlusive dressing if ordered, seal to normal skin, change q12h
• Only to dermatoses, do not use

on weeping, denuded or infected area
Perform/provide:
• Cleansing before application of drug
• Treatment for a few days after area has cleared
• Storage at room temperature
Evaluate:
• Systemic absorption: fever, infection, irritation
• Therapeutic response: absence of severe itching, patches on skin, flaking
Teach patient/family:
• To avoid sunlight on affected area, burns may occur

---

flurandrenolide

(flure-an-dren'oh-lide)

Cordan, Cordran SP, Cordran Tape

Func. class.: Topical corticosteroid
Chem. class.: Synthetic fluorinated agent, group III potency (0.05%), group IV potency (0.025%)

Action: Possesses antipruritic, antiinflammatory actions
Uses: Psoriasis, eczema, contact dermatitis, pruritus
Dosage and routes:
• *Adult and child:* Apply to affected area tid-qid, apply tape q12h
Available forms include: Oint 0.025%, 0.05%; cream 0.025%, 0.05%; lotion 0.05%, tape 4 μg/cm²
Side effects/adverse reactions:
INTEG: Burning, dryness, itching, irritation, acne, folliculitis, hypertrichosis, perioral dermatitis, hypopigmentation, atrophy, striae, miliaria, allergic contact dermatitis, secondary infection
Contraindications: Hypersensitivity to corticosteroids, fungal infections
Precautions: Pregnancy (C), lac-

---

italics = common side effects   ***bold italic*** = life threatening reactions

tation, viral infections, bacterial infections

Interactions/incompatibilities:
None known

Assess:

• Temperature; if fever develops, drug should be discontinued

Administer:

• Only to affected areas; do not get in eyes

• Medication, then cover with occlusive dressing (only if prescribed), seal to normal skin, change q12h

• Only to dermatoses; do not use on weeping, denuded, or infected area

Perform/provide:

• Cleansing before application of drug

• Treatment for a few days after area has cleared

• Storage at room temperature

Evaluate:

• Therapeutic response: absence of severe itching, patches on skin, flaking

Teach patient/family:

• To avoid sunlight on affected area; burns may occur

---

flurazepam HCl

(flure-az′e-pam)
Dalmane, Durapam, Somnol*

Func. class.: Sedative-hypnotic
Chem. class.: Benzodiazepine derivative

Controlled Substance Schedule IV (USA), Schedule F (Canada)
Action: Produces CNS depression at the limbic, thalamic, hypothalamic levels of CNS; may be mediated by neurotransmitter gamma aminobutyric (GABA); results are sedation, hypnosis, skeletal muscle relaxation, anticonvulsant activity, anxiolytic action

Uses: Insomnia

Dosage and routes:

• *Adult:* PO 15-30 mg hs, may repeat dose once if needed

• *Geriatric:* PO 15 mg hs, may increase if needed

Available forms include: Caps 15, 30 mg

Side effects/adverse reactions:

HEMA: **Leukopenia, granulocytopenia** (rare)

CNS: Lethargy, drowsiness, daytime sedation, dizziness, confusion, lightheadedness, headache, anxiety, irritability

GI: Nausea, vomiting, diarrhea, heartburn, abdominal pain, constipation

CV: Chest pain, pulse changes

Contraindications: Hypersensitivity to benzodiazepines, pregnancy, lactation, intermittent porphyria

Precautions: Anemia, hepatic disease, renal disease, suicidal individuals, drug abuse, elderly, psychosis, child <15 yr

Pharmacokinetics:

PO: Onset 15-45 min, duration 7-8 hr; metabolized by liver, excreted by kidneys (inactive/active metabolites), crosses placenta, excreted in breast milk; half-life 47-100 hr, additional 100 hr for active metabolites

Interactions/incompatibilities:

• Increased effects of this drug: cimetidine, disulfiram

• Increased or decreased effects of this drug: oral contraceptives

• Increased action of both drugs: alcohol

• Decreased effect of this drug: antacids

Assess:

• Blood studies: Hct, Hgb, RBCs (if on long-term therapy)

• Hepatic studies: AST, ALT, bilirubin

Administer:

• After removal of cigarettes, to prevent fires

• After trying conservative measures for insomnia

• ½-1 hr before hs for sleeplessness

• On empty stomach fast onset, but may be taken with food if GI symptoms occur

Perform/provide:

• Assistance with ambulation after receiving dose

• Safety measure: siderails, nightlight, callbell within easy reach

• Checking to see PO medication has been swallowed

• Storage in tight container in cool environment

Evaluate:

• Therapeutic response: ability to sleep at night, decreased amount of early morning awakening if taking drug for insomnia

• Mental status: mood, sensorium, affect, memory (long, short)

• Blood dyscrasias: fever, sore throat, bruising, rash, jaundice, epistaxis (rare)

• Type of sleep problem: falling asleep, staying asleep

Teach patient/family:

• To avoid driving or other activities requiring alertness until drug is stabilized

• To avoid alcohol ingestion or CNS depressants; serious CNS depression may result

• That effects may take 2 nights for benefits to be noticed

• Alternate measures to improve sleep: reading, exercise several hours before hs, warm bath, warm milk, TV, self-hypnosis, deep breathing

• That hangover is common in elderly, but less common than with barbiturates

Lab test interferences:

Increase: AST/ALT, serum bilirubin

False increase: Urinary 17-OHCS
Decrease: RAI uptake

Treatment of overdose: Lavage, activated charcoal, monitor electrolytes, vital signs

---

folic acid (vitamin B₉)

Folvite, Novofolacid*

Func. class.: Vitamin B complex group

Action: Needed for erythropoiesis; increases RBC, WBC, and platelet formation in megaloblastic anemias

Uses: Megaloblastic or macrocytic anemia caused by folic acid deficiency; liver disease, alcoholism, hemolysis, intestinal obstruction

Dosage and routes:
Supplement

• *Adult:* PO/IM/SC 0.1 mg qd

• *Child:* PO 0.05 mg qd

Megaloblastic/macrocytic anemia

• *Adult and child >4 yr:* PO/SC/IM 1 mg qd × 4-5 days

• *Child <4 yr:* PO/SC/IM 0.3 mg or less qd

• *Pregnancy/lactation:* PO/SC/IM 0.8 mg qd

Prevention of megaloblastic/macrocytic anemia

• *Pregnancy:* PO/SC/IM 1 mg qd

Available forms include: Tabs 0.1, 0.4, 0.8, 1 mg; inj SC, IM 5, 10 mg/ml

Side effects/adverse reactions:
RESP: Bronchospasm

Contraindications: Hypersensitivity, anemias other than megaloblastic/macrocytic anemia

Pharmacokinetics:

PO: Peak ½-1 hr, bound to plasma proteins, excreted in breast milk, methylated in liver, excreted in urine (small amounts)

Interactions/incompatibilities:
• Decreased folate levels: chloramphenicol
• Increased metabolism of: phenobarbitol, hydantoins

NURSING CONSIDERATIONS
Assess:
• Folate levels: 6-15 µg/ml
Perform/provide:
• Storage in light-resistant container
Evaluate:
• Therapeutic response: increased weight, oriented well-being, absence of fatigue
• Nutritional status: bran, yeast, dried beans, nuts, fruits, fresh vegetables, asparagus
• Drugs currently taken: alcohol, hydantoins, trimethoprim, these drugs may cause increased folic acid use by body
Teach patient/family:
• To take drug exactly as prescribed
• To notify physician of side effects

---

fructose (levulose)

Func. class.: Caloric
Chem. class.: Sugar, carbohydrate

Action: Needed for adequate utilization of amino acids, decreases protein/nitrogen loss, prevents ketosis
Uses: Increased intake of calories, increased fluids in patients unable to take adequate fluids and calories orally
Dosage and routes:
• *Adult and child:* IV not to exceed 1 g/kg/hr
Available forms include: Inj IV 10%
Side effects/adverse reactions:
CNS: Confusion, loss of consciousness, dizziness
CV: Hypertension, ***CHF, pulmonary edema***

GU: Glycosuria, osmotic diuresis
ENDO: Hyperglycemia, rebound hypoglycemia, hyperosmolar syndrome, hyperosmolar hyperglycemic nonketotic syndrome
INTEG: Chills, flushing, warm feeling, rash, urticaria, extravasation necrosis
Contraindications: Hypersensitivity, gout, hyperglycemia
Precautions: Cardiac, renal disease, urinary tract obstruction
Interactions/incompatibilities:
None known

NURSING CONSIDERATIONS
Assess:
• Electrolytes (K, Na, Ca, Cl, Mg), blood glucose, ammonia, phosphate
• Renal, liver function studies: BUN, creatinine, ALT, AST, bilirubin
• Injection site for extravasation: redness along vein, edema at site, necrosis pain, hard tender area; site should be changed immediately
• Monitor respiratory function q4h: auscultate lung fields bilaterally for rales, respirations, quality, rate, rhythm
• Monitor temperature q4h for increased fever, indicating infection; if infection suspected, infusion is discontinued, tubing, bottle cultured
• Urine glucose q6h using Tes-Tape, Clinistix, Keto-Diastix, which are not affected by infusion substances
Administer:
• After changing IV catheter, dressing q24h using aseptic technique
Evaluate:
• Therapeutic response: increased weight
• Nutritional status: calorie count by dietician
Teach patient/family
• Reason for dextrose infusion

furazolidone

(fur-a-zoe'li-done)
Furoxone

Func. class.: Antibacterial
Chem. class.: Nitrofuran

Action: Interferes with enzyme systems in bacteria

Uses: Gastroenteritis, cholera (as an adjunctive)

Dosage and routes:
• *Adult:* PO 100 mg qid
• *Child 5-12 yr:* PO 25-50 mg qid
• *Child 1-4 yr:* PO 17-25 mg qid
• *Child 1 mo-1 yr:* PO 8-17 mg qid, not to exceed 8.8 mg/kg/day

Available forms include: Tabs 100 mg; liq 50 mg/15 ml

Side effects/adverse reactions:
INTEG: Urticaria, angioedema, rash
CNS: Headache, malaise, fever
GI: Nausea, vomiting, anorexia, diarrhea, abdominal pain

Contraindications: Hypersensitivity, infant <1 mo

Precautions: Pregnancy, lactation, G-6-PD deficiency

Pharmacokinetics: Metabolized, inactivated in intestine, only 5% in urine

Interactions/incompatibilities:
• Avoid use with alcohol, MAOIs, narcotics, indirect-acting sympathomimetic amines, ephedrine, phenylephrine, tramine, other CNS depressants
• Increased hypoglycemic effect: insulin, sulfonylureas
• Disulfiram-like reaction: alcohol

NURSING CONSIDERATIONS

Assess:
• C&S before drug therapy; drug may be taken as soon as culture is taken
• Electrolytes: K, Na, Cl

Administer:
• With full glass of water

Perform/provide:
• Storage protected from light in tight container
• Adequate intake of fluids (2000 ml) during diarrhea episodes

Evaluate:
• Bowel pattern before, during treatment
• Skin eruptions, itching
• Allergies before treatment, reaction of each medication; place allergies on chart, Kardex in bright red letters, notify all people giving drugs
• Nausea, vomiting; if severe may require decrease in dosage

Teach patient/family:
• To avoid alcohol during, for 4 days after completion of therapy
• Urine may turn brown
• To avoid high tyramine foods: pickled products, aged cheese, figs, bananas, chocolate, yeast products

Treatment of overdose: Withdraw drug, maintain airway, administer epinephrine, aminophylline, O_2, IV corticosteroids

furosemide

(fur-oh'se-mide)
Lasix, Novosemide,* Uritol*

Func. class.: Loop diuretic
Chem. class.: Sulfonamide derivative

Action: Acts on loop of Henle by increasing excretion of chloride, sodium

Uses: Pulmonary edema, edema in CHF, liver disease, renal disease, antihypertension

Dosage and routes:
• *Adult:* PO 20-80 mg/day in AM, may give another dose in 6 hr, up to 600 mg/day; IM/IV 20-40 mg, increased by 20 mg q2h until desired response
• *Child:* PO/IM/IV 2 mg/kg, may

---

increase by 1-2 mg/kg/q6-8h up to 6 mg/kg

Pulmonary edema

• *Adult:* IV 40 mg given over several minutes, repeated in 1 hr; increase to 80 mg if needed

Available forms include: Tabs 20, 40, 80 mg; oral sol 10 mg/ml; inj IM, IV 10 mg/ml

Side effects/adverse reactions:

GU: Polyuria, gynecomastia, ejaculatory problems, *renal failure,* glycosuria

ELECT: Hypokalemia, hypochloremic alkalosis, hypomagnesemia, hyperuricemia, hypocalcemia, hyponatremia

CNS: Headache, fatigue, weakness, vertigo, paresthesias

GI: Nausea, diarrhea, dry mouth, vomiting, anorexia, cramps, oral, gastric irritations

EENT: Loss of hearing, ear pain, tinnitus, blurred vision

INTEG: Rash, pruritus, purpura, Stevens-Johnson syndrome, sweating, photosensitivity, urticaria

MS: Cramps, arthritis, stiffness

ENDO: Hyperglycemia

HEMA: Thrombocytopenia, agranulocytosis, leukopenia, neutropenia, anemia

CV: Orthostatic hypotension

Contraindications: Hypersensitivity to sulfonamides, anuria, hypovolemia, infants, lactation, electrolyte depletion

Precautions: Diabetes mellitus, dehydration, ascites, severe renal disease, pregnancy (C)

Pharmacokinetics:

PO: Onset 1 hr, peak 1-2 hr, duration 6-8 hr

IV: Onset 5 min, peak ½ hr, duration 2 hr

Excreted in urine, feces, crosses placenta, excreted in breast milk

Interactions/incompatibilities:

• Increased toxicity: lithium, nondepolarizing skeletal muscle relaxants, succinycholine, digitalis

• Decreased effects of: antidiabetics, tubocurarine

• Increased anticoagulant activity: anticoagulants

• Increased action of: antihypertensives, theophyllines

• Increased orthostatic hypotension: alcohol, barbiturates, narcotics

• Decreased antihypertensive effect of furosemide: indomethacin, phenytoin

NURSING CONSIDERATIONS

Assess:

• Weight, I&O daily to determine fluid loss; effect of drug may be decreased if used qd

• Rate, depth, rhythm of respiration, effect of exertion

• B/P lying, standing; postural hypotension may occur

• Electrolytes: potassium, sodium, chloride; include BUN, blood sugar, CBC, serum creatinine, blood pH, ABGs

• Glucose in urine if patient is diabetic

Administer:

• In AM to avoid interference with sleep if using drug as a diuretic

• Potassium replacement if potassium is less than 3.0

• With food, if nausea occurs, absorption may be decreased slightly

Evaluate:

• Improvement in edema of feet, legs, sacral area daily if medication is being used in CHF

• Improvement in CVP q8h

• Signs of metabolic acidosis: drowsiness, restlessness

• Signs of hypokalemia: postural hypotension, malaise, fatigue, tachycardia, leg cramps, weakness

• Rashes, temperature elevation qd

• Confusion, especially in elderly, take safety precautions if needed

Teach patient/family:

• To increase fluid intake 2-3 L/

day unless contraindicated, to rise slowly from lying or sitting position
• Adverse reactions: muscle cramps, weakness, nausea, dizziness
• Take with food or milk for GI symptoms
• Take early in day to prevent nocturia
Lab test interferences:
Interfere: GTT
Treatment of overdose: Lavage if taken orally, monitor electrolytes, administer dextrose in saline

---

gallamine triethiodide

(gal′a-meen)
Flaxedil
Func. class.: Neuromuscular blocker (nondepolarizing)

Action: Inhibits transmission of nerve impulses by binding with cholinergic receptor sites, antagonizing action of acetylcholine
Uses: Facilitation of endotracheal intubation, skeletal muscle relaxation during mechanical ventilation, surgery, or general anesthesia
Dosage and routes:
• *Adult and child >1 mo:* IV 1 mg/kg, not to exceed 100 mg, then 0.5-1 mg/kg q30-40 min
• *Child <1 mo, >5 kg:* IV 0.25-0.75 mg/kg, then 0.01-0.05 mg/kg q30-40 min
Available forms include: Inj IV 20 mg/ml
Side effects/adverse reactions:
CV: Bradycardia, tachycardia, increased, decreased B/P
*RESP: Prolonged apnea, **bronchospasm, cyanosis, respiratory depression***
EENT: Increased secretions
INTEG: Rash, flushing, pruritus, urticaria
CNS: Malignant hyperthermia
GI: Decreased motility

Contraindications: Hypersensitivity to iodides
Precautions: Pregnancy, thyroid disease, collagen disease, cardiac disease, lactation, children <2 yr, electrolyte imbalances, dehydration, neuromuscular disease (myasthenia gravis), respiratory disease
Pharmacokinetics:
IV: Onset 2 min, duration 20-60 min; half-life 2 min, 29 min (terminal), excreted in urine, feces (metabolites), crosses placenta
Interactions/incompatibilities:
• Increased neuromuscular blockade: aminoglycosides, clindamycin, lincomycin, quinidine, local anesthetics, polymyxin antibiotics, lithium, narcotic analgesics, thiazides, enflurane, isoflurane
• Dysrhythmias: theophylline
• Do not mix with barbiturates in solution or syringe
NURSING CONSIDERATIONS
Assess:
• For electrolyte imbalances (K, Mg); may lead to increased action of this drug
• Vital signs (B/P, pulse, respirations, airway) until fully recovered; rate, depth, pattern of respirations, strength of hand grip
• I&O ratio; check for urinary retention, frequency, hesitancy
Administer:
• Using nerve stimulator by anesthesiologist to determine neuromuscular blockade
• Anticholinesterase to reverse neuromuscular blockade
• By slow IV over 1-2 min (only by qualified person, usually an anesthesiologist)
• Only slight discolored solution
Perform/provide:
• Storage in light-resistant area
• Reassurance if communication is difficult during recovery from neuromuscular blockade

G

---

italics = common side effects   ***bold italic*** = life threatening reactions

Evaluate:

• Therapeutic response: paralysis of jaw, eyelid, head, neck, rest of body

• Recovery: decreased paralysis of face, diaphragm, leg, arm, rest of body

• Allergic reactions: rash, fever, respiratory distress, pruritus; drug should be discontinued

Treatment of overdose: Edrophonium or neostigmine, atropine, monitor VS; may require mechanical ventilation

---

gemfibrozil

(gem-fi'broe-zil)

Lopid

Func. class.: Antilipemic

Chem. class.: Aryloxisobutyric acid derivative

Action: Inhibits biosynthesis of VLDL, LDL, which are responsible for cholesterol development

Uses: Hyperlipidemia, xanthoma tuberosum, type III hyperlipidemia

Dosage and routes:

• *Adult:* PO 1200 mg in divided doses bid

Available forms include: Caps 500 mg

Side effects/adverse reactions:

GI: Nausea, vomiting, dyspepsia, increased liver enzymes, stomatitis, flatulence, hepatomegaly, gastritis

INTEG: Rash, urticaria, pruritus, dry hair and skin, alopecia

HEMA: Leukopenia, anemia, eosinophilia

CNS: Fatigue, weakness, headache

GU: Decreased libido, impotence, dysuria, proteinuria, oliguria

MS: Myalgias, arthralgias

CV: Angina, dysrhythmias, thrombophlebitis, *pulmonary emboli*

Contraindications: Severe hepatic disease, severe renal disease, primary biliary cirrhosis, pregnancy (B), lactation

Precautions: Peptic ulcer

Pharmacokinetics:

PO: Peak 2-6 hr, plasma protein binding >90%, half-life 6-25 hr, excreted in urine, metabolized in liver

Interactions/incompatibilities:

• May increase effect of sulfonylureas used with this drug

• May increase toxicity: probenecid

• May increase anticoagulant properties of oral anticoagulants

• Decreased effect: rifampin

NURSING CONSIDERATIONS

Assess:

• Renal, hepatic levels if patient is on long-term therapy

• For signs of vitamin A, D, K deficiency

Administer:

• Drug with meals if GI symptoms occur

Evaluate:

• Bowel pattern daily; increase bulk, water in diet if constipation develops

Teach patient/family:

• Symptoms of hypothrombinemia: bleeding mucous membranes, dark tarry stools, petechiae; these symptoms should be reported immediately

• That compliance is needed since toxicity may result if doses are missed

• That risk factors should be decreased: high fat diet, smoking, alcohol consumption, absence of exercise

• That OTC preparations should be avoided unless directed by physician

• Birth control should be practiced while on this drug

• Report GU symptoms: decreased libido, impotence, dysuria, proteinuria, oliguria

Lab test interferences:
Increase: Liver function studies, CPK, BSP, thymol turbidity

---

gentamicin sulfate

(jen-ta-mye'sin)
Alcomicin,* Apogen, Cidomycin,* Garamycin, Jenamicin, U-Gencin
Func. class.: Antibiotic
Chem. class.: Aminoglycoside

Action: Interferes with protein synthesis in bacterial cell by binding to ribosomal subunit, causing misreading of genetic code; inaccurate peptide sequence forms in protein chain, causing bacterial death

Uses: Severe systemic infections of CNS, respiratory, GI, urinary tract, bone, skin, soft tissues caused by susceptible strains of *P. aeruginosa, Proteus, Klebsiella, Serratia, E. coli, Enterobacter, Acinetobacter, Citrobacter, Staphylococcus*

Dosage and routes:
Severe systemic infections
• *Adult:* IV INF 3-5 mg/kg/day in 3 divided doses q8h; dilute in 50-200 ml NS or D_5W given over 30 min-2 hr; IM 3 mg/kg/day in divided doses q8h
• *Adult:* INTRATHECAL 4-8 mg qd
• *Child:* IV/IM 2-2.5 mg/kg q8h
• *Neonates and infants:* IV/IM 2.5 mg/kg q8h
• *Neonates <1 wk:* 2.5 mg/kg q12h
• *Infants and child >3 months:* INTRATHECAL 1-2 mg qd
Dental/respiratory procedures/ GI/GU surgery (prophylaxis endocarditis)
• *Adult:* IM 1.5 mg/kg ½-1 hr before procedure with ampicillin
• *Child:* IM 2.5 mg/kg ½-1 hr before procedure with ampicillin

Available forms include: Inj IM, IV 10, 40 mg; intrathecal 2 mg/ml
Side effects/adverse reactions:
*GU: **Oliguria, hematuria, renal damage, azotemia, renal failure, nephrotoxicity***
CNS: Confusion, depression, numbness, tremors, *convulsions,* muscle twitching, *neurotoxicity*
*EENT: **Ototoxicity,** deafness, visual disturbances
*HEMA: **Agranulocytosis, thrombocytopenia,** leukopenia, eosinophilia, anemia
GI: Nausea, vomiting, anorexia, increased ALT, AST, bilirubin, hepatomegaly, ***hepatic necrosis,*** splenomegaly
CV: Hypotension, hypertension, palpitations
INTEG: Rash, burning, urticaria, photosensitivity, dermatitis
Contraindications: Severe renal disease, hypersensitivity
Precautions: Neonates, mild renal disease, pregnancy, hearing deficits, myasthenia gravis, lactation, elderly

Pharmacokinetics:
IM: Onset rapid, peak 1-2 hr
IV: Onset immediate, peak 1-2 hr
Plasma half-life 1-2 hr; duration 6-8 hr, not metabolized, excreted unchanged in urine; crosses placental barrier

Interactions/incompatibilities:
• Increased ototoxicity, neurotoxicity, nephrotoxicity: other aminoglycosides, amphotericin B, polymyxin, vancomycin, ethacrynic acid, furosemide, mannitol, methoxyflurane, cisplatin, cephalosporins
• Decreased effects of: parenteral penicillins, digoxin, vitamin B_{12}
• Do not mix in solution or syringe: carbenicillin, ticarcillin, amphotericin B, cephalothin, erythromycin, heparin

G

---

italics = common side effects **bold italic** = life threatening reactions

• Increased effects: nondepolarizing muscle relaxants

NURSING CONSIDERATIONS

Assess:

• Weight before treatment; calculation of dosage is usually done based on ideal body weight, but may be calculated on actual body weight

• I&O ratio, urinalysis daily for proteinuria, cells, casts; report sudden change in urine output

• VS during infusion, watch for hypotension, change in pulse

• IV site for thrombophlebitis including pain, redness, swelling q30 min, change site if needed; apply warm compresses to discontinued site

• Serum peak, drawn at 30-60 min after IV infusion or 60 min after IM injection, and trough level drawn just before next dose; blood level should be 2-4 times bacteriostatic level

• Urine pH if drug is used for UTI; urine should be kept alkaline

Administer:

• IM injection in large muscle mass, rotate injection sites

• Drug in evenly spaced doses to maintain blood level

• Bicarbonate to alkalinize urine if ordered for UTI, as drug is most active in alkaline environment

Perform/provide:

• Adequate fluids of 2-3 L/day unless contraindicated to prevent irritation of tubules

• Flush of IV line with NS or D_5W after infusion

• Supervised ambulation, other safety measures with vestibular dysfunction

Evaluate:

• Therapeutic effect: absence of fever, draining wounds, negative C&S after treatment

• Renal impairment by securing urine for CrCl testing, BUN, serum creatinine; lower dosage should be given in renal impairment (CrCl <80 ml/min)

• Deafness by audiometric testing, ringing, roaring in ears, vertigo; assess hearing before, during, after treatment

• Dehydration: high sp gr, decrease in skin turgor, dry mucous membranes, dark urine

• Overgrowth of infection including increased temperature, malaise, redness, pain, swelling, perineal itching, diarrhea, stomatitis, change in cough or sputum

• C&S before starting treatment to identify infecting organism

• Vestibular dysfunction: nausea, vomiting, dizziness, headache; drug should be discontinued if severe

• Injection sites for redness, swelling, abscesses; use warm compresses at site

Teach patient/family:

• To report headache, dizziness, symptoms of overgrowth of infection, renal impairment

• To report loss of hearing, ringing, roaring in ears or feeling of fullness in head

Treatment of overdose: Hemodialysis, monitor serum levels of drug

---

gentamicin sulfate (ophthalmic)

(jen-ta-mye′sin)

Garamycin Ophthalmic, Genoptic

Func. class.: Antiinfective ophthalmic

Action: Inhibits bacterial cell wall in organism by preventing amino acids and nucleotides into cell wall

Uses: Infection of external eye

Dosage and routes:

• *Adult and child:* INSTILL 1 or 2 gtts q2-4h; TOP apply oint to conjunctival sac bid-qid

Available forms include: Oint 3 mg/g; sol 3 mg/ml

Side effects/adverse reactions:
EENT: Poor corneal wound healing, temporary visual haze, overgrowth of nonsusceptible organisms

Contraindications: Hypersensitivity

Precautions: Antibiotic hypersensitivity

Interactions/incompatibilities: None known

NURSING CONSIDERATIONS

Administer:
• After washing hands, cleanse crusts or discharge from eye before application

Perform/provide:
• Storage at room temperature

Evaluate:
• Therapeutic response: absence of redness, inflammation, tearing
• Allergy: itching, lacrimation, redness, swelling

Teach patient/family:
• To use drug exactly as prescribed
• Not to use eye makeup, towels, washcloths, eye medication of others; reinfection may occur
• That drug container tip should not be touched to eye
• To report itching, increased redness, burning, stinging, swelling; drug should be discontinued
• That drug may cause blurred vision when ointment is applied

---

gentamicin sulfate (topical)

(jen-ta-mye'sin)
Garamycin

Func. class.: Local antiinfective
Chem. class.: Aminoglycoside

Action: Interferes with bacterial cell wall synthesis
Uses: Skin infections
Dosage and routes:
• *Adult and child:* TOP rub into affected area tid-qid

Available forms include: Cream, oint 0.1%

Side effects/adverse reactions:
INTEG: Rash, urticaria, stinging, burning, photosensitivity, pruritus

Contraindications: Hypersensitivity

Precautions: Pregnancy, lactation

Interactions/incompatibilities: None known

NURSING CONSIDERATIONS

Administer:
• Enough medication to completely cover lesions
• After cleansing with soap, water before each application, dry well

Perform/provide:
• Storage at room temperature in dry place

Evaluate:
• Allergic reaction: burning, stinging, swelling, redness
• Therapeutic response: decrease in size, number of lesions

Teach patient/family:
• To apply with glove to prevent further infection
• To avoid use of OTC creams, ointments, lotions unless directed by physician
• To use medical asepsis (hand washing) before, after each application
• To avoid sunlight or wear sunscreen to prevent burns

---

glipizide

(glip-i'zide)
Glucotrol

Func. class.: Antidiabetic
Chem. class.: Sulfonylurea (2nd generation)

Action: Causes functioning β-cells in pancreas to synthesize, release insulin, leading to drop in blood glucose levels; stimulation of insulin results in increased insulin

---

italics = common side effects   ***bold italic*** = life threatening reactions

binding; not effective if patient lacks functioning β-cells

Uses: Stable adult-onset diabetes mellitus (type II)

Dosage and routes:
• *Adult:* PO 5 mg initially, then increased to desired response
• *Elderly:* PO 2.5 mg initially, then increased to desired response, max 40 mg/day

Available forms include: Tabs 5, 10 mg

Side effects/adverse reactions:
CNS: Headache, weakness, dizziness, drowsiness

GI: Hepatotoxicity, cholestatic jaundice, nausea, vomiting, diarrhea, constipation, anorexia

HEMA: Leukopenia, thrombocytopenia, agranulocytosis, aplastic anemia, increased AST, ALT, alk phosphatase, *pancytopenia, hemolytic anemia*

INTEG: Rash, allergic reactions, pruritus, urticaria, eczema, photosensitivity, erythema

ENDO: Hypoglycemia

Contraindications: Hypersensitivity to sulfonylureas, juvenile or brittle diabetes, severe renal disease, severe hepatic disease

Precautions: Pregnancy (C), elderly, cardiac disease, thyroid disease

Pharmacokinetics:
PO: Completely absorbed by GI route, onset 1-1½ hr, duration 10-24 hr, half-life 2-4 hr, metabolized in liver, excreted in urine, 90%-95% is plasma protein bound

Interactions/incompatibilities:
• Increased effects: insulin, MAOIs, cimetidine
• Decreased action of this drug: calcium channel blockers, corticosteroids, oral contraceptives, thiazide diuretics, thyroid preparations, estrogens, phenothiazines, phenytoin, rifampin, isoniazide
• Disulfiram-like reaction: alcohol

NURSING CONSIDERATIONS
Assess:
• Blood, urine glucose levels during treatment to determine diabetes control

Administer:
• Drug 30 min before meals

Perform/provide:
• Storage in tight light-resistant containers at room temperature

Evaluate:
• Therapeutic response: decrease in polyuria, polydipsia, polyphagia, clear sensorium, absence of dizziness, stable gait
• Hypoglycemic/hyperglycemic reaction that can occur soon after meals

Teach patient/family:
• To check for symptoms of cholestatic jaundice: dark urine, pruritus, yellow sclera; if these occur physician should be notified
• To use a capillary blood glucose test while on this drug
• To test urine glucose levels with Chemstrip approximately 2 hr after each meal
• The symptoms of hypo/hyperglycemia, what to do about each
• That drug must be continued on daily basis; explain consequence of discontinuing drug abruptly
• To take drug in morning to prevent hypoglycemic reactions at night
• To avoid OTC medications unless prescribed by a physician
• That diabetes is a life-long illness; drug will not cure disease
• That all food included in diet plan must be eaten in order to prevent hypoglycemia
• To carry Medic-Alert ID for emergency purposes
• To test urine for glucose/ketones tid if this drug is replacing insulin
• To continue weight control, dietary restrictions, exercise, hygiene

Treatment of overdose: 10%-50% glucose solution

---

glutamic acid HCl

(gloo-tam'ik)
Acidulin
Func. class.: Digestant
Chem. class.: Amino acid

Action: Increases gastric acidity when needed for replacement
Uses: Hypoacidity
Dosage and routes:
• *Adult:* PO 1-3 caps tid ac
Available forms include: Pulvules 340 mg
Side effects/adverse reactions:
MET: Metabolic acidosis
Contraindications: Peptic ulcer disease
Precautions: Pregnancy
Pharmacokinetics: None known
Interactions/incompatibilities: None known
NURSING CONSIDERATIONS
Assess:
• Acid-base balance during treatment
Administer:
• During meals or after meals
• High alkaline diet: oranges, dark, leafy, green vegetables, as ordered
Perform/provide:
• Storage in tight container at room temperature
Evaluate:
• For achlorhydria: belching, nausea, vomiting, diarrhea, epigastric distress

---

glutethimide

(gloo-teth'i-mide)
Doriden, Rolathimide
Func. class.: Sedative-hypnotic
Chem. class.: Piperidine derivative

Controlled Substance Schedule III (USA), Schedule F (Canada)

Action: Depresses activity in brain cells primarily in reticular activating system in brainstem, also selectively depresses neurons in posterior hypothalamus, limbic structures
Uses: Insomnia, labor (stage 1), preoperatively for relaxation
Dosage and routes:
Insomnia
• *Adult:* PO 250-500 mg hs, may repeat dose >4 hr before usual awakening, not to exceed 1 g
Preoperatively
• *Adult:* PO 500 mg hs the night before surgery, then 500 mg-1 g 1 hr before surgery
Labor
• *Adult:* PO 500 mg given at the onset of labor, may repeat
Available forms include: Tabs 250, 500 mg; caps 500 mg
Side effects/adverse reactions:
HEMA: **Thrombocytopenia, aplastic anemia, leukopenia, megaloblastic anemia**
CNS: Residual sedation, dizziness, ataxia, stimulation, headache, hangover
GI: Nausea, vomiting, hiccups, diarrhea, jaundice
GU: Porphyria
INTEG: Rash, urticaria, purpura, *exfoliative dermatitis (rare)*
EENT: Dry mouth, blurred vision
Contraindications: Hypersensitivity to this drug or piperidine derivatives, severe pain, severe renal disease, porphyria
Precautions: Depression, suicidal individuals, drug abuse, cardiac dysrhythmias, narrow-angle glaucoma, prostatic hypertrophy, stenosed peptic ulcer, pyloroduodenal/bladder neck obstruction, pregnancy (C)
Pharmacokinetics:
PO: Onset 30 min, peak 1-2 hr, duration 4-8 hr; metabolized by liver, excreted by kidneys (metabolites),

G

---

crosses placenta, excreted in breast milk; half-life 4 hr, 10 hr terminal

Interactions/incompatibilities:

• Decreased hypoprothrombinemic effect: oral anticoagulants

• Increased CNS depression: alcohol

• Increased anticholinergic: tricyclic antidepressants

NURSING CONSIDERATIONS

Assess:

• Blood studies: Hct, Hgb, RBCs (if on long-term therapy)

• Hepatic studies: AST, ALT, bilirubin

Administer:

• After removal of cigarettes, to prevent fires

• After trying conservative measures for insomnia

• ½-1 hr before hs for sleeplessness

• Several hours before patient is to arise (to avoid hangover)

Perform/provide:

• Assistance with ambulation after receiving dose

• Safety measures: siderails, nightlight, callbell within easy reach

• Checking to see PO medication has been swallowed

• Storage in tight container in cool environment

Evaluate:

• Therapeutic response: ability to sleep at night, decreased amount of early morning awakening if taking drug for insomnia

• Mental status: mood, sensorium, affect, memory (long, short)

• Blood dyscrasias: fever, sore throat, bruising, rash, jaundice, epistaxis (rare)

• Type of sleep problem: falling asleep, staying asleep

Teach patient/family:

• To avoid driving or other activities requiring alertness until drug is stabilized

• To avoid alcohol ingestion or CNS depressants; serious CNS depression may result

• Not to discontinue medication quickly after long-term use, drug should be tapered over 1-2 wk

• That effects may take 2 nights for benefits to be noticed

• Alternate measures to improve sleep: reading, exercise several hours before hs, warm bath, warm milk, TV, self-hypnosis, deep breathing

• That hangover is common in elderly, but less common than with barbiturates

• Withdrawal: nausea, vomiting, anxiety, hallucinations, insomnia, tachycardia, fever, cramps, tremors, seizures

• Blood dyscrasias: fever, sore throat, bruising, rash, jaundice (rare)

• Allergic reaction: rash, discontinue drug if rash occurs

Lab test interferences:

Interferes: 17-OHCS

Treatment of overdose: Lavage, activated charcoal, monitor electrolytes, vital signs

---

glyburide

(glye'byoor-ide)
Diabeta,* Micronase

Func. class.: Antidiabetic
Chem. class.: Sulfonylurea (2nd generation)

Action: Causes functioning β-cells in pancreas to synthesize, release insulin, leading to drop in blood glucose levels; stimulation of insulin results in increased insulin binding; not effective if patient lacks functioning β-cells

Uses: Stable adult-onset diabetes mellitus (type II)

Dosage and routes:

• *Adult:* PO 2.5-5 mg initially, then increased to desired response

• *Elderly:* PO 1.25 mg initially,

then increased to desired response; max 20 mg/day, maintenance 1.25-20 mg/qd

Available forms include: Tabs 1.25, 2.5, 5 mg

Side effects/adverse reactions:

CNS: Headache, weakness, paresthesia

GI: Nausea, fullness, heartburn, *hepatotoxicity, cholestatic jaundice*

HEMA: Leukopenia, thrombocytopenia, agranulocytosis, aplastic anemia, increased AST, ALT, alk phosphatase

INTEG: Rash, allergic reactions, pruritus, urticaria, eczema, photosensitivity, erythema

ENDO: Hypoglycemia

MS: Joint pains

Contraindications: Hypersensitivity to sulfonylureas, juvenile or brittle diabetes, severe renal disease, severe hepatic disease

Precautions: Pregnancy (B), elderly, cardiac disease, thyroid disease, severe hypoglycemic reactions

Pharmacokinetics:

PO: Completely absorbed by GI route, onset 15-60 min, peak 2-8 hr, duration 10-24 hr; half-life 2-5 hr, metabolized in liver, excreted in urine, feces (metabolites), crosses placenta, 90%-95% is plasma protein bound

Interactions/incompatibilities:

• Increased effects: insulin, MAOIs, cimetidine

• Decreased action of this drug: calcium channel blockers, corticosteroids, oral contraceptives, thiazide diuretics, thyroid preparations, estrogens, phenothiazines, phenytoin, rifampin, isoniazide

• Disulfiram-like reaction: alcohol

NURSING CONSIDERATIONS

Administer:

• Drug 30 min before meals

Perform/provide:

• Storage in tight container in cool environment

Evaluate:

• Therapeutic response: decrease in polyuria, polydipsia, polyphagia, clear sensorium, absence of dizziness, stable gait

• Hypoglycemic/hyperglycemic reaction that can occur soon after meals

Teach patient/family:

• To check for symptoms of cholestatic jaundice: dark urine, pruritus, yellow sclera; if these occur a physician should be notified

• To use a capillary blood glucose test while on this drug

• To test urine glucose levels with Chemstrip approximately 2 hr after each meal

• The symptoms of hypo/hyperglycemia, what to do about each

• That drug must be continued on daily basis; explain consequence of discontinuing drug abruptly

• To take drug in morning to prevent hypoglycemic reactions at night

• To avoid OTC medications unless prescribed by a physician

• That diabetes is a life-long illness, drug will not cure disease

• That all food included in diet plan must be eaten in order to prevent hypoglycemia

• To carry a Medic-Alert ID for emergency purposes

Treatment of overdose: 10%-50% glucose solution

glycerin

(gli′ser-in)

Func. class.: Laxative, hyperosmotic

Chem. class.: Trihydric alcohol

Action: Increases osmotic pressure, draws fluid into colon

Uses: Constipation

Dosage and routes:

• *Adult and child >6 yr:* REC SUPP 3 g; ENEMA 5-15 ml

• *Child <6 yr:* REC SUPP 1-1.5 g; ENEMA 2-5 ml

Available forms include: Rec sol 4 ml/applicator; supp

Side effects/adverse reactions: None known

Contraindications: Hypersensitivity

Interactions/incompatibilities: None known

NURSING CONSIDERATIONS

Administer:

• In morning or evening (oral dose)

Perform/provide:

• Storage in cool environment, do not freeze

Evaluate:

• Therapeutic response: decrease in constipation

• Cause of constipation; identify whether fluids, bulk, or exercise is missing from lifestyle

• Cramping, rectal bleeding, nausea, vomiting; if these symptoms occur, drug should be discontinued

Teach patient/family:

• Not to use laxatives for long-term therapy; bowel tone will be lost

• That normal bowel movements do not always occur daily

• Do not use in presence of abdominal pain, nausea, vomiting

• Notify physician if constipation unrelieved or if symptoms of electrolyte imbalance occur: muscle cramps, pain, weakness, dizziness

---

glycerin, anhydrous

(gli′ser-in)

Ophthalgan

Func. class.: Opthalmic

Chem. class.: Trihydric alcohol

Action: Reduces corneal edema by osmosis of water through corneal epithelium which is semipermeable

Uses: Reduce corneal edema

Dosage and routes:

• *Adult:* INSTILL 1-2 gtts after local anesthetic

Available forms include: Sol

Side effects/adverse reactions:

EENT: Eye pain

Contraindications: Hypersensitivity

Pharmacokinetics: Onset 10 min, peak 20 min, duration 6-8 hr

Interactions/incompatibilities: None known

NURSING CONSIDERATIONS

Administer:

• Anesthetic (tetracaine or proparacaine) before instillation to decrease pain

Perform/provide:

• Storage in tight container

Teach patient/family:

• Method of instillation, including pressure on lacrimal sac for 1 min, and not to touch dropper to eye

---

glycopyrrolate

(glye-koe-pye′roe-late)

Robinul, Robinul Forte

Func. class.: Cholinergic blocker

Chem. class.: Quaternary ammonium compound

Action: Inhibits acetylcholine at receptor sites in autonomic nervous system, which controls secretions, free acids in stomach

Uses: Decreased secretions before surgery, reversal of neuromuscular blockage, peptic ulcer disease, irritable bowel syndrome

Dosage and routes:

Preoperatively

• *Adult:* IM 0.002 mg/lb ½-1 hr before surgery

Reversal of neuromuscular blockage

• *Adult:* IV 0.2 mg for each 1 mg

of neostigmine or equal dose of pyridostigmine

GI disorders

• *Adult:* PO 1-2 mg tid; IM 0.1 mg tid-qid, titrated to patient response

Available forms include: Tabs 1, 2 mg; inj 0.2 mg/ml

Side effects/adverse reactions:

CNS: Confusion, anxiety, restlessness, irritability, delusions, hallucinations, headache, sedation, depression, incoherence, dizziness

EENT: Blurred vision, photophobia, dilated pupils, difficulty swallowing

CV: Palpitations, tachycardia, postural hypotension

GI: Dryness of mouth, constipation, nausea, vomiting, abdominal distress, paralytic ileus

GU: Hesitancy, retention

Contraindications: Hypersensitivity, narrow-angle glaucoma, myasthenia gravis, GI/GU obstruction, child <3 yr

Precautions: Pregnancy (C), elderly, lactation, tachycardia, prostatic hypertrophy

Pharmacokinetics:

PO: Peak 1 hr, duration 6 hr

SC/IM: Peak 30-45 min, duration 7 hr

IV: Peak 10-15 min, duration 4 hr Excreted in urine, bile, feces (unchanged)

Interactions/incompatibilities:

• Increased anticholinergic effect: alcohol, antihistamines, phenothiazines, amantadine

• Do not mix with diazepam, chloramphenicol, pentobarbital, sodium bicarbonate in syringe or solution

NURSING CONSIDERATIONS

Assess:

• I&O ratio; retention commonly causes decreased urinary output

Administer:

• Parenteral dose with patient recumbent to prevent postural hypotension

• With or after meals to prevent GI upset; may give with fluids other than water

• Parenteral dose slowly; keep in bed for at least 1 hr after dose

Perform/provide:

• Storage at room temperature

• Hard candy, frequent drinks, sugarless gum to relieve dry mouth

Evaluate:

• Urinary hesitancy, retention: palpate bladder if retention occurs

• Constipation; increase fluids, bulk, exercise if this occurs

• For tolerance over long-term therapy; dose may need to be increased or changed

• Mental status: affect, mood, CNS depression, worsening of mental symptoms during early therapy

Teach patient/family:

• Not to discontinue this drug abruptly; to taper off over 1 wk

• To avoid driving or other hazardous activities; drowsiness may occur

• To avoid OTC medication: cough, cold preparations with alcohol, antihistamines unless directed by physician

---

gonadorelin HCl

(goe-nad-oh-rell′in)

Factrel

Func. class.: Gonadotropin

Chem. class.: Synthetic luteinizing hormone–releasing hormone

---

Action: Combination luteinizing hormone (releasing hormone) that acts on anterior pituitary

Uses: Evaluation of response of gonadotropic hormone

Dosage and routes:

• *Adult:* SC/IV 100 µg usually given between day 1-7 of menstrual cycle

Available forms include: Powder for inj SC, IV 100, 500 µg/vial

---

italics = common side effects **bold italic** = life threatening reactions

Side effects/adverse reactions:
CNS: Dizziness, headache, flushing
GI: Nausea
INTEG: Inflammation at injection site

Contraindications: Hypersensitivity

Precautions: Pregnancy

Pharmacokinetics: Excreted by kidneys

Interactions/incompatibilities:
• Increased level of this drug: levodopa, spironolactone
• Decreased level of this drug: digoxin, oral contraceptives
• May produce false test results when used with androgens, glucocorticoids, estrogens, progestins

NURSING CONSIDERATIONS
Assess:
• Test result: pituitary/hypothalamus dysfunction (decreased LH); postmenopausal (increased LH)
Administer:
• After reconstituting with sterile diluent (1 ml) enclosed in package
• Repeated doses may be necessary to elevate pituitary gonadotropin reserve
Perform/provide:
• Storage at room temperature; use prepared solution within 24 hr

---

griseofulvin microsize/ griseofulvin ultramicrosize

(gri-see-oh-ful'vin)
Fulvicin-U/F, Grifulvin-V, Grasactin, Grisovin-FP, Fulvicin P/G, Grisactin-Ultra, Gris-PEG

Func. class.: Antifungal
Chem. class.: Penicillium griseofulvum derivative

Action: Arrests fungal cell division at metaphase of development, binds to human keratin making it resistant to disease

Uses: Mycotic infections: Tinea corporis, pedis, cruris, barbae, capitis, unguium if caused by *Epidermophyton, Microsporum, Trichophyton*

Dosage and routes:
• *Adult:* PO 500-1000 mg qd in single or divided doses (microsize), 125-165 mg bid (ultramicrosize) or 250-330 mg qd; may need 500-660 mg in divided doses for severe infections
• *Child:* PO 10 mg/kg/day or 30 mg/m²/day (microsize) or 5 mg/kg/day (ultramicrosize)

Available forms include: Microcaps 125, 250 mg; tabs 250, 500 mg; oral susp 125 mg/ml; ultratabs 125, 165, 250, 330 mg

Side effects/adverse reactions:
INTEG: Rash, urticaria, photosensitivity, lichen planus, angioedema
CNS: Headache, peripheral neuritis, paresthesias, confusion, dizziness, fatigue, insomnia, psychosis
EENT: Blurred vision, oral candidiasis, furred tongue, transient hearing loss
GU: Proteinuria, cylinduria, precipitate porphyria, increased thirst
GI: Nausea, vomiting, anorexia, diarrhea, cramps, dry mouth, flatulence
*HEMA: **Leukopenia, granulocytopenia, neutropenia, monocytosis***

Contraindications: Hypersensitivity, porphyria, hepatic disease, lupus erythematosus

Precautions: Penicillin sensitivity
Pharmacokinetics:
PO: Peak 4 hr, half-life 9-24 hr, metabolized in liver, excreted in urine (inactive metabolites), feces, perspiration

Interactions/incompatibilities:
• Tachycardia: alcohol
• Decreased action of this drug: barbiturates

• Decreased action of: warfarin, anticoagulants (oral)

NURSING CONSIDERATIONS

Assess:
• I&O ratio
• Liver studies q wk (ALT, AST, bilirubin, alk phosphatase)
• Renal studies: BUN, serum creatinine
• Blood studies: CBC, platelets, q2 wk
• Drug level during treatment

Administer:
• Drug carefully, making sure there is no confusion with dosage form (microsize vs ultrasize)
• With meals (high fat content) to decrease GI symptoms
• Until 3 separate cultures are negative for infective organism

Perform/provide:
• Storage in tight, light-resistant containers at room temperature

Evaluate:
• Therapeutic response: decreased fever, malaise, rash, negative C&S for infecting organism
• For history of penicillin allergy; may be cross-sensitive to this drug
• For renal toxicity: increasing BUN, serum creatinine, proteinuria, cylinduria
• For hepatotoxicity: increasing ALT, AST, bilirubin, alk phosphatase
• For blood dyscrasias: fatigue, malaise, dark urine, bruising

Teach patient/family:
• That long-term therapy may be needed to clear infection (2 wk-6 mo depending on organism)
• Proper hygiene: handwashing technique, nail care, use of concomitant topical agents if prescribed
• Stress compliance even after feeling better
• To avoid alcohol since nausea, vomiting, hypertension may occur
• To use sunscreen or avoid direct sunlight to prevent photosensitivity
• To notify physician of sore throat, fever, skin rash, which may indicate overgrowth of organisms

---

guaifenesin

(gwye-fen′e-sin)

Anti-Tuss, Balminil,* Bowtussin, Breonesin, Colrex, Cosin-GG, Dilyn, Glycotuss, Gly-O-Tussin, Glytuss, G-Tussin, Hytuss, Malotuss, Nortussin Proco, Recsei-Tuss, Resyl,* Robitussin, Tursen, Wal-Tussin DM

Func. class.: Expectorant

Action: Increases respiratory tract fluid by decreasing surface tension, adhesiveness, which increases removal of mucus

Uses: Dry, nonproductive cough

Dosage and routes:
• *Adult:* PO 100-400 mg q4-6h, not to exceed 1.2 g/day
• *Child:* PO 12 mg/kg/day in 6 divided doses

Available forms include: Tabs 100, 200 mg; caps 200 mg; syr 100 mg/5 ml

Side effects/adverse reactions:
CNS: Drowsiness
GI: Nausea, anorexia, vomiting

Contraindications: Hypersensitivity, persistent cough

Pharmacokinetics: Not known

Interactions/incompatibilities: None known

NURSING CONSIDERATIONS

Perform/provide:
• Storage at room temperature
• Increased fluids, room humidification to liquefy secretions

Evaluate:
• Therapeutic response: absence of cough
• Cough: type, frequency, character including sputum

Teach patient/family:
• Avoid driving, other hazardous

---

italics = common side effects   **bold italic** = life threatening reactions

activities if drowsiness occurs (rare)

• Avoid smoking, smoke-filled room, perfumes, dust, environmental pollutants, cleansers

---

guanabenz acetate

(gwan'a-benz)

Wytensin

Func. class.: Antihypertensive

Chem. class.: Central α-adrenergic agonist

Action: Stimulates central α-adrenergic receptors resulting in decreased sympathetic outflow from brain

Uses: Hypertension

Dosage and routes:

• *Adult:* PO 4 mg bid, increasing in increments of 4-8 mg/day q1-2 wk, not to exceed 32 mg bid

Available forms include: Tabs 4, 8 mg

Side effects/adverse reactions:

CV: Severe rebound hypertension, chest pain, dysrhythmias, palpitations

CNS: Drowsiness, dizziness, sedation, headache, depression, weakness

EENT: Dry mouth, nasal congestion, blurred vision

GI: Nausea, diarrhea, constipation

GU: Impotence

Contraindications: Hypersensitivity to guanabenz

Precautions: Pregnancy (C), lactation, children <12 yr, severe coronary insufficiency, recent myocardial infarction, cerebrovascular disease, severe hepatic or renal failure

Pharmacokinetics:

PO: Peak 2-4 hr; half-life 6 hr, excreted in urine

Interactions/incompatibilities:

• Increased sedation: CNS depressants

NURSING CONSIDERATIONS

Assess:

• Renal studies: protein, BUN, creatinine, watch for increased levels; may indicate nephrotic syndrome

• Baselines in renal, liver function tests before therapy begins

• K levels, although hyperkalemia rarely occurs

• Dip-stick of urine for protein qd in first morning specimen, if protein is increased a 24 hr urinary protein should be collected

• B/P during beginning treatment, periodically thereafter

Perform/provide:

• Storage of patches in cool environment, tablets in tight containers

Evaluate:

• Therapeutic response: decrease in B/P in hypertensives

• Edema in feet and legs daily

• Allergic reaction: rash, fever, pruritus, urticaria; drug should be discontinued if antihistamines fail to help

• Allergic reaction from patches: rash, urticaria, angioedema; should not continue to use

• Renal symptoms: polyuria, oliguria, frequency

Teach patient/family:

• To avoid hazardous activities

• Not to discontinue drug abruptly or withdrawal symptoms may occur: anxiety, increased B/P, headache, insomnia, increased pulse, tremors, nausea, sweating

• Not to use OTC (cough, cold, or allergy) products unless directed by physician

• Stress patient compliance with dosage schedule even if feeling better

• Notify physician of: swelling of hands or feet, irregular heartbeat, chest pain

• Excessive perspiration, dehydration, vomiting, diarrhea; may lead to fall in blood pressure—consult

---

*Available in Canada only

physician if these occur
• May cause dizziness, fainting; light-headedness may occur during 1st few days of therapy
• That compliance is necessary, not to skip or stop drug unless directed by physician
• May cause skin rash or impaired perspiration
Treatment of overdose: Administer vasopressor, discontinue drug, supine position

guanadrel sulfate

(gwahn'a-drel)
Hylorel

Func. class.: Antihypertensive
Chem. class.: Adrenergic blocker, guinidine derivative

Action: Inhibits sympathetic vasoconstriction by release of norepinephrine, depletes norepinephrine stores in adrenergic nerve endings

Uses: Hypertension

Dosage and routes:
• *Adult:* PO 5 mg bid, adjusted to desired response, may need 20-75 mg/day in divided doses

Available forms include: Tabs 10, 25 mg

Side effects/adverse reactions:
CV: Orthostatic hypotension, bradycardia, CHF, palpitations, chest pain, tachycardia, dysrhythmias

CNS: Drowsiness, fatigue, weakness, feeling of faintness, insomnia, dizziness, mental changes, memory loss, hallucinations, *depression,* anxiety, *confusion, paresthesias, headache*

GI: Nausea, cramps, diarrhea, constipation, dry mouth, anorexia, indigestion

INTEG: Rash, purpura, alopecia
*HEMA: **Agranulocytosis***
EENT: Nasal stuffiness, tinnitus, vi-

sual changes, sore throat, double vision, dry burning eyes
GU: Ejaculation failure, impotence, dysuria, nocturia, headache, frequency
RESP: ***Bronchospasm,*** dyspnea, cough, rales, SOB
MS: Leg cramps, aching, pain, inflammation

Contraindications: Hypersensitivity, pregnancy (B), pheochromocytoma, lactation, CHF, child <18 yr

Precautions: Elderly, bronchial asthma, peptic ulcer, electrolyte imbalances, vascular disease

Pharmacokinetics:
PO: Onset 0.5-2 hr, peak 3-5 hr, duration 4-14 hr; half-life 10-12 hr, excreted in urine (50% unchanged)

Interactions/incompatibilities:
• Increased hypotension: diuretics, other antihypertensives
• Do not use with MAOIs
• Increased orthostatic hypotension: alcohol
• Decreased hypotensive effect: tricyclic antidepressants, phenothiazines, ephedrine, phenylpropanolamine

NURSING CONSIDERATIONS

Assess:
• Renal function studies in renal impairment (BUN, creatinine)
• Bleeding time, check for ecchymosis, thrombocytopenia, purpura
• I&O in renal disease patient

Evaluate:
• Cardiac status: B/P, pulse, watch for hypotension
• Edema in feet, legs daily; take weight daily
• Skin turgor, dryness of mucous membranes for hydration status
• Symptoms of CHF: edema, dyspnea, wet rales

Teach patient/family:
• To avoid driving, hazardous activities if drowsiness occurs
• Not to discontinue drug abruptly

---

italics = common side effects   ***bold italic*** = life threatening reactions

• Not to use OTC products unless directed by physician: cough, cold preparations

• To report bradycardia, dizziness, confusion, depression, fever or sore throat

• That impotence, gynecomastia may occur but are reversible

• To rise slowly to sitting or standing position to minimize orthostatic hypotension

• That therapeutic effect may take 2-4 wk

---

guanethidine monosulfate

(gwahn-eth'i-deen)
Ismelin

Func. class.: Antihypertensive
Chem. class.: Antiadrenergic agent

Action: Inhibits norepinephrine release, depleting norepinephrine stores in adrenergic nerve endings
Uses: Hypertension
Dosage and routes:
• *Adult:* PO 10 mg qd, increase by 10 mg qwk at monthly intervals; may require 25-50 mg qd up to 300 mg
• *Adult:* (Hospitalized) 25-50 mg; may increase by 25-50 mg/day or every other day
• *Child:* PO 200 μg/kg/day; increase q7-10 days, not to exceed 3000 μg/kg/24 hr
Available forms include: Tabs 10, 25 mg
Side effects/adverse reactions:
CV: Orthostatic hypotension, dizziness, weakness, lassitude, bradycardia, CHF, fatigue, angina, heart block, chest paresthesia
CNS: Depression
GI: Nausea, vomiting, *diarrhea,* constipation, dry mouth, weight gain, anorexia
INTEG: Dermatitis, loss of scalp hair

HEMA: Thrombocytopenia, leukopenia
EENT: Nasal congestion, ptosis, blurred vision
GU: Ejaculation failure, impotence, nocturia, edema, retention, increased BUN
RESP: Dyspnea
Contraindications: Hypersensitivity, pheochromocytoma, recent MI, CHF, cardiac failure
Precautions: Pregnancy (B), lactation, peptic ulcer, asthma
Pharmacokinetics:
PO: Therapeutic level: 1-3 wk; half-life 5 days, metabolized by liver, excreted in urine (metabolites), breast milk
Interactions/incompatibilities:
• Increased hypotension: diuretics, other antihypertensives
• Do not use with MAOIs
• Increased orthostatic hypotension: alcohol
• Decreased hypotensive effect: tricyclic antidepressants, phenothiazines, ephedrine, phenylpropanolamine, oral contraceptives, thiothixine, doxepin, haloperidol, amphetamines
NURSING CONSIDERATIONS
Assess:
• Renal function studies in renal impairment (BUN, creatinine)
• Bleeding time, check for ecchymosis, thrombocytopenia, purpura
• I&O in renal disease patient
Evaluate:
• Cardiac status: B/P, pulse, watch for hypotension
• Edema in feet, legs daily; take weight daily
• Skin turgor, dryness of mucous membranes for hydration status
• Symptoms of CHF: edema, dyspnea, wet rales
Teach patient/family:
• To avoid driving, hazardous activities if drowsiness occurs
• Not to discontinue drug abruptly

• Not to use OTC products unless directed by physician: cough, cold preparations
• To report bradycardia, dizziness, confusion, depression, fever, sore throat
• That impotence, gynecomastia may occur, but are reversible
• To rise slowly to sitting or standing position to minimize orthostatic hypotension
• That therapeutic effect may take 2-4 wk

Lab test interferences:
Increase: BUN
Decrease: Blood glucose, VMA excretion, urinary norepinephrine
Treatment of overdose: Lavage, vasopressors given cautiously

---

haemophilus b polysaccharide vaccine

b-Capsa I
Func. class.: Vaccine

Action: Stimulates antibody production to *Haemophilus influenzae* b
Uses: Prevention of *Haemophilus influenzae* b
Dosage and routes:
• *Child 2-6 yr:* IM/SC 0.5 ml in 1 dose
Available forms include: Inj SC 25, 125, 250 μg
Side effects/adverse reactions:
CNS: Fever, irritability
INTEG: Skin abscess, urticaria, induration, warmth at site
SYST: **Anaphylaxis**
Contraindications: Hypersensitivity, active infection, poliomyelitis outbreak, immunosuppression
Precautions: Pregnancy
NURSING CONSIDERATIONS
Assess:
• For skin reactions: swelling, rash, urticaria

Administer:
• After diluting with 0.6 ml diluent, which will yield 10 doses of 0.5 ml
• Only with epinephrine 1 : 1000 on unit to treat laryngospasm
• Only by SC or IM route
Perform/provide:
• Storage in refrigerator
Evaluate:
• For history of allergies, skin conditions (eczema, psoriasis, dermatitis), reactions to vaccinations
• For anaphylaxis: inability to breathe, bronchospasm
Teach patient/family:
• That usually one dose is required
Lab test interferences:
Interfere: Latex agglutination, countercurrent immunoelectrophoresis

---

halazepam

(hal-az'e-pam)
Paxipam
Func. class.: Antianxiety
Chem. class.: Benzodiazepine

Controlled Substance Schedule IV
Action: Depresses subcortical levels of CNS, including limbic system, reticular formation
Uses: Anxiety
Dosage and routes:
• *Adult:* PO 20-40 mg tid-qid
• *Geriatric:* PO 20 mg qd-bid
Available forms include: Tabs 20, 40 mg
Side effects/adverse reactions:
CNS: Dizziness, drowsiness, confusion, headache, anxiety, tremors, stimulation, fatigue, depression, insomnia, hallucinations
GI: Constipation, dry mouth, nausea, vomiting, anorexia, diarrhea
INTEG: Rash, dermatitis, itching
CV: Orthostatic hypotension, **ECG**

---

italics = common side effects   **bold italic** = life threatening reactions

changes, tachycardia, hypotension

EENT: Blurred vision, tinnitus, mydriasis

Contraindications: Hypersensitivity to benzodiazepines, narrowangle glaucoma, psychosis, pregnancy (D), child <18 yr

Precautions: Elderly, debilitated, hepatic disease, renal disease

Pharmacokinetics:

PO: Peak 1-3 hr, duration 3-6 hr, metabolized by liver, excreted by kidneys, crosses placenta, breast milk, half-life 14 hr

Interactions/incompatibilities:

• Decreased effects of this drug: oral contraceptives, rifampin, valproic acid

• Increased effects of this drug: CNS depressants, alcohol, cimetidine, disulfiram, oral contraceptives

NURSING CONSIDERATIONS

Assess:

• B/P (↓lying, standing), pulse; if systolic B/P drops 20 mm Hg, hold drug, notify physician, respirations q5-15 min if given IV

• Blood studies: CBC during longterm therapy, blood dyscrasias have occurred rarely

• Hepatic studies: AST, ALT, bilirubin, creatinine, LDH, alk phosphatase

Administer:

• With food or milk for GI symptoms

• Crushed if patient is unable to swallow medication whole

• Sugarless gum, hard candy, frequent sips of water for dry mouth

Perform/provide:

• Assistance with ambulation during beginning therapy, since drowsiness/dizziness occurs

• Safety measures, including siderails

• Check to see PO medication has been swallowed

Evaluate:

• Therapeutic response: decreased anxiety, restlessness, sleeplessness

• Mental status: mood, sensorium, affect, sleeping pattern, drowsiness, dizziness

• Physical dependency, withdrawal symptoms: headache, nausea, vomiting, muscle pain, weakness after long-term use

• Suicidal tendencies

Teach patient/family:

• That drug may be taken with food

• Not to be used for everyday stress or used longer than 4 mo, unless directed by physician

• Avoid OTC preparations (hay fever, cough, cold) unless approved by physician

• To avoid driving or other activities that require alertness; drowsiness may occur

• To avoid alcohol ingestion or other psychotropic medications, unless prescribed by physician

• Not to discontinue medication abruptly after long-term use

• To rise slowly or fainting may occur

• That drowsiness might worsen at beginning of treatment

Lab test interferences:

Increase: AST/ALT, serum bilirubin

False increase: 17-OHCS

Decrease: RAIU

Treatment of overdose: Lavage, VS, supportive care

---

halcinonide

(hal-sin'oo-nide)

Halog

Func. class.: Corticosteroid, synthetic

Chem. class.: Fluorinated corticosteroid

Action: Antiinflammatory, antipruritic, vasoconstrictor actions

---

Uses: Inflammation of corticosteroid-responsive dermatoses

Dosage and routes:
• *Adult:* TOP apply to affected area bid-tid

Available forms include: Cream 0.025%, 0.1%; oint 0.1%; sol 0.1%

Side effects/adverse reactions:
INTEG: Acne, atrophy, epidermal thinning, purpura, striae

Contraindications: Hypersensitivity, viral infections, fungal infections

Precautions: Pregnancy

Interactions/incompatibilities: None known

NURSING CONSIDERATIONS

Administer:
• Using an occlusive dressing
• For 3-5 days after lesions are gone

Perform/provide:
• Washing of skin before application
• Dressing change qd, check area for redness, rash, inflammation, discoloration; do not leave dressing in place over 16 hr

Evaluate:
• Therapeutic response: decreased inflammation
• Infection: increased temperature, WBC, even after withdrawal of medication; keep in mind these may be systemically absorbed

Teach patient/family:
• Not to get drug in eyes or mucous membranes

haloperidol/haloperidol decanoate

(ha-loe-per'idole)

Haldol, Haldol Enthante, Peridol/ Haloperidol Decanoate

Func. class.: Antipsychotic/neuroleptic

Chem. class.: Butyrophenone

Action: Depresses cerebral cortex, hypothalamus, limbic system, which control activity and aggression; blocks neurotransmission produced by dopamine at synapse; exhibits strong α-adrenergic, anticholinergic blocking action; mechanism for antipsychotic effects is unclear.

Uses: Psychotic disorders, control of tics, vocal utterances in Tourette syndrome, short-term treatment of hyperactive children showing excessive motor activity, prolonged parenteral therapy in chronic schizophrenia

Dosage and routes:

Psychosis
• *Adult:* PO 0.5-5 mg bid or tid initially depending on severity of condition; dose is increased to desired dose, max 100 mg/day; IM 2-5 mg q4-8h
• *Child 3-12 yr:* PO/IM 0.05-0.15 mg/kg/day

Chronic schizophrenia
• *Adult:* IM 10-15 times the PO dose q4 wk (decanoate)
• *Child 3-12 yr:* PO/IM 0.05-0.15 mg/kg/day

Tics/vocal utterances
• *Adult:* PO 0.5-5 mg bid or tid increased until desired response occurs
• *Child 3-12 yr:* PO 0.05-0.075 mg/kg/day

Hyperactive Children
• *Child 3-12 yr:* PO 0.05-0.075 mg/kg/day

H

---

italics = common side effects   ***bold italic*** = life threatening reactions

Available forms include: Tabs 0.5, 1, 2, 5, 10, 20 mg; conc 2 mg/ml; inj IM 50 mg/ml

Side effects/adverse reactions:

*RESP: **Laryngospasm,** dyspnea, **respiratory depression***

*CNS: Extrapyramidal symptoms: pseudoparkinsonism, akathisia, dystonia, tardive dyskinesia, drowsiness, headache, **seizures***

INTEG: Rash, photosensitivity, dermatitis

EENT: Blurred vision, glaucoma

GI: Dry mouth, nausea, vomiting, anorexia, constipation, diarrhea, jaundice, weight gain

GU: Urinary retention, urinary frequency, enuresis, impotence, amenorrhea, gynecomastia

CV: Orthostatic hypotension, hypertension, **cardiac arrest,** ECG changes, **tachycardia**

Contraindications: Hypersensitivity, blood dyscrasias, coma, child <3 yr, brain damage, bone marrow depression, alcohol and barbiturate withdrawal states

Precautions: Pregnancy, lactation, seizure disorders, hypertension, hepatic disease, cardiac disease

Pharmacokinetics:

PO: Onset erratic, peak 2-6 hr, half-life 24 hr

IM: Onset 15-30 min, peak 15-20 min, half-life 21 hr

IM (Decanoate): Peak 4-11 days, half-life 3 wk

Metabolized by liver, excreted in urine, bile, crosses placenta, enters breast milk

Interactions/incompatibilities:

• Oversedation: other CNS depressants, alcohol, barbiturate anesthetics

• Toxicity: epinephrine

• Decreased effects of: lithium, levodopa

• Increased effects of both drugs: β-adrenergic blockers, alcohol

• Increased anticholinergic effects: anticholinergics

NURSING CONSIDERATIONS

Assess:

• Swallowing of PO medication; check for hoarding or giving of medication to other patients

• I&O ratio; palpate bladder if low urinary output occurs

• Bilirubin, CBC, liver function studies monthly

• Urinalysis is recommended before and during prolonged therapy

Administer:

• Antiparkinsonian agent, to be used if EPS occur

• IM injection into large muscle mass

Perform/provide:

• Decreased noise input by dimming lights, avoiding loud noises

• Supervised ambulation until stabilized on medication; do not involve in strenuous exercise program because fainting is possible; patient should not stand still for long periods of time

• Increased fluids to prevent constipation

• Sips of water, candy, gum for dry mouth

• Storage in tight, light-resistant container

Evaluate:

• Therapeutic response: decrease in emotional excitement, hallucinations, delusions, paranoia, reorganization of patterns of thought, speech

• Affect, orientation, LOC, reflexes, gait, coordination, sleep pattern disturbances

• B/P standing and lying; take pulse and respirations q4h during initial treatment; establish baseline before starting treatment; report drops of 30 mm Hg

• Dizziness, faintness, palpitations, tachycardia on rising

• EPS including akathisia (inability

to sit still, no pattern to movements), tardive dyskinesia (bizarre movements of jaw, mouth, tongue, extremities), pseudoparkinsonism (rigidity, tremors, pill rolling, shuffling gait)
• Skin turgor daily
• Constipation, urinary retention daily; if these occur, increase bulk, water in diet

Teach patient/family:
• That orthostatic hypotension occurs often, and to rise from sitting or lying position gradually
• To remain lying down after IM injection for at least 30 min
• To avoid hot tubs, hot showers, or tub baths since hypotension may occur
• To avoid abrupt withdrawal of this drug or EPS may result; drug should be withdrawn slowly
• To avoid OTC preparations (cough, hayfever, cold) unless approved by physician since serious drug interactions may occur; avoid use with alcohol or CNS depressants, increased drowsiness may occur
• To use a sunscreen during sun exposure to prevent burns
• Regarding compliance with drug regimen
• About EPS and necessity for meticulous oral hygiene since oral candidiasis may occur
• To report impaired vision, jaundice, tremors, muscle twitching
• In hot weather, heat stroke may occur; take extra precautions to stay cool

Lab test interferences:
Increase: Liver function tests, cardiac enzymes, cholesterol, blood glucose, prolactin, bilirubin, PBI, cholinesterase, ^{131}I
Decrease: Hormones (blood, urine)
False positive: Pregnancy tests, PKU

False negative: Urinary steroids
Treatment of overdose: Lavage, if orally injested, provide an airway; *do not induce vomiting*

haloprogin (topical)

(ha-loe-proe′jin)
Halotex
Func. class.: Local antiinfective
Chem. class.: Iodinated phenolic ester

Action: Interferes with fungal DNA replication
Uses: Tinea pedis, tinea cruris, tinea corporis, tinea manus, tinea versicolor
Dosage and routes:
• *Adult and child:* TOP apply to affected area bid × 14-21 days
Available forms include: Cream, sol 1%
Side effects/adverse reactions:
INTEG: Rash, urticaria, stinging, burning, vesiculation, maceration, pruritus
Contraindications: Hypersensitivity
Precautions: Pregnancy (B), lactation
Interactions/incompatibilities: None known
NURSING CONSIDERATIONS
Administer:
• Enough medication to completely cover lesions
• After cleansing with soap, water before each application, dry well
Perform/provide:
• Storage at room temperature in dry place
Evaluate:
• Allergic reaction: burning, stinging, swelling, redness
• Therapeutic response: decrease in size, number of lesions
Teach patient/family:
• To apply with glove to prevent further infection

- To avoid use of OTC creams, ointments, lotions unless directed by physician
- To use medical asepsis (hand washing) before, after each application
- To avoid contact with eyes

---

heparin calcium/heparin sodium

(hep'a-rin)

Calciparine, Calcilean*/Hepalean,* Hep Lock

Func. class.: Anticoagulant

Action: Prevents conversion of fibrinogen to fibrin

Uses: Deep vein thrombosis, pulmonary emboli, myocardial infarction, open heart surgery, disseminated intravascular clotting syndrome, atrial fibrillation with embolization

Dosage and routes:

Deep vein thrombosis/MI

- *Adult:* IV PUSH 5000-7000 U, then titrated to PTT level q4h; IV BOL 5000-7500 U, then IV INF; IV INF After bolus dose, then 1000 U/hr titrated to PTT level
- *Child:* IV INF 50 U/kg, maintenance 100 U/kg q4h or 20,000 U/m² qd

Pulmonary embolism

- *Adult:* IV PUSH 7500-10,000, then titrated to PTT level q4h; IV BOL 7500-10,000 U, then IV INF; IV INF After bolus dose, then 1000 U/hr titrated to PTT level
- *Child:* IV INF 50 U/kg, maintenance 100 U/kg q4h or 20,000 U/m² qd

Open heart surgery

- *Adult:* IV INF 150-300 U/kg

Available forms include: (Heparin sodium) inj 1000, 5000, 20,000, 40,000 U/ml; (Heparin calcium) inj 5000, 12,500, 20,000 U/dose

Side effects/adverse reactions:

GI: Diarrhea, nausea, vomiting, anorexia, stomatitis, abdominal cramps, *hepatitis*

GU: Hematuria

INTEG: Rash, dermatitis, urticaria, alopecia, pruritus

CNS: Fever

HEMA: Hemorrhage, agranulocytosis, leukopenia

Contraindications: Hypersensitivity, hemophilia, leukemia with bleeding, peptic ulcer disease, thrombocytopenic purpura, hepatic disease (severe), renal disease (severe), blood dyscrasias, pregnancy, severe hypertension, subacute bacterial endocarditis, acute nephritis

Precautions: Alcoholism, elderly

Pharmacokinetics:

IV: Peak 5 min, duration 2-6 hr

SC: Onset 20-60 min, duration 8-12 hr

Half-life 1½ hr, excreted in urine

Interactions/incompatibilities:

- Increased action: oral anticoagulants, salicylates, digitalis, dextran, steroids, indomethacin, ibuprofen, antigout drugs, probenecid, dipyridamole, oral contraceptives

NURSING CONSIDERATIONS

Assess:

- Blood studies (Hct, platelets, occult blood in stools) q3 mo
- Partial prothrombin time, which should be 1½-2 × control, PTT; often done qd
- B/P, watch for increasing signs of hypertension

Administer:

- At same time each day to maintain steady blood levels
- Alone, do not give with water
- Avoiding all IM injections that may cause bleeding

Perform/provide:

- Storage in tight container

Evaluate:

- Therapeutic response: decrease of deep vein thrombosis

• Bleeding gums, petecchiae, ecchymosis, black tarry stools, hematuria
• Fever, skin rash, urticaria
• Needed dosage change q 1-2 wk

Teach patient/family:
• To avoid OTC preparations that may cause serious drug interactions unless directed by physician
• That urine may turn orange/red
• Drug may be held during active bleeding (menstruation)
• To use soft-bristle toothbrush to avoid bleeding gums
• To carry a Medic-Alert ID identifying drug taken
• Stress patient compliance
• On all aspects of adjustments: dosage, route, action, side effects, when to notify physician
• To report any signs of bleeding: gums, under skin, urine, stools
• To avoid hazardous activities (football, hockey, skiing) or dangerous work

Lab test interferences:
Increase: T_3 uptake
Decrease: Uric acid

Treatment of overdose:
Protamine SO_4

---

heparin sodium/dihydroergotamine mesylate

(hep'a-rin)
Embolex

Func. class.: Anticoagulant
Chem. class.: Anionic

Action: Dihydroergotamine directly stimulates smooth muscle of peripheral blood vessels; heparin prevents conversion of fibrinogen to fibrin

Uses: Deep vein thrombosis, pulmonary emboli in patients undergoing major surgery

Dosage and routes:
• *Adult:* SC 1 amp 2 hr before surgery, q12 hr if needed × 5-7 days
Available forms include: Inj 5000 U heparin, 0.5 mg dihydroergotamine, 7.46 lidocaine HCl/0.7 ml

Side effects/adverse reactions:
GI: Nausea, vomiting, anorexia, abdominal pain
GV: Chest pain, tachycardia, bradycardia, hypertension
GU: Hematuria
INTEG: Rash, dermatitis, urticaria, ecchymosis, hematoma at injection site
CNS: Fever
HEMA: Hemorrhage

Contraindications: Hypersensitivity, hemophilia, leukemia with bleeding, peptic ulcer disease, thrombocytopenic purpura, hepatic disease (severe), renal disease (severe), severe hypertension, blood dyscrasias, pregnancy, subacute bacterial endocarditis, acute nephritis

Precautions: Alcoholism, elderly

Pharmacokinetics:
SC: Peak 4 hr, half-life 3-5 hr (heparin) 1-2 hr (DHE)

Interactions/incompatibilities:
• Decreased platelet aggregation with salicylates, dextran, phenylbutazone, ibuprofen, indomethacin, dipyridamole, hydroxychloroquine

NURSING CONSIDERATIONS
Assess:
• Blood studies (Hct, platelets, occult blood in stools) q3 mo
• Prothrombin time, which should be 1½-2 × control, PT; often done qd
• B/P, watch for increasing signs of hypertension

Administer:
• At same time each day to maintain steady blood levels
• Alone, do not give with food

H

• Avoiding all IM injections that may cause bleeding
Perform/provide:
• Storage in tight container
Evaluate:
• Therapeutic response: decrease of deep vein thrombosis
• Bleeding gums, petechiae, ecchymosis, black tarry stools, hematuria
• Fever, skin rash, urticaria
• Needed dosage change q1-2 wk
Teach patient/family:
• To avoid OTC preparations (aspirin-containing products) that may cause serious drug interactions, unless directed by physician
• That urine may turn orange/red
• Drug may be held during active bleeding (menstruation)
• To use soft-bristle toothbrush to avoid bleeding gums
• To carry a Medic-Alert ID identifying drug taken
• Stress patient compliance
• On all aspects of adjustments: dosage, route, action, side effects, when to notify physician
• To report any signs of bleeding: gums, under skin, urine, stools
• To avoid hazardous activities (football, hockey, skiing) or dangerous work
Lab test interferences:
Increase: Liver function studies
Treatment of overdose: Discontinue drug, administer vasodilators, protamine sulfate

---

hepatitis B vaccine
Heptavax-B
Func. class.: Vaccine

Action: Provides active immunity to hepatitis B
Uses: Prevention of hepatitis B virus
Dosage and routes:
• *Adult and child >10 yr:* IM 1 ml,

then 1 ml after 1 mo, then 1 ml 6 mo after initial dose
• *Child 3 mo-10 yr:* IM 0.5 ml, then 0.5 ml after 1 mo, then 0.5 ml 6 mo after initial dose
• *Patients with decreased immunity:* IM 2 ml, then 2 ml after 1 mo, then 2 ml 6 mo after initial dose
Available forms include: Inj IM 10 mg/0.5 ml, 20 μg/ml
Side effects/adverse reactions:
INTEG: Soreness at injection site, urticaria, erythema, swelling
SYST: Induration
CNS: Headache, dizziness, fever
GI: Nausea, vomiting
Contraindications: Hypersensitivity
Precautions: Pregnancy, elderly, lactation, children
NURSING CONSIDERATIONS
Assess:
• For skin reactions: rash, induration, urticaria
Administer:
• After rotating vial, do not shake
• Only with epinephrine 1:1000 on unit to treat laryngospasm
• In deltoid for better protection
Evaluate:
• For history of allergies, skin conditions (eczema, psoriasis, dermatitis), reactions to vaccinations
• For anaphylaxis: inability to breathe, bronchospasm

---

hetacillin
(het-a-sill'in)
Versapen, Versapen K
Func. class.: Broad-spectrum antibiotic
Chem. class.: Penicillin

Action: Interferes with cell wall replication of susceptible organisms; osmotically unstable cell wall swells, bursts from osmotic pressure; it is an inactive compound that is converted to ampicillin

Uses: Effective for gram-positive cocci (*S. aureus, S. faecalis, S. pneumoniae*), gram-negative cocci (*N. gonorrhoeae, N. meningitis*), gram-positive bacilli (*B. anthracis, C. perfringens, C. tetani, L. monocytogenes*), gram-negative bacilli (*E. coli*), *P. mirabilis, H. influenzae, Salmonella, Shigella*

Dosage and routes:
• *Adult:* PO 225-450 mg q6h
• *Child:* PO 22.5-45 mg/kg/day in divided doses q6h

Available forms include: Caps 225 mg; powder for oral susp 112.5, 225 mg/5 ml

Side effects/adverse reactions:
HEMA: Anemia, increased bleeding time, **bone marrow depression, granulocytopenia**

GI: Nausea, vomiting, diarrhea, increased AST, ALT, abdominal pain, glossitis, colitis

GU: Oliguria, proteinuria, hematuria, *vaginitis, moniliasis,* **glomerulonephritis**

CNS: Lethargy, hallucinations, anxiety, depression, twitching, **coma, convulsions**

META: Hyperkalemia, hypokalemia, alkalosis, hypernatremia

Contraindications: Hypersensitivity to penicillins; neonates

Precautions: Hypersensitivity to cephalosporins

Pharmacokinetics:
PO: Peak 2 hr, duration 8-10 hr; partially metabolized in liver, excreted in urine, bile, breast milk, crosses placenta

Interactions/incompatibilities:
• Decreased antimicrobial effectiveness of this drug: tetracyclines, erythromycins
• Increased penicillin concentrations when used with: aspirin, probenecid

NURSING CONSIDERATIONS
Assess:
• I&O ratio; report hematuria, oliguria since penicillin in high doses is nephrotoxic
• Any patient with compromised renal system since drug is excreted slowly in poor renal system function; toxicity may occur rapidly
• Liver studies: AST, ALT
• Blood studies: WBC, RBC, H&H, bleeding time
• Renal studies: urinalysis, protein, blood
• C&S before drug therapy; drug may be taken as soon as culture is taken

Administer:
• Drug after C&S has been completed

Perform/provide:
• Adrenalin, suction, tracheostomy set, endotracheal intubation equipment
• Adequate fluid intake (2000 ml) during diarrhea episodes
• Scratch test to assess allergy, after securing order from physician; usually done when penicillin is only drug of choice
• Storage in tight container

Evaluate:
• Therapeutic effectiveness: absence of fever, draining wounds
• Bowel pattern before, during treatment
• Skin eruptions after administration of penicillin to 1 wk after discontinuing drug
• Respiratory status: rate, character, wheezing, tightness in chest
• Allergies before initiation of treatment, reaction of each medication; highlight allergies on chart, Kardex

Teach patient/family:
• Aspects of drug therapy, including need to complete course of medication to ensure organism death (10-14 days); culture may be taken after completed course
• To report sore throat, fever, fa-

---

italics = common side effects   ***bold italic*** = life threatening reactions

tigue; could indicate superimposed infection

• To wear or carry Medic Alert ID if allergic to penicillins

• To notify nurse of diarrhea stools

Lab test interferences:

Decrease: Uric acid

False positive: Urine glucose, urine protein

Treatment of overdose: Withdraw drug, maintain airway, administer epinephrine, aminophylline, O_2, IV corticosteroids for anaphylaxis

---

hetastarch

(het′a-starch)

HES, Hespan, Volex

Func. class.: Plasma expander

Chem. class.: Synthetic polymer

Action: Similar to human albumin, which expands plasma volume by colloidal osmotic pressure

Uses: Plasma volume expander

Dosage and routes:

• *Adult:* IV INF 500-1000 ml, not to exceed 1500 ml/day, not to exceed 20 ml/kg/hr (hemorrhagic shock)

Available forms include: 6% hetastarch/0.9% NaCl

Side effects/adverse reactions:

HEMA: Decreased hematocrit, increased bleeding/coagulation times

INTEG: Rash, urticaria, pruritus, angioedema, chills, fever, flushing

RESP: Wheezing, dyspnea, ***bronchospasm, pulmonary edema***

GI: Nausea, vomiting

SYST: ***Anaphylaxis***

CNS: Chills, increased temperature, headache

Contraindications: Hypersensitivity, severe bleeding disorders, renal failure, CHF (severe)

Precautions: Pregnancy

Pharmacokinetics:

IV: Expands blood volume 1-

2 × amount infused, excreted in urine and feces

Interactions/incompatibilities: None known

NURSING CONSIDERATIONS

Assess:

• VS q5 min × 30 min

• CVP during infusion (5-10 sm H_2—normal range)

• Urine output q1h, watch for increase in urinary output, which is common; if output does not increase, infusion should be decreased or discontinued

• I&O ratio and specific gravity, urine osmolarity; if specific gravity is very low, renal clearance is low, drug should be discontinued

Administer:

• After crossmatch is drawn, if blood is to be given also

• Dextran 1 (Promit) to prevent anaphylaxis

Perform/provide:

• Storage at constant temperature 25° C (77° F); discard unused portions

Evaluate:

• Allergy: rash, urticaria, pruritus, wheezing, dyspnea, bronchospasm, drug should be discontinued immediately

• For circulatory overload: increased pulse, respirations, SOB, wheezing, chest tightness, chest pain

• For dehydration after infusion: decreased output, increased temperature, poor skin turgor, increased specific gravity, dry skin

Lab test interferences:

False increase: Blood glucose, urinary protein, bilirubin, total protein

Interferes: Rh test, blood typing/crossmatching

---

hexachlorophene

(hex-a-klor'oh-fenn)

Germa-Medica (MG), pHisoHex, pHisoScrub, Sept-Soft, WescoHEX

Func. class.: Disinfectant

Chem. class.: Polychlorinated phenol derivative

Action: Inhibits growth of gram-positive bacteria

Uses: Surgical scrub, bacteriostatic skin cleanser, gram-positive infection when other treatment has been ineffective

Dosage and routes:

• *Adult and child:* SOAP/EMUL Wash area

Available forms include: Soap, emul 3%

Side effects/adverse reactions:

INTEG: Irritation, dryness, dermatitis, scaling, photosensitivity (rare)

GI: Nausea, vomiting, diarrhea

CNS: Delirium, convulsions, restlessness, headache, confusion, tremors dizziness

Contraindications: Hypersensitivity, application to mucous membrane, occlusive dressings, infants, burns, denuded skin

Interactions/incompatibilities: None known

NURSING CONSIDERATIONS

Administer:

• To body areas only; do not apply to face, lips, mouth, eyes, mucous membrane, anus, meatus

• Only to adults; repeated use may lead to systemic absorption

Evaluate:

• Area of body involved: irritation, rash, breaks, dryness, scales

Teach patient/family:

• To report itching, irritation, dizziness, headache, confusion; discontinue drug immediately

Treatment of ingestion: Gastric lavage, administer vegetable oil, saline laxative, supportive treatment

hexocyclium methylsulfate

(hex-oh-sye'klee-um)

Tral

Func. class.: Gastrointestinal anticholinergic

Chem. class.: Synthetic quaternary ammonium compound

Action: Inhibits muscarinic actions of acetylcholine at postganglionic parasympathetic neuroeffector sites

Uses: Treatment of peptic ulcer disease in combination with other drugs; other GI disorders

Dosage and routes:

• *Adult:* PO 25 mg qid ac, hs; TIME REL 50 mg qd or bid

Available forms include: Tabs 25 mg; tabs time rel 50 mg

Side effects/adverse reactions:

CNS: Confusion, stimulation in elderly, headache, insomnia, dizziness, drowsiness, anxiety, weakness, hallucination

GI: Dry mouth, constipation, paralytic ileus, heartburn, nausea, vomiting, dysphagia, absence of taste

GU: Hesitancy, retention, impotence

CV: Palpitations, tachycardia

EENT: Blurred vision, photophobia, mydriasis, cycloplegia, increased ocular tension

INTEG: Urticaria, rash, pruritus, anhidrosis, fever, allergic reactions

Contraindications: Hypersensitivity to anticholinergics, narrow-angle glaucoma, GI obstruction, myasthenia gravis, paralytic ileus, GI atony, toxic megacolon

Precautions: Hyperthyroidism, coronary artery disease, dysrhythmias, CHF, ulcerative colitis, hypertension, hiatal hernia, hepatic disease, renal disease

Pharmacokinetics:

PO: Onset 1 hr, duration 3-4 hr; metabolized by liver, excreted in urine

Interactions/incompatibilities:

• Increased anticholinergic effect: amantadine, tricyclic antidepressants, MAOIs

• Increased effect of: nitrofurantoin

• Decreased effect of: phenothiazines, levodopa

NURSING CONSIDERATIONS

Assess:

• VS, cardiac status: checking for dysrhythmias, increased rate, palpitations

• I&O ratio; check for urinary retention or hesitancy

Administer:

• ½-1 hr ac for better absorption

• Decreased dose to elderly patients; their metabolism may be slowed

• Gum, hard candy, frequent rinsing of mouth for dryness of oral cavity

Perform/provide:

• Storage in tight container protected from light

• Increased fluids, bulk, exercise to patient's lifestyle to decrease constipation

Evaluate:

• Therapeutic response: absence of epigastric pain, bleeding, nausea, vomiting

• GI complaints: pain, bleeding (frank or occult), nausea, vomiting, anorexia

Teach patient/family:

• Avoid driving or other hazardous activities until stabilized on medication

• Avoid alcohol or other CNS depressants; will enhance sedating properties of drug

• To avoid hot environments,

stroke may occur, drug suppresses perspiration

• Use sunglasses when outside to prevent photophobia

---

homatropine hydrobromide (optic)

(hoe′ma-troe-peen)

Homatrocel, Isopto Homatropine, Murrocoll Homatropine

Func. class.: Mydriatic

Chem. class.: Synthetic alkaloid

Action: Blocks response of iris sphincter muscle, muscle of accommodation of ciliary body to cholinergic simulation, resulting in dilation, paralysis of accommodation

Uses: Uveitis, cycloplegic refraction

Dosage and routes:

• *Adult and child:* INSTILL 1-2 gtts repeat in 5-10 min for refraction or q3-4h for uveitis

Available forms include: Sol 2%, 5%

Side effects/adverse reactions:

CV: Tachycardia

CNS: Confusion, somnolence, flushing, fever

EENT: Blurred vision, photophobia, increased intraocular pressure, irritation, edema

Contraindications: Hypersensitivity, children <6 yr, narrow-angle glaucoma, increased intraocular pressure, infants

Precautions: Children, elderly, hypertension, hyperthyroidism, diabetes

Pharmacokinetics:

INSTILL: Peak ½-1 hr, duration 1-3 days

Interactions/incompatibilities: None known

NURSING CONSIDERATIONS

Evaluate:

• Therapeutic response: decrease in

inflammation or cycloplegic refraction

• Eye pain, discontinue use

Teach patient/family:

• To report change in vision, blurring or loss of sight, trouble breathing, sweating, flushing

• Method of instillation: pressure on lacrimal sac for 1 min, do not touch dropper to eye

• That blurred vision will decrease with repeated use of drug

• Not to engage in hazardous activities until able to see

• Wait 5 min to use other drops

• Do not blink more than usual

hyaluronidase

(hye-l-yoor-on'i-dase)

Wydase

Func. class.: Enzyme

Action: Hydrolyzes hyaluronic within areas filled with exudates

Uses: Hypodermoclysis, subcutaneous urography, adjunct to dispersion of other drugs

Dosage and routes:

Adjunct

• *Adult and child:* INJ 150 U with other drug

Urography

• *Adult and child:* SC 75 U over scapula, then contrast medium is injected at same site

Hypodermoclysis

• *Adult and child >3 yr:* SC 150 U/L of clysis sol for 1000 ml of clysis sol

Available forms include: Inj powder 150, 1500 U; inj sol 150 U/ml

Side effects/adverse reactions:

INTEG: Rash, urticaria, itching

Contraindications: Hypersensitivity to bovine products, CHF, hypoproteinemia

NURSING CONSIDERATIONS

Administer:

• After test dose: 0.02 ml of 150

u/ml solution is injected if wheal develops, itching test is positive

• Right after mixing since solution is unstable

Evaluate:

• Therapeutic response: absence of swelling, pain after hypodermoclysis

hydralazine HCl

(hye'dral'a-zeen)

Apresoline, Hydralyn, Rolazine

Func. class.: Antihypertensive, direct-acting peripheral vasodilator

Chem. class.: Phthalazine

Action: Vasodilates arteriolar smooth muscle by direct relaxation; reduction in blood pressure with reflex increases in cardiac function

Uses: Essential hypertension; *parenteral:* severe essential hypertension

Dosage and routes:

• *Adult:* PO 10 mg qid 2-4 days, then 25 mg for rest of 1st wk, then 50 mg qid individualized to desired response, not to exceed 300 mg; IV/IM BOL 20-40 mg q4-6h, administer PO as soon as possible; IM 20-40 mg q4-6h

• *Child:* PO 0.75 mg/kg qd 0.75-3 mg/kg/day 2-4 in 4 divided doses; max 7.5 mg/kg/24 hr; IV BOL 0.1-0.2 mg/kg q4-6h; IM 0.1-0.2 mg/kg q4-6h

Available forms include: Inj IV, IM 20 mg/ml; tabs 10, 25, 50, 100 mg

Side effects/adverse reactions:

MISC: Nasal congestion, muscle cramps, *lupus-like symptoms*

CV: Palpitations, reflex tachycardia, angina, shock, edema, rebound hypertension

CNS: Headache, tremors, dizziness, anxiety, peripheral neuritis, depression

GI: Nausea, vomiting, anorexia, diarrhea, constipation

---

italics = common side effects **bold italic** = life threatening reactions

INTEG: Rash, pruritus
HEMA: **Leukopenia, agranulocytosis,** anemia
GU: Impotence, urinary retention
Contraindications: Hypersensitivity to hydralazines, coronary artery disease, mitral valvular rheumatic heart disease, rheumatic heart disease
Precautions: Pregnancy (C), CVA, advanced renal disease
Pharmacokinetics:
PO: Onset 20-30 min, peak 1 hr, duration 2-4 hr
IM: Onset 5-10 min, peak 1 hr, duration 2-4 hr
IV: Onset 5-20 min, peak 10-80 min, duration 2-6 hr
Half-life 2-8 hr, metabolized by liver, less than 10% present in urine
Interactions/incompatibilities:
• Increased tachycardia, angina: sympathomimetics (epinephrine, norepinephrine)
• Increased effects of: β-blockers
• Use MAOIs with caution in patients receiving hydralazine
• Do not mix with any drug in syringe or solution
NURSING CONSIDERATIONS
Assess:
• B/P q5 min × 2 hr, then q1h × 2 hr, then q4h
• Pulse, jugular venous distention q4h
• Electrolytes, blood studies: potassium, sodium, chloride, CO_2, CBC, serum glucose
• Weight daily, I&O
• LE prep, ANA titer before starting therapy
Administer:
• To patient in recumbent position, keep in that position for 1 hr after administration
Evaluate:
• Edema in feet, legs daily
• Skin turgor, dryness of mucous membranes for hydration status
• Rales, dyspnea, orthopnea

• IV site for extravasation, rate
• Fever, joint pain, tachycardia, palpitations, headache, nausea
• Mental status: affect, mood, behavior, anxiety; check for personality changes
Teach patient/family:
• To take with food to increase bioavailability
• To avoid OTC preparations unless directed by physician
• To notify physician if chest pain, severe fatigue, fever, muscle or joint pain occurs
Treatment of overdose: Administer vasopressors, volume expanders for shock; if PO lavage or give activated charcoal digitalization

---

hydriodic acid
(hye-drye-oo′-dick)
Func. class.: Expectorant
Chem. class.: Iodine derivative

Action: Increases respiratory tract fluid by decreasing surface tension, adhesiveness, which increases removal of mucus
Uses: Nonproductive cough associated with chronic bronchitis, bronchial asthma, bronchiectasis, emphysema
Dosage and routes:
• *Adult:* PO 1.25-5 ml bid-tid
• *Child >1 yr:* PO 1-10 gtts tid after meals
Available forms include: Sol 70 mg/5 ml
Side effects/adverse reactions:
EENT: Tooth damage
ENDO: Iodism, goiter, myxedema
*INTEG: **Angioedema***
Contraindications: Hypersensitivity to iodides, pulmonary TB, pregnancy, hyperthyroidism, hyperkalemia, acute bronchitis
Precautions: Hypothyroidism, cystic fibrosis, lactation

Pharmacokinetics: Excreted in urine

Interactions/incompatibilities:
• Increased hypothyroid effects: lithium, antithyroid drugs
• Dysrhythmias, hyperkalemia: potassium-sparing diuretics, potassium-containing medication

NURSING CONSIDERATIONS
Administer:
• Decreased dose to elderly patients; their metabolism may be slowed

Perform/provide:
• Storage at room temperature; do not use discolored solution
• Increased fluids to liquefy secretions

Evaluate:
• Therapeutic response: absence of cough
• Cough: type, frequency, character including sputum

Teach patient/family:
• To avoid smoking, smoke-filled rooms, perfumes, dust, environmental pollutants, cleaners

---

hydrochloric acid

Func. class.: Acidifier
Chem. class.: Hydrochloric acid

Action: Necessary for electrolyte balance; needed for pancreatic/hepatic functioning (conversion of pepsinogen to pepsin)
Uses: Alkalosis (metabolic)
Dosage and routes:
• *Adult:* PO 2-8 ml tid (10% sol)
Available forms include: Liquid
Side effects/adverse reactions:
EENT: Damage to teeth enamel
GI: Hyperacidity
META: Acidosis
Contraindications: Hypersensitivity, peptic ulcer disease, hyperacidity
Pharmacokinetics: Not known

Interactions/incompatibilities:
None known
NURSING CONSIDERATIONS
Assess:
• Respiratory rate, rhythm, depth, notify physician of abnormalities
• Electrolytes and CO_2 before, during treatment
• Urine pH during beginning treatment; <4.5 indicates acidosis
Administer:
• After diluting in 200-250 ml of water
Evaluate:
• Metabolic acidosis: apathy, confusion, stupor, coma, Kussmaul respirations, cardiac dysrhythmias

---

hydrochlorothiazide

(hye-droe-klor-oh-thye′a-zide)
Chlorzide, Diaqua, Diuchlor H,* Esidrix, Hydrodiuril, Hydrozide,* Hyperetic, Neo-Codema,* Novohydrazide,* Oretic, Urozide*
Func. class.: Thiazide diuretic
Chem. class.: Sulfonamide derivative

Action: Acts on distal tubule by increasing excretion of water, sodium, chloride, potassium
Uses: Edema, hypertension
Dosage and routes:
• *Adult:* PO 25-100 mg/day
• *Child >6 mo:* PO 2.2 mg/kg/day in divided doses
• *Child <6 mo:* PO up to 3.3 mg/kg/day in divided doses
Available forms include: Tabs 25, 50, 100 mg
Side effects/adverse reactions:
GU: Frequency, polyuria, uremia, glucosuria
CNS: Drowsiness, paresthesia, anxiety, depression, headache, dizziness, fatigue, weakness
GI: Nausea, vomiting, anorexia, constipation, diarrhea, cramps, pancreatitis, GI irritation, **hepatitis**

EENT: Blurred vision

INTEG: *Rash,* urticaria, purpura, photosensitivity, fever

META: *Hyperglycemia,* hyperuricemia, increased creatinine

HEMA: *Aplastic anemia, hemolytic anemia, leukopenia, agranulocytosis, thrombocytopenia*

CV: Irregular pulse, orthostatic hypotension

ELECT: *Hypokalemia,* hypercalcemia, hyponatremia, hypochloremia

Contraindications: Hypersensitivity to thiazides or sulfonamides, anuria, renal decompensation

Precautions: Hypokalemia, renal disease, pregnancy (D), hepatic disease, gout, COPD, lupus erythematosus, diabetes mellitus

Pharmacokinetics:

PO: Onset 2 hr, peak 4 hr, duration 6-12 hr; excreted unchanged by kidneys, crosses placenta, enters breast milk

Interactions/incompatibilities:

• Increased toxicity of: lithium, nondepolarizing skeletal muscle relaxants, digitalis

• Decreased effects of: antidiabetics

• Decreased absorption of thiazides: cholestyramine, colestipol

• Decreased hypotensive response: indomethacin

• Increased action of: quinidine

NURSING CONSIDERATIONS

Assess:

• Weight, I&O daily to determine fluid loss; effect of drug may be decreased if used qd

• Rate, depth, rhythm of respiration, effect of exertion

• B/P lying, standing; postural hypotension may occur

• Electrolytes: potassium, sodium, chloride; include BUN, blood sugar, CBC, serum creatinine, blood pH, ABGs

• Glucose in urine if patient is diabetic

Administer:

• In AM to avoid interference with sleep if using drug as a diuretic

• Potassium replacement if potassium is less than 3.0

• With food, if nausea occurs, absorption may be decreased slightly

Evaluate:

• Improvement in edema of feet, legs, sacral area daily if medication is being used in CHF

• Improvement in CVP q8h

• Signs of metabolic acidosis: drowsiness, restlessness

• Signs of hypokalemia: postural hypotension, malaise, fatigue, tachycardia, leg cramps, weakness

• Rashes, temperature elevation qd

• Confusion, especially in elderly; take safety precautions if needed

Teach patient/family:

• To increase fluid intake 2-3 L/day unless contraindicated; to rise slowly from lying or sitting position

• To notify physician of muscle weakness, cramps, nausea, dizziness

• Drug may be taken with food or milk

• That blood sugar may be increased in diabetics

• Take early in day to avoid nocturia

Lab test interferences:

Increase: BSP retention, calcium, amylase

Decrease: PBI, PSP

Treatment of overdose: Lavage if taken orally, monitor electrolytes, administer dextrose in saline

hydrocortisone/hydrocortisone acetate

(hye-droe-kor'ti-sone)
Cortamed,* Otall

Func. class.: Otic
Chem. class.: Synthetic steroid

Action: Antiinflammatory, antipruritic, vasoconstrictive properties

Uses: Ear canal inflammation

Dosage and routes:
• *Adult and child:* INSTILL 3-4 gtts bid-qid

Available forms include: Otic sol 0.25%, 0.5%, 1%

Side effects/adverse reactions:
EENT: Itching, irritation in ear
INTEG: Rash, urticaria

Contraindications: Hypersensitivity, perforated eardrum

Pharmacokinetics: Not known

Interactions/incompatibilities: None known

NURSING CONSIDERATIONS

Administer:
• After removing impacted cerumen by irrigation
• After cleaning stopper with alcohol
• After restraining child if necessary
• Warming solution to body temperature

Evaluate:
• Therapeutic response: decreased ear pain, inflammation
• For redness, swelling, fever, pain in ear, which indicates infection

Teach patient/family:
• Method of instillation using aseptic technique, including not touching dropper to ear
• That dizziness may occur after instillation

hydrocortisone/hydrocortisone acetate/hydrocortisone valerate

(hye-droe-kor'ti-sone)
Acticort, Aeroseb-HC, Carmol HC, Cetacort, Cort-Dome, Delacort, Dermicort, Dermolate, Proctocort, Cortaid, Cortef, Cortifoam, Epifoam, My-Cort, Proctofoam-HC, Westcort Cream

Func. class.: Topical corticosteroid
Chem. class.: Natural nonfluorinated, group IV potency (Valerate), group VI potency (acetate and plain)

Action: Possesses antipruritic, antiinflammatory actions

Uses: Psoriasis, eczema, contact dermatitis, pruritus

Dosage and routes:
• *Adult and child:* Apply to affected area qd-qid

Available forms include: Hydrocortisone—oint 0.5%, 1%, 2.5%; cream 0.25%, 0.5%, 1%, 2.5%; lotion 0.25%, 0.5%, 1%, 2%, 2.5%; gel 1%; sol 1%; aerosol/pump spray 0.5%; *acetate*—oint 0.5%, 1%, 2.5%; cream 0.5%; lotion 0.05%; aerosol 1%; *valerate*—oint 0.2%; cream 0.2% (many others)

Side effects/adverse reactions:
INTEG: Burning, dryness, itching, irritation, acne, folliculitis, hypertrichosis, perioral dermatitis, hypopigmentation, atrophy, striae, miliaria, allergic contact dermatitis, secondary infection

Contraindications: Hypersensitivity to corticosteroids, fungal infections

Precautions: Pregnancy (C), lactation, viral infections, bacterial infections

Interactions/incompatibilities: None known

NURSING CONSIDERATIONS
Assess:
• Temperature; if fever develops, drug should be discontinued
Administer:
• Only to affected areas; do not get in eyes
• Medication, then cover with occlusive dressing (only if prescribed), seal to normal skin, change q12h
• Only to dermatoses; do not use on weeping, denuded, or infected area
Perform/provide:
• Cleansing before application of drug
• Treatment for a few days after area has cleared
• Storage at room temperature
Evaluate:
• Therapeutic response: absence of severe itching, patches on skin, flaking
Teach patient/family:
• To avoid sunlight on affected area; burns may occur
• Not to use other OTC products unless approved by physician

---

hydrocortisone/hydrocortisone acetate/hydrocortisone sodium phosphate/hydrocortisone sodium succinate

(hye-dro-kor′ti-sone)
Cortef, Hydrocortone/ Cortef Acetate, Hydrocortone Acetate/Hydrocortone Phosphate/A-Hydrocort, S-Cortilean, Solu-Cortef

Func. class.: Corticosteroid
Chem. class.: Glucocorticoid, short-acting

Action: Decreases inflammation by suppression of migration of polymorphonuclear leukocytes, fibroblasts, reversal of increased capillary permeability and lysosomal stabilization

Uses: Severe inflammation, shock, adrenal insufficiency, ulcerative colitis

Dosage and routes:
Adrenal insufficiency/inflammation
• *Adult:* PO 5-30 mg bid-qid; IM/IV 100-250 mg (succinate), then 50-100 mg IM as needed; IM/IV 15-240 mg q12h (phosphate)
Shock
• *Adult:* 500 mg-2 g q2-6h, (succinate)
• *Child:* IM/IV 0.16-1 mg/kg bid-tid (succinate)
Colitis
• *Adult:* ENEMA 100 mg nightly for 21 days
Available forms include: Retention enema 100 mg/60 ml; tabs 5, 10, 20 mg; inj 25, 50 mg/ml; inj 50 mg/ml; phosphate inj 100, 250, 500, 1000 mg/vial; succinate inj 25, 50 mg/ml

Side effects/adverse reactions:
INTEG: Acne, poor wound healing, ecchymosis, petechiae
CNS: Depression, flushing, sweating, headache, mood changes
*CV: Hypotension, **circulatory collapse, thrombophlebitis, embolism**,* tachycardia
*HEMA: **Thrombocytopenia***
MS: Fractures, osteoporosis, weakness
GI: Diarrhea, nausea, abdominal distention, GI hemorrhage, increased appetite, *pancreatitis*
EENT: Fungal infections, increased intraocular pressure, blurred vision
Contraindications: Psychosis, hypersensitivity, idiopathic thrombocytopenia, acute glomerulonephritis, amebiasis, fungal infections, nonasthmatic bronchial disease, child <2 yr
Precautions: Pregnancy (C), diabetes mellitus, glaucoma, osteo-

porosis, seizure disorders, ulcerative colitis, CHF, myasthenia gravis

Pharmacokinetics:

PO: Onset 1-2 hr, peak 1 hr, duration 1-1½ days

IM/IV: Onset 20 min, peak 4-8 hr, duration 1-1½ days

REC: Onset 3-5 days

Metabolized by liver, excreted in urine (17-OHCS, 17-KS), crosses placenta

Interactions/incompatibilities:

• Decreased action of this drug: cholestyramine, colestipol, barbiturates, rifampin, ephedrine, phenytoin, theophylline

• Decreased effects of: anticoagulants, anticonvulsants, antidiabetics, ambenonium, neostigmine, isoniazid, toxoids, vaccines

• Increased side effects: alcohol, salicylates, indomethacin, amphotericin B, digitalis preparations

• Increased action of this drug: salicylates, estrogens, indomethacin

NURSING CONSIDERATIONS

Assess:

• Potassium, blood sugar, urine glucose while on long-term therapy; hypokalemia and hyperglycemia

• Weight daily, notify physician of weekly gain >5 lb

• B/P q4h, pulse, notify physician if chest pain occurs

• I&O ratio, be alert for decreasing urinary output and increasing edema

• Plasma cortisol levels during long-term therapy (normal level: 138-635 nmol/L SI units when drawn at 8 AM)

Administer:

• After shaking suspension (parenteral)

• Titrated dose, use lowest effective dose

• IM inj deeply in large mass, ro-

tate sites, avoid deltoid, use 19G needle

• In one dose in AM to prevent adrenal suppression, avoid SC administration, damage may be done to tissue

• With food or milk to decrease GI symptoms

Perform/provide:

• Assistance with ambulation in patient with bone tissue disease to prevent fractures

Evaluate:

• Therapeutic response: ease of respirations, decreased inflammation

• Infection: increased temperature, WBC, even after withdrawal of medication; drug masks symptoms of infection

• Potassium depletion: paresthesias, fatigue, nausea, vomiting, depression, polyuria, dysrhythmias, weakness

• Edema, hypotension, cardiac symptoms

• Mental status: affect, mood, behavioral changes, aggression

Teach patient/family:

• That ID as steroid user should be carried

• To notify physician if therapeutic response decreases; dosage adjustment may be needed

• Not to discontinue this medication abruptly or adrenal crisis can result

• To avoid OTC products: salicylates, alcohol in cough products, cold preparations unless directed by physician

• Teach patient all aspects of drug use, including Cushingoid symptoms

• Symptoms of adrenal insufficiency: nausea, anorexia, fatigue, dizziness, dyspnea, weakness, joint pain

Lab test interferences:

Increase: Cholesterol, sodium,

---

blood glucose, uric acid, calcium, urine glucose

Decrease: Calcium, potassium, T_4, T_3, thyroid ^{131}I uptake test, urine 17-OHCS, 17-KS, PBI

False negative: Skin allergy tests

---

hydroflumethiazide

(hye-droe-floo-meth-eye'a-zide)
Diucardin, Saluron

Func. class.: Thiazide diuretic
Chem. class.: Sulfonamide derivative

Action: Acts on distal tubule by increasing excretion of water, sodium, chloride, potassium

Uses: Edema, hypertension

Dosage and routes:
• *Adult:* PO 25-200 mg/day in divided doses

Available forms include: Tabs 50 mg

Side effects/adverse reactions:
GU: Frequency, polyuria, uremia, glucosuria

CNS: Drowsiness, paresthesia, anxiety, depression, headache, dizziness, fatigue, weakness

GI: Nausea, vomiting, anorexia, constipation, diarrhea, cramps, pancreatitis, GI irritation, *hepatitis*

EENT: Blurred vision

INTEG: Rash, urticaria, purpura, photosensitivity, fever

META: Hyperglycemia, hyperuricemia, increased creatinine

HEMA: Aplastic anemia, hemolytic anemia, leukopenia, agranulocytosis, thrombocytopenia

CV: Irregular pulse, orthostatic hypotension

ELECT: Hypokalemia, hypercalcemia, hyponatremia, hypochloremia

Contraindications: Hypersensitivity to thiazides or sulfonamides, anuria, renal decompensation

Precautions: Hypokalemia, renal disease, pregnancy (D), hepatic disease, gout, COPD, lupus erythematosus, diabetes mellitus

Pharmacokinetics:
PO: Onset 1-2 hr, peak 3-4 hr, duration 18-24 hr; excreted unchanged by kidneys, crosses placenta, enters breast milk

Interactions/incompatibilities:
• Increased toxicity of: lithium, nondepolarizing skeletal muscle relaxants, digitalis

• Decreased effects of: antidiabetics

• Decreased absorption of thiazides: cholestyramine, colestipol

• Decreased hypotensive response: indomethacin

• Increased action of: quinidine

NURSING CONSIDERATIONS

Assess:
• Weight, I&O daily to determine fluid loss; effect of drug may be decreased if used qd

• Rate, depth, rhythm of respiration, effect of exertion

• B/P lying, standing; postural hypotension may occur

• Electrolytes: potassium, sodium, chloride; include BUN, blood sugar, CBC, serum creatinine, blood pH, ABGs

• Glucose in urine if patient is diabetic

Administer:
• In AM to avoid interference with sleep if using drug as a diuretic

• Potassium replacement if potassium is less than 3.0

• With food if nausea occurs, absorption may be decreased slightly

Evaluate:
• Improvement in edema of feet, legs, sacral area daily if medication is being used in CHF

• Improvement in CVP q8h

• Signs of metabolic acidosis: drowsiness, restlessness

• Signs of hypokalemia: postural hypotension, malaise, fatigue, tachycardia, leg cramps, weakness

• Rashes, temperature elevation qd
• Confusion, especially in elderly; take safety precautions if needed

Teach patient/family:

• To increase fluid intake 2-3 L/day unless contraindicated; to rise slowly from lying or sitting position
• To notify physician of muscle weakness, cramps, nausea, dizziness
• Drug may be taken with food or milk
• That blood sugar may be increased in diabetics
• Take early in day to avoid nocturia

Lab test interferences:

Increase: BSP retention, calcium, amylase

Decrease: PBI, PSP

Treatment of overdose: Lavage if taken orally, monitor electrolytes, administer dextrose in saline

---

hydrogen peroxide

(per-ox′ide)

Func. class.: Disinfectant
Chem. class.: Oxidizing drug

Action: Destroys bacteria by mechanical action

Uses: Douche, cleansing wounds, mouthwash for Vincent's stomatitis, removal of ear wax

Dosage and routes:

• *Adult and child:* SOL Use as needed

Available forms include: Top sol 1.5%, 3%

Side effects/adverse reactions:

CV: Oxygen emboli

INTEG: Irritation

EENT: Black hairy tongue, decalcification of tooth enamel

Contraindications: Hypersensitivity to this drug, closed wounds

Precautions: 3rd-degree burns, deep wounds

Pharmacokinetics:

TOP: Duration to end of bubbling

Interactions/incompatibilities:
None known

NURSING CONSIDERATIONS

Administer:

• To ear canal to facilate removal of cerumen
• As mouthwash for Vincent's stomatitis; do not use everyday mouthwash
• After dilution with water or salt water solution
• Only when oxygen can flow in and out of wound; emboli may result

Evaluate:

• Area of body involved: irritation, rash, breaks, dryness, scales

Lab test interferences:

False positive: Urine glucose (Clinitest or Labstix)

H

---

hydromorphone HCl

(hye-droe-mor′fone)
Dilaudid

Func. class.: Narcotic analgesics
Chem. class.: Opiate, semisynthetic phenanthrene

Controlled Substance Schedule II

Action: Inhibits ascending pain pathways in CNS, increases pain threshold, alters pain perception

Uses: Moderate to severe pain

Dosage and routes:

• *Adult:* PO 1-6 mg q4-6h prn; IM/SC/IV 2-4 mg q4-6h; REC 3 mg hs prn

Available forms include: Inj IM, IV 1, 2, 3, 4 mg/ml; tabs 1, 2, 3, 4 mg; rec supp 3 mg

Side effects/adverse reactions:

CNS: Drowsiness, dizziness, confusion, headache, sedation, euphoria

GI: Nausea, vomiting, anorexia, constipation, cramps

GU: Increased urinary output, dysuria

INTEG: Rash, urticaria, bruising, flushing, diaphoresis, pruritus

EENT: Tinnitus, blurred vision, miosis, diplopia

CV: Palpitations, bradycardia, change in B/P

RESP: Respiratory depression

Contraindications: Hypersensitivity, addiction (narcotic)

Precautions: Addictive personality, pregnancy (C), lactation, increased intracranial pressure, MI (acute), severe heart disease, respiratory depression, hepatic disease, renal disease, child <18 yr

Pharmacokinetics:

Onset 15-30 min, peak ½-1½ hr, duration 4-5 hr; metabolized by liver, excreted by kidneys, crosses placenta, excreted in breast milk

Interactions/incompatibilities:

• Effects may be increased with other CNS depressants: alcohol, narcotics, sedative/hypnotics, antipsychotics, skeletal muscle relaxants

NURSING CONSIDERATIONS

Assess:

• I&O ratio; check for decreasing output; may indicate urinary retention

Administer:

• With antiemetic if nausea, vomiting occur

• When pain is beginning to return; determine dosage interval by patient response

Perform/provide:

• Storage in light-resistant area at room temperature

• Assistance with ambulation

• Safety measures: siderails, night light, call bell within easy reach

Evaluate:

• Therapeutic response: decrease in pain

• CNS changes: dizziness, drowsiness, hallucinations, euphoria, LOC, pupil reaction

• Allergic reactions: rash, urticaria

• Respiratory dysfunction: respiratory depression, character, rate, rhythm; notify physician if respirations are <12/min

• Need for pain medication, physical dependence

Teach patient/family:

• To report any symptoms of CNS changes, allergic reactions

• That physical dependency may result when used for extended periods of time

• Withdrawal symptoms may occur: nausea, vomiting, cramps, fever, faintness, anorexia

Lab test interferences:

Increase: Amylase

Treatment of overdose: Narcan 0.2-0.8 IV, O₂, IV fluids, vasopressors

---

hydromorphone HCl

(hye-droe-mor'fone)

Dilaudid Cough Syrup

Func. class.: Antitussive, narcotic

Chem. class.: Phenanthrene derivative, guaifenesin

Controlled Substance Schedule II

Action: Increases respiratory tract fluid by decreasing surface tension, adhesiveness, which increases removal of mucus; possesses analgesic, antitussive properties

Uses: Cough

Dosage and routes:

• *Adult:* PO 1 mg q3-4h prn

• *Child 6-12 yr:* PO 0.5 mg q3-4h prn

Available forms include: Syr 1 mg/5 ml

Side effects/adverse reactions:

CNS: Dizziness, drowsiness

GI: Nausea, constipation, vomiting, anorexia

CV: Hypotension

INTEG: Urticaria, rash

*RESP: **Respiratory depression***
Contraindications: Hypersensitivity, increased intracranial pressure, status asthmaticus
Precautions: Hypothyroidism, Addison's disease, CNS depression, brain tumor, asthma, hepatic disease, renal disease, COPD, psychosis, alcoholism, convulsive disorders, pregnancy (C)
Pharmacokinetics: Metabolized by liver, half-life 2-4 hr
Interactions/incompatibilities:
• Enhanced CNS depression: barbiturates, narcotics, antipsychotics, antidepressants
NURSING CONSIDERATIONS
Assess:
• VS, cardiac status including hypotension
• Respiratory rate, depth
Administer:
• Decreased dose to elderly patients; their metabolism may be slowed
Perform/provide:
• Storage at room temperature
• Increased fluids, bulk, exercise to patient's lifestyle to decrease constipation
Evaluate:
• Therapeutic response: absence of cough
• Cough: type, frequency, character including sputum
Teach patient/family:
• Avoid driving, other hazardous activities until patient is stabilized on this medication if drowsiness occurs
• Avoid alcohol, other CNS depressants; will enhance sedating properties of this drug

hydroquinone
(hye′droe-kwin-one)
Derma-Blanch, Eldopaque, Eldoquin, Esoterica Medicated Cream, Melanex, Quinnone, Porcelana, Solaquin
Func. class.: Depigmenting agent
Chem. class.: Enzyme inhibitor

Action: Inhibits production of tyrosine, which is needed in formation of melanin
Uses: Bleaching skin, including old-age spots, freckles, lentigo, chloasma
Dosage and routes:
• *Adult and child:* TOP apply to affected area qd-bid
Available forms include: Top cream 2%, 4%; top lotion 2%; gel 4%; sol 3%
Side effects/adverse reactions:
INTEG: Rash, dryness, fissures, stinging, contact dermatitis, erythema, irritation
Contraindications: Hypersensitivity, inflamed skin, prickly heat, sunburn
Precautions: Pregnancy (C), lactation, child <1 yr
Interactions/incompatibilities:
None known
NURSING CONSIDERATIONS
Administer:
• Topical corticosteroid for irritation
• Test dose to be applied to area 25 mm in diameter, check site after 24 hr; if itching or excessive inflammation occurs, drug should not be used
Perform/provide:
• Storage at room temperature in tight container
Evaluate:
• Therapeutic response: fading of spots over time

• Area of body involved, including time involved, what helps or aggravates condition
Teach patient/family:
• To avoid application on normal skin or getting cream in eyes
• To use opaque sunscreen during day on exposed areas or bleaching effect may be reversed
• That minor redness is not a contraindication
• To continue to use sunscreen after bleaching is complete

---

hydroxocobalamin (vitamin B₁₂)

Alpha Redisol, Alpha-Ruvite, Codrozomin, Droxomin, Neo-Betalin 12, Rubesol-LA

Func. class.: Vitamin
Chem. class.: B_{12}—fat-soluble vitamin

Action: Needed for adequate nerve functioning, protein and carbohydrate metabolism, normal growth, RBC development
Uses: Vitamin B_{12} deficiency, pernicious anemia, vitamin B_{12} malabsorption syndrome, Schilling test
Dosage and routes:
• *Adult:* PO 25 μg qd × 5-10 days, maintenance 100-200 mg IM q mo; IM/SC 30-100 μg qd × 5-10 days, maintenance 100-200 mg IM q mo
• *Child:* PO 1 μg qd × 5-10 days, maintenance 60 μg IM q mo or more; IM/SC 1-30 μg qd × 5-10 days, maintenance 60 μg IM q mo or more
Pernicious anemia/malabsorption syndrome
• *Adult:* IM 100-1000 μg qd × 2 wk, then 100-1000 μg IM q mo
• *Child:* IM 1000-5000 μg × 2 wk or more given in 100-500 μg doses, then 60 μg IM/SC mo

Schilling test
• *Adult and child:* IM 1000μg in one dose
Available forms include: Tabs 25, 50, 100, 250, 500, 1000 μg; inj IM 100, 120, 1000 μg/ml
Side effects/adverse reactions:
CNS: Flushing, optic nerve atrophy
GI: Diarrhea
CV: CHF, peripheral vascular thrombosis, pulmonary edema
INTEG: Itching, rash
Contraindications: Hypersensitivity, optic nerve atrophy
Precautions: Pregnancy, lactation, children
Pharmacokinetics: Stored in liver, kidneys, stomach; 50%-90% excreted in urine, crosses placenta, breast milk
Interactions/incompatibilities:
• Decreased absorption of this drug: aminoglycosides, anticonvulsants, colchicine, chloramphenicol, aminosalicylic acid, potassium preparations
• Increased absorption of this drug: prednisone
NURSING CONSIDERATIONS
Assess:
• Potassium levels during beginning treatment
• CBC for increased reticulocyte count during 1st week of therapy, then increase RBC and hemoglobin after that
Administer:
• With fruit juice to disguise taste
• With meals if possible for better absorption
• By IM inj for pernicious anemia unless contraindicated
Evaluate:
• Therapeutic response: decreased anorexia, dyspnea on excretion, palpitations, paresthesias, psychosis, visual disturbances
• Nutritional status: egg yolks, fish, organ meats, dairy products, clams, oysters, which are good

---

sources for Vitamin B$_{12}$
• For pulmonary edema, or worsening of CHF in cardiac patients
Teach patient/family
• That treatment must continue for life if diagnosed as having pernicious anemia
Lab test interferences:
False positive: Intrinsic factor

---

hydroxychloroquine sulfate

(hye-drox-ee-klor'oh-kwin)
Plaquenil Sulfate
Func. class.: Antimalarial
Chem. class.: 4-aminoquinoline derivative

Action: Inhibits parasite replications, transcription of DNA to RNA by forming complexes with DNA of parasite
Uses: Malaria caused by *Plasmodium vivax, P. malariae, P. ovale, P. falciparum* (some strains)
Dosage and routes:
Malaria
• *Adult and child:* PO 5 mg/kg/wk on same day of week, not to exceed 300 mg; treatment should begin 2 wk before entering endemic area, continue 8 wk after leaving; if treatment begins after exposure, 600 mg for adult, 10 mg/kg for children in 2 divided doses 6 hr apart
Lupus erythematosus
• *Adult:* PO 400 mg qd-bid, length depends on patient response; maintenance 200-400 mg qd
Rheumatoid arthritis
• *Adult:* PO 400-600 mg qd, then 200-300 mg qd after good response
Available forms include: Tabs 200 mg
Side effects/adverse reactions:
CV: Hypotension, heart block, asystole with syncope
INTEG: Pruritus, pigmentary changes, skin eruptions, lichen planus–like eruptions, eczema, *exfoliative dermatitis,* alopecia
CNS: Headache, stimulation, fatigue, irritability, convulsion, bad dreams, dizziness, confusion, psychosis, decreased reflexes
EENT: Blurred vision, corneal changes, retinal changes, difficulty focusing, tinnitus, vertigo, deafness, photophobia, corneal edema
GI: Nausea, vomiting, anorexia, diarrhea, cramps
*HEMA: **Thrombocytopenia, agranulocytosis, hemolytic anemia, leukopenia***
Contraindications: Hypersensitivity, retinal field changes, prophyria, children (long-term)
Precautions: Blood dyscrasias, severe GI disease, neurologic disease, alcoholism, hepatic disease, G-6-PD deficiency, psoriasis, eczema, pregnancy
Pharmacokinetics:
PO: Peak 1-2 hr, half-life 3-5 days, metabolized in liver, excreted in urine, feces, breast milk, crosses placenta
Interactions/incompatibilities:
• Decreased action of this drug: magnesium or aluminum compounds

NURSING CONSIDERATIONS
Assess:
• Ophthalmic test if long-term treatment or drug dosage >150 mg/day
• Liver studies q wk: AST, ALT, bilirubin
• Blood studies: CBC, since blood dyscrasias occur
• For decreased reflexes: knee, ankle; watch for depression of T waves, widening of QRS complex
• ECG during therapy
Administer:
• Before or after meals at same time each day to maintain drug level
• IM after aspirating to avoid in-

---

jection into blood system, which may cause hypotension, asystole, heart block; rotate injection sites

Perform/provide:
• Storage in tight, light-resistant containers at room temperature; injection should be kept in cool environment

Evaluate:
• Allergic reactions: pruritus, rash, urticaria
• Blood dyscrasias: malaise, fever, bruising, bleeding (rare)
• For ototoxicity (tinnitus, vertigo, change in hearing); audiometric testing should be done before, after treatment
• For toxicity: blurring vision, difficulty focusing, headache, dizziness, knee, ankle reflexes; drug should be discontinued immediately

Teach patient/family:
• To use sunglasses in bright sunlight to decrease photophobia
• That urine may turn rust or brown color
• To report hearing, visual problems, fever, fatigue, bruising, bleeding, which may indicate blood dyscrasias

Treatment of overdose: Induce vomiting, gastric lavage, administer barbiturate (ultrashort-acting), vasopressin; tracheostomy may be necessary

---

hydroxyprogesterone caproate

(hye-drox-ee-proe-jess'te-rone)
Delalutin, Dura-lutin

Func. class.: Progestogen, hormone

Action: Inhibits secretion of pituitary gonadotropins, which prevents follicular maturation, ovulation, stimulates growth of mammary tissue, antineoplastic action against endometrial cancer

Uses: Uterine cancer, menstrual disorders

Dosage and routes:
• *Adult:* IM 125-375 mg q4 wk, discontinue after 4 cycles
Uterine cancer
• *Adult:* IM 1-5 g/wk

Available forms include: Inj IM 125, 250 mg/ml

Side effects/adverse reactions:
CNS: Dizziness, headache, migraines, depression, fatigue

CV: Hypotension, thrombophlebitis, edema, ***thromboembolism, stroke, pulmonary embolism, myocardial infarction***

GI: Nausea, vomiting, anorexia, cramps, increased weight, ***cholestatic jaundice***

EENT: Diplopia

GU: Amenorrhea, cervical erosion, breakthrough bleeding, dysmenorrhea, vaginal candidiasis, breast changes, *gynecomastia, testicular atrophy, impotence,* endometriosis, ***spontaneous abortion***

INTEG: Rash, urticaria, acne, hirsutism, alopecia, oily skin, seborrhea, purpura, melasma, photosensitivity

META: Hyperglycemia

Contraindications: Breast cancer, hypersensitivity, thromboembolic disorders, reproductive cancer, genital bleeding (abnormal, undiagnosed)

Precautions: Pregnancy, lactation, hypertension, asthma, blood dyscrasias, gallbladder disease, HF, diabetes mellitus, bone disease, depression, migraine headache, convulsive disorders, hepatic disease, renal disease, family history of breast or reproductive tract cancer

Pharmacokinetics:
IM: Half-life 5 min, duration 24 hr, excreted in urine, feces, metabolized in liver

---

Interactions/incompatibilities:
None known

NURSING CONSIDERATIONS
Assess:
• Weight daily, notify physician of weekly weight gain >5 lb
• B/P at beginning of treatment and periodically
• I&O ratio; be alert for decreasing urinary output, increasing edema
• Liver function studies: ALT, AST, bilirubin, periodically during long-term therapy
Administer:
• Titrated dose, use lowest effective dose
• Oil solution deeply in large muscle mass (IM), rotate sites
• In one dose in AM
• With food or milk to decrease GI symptoms
• After warming to dissolve crystals
Perform/provide:
• Storage in dark area
Evaluate:
• Therapeutic response: decreased abnormal uterine bleeding, absence of amenorrhea
• Edema, hypertension, cardiac symptoms, jaundice
• Mental status: affect, mood, behavioral changes, depression
• Hypercalcemia
Teach patient/family:
• To avoid sunlight or use sunscreen; photosensitivity can occur
• All aspects of drug usage, including cushingoid symptoms
• To report breast lumps, vaginal bleeding, edema, jaundice, dark urine, clay-colored stools, dyspnea, headache, blurred vision, abdominal pain, numbness or stiffness in legs, chest pain; male to report impotence or gynecomastia
• To report suspected pregnancy
Lab test interferences:
Increase: Alk phosphatase, nitro-

gen (urine), pregnanediol, amino acids
Decrease: GTT, HDL

---

hydroxyurea

(hye-drox'ee-yoo-ree-ah)
Hydrea
Func. class.: Antineoplastic-antimetabolite
Chem. class.: Synthetic urea analog

Action: Acts by inhibiting DNA synthesis without interfering with RNA or protein synthesis; incorporates thymidine into DNA, causing direct damage to DNA strands
Uses: Melanoma, chronic myelocytic leukemia, recurrent or metastatic ovarian cancer
Dosage and routes:
Solid tumors
• *Adult:* PO 80 mg/kg as a single dose q3 days or 20-30 mg/kg as a single dose qd
In combination with radiation
• *Adult:* PO 80 mg/kg as a single dose q3 days
Resistant chronic myelocytic leukemia
• *Adult:* PO 20-30 mg/kg/day as a single daily dose
Available forms include: Caps 500 mg
Side effects/adverse reactions:
*HEMA: **Leukopenia, anemia, thrombocytopenia***
GI: Nausea, vomiting, anorexia, diarrhea, stomatitis, constipation
GU: Increased BUN, uric acid, creatinine, temporary renal function impairment
INTEG: Rash, urticaria, pruritus, dry skin, alopecia (rare)
CV: Angina, ischemia
CNS: Headache, confusion, hallucinations, dizziness, ***convulsions***
Contraindications: Hypersensitivity, leukopenia (<2500/mm^3),

thrombocytopenia (<100,000/ mm³), anemia (severe), pregnancy
Precautions: Renal disease (severe)

Pharmacokinetics: Readily absorbed when taken orally, peak level in 2 hr, degraded in liver, excreted in urine, almost totally eliminated in 24 hr; readily crosses blood-brain barrier

Interactions/incompatibilities:
• Increased toxicity: radiation or other antineoplastics

NURSING CONSIDERATIONS
Assess:
• CBC, differential, platelet count weekly; withhold drug if WBC is <3500/mm³ or platelet count is <100,000/mm³; notify physician of these results; drug should be discontinued
• Renal function studies: BUN, serum uric acid, urine CrCl, electrolytes before, during therapy
• I&O ratio, report fall in urine output to <30 ml/hr
• Monitor temperature q4h; fever may indicate beginning infection
• Liver function tests before, during therapy: bilirubin, alk phosphatase, AST, ALT, LDH; as needed or monthly
• B/P q3-4h; check for chest pain; angina, ischemia may occur

Administer:
• Medications by oral route if possible; avoid IM, SC, IV routes to prevent infections
• Antiemetic 30-60 min before giving drug to prevent vomiting
• Antibiotics for prophylaxis of infection
• Topical or systemic analgesics for pain
• Transfusion for anemia

Perform/provide:
• Liquid diet: carbonated beverage, Jello; dry toast, crackers may be added when patient is not nauseated or vomiting

• Rinsing of mouth tid-qid with water, hydrogen peroxide; brushing of teeth bid-tid with soft brush or cotton-tipped applicators for stomatitis; use unwaxed dental floss
• Nutritious diet with iron, vitamin supplements as ordered

Evaluate:
• Bleeding: hematuria, guaiac, bruising or petechiae, mucosa or orifices q8h
• Food preferences; list likes, dislikes
• Effects of alopecia on body image, discuss feelings about body changes
• Inflammation of mucosa, breaks in skin
• Buccal cavity q8h for dryness, sores or ulceration, white patches, oral pain, bleeding, dysphagia
• Symptoms indicating severe allergic reaction: rash, urticaria, itching, flushing
• Neurotoxicity: headaches, hallucinations, convulsions, dizziness

Teach patient/family:
• To report any complaints, side effects to nurse or physician
• That hair may be lost during treatment, and wig or hair piece may make patient feel better; tell patient that new hair may be different in color, texture
• To avoid foods with citric acid, hot or rough texture if stomatitis is present
• To report stomatitis: any bleeding, white spots, ulcerations in the mouth; tell patient to examine mouth qd, report symptoms
• Contraceptive measures are recommended during therapy
• To drink 10-12 glasses of fluid/ day
• Notify physician of fever, chills, sore throat, nausea, vomiting, anorexia, diarrhea, bleeding, bruising; may indicate blood dyscrasias

---

*Available in Canada only

Lab test interferences:
Increase: Renal function studies

---

hydroxyzine HCl/
hydroxyzine pamoate

(hye-drox'i-zeen)
Atarax, Durrax, Orgatrax, Quiess, Vistaril/Vistaril IM

Func. class.: Antianxiety
Chem. class.: Piperazine derivative

Action: Depresses subcortical levels of CNS, including limbic system, reticular formation

Uses: Anxiety, hyperkinesia, preoperatively, postoperatively to prevent nausea, vomiting, to potentiate narcotic analgesics

Dosage and routes:
• *Adult:* PO 25-100 mg tid-qid
• *Child >6 yr:* 50-100 mg/day in divided doses
• *Child <6 yr:* 50 mg/day in divided doses

Preoperatively/postoperatively
• *Adult:* IM 25-100 mg q4-6h
• *Child:* IM 1.1 mg/kg q4-6h

Available forms include: Tabs 10, 25, 50, 100 mg; caps 25, 50, 100 mg; syrup 10 mg/5 ml; oral susp 25 mg/5 ml; IM inj

Side effects/adverse reactions:
CNS: Dizziness, drowsiness, confusion, headache, anxiety, tremors, stimulation, fatigue, depression, insomnia, hallucinations

GI: Constipation, dry mouth, nausea, vomiting, anorexia, diarrhea

INTEG: Rash, dermatitis, itching

CV: Orthostatic hypotension, ECG changes, tachycardia, hypotension

EENT: Blurred vision, tinnitus, mydriasis

Contraindications: Hypersensitivity to benzodiazepines, narrowangle glaucoma, psychosis, pregnancy (D), child <18 yr

Precautions: Elderly, debilitated, hepatic disease, renal disease

Pharmacokinetics:
PO: Onset 15-30 min, duration 4-6 hr, half-life 3 hr

Interactions/incompatibilities:
• Increased CNS depressant effect: barbiturates, narcotics, analgesics

NURSING CONSIDERATIONS

Assess:
• B/P (lying, standing), pulse; if systolic B/P drops 20 mm Hg, hold drug, notify physician
• Blood studies: CBC
• Hepatic studies: AST, ALT, bilirubin, creatinine

Administer:
• By Z-track injection for IM to decrease pain, chance of necrosis
• With food or milk for GI symptoms
• Crushed if patient is unable to swallow medication whole
• Gum, hard candy, frequent sips of water for dry mouth

Perform/provide:
• Assistance with ambulation during beginning therapy, since drowsiness/dizziness occurs
• Safety measures, including siderails
• Checking to see PO medication has been swallowed

Evaluate:
• Mental status: mood, sensorium, affect
• Physical dependency and withdrawal symptoms: headache, nausea, vomiting, muscle pain, weakness after long-term use
• Increased sedation

Teach patient/family:
• Not to be used for everyday stress or used longer than 4 mo
• Avoid OTC preparations (cold, cough, hay fever) unless approved by physician
• To avoid driving, activities that require alertness
• To avoid alcohol ingestion, or

H

---

italics = common side effects   ***bold italic*** = life threatening reactions

other psychotropic medications
• Not to discontinue medication quickly after long-term use
• To rise slowly or fainting may occur

Lab test interferences:
False increase: 17-OHCS
Treatment of overdose: Lavage if orally ingested; VS, supportive care; IV norepinephrine for hypotension

---

hyoscyamine sulfate

(hye-oh-sye′a-meen)
Anaspaz, Levsin, Levsinex
Func. class.: Gastrointestinal anticholinergic
Chem. class.: Belladonna alkaloid

Action: Inhibits muscarinic actions of acetylcholine at postganglionic parasympathetic neuroeffector sites
Uses: Treatment of peptic ulcer disease in combination with other drugs; other GI disorders

Dosage and routes:
• *Adult:* PO/SL 0.125-0.25 mg tid-qid ac, hs; TIME REL 0.375 q12h; IM/SC/IV 0.25-0.5 mg q6h
• *Child 2-10 yr:* ½ adult dose
• *Child <2 yr:* ¼ adult dose
Available forms include: Tabs 0.125, 0.13, 0.15 mg; caps time rel 0.375 mg; sol 0.125 mg/ml; elix 0.125 mg/5 ml; inj IM, IV, SC 0.5 mg/ml

Side effects/adverse reactions:
CNS: Confusion, stimulation in elderly, headache, insomnia, dizziness, drowsiness, anxiety, weakness, hallucination
GI: Dry mouth, constipation, paralytic ileus, heartburn, nausea, vomiting, dysphagia, absence of taste
GU: Hesitancy, retention, impotence
CV: Palpitations, tachycardia
EENT: Blurred vision, photophobia, mydriasis, cycloplegia, increased ocular tension
INTEG: Urticaria, rash, pruritus, anhidrosis, fever, allergic reactions
Contraindications: Hypersensitivity to anticholinergics, narrow-angle glaucoma, GI obstruction, myasthenia gravis, paralytic ileus, GI atony, toxic megacolon
Precautions: Hyperthyroidism, coronary artery disease, dysrhythmias, CHF, ulcerative colitis, hypertension, hiatal hernia, hepatic disease, renal disease

Pharmacokinetics:
PO: Duration 4-6 hr; metabolized by liver, excreted in urine, half-life 13-38 hr

Interactions/incompatibilities:
• Increased anticholinergic effect: amantadine, tricyclic antidepressants, MAOIs
• Increased effect of: nitrofurantoin
• Decreased effect of: phenothiazines, levodopa

NURSING CONSIDERATIONS
Assess:
• VS, cardiac status: checking for dysrhythmias, increased rate, palpitations
• I&O ratio; check for urinary retention or hesitancy
Administer:
• ½ hr ac for better absorption
• Decreased dose to elderly patients; their metabolism may be slowed
• Gum, hard candy, frequent rinsing of mouth for dryness of oral cavity
Perform/provide:
• Storage is tight container protected from light
• Increased fluids, bulk, exercise to patient's lifestyle to decrease constipation
Evaluate:
• Therapeutic response: absence of epigastric pain, bleeding, nausea, vomiting

---

• GI complaints: pain, bleeding (frank or occult), nausea, vomiting, anorexia

Teach patient/family:

• Avoid driving or other hazardous activities until stabilized on medication

• Avoid alcohol or other CNS depressants; will enhance sedating properties of this drug

• To avoid hot environments, stroke may occur, drug suppresses perspiration

• Use sunglasses when outside to prevent photophobia

---

ibuprofen

(eye-byoo′proe-fen)

Amersol, Motrin, Rufen

Func. class.: Nonsteroidal

Chem. class.: Propionic acid derivative

Action: Inhibits prostaglandin synthesis by decreasing enzyme needed for biosynthesis; possesses analgesic, antiinflammatory, antipyretic properties

Uses: Rheumatoid arthritis, osteoarthritis, primary dysmenorrhea, gout, dental pain, musculoskeletal disorders

Dosage and routes:

• *Adult:* PO 200-600 mg qid

Available forms include: Tabs 200, 300, 400, 600, 800 mg

Side effects/adverse reactions:

GI: Nausea, anorexia, vomiting, diarrhea, jaundice, ***cholestatic hepatitis,*** constipation, flatulence, cramps, dry mouth, peptic ulcer

CNS: Dizziness, drowsiness, fatigue, tremors, confusion, insomnia, anxiety, depression

CV: Tachycardia, peripheral edema, palpitations, dysrhythmias

INTEG: Purpura, rash, pruritus, sweating

GU: ***Nephrotoxicity:*** dysuria, hematuria, oliguria, azotemia

HEMA: ***Blood dyscrasias***

EENT: Tinnitus, hearing loss, blurred vision

Contraindications: Hypersensitivity, asthma, severe renal disease, severe hepatic disease

Precautions: Pregnancy, lactation, children, bleeding disorders, GI disorders, cardiac disorders, hypersensitivity to other antiinflammatory agents

Pharmacokinetics:

PO: Peak 1-2 hr, half-life 2-4 hr, metabolized in liver (inactive metabolites), excreted in urine (inactive metabolites)

Interactions/incompatibilities:

• May increase action of coumarin, phenytoin, sulfonamides

NURSING CONSIDERATIONS

Assess:

• Renal, liver, blood studies: BUN, creatinine, AST, ALT, Hgb, before treatment, periodically thereafter

• Audiometric, ophthalmic exam before, during, after treatment

Administer:

• With food to decrease GI symptoms; however, best to take on empty stomach to facilitate absorption

Perform/provide:

• Storage at room temperature

Evaluate:

• Therapeutic response: decreased pain, stiffness in joints, decreased swelling in joints, ability to move more easily

• For eye, ear problems: blurred vision, tinnitus; may indicate toxicity

Teach patient/family:

• To report blurred vision, ringing, roaring in ears; may indicate toxicity

• To avoid driving, other hazardous activities if dizziness, drowsiness occurs

• To report change in urine pattern, increased weight, edema, increased

---

pain in joints, fever, blood in urine; indicate nephrotoxicity
• That therapeutic effects may take up to 1 mo
• To avoid alcohol, salicylates; bleeding may occur

---

idoxuridine-IDU (oph-thalmic)

Herplex, Stoxil

Func. class.: Antiviral
Chem. class.: Pyrimidine nucleoside

Action: Inhibits bacterial cell wall in organism by preventing amino acids and nucleotides into cell wall
Uses: Herpes simplex keratitis alone or with corticosteroids
Dosage and routes:
• *Adult and child:* INSTILL 1 gtt q1h and 2 hr during night; TOP apply oint q4h × 1 wk, if no response, discontinue
Available forms include: Oint 0.5%, sol 0.1%
Side effects/adverse reactions:
EENT: Poor corneal wound healing, temporary visual haze, overgrowth of nonsusceptible organisms
Contraindications: Hypersensitivity
Precautions: Antibiotic hypersensitivity
Interactions/incompatibilities:
• Do not use boric acid with this drug
NURSING CONSIDERATIONS
Administer:
• After washing hands, cleanse crusts or discharge from eye before application
Perform/provide:
• Storage in refrigerator until used
Evaluate:
• Therapeutic response: absence of redness, inflammation, tearing

• Allergy: itching, lacrimation, redness, swelling
Teach patient/family:
• To use drug exactly as prescribed
• Not to use eye makeup, towels, washcloths, eye medication of others; reinfection may occur
• That drug container tip should not be touched to eye
• To report itching, increased redness, burning, stinging, swelling; drug should be discontinued
• That drug may cause blurred vision when ointment is applied

---

imipramine HCl

(im-ip'ra-meen)

Impril,* Janimine, Novopramine,* Presamine, Ropramine, Tipramine, Tofranil

Func. class.: Antidepressant—tricyclic
Chem. class.: Dibenzazepine—tertiary amine

Action: Blocks reuptake of norepinephrine, serotonin into nerve endings, increasing action of norepinephrine, serotonin in nerve cells
Uses: Depression, enuresis in children
Dosage and routes:
• *Adult:* PO/IM 75-100 mg/day in divided doses, may increase by 25-50 mg to 200 mg, not to exceed 300 mg/day; may give daily dose hs
• *Child:* PO 25-75 mg/day
Available forms include: Tabs 10, 25, 50 mg; inj IM 25 mg/2 ml
Side effects/adverse reactions:
HEMA: Agranulocytosis, thrombocytopenia, eosinophilia, leukopenia
CNS: Dizziness, drowsiness, confusion, headache, anxiety, tremors, stimulation, weakness, insomnia,

nightmares, EPS (elderly), increased psychiatric symptoms, paresthesia

GI: Diarrhea, dry mouth, nausea, vomiting, ***paralytic ileus,*** increased appetite, cramps, epigastric distress, jaundice, ***hepatitis,*** stomatitis

GU: Retention, ***acute renal failure***
INTEG: Rash, urticaria, sweating, pruritus, photosensitivity

CV: Orthostatic hypotension, ECG changes, tachycardia, ***hypertension,*** palpitations

EENT: Blurred vision, tinnitus, mydriasis

Contraindications: Hypersensitivity to tricyclic antidepressants, recovery phase of myocardial infarction, convulsive disorders, prostatic hypertrophy

Precautions: Suicidal patients, severe depression, increased intraocular pressure, narrow-angle glaucoma, urinary retention, cardiac disease, hepatic disease, hyperthyroidism, electroshock therapy, elective surgery, elderly, pregnancy (C)

Pharmacokinetics:

PO: Steady state 2-5 days; metabolized by liver, excreted by kidneys, feces, crosses placenta, excreted in breast milk, half-life 6-20 hr

Interactions/incompatibilities:

• Decreased effects of: guanethidine, clonidine, indirect acting sympathomimetics (ephedrine)

• Increased effects of: direct acting sympathomimetics (epinephrine), alcohol, barbiturates, benzodiazepines, CNS depressants

• Hyperpyretic crisis, convulsions, hypertensive episode: MAOI (pargyline [Eutonyl])

NURSING CONSIDERATIONS
Assess:

• B/P (lying, standing), pulse q4h; if systolic B/P drops 20 mm Hg

hold drug, notify physician; take vital signs q4h in patients with cardiovascular disease

• Blood studies: CBC, leukocytes, differential, cardiac enzymes if patient is receiving long-term therapy

• Hepatic studies: AST, ALT, bilirubin, creatinine

• Weight qwk, appetite may increase with drug

• ECG for flattening of T wave, bundle branch block, AV block, dysrhythmias in cardiac patients

Administer:

• Increased fluids, bulk in diet if constipation, urinary retention occur

• With food or milk for GI symptoms

• Dosage hs if over-sedation occurs during day; may take entire dose hs; elderly may not tolerate once/day dosing

• Gum, hard candy, or frequent sips of water for dry mouth

Perform/provide:

• Storage in tight container at room temperature, do not freeze

• Assistance with ambulation during beginning therapy since drowsiness/dizziness occurs

• Safety measures including siderails primarily in elderly

• Checking to see PO medication swallowed

Evaluate:

• EPS primarily in elderly: rigidity, dystonia, akathisia

• Mental status: mood, sensorium, affect, suicidal tendencies, increase in psychiatric symptoms: depression, panic

• Urinary retention, constipation; constipation is more likely to occur in children

• Withdrawal symptoms: headache, nausea, vomiting, muscle pain, weakness; do not usually occur unless drug was discontinued abruptly

---

• Alcohol consumption; if alcohol is consumed, hold dose until morning

Teach patient/family:

• That therapeutic effects may take 2-3 wk

• Use caution in driving or other activities requiring alertness because of drowsiness, dizziness, blurred vision

• To avoid alcohol ingestion, other CNS depressants

• Not to discontinue medication quickly after long-term use, may cause nausea, headache, malaise

• To wear sunscreen or large hat since photosensitivity occurs

Lab test interferences:

Increase: Serum bilirubin, alk phosphatase, blood glucose

Decrease: 5-HIAA, VMA, urinary catecholamines

Treatment of overdose: ECG monitoring, induce emesis, lavage, activated charcoal, administer anticonvulsant

---

Immune globulin

Gamastan, Gamimune, Gammar, Immuglobin, Sandoglobulin

Func. class.: Immune serum
Chem. class.: IgG

Action: Provides passive immunity to hepatitis A, measles, varicella, rubella, immune globulin deficiency

Uses: Agammaglobulinemia, hepatitis A exposure, measles exposure, measles vaccine complications, purpura, rubella exposure, chicken pox exposure

Dosage and routes:

• *Adult:* IM 30-50 ml q mo; IV 100 mg/kg q mo, 0.01-0.02 ml/kg/min × ½ hr (Gamimune); IV 200 mg/kg q, 0.05-1 ml/min × 15-30 min, then increase to 1.5-2.5 ml/min (Sandoglobulin)

• *Child:* IM 20-40 ml q mo

Hepatitis A exposure

• *Child and adult:* IM 0.02-0.04 ml/kg or 0.1 mg/kg if treatment is delayed

Hepatitis B exposure

• *Adult and child:* IM 0.06 ml/kg within 1 wk, q month

Measles

• *Child:* IM 0.25 ml/kg within 6 days

Immunoglobulin deficiency

• *Child:* IM 1.3 ml/kg, then 0.66 ml/kg after 2-4 wk and q2-4 wk thereafter

Idiopathic thrombocytopenia purpura

• *Adult:* IV 0.4 g/kg × 5 days

Available forms include: IV, IM inj 2, 10 ml/vial

Side effects/adverse reactions:

INTEG: Pain at injection site, rash, pruritus

MS: Arthralgia

SYST: Lymphadenopathy, *anaphylaxis*

CNS: Headache, fatigue, malaise

GI: Abdominal pain

Contraindications: Hypersensitivity

Interactions/incompatibilities:

• Do not administer live virus vaccines within 3 mo of this drug

NURSING CONSIDERATIONS

Administer:

• IM 3 ml or < in one site, use large muscle mass

• Only after epinephrine 1:1000, resuscitative equipment are available

• Only within 6 wk of exposure to hepatitis A

---

indapamide

(in-dap′a-mide)
Lozol
Func. class.: Diuretic
Chem. class.: Indoline

Action: Acts on proximal section of distal renal tubule by inhibiting reabsorption of sodium; may act by direct vasodilation caused by blocking of calcium channel

Uses: Edema, hypertension

Dosage and routes:
• *Adult:* PO 2.5 mg qd in AM, may be increased to 5 mg qd if needed
Available forms include: Tabs 2.5 mg

Side effects/adverse reactions:
GU: Polyuria, gynecomastia, ejaculatory problems, dysuria, frequency, impotence
ELECT: Hypochloremic alkalosis, hypomagnesemia, hyperuricemia, hypocalcemia, hyponatremia, hyperkalemia
CNS: Headache, dizziness, fatigue, weakness, paresthesias
GI: Nausea, diarrhea, dry mouth, vomiting, anorexia, cramps, constipation, pancreatitis, abdominal pain
EENT: Loss of hearing, tinnitus, blurred vision, nasal congestion, increased intraocular pressure
INTEG: Rash, pruritus, photosensitivity, alopecia, urticaria
MS: Cramps
HEMA: Thrombocytopenia, agranulocytosis, leukopenia, neutropenia, anemia
CV: Orthostatic hypotension

Contraindications: Hypersensitivity, anuria

Precautions: Hypokalemia, dehydration, ascites, hepatic disease, severe renal disease, pregnancy (B)

Pharmacokinetics:
PO: Onset 1-2 hr, peak 2 hr, duration up to 36 hr; excreted in urine, feces, half-life 14-18 hr

Interactions/incompatibilities:
• Increased effects: MAOIs, alcohol, narcotics, barbiturates, antihypertensives, anticoagulants, muscle relaxants, steroids

NURSING CONSIDERATIONS

Assess:
• Weight daily, I&O daily to determine fluid loss; effect of drug may be decreased if used qd
• Rate, depth, rhythm of respiration, effect of exertion
• B/P lying, standing; postural hypotension may occur
• Electrolytes: potassium, sodium, chloride; include BUN, CBC, serum creatinine, blood pH, ABGs

Administer:
• In AM to avoid interference with sleep
• With food, if nausea occurs, absorption may be decreased slightly

Evaluate:
• Improvement in edema of feet, legs, sacral area daily if medication is being used in CHF
• Improvement in CVP q8h
• Signs of metabolic alkalosis
• Signs of hyperkalemia
• Rashes, temperature elevation qd
• Confusion, especially in elderly; take safety precautions if needed
• Hydration: skin turgor, thirst, dry mucous membranes

Teach patient/family:
• To increase fluid intake 2-3 L/day unless contraindicated; to rise slowly from lying or sitting position
• Adverse reactions: muscle cramps, weakness, nausea, dizziness
• Take with food or milk for GI symptoms
• Take early in day to prevent nocturia

Treatment of overdose: Lavage if taken orally, monitor electrolytes, administer IV fluids

---

italics = common side effects   ***bold italic*** = life threatening reactions

indomethacin/ indomethacin sodium trihydrate

(in-doe-meth'a-sin)

Indocid, Indocin, Indocin SR, In-domed/Indocin IV

Func. class.: Nonsteroidal
Chem. class.: Propionic acid derivative

Action: Inhibits prostaglandin synthesis by decreasing enzyme needed for biosynthesis; possesses analgesic, antiinflammatory, antipyretic properties

Uses: Rheumatoid arthritis, ankylosing rheumatoid spondylitis, acute gouty arthritis, closure of patent ductus arteriosus in premature infants

Dosage and routes:
Arthritis
• *Adult:* PO/REC 25 mg bid-tid, may increase by 25 mg/day q1 wk, not to exceed 200 mg/day; SUS REL 75 mg qd, may increase to 75 mg bid

Acute arthritis
• *Adult:* PO/REC 50 mg tid; use only for acute attack, then reduce dose

Patent ductus arteriosus
• *Infant <2 days:* IV 0.2 mg/kg, then 0.1 mg/kg q12-24 hr
• *Infant 2-7 days:* IV 0.2 mg/kg, then 0.2 mg × 2 doses after 12, 24 hr
• *Infant >7 days:* IV 0.2 mg/kg, then 0.25 mg/kg × 2 doses after 12, 24 hr

Available forms include: Caps 25, 50 mg; caps ext rel 75 mg; susp 25 mg/5 ml; rec supp 50 mg

Side effects/adverse reactions:
GI: Nausea, anorexia, vomiting, diarrhea, jaundice, *cholestatic hepatitis,* constipation, flatulence, cramps, dry mouth, peptic ulcer

CNS: Dizziness, drowsiness, fatigue, tremors, confusion, insomnia, anxiety, depression
CV: Tachycardia, peripheral edema, palpitations, dysrhythmias
INTEG: Purpura, rash, pruritus, sweating
GU: Nephrotoxicity: dysuria, hematuria, oliguria, azotemia
HEMA: Blood dyscrasias
EENT: Tinnitus, hearing loss, blurred vision

Contraindications: Hypersensitivity, asthma, severe renal disease, severe hepatic disease

Precautions: Pregnancy, lactation, children, bleeding disorders, GI disorders, cardiac disorders, hypersensitivity to other antiinflammatory agents

Pharmacokinetics:
PO: Onset 1-2 hr, peak 3 hr, duration 4-6 hr; metabolized in liver, kidneys, excreted in urine, bile, feces, crosses placenta, excreted in breast milk

Interactions/incompatibilities:
• May increase action of coumarin, phenytoin, sulfonamides

NURSING CONSIDERATIONS
Assess:
• Renal, liver, blood studies: BUN, creatinine, AST, ALT, Hgb, before treatment, periodically thereafter
• Audiometric, ophthalmic exam before, during, after treatment

Administer:
• With food to decrease GI symptoms; however, best to take on empty stomach to facilitate absorption

Perform/provide:
• Storage at room temperature

Evaluate:
• Therapeutic response: decreased pain, stiffness in joints, decreased swelling in joints, ability to move more easily
• For eye, ear problems: blurred vision, tinnitus; may indicate toxicity

Teach patient/family:
• To report blurred vision, ringing, roaring in ears; may indicate toxicity
• To avoid driving, other hazardous activities if dizziness, drowsiness occurs
• To report change in urine pattern, increased weight, edema, increased pain in joints, fever, blood in urine; indicate nephrotoxicity
• That therapeutic effects may take up to 1 mo
• To avoid alcohol, salicylates; bleeding may occur

influenza virus vaccine, trivalent A & B (whole virus/split virus)

Fluzone, Fluogen
Func. class.: Vaccine

Action: Produces antibodies to influenza virus by production of antibodies
Uses: Prevention of Russian, Chile, Philippine influenza
Dosage and routes:
• *Adult and child >12 yr:* IM 0.5 ml in 1 dose
• *Child 3-12 yr:* IM 0.5 ml, repeat in 1 mo (split) unless 1978-1985 vaccine was given
• *Child 6 mo to 3 yr:* IM 0.25 ml, repeat in 1 mo (split) unless 1978-1985 vaccine was given
Available forms include: Inj IM 100 μg/ml
Side effects/adverse reactions:
CNS: Fever, Guillian-Barré syndrome
INTEG: Urticaria, induration, erythema
*SYST: **Anaphylaxis,** malaise*
MS: Myalgia
Contraindications: Hypersensitivity, active infection, chicken, egg allergy, Guillain-Barré syndrome

Precautions: Elderly, immunosuppression, pregnancy
NURSING CONSIDERATIONS
Assess:
• For skin reactions: rash, induration, erythema
Administer:
• Only with epinephrine 1 : 1000 on unit to treat laryngospasm
• Only IM
Evaluate:
• For history of allergies, skin conditions (eczema, psoriasis, dermatitis), reactions to vaccinations
• For anaphylaxis: inability to breathe, bronchospasm

insulin, isophane suspension (NPH)

Beef NPH Iletin II, Humulin N, Iletin NPH,* Insulatard NPH, NPH,* NPH Iletin I, Pork NPH Iletin II, Protaphane NPH, Novolin N

Func. class.: Antidiabetic
Chem. class.: Exogenous unmodified insulin

Action: Decreases blood sugar, increases blood pyruvate, lactate, decreases phosphate, potassium
Uses: Adult-onset diabetes, juvenile diabetes, ketoacidosis
Dosage and routes:
• *Adult:* SC dosage individualized by blood, urine glucose, usual dose 7-26 U, may increase by 2-10 U/day if needed; do not give IV
Available forms include: SC 40, 100 U
Side effects/adverse reactions:
CNS: Headache, lethargy, tremors, weakness, fatigue, delirium, sweating
CV: Tachycardia, palpitations
EENT: Blurred vision
GI: Hunger, nausea
META: Hypoglycemia

INTEG: Flushing, rash, urticaria, warmth

*SYST: **Anaphylaxis***

Contraindications: Hypersensitivity

Interactions/incompatibilities:

• Increased hypoglycemia: salicylate, alcohol, β-blockers, anabolic steroids, fenfluramine, guanethidine, oral hypoglycemics, MAOIs, tetracycline, clofibrate

• Hyperglycemia: thiazides, thyroid hormones, triamterene, phenothiazines, phenytoin, oral contraceptives, corticosteroids, estrogens, lithium

Pharmacokinetics:

SC: Onset 1-2 hr, peak 8-12 hr, duration 18-24 hr, half-life 4 hr

IV: Onset 1 min, peak 30-60 min, duration 1-2 hr, half-life 3-5 min

Metabolized by liver, muscle, kidneys; excreted in urine

NURSING CONSIDERATIONS

Assess:

• Fasting blood glucose, 2 hr PP (60-100 mg/dl normal fasting level) (70-130 mg/dl-normal 2 hr level)

Administer:

• After warming to room temperature by rotating in palms to prevent lipodystrophy from injecting cold insulin

• Increased doses if tolerance occurs

• Human insulin to those allergic to beef or pork

Perform/provide:

• Storage at room temperature for <1 mo, refrigerate all other supply, do not use discolored or cloudy solution

• Rotation of injection sites: abdomen, upper back, thighs, upper arm, buttocks; keep record of sites

Evaluate:

• Therapeutic response: decrease in polyuria, polydipsia, polyphagia, clear sensorium, absence of dizziness, stable gait

• Hypoglycemic / hyperglycemic reaction that can occur soon after meals

Teach patient/family:

• That blurred vision occurs, not to change corrective lens until vision is stabilized 1-2 mo

• To keep insulin, equipment available at all times

• That drug does not cure diabetes, but controls symptoms

• To carry Medic Alert ID as diabetic

• Hypoglycemia reaction: headache, tremors, fatigue, weakness

• Dosage, route, mixing instructions, if any diet restrictions, disease process

• To carry candy or lump sugar to treat hypoglycemia

• Symptoms of ketoacidosis: nausea, thirst, polyuria, dry mouth, decreased B/P, dry, flushed skin, acetone breath, drowsiness, Kussmaul respirations

• That a plan is necessary for diet, exercise; all food on diet should be eaten, exercise routine should not vary

• Urine glucose testing, make sure patient is able to determine glucose, acetone levels

• The pregnant patient to use glucose oxidase reagents

• To avoid OTC drugs unless directed by physician

Lab test interferences:

Increase: VMA

Decrease: Potassium, calcium

Interference: Liver function studies, thyroid function studies

Treatment of overdose: 10%-50% glucose PO if conscious or IV if comatose

insulin, isophane suspension and regular insulin

Mixtard

Func. class.: Antidiabetic
Chem. class.: Exogenous unmodified insulin

Action: Decreases blood sugar, increases blood pyruvate, lactate, decreases phosphate, potassium
Uses: Adult-onset diabetes, juvenile diabetes, ketoacidosis
Dosage and routes:
• *Adult:* SC individualized dose
Available forms include: 70 units/ml with 30 units/ml regular insulin = 100 units/ml
Side effects/adverse reactions:
CNS: Headache, lethargy, tremors, weakness, fatigue, delirium, sweating
CV: Tachycardia, palpitations
EENT: Blurred vision
GI: Hunger, nausea
META: Hypoglycemia
INTEG: Flushing, rash, urticaria, warmth
*SYST: **Anaphylaxis***
Contraindications: Hypersensitivity
Interactions/incompatibilities:
• Increased hypoglycemia: salicylate, alcohol, β-blockers, anabolic steroids, fenfluramine, guanethidine, oral hypoglycemics, MAOIs, tetracycline, clofibrate
• Hyperglycemia: thiazides, thyroid hormones, triamterene, phenothiazines, phenytoin, oral contraceptives, corticosteroids, estrogens, lithium
Pharmacokinetics:
SC: Onset 30 min, peak 4-8 hr, duration 12-24 hr, half-life 4 hr
IV: Onset 10-30 min, peak 30-60 min, duration 1-2 hr, half-life 3-5 min

Metabolized by liver, muscle, kidneys; excreted in urine
NURSING CONSIDERATIONS
Assess:
• Fasting blood glucose, 2 hr PP (60-100 mg/dl normal fasting level) (70-130 mg/dl-normal 2 hr level)
Administer:
• After warming to room temperature by rotating in palms to prevent lipodystrophy from injecting cold insulin
• Increased doses if tolerance occurs
• Human insulin to those allergic to beef or pork
Perform/provide:
• Storage at room temperature for <1 mo, refrigerate all other supply, do not use discolored or cloudy solution
• Rotation of injection sites: abdomen, upper back, thighs, upper arm, buttocks, keep record of sites
Evaluate:
• Therapeutic response: decrease in polyuria, polydipsia, polyphagia, clear sensorium, absence of dizziness, stable gait
• Hypoglycemic/hyperglycemic reaction that can occur soon after meals
Teach patient/family:
• That blurred vision occurs, not to change corrective lens until vision is stabilized 1-2 mo
• To keep insulin, equipment available at all times
• That drug does not cure diabetes, but controls symptoms
• To carry Medic Alert ID as diabetic
• Hypoglycemia reaction: headache, tremors, fatigue, weakness
• Dosage, route, mixing instructions, if any diet restrictions, disease process
• To carry candy or lump sugar to treat hypoglycemia

• Symptoms of ketoacidosis: nausea, thirst, polyuria, dry mouth, decreased B/P, dry, flushed skin, acetone breath, drowsiness, Kussmaul respirations

• That a plan is necessary for diet, exercise; all food on diet should be eaten, exercise routine should not vary

• Urine glucose testing, make sure patient is able to determine glucose, acetone levels

• The pregnant patient to use glucose oxidase reagents

• To avoid OTC drugs unless directed by physician

Lab test interferences:

Increase: VMA

Decrease: Potassium, calcium

Interference: Liver function studies, thyroid function studies

Treatment of overdose: 10%-50% glucose PO if conscious or IV if comatose

---

Insulin, protamine zinc suspension (PZI)

Beef Protamine Zinc Iletin II, Iletin PZI,* Pork Protamine Zinc Iletin II, Protamine Zinc Iletin I

Func. class.: Antidiabetic

Chem. class.: Exogenous unmodified insulin

Action: Decreases blood sugar, increases blood pyruvate, lactate, decreases phosphate, potassium

Uses: Adult-onset diabetes, juvenile diabetes, ketoacidosis

Dosage and routes:

• *Adult:* SC 7-26 U q30-60 min before breakfast, individualized

Available forms include: SC 40, 100 U

Side effects/adverse reactions:

CNS: Headache, lethargy, tremors, weakness, fatigue, delirium, sweating

CV: Tachycardia, palpitations

EENT: Blurred vision

GI: Hunger, nausea

META: Hypoglycemia

INTEG: Flushing, rash, urticaria, warmth

*SYST: **Anaphylaxis***

Contraindications: Hypersensitivity

Interactions/incompatibilities:

• Increased hypoglycemia: salicylate, alcohol, β-blockers, anabolic steroids, fenfluramine, guanethidine, oral hypoglycemics, MAOIs, tetracycline, clofibrate

• Hyperglycemia: thiazides, thyroid hormones, triamterene, phenothiazines, phenytoin, oral contraceptives, corticosteroids, estrogens, lithium

Pharmacokinetics:

SC: Onset 4-8 hr, peak 14-20 hr, duration 24-36 hr, half-life 4 hr

IV: Onset 10-30 min, peak 30-60 min, duration 1-2 hr, half-life 3-5 min

Metabolized by liver, muscle, kidneys; excreted in urine

NURSING CONSIDERATIONS

Assess:

• Fasting blood glucose, 2 hr PP (60-100 mg/dl normal fasting level) (70-130 mg/dl-normal 2 hr level)

Administer:

• After warming to room temperature by rotating in palms to prevent lipodystrophy from injecting cold insulin

• Increased doses if tolerance occurs

• Human insulin to those allergic to beef or pork

Perform/provide:

• Storage at room temperature for <1 mo, refrigerate all other supply, do not use discolored or cloudy solution

• Rotation of injection sites: abdomen, upper back, thighs, upper arm, buttocks; keep record of sites

Evaluate:
• Therapeutic response: decrease in polyuria, polydipsia, polyphagia, clear sensorium, absence of dizziness, stable gait
• Hypoglycemic/hyperglycemic reaction that can occur soon after meals

Teach patient/family:
• That blurred vision occurs, not to change corrective lens until vision is stabilized 1-2 mo
• To keep insulin, equipment available at all times
• That drug does not cure diabetes, but controls symptoms
• To carry Medic Alert ID as diabetic
• Hypoglycemia reaction: headache, tremors, fatigue, weakness
• Dosage, route, mixing instructions, if any diet restrictions, disease process
• To carry candy or lump sugar to treat hypoglycemia
• Symptoms of ketoacidosis: nausea, thirst, polyuria, dry mouth, decreased B/P, dry, flushed skin, acetone breath, drowsiness, Kussmaul respirations
• That a plan is necessary for diet, exercise; all food on diet should be eaten, exercise routine should not vary
• Urine glucose testing; make sure patient is able to determine glucose, acetone levels
• The pregnant patient to use glucose oxidase reagents
• To avoid OTC drugs unless directed by physician

Lab test interferences:
Increase: VMA
Decrease: Potassium, calcium
Interference: Liver function studies, thyroid function studies
Treatment of overdose: 10%-50% glucose PO if conscious or IV if comatose

Insulin, zinc suspension

Beef Lente Iletin II, Lente Iletin I, Lente Insulin, Pork Lente Iletin II, Lentard Monotard, Novolin L, Humulin L

Func. class.: Antidiabetic
Chem. class.: Exogenous unmodified insulin

Action: Decreases blood sugar, increases blood pyruvate, lactate, decreases phosphate, potassium
Uses: Adult-onset diabetes, juvenile diabetes, ketoacidosis
Dosage and routes:
• *Adult:* SC individualized; do not give IV
Available forms include: SC 40, 100 U
Side effects/adverse reactions:
CNS: Headache, lethargy, tremors, weakness, fatigue, delirium, sweating
CV: Tachycardia, palpitations
EENT: Blurred vision
GI: Hunger, nausea
META: Hypoglycemia
INTEG: Flushing, rash, urticaria, warmth
SYST: **Anaphylaxis**
Contraindications: Hypersensitivity
Interactions/incompatibilities:
• Increased hypoglycemia: salicylate, alcohol, β-blockers, anabolic steroids, fenfluramine, guanethidine, oral hypoglycemics, MAOIs, tetracycline, clofibrate
• Hyperglycemia: thiazides, thyroid hormones, triamterene, phenothiazines, phenytoin, oral contraceptives, corticosteroids, estrogens, lithium
Pharmacokinetics:
SC: Onset 2-4 min, peak 6-8 hr, duration 12-24 hr, half-life 4 hr
IV: Onset 10-30 min, peak 30-60

min, duration 1-2 hr, half-life 3-5 min

Metabolized by liver, muscle, kidneys; excreted in urine

NURSING CONSIDERATIONS

Assess:

• Fasting blood glucose, 2 hr PP (60-100 mg/dl normal fasting level) (70-130 mg/dl-normal 2 hr level)

Administer:

• After warming to room temperature by rotating in palms to prevent lipodystrophy from injecting cold insulin

• Increased doses if tolerance occurs

• Human insulin to those allergic to beef or pork

Perform/provide:

• Storage at room temperature for <1 mo, refrigerate all other supply, do not use discolored or cloudy solution

• Rotation of injection sites: abdomen, upper back, thighs, upper arm, buttocks; keep record of sites

Evaluate:

• Therapeutic response: decrease in polyuria, polydipsia, polyphagia, clear sensorium, absence of dizziness, stable gait

• Hypoglycemic/hyperglycemic reaction that can occur soon after meals

Teach patient/family:

• That blurred vision occurs, not to change corrective lens until vision is stabilized 1-2 mo

• To keep insulin, equipment available at all times

• That drug does not cure diabetes, but controls symptoms

• To carry Medic Alert ID as diabetic

• Hypoglycemia reaction: headache, tremors, fatigue, weakness

• Dosage, route, mixing instructions, if any diet restrictions, disease process

• To carry candy or lump sugar to treat hypoglycemia

• Symptoms of ketoacidosis: nausea, thirst, polyuria, dry mouth, decreased B/P, dry, flushed skin, acetone breath, drowsiness, Kussmaul respirations

• That a plan is necessary for diet, exercise; all food on diet should be eaten, exercise routine should not vary

• Urine glucose testing, make sure patient is able to determine glucose, acetone levels

• The pregnant patient to use glucose oxidase reagents

• To avoid OTC drugs unless directed by physician

Lab test interferences:

Increase: VMA

Decrease: Potassium, calcium

Interference: Liver function studies, thyroid function studies

Treatment of overdose: 10%-50% glucose PO if conscious or IV if comatose

---

insulin, zinc suspension extended

Iletin Ultralente,* Ultralente,* Ultralente Iletin I, Ultralente Insulin, Ultralente Purified Beef

Func. class.: Antidiabetic

Chem. class.: Exogenous unmodified insulin

Action: Decreases blood sugar, increases blood pyruvate, lactate, decreases phosphate, potassium

Uses: Adult-onset diabetes, juvenile diabetes, ketoacidosis

Dosage and routes:

• *Adult:* SC individualized; do not give IV

Available forms include: SC 40, 100 U

Side effects/adverse reactions:

CNS: Headache, lethargy, tremors,

weakness, fatigue, delirium, sweating

CV: Tachycardia, palpitations

EENT: Blurred vision

GI: Hunger, nausea

META: Hypoglycemia

INTEG: Flushing, rash, urticaria, warmth

SYST: Anaphylaxis

Contraindications: Hypersensitivity

Interactions/incompatibilities:

• Increased hypoglycemia: salicylate, alcohol, β-blockers, anabolic steroids, fenfluramine, guanethidine, oral hypoglycemics, MAOIs, tetracycline, clofibrate

• Hyperglycemia: thiazides, thyroid hormones, triamterene, phenothiazines, phenytoin, oral contraceptives, corticosteroids, estrogens, lithium

Pharmacokinetics:

SC: Onset 4-8 hr, peak 16-18 hr, duration 24-36 hr, half-life 4 hr

IV: Onset 10-30 min, peak 30-60 min, duration 1-2 hr, half-life 3-5 min

Metabolized by liver, muscle, kidneys, excreted in urine

NURSING CONSIDERATIONS

Assess:

• Fasting blood glucose, 2 hr PP (60-100 mg/dl normal fasting level) (70-130 mg/dl-normal 2 hr level)

Administer:

• After warming to room temperature by rotating in palms to prevent lipodystrophy from injecting cold insulin

• Increased doses if tolerance occurs

• Human insulin to those allergic to beef or pork

Perform/provide:

• Storage at room temperature for <1 mo, refrigerate all other supply, do not use discolored or cloudy solution

• Rotation of injection sites: abdomen, upper back, thighs, upper arm, buttocks, keep record of sites

Evaluate:

• Therapeutic response: decrease in polyuria, polydipsia, polyphagia, clear sensorium, absence of dizziness, stable gait

• Hypoglycemic/hyperglycemic reaction that can occur soon after meals

Teach patient/family:

• That blurred vision occurs, not to change corrective lens until vision is stabilized 1-2 mo

• To keep insulin, equipment available at all times

• That drug does not cure diabetes, but controls symptoms

• To carry Medic Alert ID as diabetic

• Hypoglycemia reaction: headache, tremors, fatigue, weakness

• Dosage, route, mixing instructions, if any diet restrictions, disease process

• To carry candy or lump sugar to treat hypoglycemia

• Symptoms of ketoacidosis: nausea, thirst, polyuria, dry mouth, decreased B/P, dry, flushed skin, acetone breath, drowsiness, Kussmaul respirations

• That a plan is necessary for diet, exercise; all food on diet should be eaten, exercise routine should not vary

• Urine glucose testing, make sure patient is able to determine glucose, acetone levels

• The pregnant patient to use glucose oxidase reagents

• To avoid OTC drugs unless directed by physician

Lab test interferences:

Increase: VMA

Decrease: Potassium, calcium

Interference: Liver function studies, thyroid function studies

Treatment of overdose: 10%-50%

glucose PO if conscious or IV if comatose

Insulin, zinc suspension, prompt (semilente)

Semilente Iletin I, Semilente Insulin, Semilente Purified Pork

Func. class.: Antidiabetic
Chem. class.: Exogenous unmodified insulin

Action: Decreases blood sugar, increases blood pyruvate, lactate, decreases phosphate, potassium
Uses: Adult-onset diabetes, juvenile diabetes, ketoacidosis
Dosage and routes:
• *Adult:* SC dosage individualized by blood, urine glucose qd-tid
Available forms include: SC 40, 100 U
Side effects/adverse reactions:
CNS: Headache, lethargy, tremors, weakness, fatigue, delirium, sweating
CV: Tachycardia, palpitations
EENT: Blurred vision
GI: Hunger, nausea
META: Hypoglycemia
INTEG: Flushing, rash, urticaria, warmth
SYST: Anaphylaxis
Contraindications: Hypersensitivity
Pharmacokinetics:
SC: Onset 30-60 min, peak 4-7 hr, duration 12-16 hr, half-life 4 hr
IV: Onset 10-30 min, peak 4-7 min, duration 12-16 hr, half-life 3-5 min
Metabolized by liver, muscle, kidneys; excreted in urine
Interactions/incompatibilities:
• Increased hypoglycemia: salicylate, alcohol, β-blockers, anabolic steroids, fenfluramine, guanethidine, oral hypoglycemics, MAOIs, tetracycline, clofibrate
• Hyperglycemia: thiazides, thyroid hormones, triamterene, phenothiazines, phenytoin, oral contraceptives, corticosteroids, estrogens, lithium

NURSING CONSIDERATIONS
Assess:
• Fasting blood glucose, 2 hr PP (60-100 mg/dl normal fasting level) (70-130 mg/dl-normal 2 hr level)
Administer:
• After warming to room temperature by rotating in palms, to prevent lipodystrophy from injecting cold insulin
• Increased doses if tolerance occurs
• Human insulin to those allergic to beef or pork
Perform/provide:
• Storage at room temperature for <1 mo, refrigerate all other supply, do not use discolored or cloudy solution
• Rotation of injection sites: abdomen, upper back, thighs, upper arm, buttocks; keep record of sites
Evaluate:
• Therapeutic response: decrease in polyuria, polydipsia, polyphagia, clear sensorium, absence of dizziness, stable gait
• Hypoglycemic / hyperglycemic reaction that can occur soon after meals
Teach patient/family:
• That blurred vision occurs, not to change corrective lens until vision is stabilized 1-2 mo
• To keep insulin, equipment available at all times
• That drug does not cure diabetes, but controls symptoms
• To carry Medic Alert ID as diabetic
• Hypoglycemia reaction: headache, tremors, fatigue, weakness
• Dosage, route, mixing instructions, if any diet restrictions, disease process
• To carry candy or lump sugar to

---

*Available in Canada only

treat hypoglycemia

• Symptoms of ketoacidosis: nausea, thirst, polyuria, dry mouth, decreased B/P, dry, flushed skin, acetone breath, drowsiness, Kussmaul respirations

• That a plan is necessary for diet, exercise; all food on diet should be eaten, exercise routine should not vary

• Urine glucose testing, make sure patient is able to determine glucose, acetone levels

• The pregnant patient to use glucose oxidase reagents

• To avoid OTC drugs unless directed by physician

Lab test interferences:

Increase: VMA

Decrease: Potassium, calcium

Interference: Liver function studies, thyroid function studies

Treatment of overdose: 10%-50% glucose PO if conscious or IV if comatose

---

invert sugar

Travert

Func. class.: Caloric

Chem. class.: Carbohydrate

Action: Needed for adequate utilization of amino acids, decreases protein/nitrogen loss, prevents ketosis

Uses: Increase calorie intake, nonelectrolyte fluid replacement

Dosage and routes:

• *Adult and child:* IV not to exceed 1 g/kg/hr

Available forms include: Inj IV 10%

Side effects/adverse reactions:

CNS: Confusion

CV: Hypertension, *CHF, pulmonary edema*

GI: Nausea, vomiting, liver fat deposits

GU: Glycosuria, osmotic diuresis

ENDO: Hyperglycemia, rebound hypoglycemia

INTEG: Extravasation necrosis at injection site

Contraindications: Hyperglycemia, delirum tremens, hemorrhage (cranial/spinal), CHF

Precautions: Renal, liver, cardiac disease

Interactions/incompatibilities: None known

NURSING CONSIDERATIONS

Assess:

• Electrolytes (K, Na, Ca, Cl, Mg), blood glucose, ammonia, phosphate

• Renal, liver function studies: BUN, creatinine, ALT, AST, bilirubin

• Injection site for extravasation: redness along vein, edema at site, necrosis, pain, hard tender area; site should be changed immediately

• Monitor respiratory function q4h: auscultate lung fields bilaterally for rales, respirations, quality, rate, rhythm

• Monitor temperature q4h for increased fever, indicating infection; if infection suspected, infusion is discontinued, tubing, bottle cultured

• Urine glucose q6h using Tes-Tape, Clinistix, Keto-Diastix, which are not affected by infusion substances

Administer:

• After changing IV catheter, dressing q24h using aseptic technique

Evaluate:

• Therapeutic response: increased weight

• Nutritional status: calorie count by dietician

Teach patient/family

• Reason for dextrose infusion

---

italics = common side effects   ***bold italic*** = life threatening reactions

iodinated glycerol

Organidin, Isophen Elixir

Func. class.: Expectorant
Chem. class.: Iodopropylidene glycerol isom

Action: Increases respiratory tract fluid by decreasing surface tension, adhesiveness, which increases removal of mucus

Uses: Bronchial asthma, emphysema, bronchitis

Dosage and routes:
• *Adult:* PO 60 mg qid; SOL 20 gtts qid; ELIX 5 ml qid
• *Child:* PO up to half adult dose, depending on weight

Available forms include: Tabs 30 mg; sol 50 mg/ml, 60 mg/5 ml

Side effects/adverse reactions:
EENT: Burning mouth, throat, eye irritation, swelling of eyelids
GI: Gastric irritation
ENDO: Iodism, goiter, myxedema
RESP: Pulmonary edema
INTEG: Angioedema, rash
CNS: Frontal headache, *CNS depression,* fever, parkinsonism

Contraindications: Hypersensitivity to iodides, pulmonary TB, pregnancy (X), hyperthyroidism, hyperkalemia, newborns, lactation, acute bronchitis

Precautions: Hypothyroidism, cystic fibrosis, lactation

Pharmacokinetics: Excreted in urine

Interactions/incompatibilities:
• Increased hypothyroid effects: lithium, antithyroid drugs
• Dysrhythmias, hyperkalemia: potassium-sparing diuretics, potassium-containing medication

NURSING CONSIDERATIONS
Administer:
• Orally in solution or tablet form

Perform/provide:
• Increased fluids to liquefy secretions

Evaluate:
• Therapeutic response: absence of cough
• Cough: type, frequency, character including sputum

Teach patient/family:
• Not to use if pregnant
• Symptoms of iodism: eruptions, burning of oral cavity, eye irritation
• Symptoms of hyperthyroidism: CNS depression, fever, glomerulonephritis

iodochlorhydroxyquin (clioquinol) (topical)

(eye-oh-doe-klor-hye-drox'ee-kwin)

Func. class.: Local antiinfective
Chem. class.: Halogenated hydroxy quinoline

Action: Interferes with viral DNA replication

Uses: Eczema, tinea cruris, tinea pedia, tinea corporis

Dosage and routes:
• *Adult and child:* TOP apply to affected area qd-bid

Available forms include: Cream, oint 3%

Side effects/adverse reactions:
INTEG: Rash, urticaria, stinging, burning, pruritus

Contraindications: Hypersensitivity

Precautions: Pregnancy, lactation

Interactions/incompatibilities: None known

NURSING CONSIDERATIONS
Administer:
• Enough medication to completely cover lesions
• After cleansing with soap, water before each application, dry well

Perform/provide:
• Storage at room temperature in dry place

Evaluate:
• Allergic reaction: burning, stinging, swelling, redness
• Therapeutic response: decrease in size, number of lesions

Teach patient/family:
• To apply with glove to prevent further infection
• To avoid use of OTC creams, ointments, lotions unless directed by physician
• To use medical asepsis (hand washing) before, after each application

---

iodoquinol

(eye-oh-do-kwin'ole)
Diodoquin,* Yodoxin, Amebaquine

Func. class.: Amebicide
Chem. class.: Dihalogenated derivative of 8-hydroxyquinoline

Action: Direct-acting amebicide; action occurs in intestinal lumen
Uses: Intestinal amebiasis

Dosage and routes:
• *Adult:* PO 630-650 mg tid × 20 days, not to exceed 2 g/day
• *Child:* PO 30-40 mg/kg/day in 2-3 divided doses × 20 days; do not repeat treatment before 2-3 wk
Available forms include: Tabs 210, 650 mg; powder

Side effects/adverse reactions:
*HEMA: **Agranulocytosis*** (rare)
INTEG: Rash, pruritus, discolored skin, alopecia
CNS: Headache, dizziness, ataxia
EENT: Blurred vision, sore throat, retinal edema, subacute myelooptic neuropathy
GI: Nausea, vomiting, diarrhea, epigastric distress, anorexia, gastritis, constipation, abdominal cramps, rectal irritation, itching
Contraindications: Hypersensitivity to this drug or iodine, renal disease, hepatic disease, severe thyroid disease, preexisting optic neuropathy
Precautions: Pregnancy (C)

Pharmacokinetics:
PO: Not known
Interactions/incompatibilities:
None known

NURSING CONSIDERATIONS

Assess:
• Stools during entire treatment; should be clear at end of therapy, for 1 yr before patient is considered cured
• I&O, stools for number, frequency, character

Administer:
• PO after meals to avoid GI symptoms

Perform/provide:
• Storage in tight container

Evaluate:
• Iodism: skin eruption, urticaria, discoloring of hair, nails
• Allergic reaction: fever, rash, itching, chills; drug should be discontinued if these occur
• Blurred vision
• Superimposed infection; fever, monilial growth, fatigue, malaise
• Diarrhea for 2-3 days

Teach patient/family:
• Proper hygiene after BM: handwashing technique
• Avoid contact of drug with eyes, mouth, nose, other mucous membranes
• Need for compliance with dosage schedule, duration of treatment

Lab test interferences:
False positive: PKU
Increase: PBI
Decrease: [131]I uptake test

---

ipecac syrup

(ip'e-kak)

Func. class.: Emetic
Chem. class.: Cephaelis ipeca-cuanha derivative

Action: Acts on chemoreceptor trigger zone to induce vomiting, irritates gastric mucosa
Uses: In poisoning to induce vomiting
Dosage and routes:
• *Adult:* PO 15 ml, then 200-300 ml water
• *Child >1 yr:* PO 15 ml, then 200-300 ml water
• *Child <1 yr:* PO 5-10 ml, then 100-200 ml water; may repeat dose if needed
Available forms include: Liq
Side effects/adverse reactions:
CNS: Depression, convulsions, coma
GI: Nausea, vomiting, bloody diarrhea
CV: Circulatory failure, atrial fibrillation, fatal myocarditis, dysrhythmias
Contraindications: Hypersensitivity, unconscious/semiconscious, depressed gag reflex, poisoning with petroleum products, convulsions
Precautions: Lactation, pregnancy
Pharmacokinetics:
PO: Onset 15-30 min
Interactions/incompatibilities:
• Do not administer with activated charcoal; effect will be decreased
NURSING CONSIDERATIONS
Assess:
• VS, B/P; check patients with cardiac disease more often
Administer:
• Ipecac *syrup* not ipecac, which is 14 times stronger; death may occur
• Then bounce child to increase emetic effect

• Activated charcoal if this drug doesn't work; may begin lavage after 10-15 min
Evaluate:
• Type of poisoning; do not administer if petroleum products or caustic substances have been ingested: kerosene, gasoline, lye, Drano
• Respiratory status before, during, after administration of emetic; check rate, rhythm, character; respiratory depression can occur rapidly with elderly or debilitated patients

iron dextran

Dextraron, Feostat, Hematran, Hydextran, Imferon, Irodex, K-Feron, Proferdex, Rocyte, Nor-Feran

Func. class.: Hematinic
Chem. class.: Ferric hydroxide complexed with dextran

Action: Iron is carried by transferring to the bone marrow where it is incorporated into hemoglobin
Uses: Iron deficiency anemia
Dosage and routes:
• *Adult and child:* IM 0.5 ml as a test dose by Z-track, then no more than the following per day
• *Adult <50 kg:* IM 100 mg
• *Adult >50 kg:* IM 250 mg
• *Infant <5 kg:* IM 25 mg
• *Child <9 kg:* IM 50 mg
• *Adult:* IV 0.5 ml test dose then 100 mg qd after 2-3 days; IV 250/1000 ml of NaCl, give 25 mg test dose, wait 5 min, then infuse over 6-12 hr or follow equation

$$\frac{0.3 \times \text{wt (lb)} \times 100\text{-Hgb (g/dl)} \times 100}{14.8} = \text{mg iron}$$

<30 lb should be given 80% of above formula dose
Available forms include: Inj IM/IV

50 mg/ml, inj IM only 50 mg/ml

Side effects/adverse reactions:

CNS: Headache, paresthesia, dizziness, shivering, weakness, seizures

GI: Nausea, vomiting, metallic taste, abdominal pain

INTEG: Rash, pruritus, urticaria, fever, sweating, chills, brown skin discoloration at injection site, necrosis, sterile abscesses, phlebitis

CV: Chest pain, *shock,* hypotension, tachycardia

RESP: Dyspnea

HEMA: Leukocytosis

Other: Anaphylaxis

Contraindications: Hypersensitivity, all anemias excluding iron deficiency anemia, hepatic disease

Precautions: Acute renal disease, children, asthma, lactation, rheumatoid arthritis (IV), infants <4 mo

Pharmacokinetics:

IM: Excreted in feces, urine, bile, breast milk, crosses placenta

Interactions/incompatibilities:

• Not to mix with other drugs in syringe or D_5W

• Decreased reticulocyte response: chloramphenicol

• Increased toxicity: oral iron—do not use

NURSING CONSIDERATIONS

Assess:

• Blood studies: Hct, Hgb, reticulocytes, bilirubin before treatment, at least monthly

Administer:

• Only after test dose of 25 mg by preferred route; wait at least 1 hr before giving remaining portion

• IM deeply in large muscle mass, use Z-track method and a 19-20 G 2-3 inch needle; ensure needle is long enough to place drug deep in muscle

• IV, after flushing with 10 ml of NS

• IV injection requires single dose vial without preservative; verify on label IV use is approved

• IV injection only by physician; this route is not FDA approved

• Only with epinephrine available in case of anaphylactic reaction during dose

Perform/provide:

• Storage at room temperature in cool environment

• Recumbent position 30 min after injection

Evaluate:

• Allergy: *anaphylaxis*, rash, pruritus, fever, chills

• Cardiac status: chest pain, hypotension, tachycardia

• Nutrition: amount of iron in diet (meat, dark green leafy vegetables, dried beans, dried fruits, eggs)

• Cause of iron loss or anemia including salicylates, sulfonamides

Teach patient/family:

• That iron poisoning may occur if increased beyond recommended level

Lab test interferences:

False increase: Serum bilirubin

False decrease: Serum calcium

False positive: ^{99m}Tc diphosphate bone scan, iron test (large doses >2 ml)

---

isocarboxazid

(eye-soe-kar-box′a-zid)

Marplan

Func. class.: Antidepressant—MAOI

Chem. class.: Hydrazine

Action: Increases concentrations of endogenous epinephrine, norepinephrine, serotonin, dopamine in storage sites in CNS by inhibition of MAO; increased concentration reduces depression

Uses: Depression, when uncontrolled by other means

Dosage and routes:
• *Adult:* PO 30 mg/day in divided doses, reduce dose to lowest effective dose when condition improves
Available forms include: Tabs 10 mg

Side effects/adverse reactions:
HEMA: Anemia

CNS: Dizziness, drowsiness, confusion, headache, anxiety, tremors, stimulation, weakness, hyperreflexia, mania, insomnia, fatigue, weight gain

GI: Constipation, dry mouth, nausea, vomiting, *anorexia,* diarrhea, weight gain

GU: Change in libido, frequency

INTEG: Rash, flushing, increased perspiration, jaundice

CV: Orthostatic hypotension, hypertension, dysrhythmias, hypertensive crisis

EENT: Blurred vision

ENDO: SIADH-like syndrome

Contraindications: Hypersensitivity to MAOIs, elderly, hypertension, CHF, severe hepatic disease, pheochromocytoma, severe renal disease, severe cardiac disease

Precautions: Suicidal patients, convulsive disorders, severe depression, schizophrenia, hyperactivity, diabetes mellitus, pregnancy (C)

Pharmacokinetics:
PO: Duration up to 2 wk; metabolized by liver, excreted by kidneys

Interactions/incompatibilities:
• Increased pressor effects: guanethidine, clonidine, indirect acting sympathomimetics (ephedrine)
• Increased effects of: direct acting sympathomimetics (epinephrine), alcohol, barbiturates, benzodiazepines, CNS depressants
• Hyperpyretic crisis, convulsions, hypertensive episode: tricyclic antidepressants

NURSING CONSIDERATIONS
Assess:
• B/P (lying, standing), pulse; if systolic B/P drops 20 mm Hg hold drug, notify physician
• Blood studies: CBC, leukocytes, cardiac enzymes if patient is receiving long-term therapy
• Hepatic studies: ALT, AST, bilirubin, creatinine, hepatotoxicity may occur

Administer:
• Increased fluids, bulk in diet if constipation, urinary retention occur
• With food or milk for GI symptoms
• Crushed if patient is unable to swallow medication whole
• Dosage hs if over-sedation occurs during day
• Gum, hard candy, or frequent sips of water for dry mouth
• Phentolamine for severe hypertension

Perform/provide:
• Storage in tight container in cool environment
• Assistance with ambulation during beginning therapy since drowsiness/dizziness occurs
• Safety measures including siderails
• Checking to see PO medication swallowed

Evaluate:
• Toxicity: increased headache, palpitation; discontinue drug immediately; prodromal signs of hypertensive crisis
• Mental status: mood, sensorium, affect, memory (long, short), increase in psychiatric symptoms
• Urinary retention, constipation, edema, take weight weekly
• Withdrawal symptoms: headache, nausea, vomiting, muscle pain, weakness

---

*Available in Canada only

Teach patient/family:
• That therapeutic effects may take 1-4 wk
• To avoid driving or other activities requiring alertness
• To avoid alcohol ingestion, CNS depressants or OTC medications: cold, weight, hay fever, cough syrup
• Not to discontinue medication quickly after long-term use
• To avoid high tyramine foods: cheese (aged), sour cream, beer, wine, pickled products, liver, raisins, bananas, figs, avocados, meat tenderizers, chocolate, yogurt; increase caffeine
• Report headache, palpitation, neck stiffness

Treatment of overdose: Lavage, activated charcoal, monitor electrolytes, vital signs, diazepam IV, NaHCO₃

---

isoetharine HCl/
isoetharine mesylate

(eye-soe-eth′a-reen)
Beta-Z solution, Bronkosol/Bronkometer

Func. class.: Adrenergic β-blocker

Action: Causes increased contractility and heart rate by acting on β-receptors in heart; also, acts on α-receptors, causing vasoconstriction in blood vessels; when larger doses are administered, cause vasodilation in renal, intracerebral, coronary dopaminergic receptors
Uses: Bronchospasm, asthma
Dosage and routes:
• *Adult:* INH 3-7 puffs undiluted, IPPB 0.5 ml diluted 1:3 with NS
Available forms include: Sol for nebulization 0.06%, 0.08%, 0.1%, 0.125%, 0.17%, 0.2%, 0.25%, 0.5%, 10%
Side effects/adverse reactions:
CNS: Tremors, anxiety, insomnia,

headache, dizziness, stimulation
CV: Palpitations, tachycardia, hypertension, *cardiac arrest*
GI: Nausea
Contraindications: Hypersensitivity to sympathomimetics, narrow-angle glaucoma
Precautions: Pregnancy, cardiac disorders, hyperthyroidism, diabetes mellitus, prostatic hypertrophy
Pharmacokinetics:
INH: Onset immediate, peak 5-15 min, duration 1-4 hr, metabolized in liver, GI tract, lungs, excreted in urine
Interactions/incompatibilities:
• May increase effects of both drugs when combined with other sympathomimetic
• Decreased action when used with other β-blockers

NURSING CONSIDERATIONS
Assess:
• Respiratory function: vital capacity, forced expiratory volume, ABGs
Administer:
• 2 hr before hs to avoid sleeplessness
Perform/provide:
• Storage at room temperature; do not use discolored solutions
Evaluate:
• Paresthesias and coldness of extremities, peripheral blood flow may decrease
• Injection site: tissue sloughing; if this occurs, administer phentolamine mixed with NS
• Therapeutic response: increased B/P with stabilization
Teach patient/family:
• Not to use OTC medications, extra stimulation may occur
• Use of inhaler, review package insert with patient
• To avoid getting aerosol in eyes
• To wash inhaler in warm water and dry qd
• On all aspects of drug; avoid

---

italics = common side effects   *bold italic* = life threatening reactions smoking, smoke-filled rooms, persons with respiratory infections

---

isoflurophate

(eye-soe-flure'oh-fate)
Floropryl, Diisopropyl Fluorophosphate, Diflupyl

Func. class.: Miotic
Chem. class.: Cholinesterase inhibitor, irreversible

Action: Prevents breakdown of neurotransmitter acetylcholine, which then accumulates, causing enhancement, prolongation of its physiologic effects
Uses: Wide-angle glaucoma, accommodative esotropia, conditions obstructing aqueous outflow
Dosage and routes:
• *Adult and child:* INSTILL ¼ in strip of 0.25% oint in conjunctival sac q8-72 hr for glaucoma or qhs × 2 wk for esotropia
Available forms include: Only as ophthalmic ointment 0.25%
Side effects/adverse reactions:
CNS: Headache
CV: Hypotension, bradycardia, paradoxic tachycardia
RESP: Bronchospasm, dyspnea, bronchoconstriction, wheezing
EENT: Blurred vision, lacrimation, conjunctival congestion
GU: Urinary incontinence
GI: Abdominal cramps, diarrhea, increased salivation, nausea, vomiting
Contraindications: Hypersensitivity, uveal inflammation
Precautions: History of retinal detachment
Interactions/incompatibilities:
None known
NURSING CONSIDERATIONS
Administer:
• Ointment to conjunctival sac with patient supine

Teach patient/family:
• That top of tube must not come in contact with moisture; keep tube closed, dry, away from tears or cornea; to wash hands after application of ointment
• To report change in vision, blurring or loss of sight, trouble breathing, sweating, flushing
• That long-term therapy may be required
• That blurred vision will decrease with repeated use of drug
• To minimize effects of blurred vision, application should take place at bedtime
• To observe for signs/symptoms of systemic absorption (i.e., diarrhea, weakness)
• To observe eyes for irritation
• To monitor for cardiac, respiratory, or GI problems

---

isoniazid (INH)

(eye-soe-nye'a-zid)
Hyzyd, Isotamine,* Laniazid, Nydrazid, PMS-Isoniazid,* Rimifon,* Rolazid, Teebaconin

Func. class.: Antitubercular
Chem. class.: Isonicotinic acid hydrazide

Action: Bactericidal interference with lipid, nucleic acid biosynthesis
Uses: Treatment, prevention of tuberculosis
Dosage and routes:
Treatment
• *Adult:* PO/IM 5 mg/kg qd as single dose for 9 mo to 2 yr, not to exceed 300 mg/day
• *Child and infants:* PO/IM 10-20 mg/kg qd as single dose for 18-24 mo, not to exceed 500 mg/day
Prevention
• *Adult* PO 300 mg qd as single dose × 12 mo
• *Child and infants:* PO/IM 10 mg/

---

kg qd as single dose for 12 mo, not to exceed 300 mg/day

Available forms include: Tabs 50, 100, 300 mg; inj 100 mg/ml; powder

Side effects/adverse reactions:

INTEG: Dermatitis, photosensitivity

CNS: Headache, anxiety, drowsiness, tremors, *convulsions,* lethargy, depression, confusion, psychosis, aggression

EENT: Blurred vision, optic neuritis, photophobia, leukocytosis

Contraindications: Hypersensitivity, optic neuritis

Precautions: Pregnancy, renal disease, diabetic retinopathy, cataracts, ocular defects, child <13 yr

Pharmacokinetics:

PO: Peak 1-2 hr, duration 6-8 hr

IM: Peak 45-60 min

Metabolized in liver, excreted in urine (metabolites), crosses placenta, excreted in breast milk

Interactions/incompatibilities:

• Increased toxicity: alcohol, cycloserine, ethionamide, rifampin, carbamazepine

• Decreased absorption: aluminum antacids, benzodiazepines, MAOIs, phenytoin

NURSING CONSIDERATIONS

Assess:

• Temperature, if <101° F drug should be reduced

• Liver studies q wk: ALT, AST, bilirubin

• Renal status: before, q mo: BUN, creatinine, output, sp gr, urinalysis

Administer:

• With meals to decrease GI symptoms

• Antiemetic if vomiting occurs

• After C&S is completed; q mo to detect resistance

Evaluate:

• Mental status often: affect, mood, behavioral changes; psychosis may occur

• Hepatic status: decreased appetite, jaundice, dark urine, fatigue

Teach patient/family:

• That compliance with dosage schedule, length is necessary

• That scheduled appointments must be kept or relapse may occur

• Avoid alcohol while taking drug

---

isopropamide iodide

(eye-soe-proe′pa-mide)

Darbid

Func. class.: Gastrointestinal anticholinergic

Chem. class.: Synthetic quaternary ammonium antimuscarinic

Action: Inhibits muscarinic actions of acetylcholine at postganglionic parasympathetic parasympathetic neuroeffector sites

Uses: Treatment of peptic ulcer disease, irritable bowel syndrome in combination with other drugs; for other GI disorders

Dosage and routes:

• *Adult and child >12 yr:* PO 5 mg q12h; need to titrate to patient response

Available forms include: Tabs 5 mg

Side effects/adverse reactions:

CNS: Confusion, stimulation in elderly, headache, insomnia, dizziness, drowsiness, anxiety, weakness, hallucination

GI: Dry mouth, constipation, paralytic ileus, heartburn, nausea, vomiting, dysphagia, absence of taste

GU: Hesitancy, retention, impotence

CV: Palpitations, tachycardia

EENT: Blurred vision, photophobia, mydriasis, cycloplegia, increased ocular tension

INTEG: Urticaria, rash, pruritus, anhidrosis, fever, allergic reactions

Contraindications: Hypersensitivity to anticholinergics, narrowangle glaucoma, GI obstruction,

---

italics = common side effects   ***bold italic*** = life threatening reactions

myasthenia gravis, paralytic ileus, GI atony, toxic megacolon

Precautions: Hyperthyroidism, coronary artery disease, dysrhythmias, iodine hypersensitivity, CHF, ulcerative colitis, hypertension, hiatal hernia, hepatic disease, renal disease

Pharmacokinetics:

PO: Duration 4-6 hr; metabolized by liver, excreted in urine, half-life 13-38 hr

Interactions/incompatibilities:

• Increased anticholinergic effect; amantadine, tricyclic antidepressants, MAOIs

• Increased effect of: nitrofurantoin

• Decreased effect of: phenothiazines, levodopa

NURSING CONSIDERATIONS

Assess:

• VS, cardiac status: checking for dysrhythmias, increased rate, palpitations

• I&O ratio; check for urinary retention or hesitancy

Administer:

• ½-1 hr ac for better absorption

• Decreased dose to elderly patients; their metabolism may be slowed

• Gum, hard candy, frequent rinsing of mouth for dryness of oral cavity

Perform/provide:

• Storage in tight container protected from light

• Increased fluids, bulk, exercise to patient's lifestyle to decrease constipation

Evaluate:

• Therapeutic response: absence of epigastric pain, bleeding, nausea, vomiting

• GI complaints: pain, bleeding (frank or occult), nausea, vomiting, anorexia

Teach patient/family:

• Avoid driving or other hazardous activities until stabilized on medication

• Avoid alcohol or other CNS depressants; will enhance sedating properties of this drug

• To avoid hot environments, stroke may occur, drug suppresses perspiration

• Use sunglasses when outside to prevent photophobia

Lab test interferences:

Decrease level: 24 hr ^{131}I thyroid uptake test

---

isoproterenol HCl/isoproterenol sulfate

(eye-soe-proe-ter'e-nole)

Isuprel, Proternol, Norisodrine, Vapo-Iso/Iso-Autohaler, Luf-Iso Inhalation, Medihaler-Iso, Norisodrine

Func. class.: Adrenergic
Chem. class.: Catecholamine

Action: Causes increased contractility and heart rate by acting on β-receptors in heart, also acts on α-receptors, causing vasoconstriction in blood vessels; when larger doses are administered, causes vasodilation in renal, intracerebral, coronary dopaminergic receptors

Uses: Bronchospasm, asthma, heart block, ventricular dysrhythmias, shock

Dosage and routes:

Asthma, bronchospasm

• *Adult:* SL 10-20 mg q6-8h HCl; INH 1 puff, may repeat in 2-5 min, maintenance 1-2 puffs 4-6 × per day

• *Child:* SL 5-10 mg q6-8 HCl; INH 1 puff, may repeat in 2-5 min, maintenance 1-2 puffs 4-6× per day

Heart block/ventricular dysrhythmias

• *Adult:* IV 0.02-0.06, then 0.01-0.2 mg or 5 μg/min HCl; IM 0.2

mg, then 0.02-1 mg as needed HCl
• *Child:* IV/IM ½ of beginning adult dose
Shock
• *Adult and child:* IV INF 0.5-5 μg/min 1 mg/500 ml D₅W, titrate to B/P, CVP, and hourly urine output

Available forms include: Sol for nebulization 1:400 (0.25%), 1:200 (0.5%), 1:100 (1%); aerosol 0.25%, 0.2%; powd for INH 0.1 mg/cart; inj 1:5000 (0.2 mg/ml) IV, IM; glossets (SL) 10 mg

Side effects/adverse reactions:
CNS: Tremors, anxiety, insomnia, headache, dizziness, stimulation
CV: Palpitations, tachycardia, hypertension, **cardiac arrest**
GI: Nausea

Contraindications: Hypersensitivity to sympathomimetics, narrow-angle glaucoma

Precautions: Pregnancy, cardiac disorders, hyperthyroidism, diabetes mellitus, prostatic hypertrophy

Pharmacokinetics:
INH/SL: Onset 1-2 hr
SC: Onset 2 hr
REC: Onset 2-4 hr
Metabolized in liver, lungs, GI tract

Interactions/incompatibilities:
• Increased effects of both drugs: other sympathomimetics
• Decreased action when used with β-blockers

NURSING CONSIDERATIONS
Assess:
• Blood studies (CBC, WBC, differential) since blood dyscrasias may occur (rare)
• I&O ratio; check for urinary retention, frequency, hesitancy
Administer:
• With meals for GI symptoms
Perform/provide:
• Storage at room temperature, do not use discolored solutions

Evaluate:
• For paresthesias and coldness of extremities, peripheral blood flow may decrease
• Injection site: tissue sloughing; if this occurs administer phentolamine mixed with NS
• Therapeutic response: increased B/P with stabilization
Teach patient/family:
• Use of inhaler, review package insert with patient
• To avoid getting aerosol in eyes
• To wash inhaler in warm water and dry qd
• On all aspects of drug; avoid smoking, smoke-filled rooms, persons with respiratory infections
Treatment of overdose: Administer an α-blocker, then norepinephrine for severe hypotension

---

isosorbide

(eye-soe-sor′bide)
Ismotic

Func. class.: Miscellaneous ophthalmic agent

Action: Increases osmotic gradient between plasma and ocular fluids, which decreases intraocular pressure

Uses: Intraocular pressure from glaucoma and cataract

Dosage and routes:
• *Adult:* PO 1.5 g/kg, then increase to 1-3 g/kg bid-qid

Available forms include: Sol 45%

Side effects/adverse reactions:
CNS: Headache, lightheadedness, irritability, lethargy
GI: Nausea, vomiting, anorexia, diarrhea, cramps
INTEG: Rash
META: Hypernatremia, hyperosmolarity

Contraindications: Hypersensitivity, anuria, severe renal disease,

pulmonary edema, hemorrhagic glaucoma
Interactions/incompatibilities:
None known
NURSING CONSIDERATIONS
Assess:
• I&O, report decrease urinary output
• Electrolytes during treatment
Administer:
• After pouring over ice

---

isosorbide dinitrate

(eye-soe-sor'bide)
Coronex,* Isordil, Isosorb, Onset, Sorate, Sorbitrate

Func. class.: Antianginal
Chem. class.: Nitrate

Action: Decreases preload, afterload, which is responsible for decreasing left ventricular end diastolic pressure, systemic vascular resistance
Uses: Chronic stable angina pectoris, prophylaxis of angina pain
Dosage and routes:
• *Adult:* PO 5-30 mg qid; SL 2.5-10 mg, may repeat q2-3h; CHEW TAB 5-10 mg prn or q2-3h as prophylaxis
Available forms include: Caps ext rel 40 mg; tabs 5, 10, 20, 30, 40 mg; chew tabs 5, 10 mg; tabs ext rel 40 mg; SL tabs 2.5, 5, 10 mg
Side effects/adverse reactions:
CV: Postural hypotension, tachycardia, collapse
GI: Nausea, vomiting
INTEG: Pallor, sweating
CNS: Headache, flushing, dizziness
Contraindications: Hypersensitivity to this drug or nitrites, anemia, increased intracranial pressure, cerebral hemorrhage, acute MI, pregnancy, lactation
Precautions: Postural hypotension, glaucoma

Pharmacokinetics:
SUS ACTION: Duration 6-12 hr
PO: Onset 15-30 min, duration 4-6 hr
SL: Onset 2-5 min, duration 1-2 hr
CHEW TAB: Onset 3 min, duration ½-3 hr
Metabolized by liver, excreted in urine as metabolites (80%-100%)
Interactions/incompatibilities:
• Increased effects: β-blockers, narcotics, tricyclics, diuretics, antihypertensives
• Decreased effects: sympathomimetics
NURSING CONSIDERATIONS
Assess:
• B/P, pulse, respirations during beginning therapy
Administer:
• With 8 oz of water on empty stomach (oral tablet)
Evaluate:
• Pain: duration, time started, activity being performed, character
• Tolerance if taken over long period of time
• Headache, lightheadedness, decreased B/P; may indicate a need for decreased dosage
Teach patient/family:
• That drug may be taken before stressful activity (exercise, sexual activity)
• That SL may sting when drug comes in contact with mucous membranes
• To avoid hazardous activities if dizziness occurs
• Stress patient compliance with complete medical regimen
• To make position changes slowly to prevent fainting

---

isotretinoin

(eye-soe-tret′i-noyn)
Accutane

Func. class.: Dermatologic
Chem. class.: Retinoic acid isomer,
vitamin A derivative

Action: Decreases sebum secre-
tion; improves cystic acne
Uses: Severe recalcitrant cystic
acne
Dosage and routes:
• *Adult:* PO 1-2 mg/kg/day in 2
divided doses × 15-20 wk
Available forms include: Caps 10,
20, 40 mg
Side effects/adverse reactions:
*INTEG: Dry skin, pruritus, chei-
losis, joint muscle pain, hair loss,
photosensitivity,* urticariam bruising, hirsutism
MS: Spine degeneration
CV: Chest pain
*GI: Nausea, vomiting, anorexia,
increased liver enzymes,* regional
ileus
*EENT: Eye irritation, conjunctivi-
tis, epistaxis, dry nose, mouth,*
contact lens intolerance
GU: Hematuria, proteinuria, hy-
pouricemia
HEMA: **Thrombocytopenia,** decreased H&H, WBC, reticulocyte
count
CNS: Lethargy, fatigue, headache,
depression, **pseudotumor cerebri**
Contraindications: Hypersensitivity, severe renal disease, inflamed
skin, pregnancy (X)
Precautions: Lactation, diabetes,
photosensitivity
Pharmacokinetics:
PO: Peak 2.9-3.2 hr, half-life 10-
20 hr; metabolized in liver, excreted
in urine, feces
Interactions/incompatibilities:
• Additive toxic effects: vitamin A,
do not use together

• Pseudotumor cerebri: minocy-
cline or tetracycline
• Increased triglyceride levels: al-
cohol
NURSING CONSIDERATIONS
Assess:
• Triglyceride levels, AST, ALT,
alk phosphatase; before, during
treatment
• Urinalysis qwk for protein, blood
• Blood glucose in diabetics peri-
odically
Administer:
• Whole, do not crush; give with
meals
• Second course of treatment if
needed after waiting 2 mo
Perform/provide:
• Storage in tight, light-resistant
container
Evaluate:
• Therapeutic response: decrease in
size and number of lesions
• Area of body involved, including
time involved, what helps or ag-
gravates condition
• Pseudotumor cerebri: headache,
vomiting, nausea, visual distur-
bance; discontinue drug
Teach patient/family:
• To avoid sunlight or wear sun-
screen since photosensitivity may
occur
• That an increase in acne may oc-
cur during initial treatment; de-
crease in 4-6 wk
• Not to become pregnant while
taking drug
• Not to take vitamin A supple-
ments, to take drug with meals
• Regarding package insert
• Do not crush
• Minimize or eliminate alcohol
consumption
Lab test interferences:
Increase: Sedimentation rate, tri-
glyceride, liver function studies
Decrease: RBC/WBC count

---

isoxsuprine HCl

(eye-sox'syoo-preen)

Vasodilan, Voxsuprine

Func. class.: Peripheral vasodilator

Chem. class.: Nylidrin related agent

Action: α-Adrenoreceptor with β-adrenoreceptor blocker properties; may also act directly on vascular smooth muscle; causes cardiac stimulation, uterine relaxation

Uses: Symptoms of cerebrovascular insufficiency, peripheral vascular disease including arteriosclerosis obliterans, thromboangiitis obliterans, Raynaud's disease

Dosage and routes:

• *Adult:* PO 10-20 mg tid or qid

Available forms include: Tabs 10, 20 mg

Side effects/adverse reactions:

*CV: Hypotension, **tachycardia,*** palpitations, chest pain

CNS: Dizziness, weakness, tremors, anxiety

GI: Nausea, vomiting, abdominal pain, distention

INTEG: Severe rash, flushing

Contraindications: Hypersensitivity, postpartem

Precautions: Pregnancy, tachycardia

Pharmacokinetics:

PO: Peak 1 hr, duration 3 hr, half-life 1¼ hr; excreted in urine, crosses placenta

Interactions/incompatibilities:

None known

NURSING CONSIDERATIONS

Assess:

• B/P, pulse during treatment until stable; take B/P lying, standing; orthostatic hypotension is common

Administer:

• With meals to reduce GI upset

Perform/provide:

• Storage at room temperature

Evaluate:

• Therapeutic response: ability to walk without pain, increased pulse volume, increased temperature in extremities, orientation, long- and short-term memory

Teach patient/family:

• That medication is not cure, may need to be taken continuously, therapeutic response may not be evident for 2-3 mo

• That it is necessary to quit smoking to prevent excessive vasoconstriction

• To avoid hazardous activities until stabilized on medication; dizziness may occur

• To make position changes slowly, or fainting will occur

• To discontinue drug, notify physician if rash develops

• To report palpitations, flushing if severe

• To avoid changes in temperature; extremities should be kept warm to promote better circulation

kanamycin sulfate

(kan-a-mye'sin)

Anamid,* Kantrex, Klebcil

Func. class.: Antibiotic

Chem. class.: Aminoglycoside

Action: Interferes with protein synthesis in bacterial cell by binding to ribosomal subunit, causing inaccurate peptide sequence to form in protein chain, causing bacterial death

Uses: Severe systemic infections of CNS, respiratory, GI, urinary tract, bone, skin, soft tissues caused by *E. coli, Enterobacter, Acinetobacter, Proteus, K. pneumoniae, S. marcescens, Staphylococcus;* also used as adjunct in hepatic coma, peritonitis, preoperatively to sterilize bowel

Dosage and routes:

Severe systemic infections

• *Adult and child:* IV INF 15 mg/kg/day in divided doses q8-12h; diluted 500 mg/200 ml of NS or D₅W given over 60-80 gtts/min, not to exceed 1.5 g/day; IM 15 mg/kg/day in divided doses q8-12h, not to exceed 1.5 g/day

Hepatic coma

• *Adult:* PO 8-12 g/day in divided doses

Preoperative bowel sterilization

• *Adult:* PO 1 g qlh × 4 doses, then q6h × 36-72 hr

Available forms include: Inj IM, IV 37.5, 250, 333 mg/ml; cap 500 mg

Side effects/adverse reactions:

GU: Oliguria, hematuria, renal damage, azotemia, renal failure, nephrotoxicity

CNS: Confusion, depression, numbness, tremors, *convulsions,* muscle twitching, *neurotoxicity*

EENT: Ototoxicity, deafness, visual disturbances

HEMA: Agranulocytosis, thrombocytopenia, leukopenia, eosinophilia, anemia

GI: Nausea, vomiting, anorexia, increased ALT, AST, bilirubin, hepatomegaly, *hepatic necrosis,* splenomegaly

CV: Hypotension, myocarditis

INTEG: Rash, burning, urticaria, photosensitivity, dermatitis

Contraindications: Bowel obstruction, severe renal disease, hypersensitivity

Precautions: Neonates, myasthenia gravis, hearing deficits, mild renal disease, pregnancy, lactation

Pharmacokinetics:

IM: Onset rapid, peak 1-2 hr

IV: Onset immediate, peak 1-2 hr

Plasma half-life 2-3 hr; not metabolized, excreted unchanged in urine, crosses placental barrier

Interactions/incompatibilities:

• Increased ototoxicity, neurotoxicity, nephrotoxicity: other aminoglycosides, amphotericin B, polymyxin, vancomycin, ethacrynic acid, furosemide, mannitol, methoxyflurane, cisplatin, cephalosporins

• Decreased effects of: parenteral penicillins, digoxin, vitamin B₁₂

• Do not mix in solution or syringe: carbenicillin, ticarcillin, amphotericin B, cephalothin, erythromycin, heparin

• Increased effects: nondepolarizing muscle relaxants

• Decreased effects of: oral anticoagulants

NURSING CONSIDERATIONS **K**

Assess:

• Weight before treatment; calculation of dosage is usually done based on ideal body weight, but may be calculated on actual body weight

• I&O ratio, urinalysis daily for proteinuria, cells, casts; report sudden change in urine output

• VS during infusion, watch for hypotension, change in pulse

• IV site for thrombophlebitis including pain, redness, swelling q30 min, change site if needed; apply warm compresses to discontinued site

• Serum peak, drawn at 30-60 min after IV infusion or 60 min after IM injection; trough level drawn just before next dose; blood level should be 2-4 times bacteriostatic level

• Urine pH if drug is used for UTI; urine should be kept alkaline

Administer:

• IM injection in large muscle mass, rotate injection sites

• Drug in evenly spaced doses to maintain blood level

• Bicarbonate to alkalinize urine if ordered in treating UTI, as drug is most active in alkaline environment

Perform/provide:

• Adequate fluids of 2-3 L/day unless contraindicated to prevent irritation of tubules

• Flush of IV line with NS or D_5W after infusion

• Supervised ambulation, other safety measures with vestibular dysfunction

Evaluate:

• Therapeutic effect: absence of fever, draining wounds, negative C&S after treatment

• Renal impairment by securing urine for CrCl testing, BUN, serum creatinine; lower dosage should be given in renal impairment (CrCl <80 ml/min)

• Deafness by audiometric testing, ringing, roaring in ears, vertigo; assess hearing before, during, after treatment

• Dehydration: high sp gr, decrease in skin turgor, dry mucous membranes, dark urine

• Overgrowth of infection: increased temperature, malaise, redness, pain, swelling, perineal itching, diarrhea, stomatitis, change in cough, sputum

• C&S before starting treatment to identify infecting organism

• Vestibular dysfunction: nausea, vomiting, dizziness, headache; drug should be discontinued if severe

• Injection sites for redness, swelling, abscesses; use warm compresses at site

Teach patient/family:

• To report headache, dizziness, symptoms of overgrowth of infection, renal impairment

• To report loss of hearing, ringing, roaring in ears or feeling of fullness in head

Treatment of overdose: Hemodialysis, monitor serum levels of drug

---

kaolin, pectin

(kay'o-lynn)

Baropectin, Kaoparin, Kaopectate, Kapectin, Keotin, Pectokay

Func. class.: Antidiarrheal
Chem. class.: Hydrous magnesium aluminum silicate

Action: Decreases gastric motility, H_2O content of stool

Uses: Diarrhea (cause undetermined)

Dosage and routes:

• *Adult:* PO 60-120 ml after each bm

• *Child >12 yr:* PO 60 ml after each bm

• *Child 6-12 yr:* PO 30-60 ml after each bm

• *Child 3-6 yr:* PO 15-30 ml after each bm

Available forms include: Susp Kaolin 0.87 g/5ml; Pectin 43 mg/5 ml; Kaolin 0.98 g/5 ml; Pectin 21.7 mg/5 ml

Side effects/adverse reactions:
None known

Pharmacokinetics:
Not known

Interactions/incompatibilities:
None known

NURSING CONSIDERATIONS

Administer:

• For 48 hr only

Evaluate:

• Therapeutic response: decreased diarrhea

• Bowel pattern before; for rebound constipation

• Dehydration in children

Teach patient/family:

• Not to exceed recommended dose

• To shake well before administration

---

ketamine HCl

(keet'a-meen)
Ketalar

Func. class.: General anesthetic
Chem. class.: Phencyclidine derivative

Action: Acts on limbic system, cortex to provide anesthesia
Uses: Short anesthesia for diagnostic/surgical procedures
Dosage and routes:
• *Adult and child:* IV 1-4.5 mg/kg over 1 min
• *Adult and child:* IM 6.5-13 mg/kg
Available forms include: Inj IM, IV 10, 50, 100 mg/vial
Side effects/adverse reactions:
CNS: Hallucinations, confusion, delirium, tremors, polyneuropathy, fasciculations, pseudoconvulsions
CV: Increased BP, hypotension, bradycardia
EENT: Diplopia, salivation, small increase in intraocular pressure
INTEG: Rash, pain at injection site
Contraindications: Hypersensitivity, CVA, increased intracranial pressure, severe hypertension, cardiac decompensation, child <2 yr
Precautions: Pregnancy, seizure disorders, elderly, psychiatric disorders
Pharmacokinetics:
IV: Peak 40 sec, duration 10 min
IM: Peak 3-8 min, duration 25 min
Interactions/incompatibilities:
• Increased action of this drug: narcotics or atropine
• Increased action of: tobocurarine
• Do not mix with barbiturates in solution or syringe
NURSING CONSIDERATIONS
Assess:
• VS q10 min during IV administration, q30 min after IM dose

Administer:
• Anticholinergic preoperatively to decrease solution
• Only with crash cart, resuscitative equipment nearby
• IV slowly only
• Narcotic, or diazepam to control recovery symptoms
Perform/provide:
• Quiet environment for recovery to decrease psychotic symptoms
Evaluate:
• Therapeutic response: maintenance of anesthesia
• Hallucinations, delusions, separation from environment
• Extrapyramidal reactions: dystonia, akathisia
• Increasing heart rate or decreasing B/P, notify physician at once

K

ketoconazole

(ke-to-con'a-zol)
Nizoral

Func. class.: Antifungal
Chem. class.: Imidazole derivative

Action: Alters cell membranes and interferes with fungal enzyme systems
Uses: Systemic candidiasis, chronic mucocandidiasis, oral thrush, candiduria, coccidioidomycosis, histoplasmosis, chromomycosis, paracoccidioidomycosis
Dosage and routes:
• *Adult and child >40 kg:* PO 200 mg qd, may increase to 400 mg qd if needed
• *Child 20-40 kg:* PO 100 mg qd
• *Child <20 kg:* PO 50 mg qd
Available forms include: Tabs 200 mg; susp 100 mg/5 ml
Side effects/adverse reactions:
GU: Gynecomastia, impotence
INTEG: Pruritus, fever, chills, photophobia, rash, dermatitis, purpura, urticaria
CNS: Headache, dizziness, leth-

argy, anxiety, insomnia, dreams, paresthesia

*SYST: **Anaphylaxis***

GI: Nausea, vomiting, anorexia, diarrhea, cramps, abdominal pain, constipation, flatulence, GI bleeding, ***hepatotoxicity***

Contraindications: Hypersensitivity, pregnancy (C), lactation, meningitis

Precautions: Renal disease, hepatic disease, achlorhydria (drug-induced)

Pharmacokinetics:

PO: Peak 1-2 hr, half-life 2 hr, terminal 8 hr, metabolized in liver, excreted in bile, feces, required acid pH for absorption, distributed poorly to CSF, highly protein bound

Interactions/incompatibilities:

• Hepatotoxicity: other hepatotoxic drugs

• Increased action of of this drug: cyclosporine

• Decreased action of: antacids, H_2-receptor antagonists (anticholinergics, antihistamines), isoniazid, rifampin

• Increased anticoagulant effect, coumarin anticoagulants

• Severe hypoglycemia; oral hypoglycemics

• Disulfuram reaction: alcohol

NURSING CONSIDERATIONS

Assess:

• I&O ratio

• Liver studies (ALT, AST, bilirubin) if on long-term therapy

Administer:

• In the presence of acid products only; do not use alkaline products or antacids within 2 hr of drug; may give coffee, tea, acidic fruit juices

• With food to decrease GI symptoms

• With hydrochloric acid if achlorhydria is present

Perform/provide:

• Storage in tight containers at room temperature

Evaluate:

• Therapeutic response: decreased fever, malaise, rash, negative C&S for infecting organism

• For allergic reaction: rash, photosensitivity, urticaria, dermatitis

• For hepatotoxicity: nausea, vomiting, jaundice, clay-colored stools, fatigue

Teach patient/family:

• That long-term therapy may be needed to clear infection (1 wk-6 mo depending on infection)

• To avoid hazardous activities if dizziness occurs

• To avoid antacids, OTC medications, alkaline products

• Stress patient compliance with drug regimen

• To notify physician if GI symptoms, signs of liver dysfunction (fatigue, nausea, anorexia, vomiting, dark urine, pale stools)

---

ketoprofen

(ke-to-proe'fen)
Orduis

Func. class.: Nonsteroidal
Chem. class.: Propionic acid derivative

Action: Inhibits prostaglandin synthesis by decreasing enzyme needed for biosynthesis; possesses analgesic, antiinflammatory, antipyretic properties

Uses: Mild to moderate pain, osteoarthritis, rheumatoid arthritis

Dosage and routes:

• *Adult:* PO 150-300 mg in divided doses tid-qid, not to exceed 300 mg/day

Available forms include: Caps 50, 75 mg

Side effects/adverse reactions:

GI: Nausea, anorexia, vomiting,

diarrhea, jaundice, ***cholestatic hepatitis,*** constipation, flatulence, cramps, dry mouth, peptic ulcer
CNS: Dizziness, drowsiness, fatigue, tremors, confusion, insomnia, anxiety, depression
CV: Tachycardia, peripheral edema, palpitations, dysrhythmias
INTEG: Purpura, rash, pruritus, sweating
GU: ***Nephrotoxicity:*** dysuria, hematuria, oliguria, azotemia
HEMA: ***Blood dyscrasias***
EENT: Tinnitus, hearing loss, blurred vision
Contraindications: Hypersensitivity, asthma, severe renal disease, severe hepatic disease
Precautions: Pregnancy (B), lactation, children, bleeding disorders, GI disorders, cardiac disorders, hypersensitivity to other antiinflammatory agents
Pharmacokinetics:
PO: Peak 2 hr, half-life 3-3½ hr, metabolized in liver, excreted in urine (metabolites), excreted in breast milk
Interactions/incompatibilities:
• May increase action of coumarin, phenytoin, sulfonamides
NURSING CONSIDERATIONS
Assess:
• Renal, liver, blood studies: BUN, creatinine, AST, ALT, Hgb, before treatment, periodically thereafter
• Audiometric, ophthalmic exam before, during, after treatment
Administer:
• With food to decrease GI symptoms; however, best to take on empty stomach to facilitate absorption
Perform/provide:
• Storage at room temperature
Evaluate:
• Therapeutic response: decreased pain, stiffness in joints, decreased swelling in joints, ability to move more easily
• For eye, ear problems: blurred vision, tinnitus; may indicate toxicity
Teach patient/family:
• To report blurred vision, ringing, roaring in ears; may indicate toxicity
• To avoid driving, other hazardous activities if dizziness, drowsiness occurs
• To report change in urine pattern, increased weight, edema, increased pain in joints, fever, blood in urine; indicate nephrotoxicity
• That therapeutic effects may take up to 1 mo

labetalol

(la-bet′a-lole)
Normodyne, Trandate
Func. class.: Antihypertensive
Chem. class.: Nonselective β-blocker

Action: Produces falls in B/P without reflex tachycardia or significant reduction in heart rate through mixture of α-blocking, β-blocking effects; elevated plasma renins are reduced
Uses: Mild to moderate hypertension
Dosage and routes:
Hypertension
• *Adult:* PO 100 mg bid, may be given with a diuretic, may increase to 200 mg bid after 2 days, may continue to increase q1-3 days
Hypertensive crisis
• *Adult:* IV INF 200 mg/200 ml D_5W, run at 2 mg/min; stop infusion after desired response obtained, repeat q6-8h as needed; IV BOL 20 mg over 2 min, may repeat 40-80 mg q10 min, not to exceed 300 mg
Available forms include: Tabs 100, 200, 300 mg

Side effects/adverse reactions:

*CV: Orthostatic hypotension, bradycardia, **CHF,** chest pain, **ventricular dysrhythmias**,* AV block

CNS: Dizziness, mental changes, drowsiness, fatigue, headache, catatonia, depression, anxiety, nightmares, paresthesias, lethargy

GI: Nausea, vomiting, diarrhea

INTEG: Rash, alopecia, urticaria, pruritus, fever

*HEMA: **Agranulocytosis, thrombocytopenia, purpura*** (rare)

EENT: Tinnitus, visual changes, sore throat, double vision, dry burning eyes

GU: Impotence, dysuria, ejaculatory failure

*RESP: **Bronchospasm,*** dyspnea, wheezing

Contraindications: Hypersensitivity to β-blockers, cardiogenic shock, heart block (2nd, 3rd degree), sinus bradycardia, CHF, bronchial asthma

Precautions: Major surgery, pregnancy, lactation, diabetes mellitus, renal disease, thyroid disease, COPD, well compensated heart failure, CAD, nonallergic bronchospasm

Pharmacokinetics:

PO: Onset 1-2 hr, peak 2-4 hr, duration 8-12 hr

IV: Peak 5 min

Half-life 6-8 hr, metabolized by liver (metabolites inactive), excreted in urine, bile, crosses placenta, excreted in breast milk

Interactions/incompatibilities:

• Increased hypotension: diuretics, other antihypertensives, halothane, cimetidine, nitroglycemia

• Decreased effects: sympathomimetics, lidocaine, indomethacin, theophylline

• Increased hypoglycemia: insulin

NURSING CONSIDERATIONS

Assess:

• I&O, weight daily

• B/P, pulse q4h; note rate, rhythm, quality

• Apical/radial pulse before administration; notify physician of any significant changes

• Baselines in renal, liver function tests before therapy begins

Administer:

• PO ac, hs, tablet may be crushed or swallowed whole

• Reduced dosage in renal dysfunction

• IV, keep patient recumbent for 3 hr

Perform/provide:

• Storage in dry area at room temperature, do not freeze

Evaluate:

• Therapeutic response: decreased B/P after 1-2 wk

• Edema in feet, legs daily

• Skin turgor, dryness of mucous membranes for hydration status

Teach patient/family:

• Not to discontinue drug abruptly, taper over 2 wk, may cause precipitate angina

• Not to use OTC products containing α-adrenergic stimulants (nasal decongestants, OTC cold preparations) unless directed by physician

• To report bradycardia, dizziness, confusion, depression, fever

• To take pulse at home, advise when to notify physician

• To avoid alcohol, smoking, sodium intake

• To comply with weight control, dietary adjustments, modified exercise program

• To carry Medic Alert ID to identify drug you are taking, allergies

• To avoid hazardous activities if dizziness is present

• To report symptoms of CHF: difficult breathing, especially on exertion or when lying down, night cough, swelling of extremities

• Take medication at bedtime to maintain effect of orthostatic hypotension

• Wear support hose to minimize effects of orthostatic hypotension

Lab test interferences:

False increase: Urinary catecholamines

Treatment of overdose: Lavage, IV atropine for bradycardia, IV theophylline for bronchospasm, digitalis, O_2, diuretic for cardiac failure; hemodialysis is useful for removal, hypotension; administer vasopressor (norepinephrine)

---

lactobacillus

(lak′too-ba-sill-us)

Bacid, DoFUS, Lactinex

Func. class.: Antidiarrheal

Chem. class.: Viable bacterial culture

Action: Decreases growth of organisms causing diarrhea in bowel

Uses: Diarrhea (cause undetermined), diarrhea caused by antibiotics

Dosage and routes:

• *Adult:* PO 2 caps bid-qid (Bacid), 4 tabs tid-qid (Lactinex), 1 tab qd ac (DoFUS); powder 1 pkg tid-qid (Lactinex)

Available forms include: Caps, granules 1 g/pkg, chew tabs

Side effects/adverse reactions:

GI: Flatus

Contraindications: Hypersensitivity, fever, child <3 yr, milk allergy

Pharmacokinetics:

Not known

Interactions/incompatibilities:

None known

NURSING CONSIDERATIONS

Administer:

• With water, fruit juice, or milk

• For antibiotic-induced diarrhea

• Granules or tabs with cereal, food, milk, fruit juice, water

Evaluate:

• Therapeutic response: decreased diarrhea

• Bowel pattern before; for rebound constipation

• Response after 48 hr; if no response, drug should be discontinued

• Dehydration in children; do not use in infants or children <3 yr

Teach patient/family:

• Not to exceed recommended dose

• To store in refrigerator

---

lactulose

(lak′tyoo-lose)

Cephulac, Chronulac

Func. class.: Ammonia detoxicant

Chem. class.: Lactose synthetic derivative

Action: Prevents absorption of ammonia in colon

Uses: Constipation, portal-systemic encephalopathy in patients with hepatic disease

Dosage and routes:

Constipation

• *Adult:* PO 15-60 ml qd

Encephalopathy

• *Adult:* PO 20-30 g tid or qid until stools are soft × 3 days; RET ENEMA 30-45 ml in 100 ml of fluid

Available forms include: Oral sol, rec sol 3.33 g/5 ml

Side effects/adverse reactions:

GI: Nausea, vomiting, anorexia, cramps, diarrhea, flatulence

Contraindications: Hypersensitivity

Precautions: Pregnancy, lactation, diabetes mellitus

Pharmacokinetics: Metabolized in intestine, excreted by kidneys

Interactions/incompatibilities:
• May decrease effects of this drug when used with neomycin

NURSING CONSIDERATIONS
Assess:
• Blood ammonia level (30-70 mg/100 ml)
• Blood, urine electrolytes if drug is used often by patient
• I&O ratio to identify fluid loss

Administer:
• Retention enema by diluting 300 ml lactose/700 ml of water; administer by rectal balloon catheter
• Increase fluids to 2 L/day

Evaluate:
• Therapeutic response: decreased constipation, decreased blood ammonia level
• Cause of constipation; identify whether fluids, bulk, or exercise is missing from lifestyle
• Cramping, rectal bleeding, nausea, vomiting; if these symptoms occur, drug should be discontinued
• Clearing of confusion, lethargy, restlessness, irritability

Teach patient/family:
• Not to use laxatives for long-term therapy; bowel tone will be lost

---

leucovorin calcium (citrovorum factor/folic acid)

(loo-koe-vor'in)
Calcium Folinate, Wellcovorin

Func. class.: Vitamin/folic acid antagonist antidote
Chem. class.: Tetrahydrofolic acid derivative

Action: Needed for normal growth patterns, prevents toxicity during antineoplastic therapy by protecting normal cells
Uses: Megaloblastic or macrocytic anemia caused by folic acid deficiency, overdose of folic acid antagonist, methotrexate toxicity, toxicity caused by pyrimethamine or trimethoprim, pneumocystosis, toxoplasmosis

Dosage and routes:
Megaloblastic anemia caused by enzyme deficiency
• *Adult and child:* IM 3-6 mg qd, then 1 mg PO for life
Megaloblastic anemia caused by deficiency of folate
• *Adult and child:* IM 1 mg or less qd, continued until adequate response
Methotrexate toxicity
• *Adult and child:* Given 6-36 hr after dose of methotrexate
Pyrimethamine toxicity
• *Adult and child:* PO/IM 5 mg qd
Trimethoprim toxicity
• *Adult and child:* PO IM 400 μg qd

Available forms include: Tabs 5, 25 mg; inj IM 3, 5 mg/ml; powder for inj 10 mg/ml

Side effects/adverse reactions:
RESP: Wheezing

Contraindications: Hypersensitivity, anemias other than megaloblastic not associated with B_{12} deficiency

Pharmacokinetics: Not known

Interactions/incompatibilities:
• Decreased folate levels: chloramphenicol
• Increased metabolism of: phenobarbitol, hydantoins

NURSING CONSIDERATIONS
Assess:
• Cr Cl before leucovorin rescue and qd to detect nephrotoxicity
• I&O, watch for nausea and vomiting

Administer:
• Within 1 hr of folic acid antagonist
• After reconstituting with bacteriostatic water for inj

Perform/provide:
• Increase fluid intake if used to

treat folic acid inhibitor overdose
Evaluate:
• Nutritional status: bran, yeast, dried beans, nuts, fruits, fresh vegetables, asparagus
• Therapeutic response: increased weight, oriented well-being, absence of fatigue
• Drugs currently taken: alcohol, hydantoins, trimethoprim may cause increased folic acid use by body
Teach patient/family:
• To take drug exactly as prescribed
• To notify physician of side effects

leuprolide acetate

(loo-proe′-lide)
Lupron
Func. class.: Antineoplastic hormone
Chem. class.: Gonadotropin-releasing hormone

Action: Suppresses testosterone production by stimulating FSH, then inhibiting FSH, LH
Uses: Metastatic prostate cancer
Dosage and routes:
• *Adult:* SC 1 mg/day
Available forms include: Inj SC 5 mg/ml
Side effects/adverse reactions:
GI: Nausea, vomiting, anorexia
GU: Edema
INTEG: Rash,
RESP: Emboli
Contraindications: Hypersensitivity to estradiol, thromboembolic disorders
Precautions: Edema, hepatic disease, CVA, MI, seizures, hypertension, diabetes mellitus, pregnancy
Pharmacokinetics: Not known
Interactions/incompatibilities: None known

NURSING CONSIDERATIONS
Assess:
• Pulmonary function tests, chest film before, during therapy; chest x-ray should be obtained q2 wk during treatment
• Liver function tests before, during therapy (bilirubin, AST, ALT, LDH) as needed or monthly
• RBC, Hct, Hgb since these may be decreased
Administer:
• Medications by oral route if possible; avoid IM, SC, IV routes to prevent infections
• Antacid before oral agent; give drug after evening meal before bedtime
• Antiemetic 30-60 min before giving drug to prevent vomiting
Perform/provide:
• Deep breathing exercises with patient 3-4 times/day; place in semi-Fowler's position
• Liquid diet, including cola, Jello; dry toast or crackers may be added if patient is not nauseated or vomiting
• Nutritious diet with iron, vitamin supplements as ordered
• HOB increased to facilitate breathing
• Storage in tight container at room temperature
Evaluate:
• Dyspnea, rales, unproductive cough, chest pain, tachypnea, fatigue, increased pulse, pallor, lethargy
• Food preferences; list likes, dislikes
• Edema in feet, joint, stomach pain, shaking
• Inflammation of mucosa, breaks in skin
• Yellowing of skin, sclera, dark urine, clay-colored stools, itchy skin, abdominal pain, fever, diarrhea
• Symptoms indicating severe al-

lergic reaction: rash, pruritus, urticaria, purpuric skin lesions, itching, flushing

Teach patient/family:

• To report any complaints, side effects to nurse or physician

• To report any changes in breathing, coughing

---

levodopa

(lee-voe-doe′pa)

Dopar, Larodopa, Levopa, Parda, Rio-Dopa

Func. class.: Antiparkinson agent
Chem. class.: Catecholamine

Action: Decarboxylation to dopamine, which increases dopamine levels in brain

Uses: Parkinsonism, carbon monoxide, chronic manganese intoxication, cerebral arteriosclerosis

Dosage and routes:

• *Adult:* PO 0.5-1 g qd divided bid-qid with meals, may increase by up to 0.75 g q3-7 days, not to exceed 8 g/day unless closely supervised

Available forms include: Caps 100, 250, 500 mg; tabs 100, 250, 500 mg

Side effects/adverse reactions:

HEMA: Hemolytic anemia, leukopenia, agranulocytosis

CNS: Choreiform, involuntary movements, hand tremors, fatigue, headache, anxiety, twitching, numbness, weakness, confusion, agitation, insomnia, nightmares, psychosis, hallucination, hypomania, severe depression

GI: Nausea, vomiting, anorexia, abdominal distress, dry mouth, flatulence, dysphagia, bitter taste, diarrhea, constipation

INTEG: Rash, sweating, alopecia

CV: Orthostatic hypotension, tachycardia, hypertension, palpitation

EENT: Blurred vision, diplopia, dilated pupils

Contraindications: Hypersensitivity, narrow-angle glaucoma, psychosis

Precautions: Renal disease, cardiac disease, hepatic disease, respiratory disease, MI with dysrhythmias, convulsions, peptic ulcer

Pharmacokinetics:

PO: Peak 1-3 hr, excreted in urine (metabolites)

Interactions/incompatibilities:

• Hypertensive crisis: MAOIs, sympathomimetics

• Dysrhythmias: cyclopropane, halogenated hydrocarbon anesthetics

• Increased effects of: guanethidine, methyldopa

• Decreased effects of: phenothiazines, diazepam, anticholinergics, hydantoins, reserpine, vitamin B_6, phenylbutazone

• Increased toxicity: MAOIs

NURSING CONSIDERATIONS

Assess:

• B/P, respiration

Administer:

• Drug up until NPO before surgery

• Adjust dosage depending on patient response

• With meals; limit protein taken with drug

• Only after MAOIs have been discontinued for 2 wk

Perform/provide:

• Assistance with ambulation, during beginning therapy

• Testing for diabetes mellitus, acromegaly if on long-term therapy

Evaluate:

• Mental status: affect, mood, behavioral changes, depression, complete suicide assessment

• Therapeutic response: decrease in akathesia, increased mood

Teach patient/family:

• To change positions slowly to

prevent orthostatic hypotension

• To report side effects: twitching, eye spasms; indicate overdose

• To use drug exactly as prescribed; if drug is discontinued abruptly, parkinsonian crisis may occur

• That urine, sweat may darken

• To avoid vitamin B_6 preparations, vitamin-fortified foods containing B_6; these foods can reverse effects of levodopa

Lab test interferences:

False positive: Urine ketones, urine glucose

False negative: Urine glucose (glucose oxidase)

False increase: Uric acid, urine protein

Decrease: VMA

---

levodopa-carbidopa

(lee-voe-doe′pa) (kar-bi-doe′pa)
Sinemet

Func. class.: Antiparkinson agent
Chem. class.: Catecholamine

Action: Decarboxylation to dopamine, which increases dopamine levels in brain

Uses: Parkinsonism, carbon monoxide, chronic manganese intoxication, cerebral arteriosclerosis

Dosage and routes:

• *Adult:* PO 3-6 tabs of 25 mg carbidopa/250 mg levodopa qd in divided doses, not to exceed 8 tabs/day

Available forms include: Tabs 10/100, 25/100, 25 mg carbidopa/250 mg levodopa

Side effects/adverse reactions:

*HEMA: **Hemolytic anemia, leukopenia, agranulocytosis***

CNS: Choreiform, involuntary movements, hand tremors, fatigue, headache, anxiety, twitching, numbness, weakness, confusion, agitation, insomnia, nightmares, psychosis, hallucination, hypomania, severe depression

GI: Nausea, vomiting, anorexia, abdominal distress, dry mouth, flatulence, dysphagia, bitter taste, diarrhea, constipation

INTEG: Rash, sweating, alopecia

CV: Orthostatic hypotension, tachycardia, hypertension, palpitation

EENT: Blurred vision, diplopia, dilated pupils

Contraindications: Hypersensitivity, narrow-angle glaucoma, psychosis

Precautions: Renal disease, cardiac disease, hepatic disease, respiratory disease, MI with dysrhythmias, convulsions, peptic ulcer

Pharmacokinetics:

PO: Peak 1-3 hr, excreted in urine (metabolites)

Interactions/incompatibilities:

• Hypertensive crisis: MAOIs, sympathomimetics

• Dysrhythmias: cyclopropane, halogenated hydrocarbon anesthetics

• Increased effects of: guanethidine, methyldopa

• Decreased effect of: phenothiazines, diazepam, anticholinergics, hydantoins, reserpine, vitamin B_6, phenylbutazone

• Increased toxicity: MAOIs

NURSING CONSIDERATIONS

Assess:

• B/P, respiration

Administer:

• Drug up until NPO before surgery

• Adjust dosage depending on patient response

• With meals; limit protein taken with drug

• Only after MAOIs have been discontinued for 2 wk

Perform/provide:

• Assistance with ambulation during beginning therapy

---

italics = common side effects   ***bold italic*** = life threatening reactions

• Testing for diabetes mellitus, acromegaly if on long-term therapy
Evaluate:
• Mental status: affect, mood, behavioral changes, depression, complete suicide assessment
• Therapeutic response: decrease in akathasia, increased mood
Teach patient/family:
• To change positions slowly to prevent orthostatic hypotension
• To report side effects: twitching, eye spasms; indicate overdose
• To use drug exactly as prescribed; if drug is discontinued abruptly, parkinsonian crisis may occur
• That urine, sweat may darken
Lab test interferences:
False positive: Urine ketones
False negative: Urine glucose
False increase: Uric acid, urine protein
Decrease: VMA, BUN, creatinine

---

levorphanol tartrate

(lee-vor'fa-nole)
Levo-Dromoran

Func. class.: Narcotic analgesics
Chem. class.: Opiate, synthetic morphine derivative

Controlled Substance Schedule II
Action: Inhibits ascending pain pathways in CNS, increases pain threshold, alters pain perception
Uses: Moderate to severe pain
Dosage and routes:
• *Adult:* PO/SC 2-3 mg q6-8h prn
Available forms include: Inj SC 2 mg/ml; tabs 2 mg
Side effects/adverse reactions:
CNS: Drowsiness, dizziness, confusion, headache, sedation, euphoria
GI: Nausea, vomiting, anorexia, constipation, cramps
GU: Increased urinary output, dysuria
INTEG: Rash, urticaria, bruising,

flushing, diaphoresis, pruritus
EENT: Tinnitus, blurred vision, miosis, diplopia
CV: Palpitations, bradycardia, change in B/P
RESP: Respiratory depression
Contraindications: Hypersensitivity, addiction (narcotic)
Precautions: Addictive personality, pregnancy, lactation, increase intracranial pressure, MI (acute), severe heart disease, respiratory depression, hepatic disease, renal disease, child <18 yr
Pharmacokinetics:
SC: Peak 1-½ hr, duration 4-5 hr
IV: Peak 20 min, duration 4-5 hr
Metabolized by liver, excreted by kidneys, crosses placenta, excreted in breast milk
Interactions/incompatibilities:
• Effects may be increased with other CNS depressants: alcohol, narcotics, sedative/hypnotics, antipsychotics, skeletal muscle relaxants
NURSING CONSIDERATIONS
Assess:
• I&O ratio; check for decreasing output; may indicate urinary retention
Administer:
• With antiemetic if nausea, vomiting occur
• When pain is beginning to return; determine dosage interval by patient response
Perform/provide:
• Storage in light-resistant area at room temperature
• Assistance with ambulation
• Safety measures: siderails, night light, call bell within easy reach
Evaluate:
• Therapeutic response: decrease in pain
• CNS changes: dizziness, drowsiness, hallucinations, euphoria, LOC, pupil reaction
• Allergic reactions: rash, urticaria

• Respiratory dysfunction: respiratory depression, character, rate, rhythm; notify physician if respirations are <12/min
• Need for pain medication, physical dependence

Teach patient/family:
• To report any symptoms of CNS changes, allergic reactions
• That physical dependency may result when used for extended periods of time
• Withdrawal symptoms may occur: nausea, vomiting, cramps, fever, faintness, anorexia

Lab test interferences:
Increase: Amylase

Treatment of overdose: Narcan 0.2-0.8 IV, O_2, IV fluids, vasopressors

---

levothyroxine sodium (T_4, L-thyroxine sodium)

(lee-voe-thye-rox′een)

Eltroxin, Levoid, Levothroid, Noroxine, Synthroid

Func. class.: Thyroid hormone
Chem. class.: Levoisomer of thyroxine

Action: Increases metabolic rates, increases cardiac output, O_2 consumption, body temperature, blood volume, growth, development at cellular level

Uses: Myxedema coma, thyroid hormone replacement, cretinism

Dosage and routes:
• *Adult:* PO 0.025-0.1 mg qd, increased by 0.05-0.1 mg q1-4 wk until desired response, maintenance dose 0.1-0.4 mg qd
• *Child:* PO 0.01-0.05 qd, may increase 0.025-0.05 mg q1-4 wk until desired response

Cretinism
• *Child:* IV 0.025-0.05 mg qd, may increase by 0.05 PO q2-3 wk
Myxedema coma

• *Adult:* IV 0.2-0.5 mg, may increase by 0.1-0.3 mg after 24 hr; place on oral medication as soon as possible

Available forms include: Inj IV 20, 23, 100 µg/ml; tabs 0.025, 0.05, 0.075, 0.1, 0.125, 0.15, 0.175, 0.2, 0.3 mg

Side effects/adverse reactions:
INTEG: Sweating, alopecia
CNS: Anxiety, insomnia, tremors, headache, heat intolerance, fever, coma, thyroid storm
CV: Tachycardia, palpitations, angina, dysrhythmias, hypertension, CHF
GI: Nausea, diarrhea, increased or decreased appetite, cramps
GU: Menstrual irregularities

Contraindications: Adrenal insufficiency, myocardial infarction, thyrotoxicosis

Precautions: Elderly, angina pectoris, hypertension, ischemia, renal disease, cardiac disease

Pharmacokinetics:
IV/PO: Peak 12-48 hr, half-life 6-7 days; distributed throughout body tissues

Interactions/incompatibilities:
• Decreased absorption of this drug: colestipol, cholestyramine
• Increased tachycardia: IV phenytoin
• Increased effects of: anticoagulants, sympathomimetics, tricyclic antidepressants
• Toxicity: digitalis preparations, catecholamines

NURSING CONSIDERATIONS
Assess:
• B/P, pulse before each dose
• I&O ratio
• Weight qd in same clothing, using same scale, at same time of day
• Height, growth rate if given to a child
• T_3, T_4, which are decreased, radioimmunoassay of TSH, which is increased, radio uptake, which is

---

italics = common side effects   ***bold italic*** = life threatening reactions

decreased if patient is on too low a dose of medication

• Pro-time may require decreased anticoagulant, check for bleeding, bruising

Administer:

• In AM if possible as a single dose to decrease sleeplessness

• At same time each day, to maintain drug level

• Only for hormone imbalances, not to be used for obesity, male infertility, menstrual conditions, lethargy

• Lowest dose that relieves symptoms

Perform/provide:

• Storage in tight, light-resistant container; solutions should be discarded if not used immediately

• Removal of medication 4 wk before RAIU test

Evaluate:

• Therapeutic response: absence of depression, increased weight loss, diuresis, pulse, appetite, absence of constipation, peripheral edema, cold intolerance, pale, cool dry skin, brittle nails, alopecia, coarse hair, menorrhagia, night blindness, paresthesias, syncope, stupor, coma, carotenemia skin, rosy cheeks

• Increased nervousness, excitability, irritability, which may indicate too high dose of medication, usually after 1-3 wk of treatment

• Cardiac status: angina, palpitation, chest pain, change in VS

Teach patient/family:

• Hair loss will occur in child, is temporary

• Report excitability, irritability, anxiety, which indicate overdose

• Not to use generic products or switch brands unless approved by physician

• Drug may be discontinued after birth, thyroid panel evaluated after 1-2 mo

• That hypothyroid child will show almost immediate behavior/personality change

• That treatment drug is not to be taken to reduce weight

• To avoid OTC preparations with iodine, read labels

• To avoid iodine food, salt-iodinized, soy beans, tofu, turnips, some seafood, some bread

Lab test interferences:

Increase: CPK, LDH, AST, PBI, blood glucose

Decrease: TSH, ^{131}I uptake test, uric acid, triglycerides

---

lidocaine/lidocaine HCl (topical)

(lye'-doe-kane)
Stanacaine, Xylocaine

Func. class.: Topical anesthetic
Chem. class.: Aminoacylamide

Action: Inhibits nerve impulses from sensory nerves, which produces anesthesia

Uses: Pruritus, sunburn, toothache, sore throat, cold sores, oral pain

Dosage and routes:

• *Adult and child:* TOP apply q3-4h to affected area; INSTILL 15 ml (male) or 5 ml (female) into urethra

Available forms include: Top sol

Side effects/adverse reactions:

INTEG: Rash, irritation, sensitization

Contraindications: Hypersensitivity, application to large areas

Precautions: Sepsis, pregnancy, denuded skin

Interactions/incompatibilities: None known

NURSING CONSIDERATIONS

Administer:

• After cleansing and drying of affected area

Evaluate:

• Allergy: rash, irritation, reddening, swelling

- Therapeutic response: absence of pain, itching of affected area
- Infection: if affected area is infected, do not apply

Teach patient/family:
- To report rash, irritation, redness, swelling
- How to apply ointment

---

lidocaine HCl

(lye-doe-kane)

Lido Pen Auto-Injector, Xylocaine

Func. class.: Antidysrhythmic (Class IB)

Chem. class.: Aminoacyl amide

Action: Increases electrical stimulation threshold of ventrical, HIS Purkinge system, which stabilizes cardiac membrane

Uses: Ventricular tachycardia, ventricular dysrhythmias during cardiac surgery, myocardial infarction, digitalis toxicity, cardiac catheterization

Dosage and routes:
- *Adult:* IV BOL 50-100 mg at 25-50 mg/min, repeat q3-5 min, not to exceed 300 mg in 1 hr; begin IV INF; IV INF 1-4 mg/min; IM 200-300 mg in deltoid muscle
- *Elderly:* IV BOL give ½ adult dose
- *Child:* IV BOL 1 mg/kg, then IV INF; IV INF: 30 µg/kg/min

Available forms include: Inj 0.5%, 1%, 1.5%, 2%, 4%, 5%, 10%, 20%

Side effects/adverse reactions:

CNS: Headache, dizziness, involuntary movement, confusion, psychosis, restlessness, irritability, paresthesias, *tremor*

EENT: Tinnitus, blurred vision, hearing loss

GI: Nausea, vomiting, anorexia

CV: Hypotension, bradycardia, heart block, cardiovascular collapse, arrest

RESP: Dyspnea, *respiratory depression*

INTEG: Rash, urticaria, edema, swelling

Contraindications: Hypersensitivity to amides, blood dyscrasias, severe heart block, supraventricular dysrhythmias

Precautions: Pregnancy, lactation, children, renal disease, liver disease, CHF, respiratory depression, myasthenia gravis

Pharmacokinetics:

IV: Onset 2 min, duration 20 min

IM: Onset 5-15 min, duration 1½ hr

Half-life 8 min, 1-2 hr (terminal), metabolized in liver excreted in urine, crosses placenta

Interactions/incompatibilities:
- Increased effects of: neuromuscular blockers, tubocurarine, or polymyxin B
- Increased effects: cimetidine, phenytoin, propranolol, quinidine
- Decreased effects of this drug: barbiturates

NURSING CONSIDERATIONS

Assess:
- ECG continuously to determine increased PR or QRS segments; if these develop, discontinue immediately; watch for increased ventricular ectopic beats, may need to rebolus
- IV infusion rate using infusion pump, run at less than 4 mg/min
- Blood levels
- B/P continuously for fluctuations
- I&O ratio, electrolytes (K, Na, Cl)

Administer:
- IM injection in deltoid; aspirate to avoid intravascular administration; check site daily for infiltration or extravasation

Evaluate:
- Malignant hyperthermia: tachypnea, tachycardia, changes in B/P, increased temperature

---

italics = common side effects   **bold italic** = life threatening reactions

• Cardiac rate, respiration: rate, rhythm, character, continuously
• Respiratory status: rate, rhythm, lung fields for rales, watch for respiratory depression
• CNS effects: dizziness, confusion, psychosis, paresthesias, convulsions; drug should be discontinued
• Lung fields, bilateral rales may occur in CHF patient
• Increased respiration, increased pulse; drug should be discontinued

Teach patient/family:
• Use of automatic lidocaine injection device if ordered

Lab test interferences:
Increase: CPK

Treatment of overdose: O$_2$, artificial ventilation, ECG, administer dopamine for circulatory depression, administer diazepam or thiopental for convulsions

---

lidocaine HCl

(lye'doe-kane)

Ardecaine, Dilocaine, Dolicaine, Nervocaine, Norocaine, Rocaine, Stanacaine, Ultracaine, Xylocaine

Func. class.: Local anesthetic
Chem. class.: Amide

Action: Competes with calcium for sites in nerve membrane that control sodium transport across cell membrane; decreases rise of depolarization phase of action potential

Uses: Peripheral nerve block, caudal anesthesia, epidural, spinal, surgical anesthesia

Dosage and routes:
Varies depending on route of anesthesia

Available forms include: Inj 0.5%, 1%, 1.5%, 2%, 4%, 5%; inj with epinephrine 0.5%, 1%, 1.5%, 2%

Side effects/adverse reactions:
CNS: Anxiety, restlessness, ***con-vulsions, loss of consciousness,*** drowsiness, disorientation, tremors, shivering

*CV: **Myocardial depression, cardiac arrest, dysrhythmias,*** bradycardia, hypotension, hypertension, fetal bradycardia

GI: Nausea, vomiting

EENT: Blurred vision, tinnitus, pupil constriction

INTEG: Rash, urticaria, allergic reactions, edema, burning, skin discoloration at injection site, tissue necrosis

*RESP: **Status asthmaticus, respiratory arrest, anaphylaxis***

Contraindications: Hypersensitivity, child <12 yr, elderly, severe liver disease

Precautions: Elderly, severe drug allergies, pregnancy (C)

Pharmacokinetics:
Onset 4-17 min, duration 3-6 hr; metabolized by liver, excreted in urine (metabolites)

Interactions/incompatibilities:
• Dysrhythmias: epinephrine, halothane, enflurane
• Hypertension: MAOIs, tricyclic antidepressants, phenothiazines
• Decreased action of this drug: chloroprocaine

NURSING CONSIDERATIONS

Assess:
• B/P, pulse, respiration during treatment
• Fetal heart tones if drug is used during labor

Administer:
• Only with crash cart, resuscitative equipment nearby
• Only drugs without preservatives for epidural or caudal anesthesia

Perform/provide:
• Use of new solution, discard unused portions

Evaluate:
• Therapeutic response: anesthesia necessary for procedure

• For allergic reactions: rash, urticaria, itching
• Cardiac status: ECG for dysrhythmias, pulse, B/P during anesthesia
Treatment of overdose: Airway, O_2, vasopressor, IV fluids, anticonvulsants for seizures

---

lidocaine HCl (topical)
(lye'doe-kane)
Xylocaine, Viscous Xylocaine
Func. class.: Anesthetic, topical, local
Chem. class.: Amide

Action: Inhibits conduction of nerve impulses from sensory nerves
Uses: Oral pain, topical anesthetic for mucous membrane
Dosage and routes:
• *Adult and child:* TOP apply q3-4h to affected area
Available forms include: Oint 5%; oral sol 2%, 5%
Side effects/adverse reactions:
EENT: Swelling, burning, stinging, tissue necrosis, irritation
INTEG: Rash, urticaria, edema
Contraindications: Hypersensitivity, secondary bacterial infections, infants
Precautions: Sepsis of affected area, pregnancy (C)
Pharmacokinetics:
TOP: Peak 2-5 min, duration ½-1 hr
Interactions/incompatibilities: None known
NURSING CONSIDERATIONS
Administer:
• With swab to decrease chance of ointment on healthy skin
Perform/provide:
• Storage at room temperature in tight container

Evaluate:
• For redness, swelling, irritation; drug may need to be discontinued
Teach patient/family:
• Not to eat or rinse mouth for at least 1 hr after application
• Not to eat if area is anesthetized
• That burning/stinging may occur for a few doses

---

lincomycin HCl
(lin-koe-mye'sin)
Lincocin
Func. class.: Antibacterial
Chem. class.: Lincomycin derivative

Action: Binds to 50S subunit of bacterial ribsomes, suppresses protein synthesis
Uses: Infections caused by group A β-hemolytic streptococci, pneumococci, staphylococci (respiratory tract, skin, soft tissue, urinary tract infections, osteomyelitis, septicemia)
Dosage and routes:
• *Adult:* PO 500 mg q6-8h, not to exceed 8 g/day; IM 600 mg/day or q12h; IV 600 mg-1 g q8-12h, dilute in 100 ml IV sol, infuse over 1 hr
• *Child >1 mo:* PO 30-60 mg/kg/day in divided doses q6-8h; IM 10 mg/kg/day or divided q12h; IV 10-20 mg/kg/day in divided doses q6-8h; dilute to 100 ml IV sol, infuse over 1 hr
Available forms include: Caps 500 mg; caps pediatric 250 mg; inj IM, IV 300 mg/ml
Side effects/adverse reactions:
*HEMA: **Leukopenia, eosinophilia, agranulocytosis, thrombocytopenia***
*GI: Nausea, vomiting, abdominal pain, tenesmus, diarrhea, **pseudomembranous colitis***
GU: Increased AST, ALT, bilirubin,

alk phosphatase, jaundice, *vaginitis,* urinary frequency

EENT: Rash, urticaria, pruritus, erythema, pain, abscess at injection site

Contraindications: Hypersensitivity, ulcerative colitis/enteritis, infants <1 mo

Precautions: Renal disease, liver disease, GI disease, elderly, pregnancy, lactation

Pharmacokinetics:

PO: Peak 45 min, duration 6 hr

IM: Peak 3 hr, duration 8-12 hr

Half-life 2½ hr, metabolized in liver, excreted in urine, bile, feces as active, inactive metabolites, crosses placenta, excreted in breast milk

Interactions/incompatibilities:

• Increased neuromuscular blockage: nondepolarizing muscle relaxants

• Decreased action of: chloramphenicol, erythromycin

• Decreased rate of absorption of: opiates, diphenoxylate

NURSING CONSIDERATIONS

Assess:

• Any patient with compromised renal system; drug is excreted slowly in poor renal system function; toxicity may occur rapidly

• Liver studies: AST, ALT

• Blood studies: WBC, RBC, Hct, Hgb, platelets, serum iron, reticulocytes; drug should be discontinued if bone marrow depression occurs

• Renal studies: urinalysis, protein, blood, BUN, creatinine

• C&S before drug therapy; drug may be taken as soon as culture is taken

• Drug level in impaired hepatic, renal systems

• B/P, pulse in patient receiving drug parenterally

Administer:

• IV by infusion only; do not administer bolus dose

• IM deep injection; rotate sites

• Orally with at least 8 oz water

Perform/provide:

• Storage at room temperature (capsules) and up to 2 wk (reconstituted solution)

• Adrenalin, suction, tracheostomy set, endotracheal intubation equipment on unit

• Adequate intake of fluids (2000 ml) during diarrhea episodes

Evaluate:

• Therapeutic response: decreased temperature, negative C&S

• Bowel pattern before, during treatment

• Skin eruptions, itching, dermatitis

• Respiratory status: rate, character, wheezing, tightness in chest

• Allergies before treatment, reaction of each medication; place allergies on chart, Kardex in bright red letters; notify all people giving drugs

Teach patient/family:

• To take oral drug with full glass of water; may give with food if GI symptoms occur

• Aspects of drug therapy: need to complete entire course of medication to ensure organism death (10-14 days); culture may be taken after completed course of medication

• To report sore throat, fever, fatigue; could indicate superimposed infection

• That drug must be taken in equal intervals around clock to maintain blood levels

• To wear or carry Medic Alert ID if allergic to this drug

• To notify nurse of diarrhea stools

Lab test interferences:

Increase: Alk phosphatase, bilirubin, CPK, AST/ALT

Treatment of overdose: Withdraw drug, maintain airway, administer epinephrine, aminophylline, O_2, IV corticosteroids

---

lindane (gamma benzene hexachloride)

(lin-dane)

gBh,* Kwell, Kwellada,* Scabene, G-Well

Func. class.: Scabicide

Chem. class.: Chlorinated hydrocarbon (synthetic)

Action: Stimulates nervous system of arthropods, resulting in seizures, death of organism

Uses: Scabies, lice (head/pubic), nits

Dosage and routes:

• *Adult and child:* CREAM/LOTION wash area with soap, water, remove visible crusts, apply to skin surfaces, remove with soap, water in 8-12 hr, may reapply in 1 wk if needed; SHAMPOO using 30 ml work into lather, rub for 5 min, rinse, dry with towel; comb with fine-tooth comb to remove nits

Available forms include: Lotion, shampoo, cream (1%)

Side effects/adverse reactions:

INTEG: Pruritus, rash, irritation, contact dermatitis

GI: Nausea, vomiting, diarrhea, liver damage (inhalation of vapors)

*HEMA: **Aplastic anemia** (chronic inhalation of vapors)*

*CV: **Ventricular fibrillation** (chronic inhalation of vapors)*

*GU: **Kidney damage** (chronic inhalation of vapors)*

*CNS: Tremors, **convulsions,** stimulation, dizziness (chronic inhalation of vapors)*

Contraindications: Hypersensitivity, premature neonate, patients with known seizure disorders, inflammation of skin, abrasions, or breaks in skin

Precautions: Pregnancy, avoid contact with eyes, children, infants

Pharmacokinetics:

Stored in body fat, metabolized in liver, excreted in urine, feces

Interactions/incompatibilities:

• Oils may enhance absorption; if an oil-based hair dressing is used, shampoo, rinse, dry hair before applying lindane shampoo

NURSING CONSIDERATIONS

Administer:

• To body areas, scalp only; do not apply to face, lips, mouth, eyes, any mucous membrane, anus, or meatus

• Topical corticosteroids as ordered to decrease contact dermatitis

• Lotions of menthol or phenol to control itching

• Topical antibiotics for infection

Perform/provide:

• Isolation until areas on skin, scalp have cleared and treatment is completed

• Removal of nits by using a fine-tooth comb rinsed in vinegar after treatment

Evaluate:

• Area of body involved, including crusts, nits, brownish trails on skin, itching papules in skin folds

Teach patient/family:

• To wash all inhabitants' clothing, using insecticide; preventative treatment may be required of all persons living in same house, using lotion or shampoo to decrease spread of infection

• That itching may continue for 4-6 wk

• That drug must be reapplied if accidently washed off or treatment will be ineffective

• Do not apply to face

• Treat sexual contact simultaneously

Treatment of ingestion: Gastric lavage, saline laxatives, IV valium for convulsions

L

---

italics = common side effects   ***bold italic*** = life threatening reactions

liothyronine sodium (T₃)

(lye-oh-thye'roe-neen)

Cytomel, Cyronine, Tertoxin*

Func. class.: Thyroid hormone

Chem. class.: Levoisomer of thyroxine

Action: Increases metabolic rates, increases cardiac output, O_2 consumption, body temperature, blood volume, growth, development at cellular level

Uses: Myxedema coma, thyroid hormone replacement, cretinism

Dosage and routes:

• *Adult:* PO 25 μg qd, increased by 12.5-25 μg q1-2 wk until desired response, maintenance dose 25-75 μg qd

Cretinism

• *Child >3 yr:* PO 50-100 μg qd

• *Child <3 yr:* PO 5 μg qd, increased by 5 μg q3-4 days titrated to response

Myxedema

• *Adult:* PO 5 μg qd, may increase by 5-10 μg q1-2 wk, maintenance dose 50-100 μg qd

Nontoxic goiter

• *Adult:* PO 5 μg qd, increased by 12.5-25 μg q1-2 wk, maintenance dose 75 μg qd

Suppression test

• *Adult:* PO 75-100 μg qd × 1 wk

Available forms include: Tabs 5, 25, 50 μg

Side effects/adverse reactions:

INTEG: Sweating, alopecia

CNS: Anxiety, insomnia, tremors, headache, heat intolerance, fever, coma thyroid storm

CV: Tachycardia, palpitations, angina, dysrhythmias, hypertension, CHF

GI: Nausea, diarrhea, increased or decreased appetite, cramps

GU: Menstrual irregularities

Contraindications: Adrenal insufficiency, myocardial infarction, thyrotoxicosis

Precautions: Elderly, angina pectoris, hypertension, ischemia, renal disease, cardiac disease

Pharmacokinetics:

PO: Peak 12-48 hr, half-life 6-7 days

Interactions/incompatibilities:

• Decreased absorption of this drug: colestipol, cholestyramine

• Increased tachycardia: IV phenytoin

• Increased effects of: anticoagulants, sympathomimetics, tricyclic antidepressants

• Toxicity: digitalis preparations, catecholamines

NURSING CONSIDERATIONS

Assess:

• B/P, pulse before each dose

• I&O ratio

• Weight qd in same clothing, using same scale, at same time of day

• Height, growth rate if given to a child

• T_3, T_4, which are decreased, radioimmunoassay of TSH, which is increased, radio uptake, which is decreased if patient is on too low a dose of medication

• Pro-time may require decreased anticoagulant, check for bleeding, bruising

Administer:

• In AM if possible as a single dose to decrease sleeplessness

• At same time each day to maintain drug level

• Only for hormone imbalances, not to be used for obesity, male infertility, menstrual conditions, lethargy

• Lowest dose that relieves symptoms

Perform/provide:

• Removal of medication 4 wk before RAIU test

Evaluate:

• Therapeutic response: absence of

depression, increased weight loss, diuresis, pulse, appetite, absence of constipation, peripheral edema, cold intolerance, pale, cool dry skin, brittle nails, alopecia, coarse hair, menorrhagia, night blindness, paresthesia, snycope, stupor, coma, carotenemia skin, rosy cheeks

• Increased nervousness, excitability, irritability, which may indicate too high dose of medication usually after 1-3 wk of treatment

• Cardiac status: angina, palpitation, chest pain, change in VS

Teach patient/family:

• Hair loss will occur in child, is temporary

• Report excitability, irritability, anxiety, which indicates overdose

• Not to use generic products or switch brands unless approved by physician

• That hypothyroid child will show almost immediate behavior/personality change

• That treatment drug is not to be taken to reduce weight

• To avoid OTC preparations with iodine, read labels

• To avoid iodine food, salt-iodinized, soy beans, tofu, turnips, some seafood, some bread

Lab test interferences:

Increase: CPK, LDH, AST, PBI, blood glucose

Decrease: TSH, ^{131}I uptake test, uric acid, triglycerides

---

liotrix

(lye′oh-trix)
Euthroid, Thyrolar

Func. class.: Thyroid hormone
Chem. class.: Levothyroxine/liothyronine

Action: Increases metabolic rates, increases cardiac output, O_2 consumption, body temperature, blood volume, growth, development at cellular level

Uses: Hypothyroidism

Dosage and routes:

• *Adult and child:* PO 15-30 mg qd, increased by 15-30 mg q1-2 wk until desired response, may increase by 15-30 mg q2 wk in child

• *Geriatric:* PO 15-30 mg, double dose q6-8 wk until desired response

Available forms include: Tabs 15, 30, 60, 120, 180 mg

Side effects/adverse reactions:

INTEG: Sweating, alopecia

CNS: Anxiety, insomnia, tremors, headache, heat intolerance, fever, coma, thyroid storm

CV: Tachycardia, palpitations, angina, dysrhythmias, hypertension, CHF

GI: Nausea, diarrhea, increased or decreased appetite, cramps

GU: Menstrual irregularities

Contraindications: Adrenal insufficiency, myocardial infarction, thyrotoxicosis

Precautions: Elderly, angina pectoris, hypertension, ischemia, renal disease, cardiac disease

Pharmacokinetics:

PO: Peak 12-48 hr, half-life 6-7 days

Interactions/incompatibilities:

• Decreased absorption of this drug: colestipol, cholestyramine

• Increased tachycardia: IV phenytoin

• Increased effects of: anticoagulants, sympathomimetics, tricyclic antidepressants

• Toxicity: digitalis preparations, catecholamines

NURSING CONSIDERATIONS

Assess:

• B/P, pulse before each dose

• I&O ratio

• Weight qd in same clothing, using same scale, at same time of day

• Height, growth rate if given to a child

L

• T_3, T_4 which are decreased, radioimmunoassay of TSH, which is increased, radio uptake, which is decreased if patient is on too low a dose of medication

• Pro-time may require decreased anticoagulant, check for bleeding, bruising

Administer:

• In AM if possible as a single dose to decrease sleeplessness

• At same time each day to maintain drug level

• Only for hormone imbalances, not to be used for obesity, male infertility, menstrual conditions, lethargy

• Lowest dose that relieves symptoms

Perform/provide:

• Removal of medication 4 wk before RAIU test

Evaluate:

• Therapeutic response: absence of depression, increased weight loss, diuresis, pulse, appetite, absence of constipation, peripheral edema, cold intolerance, pale, cool dry skin, brittle nails, alopecia, coarse hair, menorrhagia, night blindness, paresthesias, syncope, stupor, coma, carotenemia skin, rosy cheeks

• Increased nervousness, excitability, irritability, which may indicate too high dose of medication usually after 1-3 wk of treatment

• Cardiac status: angina, palpitation, chest pain, change in VS

Teach patient/family:

• Hair loss will occur in child, is temporary

• Report excitability, irritability, anxiety, which indicate overdose

• Not to use generic products or switch brands unless approved by physician

• That hypothyroid child will show almost immediate behavior/personality change

• That treatment drug is not to be taken to reduce weight

• To avoid OTC preparations with iodine, read labels

• To avoid iodine food, salt-iodinized, soy beans, tofu, turnips, some seafood, some bread

Lab test interferences:

Increase: CPK, LDH, AST, PBI, blood glucose

Decrease: TSH, ^{131}I uptake test, uric acid, triglycerides

---

lithium carbonate

(li'thee-um)

Lithane, Eskalith, Lithonate, Lithotabs, Lithobid, Lithium Citrate, Lithonate-S

Func. class.: Antimanic

Chem. class.: Alkali metal ion salt

Action: May alter sodium, potassium ion transport across cell membrane in nerve, muscle cells; may balance biogenic amines of norepinephrine, serotonin in CNS areas involved in emotional responses

Uses: Manic-depressive illness (manic phase), prevention of bipolar manic depressive psychosis

Dosage and routes:

• *Adult:* PO 600 mg tid, maintenance 300 mg tid or qid; SLOW REL TABS 300 mg bid, dose should be individualized to maintain blood levels at 0.5-1.5 mEq/L

Available forms include: Caps 300 mg; tabs 300 mg; tabs ext rel 300, 450 mg; oral sol 8 mEq/5 ml

Side effects/adverse reactions:

CNS: Headache, drowsiness, dizziness, tremors, twitching, ataxia, seizure, slurred speech, restlessness, confusion, stupor, memory loss, clonic movements

GI: Dry mouth, anorexia, nausea, vomiting, diarrhea, incontinence, abdominal pain

GU: Polyuria, glycosuria, protein-

uria, albuminuria, urinary incontinence, polydipsia, edema

CV: Hypotension, ECG changes,
dysrhythmias, circulatory collapse

INTEG: Drying of hair, alopecia,
rash, pruritus, hyperkeratosis

HEMA: Leukocytosis

EENT: Tinnitus, blurred vision

ENDO: Hypothyroidism, hyponatremia

MS: Muscle weakness

Contraindications: Hepatic disease, renal disease, brain trauma,
OBS, pregnancy, lactation, children <12 yr, schizophrenia, severe
cardiac disease, severe renal disease, severe dehydration

Precautions: Elderly, thyroid disease, seizure disorders, diabetes
mellitus, systemic infection, urinary retention

Pharmacokinetics:

PO: Onset rapid, peak ½-4 hr, half-
life 18-36 hr depending on age;
crosses blood-brain barrier, metabolized by liver, excreted in urine,
crosses placenta, enters breast
milk, well absorbed by oral method

Interactions/incompatibilities:

• Brain damage may occur when
used with haloperidol

• Increased effects of: neuromuscular blocking agents

• Increased renal clearance: sodium bicarbonate, acetazolamide,
mannitol, aminophylline

• Increased toxicity: indomethacin,
thiazide diuretics

• Decreased effects of this drug:
theophyllines, urea, urinary alkalinizers

NURSING CONSIDERATIONS
Assess:

• Weight daily, check for edema in
legs, ankles, wrists; report if present

• Sodium intake; decreased sodium
intake with decreased fluid intake
may lead to lithium retention; increased sodium and fluids may decrease lithium retention

• Skin turgor at least daily

• Urine for albuminuria, glycosuria, uric acid during beginning
treatment, q2 mo thereafter

• Neuro status: LOC, gait, motor
reflexes, hand tremors

• Serum lithium levels weekly initially, then q3 mo (therapeutic
level: 0.5-1.5 mEq/L)

Administer:

• With meals to avoid GI upset

• Adequate fluids (2-3 L/day) to
prevent dehydration during initial
treatment, 1-2 L/day during maintenance

Teach patient/family:

• Symptoms of minor toxicity:
vomiting, diarrhea, poor coordination, fine motor tremors, weakness, lassitude; major toxicity:
coarse tremors, severe thirst, tinnitus, dilute urine

• Action, dosage, side effects;
when to notify physician

• To monitor urine specific gravity

• That contraception is necessary
since lithium may harm fetus

• Not to operate machinery until
lithium levels are stable

Lab test interferences:

Increase: Potassium excretion,
urine glucose, blood glucose, protein, BUN

Decrease: VMA, T_3, T_4, PBI, ^{131}I

Treatment: Lavage, maintain airway, respiratory function; dialysis
for severe intoxication

---

lomustine (CCNU)

(loe-mus'teen)
CeeNU, CCNU

Func. class.: Antineoplastic alkylating agent

Chem. class.: Nitrosourea

Action: Alkylates DNA, RNA; inhibits enzymes that allow synthesis
of amino acids in proteins; also re-

L

---

italics = common side effects   ***bold italic*** = life threatening reactions

sponsible for cross-linking DNA strands

Uses: Hodgkin's disease, lymphomas, melanomas, multiple myeloma; brain, lung, bladder, kidney, colon cancer

Dosage and routes:

• *Adult:* PO 130 mg/m² as a single dose q6wk; titrate dose to WBC level; do not give repeat dose unless WBCs are >4000/mm³, platelet count >100,000/mm³

Available forms include: Cap 10, 40, 100 mg

Side effects/adverse reactions:

*HEMA: **Thrombocytopenia, leukopenia, myelosuppression, anemia***
*GI: Nausea, vomiting, anorexia, stomatitis, **hepatotoxicity***
*GU: Azotemia, **renal failure***
INTEG: Burning at injection site
*RESP: **Fibrosis, pulmonary infiltrate***

Contraindications: Hypersensitivity, leukopenia, thrombocytopenia

Precautions: Radiation therapy, pregnancy

Pharmacokinetics:

Metabolized in liver, excreted in urine; half-life 16-48 hr, 50% protein bound, crosses blood-brain barrier, appears in breast milk

Interactions/incompatibilities:

• Increased toxicity: barbiturates, phenytoin, chloral hydrate
• Increased metabolism of this drug: phenobarbital
• Potentiation of this drug: succinylcholine
• Increased bone marrow depression: allopurinol

NURSING CONSIDERATIONS

Assess:

• CBC, differential, platelet count weekly; withhold drug if WBC is <4000 or platelet count is <75,000; notify physician of results
• Pulmonary function tests, chest x-ray films before, during therapy; chest film should be obtained q2wk during treatment
• Renal function studies: BUN, serum uric acid, urine CrCl before, during therapy
• I&O ratio; report fall in urine output of 30 ml/hr
• Monitor temperature q4h (may indicate beginning infection)
• Liver function tests before, during therapy (bilirubin, AST, ALT, LDH) as needed or monthly

Administer:

• Medications by oral route; if possible avoid IM, SC, IV routes to prevent infections
• Antiemetic 30-60 min before giving drug to prevent vomiting
• Antibiotics for prophylaxis of infection
• Slow IV infusion using 21-, 23-, 25-gauge needle
• Topical or systemic analgesics for pain
• Local or systemic drugs for infection

Perform/provide:

• Storage in tight container at room temperature
• Strict medical asepsis, protective isolation if WBC levels are low
• Special skin care
• Deep breathing exercises with patient tid-qid; place in semi-Fowler's position
• Liquid diet, including cola, Jello; dry toast or crackers may be added if patient is not nauseated or vomiting
• Increase fluid intake to 2-3 L/day to prevent urate deposits, calculi formation
• Rinsing of mouth tid-qid with water, hydrogen peroxide; brushing of teeth bid-tid with soft brush or cotton tipped applicators for stomatitis; use unwaxed dental floss
• Warm compresses at injection site for inflammation

Evaluate:

• Bleeding: hematuria, guaiac, bruising or petechiae, mucosa or orifices q8h

• Dyspnea, rales, unproductive cough, chest pain, tachypnea

• Food preferences; list likes, dislikes

• Yellowing of skin, sclera, dark urine, clay-colored stools, itchy skin, abdominal pain, fever, diarrhea

• Inflammation of mucosa, breaks in skin

• Buccal cavity q8h for dryness, sores or ulceration, white patches, oral pain, bleeding, dysphagia

• Local irritation, pain, burning, discoloration at injection site

• Symptoms indicating severe allergic reaction: rash, pruritus, urticaria, purpuric skin lesions, itching, flushing

Teach patient/family:

• Of protective isolation precautions

• To report any complaints or side effects to nurse or physician

• To report any changes in breathing or coughing

• To avoid foods with citric acid, hot or rough texture

• To report any bleeding, white spots or ulcerations in mouth to physician; tell patient to examine mouth qd

---

loperamide HCl

(loe-per′a-mide)

Imodium

Func. class.: Antidiarrheal
Chem. class.: Piperidine derivative

Action: Direct action on intestinal muscles to decrease GI peristalsis
Uses: Diarrhea (cause undetermined), chronic diarrhea, ileostomy discharge

Dosage and routes:

• *Adult:* PO 4 mg, then 2 mg after each loose stool, not to exceed 16 mg/day

• *Child 2-5 yr:* PO 5 ml tid on day 1, 0.1 mg/kg after each loose stool

• *Child 5-8 yr:* PO 10 ml bid on day 1, 0.1 mg/kg after each loose stool

• *Child 8-12 yr:* PO 10 ml tid on day 1, 0.1 mg/kg after each loose stool

Available forms include: Caps 2 mg; liq 1 mg/5 ml

Side effects/adverse reactions:

CNS: Dizziness, drowsiness, fatigue

GI: Nausea, dry mouth, vomiting, constipation, abdominal pain, anorexia, toxic megacolon

INTEG: Rash, fever

Contraindications: Hypersensitivity, severe ulcerative colitis, pseudomembranous colitis

Precautions: Pregnancy, lactation, children, liver disease, dehydration, bacterial disease

Pharmacokinetics:

PO: Onset ½-1 hr, duration 4-5 hr, half-life 7-14 hr; metabolized in liver, excreted in feces as unchanged drug, small amount in urine

Interactions/incompatibilities:

• Do not mix oral solution with other solvents

NURSING CONSIDERATIONS

Assess:

• Electrolytes (K, Na, Cl) if on long-term therapy

• Skin turgor q8h if dehydration is suspected

Administer:

• For 48 hr only

Perform/provide:

• Storage in tight containers

Evaluate:

• Therapeutic response: decreased diarrhea

L

---

italics = common side effects   ***bold italic*** = life threatening reactions

• Bowel pattern before; for rebound constipation

• Response after 48 hr; if no response, drug should be discontinued

• Dehydration in children

• Abdominal distention, toxic megacolon; may occur in ulcerative colitis

Teach patient/family:

• To avoid OTC products unless directed by physician

---

lorazepam

(lor-a′ze-pam)

Ativan

Func. class.: Antianxiety
Chem. class.: Benzodiazepine

Controlled Substance Schedule IV

Action: Depresses subcortical levels of CNS, including limbic system and reticular formation

Uses: Anxiety, irritability in psychiatric or organic disorders, preoperatively, insomnia

Dosage and routes:

Anxiety

• Adult: PO 2-6 mg/day in divided doses, not to exceed 10 mg/day

Insomnia

• Adult: PO 2-4 mg hs

Preoperatively

• Adult: IM/IV 2-4 mg

Available forms include: Tabs 0.5, 1, 2 mg; IM/IV inj

Side effects/adverse reactions:

CNS: Dizziness, drowsiness, confusion, headache, anxiety, tremors, stimulation, fatigue, depression, insomnia, hallucinations

GI: Constipation, dry mouth, nausea, vomiting, anorexia, diarrhea

INTEG: Rash, dermatitis, itching

CV: Orthostatic hypotension, ECG changes, tachycardia, hypotension

EENT: Blurred vision, tinnitus, mydriasis

Contraindications: Hypersensitivity to benzodiazepines, narrowangle glaucoma, psychosis, pregnancy (D), child <18 yr

Precautions: Elderly, debilitated, hepatic disease, renal disease

Pharmacokinetics:

PO: Peak 1-3 hr, duration 3-6 hr, metabolized by liver, excreted by kidneys, crosses placenta, breast milk, half-life 14 hr

Interactions/incompatibilities:

• Decreased effects of this drug: oral contraceptives, rifampin, valproic acid

• Increased effects of this drug: CNS depressants, alcohol, cimetidine, disulfiram, oral contraceptives

NURSING CONSIDERATIONS

Assess:

• B/P (lying, standing), pulse; if systolic B/P drops 20 mm Hg, hold drug, notify physician; respirations q5-15 min if given IV

• Blood studies: CBC during longterm therapy, blood dyscrasias have occurred rarely

• Hepatic studies: AST, ALT, bilirubin, creatinine, LDH, alk phosphatase

Administer:

• With food or milk for GI symptoms

• Crushed if patient is unable to swallow medication whole

• Sugarless gum, hard candy, frequent sips of water for dry mouth

Perform/provide:

• Assistance with ambulation during beginning therapy since drowsiness/dizziness occurs

• Safety measures, including siderails

• Check to see PO medication has been swallowed

Evaluate:

• Therapeutic response: decreased

anxiety, restlessness, insomnia
• Mental status: mood, sensorium, affect, sleeping pattern, drowsiness, dizziness
• Physical dependency, withdrawal symptoms: headache, nausea, vomiting, muscle pain, weakness after long-term use
• Suicidal tendencies

Teach patient/family:
• That drug may be taken with food
• Not to be used for everyday stress or used longer than 4 mo unless directed by physician
• Avoid OTC preparations (cough, cold, hay fever) unless approved by physician
• To avoid driving, activities that require alertness, since drowsiness may occur
• To avoid alcohol ingestion or other psychotropic medications, unless prescribed by physician
• Not to discontinue medication abruptly after long-term use
• To rise slowly or fainting may occur
• That drowsiness might worsen at beginning of treatment

Lab test interferences:
Increase: AST/ALT, serum bilirubin
Decrease: RAIU
False increase: 17-OHCS

Treatment of overdose: Lavage, VS, supportive care

---

lovastatin

(lo'va-sta-tin)
Mevacor
Func. class.: Cholesterol-lowering agent
Chem. class.: Aspergillus terreus strain derivative

Action: Reduces cholesterol by decreasing production, increasing catabolism of LDL cholesterol

Uses: As an adjunct in primary hypercholesterolemia (types IIa, IIb)

Dosage and routes:
(Patient should be placed on a cholesterol-lowering diet first)
• *Adult:* PO 20 mg qd with evening meal, may increase to 20-80 mg/day in single or divided doses, not to exceed 80 mg/day; dosage adjustments should be made q month
Available forms include: Tabs 20 mg

Side effects/adverse reactions:
GI: Nausea, constipation, diarrhea, dyspepsia, flatus, abdominal pain, heartburn, **liver dysfunction**
MS: Muscle cramps, myalgia
CNS: Dizziness, headache
INTEG: Rash, pruritus
EENT: Blurred vision, dysgeusia

Contraindications: Pregnancy (X), lactation, active liver disease
Precautions: Past liver disease, alcoholics, severe acute infections, trauma, hypotension, uncontrolled seizure disorders, severe metabolic disorders, electrolyte imbalances

Pharmacokinetics:
PO: Peak 2-4 hr, metabolized in liver (metabolites), highly protein bound, excreted in urine, feces, crosses placenta, excreted in breast milk

Interactions/incompatibilities:
• Increased effects: cholestyramine

NURSING CONSIDERATIONS

Assess:
• Cholesterol levels periodically during treatment
• Liver function studies q 1-2 mo during the first 1½ yr of treatment; AST, ALT, liver function tests may increase
• Renal function in patients with compromised renal system: BUN, creatinine, I&O ratio
• Eyes with slit lamp before and 1 mo after treatment begins, lens opacities may occur

L

Administer:
• In evening with meal; if dose is increased, take with breakfast and evening meal

Perform/provide:
• Storage in cool environment in tight container protected from light

Evaluate:
• Therapeutic response: decrease in cholesterol to desired level after 1-2 yr

Teach patient/family:
• That treatment will be ongoing for several years
• That blood work and eye exam will be necessary during treatment
• To report blurred vision, severe GI symptoms, dizziness, headache
• That previously prescribed regimen will continue: low-cholesterol diet, exercise program

Lab test interferences:
Increase: CPK

---

loxapine succinate/ loxapine HCl

(lox′a′peen)
Loxapax,* Loxitane, Loxitane-C

Func. class.: Antipsychotic/Neuroleptic
Chem. class.: Dibenzoxazepine

Action: Depresses cerebral cortex, hypothalamus, limbic system, which control activity and aggression; blocks neurotransmission produced by dopamine at synapse; exhibits strong α-adrenergic, anticholinergic blocking action; mechanism for antipsychotic effects is unclear

Uses: Psychotic disorders

Dosage and routes:
• *Adult:* PO 10 mg bid-qid initially, may be rapidly increased depending on severity of condition, maintenance 20-60 mg/day; IM 12.5-50 mg q4-6 hr or more until desired response, then start PO form

Available forms include: Caps 5, 10, 25, 50 mg; conc 25 mg/ml; inj IM 50 mg/ml

Side effects/adverse reactions:
*RESP: **Laryngospasm,** dyspnea, **respiratory depression***

CNS: Extrapyramidal symptoms: pseudoparkinsonism, akathisia, dystonia, tardive dyskinesia, drowsiness, headache, seizures

HEMA: Anemia, leukopenia, leukocytosis, **agranulocytosis**

INTEG: Rash, photosensitivity, dermatitis

EENT: Blurred vision, glaucoma

GI: Dry mouth, nausea, vomiting, anorexia, constipation, diarrhea, jaundice, weight gain

GU: Urinary retention, urinary frequency, enuresis, impotence, amenorrhea, gynecomastia

CV: Orthostatic hypotension, hypertension, **cardiac arrest,** ECG changes, **tachycardia**

Contraindications: Hypersensitivity, blood dyscrasias, coma, child, brain damage, bone marrow depression, alcohol and barbiturate withdrawal states

Precautions: Pregnancy, lactation, seizure disorders, hypertension, hepatic disease, cardiac disease

Pharmacokinetics:
PO: Onset 20-30 min, peak 2-4 hr, duration 12 hr

IM: Onset 15-30 min, peak 15-20 min, duration 12 hr

Metabolized by liver, excreted in urine, crosses placenta, enters breast milk, initial half-life 5 hr, terminal half-life 19 hr

Interactions/incompatibilities:
None known

NURSING CONSIDERATIONS

Assess:
• Swallowing of PO medication; check for hoarding or giving of medication to other patients
• I&O ratio; palpate bladder if low urinary output occurs

• Bilirubin, CBC, liver function studies monthly
• Urinalysis is recommended before and during prolonged therapy
Administer:
• Antiparkinsonian agent, to be used if EPS occurs
• IM injection into large muscle mass
• Concentrate mixed in orange or grapefruit juice
Perform/provide:
• Decreased noise input by dimming lights, avoiding loud noises
• Supervised ambulation until stabilized on medication; do not involve in strenuous exercise program because fainting is possible; patient should not stand still for long periods of time
• Increased fluids to prevent constipation
• Sips of water, candy, gum for dry mouth
• Storage in tight, light-resistant container
Evaluate:
• Therapeutic response: decrease in emotional excitement, hallucinations, delusions, paranoia, reorganization of patterns of thought, speech
• Affect, orientation, LOC, reflexes, gait, coordination, sleep pattern disturbances
• B/P standing and lying; take pulse and respirations q4h during initial treatment; establish baseline before starting treatment; report drops of 30 mm Hg
• Dizziness, faintness, palpitations, tachycardia on rising
• EPS including akathisia (inability to sit still, no pattern to movements), tardive dyskinesia (bizarre movements of the jaw, mouth, tongue, extremities), pseudoparkinsonism (rigidity, tremors, pill rolling, shuffling gait)
• Skin turgor daily

• Constipation, urinary retention daily; if these occur, increase bulk, water in diet
Teach patient/family:
• That orthostatic hypotension may occur and to rise from sitting or lying position gradually
• To remain lying down after IM injection for at least 30 min
• To avoid hot tubs, hot showers, or tub baths since hypotension may occur
• To avoid abrupt withdrawal of this drug or EPS may result; drug should be withdrawn slowly
• To avoid OTC preparations (cough, hayfever, cold) unless approved by physician since serious drug interactions may occur; avoid use with alcohol or CNS depressants, increased drowsiness may occur
• To avoid hazardous activities if drowsiness or dizziness occurs
• To use a sunscreen during sun exposure to prevent burns
• Regarding compliance with drug regimen; warn patient about avoiding OTC preparation
• About necessity for meticulous oral hygiene since oral candidiasis may occur
• To report impaired vision, jaundice, tremors, muscle twitching
• In hot weather heat stroke may occur; take extra precautions to stay cool
Treatment of overdose: Lavage if orally injested, provide an airway; *do not induce vomiting*

---

lypressin
(lye-press'in)
Diapid
Func. class.: Pituitary hormone
Chem. class.: Lysine vasopressin

Action: Promotes reabsorption of water by action on renal tubular ep-

---

ithelium, smooth muscles causing constriction with a vasopressor effect

Uses: Nonnephrogenic diabetes insipidus

Dosage and routes:
• *Adult:* INTRANASAL 1-2 sprays in one or both nostrils qid, an extra dose hs if needed

Available forms include: INTRANASAL 0.185 mg/ml

Side effects/adverse reactions:
EENT: Nasal irritation, congestion, rhinitis
CNS: Drowsiness, headache, lethargy, flushing
GU: Vulval pain
GI: Nausea, heartburn, cramps
CV: Increased B/P

Contraindications: Pregnancy, childbearing-age women, hypertension

Precautions: CAD

Pharmacokinetics:
NASAL: Onset 1 hr, duration 3-8 hr, half-life 15 min; metabolized in liver, kidneys, excreted in urine

Interactions/incompatibilities: None known

NURSING CONSIDERATIONS
Assess:
• Pulse, B/P when giving drug IV or IM
• I&O ratio; weight daily, check for edema in extremities, if water retention is severe, diuretic may be prescribed

Perform/provide:
• Storage at room temperature

Evaluate:
• Therapeutic response: absence of severe thirst, decreased urine output, osmolality
• Water intoxication: lethargy, behavioral changes, disorientation, neuromuscular excitability

Teach patient/family:
• To clear nasal passages before using drug, not to inhale spray
• To carry drug at all times

• All aspects of drug: action, side effects, dose, when to notify physician

---

mafenide acetate (topical)
(ma′fe-nide)
Sulfamylon
Func. class.: Local antiinfective
Chem. class.: Sulfonamide

Action: Interferes with bacterial cell wall synthesis

Uses: Burns (2nd, 3rd degree)

Dosage and routes:
• *Adult and child:* TOP apply to affected area qd-bid, reapply as needed

Available forms include: Cream 85 mg/g

Side effects/adverse reactions:
INTEG: Rash, urticaria, stinging, burning, bleeding, excoriation of new skin, super infections, pruritus, blisters, metabolic acidosis

Contraindications: Hypersensitivity, inhalation injury

Precautions: Pregnancy (C), impaired pulmonary function, lactation, impaired renal function

Interactions/incompatibilities: None known

NURSING CONSIDERATIONS
Administer:
• Analgesic before application if needed
• Enough medication to completely cover burns, they must be covered at all times
• After cleansing debris from burn before each application
• Using aseptic technique to debrided areas

Perform/provide:
• Storage at room temperature in dry place

Evaluate:
• Allergic reaction: burning, stinging, swelling, redness

• Therapeutic response: appearance of granulation tissue
• Fluid loss: decreased urinary output

Teach patient/family:
• That therapy will continue until area is ready for grafting

---

magaldrate (aluminum magnesium complex)

(mag' al-drate)

Lowsium Riopan, Riopan Plus

Func. class.: Antacid
Chem. class.: Aluminum/magnesium hydroxide

Action: Neutralizes gastric acidity
Uses: Antacid
Dosage and routes:
• *Adult:* PO 1-2 (400-960 mg) between meals, hs, not to exceed 20 tabs/day; CHEW TAB 1-2 (480-960 mg) between meals, hs, not to exceed 20 tabs/day; SUSP 5-10 ml (400-800 mg) with water between meals, hs, not to exceed 100 ml/day

Available forms include: Tabs 480 mg; chew tabs 480 mg; susp 540 mg/5 ml

Side effects/adverse reactions:
GI: Constipation, diarrhea
META: Hypermagnesium

Contraindications: Hypersensitivity to this drug or aluminum products

Precautions: Elderly, fluid restriction, decreased GI motility, GI obstruction, dehydration, renal disease, sodium-restricted diets

Pharmacokinetics:
PO: Duration 60 min

Interactions/incompatibilities:
• Decreased effectiveness of: tetracyclines
• Decreased absorption of: anticholinergics, chlordiazepoxide, cimetidine, corticosteroids, iron salts, phenothiazines, phenytoin, fat-soluble vitamins

NURSING CONSIDERATIONS
Administer:
• Laxatives or stool softeners if constipation occurs
• After shaking, give between meals

Evaluate:
• Therapeutic response: absence of pain, decreased acidity
• Constipation: increase bulk in diet if needed

---

magnesium carbonate

Func. class.: Antacid
Chem. class.: Magnesium product

Action: Neutralizes gastric acidity
Uses: Hyperactivity, constipation
Dosage and routes:
• *Adult:* PO 0.5-2 g between meals with water
Laxative
• *Adult:* PO 8 g with water hs
Available forms include: Powder
Side effects/adverse reactions:
GI: Diarrhea, flatulence, cramps, belching, nausea, vomiting
META: Hypermagnesia: *weakness, lethargy, depression, decreased B/P, increased pulse, **respiratory depression, coma***

Contraindications: Hypersensitivity
Precautions: Severe renal disease, GI bleeding, diarrhea, intestinal obstruction
Pharmacokinetics:
PO: Excreted in urine
Interactions/incompatibilities:
• Decreased effectiveness of: tetracyclines
• Decreased absorption of: anticholinergics, chlordiazapoxide, cimetidine, corticosteroids, iron salts

M

NURSING CONSIDERATIONS
Administer:
• Aluminum antacids if diarrhea occurs
• After mixing with water
Evaluate:
• Therapeutic response: absence of pain, decreased acidity
Teach patient/family:
• Not to change antacids unless directed by physician
Lab test interferences:
Increase: Urinary pH, gastrin
Decrease: K+

---

magnesium oxide

Mag-Ox, Maox, Par-mag, Uro-mag

Func. class.: Antacid
Chem. class.: Magnesium product

Action: Neutralizes gastric acidity
Uses: Constipation, hypomagnesemia

Dosage and routes:
• *Adult:* PO 250 mg-1 g pc, hs with water
Laxative
• *Adult:* PO 4 g with water hs
Hypomagnesemia
• *Adult:* PO 650-1.3 g qd
Available forms include: Caps 140; tabs 400, 420, 500 mg
Side effects/adverse reactions:
GI: Diarrhea, flatulence, cramps, belching, nausea, vomiting
META: Hypermagnesemia: *weakness,*
lethargy, depression, decreased B/P, increased pulse, respiratory depression, coma
Contraindications: Hypersensitivity
Precautions: Severe renal disease, GI bleeding, diarrhea, intestinal obstruction
Pharmacokinetics:
PO: Excreted in urine

Interactions/incompatibilities:
• Decreased effectiveness of: tetracyclines
• Decreased absorption of: anticholinergics, chlordiazepoxide, cimetidine, corticosteroids, iron salts, phenothiazines, phenytoin, fat-soluble vitamins
NURSING CONSIDERATIONS
Administer:
• Aluminum antacids if diarrhea occurs
Evaluate:
• Therapeutic response: absence of pain, decreased acidity
• Decreased constipation, characteristics of stools
Teach patient/family:
• Not to change antacids unless directed by physician
Lab test interferences:
Increase: Urinary pH, gastrin
Decrease: K+

---

magnesium salicylate

Analate, Arthrin, Doan's pills, Efficin, Magan, Mobidin

Func. class.: Nonnarcotic analgesic
Chem. class.: Salicylate

Action: Blocks pain impulses in CNS that occur in response to inhibition of prostaglandin synthesis; antipyretic action results from inhibition of hypothalamic heat-regulating center to produce vasodilation to allow heat dissipation
Uses: Mild to moderate pain or fever including arthritis, juvenile rheumatoid arthritis
Dosage and routes:
Arthritis
• *Adult:* PO not to exceed 9.6 g/day in divided doses
Pain/fever
• *Adult:* PO 600 mg tid or qid
Available forms include: Tabs 325, 545, 600 mg

Side effects/adverse reactions:

*HEMA: **Thrombocytopenia, agranulocytosis, leukopenia, neutropenia, hemolytic anemia,*** increased pro-time

CNS: Stimulation, drowsiness, dizziness, confusion, convulsion, headache, flushing, hallucinations, coma

GI: Nausea, vomiting, GI bleeding, diarrhea, heartburn, anorexia, **hepatitis**

INTEG: Rash, urticaria, bruising

EENT: Tinnitus, hearing loss

CV: Rapid pulse, pulmonary edema

RESP: Wheezing, hyperpnea

ENDO: Hypoglycemia, hyponatremia, hypokalemia

Contraindications: Hypersensitivity to salicylates, GI bleeding, bleeding disorders, children < 3 yr, pregnancy, lactation, vitamin K deficiency

Precautions: Anemia, hepatic disease, renal disease, Hodgkin's disease

Pharmacokinetics:

PO: Onset 15-30 min, peak 1-2 hr, duration 4-6 hr, metabolized by liver, excreted by kidneys, crosses placenta, excreted in breast milk, half-life 1-3½ hr

Interactions/incompatibilities:

• Decreased effects of this drug: antacids, steroids, urinary alkalizers

• Increased blood loss: alcohol, heparin

• Increased effects of: anticoagulants, insulin, methotrexate

• Decreased effects of: probenecid, spironolactone, sulfinpyrazone, sulfonylmides

• Toxic effects: PABA

• Decreased blood sugar levels: salicylates

NURSING CONSIDERATIONS

Assess:

• Liver function studies: AST, ALT, bilirubin, creatinine if patient is on long-term therapy

• Renal function studies: BUN, urine creatinine if patient is on long-term therapy

• Blood studies: CBC, Hct, Hgb, pro-time if patient is on long-term therapy

• I&O ratio; decreasing output may indicate renal failure (long-term therapy)

Administer:

• To patient crushed or whole; chewable tablets may be chewed

• With food or milk to decrease gastric symptoms; give 30 min before or 2 hr after meals

• With full glass of water

Perform/provide:

• Repositioning to decrease pain

• Cool cloth for fever

Evaluate:

• Hepatotoxicity: dark urine, clay-colored stools, yellowing of skin, sclera, itching, abdominal pain, fever, diarrhea if patient is on long-term therapy

• Allergic reactions: rash, urticaria; if these occur, drug may need to be discontinued

• Renal dysfunction: decreased urine output

• Ototoxicity: tinnitus, ringing, roaring in ears; audiometric testing is needed before, after long-term therapy

• Visual changes: blurring, halos, corneal and retinal damage

• Edema in feet, ankles, legs

• Prior drug history; there are many drug interactions

Teach patient/family:

• To report any symptoms of hepatotoxicity, renal toxicity, visual changes, ototoxicity, allergic reactions (long-term therapy)

• Not to exceed recommended dosage; acute poisoning may result

• To read label on other OTC drugs; many contain aspirin

M

---

italics = common side effects   ***bold italic*** = life threatening reactions

• That therapeutic response takes 2 wk (arthritis)
• To avoid alcohol ingestion; GI bleeding may occur

Lab test interferences:
Increase: Coagulation studies, liver function studies, serum uric acid, amylase, CO_2, urinary protein
Decrease: Serum potassium, PBI, cholesterol
Interfere: Urine catecholamines, pregnancy test

Treatment of overdose: Lavage, activated charcoal, monitor electrolytes, VS

---

magnesium salts

Magnesium Citrate, Magnesium Sulfate, Milk of Magnesia (MOM)
Func. class.: Laxative, saline

Action: Increases osmotic pressure, draws fluid into colon
Uses: Constipation, bowel preparation before surgery or examination

Dosage and routes:
• *Adult:* PO 30-60 ml hs (Milk of Magnesia)
• *Adult and child >6 yr:* PO 15 g in 8 oz of water (Magnesium Sulfate); PO 10-20 ml (Concentrated Milk of Magnesia); PO 5-10 oz hs (Magnesium Citrate)
• *Child 2-6 yr:* 5-15 ml (Milk of Magnesia)

Available forms include: Oral sol, susp 77.5 mg/g; tabs 300, 600 mg

Side effects/adverse reactions:
CNS: Muscle weakness, flushing, sweating, confusion, sedation, depressed reflexes, *flaccid, paralysis,* hypothermia
GI: Nausea, vomiting, anorexia, cramps
CV: Hypotension, heart block, circulatory collapse
META: Electrolyte, fluid imbalances

Contraindications: Hypersensitivity, renal diseases, abdominal pain, nausea/vomiting, obstruction, acute surgical abdomen, rectal bleeding

Pharmacokinetics:
PO: Peak 1-2 hr; excreted in feces
Interactions/incompatibilities:
• Increased CNS depression: CNS depressants, barbiturates, narcotics, anesthetics

NURSING CONSIDERATIONS
Assess:
• I&O ratio; check for decrease in urinary output
Administer:
• With 8 oz of water
Evaluate:
• Therapeutic response: decreased constipation
• Cause of constipation; identify whether fluids, bulk, or exercise is missing from lifestyle
• Cramping, rectal bleeding, nausea, vomiting; if these symptoms occur, drug should be discontinued
• Magnesium toxicity: thirst, confusion, decrease in reflexes
Teach patient/family:
• Not to use laxatives for long-term therapy; bowel tone will be lost

---

magnesium sulfate

Func. class.: Anticonvulsant
Chem. class.: Magnesium product

Action: Decreases acetylcholine in motor nerve terminals, which is responsible for anticonvulsant properties; osmotically retains fluid, which increases amount of water in feces when used as laxative; reduces SA node impulse formation, prolongs conduction time in myocardium
Uses: Hypomagnesemic seizures, control of seizures in preeclampsia/eclampsia, seizures in acute nephritis

Dosage and routes:

Hypomagnesemic seizures

• *Adult:* IV 1-2 g over 15 min, then 1 g IM q4-6h, depending on response

Nephritis

• *Child:* IM 0.2 ml/kg of 50% sol q4-6h, or 100 mg/kg of 10% solution over several min; dosage depends on response

Preeclampsia/eclampsia

• *Adult:* IV 4 g/250 ml D₅W and 4 g IM, then 4 g IM q4h prn; or 4 g IV loading dose, then 1-4 g IV INF hourly

Available forms include: Inj IV, IM 10%, 50%, 12.5%, 25%; granules,

Side effects/adverse reactions:

CNS: Sweating, depressed reflexes, flushing, drowsiness, flaccid paralysis, hypothermia, weakness, sedation

CV: Hypotension, **circulatory collapse, heart block,** decreased cardiac function

Contraindications: Hypersensitivity, myocardial infarction, renal disease, pregnancy

Pharmacokinetics:

IV: Onset 1-5 min, duration 30 min

IM: Onset 1 hr, duration 3-4 hr

Metabolized by liver, excreted by kidneys

Interactions/incompatibilities:

• Increased CNS depression: barbiturates, general anesthetics, narcotics, antipsychotics

• Increased effects of: neuromuscular blockers

NURSING CONSIDERATIONS

Assess:

• VS q15 min after IV dose; do not exceed 150 mg/min

• Cardiac function: monitoring, magnesium levels

• Time contractions, determine intensity, if using during labor

• I&O: should remain at 30 ml/hr

or more; if less than this, notify physician

Administer:

• Only after calcium gluconate is available for magnesium toxicity

• IV at less than 150 mg/min; circulatory collapse may occur

Perform/provide:

• Seizure precautions: placing in dark room with decreased stimuli, padded siderails

Evaluate:

• Mental status: mood, sensorium, affect, memory (long, short)

• Respiratory dysfunction: respiratory depression, character, rate, rhythm; hold drug if respirations are <16/min

• Hypermagnesemia: depressed patellar reflex, flushing, polydipsia, confusion, weakness, flaccid paralysis, hypothermia, dyspnea

• Respiratory rate, rhythm of newborn if drug was given 24 hr before delivery or less; check reflexes of newborn whose mother received this drug before delivery

• Reflexes: knee jerk, patellar; decrease signals Mg + + toxicity

Teach patient/family:

• On all aspects of this drug: action, route, side effects, symptoms of hypermagnesemia

Treatment of overdose: Stop drug, administer calcium gluconate, monitor reflexes, magnesium levels, reflexes

---

magnesium trisilicate

Trisomin

Func. class.: Antacid

Chem. class.: Magnesium product

Action: Neutralizes gastric acidity

Uses: Constipation, hypomagnesemia

Dosage and routes:
• *Adult:* PO 1-4 g tid with 4 oz of water
Available forms include: Powder
Side effects/adverse reactions:
GI: Diarrhea, flatulence, cramps, belching, nausea, vomiting
META: Hypermagnesemia: *weakness, lethargy, depression, decreased*
*B/P, increased pulse, **respiratory depression, coma***
Contraindications: Hypersensitivity to this drug
Precautions: Severe renal disease
Pharmacokinetics:
PO: Excreted in urine
Interactions/incompatibilities:
• Decreased effectiveness of: tetracyclines
• Decreased absorption of: anticholinergics, chlordiazepoxide, cimetidine, corticosteroids, iron salts, phenothiazines, phenytoin, fat-soluble vitamins

NURSING CONSIDERATIONS
Administer:
• Aluminum antacids if diarrhea occurs
• After mixing with water
Evaluate:
• Therapeutic response: absence of pain, decreased acidity
• Decreased constipation, characteristics of stools
Teach patient/family:
• Not to change antacids unless directed by physician
Lab test interferences:
Increase: Urinary pH, gastrin
Decrease: K+

---

mannitol
(man'i-tole)
Osmitrol, Resectial
Func. class.: Osmotic diuretic
Chem. class.: Hexahydric alcohol

Action: Acts by increasing osmolarity of glomerular filtrate, which raises osmotic pressure of fluid in renal tubules; there is a decrease in reabsorption of water, increase in urinary output
Uses: Edema, promote systemic diuresis in cerebral edema, decrease intraocular pressure, improve renal function in acute renal failure, chemical poisoning
Dosage and routes:
Oliguria, prevention
• *Adult:* IV 50-100 g of a 5%-25% sol
Oliguria, treatment
• *Adult:* IV 300-400 mg/kg of a 20%-25% sol up to 100 g of a 15%-20% sol
Intraocular pressure/intracranial pressure
• *Adult:* IV 1.5-2 g/kg of a 15%-25% sol over ½-1 hr
Renal failure
• *Adult:* IV 50-200 g/24 hr, adjusted to maintain output of 30-50 mg/hr
Available forms include: Inj IV 5%, 10%, 15%, 20%, 25%
Side effects/adverse reactions:
GU: Marked diuresis, urinary retention, thirst
CNS: Dizziness, headache, convulsions
GI: Nausea, vomiting, dry mouth
CV: Edema, thrombophlebitis, hypotension, hypertension, tachycardia, angina-like chest pains, fever, chills
RESP: Pulmonary congestion
ELECT: Fluid, electrolyte imbalances, acidosis, electrolyte loss, dehydration
EENT: Loss of hearing, blurred vision, nasal congestion, decreased intraocular pressure
Contraindications: Hypersensitivity, anuria, severe pulmonary congestion, severe dehydration
Precautions: Dehydration, pregnancy, severe renal disease

Pharmacokinetics:

IV: Onset 30-60 min for diuresis, ½-1 hr for intraocular pressure, 25 min for cerebrospinal fluid; duration 4-6 hr for intraocular pressure, 3-8 hr for cerebrospinal fluid; excreted in urine

Interactions/incompatibilities:

• Decreased effect: lithium

• Increased effects of: EDTA

• Incompatible with whole blood, in solution or syringe with any other drug or solution

NURSING CONSIDERATIONS

Assess:

• Weight, I&O daily to determine fluid loss; effect of drug may be decreased if used qd

• Rate, depth, rhythm of respiration, effect of exertion

• B/P lying, standing, postural hypotension may occur

• Electrolytes: potassium, sodium, chloride; include BUN, CBC, serum creatinine, blood pH, ABGs

Administer:

• IV in 15%-25% solutions

Evaluate:

• Improvement in edema of feet, legs, sacral area daily if medication is being used in CHF

• Improvement in CVP q8h

• Signs of metabolic acidosis: drowsiness, restlessness

• Signs of hypokalemia: postural hypotension, malaise, fatigue, tachycardia, leg cramps, weakness

• Rashes, temperature elevation qd

• Confusion, especially in elderly; take safety precautions if needed

• Hydration including skin turgor, thirst, dry mucous membranes

Teach patient/family:

• To increase fluid intake 2-3 L/day unless contraindicated; to rise slowly from lying or sitting position

Lab test interferences:

Interference: Inorganic phosphorus, ethylene glycol

Treatment of overdose: Discontinue infusion, correct fluid, electrolyte imbalances, hemodialysis

---

maprotiline HCl

(ma-proe'ti-leen)
Ludiomil
Func. class.: Antidepressant
Chem. class.: Tetracyclic

Action: Blocks reuptake of norepinephrine, serotonin into nerve endings, increasing action of norepinephrine, serotonin in nerve cells

Uses: Depression, dysthymic disorder, manic depressive—depressed, agitated depression

Dosage and routes:

• *Adult:* PO 75 mg/day in moderate depression, may increase to 150 mg/day; not to exceed 225 mg in hospitalized patients, severely depressed patients that are hospitalized may be given 300 mg/day

• *Elderly:* 50-75 mg/day

Available forms include: Tabs 25, 50, 75 mg

Side effects/adverse reactions:

*HEMA: **Agranulocytosis, thrombocytopenia, eosinophilia, leukopenia***

CNS: Dizziness, drowsiness, confusion, headache, anxiety, tremors, stimulation, weakness, insomnia, nightmares, EPS (elderly), increased psychiatric symptoms

GI: Diarrhea, dry mouth, nausea, vomiting, ***paralytic ileus,*** increased appetite, cramps, epigastric distress, jaundice, ***hepatitis,*** stomatitis

*GU: Retention, **acute renal failure***

INTEG: Rash, urticaria, sweating, pruritus, photosensitivity

*CV: Orthostatic hypotension, ECG changes, tachycardia, **hypertension,*** palpitations

EENT: Blurred vision, tinnitus, mydriasis

Contraindications: Hypersensitivity to tricyclic antidepressants, recovery phase of myocardial infarction, convulsive disorders, prostatic hypertrophy

Precautions: Suicidal patients, severe depression, increased intraocular pressure, narrow-angle glaucoma, urinary retention, cardiac disease, hepatic disease, hypothyroidism, hyperthyroidism, electroshock therapy, elective surgery, elderly, pregnancy (B)

Pharmacokinetics:

PO: Onset 15-30 min, peak 12 hr, duration up to 3 wk, steady state 6-10 days; metabolized by liver, excreted by kidneys, feces, crosses placenta, half-life 21-25 hr

Interactions/incompatibilities:

• Decreased effects of: guanethidine, clonidine, indirect acting sympathomimetics (ephedrine)

• Increased effects of: direct acting sympathomimetics (epinephrine), alcohol, barbiturates, benzodiazepines, CNS depressants

• Hyperpyretic crisis, convulsions, hypertensive episode: MAOI (pargyline [Eutonyl])

NURSING CONSIDERATIONS

Assess:

• B/P (lying, standing), pulse q4h; if systolic B/P drops 20 mm Hg hold drug, notify physician; take vital signs q4h in patients with cardiovascular disease

• Blood studies: CBC, leukocytes, differential, cardiac enzymes if patient is receiving long-term therapy

• Hepatic studies: AST, ALT, bilirubin, creatinine

• Weight qwk, appetite may increase with drug

• ECG for flattening of T wave, bundle branch block, AV block, dysrhythmias in cardiac patients

Administer:

• Increased fluids, bulk in diet if constipation, urinary retention occur

• With food or milk for GI symptoms

• Dosage hs if over-sedation occurs during day; may take entire dose hs; elderly may not tolerate once/day dosing

• Gum, hard candy, or frequent sips of water for dry mouth

• Concentrate with fruit juice, water, or milk to disguise taste

Perform/provide:

• Storage in tight container at room temperature, do not freeze

• Assistance with ambulation during beginning therapy since drowsiness/dizziness occurs

• Safety measures including siderails primarily in elderly

• Checking to see PO medication swallowed

Evaluate:

• EPS primarily in elderly: rigidity, dystonia, akathisia

• Mental status: mood, sensorium, affect, suicidal tendencies, increase in psychiatric symptoms: depression, panic

• Urinary retention, constipation; constipation is more likely to occur in children

• Withdrawal symptoms: headache, nausea, vomiting, muscle pain, weakness; do not usually occur unless drug was discontinued abruptly

• Alcohol consumption; if alcohol is consumed, hold dose until morning

Teach patient/family:

• That therapeutic effects may take 2-3 wk

• Use of caution in driving or other activities requiring alertness because of drowsiness, dizziness, blurred vision

• To avoid alcohol ingestion, other CNS depressants

• Not to discontinue medication

quickly after long-term use, may cause nausea, headache, malaise
• To wear sunscreen or large hat since photosensitivity occurs

Lab test interferences:

Increase: Serum bilirubin, blood glucose, alk phosphatase

False increase: Urinary catecholamines

Decrease: VMA, 5-HIAA

Treatment of overdose: ECG monitoring, induce emesis, lavage, activated charcoal, administer anticonvulsant

---

mazindol

(may'zin-dole)

Mazanor, Sanorex

Func. class.: Cerebral stimulant

Chem. class.: Imidazoisoindole derivative

Controlled Substance Schedule IV

Action: Increases release of norepinephrine and dopamine in cerebral cortex to reticular activating system

Uses: Exogenous obesity

Dosage and routes:

• *Adult:* PO 1 mg ac, or 2 mg 1 hr before lunch

Available forms include: Tabs 1, 2 mg

Side effects/adverse reactions:

CNS: Hyperactivity, insomnia, restlessness, dizziness, headache, stimulation, irritability, drowsiness, weakness, tremor

GI: Nausea, anorexia, dry mouth, diarrhea, constipation

GU: Impotence, change in libido, difficulty urinating

CV: Palpitations, tachycardia

INTEG: Urticaria, rash, pallor, shivering, sweating

Contraindications: Hypersensitivity to sympathomimetic amine, glaucoma, drug abuse, cardiovascular disease, alcoholism

Precautions: Diabetes mellitus, hypertension, depression

Pharmacokinetics:

PO: Onset ½-1 hr, duration 8-15 hr, metabolized by liver, excreted by kidneys

Interactions/incompatibilities:

• Hypertensive crisis: MAOIs or within 14 days of MAOIs

• Increased effect of this drug: acetazolamide, antacids, sodium bicarbonate, ascorbic acid, ammonium chloride, phenothiazines, haloperidol

• Decreased effects of this drug: barbiturates

• Decreased effects of: guanethidine, other antihypertensives

NURSING CONSIDERATIONS

Assess:

• VS, B/P since this drug may reverse antihypertensives; check patients with cardiac disease more often

• CBC, urinalysis, in diabetes: blood sugar, urine sugar; insulin changes may need to be made since eating will decrease

• Height, growth rate in children; growth rate may be decreased

Administer:

• At least 6 hr before hs to avoid sleeplessness

• For obesity only if patient is on weight reduction program including dietary changes, exercise; patient will develop tolerance, and weight loss won't occur without additional methods

• Gum, hard candy, frequent sips of water for dry mouth

• If drug is being given for obesity, 1 hr before meals

Perform/provide:

• Checking to see PO medication has been swallowed

Evaluate:

• Mental status: mood, sensorium,

affect, stimulation, insomnia, aggressiveness
• Physical dependency: should not be used for extended time; dose should be discontinued gradually
• Withdrawal symptoms: headache, nausea, vomiting, muscle pain, weakness
• Drug tolerance after long-term use
• Dosage should not be increased if tolerance develops

Teach patient/family:
• To decrease caffeine consumption (coffee, tea, cola, chocolate), which may increase irritability, stimulation
• Avoid OTC preparations unless approved by physician
• To taper off drug over several weeks, or depression, increased sleeping, lethargy may ensue
• To avoid alcohol ingestion
• To avoid hazardous activities until patient is stabilized on medication
• To get needed rest, patients will feel more tired at end of day

Treatment of overdose: Administer fluids, hemodialysis or peritoneal dialysis; antihypertensive for increased B/P; ammonium Cl for increased excretion

---

measles, mumps, and rubella virus vaccine, live
M-M-R-II

Func. class.: Vaccine

Action: Produces antibodies to measles, mumps, rubella
Uses: Prevention of measles, mumps, rubella

Dosage and routes:
• *Child 1-13 yr:* SC 1000 U
Available forms include: Inj SC measles 1000 TCID$_{50}$, mumps 5000 TCID$_{50}$, rubella 1000 TCID$_{50}$

Side effects/adverse reactions:
CNS: Fever
INTEG: Urticaria, erythema
SYST: Lymphadenitis, *anaphylaxis*
MS: Osteomyelitis

Contraindications: Hypersensitivity, blood dyscrasias, anemia, active infection, immunosuppression, egg, chicken allergy, pregnancy

Interactions/incompatibilities:
• Decreased response to: TB skin test

NURSING CONSIDERATIONS
Assess:
• For skin reactions: rash, induration, erythema

Administer:
• Only with epinephrine 1:1000 on unit to treat laryngospasm
• Only SC

Evaluate:
• For history of allergies, skin conditions (eczema, psoriasis, dermatitis), reactions to vaccinations
• For anaphylaxis: inability to breathe, bronchospasm

---

mebendazole
(me-ben'da-zole)
Vermox

Func. class.: Anthelmintic
Chem. class.: Carbamate

Action: Inhibits glucose, nutrient uptake, degeneration of cytoplasmic microtubules in the cell; interferes with absorption, secretory function
Uses: Pinworms, roundworms, hookworms, whipworms, threadworms, pork tapeworms, dwarf tapeworms, beef tapeworms, hydatid cyst

Dosage and routes:
• *Adult and child >2 yr:* PO 100 mg as a single dose or bid × 3 days, depending on type of infec-

---

tion; course may be repeated in 3 wk if needed

Available forms include: Tabs, chewable 100 mg

Side effects/adverse reactions:

CNS: Dizziness, fever

GI: Transient diarrhea, abdominal pain

Contraindications: Hypersensitivity

Precautions: Child <2 yr, lactation, pregnancy (1st trimester) (C)

Pharmacokinetics:

PO: Peak ½-7 hr, excreted in feces primarily (metabolites), small amount in urine (unchanged), highly bound to plasma proteins

Interactions/incompatibilities: None known

NURSING CONSIDERATIONS

Assess:

• Stools during entire treatment; specimens must be sent to lab while still warm

Administer:

• May be crushed, chewed if unable to swallow whole

• PO after meals to avoid GI symptoms since absorption is not altered by food

• Second course after 3 wk if needed; usually recommended

Perform/provide:

• Storage in tight container

Evaluate:

• For therapeutic response: expulsion of worms and 3 negative stool cultures after completion of treatment

• For allergic reaction: rash (rare)

• For diarrhea during expulsion of worms; prevent contamination with feces

• For infection in other family members since infection from person to person is common

Teach patient/family:

• Proper hygiene after BM including handwashing technique; tell patient to avoid putting fingers in mouth

• That infected person should sleep alone; do not shake bed linen, change bed linen qd, wash in hot water

• To clean toilet qd with disinfectant (green soap solution)

• Need for compliance with dosage schedule, duration of treatment

• To wear shoes, wash all fruits and vegetables well before eating

---

mecamylamine HCl

(mek-a-mill′a-meen)

Inversine

Func. class.: Antihypertensive

Chem. class.: Ganglionic blocker

Action: Occupies receptor site, prevents acetylcholine from attaching to postsynaptic nerve ending in sympathetic ganglia

Uses: Moderate to severe hypertension, malignant hypertension

Dosage and routes:

• *Adult:* PO 2.5 mg bid, may increase in increments of 2.5 mg × 2 days until desired response, maintenance 25 mg/day in 3 divided doses

Available forms include: Tabs 2.5 mg

Side effects/adverse reactions:

CV: Postural hypotension, irregular heart rate, CHF

CNS: Drowsiness, sedation, headache, tremors, weakness, syncope, paresthesia, dizziness, ***convulsions***

EENT: Blurred vision, nasal congestion, dry mouth, dilated pupils

GU: Impotence, urinary retention, decreased libido

GI: Anorexia, glossitis, nausea, vomiting, constipation, paralytic ileus

Contraindications: Hypersensitivity, myocardial infarction, coro-

---

nary insufficiency, renal disease, glaucoma, organic pyloric stenosis, uremia

Precautions: CVA, prostatic hypertrophy, bladder neck obstruction, urethral stricture, renal dysfunction (elevated BUN), cerebral dysfunction, pregnancy (C)

Pharmacokinetics:

PO: Onset ½-2 hr, duration 6-12 hr; excreted in urine, feces, breast milk; crosses placenta

Interactions/incompatibilities:

• Increased effects: thiazide diuretics, antihypertensives, CNS depressants (alcohol, anesthetics, MAOIs), bethanechol

NURSING CONSIDERATIONS

Assess:

• B/P, other VS throughout treatment

• Weight daily, I&O

Administer:

• Whole, do not chew or crush tablets

• With meals for better absorption

• Gum, frequent rinsing of mouth, hard candy for dry mouth

Evaluate:

• Edema in feet, legs daily

• Skin turgor, dryness of mucous membranes for hydration status

• Tolerance to drug that occurs with prolonged use

• Constipation: number of stools, consistency, give stool softener as ordered or increase bulk in diet

Teach patient/family:

• To notify physician if tremor, seizure, or signs of paralytic ileus occur

• To avoid OTC preparations unless directed by physician

• To rise slowly from sitting or lying position, orthostatic hypotension may occur

• That impotence may occur, but is reversible after discontinuing drug

Treatment of overdose: Administer gastric lavage, discontinue drug, administer small doses of pressor amines for hypotension

---

mechlorethamine HCl (nitrogen mustard)

(me-klor-eth'a-meen)

Mustargen

Func. class.: Antineoplastic alkylating agent

Chem. class.: Nitrogen mustard

Action: Alkylates DNA, RNA; inhibits enzymes that allow synthesis of amino acids in proteins; also responsible for cross-linking DNA strands

Uses: Hodgkin's disease, lymphomas, lymphosarcoma; ovarian, breast, lung cancer; neoplastic effusions

Dosage and routes:

• *Adult:* IV 0.4 mg/kg or 10 mg/m^2 as 1 dose or divided doses

Neoplastic effusions

• *Adult:* INTRACAVITY 10-20 mg

Available forms include: Inj IV, intracavity 10 mg; powder for inj

Side effects/adverse reactions:

EENT: Tinnitus, hearing loss

HEMA: ***Thrombocytopenia, leukopenia, agranulocytosis,*** anemia

GI: Nausea, vomiting, diarrhea, stomatitis, weight loss, colitis, ***hepatotoxicity***

CNS: Headache, dizziness, drowsiness, paresthesia, peripheral neuropathy, ***coma***

INTEG: Alopecia, pruritus, herpes zoster

Contraindications: Lactation, pregnancy (1st trimester) myelosuppression, acute herpes zoster

Precautions: Radiation therapy, chronic lymphocytic leukopenia

Pharmacokinetics:

Metabolized in liver, excreted in urine

Interactions/incompatibilities:
• Increased toxicity: antineoplastics, radiation

NURSING CONSIDERATIONS
Assess:
• CBC, differential, platelet count weekly; withhold drug if WBC is <4000 or platelet count is <75,000; notify physician of results
• Renal function studies: BUN, serum uric acid, urine CrCl before, during therapy
• I&O ratio, report fall in urine output of 30 ml/hr
• Monitor temperature q4h (may indicate beginning infection)
• Liver function tests before, during therapy (bilirubin, AST, ALT, LDH) as needed or monthly

Administer:
• Medications by oral route; if possible avoid IM, SC, IV routes to prevent infections
• Antiemetic 30-60 min before giving drug to prevent vomiting
• Antibiotics for prophylaxis of infection
• Slow IV infusion using 21-, 23-, 25-gauge needle
• Topical or systemic analgesics for pain
• Local or systemic drugs for infection

Perform/provide:
• Storage at room temperature in dry form
• Strict medical asepsis, protective isolation if WBC levels are low
• Special skin care
• Liquid diet, including cola, Jello; dry toast or crackers may be added if patient is not nauseated or vomiting
• Increase fluid intake to 2-3 L/day to prevent urate deposits, calculi formation
• Diet low in purines: organ meats (kidney, liver), dried beans, peas to maintain alkaline urine

• Rinsing of mouth tid-qid with water, hydrogen peroxide; brushing of teeth bid-tid with soft brush or cotton tipped applicators for stomatitis; use unwaxed dental floss
• Warm compresses at injection site for inflammation

Evaluate:
• Bleeding: hematuria, guaiac, bruising or petechiae, mucosa or orifices q8h
• Food preferences; list likes, dislikes
• Yellowing of skin, sclera, dark urine, clay-colored stools, itchy skin, abdominal pain, fever, diarrhea
• Effects of alopecia on body image; discuss feelings about body changes
• Inflammation of mucosa, breaks in skin
• Buccal cavity q8h for dryness, sores, ulceration, white patches, oral pain, bleeding, dysphagia
• Local irritation, pain, burning, discoloration at injection site
• Symptoms indicating severe allergic reaction: rash, pruritus, urticaria, purpuric skin lesions, itching, flushing

Teach patient/family:
• Of protective isolation precautions
• To report any complaints or side effects to nurse or physician
• That sterility, amenorrhea can occur; reversible after discontinuing treatment
• That hair may be lost during treatment; a wig or hairpiece may make patient feel better; new hair may be different in color, texture
• To avoid foods with citric acid, hot or rough texture
• To report any bleeding, white spots, or ulcerations in mouth to physician; tell patient to examine mouth qd

M

---

italics = common side effects   ***bold italic*** = life threatening reactions

meclizine HCl

(mek'li-zeen)

Antivert, Bonamine,* Bonine, Lamine, Roclizine, Vertol

Func. class.: Antiemetic

Chem. class.: H₁-receptor antagonist, piperazine derivative

Action: Acts centrally by blocking chemoreceptor trigger zone, which in turn acts on vomiting center

Uses: Dizziness, motion sickness

Dosage and routes:

• *Adult:* PO 25-100 mg qd in divided doses or 1 hr before traveling

Available forms include: Tabs 12.5, 25, 50 mg; chew tabs 25 mg; tabs film coated 25 mg

Side effects/adverse reactions:

CNS: Drowsiness, dizziness, fatigue, restlessness, headache, insomnia

GI: Nausea, anorexia

EENT: Dry mouth, blurred vision

Contraindications: Hypersensitivity to cyclizines, shock, lactation, pregnancy

Precautions: Children, narrow-angle glaucoma, glaucoma, urinary retention, lactation, prostatic hypertrophy, elderly, pregnancy

Pharmacokinetics:

PO: Duration 8-24 hr, half-life 6 hr

Interactions/incompatibilities:

• Increased effect of: alcohol, tranquilizers, narcotics

NURSING CONSIDERATIONS

Assess:

• VS, B/P; check patients with cardiac disease more often

Administer:

• Tablets may be swallowed whole, chewed, or allowed to dissolve

Evaluate:

• Signs of toxicity of other drugs or masking of symptoms of disease: brain tumor, intestinal obstruction

• Observe for drowsiness, dizziness

Teach patient/family:

• That a false negative result may occur with skin testing; these procedures should not be scheduled for 4 days after discontinuing use

• To avoid hazardous activities, activities requiring alertness; dizziness may occur; instruct patient to request assistance with ambulation

• Avoid alcohol, other depressants

Lab test interferences:

False negative: Allergy skin testing

meclofenamate

(me-kloe-fen-am'ate)

Meclamen

Func. class.: Nonsteroidal antiinflammatory

Chem. class.: Anthranilic acid derivative

Action: Inhibits prostaglandin synthesis by decreasing an enzyme needed for biosynthesis; possesses analgesic, antiinflammatory, antipyretic properties

Uses: Mild to moderate pain, osteoarthritis, rheumatoid arthritis

Dosage and routes:

• *Adult:* PO 200-400 mg/day in divided doses tid-qid

Available forms include: Caps 50, 100 mg

Side effects/adverse reactions:

GI: Nausea, anorexia, vomiting, diarrhea, jaundice, *cholestatic hepatitis,* constipation, flatulence, cramps, dry mouth, peptic ulcer

CNS: Dizziness, drowsiness, fatigue, tremors, confusion, insomnia, anxiety, depression

CV: Tachycardia, peripheral edema, palpitations, dysrhythmias

INTEG: Purpura, rash, pruritus, sweating

GU: Nephrotoxicity: dysuria, hematuria, oliguria, azotemia

*HEMA: **Blood dyscrasias***
EENT: Tinnitus, hearing loss, blurred vision
Contraindications: Hypersensitivity, asthma, severe renal disease, severe hepatic disease
Precautions: Pregnancy, lactation, children, bleeding disorders, GI disorders, cardiac disorders, hypersensitivity to other antiinflammatory agents
Pharmacokinetics:
PO: Peak 2 hr, half-life 3-3½ hr; metabolized in liver, excreted in urine (metabolites), excreted in breast milk
Interactions/incompatibilities:
• May increase action of coumarin, phenytoin, sulfonamides when used with this drug
NURSING CONSIDERATIONS
Assess:
• Renal, liver, blood studies: BUN, creatinine, AST, ALT, Hgb before treatment, periodically thereafter
• Audiometric and ophthalmic exam before, during, after treatment
Administer:
• With food to decrease GI symptoms; best to take on empty stomach to facilitate absorption
Perform/provide:
• Storage at room temperature
Evaluate:
• Therapeutic response: decreased pain, stiffness, swelling in joints, ability to move more easily
• For eye, ear problems: blurred vision, tinnitus (may indicate toxicity)
Teach patient/family:
• To report blurred vision, ringing, roaring in ears (may indicate toxicity)
• To avoid driving or other hazardous activities if dizziness or drowsiness occurs
• To report change in urine pattern, weight increase, edema, pain increase in joints, fever, blood in urine (indicates nephrotoxicity)
• That therapeutic effects may take up to 1 mo

---

medium-chain triglycerides
MCT Oil
Func. class.: Caloric

Action: Needed for energy in body; more rapidly hydrolyzed than fat
Uses: Inadequate dietary fat intake or absorption
Dosage and routes:
• *Adult:* PO 15ml tid-qid, not to exceed 100ml/day
Available forms include: Oil (115 calories/15ml)
Side effects/adverse reactions:
CNS: Loss of consciousness (reversible)
GI: Nausea, vomiting, anorexia, cramps, diarrhea, distention
Contraindications: Hypersensitivity, severe hepatic disease, lipoproteinemia
Precautions: Portacaval shunts
Interactions/incompatibilities:
None known
NURSING CONSIDERATIONS
Assess:
• Triglycerides, free fatty acid levels, platelet counts daily to prevent fat overload, thrombocytopenia
• Liver function: AST, ALT
Administer:
• After changing IV tubing at each infusion; infection may occur with old tubing
• With infusion pump; do not use in-line filter; clogging will occur
Perform/provide:
• Use of mixed solutions that are not separated or oily looking
Evaluate:
• Therapeutic response: increased weight

M

• Nutritional status: calorie count by dietician
Teach patient/family:
• Reason for use of lipids

---

medroxyprogesterone acetate

(me-drox'ee-proe-jess'te-rone)
Amen, Curretab, Depo-Provera, Provera

Func. class.: Progestogen
Chem. class.: Progesterone derivative

Action: Inhibits secretion of pituitary gonadotropins, which prevents follicular maturation and ovulation, stimulates growth of mammary tissue, antineoplastic action against endometrial cancer
Uses: Uterine bleeding (abnormal), secondary amenorrhea, endometrial cancer, renal cancer
Dosage and routes:
Secondary amenorrhea
• *Adult:* PO 5-10 mg qd × 5-10 days
Endometrial/renal cancer
• *Adult:* 1M 400-1000 mg/wk
Uterine bleeding
• *Adult:* PO 5-10 mg qd × 5-10 days starting on 16th day of menstrual cycle
Available forms include: Tabs 2.5, 10 mg; inj susp 100, 400 mg/ml
Side effects/adverse reactions:
CNS: Dizziness, headache, migraines, depression, fatigue
CV: Hypotension, thrombophlebitis, edema, *thromboembolism, stroke, pulmonary embolism, myocardial infarction*
GI: Nausea, vomiting, anorexia, cramps, increased weight, *cholestatic jaundice*
EENT: Diplopia
GU: Amenorrhea, cervical erosion, breakthrough bleeding, dysmenorrhea, vaginal candidiasis, breast changes, *gynecomastia, testicular atrophy, impotence,* endometriosis, *spontaneous abortion*
INTEG: Rash, urticaria, acne, hirsutism, alopecia, oily skin, seborrhea, purpura, melasma, photosensitivity
META: Hyperglycemia
Contraindications: Breast cancer, hypersensitivity, thromboembolic disorders, reproductive cancer, genital bleeding (abnormal, undiagnosed)
Precautions: Pregnancy, lactation, hypertension, asthma, blood dyscrasias, gallbladder disease, CHF, diabetes mellitus, bone disease, depression, migraine headache, convulsive disorders, hepatic disease, renal disease, family history of cancer of breast or reproductive tract
Pharmacokinetics:
PO: Duration 24 hr, excreted in urine and feces, metabolized in liver
Interactions/incompatibilities:
None known
NURSING CONSIDERATIONS
Assess:
• Weight daily, notify physician of weekly weight gain >5 lb
• B/P at beginning of treatment and periodically
• I&O ratio; be alert for decreasing urinary output, increasing edema
• Liver function studies: ALT, AST, bilirubin, periodically during long-term therapy
Administer:
• Titrated dose, use lowest effective dose
• Solution deeply in large muscle mass (IM), rotate sites
• In one dose in AM
• With food or milk to decrease GI symptoms
• After warming to dissolve crystals

---

*Available in Canada only

Perform/provide:
• Storage in dark area
Evaluate:
• Therapeutic response: decreased abnormal uterine bleeding, absence of amenorrhea
• Edema, hypertension, cardiac symptoms, jaundice
• Mental status: affect, mood, behavioral changes, depression
• Hypercalcemia
Teach patient/family:
• To avoid sunlight or use sunscreen; photosensitivity can occur
• All aspects of drug usage, including cushingoid symptoms
• To report breast lumps, vaginal bleeding, edema, jaundice, dark urine, clay colored stools, dyspnea, headache, blurred vision, abdominal pain, numbness or stiffness in legs, chest pain; male to report impotence or gynecomastia
• To report suspected pregnancy
Lab test interferences:
Increase: Alk phosphatase, nitrogen (urine), pregnanediol, amino acids
Decrease: GTT, HDL

---

medrysone
(med-rye-sone)
HMS Liquifilm Ophthalmic
Func. class.: Ophthalmic antiinflammatory

Action: Decreases inflammation, resulting in decreases in pain, photophobia, hyperemia, cellular infiltration
Uses: Inflammation of eye, lids, conjunctiva, cornea, uveitis, iridocyclitis, allergic condition, burns, foreign bodies
Dosage and routes:
• *Adult and child:* Instill 1-2 gtts into conjunctival sac q1h × 2 days if needed then bid-qid
Available forms include: Susp 1%

Side effects/adverse reactions:
EENT: Increased intraocular pressure, poor corneal wound healing, increased possibility of corneal infections, glaucoma exacerbation, *optic nerve damage,* decreased acuity, visual field
Contraindications: Hypersensitivity, acute superficial herpes simplex, fungal/viral diseases of the eye or conjunctiva, active diabetes mellitus, ocular TB, infections of the eye
Precautions: Corneal abrasions, glaucoma
Interactions/incompatibilities:
None known
NURSING CONSIDERATIONS
Evaluate:
• Allergic reactions: redness, itching, swelling, lacrimation
• Therapeutic response: absence of swelling, redness, exudate
Administer:
• After shaking
Perform/provide:
• Storage in tight, light-resistant container
Teach patient/family:
• Instillation method: pressure on lacrimal sac for 1 min
• Not to share eye medications with others

M

---

mefenamic acid
(me-fe-nam'-ik)
Ponstan, Ponstel
Func. class.: Nonsteroidal
Chem. class.: Anthranilic acid derivative

Action: Inhibits prostaglandin synthesis by decreasing an enzyme needed for biosynthesis; possesses analgesic, antiinflammatory, antipyretic properties
Uses: Mild to moderate pain, osteoarthritis, rheumatoid arthritis

---

italics = common side effects   **bold italic** = life threatening reactions

Dosage and routes:
• *Adult and child >14 yr:* PO 500 mg, then 250 mg q4h, use not to exceed 1 wk
Available forms include: Caps 250 mg
Side effects/adverse reactions:
GI: Nausea, anorexia, vomiting, diarrhea, jaundice, *cholestatic hepatitis,* constipation, flatulence, cramps, dry mouth, peptic ulcer
CNS: Dizziness, drowsiness, fatigue, tremors, confusion, insomnia, anxiety, depression
CV: Tachycardia, peripheral edema, palpitations, dysrhythmias
INTEG: Purpura, rash, pruritus, sweating
GU: Nephrotoxicity: dysuria, hematuria, oliguria, azotemia
HEMA: Blood dyscrasias
EENT: Tinnitus, hearing loss, blurred vision
Contraindications: Hypersensitivity, asthma, severe renal disease, severe hepatic disease
Precautions: Pregnancy, lactation, children, bleeding disorders, GI disorders, cardiac disorders, hypersensitivity to other antiinflammatory agents
Pharmacokinetics:
PO: Peak 2 hr, half-life 3-3½ hr; metabolized in liver, excreted in urine (metabolites), excreted in breast milk
Interactions/incompatibilities:
• May increase action of coumarin, phenytoin, sulfonamides when used with this drug
NURSING CONSIDERATIONS
Assess:
• Renal, liver, blood studies: BUN, creatinine, AST, ALT, Hgb before treatment, periodically thereafter
• Audiometric, ophthalmic exam before, during, after treatment
Administer:
• With food to decrease GI symptoms; best to take on empty stomach to facilitate absorption
Perform/provide:
• Storage at room temperature
Evaluate:
• Therapeutic response: decreased pain, stiffness, swelling in joints, ability to move more easily
• For eye, ear problems: blurred vision, tinnitus (may indicate toxicity)
Teach patient/family:
• To report blurred vision, or ringing, roaring in ears (may indicate toxicity)
• To avoid driving or other hazardous activities if dizziness or drowsiness occurs
• To report change in urine pattern, weight increase, edema, pain increase in joints, fever, blood in urine (indicates nephrotoxicity)
• That therapeutic effects may take up to 1 mo

---

megestrol acetate

(me-jess′trole)
Megace, Pallace
Func. class.: Antineoplastic
Chem. class.: Hormone, progestin

Action: Affects endometrium by antiluteinizing effect; this is thought to bring about cell death
Uses: Breast, endometrial cancer
Dosage and routes:
• *Adult:* PO 40-320 mg/day in divided doses
Available forms include: Tabs 20, 40 mg
Side effects/adverse reactions:
GI: Nausea, vomiting, anorexia, diarrhea, abdominal cramps
GU: Gynecomastia, fluid retention, hypercalcemia
INTEG: Alopecia, rash, pruritus, purpura, itching
CNS: Mood swings

Contraindications: Hypersensitivity, pregnancy

Pharmacokinetics:
PO: Duration 24 hr, half-life 5 min, metabolized in liver, excreted in feces, breast milk

Interactions/incompatibilities: None known

NURSING CONSIDERATIONS

Assess:
• Pulmonary function tests, chest x-ray films before, during therapy; chest film should be obtained q2wk during treatment
• I&O ratio
• Serum Ca

Administer:
• Antacid before oral agent, give drug after evening meal, before bedtime
• Antiemetic 30-60 min before giving drug to prevent vomiting
• Antispasmodic
• Diuretics for increased fluids

Perform/provide:
• Deep breathing exercises with patient tid-qid; place in semi-Fowler's position
• Liquid diet, including cola, Jello; dry toast or crackers may be added if patient is not nauseated or vomiting
• Increase fluid intake to 2-3 L/day to prevent dehydration
• Nutritious diet with iron, vitamin supplements as ordered
• Increased fluid intake to 2000 ml/day if not contraindicated
• Limitation of calcium (dairy products)
• Check VS q4h
• Storage in tight container at room temperature

Evaluate:
• Dyspnea, rales, unproductive cough, chest pain, tachypnea, fatigue, increased pulse, pallor, lethargy
• Food preferences; list likes, dislikes
• Effects of alopecia on body image; discuss feelings about body changes
• Edema in feet, joints, hands, ankles; oliguria
• Symptoms indicating severe allergic reaction: rash, pruritus, urticaria, purpuric skin lesions, itching, flushing
• Frequency of stools, characteristics: cramping, acidosis, signs of dehydration (rapid respirations, poor skin turgor, decreased urine output, dry skin, restlessness, weakness)
• Mood swings
• Anorexia, nausea, vomiting, constipation, weakness, loss of muscle tone

Teach patient/family:
• To report any complaints or side effects to nurse or physician
• That gynecomastia can occur; reversible after discontinuing treatment

Lab test interferences:
Increase: Alk phosphatase, urinary nitrogen, urinary pregnanediol, plasma amino acids
False positive: Urine glucose
Decrease: HDL, glucose tolerance test

---

melphalan

(mel'fa-lan)
Alkeran

Func. class.: Antineoplastic alkylating agent
Chem. class.: Nitrogen mustard

Action: Alkylates DNA, RNA; inhibits enzymes that allow synthesis of amino acids in proteins; also responsible for cross-linking DNA strands

Uses: Multiple myeloma, breast cancer, reticulum cell sarcoma, testicular seminoma, malignant mel-

---

anoma, advanced ovarian cancer

Dosage and routes:

• *Adult:* PO 6 mg qd × 2-3 wk, stop drug for 4 wk or until WBC level begins to rise; do not administer if WBC <3000/mm³ or platelets <100,000/mm³; may be given 0.15 mg/kg/day × 7 days; wait until platelets and WBCs rise, then 0.05 mg/kg/day

Available forms include: Tabs 2 mg

Side effects/adverse reactions:

*HEMA: **Thrombocytopenia, neutropenia,** anemia*

GI: Nausea, vomiting, stomatitis

GU: Amenorrhea, hyperuricemia

INTEG: Rash, urticaria

*RESP: **Fibrosis, dysplasia***

Contraindications: Lactation, pregnancy (D)

Precautions: Radiation therapy, bone marrow depression

Pharmacokinetics:

Metabolized in liver, excreted in urine, half-life 1½ hr

Interactions/incompatibilities:

• Increased toxicity: antineoplastics, radiation

NURSING CONSIDERATIONS

Assess:

• CBC, differential, platelet count weekly; withhold drug if WBC is <4000 or platelet count is <75,000; notify physician of results

• Renal function studies: BUN, serum uric acid, urine CrCl before, during therapy

• I&O ratio; report fall in urine output of 30 ml/hr

• Monitor temperature q4h (may indicate beginning infection)

• Liver function tests before, during therapy (bilirubin, AST, ALT, LDH) as needed or monthly

Administer:

• Medications by oral route if possible; avoid IM, SC, IV routes to prevent infections

• Antiemetic 30-60 min before giving drug to prevent vomiting

• Antibiotics for prophylaxis of infection

• Slow IV infusion using 21-, 23-, 25-gauge needle

• Topical or systemic analgesics for pain

• Local or systemic drugs for infection

Perform/provide:

• Storage in tight, light-resistant container

• Strict medical asepsis, protective isolation if WBC levels are low

• Special skin care

• Liquid diet, including cola, Jello; dry toast or crackers may be added if patient is not nauseated or vomiting

• Increase fluid intake to 2-3 L/day to prevent urate deposits, calculi formation

• Diet low in purines: organ meats (kidney, liver), dried beans, peas to maintain alkaline urine

• Rinsing of mouth tid-qid with water, hydrogen peroxide; brushing of teeth bid-tid with soft brush or cotton tipped applicators for stomatitis; use unwaxed dental floss

• Warm compresses at injection site for inflammation

Evaluate:

• Bleeding: hematuria, guaiac, bruising or petechiae, mucosa or orifices q8hr

• Food preferences; list likes, dislikes

• Yellowing of skin, sclera, dark urine, clay-colored stools, itchy skin, abdominal pain, fever, diarrhea

• Effects of alopecia on body image; discuss feelings about body changes

• Inflammation of mucosa, breaks in skin

• Buccal cavity q8h for dryness, sores, ulceration, white patches, oral pain, bleeding, dysphagia

• Local irritation, pain, burning, discoloration at injection site

• Symptoms indicating severe allergic reaction: rash, pruritus, urticaria, purpuric skin lesions, itching, flushing

Teach patient/family:

• Of protective isolation precautions

• To report any complaints or side effects to nurse or physician

• That sterility, amenorrhea can occur; reversible after discontinuing treatment

• That hair may be lost during treatment; a wig or hairpiece may make patient feel better; new hair may be different in color, texture

• To avoid foods with citric acid, hot or rough texture

• To report any bleeding, white spots, or ulcerations in mouth to physician; tell patient to examine mouth qd

---

menadione/menadiol sodium diphosphate (vitamin K₃)

(men-a-dye'one)
Synkavite,* Synkayvite
Func. class.: Vitamin, fat soluble

Action: Needed for adequate blood clotting (factors II, VII, IX, X)

Uses: Vitamin K malabsorption, hypoprothrombinemia

Dosage and routes:

• *Adult:* PO 2-10 mg (menadione)

• *Adult:* PO/IM 5-15 mg (menadiol sodium diphosphate)

Available forms include: Tabs 5 mg; inj 5, 10, 37.5 mg/ml

Side effects/adverse reactions:

CNS: Headache, *brain damage* (large doses)

GI: Nausea, decreased liver function tests

HEMA: Hemolytic anemia, hemoglobinuria, hyperbilirubinemia

INTEG: Rash, urticaria

Contraindications: Hypersensitivity, severe hepatic disease, last few weeks of pregnancy, neonates

Pharmacokinetics: Metabolized, crosses placenta

Interactions/incompatibilities:

• Decreased action of this drug: oral antibiotics, cholestyramine, mineral oil

• Decreased action of: oral anticoagulants

NURSING CONSIDERATIONS

Assess:

• Pro-time during treatment (2 sec deviation from control time, bleeding time, and clotting time)

Administer:

• Deep IM, IV slowly over 7 min

Evaluate:

• Therapeutic response: decreased bleeding tendencies, decreased pro-time, decreased clotting time

• Nutritional status: liver (beef), spinach, tomatoes, coffee, asparagus, broccoli, cabbage, lettuce, greens

Teach patient/family:

• Not to take other supplements, unless directed by physician

• Necessary foods to be included in diet

• Avoid use of mineral oil

---

menotropin

(men-oh-troe'pin)
Pergonal
Func. class.: Gonadotropin
Chem. class.: Exogenous gonadotropin

Action: In women, increases follicular growth, maturation; in men, when given with HCG, stimulates spermatogenesis

Uses: Infertility, anovulation

Dosage and routes:

Infertility

• *Adult (men):* IM 1 amp 3 × wk

with HCG 2000 U 2 × wk × 4 mo

• *Adult (women):* IM 75 IU of FSH, LH qd × 9-12 days, then 10,000 U HCG 1 day after these drugs; repeat × 2 menstrual cycles, then increase to 150 IU of FSH, LH qd × 9-12 days, then 10,000 U HCG 1 day after these drugs × 2 menstrual cycles

Anovulation

• *Adult (women):* IM 75 IU FSH, LH qd × 9-12 days, then 10,000 U HCG 1 day after last dose of these drugs; repeat × 1-3 menstrual cycles

Available forms include: Powder for inj 17 IU/amp

Side effects/adverse reactions:

CNS: Fever

CV: Hypovolemia

GI:Nausea, vomiting, diarrhea, anorexia

GU: Ovarian enlargement, abdominal distention/pain, multiple births, ovarian hyperstimulation: sudden ovarian enlargement, ascites with or without pain, pleural effusion

HEMA: Hemoperitoneum

Contraindications: Pregnancy, primary anovulation, thyroid/adrenal dysfunction, organic intracranial lesion, ovarian cysts, primary testicular failure

Pharmacokinetics: None known

Interactions/incompatibilities: None known

NURSING CONSIDERATIONS

Assess:

• Weight qod; notify physician if weight gain increases rapidly

• Estrogen excretion level; if >100 μg/24 hr, drug is withheld, hyperstimulation syndrome may occur

• I&O ratio; be alert for decreasing urinary output

Administer:

• After reconstituting with 1-2 ml

sterile saline injection; use immediately

Evaluate:

• Ovarian enlargement, abdominal distention/pain; report symptoms immediately

Teach patient/family:

• That multiple births are possible, pregnancy usually occurs in 4-6 wk after start of treatment

• To keep appointment during treatment qod × 2 wk

• That daily intercourse is necessary from day preceding administration of gonadotropin until ovulation occurs

---

mepenzolate bromide

(me-pen′zoe′late)

Cantil

Func. class.: Gastrointestinal anticholinergic

Chem. class.: Synthetic quaternary ammonium antimuscarinic

Action: Inhibits muscarinic actions of acetylcholine at postganglionic parasympathetic neuroeffector sites

Uses: Treatment of peptic ulcer disease, irritable bowel syndrome in combination with other drugs; for other GI disorders

Dosage and routes:

• *Adult:* PO 25-50 mg qid with meals, hs, titrate to patient response

Available forms include: Tabs 25 mg

Side effects/adverse reactions:

CNS: Confusion, stimulation in elderly, headache, insomnia, dizziness, drowsiness, anxiety, weakness, hallucination

GI: Dry mouth, constipation, paralytic ileus, heartburn, nausea, vomiting, dysphagia, absence of taste

GU: Hesitancy, retention, impotence

CV: Palpitations, tachycardia
EENT: Blurred vision, photophobia, mydriasis, cycloplegia, increased ocular tension
INTEG: Urticaria, rash, pruritus, anhidrosis, fever, allergic reactions
Contraindications: Hypersensitivity to anticholinergics, narrow-angle glaucoma, GI obstruction, myasthenia gravis, paralytic ileus, GI atony, toxic megacolon
Precautions: Hyperthyroidism, coronary artery disease, dysrhythmias, CHF, ulcerative colitis, hypertension, hiatal hernia, hepatic disease, renal disease
Pharmacokinetics:
PO: Onset 1 hr, duration 3-4 hr; metabolized by liver, excreted in urine, half-life (unchanged)
Interactions/incompatibilities:
• Increased anticholinergic effect: amantadine, tricyclic antidepressants, MAOIs
• Increased effect of: nitrofurantoin
• Decreased effect of: phenothiazines, levodopa
NURSING CONSIDERATIONS
Assess:
• VS, cardiac status: checking for dysrhythmias, increased rate, palpitations
• I&O ratio; check for urinary retention or hesitancy
Administer:
• ½-1 hr ac for better absorption
• Decreased dose to elderly patients; their metabolism may be slowed
• Gum, hard candy, frequent rinsing of mouth for dryness of oral cavity
Perform/provide:
• Storage in tight container protected from light
• Increased fluids, bulk, exercise to patient's lifestyle to decrease constipation
Evaluate:
• Therapeutic response: absence of

epigastric pain, bleeding, nausea, vomiting
• GI complaints: pain, bleeding (frank or occult), nausea, vomiting, anorexia
Teach patient/family:
• Avoid driving or other hazardous activities until stabilized on medication
• Avoid alcohol or other CNS depressants; will enhance sedating properties of this drug
• To avoid hot environments, stroke may occur, drug suppresses perspiration
• Use sunglasses when outside to prevent photophobia

---

meperidine HCl

(me-per'i-deen)
Demer-Idine,* Demerol

Func. class.: Narcotic analgesics
Chem. class.: Opiate, phenylpiperidine derivative

Controlled Substance Schedule II
Action: Inhibits ascending pain pathways in CNS, increases pain threshold, alters pain perception
Uses: Moderate to severe pain, preoperatively
Dosage and routes:
Pain
• *Adult:* PO/SC/IM 50-150 mg q3-4h prn
• *Child:* PO/SC/IM 1 mg/kg q4-6h prn, not to exceed 100 mg q4h
Preoperatively
• *Adult:* IM/SC 50-100 mg q30-90 min before surgery
• *Child:* IM/SC 1-2.2 mg/kg 30-90 min before surgery
Available forms include: Inj SC, IM, IV 25, 50, 75, 100 mg/ml; tabs 50, 100 mg; syr 50 mg/5 ml
Side effects/adverse reactions:
CNS: Drowsiness, dizziness, confusion, headache, sedation, euphoria

GI: Nausea, vomiting, anorexia, constipation, cramps

GU: Increased urinary output, dysuria

INTEG: Rash, urticaria, bruising, flushing, diaphoresis, pruritus

EENT: Tinnitus, blurred vision, miosis, diplopia

CV: Palpitations, bradycardia, change in B/P

*RESP: **Respiratory depression***

Contraindications: Hypersensitivity, addiction (narcotic)

Precautions: Addictive personality, pregnancy, lactation, increased intracranial pressure, MI (acute), severe heart disease, respiratory depression, hepatic disease, renal disease, child <18 yr

Pharmacokinetics:

PO: Onset 15 min, peak 1 hr, duration 2-4 hr

SC/IM: Onset 10 min, peak 1 hr, duration 2-4 hr

IV: Onset 5 min, duration 2 hr

Metabolized by liver (to active/inactive metabolites), excreted by kidneys, crosses placenta, excreted in breast milk

Interactions/incompatibilities:

• Effects may be increased with other CNS depressants: alcohol, narcotics, sedative/hypnotics, antipsychotics, skeletal muscle relaxants

NURSING CONSIDERATIONS

Assess:

• I&O ratio; check for decreasing output; may indicate urinary retention

Administer:

• With antiemetic if nausea, vomiting occur

• When pain is beginning to return; determine dosage interval by patient response

Perform/provide:

• Storage in light-resistant area at room temperature

• Assistance with ambulation

• Safety measures: siderails, night light, call bell within easy reach

Evaluate:

• Therapeutic response: decrease in pain

• CNS changes: dizziness, drowsiness, hallucinations, euphoria, LOC, pupil reaction

• Allergic reactions: rash, urticaria

• Respiratory dysfunction: respiratory depression, character, rate, rhythm; notify physician if respirations are <12/min

• Need for pain medication, physical dependence

Teach patient/family:

• To report any symptoms of CNS changes, allergic reactions

• That physical dependency may result when used for extended periods of time

• Withdrawal symptoms may occur: nausea, vomiting, cramps, fever, faintness, anorexia

Lab test interferences:

Increase: Amylase

Treatment of overdose: Narcan 0.2-0.8 IV, O_2, IV fluids, vasopressors

---

mephentermine sulfate

(me-fen′ter-meen)

Wyamine

Func. class.: Adrenergic, direct and indirect acting

Chem. class.: Substituted phenylethylamine

Action: Causes increased contractility and heart rate by acting on β-receptors in heart; also, acts on α-receptors, causing vasoconstriction in blood vessels; when larger doses are administered, causes vasodilation in renal, intracerebral, coronary dopaminergic receptors

Uses: Shock and hypotension following variety of procedures

Dosage and routes:
Hypotension
• *Adult:* IV 15-45 mg depending on procedure
Hypotension/shock
• *Adult:* IV 0.5 mg/kg
• *Child:* IV 0.4 mg/kg
Available forms include: Inj IV 15, 30 mg/ml

Side effects/adverse reactions:
CNS: Anxiety, headache, dizziness
CV: Palpitations, tachycardia, hypertension, PVCs, angina
GI: Heartburn, nausea, vomiting
MS: Muscle cramps (leg)

Contraindications: Hypersensitivity to sympathomimetics, narrowangle glaucoma

Precautions: Pregnancy, cardiac disorders, hyperthyroidism, diabetes mellitus, prostatic hypertrophy

Pharmacokinetics:
IV: Onset immediate, duration ½-1 hr; metabolized in liver, excreted in urine

Interactions/incompatibilities:
• Do not use with MAOIs or tricyclic antidepressants; hypertensive crisis may occur
• Decreased effect of this drug: methyldopa, urinary acidifiers, rauwolfia alkaloids
• Increased effect of this drug: urinary alkalizers

NURSING CONSIDERATIONS
Assess:
• I&O ratio
• ECG during administration continuously; if B/P increases, drug is decreased
• B/P, pulse q5 min after parenteral route
• CVP or PWP during infusion if possible

Administer:
• Plasma expanders for hypovolemia
• Parenteral IV dose slowly, after reconstituting with 500 ml of D_5W

Perform/provide:
• Storage of reconstituted solution if refrigerated for no longer than 24 hr
• Do not use discolored solutions

Evaluate:
• Paresthesias and coldness of extremities, peripheral blood flow may decrease
• Injection site: tissue sloughing; if this occurs, administer phentolamine mixed with NS
• Therapeutic response: increased B/P with stabilization

Teach patient/family:
• Reason for drug administration

Treatment of overdose: Administer an α-blocker, then norepinephrine for severe hypotension

---

mephenytoin

(me-fen′i-toyn)
Mesantoin

Func. class.: Anticonvulsant
Chem. class.: Hydantoin derivative

Action: Reduces electrical discharges in motor cortex, reducing seizures; increases AV conduction velocity, prolongs refractory period

Uses: Generalized tonic-clonic, complex-partial seizures

Dosage and routes:
• *Adult:* PO 50-100 mg/day, may increase by 50-100 mg q7 days, up to 200 mg tid
• *Child:* PO 50-100 mg/day or 100-450 mg/m²/day in 3 divided doses, initially; then increase 50-100 mg q7 days, up to 200 mg tid in divided doses q8h

Available forms include: Tabs 100 mg

Side effects/adverse reactions:
HEMA: Agranulocytosis, leukopenia, neutropenia, pancytopenia, eosinophilia, lymphadenopathy
CNS: Drowsiness, dizziness, fa-

---

tigue, irritability, tremors, insomnia

GI: Nausea, vomiting
INTEG: Rash, exfoliative dermatitis
EENT: Photophobia, conjunctivitis, nystagmus, diplopia
RESP: Pulmonary fibrosis

Contraindications: Hypersensitivity to hydantoins, sinus bradycardia, heart block, Adams-Stokes syndrome

Precautions: Alcoholism, hepatic disease, renal disease, blood dyscrasias, CHF, elderly, pregnancy, respiratory depression, diabetes mellitus

Pharmacokinetics:
PO: Onset 30 min, duration 24-48 hr, metabolized by liver, excreted by kidneys, half-life 144 hr

Interactions/incompatibilities:
• Decreased effects: rifampin, chronic alcohol use, barbiturates, antihistamines, antacids, other anticonvulsants antineoplastics, calcium products, folic acid, oxacillin
• Increased effects: benzodiazepines, cimetidine, salicylates, sulfonamide, pyrazolones, phenothiazines, estrogens, disulfiram, chloramphenicol, anticoagulants
• Seizures: valproic acid
• Myocardial depression: lidocaine, propanolol, sympathomimetics

NURSING CONSIDERATIONS
Assess:
• Blood studies: CBC, platelets q2 wk until stabilized, then q mo × 12, then q3 mo; discontinue drug if neutrophils are <1600/mm³
• Drug level: therapeutic level 25-40 µg/ml

Evaluate:
• Therapeutic response: decreased seizure activity
• Mental status: mood, sensorium, affect, behavioral changes; if mental status changes, notify physician
• Eye problems: need for ophthalmic examinations before, during, after treatment (slit lamp, fundoscopy, tonometry)
• Allergic reaction: red raised rash; if this occurs, drug should be discontinued
• Blood dyscrasias: fever, sore throat, bruising, rash, jaundice
• Toxicity: bone marrow depression, nausea, vomiting, ataxia, diplopia, cardiovascular collapse, Stevens-Johnson syndrome

Teach patient/family:
• All aspects of this drug: action, route, side effects

---

mephobarbital
(me-foe-bar'bi-tal)
Mebaral, Mentabal, Mephoral
Func. class.: Anticonvulsant
Chem. class.: Barbiturate

Controlled Substance Schedule IV

Action: Depresses sensory cortex, motor activity; inhibits ascending conduction in reticular formation of thalamus.

Uses: Generalized tonic-clonic, absence seizures

Dosage and routes:
• *Adult:* PO 400-600 mg/day or in divided doses
• *Child:* PO 6-12 mg/kg/day in divided doses q6-8h

Available forms include: Tabs 32, 50, 100, 200 mg

Side effects/adverse reactions:
HEMA: Thrombocytopenia, agranulocytosis, megaloblastic anemia
CNS: Dizziness, headache, hangover, stimulation, drowsiness, increased pain
GI: Nausea, vomiting, epigastric pain
INTEG: Rash, urticaria, purpara, erythema multiforme, facial edema
EENT: Tinnitus, hearing loss
CV: Hypotension

RESP: Wheezing, hyperpnea

ENDO: Hypoglycemia, hyponatremia, hypokalemia

Contraindications: Hypersensitivity to barbiturates

Precautions: Pregnancy, hepatic disease, renal disease, lactation, alcoholism, drug abuse, hyperthyroidism

Pharmacokinetics:

PO: Onset 20-60 min, duration 6-8 hr

REC: Onset slow, duration 4-6 hr Metabolized by liver, excreted by kidneys, half-life 34 hr

Interactions/incompatibilities:

• Increased effects: CNS depressants, chloramphenicol, valproic acid, disulfiram, nondepolarizing skeletal muscle relaxants, sulfonamides

• Increased orthostatic hypotension: furosemide

NURSING CONSIDERATIONS
Assess:

• Drug level

Evaluate:

• Mental status: mood, sensorium, affect, memory (long, short)

• Respiratory depression: respiration <10/min, shallow

• Blood dyscrasias: fever, sore throat, bruising, rash, jaundice

Teach patient/family:

• All aspects of drug usage: action, side effects, dose, when to notify physician

Treatment of overdose: Administer calcium gluconate IV

---

mepivacaine HCl

(meep-ee-va-kane)

Carbocaine, Cavacaine, Isocaine

Func. class.: Local anesthetic

Chem. class.: Amide

Action: Competes with calcium for sites in nerve membrane that control sodium transport across cell membrane; decreases rise of depolarization phase of action potential

Uses: Nerve block, caudal anesthesia, epidural, pain relief, paracervical block, transvaginal block or infiltration

Dosage and routes:

Varies depending on route of anesthesia

Available forms include: Inj 1%, 1.5%, 2%, 3%

Side effects/adverse reactions:

CNS: Anxiety, restlessness, *convulsions, loss of consciousness,* drowsiness, disorientation, tremors, shivering

CV: Myocardial depression, cardiac arrest, dysrhythmias, bradycardia, hypotension, hypertension, fetal bradycardia

GI: Nausea, vomiting

EENT: Blurred vision, tinnitus, pupil constriction

INTEG: Rash, urticaria, allergic reactions, edema, burning, skin discoloration at injection site, tissue necrosis

RESP: Status asthmaticus, respiratory arrest, anaphylaxis

Contraindications: Hypersensitivity, child <12 yr, elderly, severe liver disease

Precautions: Elderly, severe drug allergies

Pharmacokinetics:

Onset 15 min, duration 3 hr; metabolized by liver, excreted in urine (metabolites)

Interactions/incompatibilities:

• Dysrhythmias: epinephrine, halothane, enflurane

• Hypertension: MAOIs, tricyclic antidepressants, phenothiazines

• Decreased action of this drug: chloroprocaine

NURSING CONSIDERATIONS
Assess:

• B/P, pulse, respiration during treatment

M

• Fetal heart tones if drug is used during labor

Administer:

• Only with crash cart, resuscitative equipment nearby

• Only drugs without preservatives for epidural or caudal anesthesia

Perform/provide:

• Use of new solution, discard unused portions

Evaluate:

• Therapeutic response: anesthesia necessary for procedure

• Allergic reactions: rash, urticaria, itching

• Cardiac status: ECG for dysrhythmias, pulse, B/P during anesthesia

Treatment of overdose: Airway, O_2, vasopressor, IV fluids, anticonvulsants for seizures

---

meprobamate

(me-proe-ba'mate)

Arcoban, Equanil, Kalmm, Meditran, Meprocon, Meprotabs, Meribam, Miltown, Neo-Tran,* Novomepro,* Saronil, Tranmep

Func. class.: Antianxiety

Chem. class.: Propanediol carbamate derivative

Controlled Substance Schedule IV

Action: Blocks impulses from cortex to thalamus in CNS

Uses: Anxiety

Dosage and routes:

• *Adult:* PO 1.2-1.6 g in 2-3 divided doses, not to exceed 2.4 g/day

• *Child 6-12 yr:* PO 100-200 mg bid-tid

Available forms include: Tabs 200, 400, 600 mg; caps 400 mg sust rel caps 200, 400 mg

Side effects/adverse reactions:

HEMA: Thrombocytopenia, leukopenia, eosinophilia

CNS: Dizziness, drowsiness, headache

GI: Nausea, vomiting, anorexia, diarrhea, stomatitis

INTEG: Urticaria, pruritus, maculopapular rash

CV: Hypotension, tachycardia, palpitations

EENT: Blurred vision, tinnitus, mydriasis, slurred speech

Contraindications: Hypersensitivity, renal failure, porphyria

Precautions: Suicidal patients, severe depression, renal disease, hepatic disease, elderly

Pharmacokinetics:

PO: Onset 1 hr, metabolized by liver, excreted by kidneys, in feces, crosses placenta, breast milk, half-life 6-16 hr

Interactions/incompatibilities:

• Increased effects of this drug; CNS depressants, alcohol, tricyclic antidepressants

NURSING CONSIDERATIONS

Assess:

• B/P (lying, standing), pulse; if systolic B/P drops 20 mm Hg, hold drug, notify physician; respirations q5-15 min if given IV

• Blood studies: CBC during long-term therapy, blood dyscrasias have occurred rarely

• Hepatic studies: AST, ALT, bilirubin, creatinine, LDH, alk phosphatase

Administer:

• With food or milk for GI symptoms

• Crushed if patient is unable to swallow medication whole

• Sugarless gum, hard candy, frequent sips of water for dry mouth

Perform/provide

• Assistance with ambulation during beginning therapy since drowsiness/dizziness occurs

• Safety measures, including siderails

• Check to see PO medication has been swallowed
Evaluate:
• Therapeutic response: decreased anxiety, restlessness, insomnia
• Mental status: mood, sensorium, affect, sleeping pattern, drowsiness, dizziness
• Physical dependency, withdrawal symptoms: headache, nausea, vomiting, muscle pain, weakness after long-term use
• Suicidal tendences
Teach patient/family:
• That drug may be taken with food
• Not to be used for everyday stress or used longer than 4 months, unless directed by physician
• Avoid OTC preparations (alcohol, cold, hay fever) unless approved by physician
• To avoid driving, activities that require alertness, since drowsiness may occur
• To avoid alcohol ingestion or other psychotropic medications, unless prescribed by physician
• Not to discontinue medication abruptly after long-term use
• To rise slowly or fainting may occur
• That drowsiness might worsen at beginning of treatment
Lab test interferences:
False increase: 17-OHCS
Treatment of overdose: Lavage, VS, supportive care

merbromin
Mercurochrome
Func. class.: Disinfectant
Chem. class.: Polychlorinated phenol derivative

Action: Inhibits growth of gram-positive bacteria
Uses: Surgical scrub, bacteriostatic skin cleanser, gram-positive infec-

tion when other treatment has been ineffective
Dosage and routes:
• *Adult and child:* Use prn
Available forms include: Top soap, emul
Side effects/adverse reactions:
INTEG: Irritation, dryness, dermatitis, scaling
GI: Nausea, vomiting, diarrhea
CNS: Delirium, convulsions, restlessness, headache, confusion, tremors, dizziness
Contraindications: Hypersensitivity, occlusive dressings, infants, burns
Interactions/incompatibilities:
None known
NURSING CONSIDERATIONS
Administer:
• To body areas only; do not apply to face, lips, mouth, eyes, mucous membrane, anus, meatus
• Only to adults; repeated use may lead to systemic absorption
Evaluate:
• Area of the body involved: irritation, rash, breaks, dryness, scales
Teach patient/family:
• To report itching, irritation, dizziness, headache, confusion, discontinue drug immediately
Treatment of ingestion: Gastric lavage, administer vegetable oil, saline laxative, supportive treatment

mercaptopurine (6-MP)
(mer-kap-toe-pyoor'een)
Purinethol
Func. class.: Antineoplastic-antimetabolite
Chem. class.: Purine analog

Action: Inhibits purine metabolism by blocking inosinic acid conversion to adenine, which is responsible for DNA, RNA synthesis
Uses: Chronic myelocytic leuke-

mia, acute lymphoblastic leukemia in children, acute myelogenous leukemia

Dosage and routes:
• *Adult and child:* PO 2.5 mg/kg/day, not to exceed 5 mg/kg/day; maintenance 1.5-2.5 mg/kg/day
• *Child:* 70 mg/m²/day

Available forms include: Tabs 50 mg

Side effects/adverse reactions:
CNS: Fever, headache, weakness
HEMA: **Thrombocytopenia, leukopenia, myelosuppression, anemia**
GI: Nausea, vomiting, anorexia, diarrhea, stomatitis, **hepatotoxicity** (with high doses), jaundice, gastritis
GU: **Renal failure,** hyperuricemia, oliguria, crystalluria, **hematuria**
INTEG: Rash, alopecia (rare), dry skin, urticaria

Contraindications: Patients with prior drug resistance, leukopenia (<2500/mm³), thrombocytopenia (<100,000/mm³), anemia, pregnancy

Precautions: Renal disease

Pharmacokinetics: Incompletely absorbed when taken orally, metabolized in liver, excreted in urine

Interactions/incompatibilities:
• Increased toxicity: radiation or other antineoplastics
• Increased bone marrow depression: allopurinol
• Reversal of neuromuscular blockade: nondepolarizing muscle relaxants

NURSING CONSIDERATIONS
Assess:
• CBC, differential, platelet count weekly; withhold drug if WBC is <3500 or platelet count is <100,000; notify physician of these results; drug should be discontinued
• Renal function studies: BUN, serum uric acid, urine CrCl, electrolytes before, during therapy

• I&O ratio; report fall in urine output to <30 ml/hr
• Monitor temperature q4h; fever may indicate beginning infection
• Liver function tests before, during therapy: bilirubin, alk phosphatase, AST, ALT, q wk during beginning therapy

Administer:
• Medications by oral route if possible; avoid IM, SC, IV routes to prevent infections
• Antacid before oral agent; give drug after evening meal before bedtime
• Antiemetic 30-60 min before giving drug to prevent vomiting
• Allopurinol or sodium bicarbonate to maintain uric acid levels, alkalinization of urine
• Antibiotics for prophylaxis of infection
• Topical or systemic analgesics for pain
• Transfusion for anemia

Perform/provide:
• Strict medical asepsis, protective isolation if WBC levels are low
• Liquid diet: carbonated beverage, Jello; dry toast, crackers may be added when patient is not nauseated or vomiting
• Increase fluid intake to 2-3 L/day to prevent urate deposits, calculi formation, unless contraindicated
• Diet low in purines: absence of organ meats (kidney, liver), dried beans, peas to maintain alkaline urine
• Rinsing of mouth tid-qid with water, hydrogen peroxide; brushing of teeth bid-tid with soft brush or cotton-tipped applicators for stomatitis; use unwaxed dental floss
• Nutritious diet with iron, vitamin supplements as ordered
• Storage in tightly closed container in cool environment

Evaluate:
• Bleeding: hematuria, guaiac,

bruising, petechiae, mucosa or orifices q8h

• Food preferences; list likes, dislikes

• Effects of alopecia on body image; discuss feelings about body changes

• Inflammation of mucosa, breaks in skin

• Buccal cavity q8h for dryness, sores, ulceration, white patches, oral pain, bleeding, dysphagia

• Symptoms indicating severe allergic reaction: rash, urticaria, itching, flushing

Teach patient/family:

• To report any complaints, side effects to nurse or physician

• That hair may be lost during treatment and wig or hairpiece may make patient feel better; tell patient that new hair may be different in color, texture (alopecia is rare)

• To avoid foods with citric acid, hot or rough texture if stomatitis is present

• To report stomatitis: any bleeding, white spots, ulcerations in mouth; tell patient to examine mouth qd, report symptoms

• Contraceptive measures are recommended during therapy

• To drink 10-12 glasses of fluid/day

• Notify physician of fever, chills, sore throat, nausea, vomiting, anorexia, diarrhea, bleeding, bruising, which may indicate blood dyscrasias

---

mesoridazine besylate

(mez-oh-rid′a-zeen)
Serentil

Func. class.: Antipsychotic/neuroleptic
Chem. class.: Phenothiazine, piperidine

Action: Depresses cerebral cortex, hypothalamus, limbic system, which control activity, aggression; blocks neurotransmission produced by dopamine at synapse; exhibits strong α-adrenergic, anticholinergic blocking action; mechanism for antipsychotic effects is unclear

Uses: Psychotic disorders, schizophrenia, anxiety, alcoholism, behavioral problems in mental deficiency, chronic brain syndrome

Dosage and routes:
Schizophrenia
• *Adult:* PO 50 mg tid, optimum dose 100-400 mg/day; IM 25 mg may repeat ½-1 hr; dosage range 25-200 mg/day
Behavior problems
• *Adult:* PO 25 mg tid; optimum dose 75-300 mg/day;
Alcoholism
• *Adult:* PO 25 mg bid; optimum dose 50-200 mg/day
Psychoneurosis
• *Adult:* PO 10 mg tid; optimum dose 30-150 mg/day
Available forms include: Tabs 10, 25, 50, 100 mg; conc 25 mg/ml; inj IM 25 mg/ml

Side effects/adverse reactions:
RESP: **Laryngospasm,** dyspnea, **respiratory depression**
CNS: Extrapyramidal symptoms: pseudoparkinsonism, akathisia, dystonia, tardive dyskinesia, drowsiness, headache,
HEMA: Anemia, leukopenia, leukocytosis, **agranulocytosis**
INTEG: Rash, photosensitivity, dermatitis
EENT: Blurred vision, glaucoma
GI: Dry mouth, nausea, vomiting, anorexia, constipation, diarrhea, jaundice, weight gain
GU: Urinary retention, urinary frequency, enuresis, impotence, amenorrhea, gynecomastia
CV: Orthostatic hypotension, hypertension, **cardiac arrest,** ECG changes, **tachycardia**

M

italics = common side effects   **bold italic** = life threatening reactions

Contraindications: Hypersensitivity, circulatory collapse, liver damage, cerebral arteriosclerosis, coronary disease, severe hypertension/hypotension, blood dyscrasias, coma, brain damage, bone marrow depression

Precautions: Pregnancy, lactation, seizure disorders, hypertension, hepatic disease, cardiac disease

Pharmacokinetics:

PO: Onset erratic, peak 2 hr, duration 4-6 hr

IM: Onset 15-30 min, peak 30 min, duration 6-8 hr

Metabolized by liver, excreted in urine, crosses placenta, enters breast milk

Interactions/incompatibilities:

• Oversedation: other CNS depressants, alcohol, barbiturate anesthetics

• Toxicity: epinephrine

• Decreased absorption: aluminum hydroxide or magnesium hydroxide antacids

• Decreased effects of: lithium, levodopa

• Increased effects of both drugs: β-adrenergic blockers, alcohol

• Increased anticholinergic effects: anticholinergics

NURSING CONSIDERATIONS

Assess:

• Swallowing of PO medication; check for hoarding or giving of medication to other patients

• I&O ratio; palpate bladder if low urinary output occurs

• Bilirubin, CBC, liver function studies monthly

• Urinalysis is recommended before, during prolonged therapy

Administer:

• Antiparkinsonian agent, after securing order from physician to be used if EPS occur

• Concentrate mixed in distilled water, orange, grape juice; do not prepare, store bulk dilutions

• IM injection into large muscle mass

Perform/provide:

• Decreased noise input by dimming lights, avoiding loud noises

• Supervised ambulation until stabilized on medication; do not involve in strenuous exercise program because fainting is possible; patient should not stand still for long periods of time

• Increased fluids to prevent constipation

• Sips of water, candy, gum for dry mouth

• Storage in tight, light-resistant container

Evaluate:

• Therapeutic response: decrease in emotional excitement, hallucinations, delusions, paranoia, and reorganization of patterns of thought, speech

• Affect, orientation, LOC, reflexes, gait, coordination, sleep pattern disturbances

• B/P standing and lying; also include pulse and respirations; take these q4h during initial treatment; establish baseline before starting treatment; report drops of 30 mm Hg

• Dizziness, faintness, palpitations, tachycardia on rising

• EPS including akathisia (inability to sit still, no pattern to movements), tardive dyskinesia (bizarre movements of jaw, mouth, tongue, extremities), pseudoparkinsonism (rigidity, tremors, pill rolling, shuffling gait)

• Skin turgor daily

• Constipation, urinary retention daily; if these occur increase bulk, water in diet

Teach patient/family:

• That orthostatic hypotension occurs frequently, and to rise from sitting or lying position gradually

• To remain lying down after IM

injection for at least 30 min

• To avoid hot tubs, hot showers, or tub baths since hypotension may occur

• To avoid abrupt withdrawal of this drug or EPS may result; drugs should be withdrawn slowly

• To avoid OTC preparations (cough, hayfever, cold) unless approved by physician since serious drug interactions may occur; avoid use with alcohol or CNS depressants, increased drowsiness may occur

• To use sunscreen during sun exposure to prevent burns

• Regarding compliance with drug regimen

• About necessity for meticulous oral hygiene since oral candidiasis may occur

• To report sore throat, malaise, fever, bleeding, mouth sores; if these occur, a CBC should be drawn and drug discontinued

• In hot weather heat stroke may occur; take extra precautions to stay cool

Lab test interferences:

Increase: Liver function tests, cardiac enzymes, cholesterol, blood glucose, prolactin, bilirubin, PBI, cholinesterase, ^{131}I

Decrease: Hormones (blood, urine)

False positive: Pregnancy tests, PKU

False negative: Urinary steroids, 17-OHCS

Treatment of overdose: Lavage if orally injested, provide an airway; *do not induce vomiting*

---

metaproterenol sulfate

(met-a-proe-ter′e-nole)
Alupent, Metaprel
Func. class.: Adrenergic

Action: Relaxes bronchial smooth

muscle by direct action on β-adrenergic receptors

Uses: Bronchial asthma, bronchospasm

Dosage and routes:

• *Adult and child>12 yr:* INH 2-3 puffs, may repeat q 3-4h, not to exceed 12 puffs/day

Asthma/bronchospasm

• *Adult:* PO 20 mg q6-8h

• *Child >9 yr or >27 kg:* PO 20 mg q6-8h or 0.4-0.9 mg/kg/dose tid

• *Child 6-9 yr or <27 kg:* PO 10 mg q6-8h or 0.4-0.9 mg/kg/dose tid

Available forms include: Tabs 10, 20 mg; aerosol 0.65 mg/dose; syrup 10 mg/5 ml; sol nebulizer 0.6%, 5%

Side effects/adverse reactions:

CNS: Tremors, anxiety, insomnia, headache, dizziness, stimulation

CV: Palpitations, tachycardia, hypertension, *cardiac arrest*

GI: Nausea

Contraindications: Hypersensitivity to sympathomimetics, narrowangle glaucoma

Precautions: Pregnancy, cardiac disorders, hyperthyroidism, diabetes mellitus, prostatic hypertrophy

Pharmacokinetics:

PO: Onset 2-15 min, peak 1 hr, duration 4 hr, excreted in urine as metabolites

Interactions/incompatibilities:

• Increased effects of both drugs: other sympathomimetics

• Decreased action: β-blockers

NURSING CONSIDERATIONS

Assess:

• Respiratory function: vital capacity, forced expiratory volume, ABGs

Administer:

• 2 hr before hs to avoid sleeplessness

Perform/provide:
• Storage at room temperature, do not use discolored solutions
Evaluate:
• Therapeutic response: absence of dyspnea, wheezing
• Tolerance over long-term therapy, dose may need to be increased or changed
Teach patient/family:
• Not to use OTC medications, extra stimulation may occur
• Use of inhaler, review package insert with patient
• To avoid getting aerosol in eyes
• To wash inhaler in warm water and dry qd
• On all aspects of drug; avoid smoking, smoke-filled rooms, persons with respiratory infections

---

metaraminol bitartrate

(met-a-ram′i-nole)
Aramine

Func. class.: Adrenergic
Chem. class.: Substituted β-phenylethylamine

Action: Both direct and indirect effects on sympathetic terminals; inhibits GI, smooth muscle and vascular smooth muscle supplying skeletal muscle; cardiac excitatory effects; increases heart rate and force of heart muscle contraction
Uses: Hypotension, shock
Dosage and routes:
Hypotension
• *Adult:* IM/SC 2-10 mg
• *Child:* IV 0.01 mg/kg; IV INF 1 mg/25 ml D_5W, titrated to B/P
Shock
• *Adult:* IV 0.5-5 mg, then IV infusion of 15-100 mg/500 ml sol
• *Child:* IV 0.01 mg/kg; IV INF 1 mg/25 ml D_5W, titrated to B/P
Available forms include: Inj IV, SC, IM 10 mg/ml 1%

Side effects/adverse reactions:
CNS: Headache
CV: Palpitations, tachycardia, hypotension, ectopic beats, angina
GI: Nausea, vomiting
INTEG: Necrosis, tissue sloughing with extravasation, *gangrene*
Contraindications: Hypersensitivity, ventricular fibrillation, tachydysrhythmias, pheochromocytoma
Precautions: Pregnancy, lactation, arterial embolism, peripheral vascular disease
Pharmacokinetics:
IV: Onset 1-2 min
IM: Onset 10 min
Interactions/incompatibilities:
• Do not use within 2 wk of MAOIs, or hypertensive crisis may result
• Dysrhythmias: general anesthetics
• Decreased action of this drug: other β-blockers
• Increased B/P: oxytocics
• Increased pressor effect: tricyclic antidepressant, MAOIs
• Incompatible with alkaline solutions: Na, HCO_3

NURSING CONSIDERATIONS
Assess:
• I&O ratio
• ECG during administration continuously, if B/P increases, drug is decreased
• B/P and pulse q5 min after parenteral route
• CVP or PWP during infusion if possible
Administer:
• Plasma expanders for hypovolemia
• Parenteral IV dose slowly, after reconstituting with 500 ml of D_5W or NS
Perform/provide:
• Storage of reconstituted solution if refrigerated for no longer than 24 hr

---

• Do not use discolored solutions
Evaluate:
• For paresthesias and coldness of extremities, peripheral blood flow may decrease
• Injection site: tissue sloughing; if this occurs, administer phentolamine mixed with NS
• Therapeutic response: increased B/P with stabilization
Teach patient/family:
• Reason for drug administration
Treatment of overdose: Administer an α-blocker, then norepinephrine for severe hypotension

---

methadone HCl

(meth′a-done)
Dolophine, Methadone HCl Oral Solution

Func. class.: Narcotic analgesics
Chem. class.: Opiate, synthetic diphenylheptane derivative

Controlled Substance Schedule II
Action: Inhibits ascending pain pathways in CNS, increases pain threshold, alters pain perception
Uses: Severe pain, narcotic withdrawal
Dosage and routes:
Pain
• *Adult:* PO/SC/IM 2.5-10 mg q4-12h prn
Narcotic withdrawal
• *Adult:* PO 15-40 mg/day individualized initially, then 20-120 mg/day titrated to patient response
Available forms include: Inj SC, IM 10 mg/ml; tabs 5, 10 mg; oral sol 5, 10 mg/5 ml; dispersible tabs 40 mg
Side effects/adverse reactions:
CNS: Drowsiness, dizziness, confusion, headache, sedation, euphoria
GI: Nausea, vomiting, anorexia, constipation, cramps

GU: Increased urinary output, dysuria
INTEG: Rash, urticaria, bruising, flushing, diaphoresis, pruritus
EENT: Tinnitus, blurred vision, miosis, diplopia
CV: Palpitations, bradycardia, change in B/P
RESP: Respiratory depression
Contraindications: Hypersensitivity, addiction (narcotic)
Precautions: Addictive personality, pregnancy, lactation, increased intracranial pressure, MI (acute), severe heart disease, respiratory depression, hepatic disease, renal disease, child <18 yr
Pharmacokinetics:
PO: Onset 30-60 min, duration 6-8 hr
SC/IM: Onset 10-20 min, peak 1 hr, duration 6-8 hr, cumulative 22-48 hr
Metabolized by liver, excreted by kidneys, crosses placenta, excreted in breast milk, half-life 15-25 hr
Interactions/incompatibilities:
• Effects may be increased with other CNS depressants: alcohol, narcotics, sedative/hypnotics, antipsychotics, skeletal muscle relaxants
NURSING CONSIDERATIONS
Assess:
• I&O ratio; check for decreasing output; may indicate urinary retention
Administer:
• With antiemetic if nausea, vomiting occur
• When pain is beginning to return; determine dosage interval by patient response
Perform/provide:
• Storage in light-resistant area at room temperature
• Assistance with ambulation
• Safety measures: siderails, night light, call bell within easy reach

M

Evaluate:

• Therapeutic response: decrease in pain

• CNS changes: dizziness, drowsiness, hallucinations, euphoria, LOC, pupil reaction

• Allergic reactions: rash, urticaria

• Respiratory dysfunction: respiratory depression, character, rate, rhythm; notify physician if respirations are <12/min

• Need for pain medication, physical dependence

Teach patient/family:

• To report any symptoms of CNS changes, allergic reactions

• That physical dependency may result when used for extended periods of time

• Withdrawal symptoms may occur: nausea, vomiting, cramps, fever, faintness, anorexia

Lab test interferences:

Increase: Amylase

Treatment of overdose: Narcan 0.2-0.8 IV, O_2, IV fluids, vasopressors

---

methamphetamine HCl

(meth-am-fet′a-meen)

Mazanor, Sanorex

Func. class.: Cerebral stimulants
Chem. class.: Amphetamine

Controlled Substance Schedule II

Action: Increases release of norepinephrine and dopamine in cerebral cortex to reticular activating system

Uses: Exogenous obesity, minimal brain dysfunction

Dosage and routes:

Minimal brain dysfunction

• *Child >6 yr:* 2.5-5 mg qd or bid increasing by 5 mg/wk

Obesity

• *Adult:* PO 2.5-5 mg qd-tid 30 min ac or 5-15 mg long-acting tab qd in AM

Available forms include: Tabs 5, 10 mg; tabs long-acting 5, 10, 15 mg

Side effects/adverse reactions:

CNS: Hyperactivity, insomnia, restlessness, talkativeness, dizziness, headache, chills, stimulation, dysphoria, irritability, aggressiveness

GI: Nausea, vomiting, anorexia, dry mouth, diarrhea, constipation, weight loss, metallic taste, cramps

GU: Impotence, change in libido

CV: Palpitations, tachycardia, hypertension, hypotension

INTEG: Urticaria

Contraindications: Hypersensitivity to sympathomimetic amines, hyperthyroidism, hypertension, glaucoma hypertrophy, severe arteriosclerosis, nephritis, angina pectoris, parkinsonism, drug abuse, cardiovascular disease, anxiety

Precautions: Gilles de la Tourette's disorder, pregnancy (C), lactation, child <3 years, diabetes mellitus, elderly

Pharmacokinetics:

PO: Duration 3-6 hr, metabolized by liver, excreted by kidneys, crosses blood-brain barrier

Interactions/incompatibilities:

• Hypertensive crisis: MAOIs or within 14 days of MAOIs

• Increased effect of this drug: acetazolamide, antacids, sodium bicarbonate, ascorbic acid, ammonium chloride, phenothiazines, haloperidol

• Decreased effects of this drug: barbiturates

• Decreased effects of: guanethidine, other antihypertensives

NURSING CONSIDERATIONS

Assess:

• VS, B/P since this drug may reverse antihypertensives; check patients with cardiac disease more often

• CBC, urinalysis, in diabetes:

blood sugar, urine sugar; insulin changes may need to be made since eating will decrease

• Height, growth rate in children; growth rate may be decreased

Administer:

• At least 6 hr before hs to avoid sleeplessness

• For obesity only if patient is on weight reduction program including dietary changes, exercise; patient will develop tolerance, loss of weight won't occur without additional methods

• Gum, hard candy or frequent sips of water for dry mouth

• If drug is being given for obesity, 1 hr before meals

Perform/provide:

• Checking to see PO medication has been swallowed

Evaluate:

• Mental status: mood, sensorium, affect, stimulation, insomnia, aggressiveness

• Physical dependency: should not be used for extended time; dose should be discontinued gradually

• Withdrawal symptoms: headache, nausea, vomiting, muscle pain, weakness

• Drug tolerance after long-term use

• Dosage should not be increased if tolerance develops

Teach patient/family:

• To decrease caffeine consumption (coffee, tea, cola, chocolate), which may increase irritability, stimulation

• Avoid OTC preparations unless approved by physician

• To taper off drug over several weeks, or depression, increased sleeping, lethargy may ensue

• To avoid alcohol ingestion

• To avoid hazardous activities until patient is stabilized on medication

• To get needed rest; patients will

feel more tired at end of day

Treatment of overdose: Administer fluids, hemodialysis or peritoneal dialysis; antihypertensive for increased B/P; ammonium Cl for increased excretion.

methantheline bromide

(meth-an'tha-leen)

Banthine

Func. class.: Gastrointestinal anticholinergic

Chem. class.: Synthetic quaternary ammonium antimuscarinic

Action: Inhibits muscarinic actions of acetylcholine at postganglionic parasympathetic neuroeffector sites

Uses: Treatment of peptic ulcer disease, irritable bowel syndrome, pancreatitis, gastritis, biliary dyskinesia, pylorospasm, reflex neurogenic bladder in children

Dosage and routes:

• *Adult:* PO 50-100 mg q6h

• *Child >1 yr:* PO 12.5-50 mg qid

• *Child <1 yr:* PO 12.5-25 mg qid

• *Neonate:* PO 12.5 mg bid-tid

Available forms include: Tabs 50 mg

Side effects/adverse reactions:

CNS: Confusion, stimulation in elderly, headache, insomnia, dizziness, drowsiness, anxiety, weakness, hallucination

GI: Dry mouth, constipation, paralytic ileus, heartburn, nausea, vomiting, dysphagia, absence of taste

GU: Hesitancy, retention, impotence

CV: Palpitations, tachycardia

EENT: Blurred vision, photophobia, mydriasis, cycloplegia, increased ocular tension

INTEG: Urticaria, rash, pruritus, anhidrosis, fever, allergic reactions

Contraindications: Hypersensitivity to anticholinergics, narrow-angle glaucoma, GI obstruction, myasthenia gravis, paralytic ileus, GI atony, toxic megacolon

Precautions: Hyperthyroidism, coronary artery disease, dysrhythmias, CHF, ulcerative colitis, hypertension, hiatal hernia, hepatic disease, renal disease

Pharmacokinetics:

PO: Onset 30-45 min, duration 4-6 hr; metabolized by liver, excreted in urine, bile

Interactions/incompatibilities:

• Increased anticholinergic effect: amantadine, tricyclic antidepressants, MAOIs

• Increased effect of: nitrofurantoin

• Decreased effect of: phenothiazines, levodopa

NURSING CONSIDERATIONS

Assess:

• VS, cardiac status: checking for dysrhythmias, increased rate, palpitations

• I&O ratio; check for urinary retention, hesitancy

Administer:

• ½-1 hr ac for better absorption

• Decreased dose to elderly patients; their metabolism may be slowed

• Gum, hard candy, frequent rinsing of mouth for dryness of oral cavity

Perform/provide:

• Storage in tight container protected from light

• Increased fluids, bulk, exercise to patient's lifestyle to decrease constipation

Evaluate:

• Therapeutic response: absence of epigastric pain, bleeding, nausea, vomiting

• GI complaints: pain, bleeding (frank or occult), nausea, vomiting, anorexia

Teach patient/family:

• Avoid driving or other hazardous activities until stabilized on medication

• Avoid alcohol or other CNS depressants; will enhance sedating properties of this drug

---

metharbital

(meth-ar′bi-tal)

Gemonil, Metharbitone

Func. class.: Anticonvulsant

Chem. class.: Barbiturate derivative

Controlled Substance Schedule III

Uses: Generalized tonic-clonic, absence, myoclonic, mixed seizures

Dosage and routes:

• *Adult:* PO 100 mg qd-tid, may increase to 800 mg/day in divided doses

• *Child:* PO 5-15 mg/kg/day in divided doses tid; may increase to 50-100 mg bid or tid

Available forms include: Tabs 100 mg

Side effects/adverse reactions:

*HEMA: **Thrombocytopenia, agranulocytosis, megaloblastic anemia***

CNS: Dizziness, headache, hangover, stimulation, drowsiness, increased pain

GI: Nausea, vomiting, epigastric pain

INTEG: Rash, urticaria, purpara, erythema multiforme, facial edema

EENT: Tinnitus, hearing loss

CV: Hypotension

RESP: Wheezing, hyperpnea

ENDO: Hypoglycemia, hyponatremia, hypokalemia

Contraindications: Hypersensitivity to barbiturates

Precautions: Pregnancy, hepatic disease, renal disease, lactation, alcoholism, drug abuse, hyperthyroidism

Pharmacokinetics:

PO: Onset 2-4 hr, duration 6-12 hr

REC: Onset slow, duration 4-6 hr
Metabolized by liver, excreted by kidneys

Interactions/incompatibilities:
• Increased effects: CNS depressants, chloramphenicol, valproic acid, disulfiram, nondepolarizing skeletal muscle relaxants, sulfonamides
• Increased orthostatic hypotension: furosemide

NURSING CONSIDERATIONS
Assess:
• Drug level
Evaluate:
• Mental status: mood, sensorium, affect, memory (long, short)
• Respiratory depression
• Blood dyscrasias: fever, sore throat, bruising, rash, jaundice
Teach patient/family:
• All aspects of drug administration: action, dose, route, when to notify physician
Treatment of overdose: Administer calcium gluconate IV

---

methazolamide
(meth-a-zoe'la-mide)
Neptazane
Func. class.: Carbonic anhydrase inhibitor diuretic
Chem. class.: Sulfonamide derivative

Action: Decreases production of aqueous humor in eye, which lowers intraocular pressure
Uses: Open-angle glaucoma or preoperatively in narrow-angle glaucoma
Dosage and routes:
• *Adult:* PO 50-100 mg bid or tid
Available forms include: Tabs 50 mg
Side effects/adverse reactions:
GU: Frequency, hypokalemia, polyuria, uremia, glucosuria, hematuria, decreases libido, impotence
CNS: Drowsiness, paresthesia, anxiety, depression, headache, dizziness, confusion, stimulation, fatigue, *convulsions*
GI: Nausea, vomiting, anorexia, constipation, diarrhea, melena, weight loss, hepatic insufficiency
EENT: Myopia, tinnitus
INTEG: Rash, pruritus, urticaria, fever, photosensitivity
ENDO: Hypoglycemia
HEMA: Hyperchloremia, *aplastic anemia, hemolytic anemia, leukopenia, agranulocytosis, thrombocytopenia, purpura, pancytopenia*
Contraindications: Hypersensitivity to sulfonamides, severe renal disease, severe hepatic disease, electrolyte imbalances (hyponatremia, hypokalemia), hypochloremic acidosis, Addison's disease
Precautions: Hypercalciuria, pregnancy, COPD
Pharmacokinetics:
PO: Onset 2-4 hr, peak 6-8 hr, duration 10-18 hr; excreted in urine, crosses placenta
Interactions/incompatibilities:
• Increased action of: amphetamines, procainamide, quinidine, tricyclics, digitalis
• Decreased effects of: salicylates, lithium, barbiturates, methotrexate, chlorpropamide
• Hypokalemia: with other diuretics, corticosteroids, amphotericin B

NURSING CONSIDERATIONS
Assess:
• Weight, I&O daily to determine fluid loss; effect of drug may be decreased if used qd
• Rate, depth, rhythm of respiration, effect of exertion
• B/P lying, standing; postural hypotension may occur
• Electrolytes: potassium, sodium,

M

---

chloride; include BUN, blood sugar, CBC, serum creatinine, blood pH, ABGs

Administer:

• In AM to avoid interference with sleep if using drug as a diuretic

• Potassium replacement if potassium is less than 3.0

• With food, if nausea occurs, absorption may be decreased slightly

Evaluate:

• Therapeutic response: improvement in edema of feet, legs, sacral area daily if medication is being used in CHF; or decrease in aqueous humor if medication is being used in glaucoma

• Improvement in CVP q8h

• Signs of metabolic acidosis: drowsiness, restlessness

• Signs of hypokalemia: postural hypotension, malaise, fatigue, tachycardia, leg cramps, weakness

• Rashes, temperature elevation qd

• Confusion, especially in elderly; take safety precautions if needed

Teach patient/family:

• To increase fluid intake 2-3 L/ day unless contraindicated; to rise slowly from lying or sitting position

• To notify physician if sore throat, unusual bleeding, bruising, paresthesias, tremors, flank pain, or skin rash occurs

• To avoid hazardous activities if drowsiness occurs

Lab test interferences:

False positive: Urinary protein

Treatment of overdose: Lavage if taken orally, monitor electrolytes, administer dextrose in saline

methdilazine HCl

(meth-dill′a-zeen)

Dilosyn,* Tacaryl

Func. class.: Antihistamine

Chem. class.: Phenothiazine derivative, H₁-receptor antagonist

Action: Acts on blood vessels, GI, respiratory system by competing with histamine for H_1-receptor site; decreases allergic response by blocking histamine

Uses: Pruritus

Dosage and routes:

• *Adult:* PO 8 mg bid-qid; CHEW TAB 8 mg bid-qid

• *Child >3 yr:* PO 4 mg bid-qid; CHEW TAB 4 mg bid-qid

Available forms include: Tabs 8 mg; tabs, chewable 4 mg; syr 4 mg/ 5 ml

Side effects/adverse reactions:

CNS: Dizziness, drowsiness, poor coordination, fatigue, anxiety, euphoria, confusion, paresthesia, neuritis

CV: Hypotension, palpitations, tachycardia

RESP: Increased thick secretions, wheezing, chest tightness

GI: Dry mouth, nausea, vomiting, anorexia, constipation, diarrhea

INTEG: Rash, urticaria, photosensitivity

GU: Retention, dysuria, frequency

EENT: Blurred vision, dilated pupils, tinnitus, nasal stuffiness, dry nose, throat, mouth

Contraindications: Hypersensitivity to H_1-receptor antagonist, acute asthma attack, lower respiratory tract disease

Precautions: Increased intraocular pressure, renal disease, cardiac disease, hypertension, bronchial asthma, seizure disorder, stenosed peptic ulcers, hyperthyroidism, prostatic hypertrophy, bladder neck obstruction, pregnancy

Pharmacokinetics:

PO: Onset 20 min, duration 4-6 hr, metabolized in liver, excreted by kidneys, GI tract (inactive metabolites)

Interactions/incompatibilities:

• Increased CNS depression: barbiturates, narcotics, hypnotics, tricyclic antidepressants, alcohol

• Decreased effect of: oral anticoagulants, heparin

• Increased effect of this drug: MAOIs

NURSING CONSIDERATIONS

Assess:

• I&O ratio; be alert for urinary retention, frequency, dysuria; drug should be discontinued if these occur

• CBC during long-term therapy

Administer:

• Coffee, tea, cola (caffeine) to decrease drowsiness

• With meals if GI symptoms occur, absorption may slightly decrease

Perform/provide:

• Hard candy, gum, frequent rinsing of mouth for dryness

• Storage in tight container at room temperature

Evaluate:

• Therapeutic response: absence of running or congested nose or rashes

• Respiratory status: rate, rhythm, increase in bronchial secretions, wheezing, chest tightness

• Cardiac status: palpitations, increased pulse, hypotension

Teach patient/family:

• All aspects of drug use; to notify physician if confusion, sedation, hypotension occurs

• To avoid driving or other hazardous activity if drowsiness occurs

• To avoid concurrent use of alcohol or other CNS depressants

Lab test interferences:

False positive: Pregnancy test (urinary)

False negative: Skin allergy tests

Increase: Blood glucose

Interfere: Blood grouping

Treatment of overdose: Administer ipecac syrup or lavage, diazepam, vasopressors, barbiturates (short-acting)

---

methenamine hippurate/methenamine mandelate

(meth-en'a-meen) (hip'yoo-rate)
Hiprex, Hip-Rex,* Urex/Mandelamine, Sterine*

Func. class.: Urinary antiinfective
Chem. class.: Methenamine, mandelic acid

Action: In acid urine, it is hydrolyzed to ammonia, formaldehyde, which are bactericidal

Uses: Urinary tract infections caused by *E. coli, Klebsiella, Enterobacter, P. mirabilis, P. morganii, Serratia, Citrobacter*

Dosage and routes:

• *Adult and child >12 yr:* PO 1 g q12h, maximum: 4 g/24 hr

• *Child 6-12 yr:* PO 500 mg-1g q12h

Neurogenic bladder

• *Adult:* PO 1 g qid pc

• *Child 6-12 yr:* PO 500 mg qid pc

• *Child <6 yr:* PO 50 mg/kg in 4 divided doses pc

Available forms include: Tabs 500 mg, 1 g; oral sol 500 mg, 1 g; susp 250, 500 mg/5 ml; tabs, enteric-coated 250, 500 mg, g; tabs, film-coated 500 mg, 1g

Side effects/adverse reactions:

CNS: Headache

INTEG: Pruritus, rash, urticaria

GI: Nausea, vomiting, anorexia,

M

---

abdominal pain, increase AST, ALT

GU: Dysuria, bladder irritation, albuminuria, hematuria, crystalluria
EENT: Tinnitus, stomatitis

Contraindications: Hypersensitivity, severe dehydration, renal insufficiency

Precautions: Renal disease, pregnancy, lactation

Pharmacokinetics:
PO: Excreted in urine, half-life 4 hr

Interactions/incompatibilities:
• Insoluble precipitate in urine: sulfonamides may form
• Do not use with silver, iron, mercury salts

NURSING CONSIDERATIONS

Assess:
• I&O ratio, urine pH <5.5 is ideal
• Periodic liver function test: AST, ALT, alk phosphatase
• C&S before treatment, after completion

Administer:
• After clean-catch urine is obtained for C&S
• Two daily doses if urine output is high or if patient has diabetes
• Up to 12 g of Vitamin C if needed to acidify urine; cranberry, prune juice may be used

Perform/provide:
• Storage protected from high temperature
• Limited intake of alkaline foods or drugs: milk, dairy products, peanuts, vegetables, alkaline antacids, sodium bicarbonate

Evaluate:
• Therapeutic response: decreased pain, frequency, urgency, negative C&S absence of infection
• Allergy: fever, flushing, rash, urticaria, pruritus

Teach patient/family:
• Keep urine acidic by eating food that acidifies urine (meats, eggs, fish, gelatin products, prunes, plums, cranberries)

• Fluids must be increased to 3 L/day to avoid crystallization in kidneys
• Complete full course of drug therapy; take drug at evenly spaced intervals around clock for best results

Lab test interferences:
Interfere: VMA, urinary catecholamines
False decrease: Urine estriol, 5HIAA
False increase: 17-OHCS

---

methicillin sodium

(meth-i-sill'in)
Celbenin, Staphcillin

Func. class.: Broad-spectrum antibiotic
Chem. class.: Penicillinase-resistant penicillin

Action: Interferes with cell wall replication of susceptible organisms; osmotically unstable cell wall swells, bursts from osmotic pressure

Uses: Effective for gram-positive cocci *(S. aureus, S. pyogenes, S. viridans, S. faecalis, S. bovis, S. pneumoniae),* infections caused by penicillinase-producing *Staphylococcus*

Dosage and routes:
• *Adult:* IM/IV 4-6 g/day in divided doses q4-6h
• *Child:* IM/IV 100-200 mg/kg/day in divided doses q4-6h
Available forms include: Powder for inj IM, IV 1, 4, 6, 10 g; IV INF only 1, 4 g

Side effects/adverse reactions:
HEMA: Anemia, increased bleeding time, *bone marrow depression, granulocytopenia*
GI: Nausea, vomiting, diarrhea, increased AST, ALT, abdominal pain, glossitis, colitis
GU: Oliguria, proteinuria, hema-

turia, *vaginitis, moniliasis,* **glomerulonephritis**
CNS: Lethargy, hallucinations, anxiety, depression, twitching, **coma, convulsions**
META: Hyperkalemia, hypokalemia, alkalosis, hypernatremia
Contraindications: Hypersensitivity to penicillins
Precautions: Pregnancy (B), hypersensitivity to cephalosporins, neonates
Pharmacokinetics:
IM: Peak ½-1 hr, duration 4 hr
IV: Peak 15 min, duration 2 hr
Metabolized in liver, excreted in urine, bile, breast milk, crosses placenta
Interactions/incompatibilities:
• Decreased antimicrobial effectiveness of this drug: tetracyclines, erythromycins
• Increased penicillin concentrations when used with: aspirin, probenecid

NURSING CONSIDERATIONS
Assess:
• I&O ratio; report hematuria, oliguria since penicillin in high doses is nephrotoxic
• Any patient with compromised renal system since drug is excreted slowly in poor renal system function; toxicity may occur rapidly
• Liver studies: AST, ALT
• Blood studies: WBC, RBC, H&H, bleeding time
• Renal studies: urinalysis, protein, blood
• C&S before drug therapy; drug may be taken as soon as culture is taken
Administer:
• Drug after C&S has been completed
Perform/provide:
• Adrenalin, suction, tracheostomy set, endotracheal intubation equipment
• Adequate fluid intake (2000 ml) during diarrhea episodes
• Scratch test to assess allergy after securing order from physician; usually done when penicillin is only drug of choice
• Storage at room temperature; reconstituted solution is stable for 8 hr or piggyback for 24 hr
Evaluate:
• Therapeutic effectiveness: absence of fever, draining wounds
• Bowel pattern before, during treatment
• Skin eruptions after administration of penicillin to 1 wk after discontinuing drug
• Respiratory status: rate, character, wheezing, tightness in chest
• Allergies before initiation of treatment, reaction of each medication; highlight allergies on chart, Kardex
Teach patient/family:
• Culture may be taken after completed course of medication
• To report sore throat, fever, fatigue; could indicate superimposed infection
• To wear or carry Medic Alert ID if allergic to penicillins
• To notify nurse of diarrhea stools
Lab test interferences:
Decrease: Uric acid
False positive: Urine glucose, urine protein
Treatment of overdose: Withdraw drug, maintain airway, administer epinephrine, aminophylline, O_2, IV corticosteroids for anaphylaxis

methimazole

(meth-im′a-zole)
Tapazole
Func. class.: Antithyroid hormone
Chem. class.: Thioamide

Action: Inhibits synthesis of thyroid hormones by decreasing iodine use in manufacture of thyroglobin and iodothyronine; does not affect already formed hormones

Uses: Hyperthyroidism, preparation for thyroidectomy, thyrotoxic crisis

Dosage and routes:
Hyperthyroidism
• *Adult:* PO 5-20 mg tid depending on severity of condition, continue until euthyroid, maintenance dose 5 mg qd-tid, maximal dose 150 mg qd
• *Child:* PO 0.4 mg/kg/day in divided doses q8h, continue until euthyroid maintenance dose 0.2 mg/kg/day in divided doses q8h

Preparation for thyroidectomy
• *Adult and child:* PO same as above; iodine may be added × 10 days before surgery

Thyrotoxic crisis
• *Adult and child:* PO same as hyperthyroidism with iodine and propranolol

Available forms include: Tabs 5, 10 mg

Side effects/adverse reactions:
ENDO: Enlarged thyroid
INTEG: Rash, urticaria, pruritus, alopecia, hyperpigmentation, lupuslike syndrome
GU: Irregular menses, ***nephritis***
CNS: Drowsiness, headache, vertigo, fever, paresthesias, neuritis
*HEMA: **Agranulocytosis, leukopenia, thrombocytopenia, hypothrombinemia, lymphadenopathy***
*GI: Nausea, diarrhea, vomiting, **jaundice, hepatitis,** loss of taste*
MS: Myalgia, arthralgia, nocturnal muscle cramps

Contraindications: Hypersensitivity, pregnancy (3rd trimester), lactation

Precautions: Infection, bone marrow depression, hepatic disease, pregnancy (1st, 2nd trimester)

Pharmacokinetics:
PO: Onset 30-40 min, duration 2-4 hr, half-life 1-2 hr, excreted in urine, bile, breast milk, crosses placenta

Interactions/incompatibilities:
• Increased anticoagulant effect of heparin, oral anticoagulants

NURSING CONSIDERATIONS
Assess:
• Pulse, B/P, temperature
• I&O ratio, check for edema: puffy hands, feet, periorbit; indicate hypothyroidism
• Weight qd; same clothing, scale, time of day
• T_3, T_4, which are increased; serum TSH, which is decreased; free thyroxine index, which is increased if dosage is too low; discontinue drug 3-4 wk before RAIU
• Blood work: CBC for blood dyscrasias: leukopenia, thrombocytopenia, agranulocytosis

Administer:
• With meals to decrease GI upset
• At same time each day, to maintain drug level
• Lowest dose that relieves symptoms

Perform/provide:
• Storage in light-resistant container
• Fluids to 3-4 L/day, unless contraindicated

Evaluate:
• Therapeutic effect: weight gain, decreased pulse, decreased T_4, B/P
• Overdose: peripheral edema, heat intolerance, diaphoresis, palpitations, dysrhythmias, severe tachycardia, increased temperature, delirium, CNS irritability
• Hypersensitivity: rash, enlarged cervical lymph nodes; drug may need to be discontinued
• Hypoprothrombinemia: bleeding, petechiae, ecchymosis
• Clinical response: after 3 wk should include increased weight, pulse; decreased T_4

• Bone marrow depression: sore throat, fever, fatigue

Teach patient/family:

• To abstain from breast feeding after delivery

• To take pulse daily

• Report redness, swelling, sore throat, mouth lesions, which indicate blood dyscrasias

• To keep graph of weight, pulse, mood

• Avoid OTC products that contain iodine

• That seafood, other iodine products may be restricted

• Not to discontinue this medication abruptly; thyroid crisis may occur; stress patient response

• That response may take several months if thyroid is large

• Symptoms/signs of overdose: periorbital edema, cold intolerance, mental depression

• Symptoms of inadequate dose: tachycardia, diarrhea, fever, irritability

Lab test interferences:

Increase: Pro-time, AST/ALT, alk phosphatase

---

methocarbamol

(meth-oh-kar'ba-mole)

Delaxin, Forbaxin, Robamol, Robaxin, Romethocarb, Spenaxin

Func. class.: Skeletal muscle relaxant

Chem. class.: Carbamate derivative

Action: CNS depressant; action may be from sedative action; precise mechanism of action is unknown

Uses: Pain in musculoskeletal conditions, tetanus management

Dosage and routes:

Pain

• *Adult:* PO 1.5 g × 2-3 days, then 1 g qid; IM 500 mg in each gluteal region, may repeat q8h; IV BOL 1-3 g/day at 3 ml/min; IV INF 1 gm/250 ml D₅W or NS, not to exceed 3 g/day

Tetanus

• *Adult:* IV INF 1-3 g/L of solution q6h; IV BOL 1-2 g injected into running IV

• *Child:* IV 15 mg/kg q6h

Available forms include: Tabs 500, 750 mg; inj IM, IV 100 mg/ml

Side effects/adverse reactions:

CNS: Dizziness, weakness, drowsiness, headache, tremor, depression, insomnia, seizures

EENT: Diplopia, temporary loss of vision, blurred vision, nystagmus

CV: Postural hypotension, tachycardia

GI: Nausea, vomiting, hiccups, anorexia, metallic taste

INTEG: Rash, pruritus, fever, facial flushing, urticaria

Contraindications: Hypersensitivity, child <12 yr, intermittent porphyria

Precautions: Renal disease, hepatic disease, addictive personalities

Pharmacokinetics:

PO: Onset ½ hr, peak 1-2 hr, half-life 1-2 hr, metabolized in liver, excreted in urine (unchanged), crosses placenta

Interactions/incompatibilities:

• Increased CNS depression: alcohol, tricylic antidepressants, narcotics, barbiturates, sedatives, hypnotics

NURSING CONSIDERATIONS

Assess:

• Blood studies: CBC, WBC, differential; blood dyscrasias may occur

• Liver function studies: AST, ALT, alk phosphatase; hepatitis may occur

• ECG in epileptic patients; poor seizure control has occurred with patients taking this drug

M

Administer:
• With meals for GI symptoms
• By slow IV to prevent phlebitis <300 mg/min
• IM deeply in large muscle mass; rotate sites

Perform/provide:
• Storage in tight container at room temperature
• Assistance with ambulation if dizziness, drowsiness occurs

Evaluate:
• Therapeutic response: decreased pain, spasticity
• Allergic reactions: rash, fever, respiratory distress
• Severe weakness, numbness in extremities
• Psychologic dependency: increased need for medication, more frequent requests for medication, increased pain
• CNS depression: dizziness, drowsiness, psychiatric symptoms

Teach patient/family:
• Not to discontinue medication quickly; insomnia, nausea, headache, spasticity, tachycardia will occur, drug should be tapered off over 1-2 wk
• Not to take with alcohol, other CNS depressants
• To avoid altering activities while taking this drug
• To avoid hazardous activities if drowsiness, dizziness occurs
• To avoid using OTC medication: cough preparations, antihistamines, unless directed by physician

Lab test interferences:
False increase: VMA, urinary 5-HIAA

Treatment of overdose: Induce emesis of conscious patient, lavage, dialysis

---

methohexital sodium

(meth-oh-hex′i-tal)
Brevital Sodium, Brietal Sodium*
Func. class.: General anesthetic
Chem. class.: Barbiturate

Controlled Substance Schedule IV

Action: Acts in reticular-activating system to produce anesthesia

Uses: General anesthesia, for electroshock therapy, reduction of fractures

Dosage and routes:
• *Adult and child:* IV 50-100 mg given 1 ml/5 sec

Maintenance
• *Adult and child:* IV 20-40 mg q4-7 min of a 0.1% solution; CONT IV 1 gtt/sec of a 0.2% solution

Available forms include: Inj IV 500 mg, 2.5, 5g

Side effects/adverse reactions:
RESP: Respiratory depression, bronchospasm
CNS: Retrograde amnesia, prolonged somnolence
CV: Tachycardia, hypotension, *myocardial depression, dysrhythmias*
EENT: Sneezing, coughing
INTEG: Chills, *shivering,* necrosis, pain at injection site
MS: Muscle irritability

Contraindications: Hypersensitivity, status asthmaticus, hepatic/intermittent porphyrias

Precautions: Severe cardiovascular disease, renal disease, hypotension, liver disease, myxedema, myasthenia gravis, asthma, increased intracranial pressure

Pharmacokinetics:
IV: Onset 30-40 sec; half-life 11.5 hr, crosses placenta

Interactions/incompatibilities:
• Increased action: CNS depressants

• Do not mix with atropine or silicone in solution or syringe

NURSING CONSIDERATIONS
Assess:
• VS q3-5 min during IV administration, after dose, q4 hr postoperatively
Administer:
• After preparation with sterile water of 0.9% or 5% dextrose
• Only with crash cart, resuscitative equipment nearby
• IV slowly only
Evaluate:
• Extravasation, if it occurs use nitroprusside or chloroprocaine to decrease pain, increase circulation
• Dysrhythmias or myocardial depression

---

methotrexate/methotrexate sodium (amethopterin, MTX)

(meth-oh-trex′ate)
Folex, Mexate
Func. class.: Antineoplastic-antimetabolite
Chem. class.: Folic acid antagonist

Action: Inhibits an enzyme that reduces folic acid, which is needed for nucleic acid synthesis in cancerous cells
Uses: Acute lymphocytic leukemia, in combination for breast, lung, head, neck cancer, lymphosarcoma, psoriasis, gestational choriocarcinoma, hydatidiform mole
Dosage and routes:
Leukemia
• *Adult and child:* PO 3.3 mg/m²/qd; maintenance 30 mg/m²/day 2×/wk; IV 2.5 mg/kg q2 wk
Choriocarcinoma
• *Adult and child:* PO 15-30 mg/m² qd × 5 days, then off 1 wk; may repeat
Available forms include: Tabs, 2.5 mg; inj IV 25 mg/ml; powder for

inj IV 20, 25, 50, 100, 250 mg; sodium inj IV 2.5, 25 mg/ml
Side effects/adverse reactions:
HEMA: **Leukopenia, thrombocytopenia, myelosuppression, anemia**
GI: Nausea, vomiting, anorexia, diarrhea, stomatitis, **hepatotoxicity,** cramps, ulcer, gastritis, **GI hemorrhage,** abdominal pain, **hematemesis**
GU: Urinary retention, **renal failure,** menstrual irregularities, defective spermatogenesis, hematuria, **azotemia, uric acid nephropathy**
INTEG: Rash, alopecia, dry skin, urticaria, photosensitivity, folliculitis, vasculitis, petechiae, ecchymosis, acne, alopecia
CNS: Dizziness, **convulsions,** headache, confusion, hemiparesis, malaise, fatigue, chills, fever
Contraindications: Hypersensitivity, leukopenia (<2500/mm³), thrombocytopenia (<100,000/mm³), anemia, psoriatic patients with severe renal/hepatic disease, pregnancy
Precautions: Renal disease, lactation
Pharmacokinetics:
PO: Readily absorbed when taken orally, peak 1-4 hr
IV/IM: Peak ½-2 hr
Not metabolized, excreted in urine (unchanged), crosses placenta, blood-brain barrier, 50% plasma protein bound
Interactions/incompatibilities:
• Increased toxicity: aspirin, sulfa drugs, other antineoplastics, radiation, alcohol, probenecid, phenytoin, phenylbutazone, pyrimethamine
• Decreased effect of: oral digoxin
• Increased hypoprothrombinemia: oral anticoagulants
• Decreased effect of this drug: folic acid supplements

NURSING CONSIDERATIONS
Assess:
• CBC, differential, platelet count weekly; withhold drug if WBC is <3500/mm³ or platelet count is <100,000/mm³; notify physician of these results; drug should be discontinued
• Renal function studies: BUN, serum uric acid, urine CrCl, electrolytes before, during therapy
• I&O ratio; report fall in urine output to <30 ml/hr
• Monitor temperature q4h; fever may indicate beginning infection
• Liver function tests before and during therapy: bilirubin, alk phosphatase, AST, ALT; liver biopsy should be done before start of therapy (psoriasis patients)
• Bleeding time, coagulation time during treatment

Administer:
• Medications by oral route if possible; avoid IM, SC, IV routes to prevent infections
• Antacid before oral agent; give drug after evening meal before bedtime
• Antiemetic 30-60 min before giving drug to prevent vomiting
• Allopurinol or sodium bicarbonate to maintain uric acid levels, alkalinization of urine
• Antibiotics for prophylaxis of infection
• Topical or systemic analgesics for pain
• Transfusion for anemia

Perform/provide:
• Strict medical asepsis and protective isolation if WBC levels are low
• Liquid diet: carbonated beverage, Jello; dry toast, crackers may be added when patient is not nauseated or vomiting
• Increased fluid intake to 2-3 L/day to prevent urate deposits, calculi formation, unless contraindicated

• Diet low in purines: absence of organ meats (kidney, liver), dried beans, peas to maintain alkaline urine
• Rinsing of mouth tid-qid with water, hydrogen peroxide; brushing of teeth bid-tid with soft brush or cotton-tipped applicators for stomatitis; use unwaxed dental floss
• Nutritious diet with iron, vitamin supplements
• Storage in tightly closed container in cool environment; store injection, powder for injection in dark, dry area

Evaluate:
• Bleeding: hematuria, guaiac, bruising or petechiae, mucosa or orifices q8h
• Food preferences; list likes, dislikes
• Effects of alopecia on body image; discuss feelings about body changes
• Hepatotoxicity: yellowing of skin, sclera, dark urine, clay-colored stools, pruritus, abdominal pain, fever, diarrhea
• Buccal cavity q8h for dryness, sores, ulceration, white patches, oral pain, bleeding, dysphagia
• Symptoms indicating severe allergic reaction: rash, urticaria, itching, flushing

Teach patient/family:
• Why protective isolation precautions are needed
• To report any complaints, side effects to nurse or physician: black tarry stools, chills, fever, sore throat, bleeding, bruising, cough, shortness of breath, dark or bloody urine
• That hair may be lost during treatment and wig or hairpiece may make patient feel better; tell patient that new hair may be different in color, texture (alopecia is rare)
• To avoid foods with citric acid,

---

hot or rough texture if stomatitis is present

• To report stomatitis: any bleeding, white spots, ulcerations in mouth to physician; tell patient to examine mouth qd, report symptoms to nurse

• Contraceptive measures are recommended during therapy for at least 8 wk following cessation of therapy

• To drink 10-12 glasses of fluid/day

• To avoid alcohol, salicylates

---

methotrimeprazine HCl

(meth-oh-trye-mep′ra-zeen)
Levoprome, Nozinan*

Func. class.: Sedative-hypnotic
Chem. class.: Aliphatic (propyl-amine-phenothiazine derivative)

Controlled Substance Schedule III (USA), Schedule F (Canada)
Action: Depresses cerebral cortex, hypothalamus, limbic system; blocks neurotransmission produced by dopamine at synapse; exhibits strong α-adrenergic, anticholinergic blocking action
Uses: Sedation, analgesia, preoperative and postoperative analgesia, obstetric analgesia
Dosage and routes:
Analgesia/sedation
• *Adult and child >12 yr:* IM 10-20 mg q4-6h prn
• *Elderly:* IM 5-10 mg q4-6h
Preoperative medication
• *Adult and child >12 yr:* IM 2-20 mg 45 min to 3 hr before surgery
Postoperative medication
• *Adult and child >12 yr:* IM 2.5-7.5 mg q4-6h titrated to patient's needs
Available forms include: Inj IM 20 mg/ml
Side effects/adverse reactions:
*HEMA: **Thrombocytopenia, agran-ulocytosis, leukopenia, neutropenia, hemolytic anemia*** (long-term, high dose), increased protime
CNS: Weakness, dizziness, drowsiness, confusion, delirium, euphoria, headache, sedation, EPS
GI: Nausea, vomiting, abdominal pain, dry mouth, jaundice (long-term use)
GU: Hematuria, dysuria, hesitancy, retention, uterine inertia (rare)
INTEG: Pain, edema at injection site, fever, chills
EENT: Nasal congestion, blurred vision, slurred speech
CV: Orthostatic hypotension, palpitations, tachycardia, bradycardia
Contraindications: Hypersensitivity to this drug, phenothiazines, bisulfite; seizures; severe hepatic disease; severe renal disease; severe cardiac disease; coma
Precautions: Elderly, pregnancy
Pharmacokinetics:
PO: Onset 20-30 min, peak 1-2 hr, duration 4 hr; metabolized by liver, excreted by kidneys and in feces, crosses placenta, excreted in breast milk
Interactions/incompatibilities:
• Mix only with scopolamine or atropine; not to be mixed in syringe or solution with any other drugs
• Increased sedation: CNS depressants, alcohol, barbiturates, reserpine, narcotics, general anesthetics, meprobamate
NURSING CONSIDERATIONS
Assess:
• Blood studies: CBC, ALT, AST, bilirubin
• VS q10 min for 30 min; watch for decreasing B/P with increased pulse that may occur 10-30 min after injection
• Effect on uterine contractions, fetal heart tones if using for labor

---

Administer:

• After removal of cigarettes, to prevent fires

• IM injection in deep large muscle mass to prevent tissue sloughing, rotate sites

• Lowest dose, then gradually increase; lower doses are required after general anesthesia

Perform/provide:

• Bedrest for several hours after injection if orthostatic hypotension occurs

• Safety measure: siderails, nightlight, callbell within easy reach

• Storage in darkness, expires after 5 yr

• Assistance with ambulation for 6 hr after injection

Evaluate:

• Therapeutic response: decrease in pain, grimacing, absence of change in VS, ability to cough and breathe deep after surgery

Teach patient/family:

• To avoid ambulation without assistance for 6 hr after drug is given

Treatment of overdose: Lavage, activated charcoal, monitor electrolytes, vital signs

---

methoxsalen

(meth-ox′a-len)

Oxsoralen

Func. class.: Pigmenting agent
Chem. class.: Psoralen derivative

Action: Decreases cell turnover by combining with epidermal cell DNA, causing photo damage when used with ultraviolet rays

Uses: Vitiligo, psoriasis

Dosage and routes:

• *Adult and child >12 yr:* PO 20 mg qd 2-4 hr before exposure to therapeutic ultraviolet rays; TOP apply 1-2 hr before exposure to UVA light

Available forms include: Lotion 1%; caps 10 mg; contains tartrazine

Side effects/adverse reactions:

CNS: Headache, depression, restlessness, anxiety, nervousness, vertigo

GI: Nausea, *vomiting,* anorexia, diarrhea

INTEG: Rash, pruritus, burning, peeling, erythema, edema

Contraindications: Hypersensitivity, melanoma, LE, albinism, sunburn, cataracts, squamous cell cancer, pregnancy

Precautions: Hepatic disease, cardiac disease, children, lactation

Pharmacokinetics:

PO: Duration 8 hr, half-life ½-1 hr, metabolized in liver, excreted in urine

Interactions/incompatibilities:

• May increase effects of this drug: other photosensitizing agents, phenothiazines, thiazides, tetracyclines

NURSING CONSIDERATIONS

Assess:

• Hepatic test (AST, ALT, bilirubin), renal test (BUN, protein), antinuclear antibodies during treatment

Administer:

• With food or milk to prevent GI upset

• To prevent extensive phototoxicity, qod

Perform/provide:

• Protection to eyes, lips during treatment

Evaluate:

• Therapeutic response: increased pigmentation in vitiligo, decreased psoriatic areas

Teach patient/family:

• To avoid UVA exposure for at least 24 hr after topical application, and 8 hr after PO dose

• Sunscreen may be used if exposure to sunlight occurs after treatment

methscopolamine bromide

(meth-skoe-pol′a-meen)

Pamine, Scoline

Func. class.: Gastrointestinal anticholinergic

Chem. class.: Synthetic quaternary ammonium antimuscarinic

Action: Inhibits muscarinic actions of acetylcholine at postganglionic parasympathetic neuroeffector sites

Uses: Treatment of peptic ulcer disease

Dosage and routes:

• *Adult:* PO 2.5-5 mg ½ hr ac, hs

Available forms include: Tabs 2.5 mg

Side effects/adverse reactions:

CNS: Confusion, stimulation in elderly, headache, insomnia, dizziness, drowsiness, anxiety, weakness, hallucination

GI: Dry mouth, constipation, paralytic ileus, heartburn, nausea, vomiting, dysphagia, absence of taste

GU: Hesitancy, retention, impotence

CV: Palpitations, tachycardia

EENT: Blurred vision, photophobia, mydriasis, cycloplegia, increased ocular tension

INTEG: Urticaria, rash, pruritus, anhidrosis, fever, allergic reactions

Contraindications: Hypersensitivity to anticholinergics, narrow-angle glaucoma, GI obstruction, myasthenia gravis, paralytic ileus, GI atony, toxic megacolon

Precautions: Hyperthyroidism, coronary artery disease, dysrhythmias, CHF, ulcerative colitis, hypertension, hiatal hernia, hepatic disease, renal disease

Pharmacokinetics:

PO: Onset 1 hr, duration 4-6 hr; metabolized by liver, excreted in urine

Interactions/incompatibilities:

• Increased anticholinergic effect: amantadine, tricyclic antidepressants, MAOIs

• Increased effect of: nitrofurantoin

• Decreased effect of: phenothiazines, levodopa

NURSING CONSIDERATIONS

Assess:

• VS, cardiac status: checking for dysrhythmias, increased rate, palpitations

• I&O ratio; check for urinary retention or hesitancy

Administer:

• ½-1 hr ac for better absorption

• Decreased dose to elderly patients; their metabolism may be slowed

• Gum, hard candy, frequent rinsing of mouth for dryness of oral cavity

Perform/provide:

• Storage in tight container protected from light

• Increased fluids, bulk, exercise to patient's lifestyle to decrease constipation

Evaluate:

• Therapeutic response: absence of epigastric pain, bleeding, nausea, vomiting

• GI complaints: pain, bleeding (frank or occult), nausea, vomiting, anorexia

Teach patient/family:

• Avoid driving or other hazardous activities until stabilized on medication

• Avoid alcohol or other CNS depressants; will enhance sedating properties of this drug

M

---

italics = common side effects   ***bold italic*** = life threatening reactions

methsuximide

(meth-sux'i-mide)
Celontin

Func. class.: Anticonvulsant
Chem. class.: Succinimide

Action: Inhibits spike, wave formation in absence seizures (petit mal), decreases amplitude, frequency, duration, spread of discharge in minor motor seizures

Uses: Refractory absence seizures

Dosage and routes:

• *Adult and child:* PO 300 mg/day; may increase by 300 mg/wk, not to exceed 1.2 g/day in divided doses

Available forms include: Caps, half-strength 150 mg; caps 300 mg

Side effects/adverse reactions:

HEMA: Agranulocytosis, aplastic anemia, thrombocytopenia, leukocytosis, eosinophilia, pancytopenia

CNS: Drowsiness, dizziness, fatigue, euphoria, lethargy, irritability, depression, insomnia, anxiety, aggressiveness

GI: Nausea, vomiting, heartburn, anorexia, diarrhea, abdominal pain, cramps, constipation

GU: Vaginal bleeding, *hematuria, renal damage*

INTEG: Urticaria, pruritic erythema, hirsutism, *Stevens-Johnson syndrome*

EENT: Myopia, gum hypertrophy, tongue swelling, blurred vision

Contraindications: Hypersensitivity to succinimide derivatives

Precautions: Hepatic disease, renal disease, pregnancy, lactation

Pharmacokinetics:

PO: Onset 15-30 min, peak 1-2 hr, duration 4-6 hr

REC: Onset slow, duration 4-6 hr Metabolized by liver, excreted by kidneys, half-life 2⅗-4 hr

Interactions/incompatibilities:

• Antagonist effect: tricyclic antidepressants

• Decreased effects of: estrogens, oral contraceptives

NURSING CONSIDERATIONS

Assess:

• Renal studies: urinalysis, BUN, urine creatinine

• Blood studies: CBC, Hct, Hgb, reticulocyte counts q wk for 4 wk then q mo

• Hepatic studies: ALT, AST, bilirubin, creatinine

• Drug levels during initial treatment, therapeutic range (40-80 μg/ml)

Administer:

• With food, milk to decrease GI symptoms

Perform/provide:

• Hard candy, frequent rinsing of mouth, gum for dry mouth

• Assistance with ambulation during early part of treatment; dizziness occurs

Evaluate:

• Therapeutic response: decreased seizure activity, document on patient's chart

• Mental status: mood, sensorium, affect, behavioral changes; if mental status changes notify physician

• Eye problems; need for ophthalmic exams before, during, after treatment (slit lamp, fundoscopy, tonometry)

• Allergic reaction: red raised rash; if this occurs, drug should be discontinued

• Blood dyscrasias: fever, sore throat, bruising, rash, jaundice

• Toxicity: bone marrow depression, nausea, vomiting, ataxia, diplopia

Teach patient/family:

• To carry ID card of Medic-Alert bracelet stating drugs taken, condition, physician's name, phone number

---

• To avoid driving, other activities that require alertness
• To avoid alcohol ingestion, CNS depressants; increased sedation may occur
• Not to discontinue medication quickly after long-term use
• All aspects of drug: action, use, side effects, adverse reactions, when to notify physician
• That drug may change urine to pink or brown

Lab test interferences:
Increase: Coombs' test
Treatment of overdose: Lavage, activated charcoal, monitor electrolytes, VS

---

methyclothiazide

(meth-i-kloe-thye′a-zide)
Aquatensen, Duretic,* Enduron
Func. class.: Diuretic
Chem. class.: Thiazide; sulfonamide derivative

Action: Acts on distal tubule by increasing excretion of water, sodium, chloride, potassium
Uses: Edema, hypertension
Dosage and routes:
• *Adult:* PO 2.5-10 mg/day
Available forms include: Tabs 2.5, 5 mg
Side effects/adverse reactions:
GU: Frequency, polyuria, uremia, glucosuria
CNS: Drowsiness, paresthesia, anxiety, depression, headache, dizziness, fatique, weakness
GI: Nausea, vomiting, anorexia, constipation, diarrhea, cramps, pancreatitis, GI irritation, *hepatitis*
EENT: Blurred vision
INTEG: Rash, urticaria, purpura, photosensitivity, fever
META: Hyperglycemia, hyperuricemia, increased creatinine
HEMA: Aplastic anemia, hemolytic anemia, leukopenia, agranulocy-tosis, thrombocytopenia
CV: Irregular pulse, orthostatic hypotension
ELECT: Hypokalemia, hypercalcemia, hyponatremia, hypochloremia
Contraindications: Hypersensitivity to thiazides or sulfonamides, anuria, renal decompensation
Precautions: Hypokalemia, renal disease, pregnancy, hepatic disease, gout, COPD, lupus erythematosus, diabetes mellitus
Pharmacokinetics:
PO: Onset 2 hr, peak 6 hr, duration >24 hr; excreted unchanged by kidneys, crosses placenta, enters breast milk
Interactions/incompatibilities:
• Increased toxicity of: lithium, nondepolarizing skeletal muscle relaxants, digitalis
• Decreased effects of: antidiabetics
• Decreased absorption of thiazides: cholestyramine, colestipol
• Decreased hypotensive response: indomethacin
• Increased action of: quinidine
NURSING CONSIDERATIONS
Assess:
• Weight, I&O daily to determine fluid loss; effect of drug may be decreased if used qd
• Rate, depth, rhythm of respiration, effect of exertion
• B/P lying, standing, postural hypotension may occur
• Electrolytes: potassium, sodium, chloride; include BUN, blood sugar, CBC, serum creatinine, blood pH, ABGs
• Glucose in urine if patient is diabetic
Administer:
• In AM to avoid interference with sleep if using drug as a diuretic
• Potassium replacement if potassium is less than 3.0
• With food, if nausea occurs, absorption may be decreased slightly

---

italics = common side effects   **bold italic** = life threatening reactions

Evaluate:
• Improvement in edema of feet, legs, sacral area daily if medication is being used in CHF
• Improvement in CVP q8h
• Signs of metabolic acidosis: drowsiness, restlessness
• Signs of hypokalemia: postural hypotension, malaise, fatigue, tachycardia, leg cramps, weakness
• Rashes, temperature elevation qd
• Confusion, especially in elderly; take safety precautions if needed

Teach patient/family:
• To increase fluid intake 2-3 L/day unless contraindicated, to rise slowly from lying or sitting position
• To notify physician of muscle weakness, cramps, nausea, dizziness
• Drug may be taken with food or milk
• That blood sugar may be increased in diabetics
• Take early in day to avoid nocturia

Lab test interferences:
Increase: BSP retention, calcium, amylase
Decrease: PBI, PSP

Treatment of overdose: Lavage if taken orally, monitor electrolytes, administer dextrose in saline

---

methylcellulose

(meth-ill-sell′yoo-lose)

Cellothyl, Citrucel, Cologel, Hydrolose, Syncelose,

Func. class.: Laxative, bulk
Chem. class.: Hydrophilic semisynthetic cellulose derivative

Action: Attracts water, expands in intestine to increase peristalsis; also absorbs excess water in stool; decreases diarrhea
Uses: Constipation

Dosage and routes:
• *Adult:* PO 5-20 ml tid with 8 oz of water
• *Child:* PO 5-10 ml qd or bid with water or 500 mg tid with 8 oz of water

Available forms include: Powder 105 mg/g; sol 450 mg/5 ml; tab 500 mg

Side effects/adverse reactions:
GI: Obstruction, abdominal distention

Contraindications: Hypersensitivity, GI obstruction

Pharmacokinetics:
PO: Onset 12-24 hr, peak 1-3 days

Interactions/incompatibilities:
• Decreased absorption: antibiotics, digitalis, nitrofurantoin, salicylates, tetracyclines, oral anticoagulants

NURSING CONSIDERATIONS

Assess:
• Blood, urine electrolytes if drug is used often by patient
• I&O ratio to identify fluid loss

Administer:
• Alone for better absorption; do not take within 1 hr of other drugs or within 1 hr of antacids, milk, or cimetidine
• In morning or evening (oral dose)

Evaluate:
• Therapeutic response: decrease in constipation
• Cause of constipation; identify whether fluids, bulk, or exercise is missing from lifestyle
• Cramping, rectal bleeding, nausea, vomiting; if these symptoms occur, drug should be discontinued

Teach patient/family:
• Swallow tabs whole; do not chew
• That normal bowel movements do not always occur daily
• Do not use in presence of abdominal pain, nausea, vomiting
• Notify physician if constipation unrelieved or if symptoms of elec-

trolyte imbalance occur: muscle cramps, pain, weakness, dizziness

---

methyldopa/methyldopate

(meth-ill-doe′pa)

Aldomet, Dopamet,* Medimet,* Novomedopa*

Func. class.: Antihypertensive
Chem. class.: Centrally-acting adrenergic inhibitor

Action: Stimulates central α-adrenergic receptors or acts as false transmitter, resulting in reduction of arterial pressure

Uses: Hypertension

Dosage and routes:
• *Adult:* PO 250 mg bid or tid, then adjusted q2 days as needed, 0.5-3 g qd in 2-4 divided doses (maintenance), not to exceed 3 g day; IV 250 mg-500 mg in 100 ml D$_5$W q6h, run over 30-60 min, not to exceed 1 g q6h
• *Child:* PO 10 mg/kg/day in 2-4 divided doses, not to exceed 65 mg/kg or 3 g/day, whichever is less; IV 20-40 mg/kg/day in 4 divided doses, not to exceed 65 mg/kg

Available forms include: Tabs 125, 250, 500 mg; oral susp 250 mg/5ml; inj IV 50 mg/ml

Side effects/adverse reactions:
GI: Nausea, vomiting, diarrhea, constipation, hepatic dysfunction
CV: Bradycardia, myocarditis, orthostatic hypotension, angina, edema, weight gain
CNS: Drowsiness, weakness, dizziness, sedation, headache, depression, psychosis
EENT: Nasal congestion, eczema
*HEMA: **Leukopenia, thrombocytopenia,*** anemia, positive Coombs' test
INTEG: Lupus-like syndrome
GU: Impotence, failure to ejaculate

Contraindications: Active hepatic disease, hypersensitivity, blood dyscrasias

Precautions: Pregnancy, liver disease, eclampsia, severe cardiac disease

Pharmacokinetics:
PO: Peak 2-4 hr, duration 12-24 hr
IV: Peak 2 hr, duration 10-16 hr
Metabolized by liver, excreted in urine

Interactions/incompatibilities:
• Increased hypoglycemia: talbutal
• Increased pressor effect: sympathomimetic amines (norepinephrine, phenylpropanolamine)
• Increased hypotension: levodopa
• Increased sedation: haloperidol
• Increased action of: anesthetics

NURSING CONSIDERATIONS

Assess:
• Blood studies: neutrophils, decreased platelets
• Renal studies: protein, BUN, creatinine, watch for increased levels, may indicate nephrotic syndrome
• Baselines in renal, liver function tests before therapy begins
• K levels, although hyperkalemia rarely occurs
• B/P during beginning treatment, periodically thereafter

Perform/provide:
• Storage of tablets in tight containers

Evaluate:
• Therapeutic response: decrease in B/P in hypertension
• Allergic reaction: rash, fever, pruritus, urticaria; drug should be discontinued if antihistamines fail to help
• Symptoms of CHF: edema, dyspnea, wet rales, B/P
• Renal symptoms: polyuria, oliguria, frequency

Teach patient/family:
• To avoid hazardous activities
• Administer 1 hr before meals
• Not to discontinue drug abruptly

---

italics = common side effects   ***bold italic*** = life threatening reactions

or withdrawal symptoms may occur: anxiety, increased B/P, headache, insomnia, increased pulse, tremors, nausea, sweating

• Not to use OTC (cough, cold, allergy) products unless directed by physician

• Tell patient to avoid sunlight or wear sunscreen if in sunlight, photosensitivity may occur

• Stress patient compliance with dosage schedule even if feeling better

• To rise slowly to sitting or standing position to minimize orthostatic hypotension

• Notify physician of: mouth sores, sore throat, fever, swelling of hands or feet, irregular heartbeat, chest pain, signs of angioedema

• Excessive perspiration, dehydration, vomiting, diarrhea may lead to fall in blood pressure; consult physician if these occur

• Dizziness, fainting, light-headedness may occur during 1st few days of therapy

• That compliance is necessary, not to skip or stop drug unless directed by physician

• May cause skin rash or impaired perspiration

---

methylergonovine maleate

(meth-ill-er-goe-noe'veen)
Methergine
Func. class.: Oxytocic
Chem. class.: Ergot alkaloid

Action: Stimulates uterine contractions, decreases bleeding
Uses: Treatment of hemorrhage associated with postpartum or postabortion
Dosage and routes:
• *Adult:* IM 0.2 mg q2-5h, not to exceed 5 doses; IV 0.2 mg given over 1 min; PO 0.2-0.4 mg q6-

12h × 2-7 days after initial IM or IV dose
Available forms include: Inj IM, IV 0.2 mg/ml; tabs 0.2 mg
Side effects/adverse reactions:
CNS: Headache, dizziness
GI: Nausea, vomiting
CV: Chest pain, palpitation, hypertension
EENT: Tinnitus
INTEG: Sweating, rash
Contraindications: Hypersensitivity to ergot preparations, indication of labor, delivery of placenta, hypertension, PID, respiratory disease, cardiac disease
Precautions: Severe hepatic disease, severe renal disease, jaundice, diabetes mellitus, convulsive disorders
Pharmacokinetics:
PO: Onset 5-25 min, duration 3 hr
IM: Onset 2-5 min, duration 3 hr
IV: Onset immediate, duration 45 min
Metabolized in liver, excreted in urine
Interactions/incompatabilities: None known
NURSING CONSIDERATIONS
Assess:
• B/P, pulse; watch for changes that may indicate hemorrhage
• Respiratory rate, rhythm, depth; notify physician of abnormalities
Administer:
• IM in deep muscle mass; rotate injection sites if additional doses are given
• After having crash cart available on unit
Evaluate:
• For length, duration of contraction; notify physician of contractions lasting over 1 min or absence of contractions
Teach patient/family:
• To report increased blood loss, abdominal cramps, increased temperature or foul-smelling lochia

methylene blue

(meth'i-leen)

MG-Blue, Urolene Blue, Wright's Stain

Func. class.: Urinary tract antiseptic

Chem. class.: Antiseptic dye

Action: Oxidation reduction; has opposite action on hemoglobin depending on concentration; with increased concentration, converts ferrous ion of reduced hemoglobin to ferric form, methemoglobin is thus produced; prolonged administration accelerates destruction of erythrocytes.

Uses: Urinary tract infections caused by *E. coli, Klebsiella, Enterobacter, P. mirabilis, P. vulgaris, P. morganii, Serratia, Citrobacter*

Dosage and routes:

• *Adult:* PO 65-130 mg pc with full glass of water

Cyanide poisoning/methemoglobinemia

• *Adult and child:* IV 1-2 mg/kg of 1% sol, inject slowly over 5 min or more

Available forms include: Tabs 65 mg, inj 10 mg/ml

Side effects/adverse reactions:

CV: Cyanosis, CV abnormalities

INTEG: Pruritus, rash, urticaria, photosensitivity, profuse sweating

CNS: Dizziness, headache, drowsiness, mental confusion

GI: Nausea, vomiting, abdominal pain, diarrhea

GU: Bladder irritation

Contraindications: Hypersensitivity to this drug, renal insufficiency

Precautions: Anemia, renal disease, hepatic disease, G-6-PD deficiency

Pharmacokinetics:

PO/IV: Excreted in urine, bile, feces

Interactions/incompatibilities:
None known

NURSING CONSIDERATIONS

Assess:

• For cyanosis

• I&O ratio, urine pH <5.5 is ideal

• Hct, Hgb

Administer:

• After clean-catch urine is obtained for C&S

• Two daily doses if urine output is high or if patient has diabetes

Perform/provide:

• Limited intake of alkaline foods, drugs: milk, dairy products, peanuts, vegetables, alkaline antacids, sodium bicarbonate

Evaluate:

• Therapeutic response: decreased pain, frequency, urgency, C&S absence of infection

• CNS symptoms: insomnia, headache, drowsiness, confusion

• Allergic reactions: fever, flushing, rash, urticaria, pruritus

Teach patient/family:

• Instruct patient that anemia may result with continued administration

• Instruct patient that drug turns urine, sometimes stool, blue green

• If symptoms do not improve, or become worse, notify physician

• Notify physician of any sign/symptoms of side effects or adverse reactions

methylphenidate HCl

(meth-ill-fen'i-date)

Methidate, Ritalin, Ritalin SR

Func. class.: Cerebral stimulant

Chem. class.: Piperidine derivative

Controlled Substance Schedule II

Action: Increases release of norepinephrine, dopamine in cerebral

M

---

cortex to reticular activating system
Uses: Attention deficit disorder with hyperactivity, narcolepsy
Dosage and routes:
Attention deficit disorder
• *Child >6 yr:* 5-10 mg before breakfast and lunch, increasing by 5-10 mg/wk, not to exceed 60 mg/day
Narcolepsy
• *Adult:* PO 10 mg bid-tid, 30 min before meals
Available forms include: Tabs 5, 10, 20 mg; tabs susp rel 20 mg
Side effects/adverse reactions:
CNS: Hyperactivity, insomnia, restlessness, talkativeness, dizziness, headache, akathisia, dyskinesia, Tourette's disease
GI: Nausea, vomiting, anorexia, dry mouth, diarrhea, constipation, weight loss, abdominal pain
CV: Palpitations, tachycardia
INTEG: Exfoliative dermatitis, urticaria, rash, erythema-multiforme
ENDO: Growth retardation
EENT: Blurred vision
Contraindications: Hypersensitivity to sympathomimetic amines, glaucoma, drug abuse, cardiovascular disease, alcoholism
Precautions: Diabetes mellitus, hypertension, depression
Pharmacokinetics:
PO: Onset ½-1 hr, duration 8-15 hr, metabolized by liver, excreted by kidneys
Interactions/incompatibilities:
• Hypertensive crisis: MAOIs or within 14 days of MAOIs
• Increased effect of acetazolamide, antacids, sodium bicarbonate, ascorbic acid, ammonium chloride, phenothiazines, haloperidol
• Decreased effects of this drug: barbiturates
• Decreased effects of: guanethidine, other antihypertensives

NURSING CONSIDERATIONS
Assess:
• VS, B/P since this drug may reverse antihypertensives; check patients with cardiac disease more often
• CBC, urinalysis, in diabetes: blood sugar, urine sugar; insulin changes may need to be made since eating will decrease
• Height, growth rate in children; growth rate may be decreased
Administer:
• At least 6 hr before hs to avoid sleeplessness
• For obesity only if patient is on weight reduction program including dietary changes, exercise; patient will develop tolerance, and weight loss won't occur without additional methods
• Gum, hard candy, frequent sips of water for dry mouth
• If drug is being given for obesity, 1 hr before meals
Perform/provide:
• Check to see PO medication has been swallowed
Evaluate:
• Mental status: mood, sensorium, affect, stimulation, insomnia, aggressiveness
• Physical dependency: should not be used for extended time; dose should be discontinued gradually
• Withdrawal symptoms: headache, nausea, vomiting, muscle pain, weakness
• Drug tolerance after long-term use
• Dosage should not be increased if tolerance develops
Teach patient/family:
• To decrease caffeine consumption (coffee, tea, cola, chocolate); may increase irritability, stimulation
• Avoid OTC preparations unless approved by physician
• To taper off drug over several

weeks, or depression, increased sleeping, lethargy will ensue

• To avoid alcohol ingestion

• To avoid hazardous activities until patient is stabilized on medication

• To get needed rest; patients will feel more tired at end of day

Treatment of overdose: Administer fluids, hemodialysis or peritoneal dialysis; Antihypertensive for increased B/P, ammonium Cl for increased excretion

---

methylprednisolone/methylprednisolone acetate/methylprednisolone sodium succinate

(meth-ill-pred-niss'oh-lone)
Medrol/Depo-Medrol, Duralone, Medralone, Per-Dep, Rep-Pred/A-Methapred, Solu-Medrol

Func. class.: Corticosteroid
Chem. class.: Glucocorticoid, immediate acting

Action: Decreases inflammation by suppression of migration of polymorphonuclear leukocytes, fibroblasts, reversal of increased capillary permeability and lysosomal stabilization

Uses: Severe inflammation, shock, adrenal insufficiency

Dosage and routes:

Adrenal insufficiency/inflammation

• *Adult:* PO 2-60 mg in 4 divided doses; IM 40-80 mg (acetate); IM/IV 10-250 mg (succinate); INTRA-ARTICULAR: 4-30 mg (acetate)

• *Child:* IV 117 μg-1.66 mg/kg in 3-4 divided doses (succinate)

Shock

• *Adult:* IV 100-250 mg q2-6h, (succinate)

Available forms include: Tabs 2, 4, 6, 8, 16, 24, 32 mg; inj 20, 40, 80 mg/ml acetate; inj 40, 125, 500, 1000 mg/vial succinate

Side effects/adverse reactions:

INTEG: Acne, poor wound healing, ecchymosis, petechiae

CNS: Depression, flushing, sweating, headache, mood changes

*CV: Hypotension, **circulatory collapse, thrombophlebitis, embolism**,* tachycardia

*HEMA: **Thrombocytopenia***

MS: Fractures, osteoporosis, weakness

*GI: Diarrhea, nausea, abdominal distention, GI hemorrhage, increased appetite, **pancreatitis***

EENT: Fungal infections, increased intraocular pressure, blurred vision

Contraindications: Psychosis, hypersensitivity, idiopathic thrombocytopenia, acute glomerulonephritis, amebiasis, fungal infections, nonasthmatic bronchial disease, child <2 yr

Precautions: Pregnancy, diabetes mellitus, glaucoma, osteoporosis, seizure disorders, ulcerative colitis, CHF, myasthenia gravis

Pharmacokinetics:

PO: Peak 1-2 hr
IM: Peak 4-8 days
INTRAARTICULAR: Peak 1-5 wk
Half-life >3½ hr

Interactions/incompatibilities:

• Decreased action of this drug: cholestyramine, colestipol, barbiturates, rifampin, ephedrine, phenytoin, theophylline

• Decreased effects of: anticoagulants, anticonvulsants, antidiabetics, ambenonium, neostigmine, isoniazid, toxoids, vaccines

• Increased side effects: alcohol, salicylates, indomethacin, amphotericin B, digitalis preparations

• Increased action of this drug: salicylates, estrogens, indomethacin

NURSING CONSIDERATIONS

Assess:

• Potassium, blood sugar, urine

M

---

glucose while on long-term therapy; hypokalemia and hyperglycemia

• Weight daily, notify physician of weekly gain >5 lb

• B/P q4h, pulse, notify physician if chest pain occurs

• I&O ratio, be alert for decreasing urinary output and increasing edema

• Plasma cortisol levels during long-term therapy (normal level: 138-635 nmol/L SI units when drawn at 8 AM)

Administer:

• After shaking suspension (parenteral)

• Titrated dose, use lowest effective dose

• IM inj deeply in large mass, rotate sites, avoid deltoid, use 19G needle

• In one dose in AM to prevent adrenal suppression, avoid SC administration, damage may be done to tissue

• With food or milk to decrease GI symptoms

Perform/provide:

• Assistance with ambulation in patient with bone tissue disease to prevent fractures

Evaluate:

• Therapeutic response: ease of respirations, decreased inflammation

• Infection: increased temperature, WBC, even after withdrawal of medication; drug masks symptoms of infection

• Potassium depletion: paresthesias, fatigue, nausea, vomiting, depression, polyuria, dysrhythmias, weakness

• Edema, hypotension, cardiac symptoms

• Mental status: affect, mood, behavioral changes, aggression

Teach patient/family:

• That ID as steroid user should be carried

• To notify physician if therapeutic response decreases; dosage adjustment may be needed

• Not to discontinue this medication abruptly or adrenal crisis can result

• To avoid OTC products: salicylates, alcohol in cough products, cold preparations unless directed by physician

• Teach patient all aspects of drug use, including Cushingoid symptoms

• Symptoms of adrenal insufficiency: nausea, anorexia, fatigue, dizziness, dyspnea, weakness, joint pain

Lab test interferences:

Increase: Cholesterol, sodium, blood glucose, uric acid, calcium, urine glucose

Decrease: Calcium, potassium, T_4, T_3, thyroid ^{131}I uptake test, urine 17-OHCS, 17-KS, PBI

False negative: Skin allergy tests

methylprednisolone acetate

(meth-ill-pred-niss'oh-lone)
Medrol

Func. class.: Topical corticosteroid
Chem. class.: Synthetic fluorinated agent

Action: Possesses antipruritic, antiinflammatory actions

Uses: Corticosteroid-responsive dermatoses

Dosage and routes:

• *Adult and child:* TOP apply to affected area qd-qid

Available forms include: Oint 0.25%, 1%

Side effects/adverse reactions:

INTEG: Burning, dryness, itching, irritation, acne, folliculitis, hypertrichosis, perioral dermatitis, hypopigmentation, atrophy, striae, miliaria, allergic contact dermatitis, secondary infection

Contraindications: Hypersensitivity to corticosteroids, fungal infections, viral infections

Precautions: Pregnancy (C), lactation, viral infections, bacterial infections

Pharmacokinetics: Not known

Interactions/incompatibilities: None known

NURSING CONSIDERATIONS

Assess:

• Temperature, if fever develops drug should be discontinued

Administer:

• Only to affected areas, do not get in eyes

• Then cover with occlusive dressing if ordered, seal to normal skin, change q12h

• Only to dermatoses, do not use on weeping, denuded or infected area

Perform/provide:

• Cleansing before application of drug

• Treatment for a few days after area has cleared

• Storage at room temperature

Evaluate:

• Systemic absorption: fever, infection, irritation

• Therapeutic response: absence of severe itching, patches on skin, flaking

Teach patient/family:

• To avoid sunlight on affected area, burns may occur

---

methylprednisolone acetate

(meth-ill-pred-niss'oh-lone)

Medrol

Func. class.: Topical corticosteroid
Chem. class.: Synthetic nonfluorinated agent, group VI potency

Action: Possesses antipruritic, antiinflammatory actions

Uses: Psoriasis, eczema, contact dermatitis, pruritus

Dosage and routes:

• *Adult and child:* Apply to affected area qd-qid

Available forms include: Oint 0.25%, 1%

Side effects/adverse reactions:

INTEG: Burning, dryness, itching, irritation, acne, folliculitis, hypertrichosis, perioral dermatitis, hypopigmentation, atrophy, striae, miliaria, allergic contact dermatitis, secondary infection

Contraindications: Hypersensitivity to corticosteroids, fungal infections

Precautions: Pregnancy (C), lactation, viral infections, bacterial infections

Interactions/incompatibilities: None known

NURSING CONSIDERATIONS

Assess:

• Temperature; if fever develops, drug should be discontinued

Administer:

• Only to affected areas; do not get in eyes

• Medication, then cover with occlusive dressing (only if prescribed), seal to normal skin, change q12h

• Only to dermatoses; do not use on weeping, denuded, or infected area

Perform/provide:

• Cleansing before application of drug

• Treatment for a few days after area has cleared

• Storage at room temperature

Evaluate:

• Therapeutic response: absence of severe itching, patches on skin, flaking

Teach patient/family:

• To avoid sunlight on affected area, burns may occur

---

italics = common side effects   ***bold italic*** = life threatening reactions

methyltestosterone

(meth-ill-tess-toss'te-rone)

Android-5, Android-10, Metandren, Oreton-Methyl, Testred, Virilon

Func. class.: Androgenic anabolic steroid

Chem. class.: Halogenated testosterone derivative

Action: Increases weight by building body tissue, increases potassium, phosphorus, chloride, nitrogen levels, increases bone development

Uses: Breast cancer in postmenopausal women, breast engorgement, eunuchoidism, eunuchism, male climacteric, cryptorchidism (postpubertal)

Dosage and routes:

Breast cancer

• *Adult:* PO 200 mg qd, BUC 100 mg qd

Breast engorgement

• *Adult:* PO 80 mg qd × 3-5 days, BUC 40 mg qd × 3-5 days

Eunuchoidism/eunuchism/male climacteric

• *Adult:* PO 10-40 mg qd, BUC 5-20 mg qd

Cryptorchidism

• *Adult:* PO 30 mg qd, BUC 15 mg qd

Available forms include: Tabs 10, 25 mg; tabs buccal 5, 10 mg; caps 10 mg

Side effects/adverse reactions:

INTEG: Rash, acneiform lesions, oily hair, skin, flushing, sweating, acne vulgaris, alopecia, hirsutism

CNS: Dizziness, headache, fatigue, tremors, paresthesias, flushing, sweating, anxiety, lability, insomnia

MS: Cramps, spasms

CV: Increased B/P

GU: Hematuria, amenorrhea, vaginitis, decreased libido, decreased breast size, clitoral hypertrophy, testicular atrophy

GI: Nausea, vomiting, constipation, weight gain, *cholestatic jaundice*

EENT: Carpal tunnel syndrome, conjunctional edema, nasal congestion

ENDO: Abnormal GTT

Contraindications: Severe renal disease, severe cardiac disease, severe hepatic disease, hypersensitivity, pregnancy, lactation, genital bleeding (abnormal)

Precautions: Diabetes mellitus, CV disease, MI

Pharmacokinetics:

PO, BUC: Metabolized in liver, excreted in urine, breast milk, crosses placenta

Interactions/incompatibilities:

• Increased effects of: oral antidiabetics, oxyphenbutazone

• Increased PT with anticoagulants

• Edema: ACTH, adrenal steroids

• Decreased effects of: insulin

NURSING CONSIDERATIONS

Assess:

• Weight daily, notify physician if weekly weight gain is >5 lb

• B/P q4h

• I&O ratio; be alert for decreasing urinary output and increasing edema

• Growth rate in children since growth rate may be uneven (linear/bone growth) when used for extended periods of time

• Electrolytes: K, Na, Cl, Ca+; cholesterol

• Liver function studies: ALT, AST, bilirubin

Administer:

• Titrated dose, use lowest effective dose

• With food or milk to decrease GI symptoms; decrease Na if edema occurs

Perform/provide:
• Diet with increased calories, protein; decrease sodium if edema occurs

Evaluate:
• Therapeutic response: increased appetite, increased stamina
• Edema, hypertension, cardiac symptoms, jaundice
• Mental status: affect, mood, behavioral changes, aggression
• Signs of masculinization in female: increased libido, deepening of voice, breast tissue, enlarged clitoris, menstrual irregularities; male: gynecomastia, impotence, testicular atrophy
• Hypercalcemia: lethargy, polyuria, polydipsia, nausea, vomiting, constipation, drug may need to be decreased
• Hypoglycemia in diabetics; oral anticoagulant action is decreased

Teach patient/family:
• Drug needs to be combined with complete health plan: diet, rest, exercise
• To notify physician if therapeutic response decreases
• Not to discontinue medication abruptly
• Teach patient all aspects of drug usage, including sex characteristics change
• Females to report menstrual irregularities
• That 1-3 mo course is necessary for response in breast cancer
• Procedure for use of buccal tablets: requires 30-60 min to dissolve, change absorption site with each dose; do not eat, drink, chew, or smoke while tablet is in place

Lab test interferences:
Increase: Serum cholesterol, blood glucose, urine glucose
Decrease: Serum calcium, serum potassium, T_4, T_3, thyroid ^{131}I uptake test, urine 17-OHCS, 17-KS, PBI, BSP

methyprylon

(meth-i-prye'lon)
Noludar

Func. class.: Sedative-hypnotic
Chem. class.: Piperidine derivative

Controlled Substance Schedule III (USA), Schedule F (Canada)
Action: Acts at level of thalamus to produce CNS mood alterations by interfering with nerve impulse transmission in sensory cortex by increasing threshold of arousal centers

Uses: Insomnia

Dosage and routes:
• *Adult:* PO 200-400 mg 15 min before hs
• *Child >3 mo:* PO 50 mg hs, may increase to 200 mg if needed, not to exceed 400 mg/day

Available forms include: Caps 300 mg, tabs 50, 200 mg

Side effects/adverse reactions:
CNS: Residual sedation, dizziness, ataxia, stimulation, headache, pyrexia, nightmares, depression
GI: Nausea, vomiting, diarrhea, esophagitis, constipation
INTEG: Rash, pruritus

Contraindications: Hypersensitivity to piperidine derivatives, severe pain, severe renal disease, porphyria

Precautions: Depression, suicidal individuals, drug abuse, cardiac dysrhythmias, narrow-angle glaucoma, prostatic hypertrophy, stenosed peptic ulcer, pyloroduodenal/bladder neck obstruction

Pharmacokinetics:
PO: Onset 45 min, peak 1-2 hr, duration 5-8 hr; metabolized by the liver, excreted by the kidneys, crosses placenta, excreted in breast milk; half-life 3-6 hr

M

Interactions/incompatibilities:
• Increased CNS depression: alcohol, barbiturates, narcotics

NURSING CONSIDERATIONS
Assess:
• Blood studies: Hct, Hgb, RBCs (long-term therapy)
• Hepatic studies: AST, ALT, bilirubin (long-term therapy)
Administer:
• After removal of cigarettes to prevent fires
• After trying conservative measures for insomnia
• ½-1 hr before hs for sleeplessness
• On empty stomach fast onset, but may be taken with food if GI symptoms occur
Perform/provide:
• Assistance with ambulation after receiving dose
• Safety measures: siderails, nightlight, callbell within easy reach
• Checking to see PO medication has been swallowed
• Storage in tight, light-resistant container in cool environment
Evaluate:
• Therapeutic response: ability to sleep at night, decreased amount of early morning awakening if taking drug for insomnia
• Mental status: mood, sensorium, affect, memory (long, short)
• Type of sleep problem: falling asleep, staying asleep
• Physical dependency including more frequent requests for medication, shakes, anxiety
• Withdrawal: nausea, vomiting, anxiety, hallucinations, insomnia, tachycardia, fever, cramps, tremors, seizures
• Allergic reaction: rash; discontinue drug if rash occurs
Teach patient/family:
• To avoid driving or other activities requiring alertness until drug stabilized
• To avoid alcohol ingestion or CNS depressants; serious CNS depression may result
• Not to discontinue medication quickly after long-term use; drug should be tapered over 1-2 wk
• That effects may take 2 nights for benefits to be noticed
• Alternate measures to improve sleep: reading, exercise several hours before hs, warm bath, warm milk, TV, self-hypnosis, deep breathing
• That hangover is common in elderly, but less common than with barbiturates

Treatment of overdose: Lavage, activated charcoal, monitor electrolytes, vital signs

---

methysergide maleate

(meth-i-ser'jide)
Sansert

Func. class.: Adrenergic blocker
Chem. class.: Ergot derivative

Action: May decrease serotonin levels in CNS leading to decreased vasoconstriction

Uses: Headache (vascular, migraine), prophylaxis, diarrhea in carcinoid disease

Dosage and routes:
• *Adult:* PO 2 mg bid with meals
Available forms include: Tabs 2 mg

Side effects/adverse reactions:
CV: Retroperitoneal fibrosis, valvular thickening
CNS: Tremors, anxiety, insomnia, headache, dizziness, euphoria, confusion, depersonalization, hallucination, paresthesias
CV: Palpitations, tachycardia, postural hypertension, angina, thrombophlebitis, ECG changes, *cardiac fibrosis*
GI: Nausea, vomiting
MS: Arthralgia, myalgia
INTEG: Flushing, rash, alopecia

Contraindications: Hypersensitivity to ergot tartrazine, pregnancy, occlusion (peripheral, vascular), CAD, hepatic disease, renal disease, peptic ulcer, hypertension
Precautions: Pregnancy, lactation, children
Pharmacokinetics:
PO: Half-life 10 hr, metabolized by liver, excreted in urine (metabolites/unchanged drug)
Interactions/incompatibilities:
• Increased vasoconstriction: beta blockers

NURSING CONSIDERATIONS
Assess:
• Weight daily, check for peripheral edema in feet, legs
Administer:
• IM dose, which takes 20 min for effect, or use IV for immediate effect
• At beginning of headache, dose must be titrated to patient response
• Give with meals or after meals to avoid GI symptoms
• Only to women who are not pregnant, harm to fetus may occur
Perform/provide:
• Storage in dark area, do not use discolored solutions
• Quiet, calm environment with decreased stimulation for noise, bright light, or excessive talking
Evaluate:
• Therapeutic response: decrease in frequency, severity of headache
• For stress level, activity, recreation, coping mechanisms of patient
• Neurological status: LOC, blurring vision, nausea, vomiting, tingling in extremities that occur preceding headache
• Ingestion of tyramine foods (pickled products, beer, wine, aged cheese), food additives, preservatives, colorings, artificial sweeteners, chocolate, caffeine; may precipitate these types of headaches

Teach patient/family:
• Not to use OTC medications, serious drug interactions may occur
• To maintain dose at approved level, not to increase even if drug does not relieve headache
• To report side effects: increased vasoconstriction starting with cold extremities, then paresthesia, weakness
• That an increase in headaches may occur when this drug is discontinued after long-term use
• Keep drug out of reach of children, death may occur
• Report at once: dyspnea, paresthesias, urinary problems, pain in abdomen, chest, back, legs

---

metoclopramide HCl
(met-oh-kloe-pra′ mide)
Maxeran,* Reglan
Func. class.: Cholinergic
Chem. class.: Central dopamine receptor antagonist

Action: Enhances response to acetylcholine of tissue in upper GI tract, which causes contraction of gastric muscle, relaxes pyloric, duodenal segments, increases peristalsis
Uses: Prevention of nausea, vomiting induced by chemotherapy, delayed gastric emptying, gastroesophageal reflux
Dosage and routes:
Nausea/vomiting
• *Adult:* IV 2 mg/kg q2h × 5 doses 30 min before administration of chemotherapy
Delayed gastric emptying
• *Adult:* PO 10 mg 30 min ac, hs × 2-8 wk
Gastroesophageal reflux
• *Adult:* PO 10-15 mg qid 30 min ac
Available forms include: Tabs 5,

M

---

10 mg; syr 5 mg/5 ml; inj IV 5 mg/ml

Side effects/adverse reactions:

CNS: Sedation, fatigue, restlessness, headache, sleeplessness, dystonia, dizziness, drowsiness

GI: Dry mouth, constipation, nausea, anorexia, vomiting

GU: Decreased libido, prolactin secretion, amenorrhea, galactorrhea

CV: Hypotension, supraventricular tachycardia

INTEG: Urticaria, rash

Contraindications: Hypersensitivity to this drug or procaine or procainamide, seizure disorder, pheochromocytoma, breast cancer, GI obstruction

Precautions: Pregnancy, lactation, GI hemorrhage, CHF

Pharmacokinetics:

IV: Onset 1-3 min, duration 1-2 hr
PO: Onset ½-1 hr, duration 1-2 hr
IM: Onset 10-15 min, duration 1-2 hr

Metabolized by liver, excreted in urine, half-life 4 hr

Interactions/incompatibilities:

• Decreased action of this drug: anticholinergics, opiates

• Increased sedation: alcohol, other CNS depressants

NURSING CONSIDERATIONS
Administer:

• ½-1 hr before meals for better absorption

• Gum, hard candy, frequent rinsing of mouth for dryness of oral cavity

• IV infusion injection slowly

Perform/provide:

• Protect from light with aluminum foil during infusion

• Discard open ampules

Evaluate:

• Therapeutic response: absence of nausea, vomiting, anorexia, fullness

• GI complaints: nausea, vomiting, anorexia, constipation

Teach patient/family:

• Avoid driving or other hazardous activities until patient is stabilized on this medication

• Avoid alcohol or other CNS depressants that will enhance sedating properties of this drug

Lab test interferences:

Increase: Prolactin, aldosterone, thyrotropin

---

metocurine iodide

(met-oh-kyoo'reen)
Metubine Iodide

Func. class.: Neuromuscular blocker (nondepolarizing)
Chem. class.: Methyl analog of tubocurarine

Action: Inhibits transmission of nerve impulses by binding with cholinergic receptor sites, antagonizing action of acetylcholine

Uses: Facilitation of endotracheal intubation, skeletal muscle relaxation during mechanical ventilation, surgery, or general anesthesia

Dosage and routes:

• *Adult:* IV 2-4 mg if given cyclopropane as an anesthetic; 1.5-3 mg if given ether as an anesthetic; 4-7 mg if given nitrous oxide

Available forms include: Inj IV 2 mg/ml

Side effects/adverse reactions:

CV: Bradycardia, tachycardia, increased, decreased B/P

*RESP: Prolonged apnea, **bronchospasm, cyanosis, respiratory depression***

EENT: Increased secretions

INTEG: Rash, flushing, pruritus, urticaria

Contraindications: Hypersensitivity to iodides

Precautions: Pregnancy, cardiac disease, hepatic disease, renal disease, lactation, children <2 yr, electrolyte imbalances, dehydration, neuromuscular disease (myasthenia gravis), respiratory disease

Pharmacokinetics:

IV: Peak 3-5 min, duration 35-90 min; half-life 3½ hr, excreted in urine, bile (½ unchanged), crosses placenta

Interactions/incompatibilities:

• Increased neuromuscular blockade: aminoglycosides, clindamycin, lincomycin, quinidine, local anesthetics, polymyxin antibiotics, lithium, narcotic analgesics, thiazides, enflurane, isoflurane

• Dysrhythmias: theophylline

• Do not mix with barbiturates in solution or syringe

NURSING CONSIDERATIONS

Assess:

• For electrolyte imbalances (K, Mg), may lead to increased action of this drug

• Vital signs (B/P, pulse, respirations, airway) until fully recovered; rate, depth, pattern of respirations, strength of hand grip

• I&O ratio, check for urinary retention, frequency, hesitancy

Administer:

• Using nerve stimulator by anesthesiologist to determine neuromuscular blockade

• Anticholinesterase to reverse neuromuscular blockade

• By slow IV over 1-2 min (only by qualified person, usually an anesthesiologist)

• Only slightly discolored solution

Perform/provide:

• Storage in light-resistant area

• Reassurance if communication is difficult during recovery from neuromuscular blockade

Evaluate:

• Therapeutic response: paralysis of jaw, eyelid, head, neck, rest of body

• Recovery: decreased paralysis of face, diaphragm, leg, arm, rest of body

• Allergic reactions: rash, fever, respiratory distress, pruritus; drug should be discontinued

Treatment of overdose: Edrophonium or neostigmine, atropine, monitor VS; may require mechanical ventilation

---

metolazone

(me-tole'a-zone)

Diulo, Zaroxolyn

Func. class.: Diuretic

Chem. class.: Thiazide-like; quinazoline derivative

Action: Acts on distal tubule by increasing excretion of water, sodium, chloride, potassium

Uses: Edema, hypertension

Dosage and routes:

Edema

• *Adult:* PO 5-20 mg/day

Hypertension

• *Adult:* PO 2.5-5 mg/day

Available forms include: Tabs 2.5, 5, 10 mg

Side effects/adverse reactions:

GU: Frequency, polyuria, uremia, glucosuria

CNS: Drowsiness, paresthesia, anxiety, depression, headache, dizziness, fatigue, weakness

GI: Nausea, vomiting, anorexia, constipation, diarrhea, cramps, pancreatitis, GI irration, *hepatitis*

EENT: Blurred vision

INTEG: Rash, urticaria, purpura, photosensitivity, fever

META: Hyperglycemia, hyperuricemia, increased creatinine

HEMA: Aplastic anemia, hemolytic anemia, leukopenia, agranulocytosis, thrombocytopenia

CV: Irregular pulse, orthostatic hypotension

ELECT: Hypokalemia, hypercalce-

M

---

mia, hyponatremia, hypochloremia

Contraindications: Hypersensitivity to thiazides or sulfonamides, anuria, renal decompensation

Precautions: Hypokalemia, renal disease, pregnancy, hepatic disease, gout, COPD, lupus erythematosus, diabetes mellitus

Pharmacokinetics:

PO: Onset 1 hr, peak 2 hr, duration 12-24 hr; excreted unchanged by kidneys, crosses placenta, enters breast milk, half-life 8 hr

Interactions/incompatibilities:

• Increased toxicity of: lithium, nondepolarizing skeletal muscle relaxants, digitalis

• Decreased effects of: antidiabetics

• Decreased absorption of thiazides: cholestyramine, colestipol

• Decreased hypotensive response: indomethacin

• Increased action of: quinidine

NURSING CONSIDERATIONS

Assess:

• Weight, I&O daily to determine fluid loss; effect of drug may be decreased if used qd

• Rate, depth, rhythm of respiration, effect of exertion

• B/P lying, standing, postural hypotension may occur

• Electrolytes: potassium, sodium, chloride; include BUN, blood sugar, CBC, serum creatinine, blood pH, ABGs

• Glucose in urine if patient is diabetic

Administer:

• In AM to avoid interference with sleep if using drug as a diuretic

• Potassium replacement if potassium is less than 3.0

• With food, if nausea occurs, absorption may be decreased slightly

Evaluate:

• Improvement in edema of feet, legs, sacral area daily if medication is being used in CHF

• Improvement in CVP q8h

• Signs of metabolic acidosis: drowsiness, restlessness

• Signs of hypokalemia: postural hypotension, malaise, fatigue, tachycardia, leg cramps, weakness

• Rashes, temperature elevation qd

• Confusion, especially in elderly; take safety precautions if needed

Teach patient/family:

• To increase fluid intake 2-3 L/day unless contraindicated, to rise slowly from lying or sitting position

• To notify physician of muscle weakness, cramps, nausea, dizziness

• Drug may be taken with food or milk

• That blood sugar may be increased in diabetics

• Take early in day to avoid nocturia

Lab test interferences:

Increase: BSP retention, calcium, amylase

Decrease: PBI, PSP

Treatment of overdose: Lavage if taken orally, monitor electrolytes, administer dextrose in saline

---

metoprolol tartrate

(met-oh′proe-lole)

Betaloc,* Lopresor,* Lopressor

Func. class.: Antihypertensive

Chem. class.: β_1-blocker

Action: Produces falls in B/P without reflex tachycardia or significant reduction in heart rate through β-blocking effects; elevated plasma renins are reduced; blocks β_2-adrenergic receptors in bronchial, vascular smooth muscle only at high doses (decreases rate of SA node)

Uses: Mild to moderate hypertension, acute myocardial infarction to reduce cardiovascular mortality

Dosage and routes:
Hypertension
• *Adult:* PO 50 mg bid, or 100 mg qd, may give up to 200-450 mg in divided doses

Myocardial infarction
• *Adult:* (Early treatment) IV BOL 5 mg q 2 min × 3, then 50 mg PO 15 min after last dose and q6h × 48 hr; (late treatment) PO maintenance 100 mg bid for 3 mo

Available forms include: Tabs 50, 100 mg; inj IV 1 mg/ml

Side effects/adverse reactions:

CV: Hypotension, *bradycardia, CHF: Palpitations,* dysrhythmias, *cardiac arrest, AV block*

CNS: Insomnia, dizziness, mental changes, hallucinations, *depression,* anxiety, headaches, nightmares, confusion, fatigue

GI: Nausea, vomiting, colitis, cramps, *diarrhea,* constipation, flatulence, dry mouth, *hiccups*

INTEG: Rash, purpura, alopecia, dry skin, urticaria, pruritus

HEMA: Agranulocytosis, eosinophilia, thrombocytopenia, purpura

EENT: Sore throat, dry burning eyes

GU: Impotence

RESP: Bronchospasm, dyspnea, wheezing

Contraindications: Hypersensitivity to β-blockers, cardiogenic shock, heart block (2nd, 3rd degree), sinus bradycardia, CHF, bronchial asthma

Precautions: Major surgery, pregnancy (C), lactation, diabetes mellitus, renal disease, thyroid disease, COPD, heart failure, CAD, nonallergic bronchospasm, hepatic disease

Pharmacokinetics:
PO: Peak 2-4 hr, duration 13-19 hr; half-life 3-4 hr, metabolized in liver (metabolites), excreted in urine, crosses placenta, enters breast milk

Interactions/incompatibilities:
• Increased hypotension, bradycardia: reserpine, hydralazine, methyldopa, prazosin, anticholinergics
• Decreased antihypertensive effects: indomethacin, sympathomimetics
• Increased hypoglycemic effects: insulin
• Decreased bronchodilation: theophyllines

NURSING CONSIDERATIONS
Assess:
• ECG, directly when giving IV during initial treatment
• I&O, weight daily
• B/P, pulse q4h; note rate, rhythm, quality
• Apical/radial pulse before administration; notify physician of any significant changes
• Baselines in renal, liver function tests before therapy begins

Administer:
• PO ac, hs, tablet may be crushed or swallowed whole
• Reduced dosage in renal dysfunction
• IV, keep patient recumbent for 3 hr

Perform/provide:
• Storage in dry area at room temperature, do not freeze

Evaluate:
• Therapeutic response: decreased B/P after 1-2 wk
• Edema in feet, legs daily
• Skin turgor, dryness of mucous membranes for hydration status

Teach patient/family:
• Take with or immediately after meals
• Not to discontinue drug abruptly, taper over 2 wk, may cause precipitate angina
• Not to use OTC products containing α-adrenergic stimulants (nasal decongestants, OTC cold preparations) unless directed by physician

---

• To report bradycardia, dizziness, confusion, depression, fever, sore throat, shortness of breath to physician

• To take pulse at home, advise when to notify physician

• To avoid alcohol, smoking, sodium intake

• To comply with weight control, dietary adjustments, modified exercise program

• To carry Medic Alert ID to identify drug you are taking, allergies

• To avoid hazardous activities if dizziness is present

• To report symptoms of CHF: difficult breathing, especially on exertion or when lying down, night cough, swelling of extremities

• Take medication hs to maintain effect of orthostatic hypotension

• Wear support hose to minimize effects of orthostatic hypotension

Lab test interferences:

Increase: Liver function tests, renal function tests

Treatment of overdose: Lavage, IV atropine for bradycardia, IV theophylline for bronchospasm, digitalis, O_2, diuretic for cardiac failure, hemodialysis, hypotension administer vasopressor (norepinephrine)

---

metronidazole/metronidazole HCl

(me-troe-ni'da-zole)

Apo-Metronidazole,* Flagyl, Metryl, Neo-Tric,* Novonidazole,* PMS-Metronidazole,* Satric, Trikacide,* Flagyl IV, Flagyl IV RTU, Metro IV, Femazole, Metric, Metronid, Protostat

Func. class.: Trichomonacide, amebicide

Chem. class.: Nitroimidazole derivative

Action: Direct-acting amebicide/ trichomonacid binds, degrades DNA inside, outside organism

Uses: Intestinal amebiasis, amebic abscess, trichomoniasis, refractory trichomoniasis, bacterial anaerobic infections, giardiasis

Dosage and routes:

Trichomoniasis

• *Adult:* PO 250 mg tid × 7 days, or 2 g in single dose; do not repeat treatment for 2-3 wk

Refractory trichomoniasis

• *Adult:* PO 250 mg bid × 10 days

Amebic abscess

• *Adult:* PO 500-750 mg tid × 5-10 days

• *Child:* PO 35-50 mg/kg/day in 3 divided doses × 10 days

Intestinal amebiasis

• *Adult:* PO 750 mg tid × 5-10 days

• *Child:* PO 35-50 mg/kg/day in 3 divided doses × 10 days; then give oral iodoquinol

Anerobic bacterial infections

• *Adult:* IV INF 15 mg/kg over 1 hr, then 7.5 mg/kg IV or PO q6h, not to exceed 4 g/day

Giardiasis

• *Adult:* PO 250 mg tid × 5 days

• *Child:* PO 5 mg/kg tid × 5 days

Available forms include: Tabs 250, 500 mg; film-coated tabs 250, 1500 mg; inj IV 5 mg/vial; HCl inj IV 500 mg

Side effects/adverse reactions:

CV: Flat T waves

HEMA: Leukopenia, bone marrow aplasia

INTEG: Rash, pruritus, urticaria, flushing

CNS: Headache, dizziness, confusion, depression, fatigue, drowsiness, insomnia, paresthesia, peripheal neuropathy, *convulsions,* incoordination, depression

EENT: Blurred vision, sore throat, retinal edema, dry mouth, bitter taste, furry tongue, glossitis, stomatitis

GI: Nausea, vomiting, diarrhea, epigastric distress, anorexia, constipation, abdominal cramps, metallic taste, ***pseudomembranous colitis***

GU: Polyuria, albuminuria, dysuria, cystitis, decreased libido, ***nephrotoxicity,*** incontinence, dyspareunia

Contraindications: Hypersensitivity to this drug, renal disease, hepatic disease, contracted visual or color fields, blood dyscrasias, pregnancy (1st trimester), lactation, CNS disorders

Precautions: *Candida* infections, pregnancy (2nd, 3rd trimesters) (B)

Pharmacokinetics:

IV/PO: Peak 1-2 hr, half-life 6⅓-11½ hr, crosses placenta, excreted in feces

Interactions/incompatibilities:

• Disulfiramic reaction: alcohol
• May increase action: warfarin
• Psychosis: disulfiram
• Decreased action of this drug: phenobarbital

NURSING CONSIDERATIONS

Assess:

• Stools during entire treatment; should be clear at end of therapy, for 1 yr before patient is considered cured (amebiasis)
• Vision by ophthalmalogic exam during, after therapy; vision problems occur often
• I&O, stools for number, frequency, character

Administer:

• PO after meals to avoid GI symptoms, metallic taste

Perform/provide:

• Storage in light-resistant container

Evaluate:

• Neurotoxicity: peripheral neuropathy, seizures, dizziness, incoordination, pruritus, joint pains; may be discontinued
• Allergic reaction: fever, rash,

itching, chills; drug should be discontinued if these occur
• Superimposed infection: fever, monilial growth, fatigue, malaise
• Renal and reproductive dysfunction: dysuria, polyuria, impotence, dyspareunia, decreased libido

Teach patient family:

• Urine may turn dark reddish brown
• Proper hygiene after BM: handwashing technique
• Need for compliance with dosage schedule, duration of treatment
• To use condoms if treatment for trichomoniasis or cross contamination may occur
• Treatment of both partners is necessary

Lab test interferences:

Decrease: AST, ALT

---

metyrosine

(me-tye′roe-seen)
Demser

Func. class.: Antihypertensive
Chem. class.: Adrenergic blocker

Action: Inhibits enzyme tyrosine hydroxylase, resulting in decreased levels of catecholamines

Uses: Pheochromocytoma

Dosage and routes:

• *Adult and child >12 yr:* PO 250 mg qid, may increase by 250-500 mg qd to a max of 4 g/day in divided doses

Available forms include: Caps 250 mg

Side effects/adverse reactions:

CV: Severe rebound hypertension
CNS: Sedation, drowsiness, dizziness, headache, depression, EPS, hallucinations, psychosis, agitation
INTEG: Rash, urticaria
EENT: Dry mouth
GU: Dysuria, oliguria, hematuria, enuresis, impotence
GI: Nausea, vomiting, anorexia,

diarrhea, abdominal pain

MISC: Breast swelling, nasal stuffiness

Contraindications: Hypersensitivity, essential hypertension, children <12 yr

Precautions: Pregnancy (C), lactation, hepatic disease, renal disease

Pharmacokinetics:

PO: Onset 2 days, duration 3-4 days; half-life 3.4-3.7 hr, excreted in urine

Interactions/incompatibilities:

• Increased sedation: CNS depressants: alcohol, barbiturates, antipsychotics

• Decreased effects of: levodopa

• Extrapyramidal effects: phenothiazines, haloperidol

NURSING CONSIDERATIONS

Assess:

• Electrolytes: K, Na, Cl, CO_2

• Renal function studies: catecholamines, BUN, creatinine

• Hepatic function studies: AST, ALT, alk phosphatase

• ECG, BMR

• B/P, other VS throughout treatment

• Weight daily, I&O

Administer:

• Antiemetic or antidiarrheals for vomiting, diarrhea

Perform/provide:

• Fluids to 2 L/day to prevent crystallization by kidneys

Evaluate:

• Change in behavior or personality: psychosis, anxiety, hallucinations, EPS

• Nausea, vomiting, diarrhea

• Edema in feet, legs daily

• Skin turgor, dryness of mucous membranes for hydration status

Teach patient/family:

• Take each dose with a full glass of water; maintain sufficient daily intake

• Not to drive or perform hazardous tasks if behavioral changes, dizziness, or drowsiness occurs

• Avoid alcohol or other CNS depressants

• Notify physician if any of following occur: jaw stiffness, drooling, speech difficulty, tremors, disorientation, diarrhea, painful urination

Lab test interferences:

False increase: Urinary catecholamines

Treatment of overdose: Administer vasopressors, discontinue drug

---

mexiletine HCl

(mex-il'e-teen)

Mexitil

Func. class.: Antidysrhythmic (Class IB)

Chem. class.: Lidocaine analog

Action: Increases electrical stimulation threshold of ventrical, HIS Purkinge system, which stabilizes cardiac membrane

Uses: Ventricular tachycardia, ventricular dysrhythmias during cardiac surgery, myocardial infarction

Dosage and routes:

• *Adult:* IV BOL 150-250 mg over 3-5 min, then begin IV INF; IV INF 0.5-1.5 mg/min; PO maintenance dose 200-400 mg q8h

Available forms include: Caps 150, 200, 250 mg; inj

Side effects/adverse reactions:

CNS: Headache, dizziness, confusion, convulsions

EENT: Blurred vision, hearing loss

GI: Nausea, vomiting, anorexia, diarrhea, abdominal pain, *hepatitis,* dry mouth

CV: Hypotension, bradycardia, angina, PVCs, *heart block, cardiovascular collapse, arrest,* sinus node slowing, *left ventricular failure*

RESP: Dyspnea, ***fibrosis, embolism,*** pneumonia
INTEG: Rash, alopecia
HEMA: ***Thrombocytopenia, leukopenia, agranulocytosis, hypoplastic anemia,*** SLE syndrome
GU: Urinary hesitancy, decreased libido
Contraindications: Hypersensitivity to amides, cardiogenic shock, blood dyscrasias, severe heart block, supraventricular dysrhythmias
Precautions: Pregnancy, lactation, children, renal disease, liver disease, CHF, respiratory depression, myasthenia gravis
Pharmacokinetics:
PO: Peak 1 hr; half-life 12 hr, metabolized by liver, excreted unchanged by kidneys (10%), excreted in breast milk
Interactions/incompatibilities:
• Increased effects: cimetidine, phenytoin, propranolol, quinidine
NURSING CONSIDERATIONS
Assess:
• ECG continuously to determine increased PR or QRS segments; if these develop, discontinue immediately; watch for increased ventricular ectopic beats, may need to rebolus
• IV infusion rate using infusion pump, run at less than 4 mg/min
• Blood levels (therapeutic level 1-2 μg/ml)
• B/P continuously for fluctuations
• I&O ratio, electrolytes (K, Na, Cl)
Administer:
• IM injection in deltoid; aspirate to avoid intravascular administration; check site daily for infiltration or extravasation
Evaluate:
• Malignant hyperthermia: tachypnea, tachycardia, changes in B/P, increased temperature
• Cardiac rate, respiration: rate, rhythm, character, continuously
• Respiratory status: rate, rhythm, lung fields for rales, watch for respiratory depression
• CNS effects: dizziness, confusion, psychosis, paresthesias, convulsions; drug should be discontinued
• Lung fields, bilateral rales may occur in CHF patient
• Increased respiration, increased pulse, drug should be discontinued
Lab test interferences:
Increase: CPK
Treatment of overdose: O_2, artificial ventilation, ECG, administer dopamine for circulatory depression, administer diazepam or thiopental for convulsions

---

mezlocillin sodium

(mez-loe-sill′in)
Mezlin
Func. class.: Broad-spectrum antibiotic
Chem. class.: Extended-spectrum penicillin

Action: Interferes with cell wall replication of susceptible organisms; osmotically unstable cell wall swells, bursts from osmotic pressure
Uses: Effective for gram-positive cocci (*S. aureus, S. viridans, S. faecalis, S. pneumoniae*), gram-negative cocci (*N. gonorrhoeae*), gram-positive bacilli, *C. perfringens, C. tetani,* gram-negative bacilli (*Bacteroides, E. coli, H. influenzae, Klebsiella, P. mirabilis, Peptococcus, Peptostreptococcus, M. morganii, Enterobacter, Serratia, Pseudomonas, P. vulgaris, P. rettgeri, Shigella, Citrobacter, Veillonella*)
Dosage and routes:
• *Adult:* IM/IV 200-300 mg/kg/day in divided doses q4-6h, may

give up to 24 g/day for severe infections

• *Child:* IM/IV 50 mg/kg in divided doses q4-6h

• *Infants >7 days:* >2000 g 75 mg/kg q6h; ≤2000 g 75 mg/kg q8h

• *Infants ≤7 days:* 75 mg/kg q12h

Available forms include: Powder for inj IM, IV 1, 2, 3, 4 g; IV INF 2, 3, 4 g

Side effects/adverse reactions:

HEMA: Anemia, increased bleeding time, *bone marrow depression, granulocytopenia*

GI: Nausea, vomiting, diarrhea, increased AST, ALT, abdominal pain, glossitis, colitis

GU: Oliguria, proteinuria, hematuria, (vaginitis, moniliasis), *glomerulonephritis*

CNS: Lethargy, hallucinations, anxiety, depression, twitching, *coma, convulsions*

META: Hyperkalemia, hypokalemia, alkalosis, hypernatremia

Contraindications: Hypersensitivity to penicillins

Precautions: Pregnancy (B), hypersensitivity to cephalosporins, neonates

Pharmacokinetics:

IM: Peak 45 min

IV: Peak 5 min

Half-life 50-55 min, partially metabolized in liver, excreted in urine, bile, breast milk (small amount), crosses placenta

Interactions/incompatibilities:

• Decreased antimicrobial effectiveness of this drug: tetracyclines, erythromycins, aminoglycosides IV

• Increased penicillin concentrations when used with: aspirin, probenecid

NURSING CONSIDERATIONS

Assess:

• I&O ratio; report hematuria, oliguria since penicillin in high doses is nephrotoxic

• Any patient with compromised renal system since drug is excreted slowly in poor renal system function; toxicity may occur rapidly

• Liver studies: AST, ALT

• Blood studies: WBC, RBC, H&H, bleeding time

• Renal studies: urinalysis, protein, blood

• C&S before drug therapy; drug may be taken as soon as culture is taken

Administer:

• Drug after C&S has been completed

Perform/provide:

• Adrenalin, suction, tracheostomy set, endotracheal intubation equipment

• Adequate fluid intake (2000 ml) during diarrhea episodes

• Scratch test to assess allergy, after securing order from physician; usually done when penicillin is only drug of choice

• Storage at room temperature; reconstituted solution is stable for 24 hr refrigerated

Evaluate:

• Therapeutic effectiveness: absence of fever, draining wounds

• Bowel pattern before and during treatment

• Skin eruptions after administration of penicillin to 1 wk after discontinuing drug

• Respiratory status: rate, character, wheezing, and tightness in chest

• Allergies before initiation of treatment, and reaction of each medication; highlight allergies on chart, Kardex

Teach patient/family:

• Culture may be taken after completed course of medication

• To report sore throat, fever, fa-

tigue; could indicate superimposed infection
• To wear or carry Medic Alert ID if allergic to penicillins
• To notify nurse of diarrhea stools
Lab test interferences:
Decrease: Uric acid
False positive: Urine glucose, urine protein
Treatment of overdose: Withdraw drug, maintain airway, administer epinephrine, aminophylline, O_2, IV corticosteroids for anaphylaxis

---

miconazole

(mi-kon′a-zole)
Monistat, Monistat IV
Func. class.: Antifungal
Chem. class.: Imidazole

Action: Alters cell membranes and interferes with fungal enzyme systems
Uses: Coccidioidomycosis, candidiasis, cryptococcosis, paracoccidioidomycosis, chronic mucocutaneous candidiasis, fungal meningitis; IV used for severe infections only
Dosage and routes:
• *Adult:* IV INF 200-3600 mg/day; may be divided in 3 infusions 200-1200 mg/infusion; may need to repeat course; INTRATHECAL 20 mg given simultaneously with IV for fungal meningitis q3-7 days
• *Adult:* TOP apply to affected areas bid; VAG CREAM apply × 1 wk qhs or × 3 days (Monistat 3 vs Monistat 7)
• *Child:* IV 20-40 mg/kg/day, not to exceed 15 mg/kg/inf
Available forms include: Inj IV 10 mg/ml; aerosol 2%; cream, lotion, powder, vaginal cream (2%); supp, vaginal 100, 200 mg
Side effects/adverse reactions:
CV: Tachycardia, dysrhythmias (rapid IV)

INTEG: Pruritus, rash, fever, flushing, anaphylaxis, hives
CNS: Drowsiness, headache
GU: Valvovaginal burning, itching, hyponatremia, pelvic cramps (topical forms)
GI: Nausea, vomiting, anorexia, diarrhea, cramps
HEMA: Decreased Hct, **thrombocytopenia,** hyperlipidemia
Contraindications: Hypersensitivity
Precautions: Renal disease, hepatic disease
Pharmacokinetics:
IV: Half-life triphasic 0.4, 2.1, 24.1 hr, metabolized in liver, excreted in feces, urine (inactive metabolites), >90% protein binding
Interactions/incompatibilities:
• Increased action of: anticoagulants
• Decreased action of both drugs: amphotericin
NURSING CONSIDERATIONS
Assess:
• Cardiac system: B/P, pulse, ECG; watch for increasing pulse, cardiac dysrhythmias; drug should be discontinued if these occur
• Blood studies: Hct, Ca, cholesterol, triglycerides, platelets, sodium
Administer:
• After C&S is obtained to identify causative organism
• Antiemetic for nausea and vomiting as ordered
• After test dose of 200 mg is given by physician; watch for allergic reactions
• IV over ½-1 hr, dilute in 200 ml isotonic saline or D_5W
• IV after diluting with NS if hyponatremia has occurred
• Topical by rubbing into affected area
Evaluate:
• Therapeutic response: decreased fever, malaise, rash, negative C&S

for infecting organism

• For phlebitis, pruritus; may need benadryl IV, continue unless reaction is severe

• Allergic reaction after test dose; have epinephrine available

Perform/provide:

• Storage of diluted preparations at room temperature for 24 hr

Teach patient/family:

• That long-term therapy may be needed to clear infection (1 wk-1 mo)

• Proper hygiene: handwashing techniques, nail care

• Report vaginitis; use light-day pad for vaginal dose

• Avoid contact with eyes, nose

• Avoid sexual contact during treatment; reinfection may occur

---

miconazole nitrate (topical)

(mi-kon'a-zole)

Micatin, Monistat-Derm, Monistat

Func. class.: Local antiinfective
Chem. class.: Antifungal

Action: Interferes with fungal DNA replication; binds sterols in fungal cell membrane, which increases permeability, leaking of nutrients

Uses: Tinea pedis, tinea cruris, tinea corporis, tinea versicolor, vaginal or vulvae candida albicans

Dosage and routes:

• *Adult and child:* TOP apply to affected area bid × 2-4 wk

• *Adult:* INTRA VAG give 1 applicator or suppository × 7 days hs

Available forms include: Cream, lotion, powder, spray 2%; vag cream 2%; vag supp 100, 200 mg

Side effects/adverse reactions:

GU: Vulvovaginal burning, itching, pelvic cramps

INTEG: Rash, urticaria, stinging, burning

Contraindications: Hypersensitivity

Precautions: Child <2 yr, pregnancy, lactation

Interactions/incompatibilities: None known

NURSING CONSIDERATIONS

Administer:

• Enough medication to completely cover lesions

• After cleansing with soap, water before each application, dry well

Perform/provide:

• Storage at room temperature in dry place

Evaluate:

• Allergic reaction: burning, stinging, swelling, redness

• Therapeutic response: decrease in size, number of lesions

Teach patient/family:

• To apply with glove to prevent further infection

• To avoid use of OTC creams, ointments, lotions unless directed by physician

• To use medical asepsis (hand washing) before, after each application

• To avoid contact with eyes

---

microfibrillar collagen hemostat

Avitene, MCH

Func. class.: Hemostatic
Chem. class.: Purified cattle collagen

Action: Platelets adhere to hemostat, cause aggregation to form thrombi

Uses: For hemostasis in surgery

Dosage and routes:

• *Adult and child:* TOP apply to bleeding area after drying with sponge, compress for 1-5 min, may reapply if needed

---

Side effects/adverse reactions:
INTEG: Rash, abscess, allergic reactions
HEMA: Hematoma
Contraindications: Hypersensitivity, closure of skin incision, contaminated wounds
Precautions: Pregnancy (C)
Interactions/incompatibilities:
None known
NURSING CONSIDERATIONS
Administer:
• Using gloves with forceps; area must be dry for drug to work
• Only new product; do not resterilize
Evaluate:
• Allergy: fever, rash, itching, jaundice
• Bleeding: mucous membranes, epistaxis, ecchymosis, petechiae, hematuria, hematemesis

mineral oil

Agoral Plain, Fleet Mineral Oil Enema, Kondremul, Neo-Cultol, Petrogalar Plain, Zymenol

Func. class.: Laxative
Chem. class.: Petroleum hydrocarbon

Action: Eases passage of stool by decreasing water absorption from feces
Uses: Constipation, preparation for bowel surgery or examination
Dosage and routes:
• *Adult:* PO 15-30 ml hs; ENEMA 4 oz
• *Child:* PO 5-15 ml hs; ENEMA 1-2 oz
Available forms include: Oil, enema; jelly 55%; susp 1.4, 2.5, 2.75 mg/5 ml
Side effects/adverse reactions:
CNS: Muscle weakness
GI: Nausea, vomiting, anorexia, diarrhea, pruritus ani, hepatic infiltration

META: Hypoprothrombinemia
RESP: Lipoid pneumonia
Contraindications: Hypersensitivity, intestinal obstruction, abdominal pain, nausea/vomiting
Precautions: Pregnancy
Pharmacokinetics: Excreted in feces
Interactions/incompatibilities:
• May increase effect of: oral anticoagulants
NURSING CONSIDERATIONS
Assess:
• Blood, urine electrolytes if drug is used often by patient
• I&O ratio to identify fluid loss
Administer:
• Alone for better absorption; do not take within 1 hr of other drugs or within 1 hr of antacids, milk, or cimetidine
• In morning or evening (oral dose)
Evaluate:
• Therapeutic response: decrease in constipation
• Cause of constipation; identify whether fluids, bulk, or exercise is missing from lifestyle
• Cramping, rectal bleeding, nausea, vomiting; if these symptoms occur, drug should be discontinued
Teach patient/family:
• Not to use laxatives for long-term therapy; bowel tone will be lost
• That normal bowel movements do not always occur daily
• Do not use in presence of abdominal pain, nausea, vomiting
• Notify physician if constipation unrelieved or if symptoms of electrolyte imbalance occur: muscle cramps, pain, weakness, dizziness

M

minocycline HCl

(mi-noe-sye'kleen)

Minocin, Vectrin, Minocin IV

Func. class.: Broad spectrum antibiotic

Chem. class.: Tetracycline

Action: Inhibits protein synthesis, phosphorylation in microorganisms by binding to 30S ribosomal subunits, reversibly binding to 50S ribosomal subunits

Uses: Syphilis, chlamydia trachomatis, gonorrhea, lymphogranuloma venereum, staphylococci

Dosage and routes:

• *Adult:* PO/IV 200 mg, then 100 mg q12h or 50 mg q6h

• *Child >8 yr:* PO/IV 4 mg/kg then 4 mg/kg/day PO in divided doses q12h; administer IV in 500-1000 ml sol over 6 hr

Gonorrhea

• *Adult:* PO 200 mg, then 100 mg q12h × 4 days

Chlamydia trachomatis

• *Adult:* PO 100 mg bid × 7 days

Syphilis

• *Adult:* PO 200 mg, then 100 mg q12h × 10-15 days

Available forms include: Tabs 50, 100 mg; oral susp 50 mg/5 ml; powder for inj IV 100 mg/vial

Side effects/adverse reactions:

CNS: Fever headache, paresthesia

HEMA: Eosinophilia, neutropenia, thrombocytopenia, leukocytosis, hemolytic anemia

EENT: Dysphagia, glossitis, decreased calcification of deciduous teeth, abdominal pain, oral candidiasis

GI: Nausea, vomiting, diarrhea, anorexia, enterocolitis, *hepatotoxicity,* flatulence, abdominal cramps, epigastric burning, stomatitis, *pseudomembranous colitis*

CV: Pericarditis

GU: Increased BUN, polyuria, polydipsia, renal failure, nephrotoxicity

INTEG: Rash, urticaria, photosensitivity, increased pigmentation, exfoliative dermatitis, pruritus, angioedema

Contraindications: Hypersensitivity to tetracyclines, children <8 yr

Precautions: Renal disease, hepatic disease, lactation, pregnancy

Pharmacokinetics:

PO: Half-life 11-17 hr; excreted in feces, crosses placenta, excreted in breast milk, 55%-88% protein bound

Interactions/incompatibilities:

• Decreased effect of this drug: antacids, $NaHCO_3$, dairy products, alkali products

• Increased effect: anticoagulants

• Decreased effect: penicillins

• Nephrotoxicity: methoxyflurane

NURSING CONSIDERATIONS

Assess:

• I&O ratio

• Blood studies: PT, CBC, AST, ALT, BUN, creatinine

Administer:

• After C&S obtained

• 2 hr before or after laxative or ferrous products; 3 hr after antacid

Perform/provide:

• Storage in tight, light-resistant container at room temperature

Evaluate:

• Therapeutic response: decreased temperature, absence of lesions, negative C&S

• Allergic reactions: rash, itching, pruritus, angioedema

• Nausea, vomiting, diarrhea; administer antiemetic, antacids as ordered

• Overgrowth of infection: increased temperature, malaise, redness, pain, swelling, drainage, perineal itching, diarrhea, changes in cough or sputum

---

Teach patient/family:
• To avoid sun exposure since burns may occur; sunscreen does not seem to decrease photosensitivity
• Of diabetic to avoid use of Clinistix, Diastix, or Tes-Tape for urine glucose testing
• That all prescribed medication must be taken to prevent superimposed infection
• To avoid milk products

Lab test interferences:
False positive: Urine glucose with Clinistix or Tes-Tape
False increase: Urinary catecholamines

---

minoxidil

(mi-nox-i-dill)

Loniten

Func. class.: Antihypertensive
Chem. class.: Vasodilator—peripheral

Action: Directly relaxes arteriolar smooth muscle, causing vasodilation

Uses: Severe hypertension not responsive to other therapy; topically to treat alopecia

Dosage and routes:
• *Adult:* PO 5 mg/day not to exceed 100 mg daily, usual range 10-40 mg/day in single doses
• *Child <12 yr:* (Initial) 0.2 mg/kg/day; (effective range) 0.25-1 mg/kg/day; (max) 50 mg/day
Alopecia
• *Adult:* Apply topically, rub into scalp daily
Available forms include: Tabs 2.5, 10 mg

Side effects/adverse reactions:
CV: Severe rebound hypertension, tachycardia, angina, increased T wave, *CHF, pulmonary edema,* edema, sodium, water retention
CNS: Drowsiness, dizziness, seda-

tion, headache, depression
GI: Nausea, vomiting
GU: Gynecomastia, breast tenderness
INTEG: Pruritus, *Stevens-Johnson syndrome,* rash, hirsutism

Contraindications: Acute myocardial infarction, dissecting aortic aneurysm, hypersensitivity, pheochromocytoma

Precautions: Pregnancy (C), lactation, children, renal disease, CAD, CHF

Pharmacokinetics:
PO: Onset 30 min, peak 2-3 hr, duration 75 hr; half-life 4.2 hr, metabolized in liver, metabolites, excreted in urine, feces

Interactions/incompatibilities:
• Orthostatic hypotension: guanethidine

NURSING CONSIDERATIONS
Monitor:
• Electrolytes: K, Na, Cl, CO_2
• Renal function studies: catecholamines, BUN, creatinine
• Hepatic function studies: AST, ALT, alk phosphatase
• B/P, other VS throughout treatment
• Weight daily, I&O

Administer:
• With meals for better absorption, to decrease GI symptoms
• With β-blocker or diuretic

Evaluate:
• Therapeutic response: decreased B/P or increased hair growth
• Nausea
• Edema in feet, legs daily
• Skin turgor, dryness of mucous membranes for hydration status
• Rales, dyspnea, orthopnea

Teach patient/family:
• That body hair will increase but is reversible after discontinuing treatment
• Not to discontinue drug abruptly
• To report pitting edema, dizziness, weight gain >5 lb, shortness

M

---

of breath, bruising or bleeding, heart rate >20 beats/min over normal, severe indigestion, dizziness, light-headedness, panting, new or aggravated symptoms of angina

• To take drug exactly as prescribed or serious side effects may occur

Lab test interferences:

Increase: Renal function studies

Decrease: Hgb/Hct/RBC

Treatment of overdose: Administer normal saline IV, phenylephrine, angiotensin II, vasopressor, dopamine may reverse hypotension

---

mitomycin

(mye-toe-mye′sin)

Mutamycin

Func. class.: Antineoplastic, antibiotic

Action: Inhibits DNA synthesis, primarily; derived from *Streptomyces caespitosus;* appears to cause cross-linking of DNA

Uses: Pancreas, stomach cancer

Dosage and routes:

• *Adult:* IV 2 mg/m²/day × 5 days, stop drug for 2 days, then repeat cycle; or 20 mg/m² as a single dose, repeat cycle in 6-8 wk; stop drug if platelets are <75,000/mm³ or WBC is <3000/mm³

Available forms include: Inj IV

Side effects/adverse reactions:

HEMA: Thrombocytopenia, leukopenia, myelosuppression, anemia

GI: Nausea, vomiting, anorexia, stomatitis, hepatotoxicity, diarrhea

GU: Urinary retention, *renal failure,* edema

INTEG: Rash, alopecia

RESP: Fibrosis, pulmonary infiltrate, dyspnea

CNS: Fever, headache, confusion, drowsiness, syncope, fatigue

EENT: Blurred vision

Contraindications: Hypersensitivity, pregnancy (1st trimester), as a single agent, thrombocytopenia, coagulation disorders

Precautions: Renal disease, bone marrow depression

Pharmacokinetics: Half-life 17 min, metabolized in liver, 10% excreted in urine (unchanged)

Interactions/incompatibilities:

• Increased toxicity: other antineoplastics or radiation

NURSING CONSIDERATIONS

Assess:

• CBC, differential, platelet count weekly; withhold drug if WBC is <4000/mm³ or platelet count is <75,000/mm³; notify physician of these results

• Pulmonary function tests, chest x-ray before, during therapy; chest x-ray should be obtained q2 wk during treatment

• Renal function studies: BUN, serum uric acid, urine CrCl, electrolytes before, during therapy

• I&O ratio; report fall in urine output to <30 ml/hr

• Monitor temperature q4h; fever may indicate beginning infection

• Liver function tests before, during therapy: bilirubin, AST, ALT, alk phosphatase as needed or monthly

Administer:

• Medications by oral route if possible; avoid IM, SC, IV routes to prevent infections

• Antiemetic 30-60 min before giving drug to prevent vomiting

• Antibiotics for prophylaxis of infection

• Slow IV infusion using 21-, 23-, 25-gauge needle; check for extravasation

• Topical or systemic analgesics for pain

• Transfusion for anemia

• Antispasmodic for GI symptoms

Perform/provide:

• Strict medical asepsis, protective

isolation if WBC levels are low

• Liquid diet: carbonated beverages, Jello; dry toast, crackers may be added if patient is not nauseated or vomiting

• Rinsing of mouth tid-qid with water, hydrogen peroxide; brushing of teeth bid-tid with soft brush or cotton-tipped applicators for stomatitis; use unwaxed dental floss

• Warm compresses at injection site for inflammation; check for extravasation

• Storage at room temperature for 1 wk after reconstituting or 2 wk refrigerated

Evaluate:

• Bleeding: hematuria, guaiac, bruising, petechiae, mucosa or orifices q8h

• Dyspnea, rales, unproductive cough, chest pain, tachypnea, fatigue, increased pulse, pallor, lethargy

• Food preferences; list likes, dislikes

• Effects of alopecia on body image; discuss feelings about body changes

• Edema in feet, joint, stomach pain, shaking

• Inflammation of mucosa, breaks in skin

• Yellowing of skin, sclera, dark urine, clay-colored stools, itchy skin, abdominal pain, fever, diarrhea

• Buccal cavity q8h for dryness, sores, ulceration, white patches, oral pain, bleeding, dysphagia

• Local irritation, pain, burning at injection site

• GI symptoms: frequency of stools, cramping

• Acidosis, signs of dehydration: rapid respirations, poor skin turgor, decreased urine output, dry skin, restlessness, weakness

Teach patient/family:

• Why protective isolation precautions are necessary

• To report any complaints, side effects to nurse or physician

• That hair may be lost during treatment and wig or hairpiece may make the patient feel better; tell patient that new hair may be different in color, texture

• To avoid foods with citric acid, hot or rough texture

• To report any bleeding, white spots, ulcerations in mouth; tell patient to examine mouth qd

---

mitotane

(mye´toe-tane)
Lysodren
Func. class.: Antineoplastic
Chem. class.: Hormone, adrenal cytotoxic agent

Action: Acts on adrenal cortex to suppress activity; a cytotoxic agent that suppresses activity rather then causing cell death

Uses: Adrenocortical carcinoma

Dosage and routes:

• *Adult:* PO 9-10 g/day in divided doses tid or qid; may need to decrease dose if severe reactions occur

Available forms include: Tabs 500 mg

Side effects/adverse reactions:

GI: Nausea, vomiting, anorexia, diarrhea

GU: Proteinuria, hematuria

INTEG: Rash

*RESP: **Fibrosis, pulmonary infiltrate***

CV: Hypertension, orthostatic hypotension

CNS: Lightheadedness, flushing, sedation, vertigo

EENT: Lethargy, blurring, retinopathy

Contraindications: Hypersensitivity

Precautions: Lactation, hepatic

M

disease, pregnancy (C)

Pharmacokinetics: Adequately absorbed orally (40%), excreted in urine, bile

Interactions/incompatibilities:

• Decreased effects of corticosteroids

NURSING CONSIDERATIONS

Assess:

• Pulmonary function tests, chest x-ray films before, during therapy; chest film should be obtained q2wk during treatment

• Renal function studies: BUN, serum uric acid, urine CrCl electrolytes before, during therapy

• I&O ratio

• Urinary 17-OHCS before, during treatment

Administer:

• Antacid before oral agent, give drug after evening meal, before bedtime

• Antiemetic 30-60 min before giving drug to prevent vomiting

• Antispasmodic

Perform/provide:

• Deep breathing exercises with patient tid-qid; place in semi-Fowler's position

• Liquid diet, including cola, Jello; dry toast or crackers may be added if patient is not nauseated or vomiting

• Increase fluid intake to 2-3 L/day to prevent dehydration

• HOB increased to facilitate breathing

• Increased fluid intake to 2000 ml/day if not contraindicated

• Nutritious diet with iron, vitamin supplements as ordered

• Storage in tight, light-resistant container

Evaluate:

• Dyspnea, rales, unproductive cough, chest pain, tachypnea, fatigue, increased pulse, pallor, lethargy

• Food preferences; list likes, dislikes

• Muscular weakness, fatigue, oliguria, hypoglycemia

• Frequency of stools, characteristics: cramping, acidosis, signs of dehydration (rapid respirations, poor skin turgor, decreased urine output, dry skin, restlessness, weakness)

• Symptoms indicating severe allergic reactions: rash, pruritus, itching, flushing

Teach patient/family:

• To report any complaints, side effects to nurse or physician

• To report any changes in breathing, coughing

• To avoid driving or other activities requiring alertness

Lab test interferences:

Decrease: PBI, urinary 17-OHCS

---

molindone HCl

(moe-lin'done)

Moban

Func. class.: Antipsychotic/neuroleptic

Chem. class.: Dihydroindolone

Action: Depresses cerebral cortex, hypothalamus, limbic system, which control activity, aggression; blocks neurotransmission produced by dopamine at synapse; exhibits strong α-adrenergic, anticholinergic blocking action; mechanism for antipsychotic effects is unclear

Uses: Psychotic disorders

Dosage and routes:

• *Adult:* PO 50-75 mg/day increasing to 225 mg/day if needed

Available forms include: Tabs 5, 10, 25, 50, 100 mg; conc 20 mg/ml

Side effects/adverse reactions:

*RESP: **Laryngospasm,** dyspnea, **respiratory depression***

CNS: Extrapyramidal symptoms:

pseudoparkinsonism, akathisia, dystonia, tardive dyskinesia, drowsiness, headache, seizures
HEMA: Anemia, leukopenia, leukocytosis, **agranulocytosis**
INTEG: Rash, photosensitivity, dermatitis
EENT: Blurred vision, glaucoma
GI: Dry mouth, nausea, vomiting, anorexia, constipation, diarrhea, jaundice, weight gain
GU: Urinary retention, urinary frequency, enuresis, impotence, amenorrhea, gynecomastia
CV: Orthostatic hypotension, hypertension, **cardiac arrest**, ECG changes, **tachycardia**
Contraindications: Hypersensitivity, blood dyscrasias, coma, child, brain damage, bone marrow depression, alcohol and barbiturate withdrawal states
Precautions: Pregnancy, lactation, seizure disorders, hypertension, hepatic disease, cardiac disease
Pharmacokinetics:
PO: Onset erratic, peak 1½ hr, duration 24-36 hr; metabolized by liver, excreted in urine, may cross placenta, enters breast milk, half-life 1½ hr
Interactions/incompatibilities:
Decreased levels of phenytoin, tetracyclines
NURSING CONSIDERATIONS
Assess:
• Swallowing of PO medication; check for hoarding or giving of medication to other patients
• I&O ratio; palpate bladder if low urinary output occurs
• Bilirubin, CBC, liver function studies monthly
• Urinalysis is recommended before, during prolonged therapy
Administer:
• Antiparkinsonian agent, after securing order from physician, to be used if EPS occur

• IM injection into large muscle mass
• Concentrate mixed in orange or grapefruit juice
Perform/provide:
• Decreased noise input by dimming lights, avoiding loud noises
• Supervised ambulation until stabilized on medication; do not involve in strenuous exercise program because fainting is possible; patient should not stand still for long periods of time
• Increased fluids to prevent constipation
• Sips of water, candy, gum for dry mouth
• Storage in tight, light-resistant container
Evaluate:
• Therapeutic response: decrease in emotional excitement, hallucinations, delusions, paranoia, reorganization of patterns of thought, speech
• Affect, orientation, LOC, reflexes, gait, coordination, sleep pattern disturbances
• B/P standing and lying; also include pulse, respirations; take these q4h during initial treatment; establish baseline before starting treatment; report drops of 30 mm Hg
• Dizziness, faintness, palpitations, tachycardia on rising
• EPS including akathisia (inability to sit still, no pattern to movements), tardive dyskinesia (bizarre movements of the jaw, mouth, tongue, extremities), pseudoparkinsonism (rigidity, tremors, pill rolling, shuffling gait)
• Skin turgor daily
• Constipation, urinary retention daily; if these occur, increase bulk and water in diet
Teach patient/family:
• That orthostatic hypotension may occur and to rise from sitting or lying position gradually

italics = common side effects   **bold italic** = life threatening reactions

• To avoid hot tubs, hot showers, or tub baths since hypotension may occur

• To avoid abrupt withdrawal of this drug or EPS may result; drugs should be withdrawn slowly

• To avoid OTC preparations (cough, hayfever, cold) unless approved by physician since serious drug interactions may occur; avoid use with alcohol or CNS depressants, increased drowsiness may occur

• To avoid hazardous activities if drowsiness or dizziness occurs

• To use sunscreen during sun exposure to prevent burns

• Regarding compliance with drug regimen

• About necessity for meticulous oral hygiene since oral candidiasis may occur

• To report impaired vision, jaundice, tremors, muscle twitching

• In hot weather, heat stroke may occur; take extra precautions to stay cool

Lab test interferences:

Increase: Liver function tests, cardiac enzymes, cholesterol, blood glucose, prolactin, bilirubin, PBI, cholinesterase, ^{131}I

Decrease: Hormones (blood, urine)

False positive: Pregnancy tests, PKU

False negative: Urinary steroids

Treatment of overdose: Lavage if orally injested, provide an airway; *do not induce vomiting*

---

morphine sulfate

(mor'feen)

Duramorph PF, MS Contin, RMS, Roxanol, Roxanol SR

Func. class.: Narcotic analgesics
Chem. class.: Opiate

Controlled Substance Schedule II

Action: Inhibits ascending pain pathways in CNS, increases pain threshold, alters pain perception

Uses: Severe pain

Dosage and routes:

• *Adult:* SC/IM 4-15 mg q4h prn; PO 30-60 mg q4h prn; EXT REL q8-12h; REC 30-60 mg q4h prn; IV 4-10 mg diluted in 4-5 ml of water for injection, over 5 min

• *Child:* SC 0.1-0.2 mg/kg, not to exceed 15 mg

Available forms include: Inj SC, IM, IV 2, 4, 5, 8, 10, 15 mg/ml; sol tabs 10, 15, 30 mg; oral sol 10, 20 mg/5 ml, 20 mg/10 ml, 20 mg/ml; oral tabs 15, 30 mg; rec supp 5, 10, 20 mg; ext rel tabs 300 mg

Side effects/adverse reactions:

CNS: Drowsiness, dizziness, confusion, headache, sedation, euphoria

GI: Nausea, vomiting, anorexia, constipation, cramps

GU: Increased urinary output, dysuria

INTEG: Rash, urticaria, bruising, flushing, diaphoresis, pruritus

EENT: Tinnitus, blurred vision, miosis, diplopia

CV: Palpitations, bradycardia, change in B/P

RESP: Respiratory depression

Contraindications: Hypersensitivity, addiction (narcotic)

Precautions: Addictive personality, pregnancy, lactation, increased intracranial pressure, MI (acute), severe heart disease, respiratory depression, hepatic disease, renal disease, child <18 yr

Pharmacokinetics:

PO: Onset variable, peak variable, duration variable

SC: Onset 15-30 min, peak 50-90 min

IV: Peak 20 min

Metabolized by liver, excreted by kidneys, crosses placenta, excreted in breast milk, half-life 2½-3 hr

---

Interactions/incompatibilities:

• Effects may be increased with other CNS depressants: alcohol, narcotics, sedative/hypnotics, antipsychotics, skeletal muscle relaxants

NURSING CONSIDERATIONS

Assess:

• I&O ratio; check for decreasing output; may indicate urinary retention

Administer:

• With antiemetic if nausea, vomiting occur

• When pain is beginning to return; determine dosage interval by patient response

Perform/provide:

• Storage in light-resistant area at room temperature

• Assistance with ambulation

• Safety measures: siderails, night light, call bell within easy reach

Evaluate:

• Therapeutic response: decrease in pain

• CNS changes: dizziness, drowsiness, hallucinations, euphoria, LOC, pupil reaction

• Allergic reactions: rash, urticaria

• Respiratory dysfunction: respiratory depression, character, rate, rhythm; notify physician if respirations are <12/min

• Need for pain medication, physical dependence

Teach patient/family:

• To report any symptoms of CNS changes, allergic reactions

• That physical dependency may result when used for extended periods of time

• Withdrawal symptoms may occur: nausea, vomiting, cramps, fever, faintness, anorexia

Lab test interferences:

Increase: Amylase

Treatment of overdose: Narcan 0.2-0.8 IV, O_2, IV fluids, vasopressors

---

moxalactam disodium

(mox'a-lak-tam)

Moxam

Func. class.: Antibiotic, broad-spectrum

Chem. class.: Cephalosporin (3rd generation)

Action: Inhibits bacterial cell wall synthesis, rendering cell wall osmotically unstable

Uses: Gram-negative bacilli: *H. influenzae, E. coli, P. mirabilis, Klebsiella, Serratia;* gram-positive organisms: *S. pneumoniae, S. pyogenes, S. aureus;* serious lower respiratory tract, urinary tract, skin, bone infections, septicemia, meningitis

Dosage and routes:

• *Adult:* IM/IV 2-4 g/day in equally divided doses q8-12h × 10-14 days

Severe infections

• *Adult:* IM/IV 4 g q8h

• *Child:* IM/IV 50 mg/kg q6-8h

• *Neonate:* IM/IV 50 mg/kg q6-8h

Available forms include: Powder for inj IM, IV 1, 2, 10 g

Side effects/adverse reactions:

CNS: Headache, dizziness, weakness, paresthesia, fever, chills

GI: Nausea, vomiting, diarrhea, anorexia, pain, glossitis, bleeding, increased AST, ALT, bilirubin, LDH, alk phosphatase, abdominal pain

GU: Proteinuria, vaginitis, pruritus, candidiasis, increased BUN, *nephrotoxicity, renal failure*

HEMA: Leukopenia, *thrombocytopenia, agranulocytosis,* anemia, neutropenia, lymphocytosis, eosinophilia, *pancytopenia, hemolytic anemia*

INTEG: Rash, urticaria, dermatitis, *anaphylaxis*

---

italics = common side effects   **bold italic** = life threatening reactions

RESP: Dyspnea

Contraindications: Hypersensitivity to cephalosporins

Precautions: Hypersensitivity to penicillins, pregnancy, lactation, renal disease

Pharmacokinetics:

IV: Peak 5 min

IM: Peak ½-2 hr

Half-life 2-2½ hr, 25% bound by plasma proteins, 80% eliminated unchanged in urine in 24 hr, crosses placenta, blood-brain barrier, excreted in breast milk, not metabolized

Interactions/incompatibilities:

• Do not mix with tetracyclines, erythromycins, calcium chloride, magnesium salts in same parenteral fluid

• Decreased effects: tetracyclines, erythromycins

• Increased toxicity: aminoglycosides, furosemides, probenecid, sulfinpyrazone, colistin, ethacrynic acid

NURSING CONSIDERATIONS

Assess:

• Nephrotoxicity: increased BUN, creatinine

• I&O daily

• Blood studies: AST, ALT, CBC, Hct, bilirubin, LDH, alk phosphatase, Coombs' test monthly if patient is on long-term therapy

• Electrolytes: potassium, sodium, chloride monthly if patient is on long-term therapy

• Bowel pattern qd; if severe diarrhea occurs, drug should be discontinued; may indicate pseudomembranous colitis

• IV site for extravasation, phlebitis; change site q72h

Administer:

• For 10-14 days to ensure organism death, prevent superimposed infection

• With food if needed for GI symptoms

• After C&S

Evaluate:

• Therapeutic response: decreased fever, malaise, chills

• Urine output: if decreasing, notify physician; may indicate nephrotoxicity

• Allergic reactions: rash, urticaria, pruritus, chills, fever, joint pain, angioedema; may occur few days after therapy begins

• Bleeding: ecchymosis, bleeding gums, hematuria, stool guaiac daily

• Overgrowth of infection: perineal itching, fever, malaise, redness, pain, swelling, drainage, rash, diarrhea, change in cough, sputum

Teach patient/family:

• To use yogurt or buttermilk to maintain intestinal flora, decrease diarrhea

• To take all medication prescribed for length of time ordered

• To report sore throat, bruising, bleeding, joint pain; may indicate blood dyscrasias (rare)

Lab test interferences:

Increase (false): Creatinine (serum urine), urinary 17-KS

False positive: Urinary protein, direct Coombs', urine glucose

Interference: Cross-matching

Treatment of overdose: Epinephrine, antihistamines, resuscitate if needed (anaphylaxis)

---

multivitamins

Many brands

Func. class.: Vitamin

Action: Needed for adequate metabolism

Uses: Prevention and treatment of vitamin deficiencies

Dosage and routes:

• *Adult and child:* PO depends on brand

Available forms include: Many forms available
Side effects/adverse reactions: None known
Pharmacokinetics: Not known
Interactions/incompatibilities:
• Check each vitamin for specific interactions
NURSING CONSIDERATIONS
Evaluate:
• Therapeutic response: check each individual vitamin for guidelines
• Vitamin deficiency: usually more than one vitamin is deficient
Teach patient/family:
• That adequate nutrition must be maintained to prevent further deficiencies
• Drug interaction that should be avoided
• Stress compliance with regimen
• To avoid using flavored multivitamins as candy; child may overdose
• Store out of children's reach

---

nadolol

(nay-doe'-lole)
Corgard
Func. class.: Antihypertensive, antianginal
Chem. class.: β-adrenergic receptor blocker

Action: Long-acting, nonselective β-adrenergic receptor blocking agent; mechanism is similar to propranolol and not generally described as calcium channel blocker
Uses: Chronic stable angina pectoris, mild to moderate hypertension
Dosage and routes:
• *Adult:* PO 40 mg qd, increase to 40-80 mg q3-7 days; maintenance 80-240 mg/day for angina, 80-320 mg/day for hypertension
Available forms include: Oral tabs 40-160 mg

Side effects/adverse reactions:
RESP: Dyspnea, respiratory dysfunction
CV: Bradycardia, hypotension, CHF, palpitations
CNS: Fatigue, dizziness, headache, paresthesia, mental changes
HEMA: Agranulocytosis, thrombocytopenia
GI: Nausea, vomiting, diarrhea, colitis, constipation, cramps, dry mouth
INTEG: Rash, pruritus, fever
CNS: Depression, hallucinations, dizziness, fatigue, lethargy, paresthesias
EENT: Sore throat, *laryngospasm*
Contraindications: Hypersensitivity to this drug, cardiac failure, cardiogenic shock, 2nd or 3rd degree heart block, bronchospastic disease
Precautions: Diabetes mellitus, pregnancy, renal disease, lactation, CHF, hyperthyroidism, COPD
Pharmacokinetics:
PO: Onset variable, peak 3-4 hr, duration 17-24 hr; half-life 16-20 hr, not metabolized, excreted in urine (unchanged), bile, breast milk
Interactions/incompatibilities:
• Increased effects: barbiturates, hypoglycemia, reserpine, levodopa, digitalis, ergots, neuromuscular blocking agents
• Decreased effects: norepinephrine, xanthines, isoproterenol
NURSING CONSIDERATIONS
Assess:
• B/P, pulse, respirations during beginning therapy
• Weight qd, report gain of 5 lb
• I&O ratio, CrCl if kidney damage is diagnosed
• qd, note need to be administered more often
Administer:
• With 8 oz water on empty stomach (oral tablet)
Evaluate:
• Pain: duration, time started, ac-

N

---

tivity being performed, character
• Tolerance if taken over long period of time
• Headache, lightheadedness, decreased B/P; may indicate a need for decreased dosage
Teach patient/family:
• That drug may be taken before stressful activity: exercise, sexual activity
• That SL may sting when drug comes in contact with mucous membranes
• To avoid hazardous activities if dizziness occurs
• Stress patient compliance with complete medical regimen
• To make position changes slowly to prevent fainting
• Decrease dosage over 2 weeks to prevent cardiac damage
Lab test interferences:
Increase: Serum potassium, serum uric acid, ALT/AST, alk phosphatase, LDH
Decrease: Blood glucose

---

nafcillin sodium

(naf-sill′-in)

Nafcil, Nallpen, Unipen

Func. class.: Broad-spectrum antibiotic

Chem. class.: Penicillinase-resistant penicillin

Action: Interferes with cell wall replication of susceptible organisms; osmotically unstable cell wall swells, bursts from osmotic pressure

Uses: Effective for gram-positive cocci *(S. aureus, S. viridans, S. pneumoniae)*, infections caused by penicillinase-producing *Staphylococcus*

Dosage and routes:
• *Adult:* IM/IV 2-3 g/day in divided doses q4-6h; PO 2-4 g/day in divided doses q4-6h

• *Child:* IM/IV 25 mg/kg/day q12h; PO 25 mg/kg/day in divided doses q6h

Available forms include: Caps 250 mg; tabs 500 mg; powder for oral susp 250 mg/5 ml; powder for inj IM, IV 500 mg, 1, 2, 10 g; IV 1, 1.5, 2, 4 g

Side effects/adverse reactions:

HEMA: Anemia, increased bleeding time, *bone marrow depression, granulocytopenia*

GI: Nausea, vomiting, diarrhea, increased AST, ALT, abdominal pain, glossitis, colitis

GU: Oliguria, proteinuria, hematuria, *vaginitis, moniliasis, glomerulonephritis*

CNS: Lethargy, hallucinations, anxiety, depression, twitching, *coma, convulsions*

META: Hyperkalemia, hypokalemia, alkalosis, hypernatremia

Contraindications: Hypersensitivity to penicillins

Precautions: Pregnancy (B), hypersensitivity to cephalosporins, neonates

Pharmacokinetics:

IM/PO: Peak 30-60 min, duration 4-6 hr, half-life 1 hr, excreted in bile, urine

Interactions/incompatibilities:

• Decreased antimicrobial effectiveness of this drug: tetracyclines, erythromycins

• Increased penicillin concentrations when used with: aspirin, probenecid

NURSING CONSIDERATIONS

Assess:

• I&O ratio; report hematuria, oliguria since penicillin in high doses is nephrotoxic

• Any patient with compromised renal system since drug is excreted slowly in poor renal system function; toxicity may occur rapidly

• Liver studies: AST, ALT

• Blood studies: WBC, RBC,

H&H, bleeding time
• Renal studies: urinalysis, protein, blood
• C&S before drug therapy; drug may be taken as soon as culture is taken
Administer:
• Drug after C&S has been completed
Perform/provide:
• Adrenalin, suction, tracheostomy set, endotracheal intubation equipment
• Adequate fluid intake (2000 ml) during diarrhea episodes
• Scratch test to assess allergy, after securing order from physician; usually done when penicillin is only drug of choice
• Storage in tight container; refrigerate reconstituted solution
Evaluate:
• Therapeutic effectiveness: absence of fever, draining wounds
• Bowel pattern before and during treatment
• Skin eruptions after administration of penicillin to 1 wk after discontinuing drug
• Respiratory status: rate, character, wheezing, and tightness in chest
• Allergies before initiation of treatment, and reaction of each medication; highlight allergies on chart, Kardex
Teach patient/family:
• Aspects of drug therapy, including need to complete course of medication to ensure organism death (10-14 days); culture may be taken after completed course
• To report sore throat, fever, fatigue; could indicate superimposed infection
• To wear or carry Medic Alert ID if allergic to penicillins
• To notify nurse of diarrhea stools
Lab test interferences:
Decrease: Uric acid

False positive: Urine glucose, urine protein
Treatment of overdose: Withdraw drug, maintain airway, administer epinephrine, aminophylline, O_2, IV corticosteroids for anaphylaxis

---

nalbuphine HCl

(nal'byoo-feen)
Nubain
Func. class.: Non-narcotic analgesics
Chem. class.: Opiate

Action: Inhibits ascending pain pathways in CNS, increases pain threshold, alters pain perception
Uses: Moderate to severe pain
Dosage and routes:
• *Adult:* SC/IM/IV 10-20 mg q3-6h prn, not to exceed 160 mg/day
Available forms include: Inj SC, IM, IV 10, 20 mg/ml
Side effects/adverse reactions:
CNS: Drowsiness, dizziness, confusion, headache, sedation, euphoria
GI: Nausea, vomiting, anorexia, constipation, cramps
GU: Increased urinary output, dysuria
INTEG: Rash, urticaria, bruising, flushing, diaphoresis, pruritus
EENT: Tinnitus, blurred vision, miosis, diplopia
CV: Palpitations, bradycardia, change in B/P
*RESP: **Respiratory depression***
Contraindications: Hypersensitivity, addiction (narcotic)
Precautions: Addictive personality, pregnancy, lactation, increased intracranial pressure, MI (acute), severe heart disease, respiratory depression, hepatic disease, renal disease
Pharmacokinetics:
SC/IM/IV: Duration 3-6 h; metab-

olized by liver, excreted by kidneys, half-life 5 hr

Interactions/incompatibilities:

• Effects may be increased with other CNS depressants: alcohol, narcotics, sedative/hypnotics, antipsychotics, skeletal muscle relaxants

NURSING CONSIDERATIONS
Assess:

• I&O ratio; check for decreasing output; may indicate urinary retention

Administer:

• With antiemetic if nausea, vomiting occur

• When pain is beginning to return; determine dosage interval by patient response

Perform/provide:

• Storage in light-resistant area at room temperature

• Assistance with ambulation

• Safety measures: siderails, night light, call bell within easy reach

Evaluate:

• Therapeutic response: decrease in pain

• CNS changes: dizziness, drowsiness, hallucinations, euphoria, LOC, pupil reaction

• Allergic reactions: rash, urticaria

• Respiratory dysfunction: respiratory depression, character, rate, rhythm; notify physician if respirations are <12/min

• Need for pain medication, physical dependence

Teach patient/family:

• To report any symptoms of CNS changes, allergic reactions

• That physical dependency may result when used for extended periods of time

• Withdrawal symptoms may occur: nausea, vomiting, cramps, fever, faintness, anorexia

Lab test interferences:

Increase: Amylase

Treatment of overdose: Narcan

0.2-0.8 IV, O_2, IV fluids, vasopressors

---

nalidixic acid

(nal-i-dix'ik)

NegGram, Nogram, Cybis, Wintomylon

Func. class.: Urinary tract antiseptic

Chem. class.: Synthetic naphthyridine derivative

Action: Appears to inhibit DNA polymerization, primary target being single-stranded DNA precursors in late stages of chromosomal replication

Uses: Urinary tract infections (acute/chronic) caused by *E. coli, Klebsiella, Enterobacter, P. mirabilis, P. vulgaris, P. morganii*

Dosage and routes:

• *Adult:* PO 1 g qid × 1-2 wk, 2 g/day for long-term treatment

• *Child >3 months:* PO 55 mg/kg/day in 4 divided doses for 1-2 wk; 33 mg/kg/day for long-term treatment

Available forms include: Tabs 100, 250, 500 mg; susp 250 mg/2 ml

Side effects/adverse reactions:

INTEG: Pruritus, rash, urticaria, photosensitivity

CNS: Dizziness, headache, drowsiness, insomnia convulsions

GI: Nausea, vomiting, abdominal pain, diarrhea

EENT: Sensitivity to light, blurred vision, change in color perception

Contraindications: Hypersensitivity, 1st trimester of pregnancy, 1st trimester of breast feeding, CNS damage, liver disease, liver failure, infants <3 months

Precautions: Elderly, renal disease, hepatic disease

Pharmacokinetics:

PO: Peak 1-2 hr, metabolized in liver, excreted in urine (unchange/

---

conjugates), crosses placenta, enters breast milk

Interactions/incompatibilities:

• Increased effects of: oral coagulants

• Decreased effects of: antacids

NURSING CONSIDERATIONS

Assess:

• Blood count for patients on chronic therapy

• I&O ratio, urine pH <5.5 is ideal

• Renal, hepatic function

• Photosensitivity: if present, drug should be discontinued

Administer:

• After clean-catch urine is obtained for C&S

• Two daily doses if urine output is high or if patient has diabetes

Perform/provide:

• Limited intake of alkaline foods, drugs: milk, dairy products, peanuts, vegetables, alkaline antacids, sodium bicarbonate

• Protection from freezing

Evaluate:

• CNS symptoms: insomnia, vertigo, headache, drowsiness, convulsions

• Allergy: fever, flushing, rash, urticaria, pruritus

Teach patient/family:

• That photosensitivity occurs; that patient should avoid sunlight or use sunscreen to prevent burns

• Take medication with food or milk to decrease GI irritation

• Instruct client to protect suspension from freezing, shake well before taking

• May cause drowsiness; instruct client to seek aid in walking, other activities; advise client not to drive or operate machinery while on medication

• Instruct clients with diabetes that Clinitest may prove false positive for glucose; therefore Tes-Tape or Clinistix should be used

Lab test interferences:

False positive: Urinary glucose

False increase: 17-OHCS, VMA

---

naloxone HCl

Narcan

Func. class.: Narcotic antagonist

Chem. class.: Thebaine derivative

Action: Competes with narcotics at narcotic receptor sites

Uses: Narcotic-induced respiratory depression including pentazocine, propoxyphene

Dosage and routes:

Narcotic-induced respiratory depression

• *Adult:* IV/SC/IM 0.4-2 mg; repeat q2-3 min, if needed

Postoperative respiratory depression

• *Adult:* IV 0.1-0.2 mg q2-3 min prn

• *Child:* IV/IM/SC 0.01 mg/kg q2-3 min prn

Asphyxia neonatorum

• *Neonates:* IV 0.01 mg/kg given into umbilical vein after delivery, may repeat in q2-3 min × 3 doses

Available forms include: Inj IV, IM, SC 0.02, 0.4, 1 mg/ml

Side effects/adverse reactions:

HEMA: ***Thrombocytopenia, agranulocytosis, leukopenia, neutropenia, hemolytic anemia,*** increased pro-time

CNS: Stimulation, drowsiness, dizziness, confusion, convulsion, headache, flushing, hallucinations, coma

GI: Nausea, vomiting, GI bleeding, diarrhea, heartburn, anorexia, ***hepatitis***

INTEG: Rash, urticaria, bruising

EENT: Tinnitus, hearing loss

CV: Rapid pulse, pulmonary edema

RESP: Wheezing, hyperpnea

ENDO: Hypoglycemia, hyponatre-

N

---

mia, hypokalemia

Contraindications: Hypersensitivity to salicylates, GI bleeding, bleeding disorders, children <3 yr, lactation, vitamin K deficiency

Precautions: Anemia, hepatic disease, renal disease, Hodgkin's disease, pregnancy (B)

Pharmacokinetics:

PO: Onset 15-30 min, peak 1-2 hr, duration 4-6 hr

REC: Onset slow, duration 4-6 hr

Metabolized by liver, excreted by kidneys, crosses placenta, excreted in breast milk, half-life 1-3½ hr

Interactions/incompatibilities:

• Decreased effects: antacids, steroids, urinary alkalizers

• Increased blood loss: alcohol, heparin

• Increased effects: anticoagulants, insulin, methotrexate

• Decreased effects: probenecid, spironolactone, sulfinpyrazone, sulfonamides

• Toxic effects: para-aminobenzoic acid

• In large doses salicylates lower blood sugar levels, deplete liver glycogens; use cautiously with diabetics

NURSING CONSIDERATIONS
Assess:

• VS q3-5 min

• ABGs including PO_2, PCO_2

Administer:

• Only if resuscitative equipment is nearby

Perform/provide:

• Storage at room temperature in darkness

Evaluate:

• Signs of withdrawal in drug-dependent individuals

• Cardiac status: tachycardia, hypertension

• Respiratory dysfunction: respiratory depression, character, rate, rhythm; if respirations are <10/ min, respiratory stimulant should be administered

Lab test interferences:

Increase: Bleeding time, pro-time, serum uric acid, bilirubin, alk phosphatase, AST, ALT, amylase, CO_2, urinary protein

Decrease: Serum potassium, PBI, cholesterol, urinary PSP

Interfere: Urine VMA, 5-HIAA, urine glucose, pregnancy test

Overdose:

Symptoms: Nausea, vomiting, tinnitus, dizziness, tachycarida, respiratory alkalosis, then respiratory acidosis respiratory depression

Treatment: Lavage, activated charcoal, monitor electrolytes, VS

---

naltrexone HCl

(nal-trex′one)

Trexan

Func. class.: Narcotic antagonist
Chem. class.: Thebaine derivative

Action: Competes with narcotics at narcotic receptor sites

Uses: Blockage of opioid analgesics

Dosage and routes:

• *Adult:* PO 25 mg, may give 25 mg after 1 hr if there are no withdrawal symptoms; 50-150 mg may be given qd depending on patient need

Available forms include: Tabs 50 mg

Side effects/adverse reactions:

HEMA: **Thrombocytopenia, agranulocytosis, leukopenia, neutropenia, hemolytic anemia,** increased pro-time

CNS: Stimulation, drowsiness, dizziness, confusion, convulsion, headache, flushing, hallucinations, coma

GI: Nausea, vomiting, GI bleeding, diarrhea, heartburn, anorexia, **hepatitis**

INTEG: Rash, urticaria, bruising
EENT: Tinnitus, hearing loss
CV: Rapid pulse, pulmonary edema
RESP: Wheezing, hyperpnea
ENDO: Hypoglycemia, hyponatremia, hypokalemia
Contraindications: Hypersensitivity to salicylates, GI bleeding, bleeding disorders, children <3 yr, lactation, vitamin K deficiency
Precautions: Anemia, hepatic disease, renal disease, Hodgkin's disease, pregnancy (C)
Pharmacokinetics:
PO: Onset 15-30 min, peak 1-2 hr, duration 4-6 hr
REC: Onset slow, duration 4-6 hr
Metabolized by liver, excreted by kidneys, crosses placenta, excreted in breast milk, half-life 1-3½ hr
Interactions/incompatibilities:
• Decreased effects: antacids, steroids, urinary alkalizers
• Increased blood loss: alcohol, heparin
• Increased effects: anticoagulants, insulin, methotrexate
• Decreased effects: probenecid, spironolactone, sulfinpyrazone, sulfonamides
• Toxic effects: para-aminobenzoic acid
• In large doses salicylates lower blood sugar levels, deplete liver glycogens; use cautiously with diabetics

NURSING CONSIDERATIONS
Assess:
• VS q3-5 min
• ABGs including PO_2, PCO_2
Administer:
• Only if resuscitative equipment is nearby
Perform/provide:
• Storage in tight container
Evaluate:
• Signs of withdrawal in drug-dependent individuals
• Cardiac status: tachycardia, hypertension

• Respiratory dysfunction: respiratory depression, character, rate, rhythm; if respirations are <10/min, respiratory stimulant should be administered
Lab test interferences:
Increase: Bleeding time, pro-time, serum uric acid, bilirubin, alk phosphatase, AST, ALT, amylase, CO_2, urinary protein
Decrease: Serum potassium, PBI, cholesterol, urinary PSP
Interfere: Urine VMA, 5-HIAA, urine glucose, pregnancy test
Overdose:
Symptoms: Nausea, vomiting, tinnitus, dizziness, tachycardia, respiratory alkalosis, then respiratory acidosis respiratory depression
Treatment: Lavage, activated charcoal, monitor electrolytes, VS

---

nandrolone decanoate/ nandrolone phenpropionate
(nan'droe-lone)
Androlone-50, Androlone-D 50, Deca-Durabolin, Hybolin Decanoate, Anabolin, Anorolone, Durabolin, Hybolin Improved, Nandrobolic, Nandrolin

Func. class.: Androgenic anabolic steroid
Chem. class.: Halogenated testosterone derivative

Action: Increases weight by building body tissue, increases potassium, phosphorus, chloride, nitrogen levels, increases bone development
Uses: Tissue building, severe disease, refractory anemias, metastatic breast cancer
Dosage and routes:
Tissue building (possibly effective)
• *Adult:* IM 50-100 mg q3-4 wk (decanoate)

• *Child 2-13 yr:* IM 25-50 mg q3-4 wk (decanoate)

Severe disease/refractory anemias
• *Adult:* IM 100-200 mg q wk (decanoate)

Breast cancer
• *Adult:* IM 50-100 mg q wk (phenpropionate)

Available forms include: Phenpropionate inj IM 25, 50 mg/ml; decanoate inj IM 50, 100, 200 mg/ml

Side effects/adverse reactions:

INTEG: Rash, acneiform lesions, oily hair, skin, flushing, sweating, acne vulgaris, alopecia, hirsutism

CNS: Dizziness, headache, fatigue, tremors, paresthesias, flushing, sweating, anxiety, lability, insomnia

MS: Cramps, spasms

CV: Increased B/P

GU: Hematuria, amenorrhea, vaginitis, decreased libido, decreased breast size, clitoral hypertrophy, testicular atrophy

GI: Nausea, vomiting, constipation, weight gain, *cholestatic jaundice*

EENT: Carpal tunnel syndrome, conjunctional edema, nasal congestion

ENDO: Abnormal GTT

Contraindications: Severe renal disease, severe cardiac disease, severe hepatic disease, hypersensitivity, pregnancy (C), lactation, abnormal genital bleeding

Precautions: Diabetes mellitus, CV disease, MI

Pharmacokinetics:

IM: Metabolized in liver, excreted in urine, crosses placenta, excreted in the breast milk

Interactions/incompatibilities:
• Increased effects of: oral antidiabetics, oxyphenbutazone
• Increased PT: anticoagulants
• Edema: ACTH, adrenal steroids
• Decreased effects of: insulin

NURSING CONSIDERATIONS

Assess:
• Weight daily, notify physician if weekly weight gain is >5 lb
• B/P q4h
• I&O ratio; be alert for decreasing urinary output, increasing edema
• Growth rate in children since growth rate may be uneven (linear/bone growth) when used for extended periods of time
• Electrolytes: K, Na, Cl, Ca; cholesterol
• Liver function studies: ALT, AST, bilirubin

Administer:
• Titrated dose, use lowest effective dose

Perform/provide:
• Diet with increased calories, protein; decrease sodium if edema occurs

Evaluate:
• Therapeutic response: increased appetite, increased stamina
• Edema, hypertension, cardiac symptoms, jaundice
• Mental status: affect, mood, behavioral changes, aggression
• Signs of masculinization in female: increased libido, deepening of voice, breast tissue, enlarged clitoris, menstrual irregularities; male: gynecomastia, impotence, testicular atrophy
• Hypercalcemia: lethargy, polyuria, polydipsia, nausea, vomiting, constipation, drug may need to be decreased
• Hypoglycemia in diabetics; since oral anticoagulant action is decreased

Teach patient/family:
• Drug needs to be combined with complete health plan: diet, rest, exercise
• To notify physician if therapeutic response decreases
• Not to discontinue medication abruptly

• Teach patient all aspects of drug usage, including changes in sex characteristics
• Females to report menstrual irregularities
• That 1-3 mo course is necessary for response in breast cancer
• Procedure for use of buccal tablets: requires 30-60 min to dissolve, change absorption site with each dose; do not eat, drink, chew, or smoke while tablet is in place

Lab test interferences:
Increase: Serum cholesterol, blood glucose, urine glucose
Decrease: Serum calcium, serum potassium, T_4, T_3, thyroid ^{131}I uptake test, urine 17-OHCS, 17-KS, PBI, BSP

---

naphazoline HCl

(naf-az′oh-leen)
Privine

Func. class.: Nasal decongestant
Chem. class.: Sympathomimetic amine

Action: Produces vasoconstriction (rapid, long-acting) of arterioles thereby decreasing fluid exudation, mucosal engorgement

Uses: Nasal congestion

Dosage and routes:
• *Adult:* INSTILL 2 gtts or sprays to nasal mucosa q3-4h
• *Child 6-12 yr:* INSTILL 1-2 gtts or sprays, repeat q3-4h prn, not to exceed 5 days

Available forms include: Sol 0.05%

Side effects/adverse reactions:
GI: Nausea, vomiting, anorexia
EENT: Irritation, burning, sneezing, stinging, dryness, rebound congestion
INTEG: Contact dermatitis
CNS: Anxiety, restlessness, tremors, weakness, insomnia, dizziness, fever, headache

Contraindications: Hypersensitivity to sympathomimetic amines

Precautions: Child <6 yr, elderly, diabetes, cardiovascular disease, hypertension, hyperthyroidism, increased ICP, prostatic hypertrophy

Interactions/incompatibilities:
• Hypertension: MAOIs, β-adrenergic blockers
• Hypotension: methyldopa, mecamylamine, reserpine

NURSING CONSIDERATIONS

Administer:
• No more than q4h
• For <4 consecutive days

Perform/provide:
• Environmental humidification to decrease nasal congestion, dryness
• Storage in light-resistant containers; do not expose to high temperatures

Evaluate:
• Redness, swelling, pain in nasal passages

Teach patient/family:
• Stinging may occur for several applications; drying of mucosa may be decreased by environmental humidification
• To notify physician if irregular pulse, insomnia, dizziness, or tremors occur
• Proper administration to avoid systemic absorption

N

---

naphazoline HCl

(naf-az′oh-leen)
AK-Con Ophthalmic, Albalon, Clear Eyes, Muro's Opcon, Nafazair, Naphcon, Vasocon

Func. class.: Ophthalmic vasoconstrictor
Chem. class.: Direct imidazoline derivative

Action: Vasoconstriction of eye arterioles; decreases eye engorgement by stimulation of α-adrenergic receptors

---

Uses: Relieves hyperemia, irritation in superficial corneal vascularity
Dosage and routes:
• *Adult:* INSTILL 1-2 gtts q3-4h
Available forms include: Sol 0.1%, 0.05%, 0.03%, 0.02%, 0.012%

Side effects/adverse reactions:
CNS: Headache, dizziness, sedation, anxiety, weakness, sweating (systemic absorption)
CV: Hypertension, dysrhythmias, tachycardia, CV collapse (systemic absorption)
EENT: Pupil dilation, increased intraocular pressure, photophobia
Contraindications: Hypersensitivity, glaucoma (narrow-angle)
Precautions: Hypertension, hyperthyroidism, elderly, severe arteriosclerosis, cardiac disease, pregnancy
Pharmacokinetics:
INSTILL: Duration 2-3 hr
Interactions/incompatibilities:
• Increased pressor effects: MAOIs, tricyclic antidepressants
NURSING CONSIDERATIONS
Perform/provide:
• Storage in tight, light-resistant container
Teach patient/family:
• To report change in vision, blurring, or loss of sight; breathing trouble, sweating, flushing, anxiety, weakness
• Method of instillation; tilt head backward, hold dropper over eye, drop medication inside lower lid, using pressure on inside corner of eye hold 1 min, do not touch dropper to eye
• That blurred vision will decrease with repeated use of drug
• To notify physician if headache, spots, redness, pain occur; discontinue use

---

naproxen/naproxen sodium

(na-prox′en)
Naprosyn/Anaprox
Func. class.: Nonsteroidal
Chem. class.: Propionic acid derivative

Action: Inhibits prostaglandin synthesis by decreasing an enzyme needed for biosynthesis; possesses analgesic, antiinflammatory, antipyretic properties
Uses: Mild to moderate pain, osteoarthritis, rheumatoid arthritis
Dosage and routes:
• *Adult:* PO 250-500 mg bid, not to exceed 1 g/day (base); 525 mg, then 275 mg q6-8h prn, not to exceed 1475 mg (sodium)
Available forms include: Tabs 250, 275, 375, 500 mg

Side effects/adverse reactions:
GI: Nausea, anorexia, vomiting, diarrhea, jaundice, *cholestatic hepatitis,* constipation, flatulence, cramps, dry mouth, peptic ulcer
CNS: Dizziness, drowsiness, fatigue, tremors, confusion, insomnia, anxiety, depression
CV: Tachycardia, peripheral edema, palpitations, dysrhythmias
INTEG: Purpura, rash, pruritus, sweating
*GU: **Nephrotoxicity:*** dysuria, hematuria, oliguria, azotemia
*HEMA: **Blood dyscrasias***
EENT: Tinnitus, hearing loss, blurred vision
Contraindications: Hypersensitivity, asthma, severe renal disease, severe hepatic disease
Precautions: Pregnancy, lactation, children, bleeding disorders, GI disorders, cardiac disorders, hypersensitivity to other antiinflammatory agents

Pharmacokinetics:
PO: Peak 2 hr, half-life 3-3½ hr; metabolized in liver, excreted in urine (metabolites), excreted in breast milk

Interactions/incompatibilities:
• May increase action of coumarin, phenytoin, sulfonamides when used with this drug

NURSING CONSIDERATIONS
Assess:
• Renal, liver, blood studies: BUN, creatinine, AST, ALT, Hgb before treatment, periodically thereafter
• Audiometric, ophthalmic exam before, during, after treatment

Administer:
• With food to decrease GI symptoms; best to take on empty stomach to facilitate absorption

Perform/provide:
• Storage at room temperature

Evaluate:
• Therapeutic response: decreased pain, stiffness, swelling in joints, ability to move more easily
• For eye, ear problems: blurred vision, tinnitus (may indicate toxicity)

Teach patient/family:
• To report blurred vision, ringing, roaring in ears (may indicate toxicity)
• To avoid driving or other hazardous activities if dizziness or drowsiness occurs
• To report change in urine pattern, weight increase, edema, pain increase in joints, fever, blood in urine (indicates nephrotoxicity)
• That therapeutic effects may take up to 1 mo

---

natamycin (ophthalmic)
(na-ta-mye′sin)
Natacyn

Func. class.: Antiinfective
Chem. class.: Tetraene polyene compound

Action: Inhibits bacterial cell wall in organism by preventing amino acids and nucleotides into cell wall
Uses: Eye infection

Dosage and routes:
• *Adult and child:* INSTILL 1 gtt q1-2h × 3-4 days, then decrease to 1 gtt 8 × /day

Available forms include: Susp 5%

Side effects/adverse reactions:
EENT: Poor corneal wound healing, temporary visual haze, overgrowth of nonsusceptible organisms

Contraindications: Hypersensitivity

Precautions: Antibiotic hypersensitivity

Interactions/incompatibilities:
None known

NURSING CONSIDERATIONS
Administer:
• After washing hands, cleanse crusts or discharge from eye before application

Perform/provide:
• Storage at room temperature

Evaluate:
• Therapeutic response: absence of redness, inflammation, tearing
• Allergy: itching, lacrimation, redness, swelling

Teach patient/family:
• To use drug exactly as prescribed
• Not to use eye makeup, towels, washcloths, eye medication of others; reinfection may occur
• That drug container tip should not be touched to eye
• To report itching, increased redness, burning, stinging, swelling; drug should be discontinued

---

italics = common side effects   ***bold italic*** = life threatening reactions

neomycin sulfate

(nee-oh-mye'sin)

Mycifradin Sulfate, Neobiotic

Func. class.: Antibiotic

Chem. class.: Aminoglycoside

Action: Inferferes with protein synthesis in bacterial cell by binding to ribosomal subunit causing inaccurate peptide sequence to form in protein chain, causing bacterial death

Uses: Severe systemic infections of CNS, respiratory, GI, urinary tract, eye, bone, skin, soft tissues caused by *P. aeruginosa, E. coli, Enterobacter, K. pneumoniae, P. vulgaris;* also used for hepatic coma, preoperatively to sterilize bowel, infectious diarrhea caused by enteropathogenic *E. coli*

Dosage and routes:

Severe systemic infections

• *Adult:* IM 15 mg/kg/day in 4 divided doses, not to exceed 1 g/day

Hepatic coma

• *Adult:* PO 4-12 g/day in divided doses × 5-6 days; REC 200 ml of 1% or 100 ml of 2% retained for ½-1 hr

• *Child:* 50-100 mg/kg/day in divided doses

Preoperative bowel sterilization

• *Adult:* PO 1 g qlh × 4 doses, then q4h × balance of 24 hr; give saline cathartic before giving this drug

Available forms include: Tabs 500 mg; top, inj IM 500 mg; ophth oint, liq 125 mg/5 ml

Side effects/adverse reactions:

GU: Oliguria, hematuria, renal damage, azotemia, renal failure, nephrotoxicity

CNS: Confusion, depression, numbness, tremors, *convulsions,* muscle twitching, *neurotoxicity*

EENT: Ototoxicity, deafness, visual disturbances

HEMA: Agranulocytosis, thrombocytopenia, leukopenia, eosinophilia, anemia

GI: Nausea, vomiting, anorexia, increased ALT, AST, bilirubin, hepatomegaly, *hepatic necrosis,* splenomegaly

CV: Hypotension, myocarditis

INTEG: Rash, burning, urticaria, photosensitivity, dermatitis

Contraindications: Bowel obstruction (oral use), severe renal disease, hypersensitivity

Precautions: Neonates, mild renal disease, pregnancy, hearing deficits, lactation, myasthenia gravis

Pharmacokinetics:

PO: Onset rapid, peak 1-2 hr

REC: Onset immediate, peak 1-2 hr

Plasma half-life 1-3 hr; not metabolized, excreted unchanged in urine, crosses placental barrier

Interactions/incompatibilities:

• Increased ototoxicity, neurotoxicity, nephrotoxicity: other aminoglycosides, amphotericin B, polymyxin, vancomycin, ethacrynic acid, furosemide, mannitol, methoxyflurane, cisplatin, cephalosporins

• Decreased effects of: parenteral penicillins, vitamin B_{12}

• Do not mix in solution or syringe: carbenicillin, ticarcillin, amphotericin B, cephalothin, erythromycin, heparin

• Increased effects: nondepolarizing muscle relaxants, oral anticoagulants when given with oral neomycin

• Decreased effects of: digoxin when given with oral neomycin

NURSING CONSIDERATIONS

Assess:

• Weight before treatment; calculation of dosage is usually done based on ideal body weight, but may be calculated on actual body weight

• I&O ratio, urinalysis daily for proteinuria, cells, casts; report sudden change in urine output

• Urine pH if drug is used for UTI; urine should be kept alkaline

Administer:

• IM injection in large muscle mass, rotate injection sites

• Drug in evenly spaced doses to maintain blood level

• Bicarbonate to alkalinize urine if ordered in treating UTI, as drug is most active in alkaline environment

Perform/provide:

• Adequate fluids of 2-3 L/day unless contraindicated to prevent irritation of tubules

• Supervised ambulation, other safety measures with vestibular dysfunction

Evaluate:

• Therapeutic effect: absence of fever, draining wounds, negative C&S after treatment

• Renal impairment by securing urine for CrCl testing, BUN, serum creatinine; lower dosage should be given in renal impairment (CrCl <80 ml/min)

• Deafness by audiometric testing, ringing, roaring in ears, vertigo; assess hearing before, during, after treatment

• Dehydration: high sp gr, decrease in skin turgor, dry mucous membranes, dark urine

• Overgrowth of infection: increased temperature, malaise, redness, pain, swelling, perineal itching, diarrhea, stomatitis, change in cough, sputum

• C&S before starting treatment to identify infecting organism

• Vestibular dysfunction: nausea, vomiting, dizziness, headache; drug should be discontinued if severe

• Injection sites for redness, swelling, abscesses; use warm compresses at site

Teach patient/family:

• To report headache, dizziness, symptoms of overgrowth of infection, renal impairment

• To report loss of hearing, ringing, roaring in ears or a feeling of fullness in head

Treatment of overdose: Hemodialysis, monitor serum levels of drug

---

neomycin sulfate

(nee-oh-mye′sin)
Drotic, Otocort
Func. class.: Otic, antibiotic

Action: Inhibits protein synthesis in susceptible microorganisms
Uses: Ear infection (external)
Dosage and routes:
• *Adult and child:* INSTILL 2-5 gtts tid-qid
Available forms include: Otic sol in combination with neomycin, hydrocortisone 0.25%, 0.5%
Side effects/adverse reactions:
EENT: Itching, irritation in ear
INTEG: Rash, urticaria
Contraindications: Hypersensitivity, perforated eardrum
Pharmacokinetics: Not known
Interactions/incompatibilities:
None known
NURSING CONSIDERATIONS
Administer:
• After removing impacted cerumen by irrigation
• After cleaning stopper with alcohol
• After restraining child if necessary
• Warming solution to body temperature
Evaluate:
• Therapeutic response: decreased ear pain
• For redness, swelling, fever, pain

N

in ear, which indicates superimposed infection

Teach patient/family:
• Method of instillation using aseptic technique, including not touching dropper to ear
• That dizziness may occur after instillation

---

neomycin sulfate (topical)

(nee-oh-mye'sin)
Mycifradin,* Myciguent, Neocin*
Func. class.: Local antiinfective
Chem. class.: Aminoglycoside

Action: Interferes with bacterial DNA replication
Uses: Skin infections
Dosage and routes:
• *Adult and child:* TOP rub into affected area bid-tid
Available forms include: Oint, cream 0.5%
Side effects/adverse reactions:
INTEG: Rash, urticaria, scaling, redness
Contraindications: Hypersensitivity, large areas
Precautions: Pregnancy, lactation
Interactions/incompatibilities: None known
NURSING CONSIDERATIONS
Administer:
• Enough medication to completely cover lesions
• After cleansing with soap, water before each application, dry well
Perform/provide:
• Storage at room temperature in dry place
Evaluate:
• Allergic reaction: burning, stinging, swelling, redness
• Therapeutic response: decrease in size, number of lesions
Teach patient/family:
• To apply with glove to prevent further infection

• To avoid use of OTC creams, ointments, lotions unless directed by physician
• To use medical asepsis (hand washing) before, after each application

---

neostigmine bromide/ neostigmine methylsulfate

(nee-oh-stig'meen)
Prostigmin Bromide/Prostigmin
Func. class.: Cholinergics
Chem. class.: Quaternary compound

Action: Inhibits destruction of acetylcholine, which increases concentration at sites where acetylcholine is released; this facilitates transmission of impulses across myoneural junction
Uses: Myasthenia gravis, tubocurarine antagonist, bladder distention, ileus postoperatively
Dosage and routes:
Myasthenia gravis
• *Adult:* PO 15-30 mg tid; IM/IV 0.5-2 mg q1-3h
• *Child:* PO 7.5-15 mg tid-qid
Tubocurarine antagonist
• *Adult:* IV 0.5-2 mg slowly, may repeat if needed or may give 0.6-1.2 mg atropine before this drug
Abdominal distention/postoperative ileus
• *Adult:* IM/SC 0.25-1 mg q4-6h depending on condition
Available forms include: Tabs 15 mg; inj IM, SC, IV 1:1000, 1:2000, 1:4000
Side effects/adverse reactions:
INTEG: Rash, urticaria
CNS: Dizziness, headache, sweating, confusion, weakness, convulsions, incoordination, paralysis
GI: Nausea, diarrhea, vomiting, cramps

CV: Tachycardia
GU: Frequency, incontinence
RESP: Respiratory depression, bronchospasm, constriction
EENT: Miosis, blurred vision, lacrimation

Contraindications: Bradycardia, hypotension, obstruction of intestine, renal system, pregnancy (C)

Precautions: Seizure disorders, bronchial asthma, coronary occlusion, hyperthyroidism, dysrhythmias, peptic ulcer, megacolon, poor GI motility

Pharmacokinetics:
PO: Onset 2-4 hr, duration 2½-4 hr
IM/IV/SC: Onset 10-30 min, duration 2½-4 hr
Metabolized in liver, excreted in urine

Interactions/incompatibilities:
• Decreased action of: gallamine, metocurine, pancuronium, tubocurarine, atropine
• Increased action of: decamethonium, succinylcholine
• Decreased action of this drug: aminoglycosides, anesthetics, procainamide, quinidine

NURSING CONSIDERATIONS
Assess:
• VS, respiration q8h
• I&O ratio; check for urinary retention or incontinence

Administer:
• Only with atropine sulfate available for cholinergic crisis
• Only after all other cholinergics have been discontinued
• Increased doses if tolerance occurs
• Larger doses after exercise or fatigue
• With food or milk to decrease GI symptoms
• On empty stomach for better absorption

Perform/provide:
• Storage at room temperature

Evaluate:
• Therapeutic response: increased muscle strength, hand grasp, improved gait, absence of labored breathing (if severe)
• Bradycardia, hypotension, bronchospasm, headache, dizziness, convulsions, respiratory depression; drug should be discontinued if toxicity occurs

Teach patient/family:
• That drug is not a cure, it only relieves symptoms
• All aspects of drug: action, side effects, dose, when to notify physician
• To wear Medic Alert ID specifying myasthenia gravis, drugs taken

---

netilmicin sulfate

(ne-til-mye′sin)
Netromycin
Func. class.: Antibiotic
Chem. class.: Aminoglycoside

N

Action: Interferes with protein synthesis in bacterial cell by binding to ribosomal subunit, causing inaccurate peptide sequence to form in protein chain, causing bacterial death

Uses: Severe systemic infections of CNS, respiratory, GI, urinary tract, bone, skin, soft tissues caused by *P. aeruginosa, E. coli, Enterobacter, Acinetobacter, Providencia, Citrobacter, Staphylococcus, K. pneumoniae, P. mirabilis, Serratia*

Dosage and routes:
Normal renal function
• *Adult and child >12 yr:* IM/IV 3-6.5 mg/kg/day; may give q8-12h for severe infections
• *Child and infant 6 wk-12 yr:* IM/IV 5.5-8 mg/kg/day in divided doses q8-12h
• *Neonate <6 wk:* IM/IV 4-6.5

mg/kg/day in divided doses q12h
Available forms include: Inj IM,
IV 10, 25, 100 mg/ml
Side effects/adverse reactions:
*GU: Oliguria, hematuria, renal
damage, azotemia, renal failure,
nephrotoxicity*
CNS: Confusion, depression,
numbness, tremors, *convulsions,*
muscle twitching, *neurotoxicity*
EENT: Ototoxicity, deafness, visual
disturbances
*HEMA: Agranulocytosis, throm-
bocytopenia,* leukopenia, eosino-
philia, anemia
GI: Nausea, vomiting, anorexia, increased ALT, AST, bilirubin, hepatomegaly, *hepatic necrosis,*
splenomegaly
CV: Hypotension, myocarditis
INTEG: Rash, burning, urticaria,
photosensitivity, dermatitis
Contraindications: Severe renal
disease, hypersensitivity
Precautions: Neonates, mild renal
disease, pregnancy, children <12
yr, lactation, myasthenia gravis,
hearing deficit
Pharmacokinetics:
IM: Onset rapid, peak 1-2 hr
IV: Onset immediate, peak 1-2 hr
Plasma half-life 2-3 hr, not metabolized, excreted unchanged in
urine, crosses placental barrier
Interactions/incompatibilities:
• Increased ototoxicity, neurotoxicity, nephrotoxicity: other aminoglycosides, amphotericin B, polymyxin, vancomycin, ethacrynic
acid, furosemide, mannitol, methoxyflurane, cisplatin, cephalosporins
• Decreased effects: parenteral
penicillins
• Do not mix in solution or syringe:
carbenicillin, ticarcillin, amphotericin B, cephalothin, erythromycin,
heparin

• Increased effects: nondepolarizing muscle relaxants
NURSING CONSIDERATIONS
Assess:
• Weight before treatment; calculation of dosage is usually done
based on ideal body weight, but
may be calculated on actual body
weight
• Daily I&O ratio, urinalysis for
proteinuria, cells, casts; report sudden change in urine output
• VS during infusion, watch for hypotension, change in pulse
• IV site for thrombophlebitis including pain, redness, swelling q30
min, change site if needed; apply
warm compresses to discontinued
site
• Serum peak, drawn at 30-60 min
after IV infusion or 60 min after IM
injection; trough level drawn just
before next dose; blood level
should be 2-4 times bacteriostatic
level
• Urine pH if drug is used for UTI;
urine should be kept alkaline
Administer:
• IM injection in large muscle
mass, rotate injection sites
• Drug in evenly spaced doses to
maintain blood level
• Bicarbonate to alkalinize urine if
ordered in treating UTI, as drug is
most active in alkaline environment
Perform/provide:
• Adequate fluids of 2-3 L/day unless contraindicated to prevent irritation of tubules
• Flush of IV line with NS or D_5W
after infusion
• Supervised ambulation, other
safety measures with vestibular
dysfuncton
Evaluate:
• Therapeutic effect: absence of fever, draining wounds, negative
C&S after treatment
• Renal impairment by securing
urine for CrCl testing, BUN, serum

creatinine; a lower dosage should be given in renal impairment (CrCl <80 ml/min)

• Deafness by audiometric testing, ringing, roaring in ears, vertigo; assess hearing before, during, after treatment

• Dehydration: high sp gr, decrease in skin turgor, dry mucous membranes, dark urine

• Overgrowth of infection: increased temperature, malaise, redness, pain, swelling, perineal itching, diarrhea, stomatitis, change in cough or sputum

• C&S before starting treatment to identify infecting organism

• Vestibular dysfunction: nausea, vomiting, dizziness, headache; drug should be discontinued if severe

• Injection sites for redness, swelling, abscesses; use warm compresses at site

Teach patient/family:

• To report headache, dizziness, symptoms of overgrowth of infection, renal impairment

• To report loss of hearing, ringing, roaring in ears or feeling of fullness in head

Treatment of overdose: Hemodialysis, monitor serum levels of drug

---

niacin (vitamin B₃/ nicotinic acid)/niacin-amide (nicotinamide)

(nye′a-sin) (nye-a-sin′a-mide)
Niac, Nico-400, Nicobid, Nicolar, Nico-Span

Func. class.: Vitamin B₃
Chem. class.: Water-soluble vitamin

Action: Needed for conversion of fats, protein, carbohydrates, by oxidation reduction; acts directly on vascular smooth muscle causing vasodilation; high doses decrease serum lipids

Uses: Pellagra, hyperlipidemias, (niacin) peripheral vascular disease (niacin)

Dosage and routes:

Adjunct in hyperlipidemia

• *Adult:* PO 1.5-3 g qd in 3 divided doses after meals, may be increased to 6 g/day

Pellagra

• *Adult:* IM/SC/PO/IV INF 10-20 mg, not to exceed 500 mg total dose

• *Child:* IM/SC/PO/IV INF 300 mg until desired response

Peripheral vascular disease

• *Adult:* PO 250-800 mg qd in divided doses

Available forms include: Nicotinic acid—tabs 20, 25, 50, 100, 500 mg; caps timed released 125, 250, 300, 400, 500 mg; tabs time released 150 mg; elix 50 mg/5 ml; inj 100 mg/ml; nicotinamide—tabs 50, 100, 500 mg; tabs timed release 1000 mg; inj IV, IM, SC 100 mg/ml

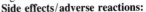

Side effects/adverse reactions:

CNS: Paresthesias, headache, dizziness, anxiety

GI: Nausea, vomiting, anorexia, flatulence, xerostomia, *jaundice,* diarrhea, peptic ulcer

GU: Hyperuricemia, glycosuria, hypoalbuminemia

CV: Postural hypotension, vasovagal attacks, dysrhythmias

EENT: Blurred vision, ptosis

INTEG: Flushing, dry skin, rash, pruritus

RESP: Wheezing

Contraindications: Hypersensitivity, pregnancy, peptic ulcer, hepatic disease, lactation, hemorrhage, severe hypotension

Precautions: Glaucoma, cardiovascular disease, CAD, diabetes mellitus, gout, schizophrenia

---

Pharmacokinetics:
PO: Peak 30-70 min, half-life 45 min, metabolized in liver, 30% excreted unchanged in urine

Interactions/incompatibilities:
• Increased action of: ganglionic blockers

NURSING CONSIDERATIONS
Assess:
• Liver function studies: AST, ALT, bilirubin, alk phosphatase; blood glucose before and during treatment
• Niacin levels while taking this drug

Administer:
• With meals for GI symptoms

Evaluate:
• Therapeutic response: decreased lipids, warm extremities, absence of numbness in extremities
• Nutritional status: liver, yeast, legumes, organ meat, lean poultry
• Liver dysfunction: clay colored stools, itching, dark urine, jaundice
• CNS symptoms: headache, paresthesias, blurred vision

Teach patient/family:
• That flushing and increase in feelings of warmth will occur several hours after taking drug (PO) or immediately (IM/IV/SC)
• To remain recumbent if postural hypotension occurs
• To abstain from alcohol if drug is prescribed for hyperlipidemia
• To avoid sunlight if skin lesions are present

Lab test interferences:
Increase: Bilirubin, alk phosphatase, liver enzymes, LDH, uric acid
Decrease: Cholesterol
False increase: Urinary catecholamines
False positive: Urine glucose

niclosamide
(ni-kloe'sa-mide)
Niclocide

Func. class.: Anthelmintic
Chem. class.: Salicylanilide derivative

Action: Inhibits synthesis in mitochondria; leads to destruction in intestine where worm may be digested, removed in feces; not effective for ova or larval stage

Uses: Regular, dwarf tapeworms

Dosage and routes:
• *Adult:* PO 2 g chewed as a single dose or × 7 days depending on type of infection
• *Child >34 kg:* PO 1.5 g chewed as a single dose or × 7 days depending on type of infection
• *Child <34 kg:* PO 1 g chewed as a single dose or 1 g on day 1, then 0.5 g × 6 days depending on type of infection

Available forms include: Tabs, chewable 500 mg

Side effects/adverse reactions:
INTEG: Rash, pruritus, pruritus ani, alopecia
CNS: Dizziness, headache, drowsiness, restlessness, sweating, fever
EENT: Bad taste, oral irritation
GI: Nausea, vomiting, anorexia, diarrhea, constipation, rectal bleeding

Contraindications: Hypersensitivity

Precautions: Child <2 yr, pregnancy (B), lactation

Pharmacokinetics: Not known

Interactions/incompatibilities: None known

NURSING CONSIDERATIONS
Assess:
• Stools during entire treatment, 1, 3 mo after treatment; specimens must be sent to lab while still warm

Administer:

• May be crushed, mixed with water if unable to swallow whole

• Laxatives if constipated; not needed for drug to work

• After breakfast, tab must be chewed, not swallowed

Perform/provide:

• Storage in tight, light-resistant container in cool environment: do not freeze

Evaluate:

• Therapeutic response: expulsion of worms, 3 negative stool cultures after completion of treatment

• For allergic reaction: rash, itching in anal area

• For diarrhea during expulsion of worms

• For infection in other family members since infection from person to person is common

Teach patient/family:

• Proper hygiene after BM including handwashing technique; tell patient to avoid putting fingers in mouth

• That infected person should sleep alone; do not shake bed linen, change bed linen qd, wash in hot water

• To clean toilet qd with disinfectant (green soap solution)

• Need for compliance with dosage schedule, duration of treatment

• To drink fruit juice to remove mucous that intestinal tapeworms burrow in, aids in explusion of worms (dwarf tapeworms only)

Treatment of overdose: Enemas, laxatives; do not induce vomiting

---

nicotine resin complex

(nik′o-teen)

Nicorette

Func. class.: Smoking deterrent
Chem. class.: Cholinergic

Action: Increase catecholamine release from adrenal medulla by stimulating receptors in CNS

Uses: Deter cigarette smoking

Dosage and routes:

• *Adult:* GUM 1 piece chewed × ½ hr as needed to abstain from smoking, not to exceed 30/day

Available forms include: Gum

Side effects/adverse reactions:

EENT: Jaw ache, irritation in buccal cavity

CNS: Dizziness, vertigo, insomnia

GI: Nausea, vomiting, anorexia, indigestion, diarrhea, abdominal pain

CV: Dysrhythmias, tachycardia, palpitations

Contraindications: Hypersensitivity, immediate post MI recovery period, severe angina pectoris, pregnancy

Precautions: Vasoplastic disease, dysrhythmias, diabetes mellitus, children

Pharmacokinetics:

Onset 15-30 min, metabolized in liver, excreted in urine, half-life 2-3 hr, 30-120 hr, (terminal)

Interactions/incompatibilities:
None known

NURSING CONSIDERATIONS

Assess:

• Adverse reaction: irritation of buccal cavity, dislike of taste, jaw ache

Evaluate:

• Therapeutic response: decrease in urge to smoke, decreased need for gum after 3-6 mo

Teach patient/family:

• To chew gum slowly for 30 min to promote buccal absorption of the drug; do not chew over 45 min

• To begin drug withdrawal after 3 mo use; not to exceed 6 mo

• All aspects of drug; give package insert to patient

• That gum will not stick to dentures, dental appliances

• That gum is as toxic as cigarette;

N

it is to be used only to deter smoking
• Not to use during pregnancy; birth defects may occur

---

nifedipine

(nye-fed'i-peen)
Adalat,* Procardia
Func. class.: Calcium channel blocker
Chem. class.: Dihydropyridine

Action: Inhibits calcium ion influx across cell membrane during cardiac depolarization; produces relaxation of coronary vascular smooth muscle, dilates coronary arteries

Uses: Chronic stable angina pectoris, vasospastic angina

Dosage and routes:
• *Adult:* PO 10 mg tid, increase in 10 mg increments q4-6h, not to exceed 180 mg or single dose of 30 mg

Available forms include: Caps 10, 20 mg

Side effects/adverse reactions:
CV: Dysrhythmia, edema, CHF, bradycardia, hypotension, palpitations

GI: Nausea, vomiting, diarrhea, gastric upset, constipation, increased liver function studies

GU: Nocturia, polyuria, *acute renal failure*

INTEG: Rash, pruritus, flushing, photosensitivity

CNS: Headache, fatigue, drowsiness, dizziness, anxiety, depression, weakness, insomnia, confusion

Contraindications: Sick sinus syndrome, 2nd or 3rd degree heart block, hypotension less than 90 mm Hg systolic

Precautions: CHF, hypotension, hepatic injury, pregnancy, lactation, children, renal disease

Pharmacokinetics:
PO: Onset 10 min, peak 30 min, half-life 2-5 hr; metabolized by liver, excreted in urine (98% as metabolites)

Interactions/incompatibilities:
• Increased effects of: barbiturates, hypoglycemia, reserpine, levodopa, digitalis, ergots, neuromuscular blocking agents
• Decreased effects: norepinephrine, xanthines, isoproterenol

NURSING CONSIDERATIONS

Assess:
• Blood levels (therapeutic levels: 0.025-0.1 μg/ml)

Administer:
• Before meals, hs

Evaluate:
• Therapeutic response: decreased anginal pain
• Cardiac status: B/P, pulse, respiration, ECG

Teach patient/family:
• How to take pulse before taking drug; record or graph should be kept
• To avoid hazardous activities until stabilized on drug, dizziness is no longer a problem
• To limit caffeine consumption
• To avoid OTC drugs unless directed by a physician
• Stress patient compliance to all areas of medical regimen: diet, exercise, stress reduction, drug therapy

Treatment of overdose: Defibrillation, atropine for AV block, vasopressor for hypotension

---

nikethamide

(ni-keth'a-mide)
Coramine
Func. class.: Cerebral stimulants
Chem. class.: Nicotinamide, diethyl derivative

Action: Direct medullary effect

causing respiratory, circulatory stimulation

Uses: CO_2 poisoning, cardiac arrest from anesthetic overdose, acute alcoholism, respiratory paralysis, respiratory depression, shock, narcosis, adjunct in neonatal asphyxia

Dosage and routes:

CO_2 poisoning
• *Adult:* IV 1.25-2.5 g, then 1.25 g q5min × 1 hr prn

Respiratory paralysis
• *Adult:* IV 3.75 g, may be repeated prn

Respiratory depression
• *Adult:* IV 1.25-2.5 g

Alcoholism
• *Adult:* IV 1.25-5 g, may repeat prn

Cardiac arrest
• *Adult:* IC 125-250 mg

Narcosis
• *Adult:* IV/IM 1 g

Neonatal asphyxia
• *Neonates:* 375 mg injected into umbilical vein

Available forms include: Inj IV, IM 25%; oral sol 25%

Side effects/adverse reactions:

CNS: Convulsions, headache, restlessness, dizziness, confusion, paresthesias, flushing, sweating, bilateral Babinski's sign, twitching, fear

GI: Nausea, vomiting, anorexia, diarrhea, hiccups

GU: Retention, incontinence

CV: Chest pain, hypertension, increase in heart rate, B/P, lowered T waves

INTEG: Pruritus, sweating, flushing, warmth

EENT: Pupil dilation, burning, itching of nose, sneezing, coughing

RESP: Laryngospasm, bronchospasm, rebound hypoventilation, increase respiratory rate

Contraindications: Hypersensitivity, seizure disorders, severe hypertension, severe bronchial asthma, severe dyspnea, severe cardiac disorders, pneumothorax, pulmonary embolism, severe respiratory disease

Precautions: Bronchial asthma, hyperthyroidism, pheochromocytoma, severe tachycardia, dysrhythmias, cerebral edema, increase cerebrospinal fluid

Pharmacokinetics:

IM: Peak ½ hr, duration 1 hr

IV: Duration 5-10 min

Excreted by kidneys, *metabolite*

Interactions/incompatibilities:
• Synergistic pressor effect: MAOIs, sympathomimetics
• Cardiac dysrhythmias: halothane, cyclopropane, enflurane
• Do not mix in alkaline solution including thiopental sodium

NURSING CONSIDERATIONS

Assess:
• B/P, HR, deep tendon reflexes, ABGs before administration
• PO_2, PCO_2, O_2 saturation during treatment

Administer:
• IV, adjust for desired respiratory response
• Only after adequate airway is established
• After oxygen, IV barbiturates, resuscitative equipment available
• Using an infusion pump IV

Perform/provide:
• Storage at room temperature
• Placing patient in Sims' position to prevent aspiration of vomitus
• Discontinue infusion if side effects occur

Evaluate:
• Hypertension, dysrhythmias, tachycardia, dyspnea, skeletal muscle hyperactivity; may indicate overdosage; discontinue if PCO_2 or O_2
• Respiratory stimulation: increased respiratory rate, abnormal rhythm

N

---

italics = common side effects   ***bold italic*** = life threatening reactions

• Extravasation, change IV site q48h

Treatment of overdose: Lavage, activated charcoal, monitor electrolytes, vital signs

---

nitrofurantoin/nitrofurantoin macrocrystals

(nye-troe-fyoor'an-toyn)

Furadantin, Furalan, Furantoin, J-Dantin, Nephronex,* Nitrex, Novofuran,* Sarodant

Func. class.: Urinary tract antiseptic

Chem. class.: Synthetic nitrofuran derivative

Action: Appears to inhibit DNA polymerization, primary target being single-stranded DNA precursors in late stages of chromosomal replication

Uses: Urinary tract infections caused by *E. coli, Klebsiella, Pseudomonas, P. vulgaris, P. morganii, Serratia, Citrobacter, S. aureus*

Dosage and routes:

• *Adult and child >12 yr:* PO 50-100 mg qid pc or 50-100 mg hs for long-term treatment

• *Adult and child >54 kg:* IV 180 mg bid

• *Adult and child <54 kg:* IV 6.6 mg/kg

• *Child 1 mo-3 yr:* PO 5-7 mg/kg/day in 4 divided doses; 33 mg/kg/day for long-term treatment

Available forms include: Caps 25, 50, 100 mg; tabs 50, 100 mg; susp 25 mg/5 ml

Side effects/adverse reactions:

INTEG: Pruritus, rash, urticaria, angioedema, alopecia, tooth staining

CNS: Dizziness, headache, drowsiness, peripheral neuropathy

GI: Nausea, vomiting, abdominal pain, diarrhea, cholestatic jaundice

Contraindications: Hypersensitivity, anuria, severe renal disease

Precautions: Pregnancy, lactation

Pharmacokinetics:

PO/IV: Half-life 20-60 min, crosses blood-brain barrier, placenta, enters breast milk, excreted as inactive metabolites in liver

Interactions/incompatibilities:

• Increased effects of: probenecid
• Antagonistic effect: nalidixic acid
• Decreased absorption of: magnesium trisilicate antacid

NURSING CONSIDERATIONS

Assess:

• Blood count for patients on chronic therapy
• I&O ratio, urine pH <5.5 is ideal
• Renal and hepatic function
• Photosensitivity: if present, drug should be discontinued

Administer:

• After clean-catch urine is obtained for C&S
• Two daily doses if urine output is high or if patient has diabetes

Perform/provide:

• Limited intake of alkaline foods or drugs: milk, dairy products, peanuts, vegetables, alkaline antacids, sodium bicarbonate
• Protection from freezing

Evaluate:

• CNS symptoms: insomnia, vertigo, headache, drowsiness, convulsions
• Allergy: fever, flushing, rash, urticaria, pruritus

Teach patient/family:

• That photosensitivity occurs; patient should avoid sunlight or use sunscreen to prevent burns
• Take medication with food or milk to decrease GI irritation
• Instruct client to protect susp from freezing and shake well before taking
• May cause drowsiness; instruct client to seek aid in walking and other activities; advise client not to

drive or operate machinery while on medication

• Instruct clients with diabetes that Clinitest may prove false-positive for glucose; and therefore Tes-Tape or Clinistix should be used

nitrofurazone (topical)

(nye-troe-fyoor′a-zone)
Furacin

Func. class.: Local antiinfective
Chem. class.: Synthetic nitrofuran

Action: Interferes with bacterial cell wall synthesis
Uses: Burns (2nd, 3rd degree)
Dosage and routes:
• *Adult and child:* TOP apply to affected area qd or qod
Available forms include: Sol, oint, cream 0.2%
Side effects/adverse reactions:
INTEG: Rash, urticaria, stinging, burning, superinfections
Contraindications: Hypersensitivity, G-6-PD deficiency
Precautions: Pregnancy (C), lactation
Interactions/incompatibilities:
None known
NURSING CONSIDERATIONS
Administer:
• Analgesic before application if needed
• Enough medication to completely cover burns
• After cleansing debris from area before each application
• Using sterile technique
Perform/provide:
• Storage at room temperature in dry place
Evaluate:
• Allergic reaction: burning, stinging, swelling, redness
• Therapeutic response: development of granulation tissue

Teach patient/family:
• That drug may be used until grafting is possible

nitroglycerin

(nye-troe-gli′ser-in)
Ang-O-Span, Cardabid, Corobid, Nitro-Bid, Nitrocap, Nitrocels, Nitrodisc, Nitro-Dur, Nitrol, Nitrospan, Nitrostabilin,* Nitrostat, Tridil

Func. class.: Vasodilatory coronary
Chem. class.: Nitrate

Action: Decreases preload, afterload, which is responsible for decreasing left ventricular end diastolic pressure, systemic vascular resistance
Uses: Chronic stable angina pectoris, prophylaxis of angina pain
Dosage and routes:
• *Adult:* SL dissolve tablet under tongue when pain begins, prn 150-500 μg q2-3h; SUS CAP q8-12h on empty stomach; TOP 1-2 q8h, increase to 4 q4h as needed; IV 5 μg/min, then increase by 5 μg/min q3-5 min; if no response after 20 μg/min, increase to 10-20 μg/min until desired response; TRANS apply a pad qd to a site free of hair
Available forms include: Buccal tabs 1, 2, 3 mg; aero 0.4 mg/meter spray; caps 2.5, 6.5, 9 mg; tabs ext rel 2.6, 6.5, 9 mg; inj 0.5, 0.8, 5 mg/ml; SL tabs 0.15, 0.3, 0.4, 0.6 mg; top oint 2%; trans derm syst 2.5, 5, 7.5, 10, 15 mg/24 hr
Side effects/adverse reactions:
CV: Postural hypotension, tachycardia, collapse
GI: Nausea, vomiting
INTEG: Pallor, sweating
CNS: Headache, flushing, dizziness
Contraindications: Hypersensitivity to this drug or nitrites, anemia, increased intracranial pressure, ce-

N

rebral hemorrhage, acute MI, pregnancy, lactation
Precautions: Postural hypotension, glaucoma
Pharmacokinetics:
SUS REL: Onset 1 hr, peak 3-4 hr, duration 8-12 hr
PO: Onset 15-60 min, peak 1-1½ hr, duration 4-12 hr
SL: Onset 1-3 min, duration 30 min
TRANS DER: Onset ½-1 hr, duration 24 hr
IV: Onset immediately, duration variable
TRANSMUC: Onset 3 min, duration 10-30 min
Metabolized by liver, excreted in urine
Interactions/incompatibilities:
• Increased effects: β-blockers, narcotics, tricyclics, diuretics, antihypertensives
• Decreased effects: sympathomimetics

NURSING CONSIDERATIONS
Assess:
• B/P, pulse, respirations during beginning therapy
Administer:
• With 8 oz of water on empty stomach (oral tablet)
Evaluate:
• Pain: duration, time started, activity being performed, character
• Tolerance if taken over long period of time
• Headache, lightheadedness, decreased B/P; may indicate a need for decreased dosage
Teach patient/family:
• That drug may be taken before stressful activity: exercise, sexual activity
• That SL may sting when drug comes in contact with mucous membranes
• To avoid hazardous activities if dizziness occurs
• Stress patient compliance with complete medical regimen

• To make position changes slowly to prevent fainting

---

nitroprusside sodium
(nye-troe-pruss'ide)
Nipride, Nitropress
Func. class.: Antihypertensive
Chem. class.: Peripheral vasodilator

Action: Directly relaxes arteriolar, venous smooth muscle; resulting in reduction in cardiac preload, afterload
Uses: Hypertensive crisis, to decrease bleeding by creating hypotension during surgery
Dosage and routes:
• *Adult:* IV INF dissolve 50 mg in 2-3 ml of D_5W, then dilute in 250-1000 ml of D_5W; run at 0.5-8 μg/kg/min
Available forms include: Inj IV 50 mg
Side effects/adverse reactions:
GI: Nausea, vomiting, abdominal pain
CNS: Dizziness, headache, agitation, twitching, decreased reflexes, loss of consciousness, restlessness
EENT: Tinnitus, blurred vision
GU: Impotence
INTEG: Pain, irritation at injection site, sweating
Contraindications: Hypersensitivity, hypertension (compensatory)
Precautions: Pregnancy, lactation, children, fluid, electrolyte imbalances, hepatic disease, renal disease, hypothyroidism, elderly
Pharmacokinetics:
IV: Onset 1-2 min, duration 1-10 min after IV done, half-life 4 days in patients with normal renal function; metabolized in liver, excreted in urine
Interactions/incompatibilities:
• Severe hypotension: ganglionic blockers, volatile liquid anesthet-

ics, halothane, enflurane, circulatory depressants

• Do not mix with any drug in syringe or solution

NURSING CONSIDERATIONS

Assess:

• Electrolytes: K, Na, Cl, CO_2

• Renal function studies: catecholamines, BUN, creatinine

• Hepatic function studies: AST, ALT, alk phosphatase

• B/P by direct means if possible, check ECG continuously

• Weight daily, I&O

• Thiocyanate levels qd if on long-term treatment

Administer:

• Depending on B/P reading q15 min

• Using an infusion pump only, wrap bottle with aluminum foil to protect from light; observe for color change in the infusion, discard if highly discolored (blue, green, dark red)

Evaluate:

• Therapeutic response: decreased B/P, absence of bleeding

• Nausea, vomiting, diarrhea

• Edema in feet, legs daily

• Skin turgor, dryness of mucous membranes for hydration status

• Rales, dyspnea, orthopnea q30 min

Treatment of overdose: Administer amyl nitrite inhalation until 3% sodium nitrate solution can be prepared for IV administration, then inject sodium thiosulfate IV, correct drop in BP with vasopressor

---

norepinephrine injection

(nor-ep-i-nef′rin)

Levophed

Func. class.: Adrenergic

Chem. class.: Catecholamine

Action: Causes increased contrac-

tility and heart rate by acting on β-receptors in heart; also, acts on α-receptors, causing vasoconstriction in blood vessels; when larger doses are administered, causes vasodilation in renal, intracerebral, coronary dopaminergic receptors

Uses: Acute hypotension

Dosage and routes:

• *Adult:* IV INF 8-12 µg/min titrated to B/P

Available forms include: Inj IV 1 mg/ml

Side effects/adverse reactions:

CNS: Headache

CV: Palpitations, tachycardia, hypotension, ectopic beats, angina

GI: Nausea, vomiting

INTEG: Necrosis, tissue sloughing with extravasation, **gangrene**

Contraindications: Hypersensitivity, ventricular fibrillation, tachydysrhythmias, pheochromocytoma

Precautions: Pregnancy, lactation, arterial embolism, peripheral vascular disease

Pharmacokinetics:

IV: Onset 1-2 min, metabolized in liver, excreted in urine (inactive metabolites), crosses placenta

Interactions/incompatibilities:

• Do not use within 2 wk of MAOIs, or hypertensive crisis may result

• Dysrhythmias: general anesthetics

• Decreased action of this drug: other β-blockers

• Increased B/P: oxytocics

• Increased pressor effect: tricyclic antidepressant, MAOIs

• Incompatible with alkaline solutions: Na, HCO_3

NURSING CONSIDERATIONS

Assess:

• I&O ratio

• ECG during administration continuously, if B/P increases, drug is decreased

N

• B/P and pulse q5 min after parenteral route

• CVP or PWP during infusion if possible

Administer:

• Plasma expanders for hypovolemia

• Using 2 bottle set up so drug may be discontinued while IV is still running

Perform/provide:

• Storage of reconstituted solution if refrigerated for no longer than 24 hr

• Do not use discolored solutions

Evaluate:

• For paresthesias and coldness of extremities, peripheral blood flow may decrease

• Injection site: tissue sloughing; if this occurs, administer phentolamine mixed with NS

• Therapeutic response: increased B/P with stabilization

Teach patient/family:

• Reason for drug administration

Treatment of overdose: Administer an α-blocker, then norepinephrine for severe hypotension

---

norethindrone

(nor-eth-in′drone)

Micronor, Norlutin, Nor-QD

Func. class.: Progestogen

Chem. class.: Progesterone derivative

Action: Inhibits secretion of pituitary gonadotropins, which prevents follicular maturation, ovulation, stimulates growth of mammary tissue, antineoplastic action against endometrial cancer

Uses: Uterine bleeding (abnormal), amenorrhea, endometriosis

Dosage and routes:

• Adult: PO 5-20 mg qd days 5-25 of menstrual cycle

Endometriosis

• Adult: PO 10 mg qd × 2 wk, then increased by 5 mg qd × 2 wk, up to 30 mg qd

Available forms include: Tabs 5 mg

Side effects/adverse reactions:

CNS: Dizziness, headache, migraines, depression, fatigue

CV: Hypotension, thrombophlebitis, edema, *thromboembolism, stroke, pulmonary embolism, myocardial infarction*

GI: Nausea, vomiting, anorexia, cramps, increased weight, *cholestatic jaundice*

EENT: Diplopia

GU: Amenorrhea, cervical erosion, breakthrough bleeding, dysmenorrhea, vaginal candidiasis, breast changes, (gynecomastia, testicular atrophy, impotence), endometriosis, *spontaneous abortion*

INTEG: Rash, urticaria, acne, hirsutism, alopecia, oily skin, seborrhea, purpura, melasma, photosensitivity

META: Hyperglycemia

Contraindications: Breast cancer, hypersensitivity, thromboembolic disorders, reproductive cancer, genital bleeding (abnormal, undiagnosed)

Precautions: Pregnancy, lactation, hypertension, asthma, blood dyscrasias, gallbladder disease, CHF, diabetes mellitus, bone disease, depression, migraine headache, convulsive disorders, hepatic disease, renal disease, family history of breast or reproductive tract cancer

Pharmacokinetics:

PO: Duration 24 hr, excreted in urine, feces, metabolized in liver

Interactions/incompatibilities:

None known

NURSING CONSIDERATIONS

Assess:

• Weight daily: notify physician of

---

weekly weight gain >5 lb
• B/P at beginning of treatment and periodically
• I&O ratio; be alert for decreasing urinary output, increasing edema
• Liver function studies: ALT, AST, bilirubin, periodically during long-term therapy

Administer:
• Titrated dose, use lowest effective dose
• Solution deeply in large muscle mass (IM), rotate sites
• In one dose in AM
• With food or milk to decrease GI symptoms
• After warming to dissolve crystals

Perform/provide:
• Storage in dark area

Evaluate:
• Therapeutic response: decreased abnormal uterine bleeding, absence of amenorrhea
• Edema, hypertension, cardiac symptoms, jaundice
• Mental status: affect, mood, behavioral changes, depression
• Hypercalcemia

Teach patient/family:
• To avoid sunlight or use sunscreen, photosensitivity can occur
• All aspects of drug usage, including cushingoid symptoms
• To report breast lumps, vaginal bleeding, edema, jaundice, dark urine, clay-colored stools, dyspnea, headache, blurred vision, abdominal pain, numbness or stiffness in legs, chest pain; male to report impotence or gynecomastia
• To report suspected pregnancy

Lab test interferences:
Increase: Alk phosphatase, nitrogen (urine), pregnanediol, amino acids
Decrease: GTT, HDL

norethindrone acetate

(nor-eth-in'drone)
Aygestin, Norlutate
Func. class.: Progestogen
Chem. class.: Progesterone derivative

Action: Inhibits secretion of pituitary gonadotropins, which prevents follicular maturation, ovulation, stimulates growth of mammary tissue, antineoplastic action against endometrial cancer
Uses: Uterine bleeding (abnormal), amenorrhea, endometriosis

Dosage and routes:
• *Adult:* PO 2.5-10 mg qd days 5-25 of menstrual cycle
Endometriosis
• *Adult:* PO 5 mg qd × 2 wk, then increased by 2.5 mg qd × 2 wk, up to 15 mg qd
Available forms include: Tabs 5 mg

Side effects/adverse reactions:
CNS: Dizziness, headache, migraines, depression, fatigue
CV: Hypotension, thrombophlebitis, edema, ***thromboembolism, stroke, pulmonary embolism, myocardial infarction***
GI: Nausea, vomiting, anorexia, cramps, increased weight, ***cholestatic jaundice***
EENT: Diplopia
GU: Amenorrhea, cervical erosion, breakthrough bleeding, dysmenorrhea, vaginal candidiasis, breast changes, *gynecomastia, testicular atrophy, impotence,* endometriosis, ***spontaneous abortion***
INTEG: Rash, urticaria, acne, hirsutism, alopecia, oily skin, seborrhea, purpura, melasma, photosensitivity
META: Hyperglycemia
Contraindications: Breast cancer, hypersensitivity, thromboembolic

N

disorders, reproductive cancer, genital bleeding (abnormal, undiagnosed), cerebral hemorrhage

Precautions: Pregnancy, lactation, hypertension, asthma, blood dyscrasias, gallbladder disease, CHF, diabetes mellitus, bone disease, depression, migraine headache, convulsive disorders, hepatic disease, renal disease, family history of breast or reproductive tract cancer

Pharmacokinetics:

PO: Duration 24 hr, excreted in urine, feces, metabolized in liver

Interactions/incompatibilities:

None known

NURSING CONSIDERATIONS

Assess:

• Weight daily; notify physician of weekly weight gain >5 lb

• B/P at beginning of treatment and periodically

• I&O ratio; be alert for decreasing urinary output, increasing edema

• Liver function studies: ALT, AST, bilirubin, periodically during long-term therapy

Administer:

• Titrated dose, use lowest effective dose

• Oil solution deeply in large muscle mass (IM), rotate sites

• In one dose in AM

• With food or milk to decrease GI symptoms

• After warming to dissolve crystals

Perform/provide:

• Storage in dark area

Evaluate:

• Therapeutic response: decreased abnormal uterine bleeding, absence of amenorrhea

• Edema, hypertension, cardiac symptoms, jaundice

• Mental status: affect, mood, behavioral changes, depression

• Hypercalcemia

Teach patient/family:

• To avoid sunlight or use sunscreen, photosensitivity can occur

• All aspects of drug usage, including cushingoid symptoms

• To report breast lumps, vaginal bleeding, edema, jaundice, dark urine, clay-colored stools, dyspnea, headache, blurred vision, abdominal pain, numbness or stiffness in legs, chest pain; male to report impotence or gynecomastia

• To monitor blood sugar, if diabetic

• To report suspected pregnancy

Lab test interferences:

Increase: Alk phosphatase, nitrogen (urine), pregnanediol, amino acids

Decrease: GTT, HDL

---

norgestrel

(nor-jess'trel)

Ovrette

Func. class.: Progestogen

Chem. class.: Progesterone derivative

Action: Inhibits secretion of pituitary gonadotropins, which prevents follicular maturation, ovulation, stimulates growth of mammary tissue, antineoplastic action against endometrial cancer

Uses: Contraception

Dosage and routes:

• *Adult:* PO 1 tablet qd

Available forms include: Tabs 0.35, 0.075 mg

Side effects/adverse reactions:

CNS: Dizziness, headache, migraines, depression, fatigue

CV: Hypotension, thrombophlebitis, edema, *thromboembolism, stroke, pulmonary embolism, myocardial infarction*

GI: Nausea, vomiting, anorexia, cramps, increased weight, *cholestatic jaundice*

EENT: Diplopia

GU: Amenorrhea, cervical erosion, breakthrough bleeding, dysmenorrhea, vaginal candidiasis, breast changes, *gynecomastia, testicular atrophy, impotence,* endometriosis, *spontaneous abortion*

INTEG: Rash, urticaria, acne, hirsutism, alopecia, oily skin, seborrhea, purpura, melasma, photosensitivity

META: Hyperglycemia

Contraindications: Breast cancer, hypersensitivity, thromboembolic disorders, reproductive cancer, genital bleeding (abnormal, undiagnosed), cerebral hemorrhage, pregnancy (X)

Precautions: Lactation, hypertension, asthma, blood dyscrasias, gallbladder disease, CHF, diabetes mellitus, bone disease, depression, migraine headache, convulsive disorders, hepatic disease, renal disease, family history of breast or reproductive tract cancer

Pharmacokinetics:

PO: Duration 24 hr, excreted in urine and feces, metabolized in liver

Interactions/incompatibilities: None known

NURSING CONSIDERATIONS
Assess:

• Weight daily; notify physician of weekly weight gain >5 lb

• B/P at beginning of treatment and periodically

• I&O ratio; be alert for decreasing urinary output, increasing edema

• Liver function studies: ALT, AST, bilirubin, periodically during long-term therapy

Administer:

• Titrated dose; use lowest effective dose

• Oil solution deeply in large muscle mass (IM), rotate sites

• In one dose in AM

• With food or milk to decrease GI symptoms

• After warming to dissolve crystals

Perform/provide:

• Storage in dark area

Evaluate:

• Therapeutic response: decreased abnormal uterine bleeding, absence of amenorrhea

• Edema, hypertension, cardiac symptoms, jaundice

• Mental status: affect, mood, behavioral changes, depression

• Hypercalcemia

Teach patient/family:

• To avoid sunlight or use sunscreen, photosensitivity can occur

• All aspects of drug usage, including cushingoid symptoms

• To report breast lumps, vaginal bleeding, edema, jaundice, dark urine, clay-colored stools, dyspnea, headache, blurred vision, abdominal pain, numbness or stiffness in legs, chest pain; male to report impotence or gynecomastia

• To report suspected pregnancy

• To monitor blood sugar, if diabetic

Lab test interferences:

Increase: Alk phosphatase, nitrogen (urine), pregnanediol, amino acids

Decrease: GTT, HDL

---

nortriptyline HCl
(nor-trip′ti-leen)

Aventyl, Pamelor

Func. class.: Antidepressant—tricyclic

Chem. class.: Dibenzocycloheptene—secondary amine

Action: Blocks reuptake of norepinephrine, serotonin into nerve endings, increasing action of nor-

N

---

epinephrine, serotonin in nerve cells

Uses: Endogenous depression

Dosage and routes:

• *Adult:* PO 25 mg tid or qid, may increase to 150 mg/day; may give daily dose hs

Available forms include: Caps 10, 25, 75 mg; sol 10 mg/5 ml

Side effects/adverse reactions:

*HEMA: **Agranulocytosis, thrombocytopenia, eosinophilia, leukopenia***

CNS: Dizziness, drowsiness, confusion, headache, anxiety, tremors, stimulation, weakness, insomnia, nightmares, EPS (elderly), increased psychiatric symptoms

GI: Constipation, dry mouth, nausea, vomiting, ***paralytic ileus,*** increased appetite, cramps, epigastric distress, jaundice, ***hepatitis,*** stomatitis

*GU: Retention, **acute renal failure***

INTEG: Rash, urticaria, sweating, pruritus, photosensitivity

*CV: Orthostatic hypotension, ECG changes, tachycardia, **hypertension,*** palpitations

EENT: Blurred vision, tinnitus, mydriasis

Contraindications: Hypersensitivity to tricyclic antidepressants, recovery phase of myocardial infarction, convulsive disorders, prostatic hypertrophy

Precautions: Suicidal patients, severe depression, increased intraocular pressure, narrow-angle glaucoma, urinary retention, cardiac disease, hepatic disease, hyperthyroidism, electroshock therapy, elective surgery, pregnancy (C)

Pharmacokinetics:

PO: Steady state 4-19 days; metabolized by liver, excreted by kidneys, crosses placenta, excreted in breast milk, half-life 18-28 hr

Interactions/incompatibilities:

• Decreased effects of: guanethi-

dine, clonidine, indirect acting sympathomimetics (ephedrine)

• Increased effects of: direct acting sympathomimetics (epinephrine), alcohol, barbiturates, benzodiazepines, CNS depressants

• Hyperpyretic crisis, convulsions, hypertensive episode: MAOI

NURSING CONSIDERATIONS

Assess:

• B/P (lying, standing), pulse q4h; if systolic B/P drops 20 mm Hg hold drug, notify physician; take vital signs q4h in patients with cardiovascular disease

• Blood studies: CBC, leukocytes, differential, cardiac enzymes if patient is receiving long-term therapy

• Hepatic studies: AST, ALT, bilirubin, creatinine

• Weight qwk, appetite may increase with drug

• ECG for flattening of T wave, bundle branch block, AV block, dysrhythmias in cardiac patients

Administer:

• Increased fluids, bulk in diet if constipation, urinary retention occur

• With food or milk for GI symptoms

• Dosage hs if over-sedation occurs during day; may take entire dose hs; elderly may not tolerate once/day dosing

• Gum, hard candy, or frequent sips of water for dry mouth

• Concentrate with fruit juice, water, or milk to disguise taste

Perform/provide:

• Storage in tight, light-resistant container at room temperature

• Assistance with ambulation during beginning therapy since drowsiness/dizziness occurs

• Safety measures including siderails primarily in elderly

• Checking to see PO medication swallowed

Evaluate:
• EPS primarily in elderly: rigidity, dystonia, akathisia
• Mental status: mood, sensorium, affect, suicidal tendencies, increase in psychiatric symptoms: depression, panic
• Urinary retention, constipation; constipation is more likely to occur in children
• Withdrawal symptoms: headache, nausea, vomiting, muscle pain, weakness; do not usually occur unless drug was discontinued abruptly
• Alcohol consumption; if alcohol is consumed, hold dose until morning

Teach patient/family:
• That therapeutic effects may take 2-3 wk
• Use caution in driving or other activities requiring alertness because of drowsiness, dizziness, blurred vision
• To avoid alcohol ingestion, other CNS depressants
• Not to discontinue medication quickly after long-term use, may cause nausea, headache, malaise
• To wear sunscreen or large hat since photosensitivity occurs

Lab test interferences:
Increase: Serum bilirubin, blood glucose, alk phosphatase
False increase: Urinary catecholamines
Decrease: VMA, 5-HIAA

Treatment of overdose: ECG monitoring, induce emesis, lavage, activated charcoal, administer anticonvulsant

novobiocin calcium, novobiocin sodium

(noe-voe-bye′o-sin)
Albamycin

Func. class.: Antibacterial
Chem. class.: Streptomyces derivative

Action: Interferes with bacterial synthesis in cell wall
Uses: Serious or life-threatening infections caused by *S. aureus,* or *Proteus* when other antibiotics cannot be used, usually used in combination with penicillin

Dosage and routes:
• *Adult:* PO 250-500 mg q6h or 500 mg-1 g q12h, not to exceed 2 g/day
• *Child:* PO 15-45 mg/kg/day in divided doses q6h

Available forms include: Caps 250 mg

Side effects/adverse reactions:
CNS: Dizziness, drowsiness, light headedness
*HEMA: **Pancytopenia, agranulocytosis, anemia, hemolytic anemia, thrombocytopenia, eosinophilia***
*RESP: **Allergic pneumonitis***
GI: Nausea, vomiting, anorexia, diarrhea, abdominal pain, jaundice, ***intestinal hemorrhage***
INTEG: Urticaria, rash, pruritus, alopecia

Contraindications: Hypersensitivity, neonate, pregnancy

Pharmacokinetics:
PO: Peak 2 hr; excreted in bile, feces, highly protein bound

Interactions/incompatibilities:
None known

NURSING CONSIDERATIONS
Assess:
• Any patient with compromised renal system; drug is excreted slowly in poor renal system func-

N

tion; toxicity may occur rapidly
• Liver studies: AST, ALT
• Blood studies: WBC, RBC, Hct, Hgb, platelets, serum iron, reticulocytes; drug should be discontinued if bone marrow depression occurs
• Renal studies: urinalysis, protein, blood, BUN, creatinine
• C&S before drug therapy; drug may be taken as soon as culture is taken
• Drug level in impaired hepatic, renal systems
Administer:
• Orally with at least 8 oz water
Perform/provide:
• Storage at room temperature (capsules), up to 2 wk (reconstituted solution)
• Adrenalin, suction, tracheostomy set, endotracheal intubation equipment on unit
• Adequate intake of fluids (2000 ml) during diarrhea episodes
Evaluate:
• Therapeutic response: decreased temperature, negative C&S
• Bowel pattern before, during treatment
• Skin eruptions, itching, dermatitis
• Respiratory status: rate, character, wheezing, tightness in chest
• Allergies before treatment, reaction of each medication; place allergies on chart, Kardex in bright red letters; notify all people giving drugs
Teach patient/family:
• To take oral drug with full glass of water; may give with food if GI symptoms occur
• Aspects of drug therapy: need to complete entire course of medication to ensure organism death (10-14 days); culture may be taken after completed course of medication
• To report sore throat, fever, fatigue; could indicate superimposed infection
• That drug must be taken in equal intervals around clock to maintain blood levels
• To wear or carry Medic Alert ID if allergic to this drug
• To notify nurse of diarrhea stools
Lab test interferences:
Increase: Alk phosphatase, bilirubin, CPK, AST/ALT
Treatment of overdose: Withdraw drug, maintain airway, administer epinephrine, aminophylline, O_2, IV corticosteroids

---

nylidrin HCl

(nye'li-drin)
Arlidin, Rolidrin
Func. class.: Peripheral vasodilator, β-adrenergic agonist
Chem. class.: β-Adrenergic agonist-phenylisopropylamine

Action: Acts on β-adrenergic receptors in arterioles, skeletal muscles; increases cardiac output
Uses: Arteriosclerosis obliterans, thromboangiitis obliterans, diabetic vascular disease, night leg cramps, Raynaud's disease, ischemic ulcer, frostbite, acrocyanosis, acroparesthesia, thrombophlebitis, primary cochlear cell ischemia, cochlear stria ischemia, muscular or ampullar ischemia, other disturbances from labyrinth artery spasm or obstruction
Dosage and routes:
• *Adult:*PO 3-12 mg tid or qid
Available forms include: Tabs 6, 12 mg
Side effects/adverse reactions:
CV: Postural hypotension, palpitations
CNS: Dizziness, anxiety, tremors, weakness
GI: Nausea, vomiting
INTEG: Flushing

Contraindications: Hypersensitivity, paroxysmal tachycardia, progressive angina pectoris, thyrotoxicosis, myocardial infarction
Precautions: CHF, pregnancy
Pharmacokinetics:
PO: Onset 10 min, peak 30 min, duration 2 hr; slowly metabolized in liver, excreted in urine, therapeutic effect may take several weeks
Interactions/incompatibilities:
• Increased hypotension: phenothiazines

NURSING CONSIDERATIONS
Assess:
• B/P, pulse during treatment until stable; take B/P lying, standing; orthostatic hypotension is common
Administer:
• With meals to reduce GI upset
Perform/provide:
• Storage at room temperature
Evaluate:
• Therapeutic response: ability to walk without pain, increased pulse volume, increased temperature in extremities or orientation, long- and short-term memory
Teach patient/family:
• That medication is not cure, may need to be taken continuously; therapeutic response may not be evident for 2-3 mo
• That it is necessary to quit smoking to prevent excessive vasoconstriction
• To avoid hazardous activities until stabilized on medication; dizziness may occur

nystatin
(nye-stat'in)
Mycostatin, Nadostine,* Nilstat, O-V Statin
Func. class.: Antifungal
Chem. class.: Amphoteric polyene macrolide

Action: Binds sterols of cell membrane in fungi, allowing intracellular components to leak
Uses: *Candida* species causing oral, vaginal, intestinal infections
Dosage and routes:
Oral infection
• *Adult:* SUSP 400,000-600,000 U qid
• *Child and infants >3 mo:* SUSP 250,000-500,000 U qid
• *Newborn and premature infants:* SUSP 100,000 U qid
GI infection
• *Adult:* PO 500,000-1,000,000 U tid
Vaginal infection
• *Adult:* VAG TAB 100,000 U inserted high into vagina qd-bid × 2 wk
Available forms include: Tabs 500,000 U; vag tabs 100,000 U; powder 50 mill, 150 mill, 500 mill, 1 bill, 2 bill, 5 bill U; susp 100,000 U; top cream, oint, powder 100,000 U
Side effects/adverse reactions:
INTEG: Rash, urticaria (rare)
GI: Nausea, vomiting, anorexia, diarrhea, cramps
Contraindications: Hypersensitivity
Precautions: Pregnancy (A)
Pharmacokinetics:
PO: Little absorption, excreted in feces
Interactions/incompatibilities:
None known

N

NURSING CONSIDERATIONS
Administer:

• Oral suspension dose by placing ½ in each cheek, then swallow

• Topical dose after cleansing area; mouth may be swabbed

Perform/provide:

• Storage in refrigerator, oral susp, tabs in tight, light-resistant containers at room temperature

Evaluate:

• For allergic reaction: rash, urticaria; drug may need to be discontinued

• For predisposing factors: antibiotic therapy, pregnancy, diabetes mellitus, sexual partner infection (vaginal infections)

Teach patient/family:

• That long-term therapy may be needed to clear infection; to complete entire course of medication

• Proper hygiene: changing socks if feet are infected, using no commercial mouthwashes for mouth infection

• Avoid getting preparation on hands

• To wear light day pad for vaginal preparations

• Avoid tight shoes, bandages when using for feet infection

• Avoid sexual contact during treatment to minimize reinfection

• Notify physician if irritation occurs; drug may need to be discontinued

• That relief from itching may occur after 24-72 hr

---

nystatin (topical)
(nye-stat'in)

Mycostatin, Nadostine, Nilstat

Func. class.: Local antiinfective
Chem. class.: Antifungal

Action: Interferes with fungal DNA replication; binds sterols in fungal cell membrane, which increases permeability, leaking of cell nutrients

Uses: Cutaneous vulvovaginal candidiasis, mucocutaneous fungal infections

Dosage and routes:

• *Adult and child:* TOP apply to affected area bid × 14 days; VAG 1-2 tabs (100,000 U each) inserted into vagina

Available forms include: Cream, oint, powder, spray, vag tabs 100,000 U

Side effects/adverse reactions:

INTEG: Rash, urticaria, stinging, burning

Contraindications: Hypersensitivity

Precautions: Pregnancy (C), lactation

Interactions/incompatibilities: None known

NURSING CONSIDERATIONS
Administer:

• Vaginal tablets by inserting high into vagina

• Enough medication to completely cover lesions

• After cleansing with soap, water before each application, dry well

Perform/provide:

• Storage at room temperature in dry place

Evaluate:

• Allergic reaction: burning, stinging, swelling, redness

• Therapeutic response: decrease in size, number of lesions, decreased itching, white patches on vulvae

Teach patient/family:

• To apply with glove to prevent further infection

• To avoid use of OTC creams, ointments, lotions unless directed by physician

• To use medical asepsis (hand washing) before, after each application

---

opium tincture/ camphorated opium tincture

(oh'pee-um)

Paregoric

Func. class.: Antidiarrheal

Chem. class.: Opium/opium and morphine

Controlled Substance Schedule III/II (depending on amount of opium)

Action: Antiperistaltic activity

Uses: Diarrhea (cause undetermined); to treat withdrawal symptoms in infants born to addicted mothers

Dosage and routes:

• *Adult:* PO 0.3-1 ml qid, not to exceed 6 ml/day (tincture) or 5-10 ml bid-qid (camphorated)

• *Child:* PO 0.25-0.5 ml/kg qd-qid (camphorated)

Withdrawal

• *Neonates:* PO 1:25 dilution, 3-6 gtt q3-6 hr (tincture), dosage adjustment is made to control symptoms

Available forms include: Liq 2 mg morphine equivalent per 5 ml

Side effects/adverse reactions:

CNS: Dizziness, drowsiness, fainting, flushing, physical dependency

CNS depression

GI: Nausea, vomiting, constipation, abdominal pain

Contraindications: Hypersensitivity

Precautions: Liver disease, addiction-prone individuals, prostatic hypertrophy (severe)

Pharmacokinetics:

PO: Duration 4 hr, half-life 2-3 hr; metabolized in liver, excreted in urine

Interactions/incompatibilities:

• Increased action of both drugs: other CNS depressants

NURSING CONSIDERATIONS

Assess:

• Electrolytes (K, Na, Cl) if on long-term therapy

• Skin turgor q8h if dehydration is suspected

Administer:

• Undiluted with water

• For 48 hr only

Evaluate:

• Therapeutic response: decreased diarrhea

• Bowel pattern before; for rebound constipation

• Response after 48 hr; if no response, drug should be discontinued

• Dehydration in children

• Abdominal distention; toxic megacolon may occur in ulcerative colitis

Teach patient/family:

• To avoid OTC products (cough, cold, hay fever preparations) unless directed by physician

• Not to exceed recommended dose

oral contraceptives

Func. class.: Hormone

Chem. class.: Estrogen/progestin combinations

Action: Prevents ovulation by suppressing follicle stimulating, luteinizing hormone

Uses: To prevent pregnancy, endometriosis, hypermenorrhea

Dosage and routes:

• *Adult:* PO 1 qd starting on day 5 of menstrual cycle; day 1 is 1st day of period

20/21 tablet packs

• *Adult:* PO 1 qd starting on day 7 of menstrual cycle; day 1 is 1st day of period, then on 20 or 21 days, off 7 days

28 tablet packs

• *Adult:* PO 1 qd continuously

Biphasic

---

italics = common side effects   ***bold italic*** = life threatening reactions

• *Adult:* 1 qd × 10 days, then next color 1 qd × 11 days

Triphasic

• *Adult:* 1 qd; check package insert for each new brand

Endometriosis

• *Adult:* PO 1 qd × 20 days from day 5 to 24 of cycle

• *Adult:* PO 1 qd; check package insert for specific instructions

Available forms include: Check specific brand

Side effects/adverse reactions:

GI: Nausea, vomiting, cramps, diarrhea, bloating, constipation, change in appetite, *cholestatic jaundice*

INTEG: Chloasma, melasma, acne, rash, urticaria, erythema, pruritus, hirsutism, alopecia, photosensitivity

CV: Increased B/P, thromboembolic conditions, fluid retention, edema

ENDO: Decreased glucose tolerance, increased TBG, PBI, T_4, T_3

GU: Breakthrough bleeding, amenorrhea, spotting, dysmenorrhea, galactorrhea, endocervical hyperplasia, vaginitis, cystitis-like syndrome, breast change

CNS: Depression, fatigue, dizziness, nervousness, anxiety, headache

EENT: Optic neuritis, retinal thrombosis, cataracts

HEMA: Increased fibrinogen, clotting factor

Contraindications: Pregnancy (X), lactation, reproductive cancer, thrombophlebitis, MI, hepatic tumors, hepatic disease, CAD, women 40 and over

Precautions: Depression, hypertension, renal disease, seizure disorders, lupus erythematosus, rheumatic disease, migraine headache, amenorrhea, irregular menses, breast cancer (fibrocystic), gallbladder disease

Pharmacokinetics: Excreted in breast milk

Interactions/incompatibilities:

• Decreased effectiveness of this drug: anticonvulsants, rifampin, analgesics, antibiotics, antihistamines, chenodiol, griseofulvin

• Decreased action of: oral anticoagulants

• Increased clotting: aminocaproic acid

NURSING CONSIDERATIONS

Monitor:

• Glucose, thyroid function, liver function tests

Evaluate:

• Therapeutic response: absence of pregnancy, endometriosis, hypermenorrhea

• Reproductive changes: change in breasts, tumors, positive Pap smear; drug should be discontinued if changes occur

Teach patient/family:

• Detection of clots using Homan's sign

• To use sunscreen or avoid sunlight; photosensitivity can occur

• To take at same time each day to ensure equal drug level

• To report GI symptoms that occur after 4 mo

• To use another birth control method during 1st week of oral contraceptive use

• To take another tablet as soon as possible if one is missed

• That after drug is discontinued, pregnancy may not occur for several months

• To report abdominal pain, change in vision, shortness of breath, change in menstrual flow, spotting, breakthrough bleeding, breast lumps, swelling

• That continuing medical care is needed: PAP smear and gynecologic examinations q6 mo

Lab test interferences:

Increase: Pro-time, clotting factors

VII, VIII, IX, X, TBG, PBI, T$_4$, platelet aggregability, BSP, triglycerides, bilirubin, AST, ALT
Decrease: T$_3$, antithrombin III, folate, metyrapone test, GTT, 17-OHCS

---

orphenadrine citrate

(or-fen'a-dreen)
Banflex, Flexon, Myolin, Norflex, Ro-Orphena, X-Otag

Func. class.: Skeletal muscle relaxant, central acting
Chem. class.: Tertiary amine

Action: Acts centrally on skeletal muscle to relax, inhibit muscle spasm
Uses: Pain in musculoskeletal conditions, Parkinson's syndrome
Dosage and routes:
• *Adult:* PO 100 mg bid; IM/IV 60 mg q12h
Available forms include: Tabs 100 mg; tabs sus rel 100 mg; inj IM, IV 30 mg/ml
Side effects/adverse reactions:
HEMA: Aplastic anemia
CNS: Dizziness, weakness, fatigue, drowsiness, headache, disorientation, insomnia, stimulation, hallucination, agitation
EENT: Nasal congestion, blurred vision, increased intraocular pressure
CV: Hypotension, tachycardia
GI: Nausea, vomiting, constipation, dry mouth
GU: Urinary frequency, hesitancy
INTEG: Rash, pruritus, urticaria
Contraindications: Hypersensitivity, narrow-angle glaucoma, GI obstruction, myasthenia gravis, stenosing peptic ulcer
Precautions: Pregnancy, children, cardiac disease
Pharmacokinetics:
PO: Peak 2 hr, duration 4-6 hr, half-life 14 hr, metabolized in liver, excreted in urine (unchanged)

Interactions/incompatibilities:
• Increased CNS effects: propoxyphene
NURSING CONSIDERATIONS
Assess:
• Blood studies: CBC, WBC, differential; blood dyscrasias may occur (rare)
• I&O ratio; check for urinary retention, frequency, hesitancy
Administer:
• With meals for GI symptoms
Perform/provide:
• Assistance with ambulation if dizziness, drowsiness occurs
Evaluate:
• Therapeutic response: decreased rigidity, spasms
• Allergic reactions: rash, fever, respiratory distress
• Blood dyscrasias: temperature, bleeding, fatigue (rare)
• CNS symptoms: dizziness, drowsiness, psychiatric symptoms
Teach patient/family:
• Not to discontinue medication quickly; insomnia, nausea, headache will occur
• Not to take with alcohol, other CNS depressants
• To avoid altering activities while taking this drug
• To avoid hazardous activities if drowsiness, dizziness occurs
• To avoid using OTC medication: cough preparations, antihistamines, unless directed by physician

---

oxacillin sodium

(ox-a-sill'in)
Bactocill, Prostaphilin

Func. class.: Broad-spectrum antibiotic
Chem. class.: Penicillinase-resistant penicillin

Action: Interferes with cell wall replication of susceptible organisms; osmotically unstable cell wall

---

swells, bursts from osmotic pressure

Uses: Effective for gram-positive cocci *(S. aureus, S. pneumoniae),* infections caused by penicillinase-producing *Staphylococcus*

Dosage and routes:

• *Adult:* PO 2-4 g/day in divided doses q6h; IM/IV 2-12 g/day in divided doses q4-6h

• *Child:* PO 50-100 mg/kg/day in divided doses q6h; IM/IV 50-100 mg/kg/day in divided doses q4-6h

Available forms include: Caps 250, 500 mg; powder for oral susp 250 mg/5 ml; powder for inj IM, IV 250, 500 mg, 1, 2, 4, 10 g; IV INF 1, 2, 4 g

Side effects/adverse reactions:

HEMA: Anemia, increased bleeding time, *bone marrow depression, granulocytopenia*

GI: Nausea, vomiting, diarrhea, increased AST, ALT, abdominal pain, glossitis, colitis

GU: Oliguria, proteinuria, hematuria, *vaginitis, moniliasis, glomerulonephritis*

CNS: Lethargy, hallucinations, anxiety, depression, twitching, *coma, convulsions*

META: Hyperkalemia, hypokalemia, alkalosis, hypernatremia

Contraindications: Hypersensitivity to penicillins

Precautions: Pregnancy (B), hypersensitivity to cephalosporins, neonates

Pharmacokinetics:

PO/IM: Peak 30-60 min, duration 4-6 hr

IV: Peak 5 min, duration 4-6 hr, half-life 30-60 min, excreted in urine, bile, breast milk, crosses placenta

Interactions/incompatibilities:

• Decreased antimicrobial effectiveness of this drug: tetracyclines, erythromycins

• Increased penicillin concentrations when used with: aspirin, probenecid

NURSING CONSIDERATIONS

Assess:

• I&O ratio; report hematuria, oliguria since penicillin in high doses is nephrotoxic

• Any patient with compromised renal system since drug is excreted slowly in poor renal system function; toxicity may occur rapidly

• Liver studies: AST, ALT

• Blood studies: WBC, RBC, H&H, bleeding time

• Renal studies: urinalysis, protein, blood

• C&S before drug therapy; drug may be taken as soon as culture is taken

Administer:

• Drug after C&S has been completed

Perform/provide:

• Adrenalin, suction, tracheostomy set, endotracheal intubation equipment

• Adequate fluid intake (2000 ml) during diarrhea episodes

• Scratch test to assess allergy, after securing order from physician; usually done when penicillin is only drug of choice

• Storage in tight container; refrigerate reconstituted solution

Evaluate:

• Therapeutic effectiveness: absence of fever, draining wounds

• Bowel pattern before and during treatment

• Skin eruptions after administration of penicillin to 1 wk after discontinuing drug

• Respiratory status: rate, character, wheezing, tightness in chest

• Allergies before initiation of treatment, and reaction of each medication; highlight allergies on chart, Kardex

---

*Available in Canada only

Teach patient/family:

• Aspects of drug therapy including need to complete course of medication to ensure organism death (10-14 days); culture may be taken after completed course

• To report sore throat, fever, fatigue; could indicate superimposed infection

• To wear or carry Medic Alert ID if allergic to penicillins

• To notify nurse of diarrhea stools

Lab test interferences:

Decrease: Uric acid

False positive: Urine glucose, urine protein

Treatment of overdose: Withdraw drug, maintain airway, administer epinephrine, aminophylline, O_2, IV corticosteroids for anaphylaxis

---

oxamniquine

(ox-am′ni-kwin)

Vansil

Func. class.: Anthelmintic

Chem. class.: Tetrahydroquinone derivative

Action: Causes paralysis, contraction, leading to dislodgement of suckers; they are carried to liver where phagocytosis takes place

Uses: Schistosomiasis

Dosage and routes:

• *Adult and child >30 kg:* PO 12-15 mg/kg as single dose

• *Child <30 kg:* PO 20 mg/kg in 2 divided doses q2-8h

Available forms include: Caps 250 mg

Side effects/adverse reactions:

INTEG: Rash, pruritus, urticaria

CNS: Dizziness, headache, drowsiness, insomnia, convulsions, hallucination, personality changes, stimulation

EENT: Bad taste, oral irritation

GI: Nausea, vomiting, anorexia, abdominal pain

HEMA: Increased sed rate, reticulocyte count, increase or decrease in leukocytes

Contraindications: Hypersensitivity

Precautions: Pregnancy (C), lactation, seizure disorders

Pharmacokinetics:

PO: Peak 1-1½ hr, half-life 1-2½ hr, excreted in urine, (unchanged/ metabolites)

Interactions/incompatibilities: None known

NURSING CONSIDERATIONS

Assess:

• Stools during entire treatment, 1, 3 mo after treatment; specimens must be sent to lab while still warm

Administer:

• PO after meals to avoid GI symptoms

Perform/provide:

• Storage in tight container, cool environment

Evaluate:

• Therapeutic response: expulsion of worms, 3 negative stool cultures after completion of treatment

• For allergic reaction: rash, itching, urticaria

• For infection in other family members since infection from person to person is common

Teach patient/family:

• Proper hygiene after BM including handwashing technique; tell patient to avoid putting fingers in mouth

• That infected person should sleep alone; do not shake bed linen, change bed linen daily, wash in hot water

• To clean toilet qd with disinfectant (green soap solution)

• Need for compliance with dosage schedule, duration of treatment

• That urine may turn orange or red

• To avoid hazardous activities since drowsiness occurs

---

italics = common side effects   ***bold italic*** = life threatening reactions

• That seizures may recur in patient who is controlled on medication
Lab test interferences:
Interferes: Urinalysis

---

oxandrolone

(ox-an′droe-lone)
Anavar

Func. class.: Androgenic anabolic steroid
Chem. class.: Halogenated testosterone derivative

Action: Increases weight by building body tissue, increases potassium, phosphorus, chloride, nitrogen levels, increases bone development
Uses: Tissue building after steroid therapy, osteoporosis, prolonged immobility
Dosage and routes:
• *Adult:* PO 2.5 mg bid-qid, not to exceed 20 mg qd × 2-3 wk
• *Child:* PO 0.25 mg/kg/day × 2-4 wk, not to exceed 3 mo
Available forms include: Tabs 2.5 mg
Side effects/adverse reactions:
INTEG: Rash, acneiform lesions, oily hair, skin, flushing, sweating, acne vulgaris, alopecia, hirsutism
CNS: Dizziness, headache, fatigue, tremors, paresthesias, flushing, sweating, anxiety, lability, insomnia
MS: Cramps, spasms
CV: Increased B/P
GU: Hematuria, amenorrhea, vaginitis, decrease libido, decreased breast size, clitoral hypertrophy, testicular atrophy
GI: Nausea, vomiting, constipation, weight gain, *cholestatic jaundice*
EENT: Carpal tunnel syndrome, conjunctional edema, nasal congestion
ENDO: Abnormal GTT

Contraindications: Severe renal disease, severe cardiac disease, severe hepatic disease, hypersensitivity, pregnancy (X), lactation, genital bleeding (abnormal)
Precautions: Diabetes mellitus, CV disease, MI
Pharmacokinetics:
PO: Metabolized in liver, excreted in urine, crosses placenta, excreted in breast milk
Interactions/incompatibilities:
• Increased effects of: oral antidiabetics, oxyphenbutazone
• Increased PT: anticoagulants
• Edema: ACTH, adrenal steroids
• Decreased effects of: insulin
NURSING CONSIDERATIONS
Assess:
• Weight daily, notify physician if weekly weight gain is >5 lb
• B/P q4h
• I&O ratio; be alert for decreasing urinary output, increasing edema
• Growth rate in children since growth rate may be uneven (linear/bone browth) when used for extended time
• Electrolytes: K, Na, Cl, Ca; cholesterol
• Liver function studies: ALT, AST, bilirubin
Administer:
• Titrated dose, use lowest effective dose
Perform/provide:
• Diet with increased calories and protein; decrease sodium if edema occurs
• Supportive drug of enemia
Evaluate:
• Therapeutic response: occurs in 4-6 wk in osteoporosis
• Edema, hypertension, cardiac symptoms, jaundice
• Mental status: affect, mood, behavioral changes, aggression
• Signs of masculinization in female: increased libido, deepening of voice, breast tissue, enlarged

clitoris, menstrual irregularities; male: gynecomastia, impotence, testicular atrophy

• Hypercalcemia: lethargy, polyuria, polydipsia, nausea, vomiting, constipation; drug may need to be decreased

• Hypoglycemia in diabetics, since oral anticoagulant action is decreased

Teach patient/family:

• Drug needs to be combined with complete health plan: diet, rest, exercise

• To notify physician if therapeutic response decreases

• Not to discontinue this medication abruptly

• Teach patient all aspects of drug usage, including change in sex characteristics

• Women to report menstrual irregularities

• That 1-3 mo course is necessary for response in breast cancer

• Procedure for use of buccal tablets (requires 30-60 min to dissolve, change absorption site with each dose; do not eat, drink, chew, or smoke while tablet is in place)

Lab test interferences:

Increase: Serum cholesterol, blood glucose, urine glucose

Decrease: Serum calcium, serum potassium, T_4, T_3, thyroid ^{131}I uptake test, urine 17-OHCS, 17-KS, PBI, BSP

---

oxazepam

(ox-a'ze-pam)
Serax

Func. class.: Antianxiety
Chem. class.: Benzodiazepine

Controlled Substance Schedule IV

Action: Depresses subcortical levels of CNS, including limbic system and reticular formation

Uses: Anxiety, alcohol withdrawal

Dosage and routes:

Anxiety

• *Adult:* PO 10-30 mg tid-qid

Alcohol withdrawal

• *Adult:* PO 15-30 mg tid-qid

Available forms include: Caps 10, 15, 30 mg, tabs 15 mg

Side effects/adverse reactions:

CNS: Dizziness, drowsiness, confusion, headache, anxiety, tremors, stimulation, fatigue, depression, insomnia, hallucinations

GI: Constipation, dry mouth, nausea, vomiting, anorexia, diarrhea

INTEG: Rash, dermatitis, itching

*CV: Orthostatic hypotension, **ECG changes, tachycardia,*** hypotension

EENT: Blurred vision, tinnitus, mydriasis

Contraindications: Hypersensitivity to benzodiazepines, narrowangle glaucoma, psychosis, pregnancy (D), child <18 yr

Precautions: Elderly, debilitated, hepatic disease, renal disease

Pharmacokinetics:

PO: Peak 2-4 hr, metabolized by liver, excreted by kidneys, half-life 3-21 hr

Interactions/incompatibilities:

• Decreased effects of this drug: oral contraceptives, rifampin, valproic acid

• Increased effects of this drug: CNS depressants, alcohol, cimetidine, disulfiram, oral contraceptives

NURSING CONSIDERATIONS

Assess:

• B/P (lying, standing), pulse; if systolic B/P drops 20 mm Hg, hold drug, notify physician; respirations q5-15 min if given IV

• Blood studies: CBC during longterm therapy, blood dyscrasias have occurred rarely

• Hepatic studies: AST, ALT, bili-

---

rubin, creatinine, LDH, alk phosphatase

Administer:

• With food or milk for GI symptoms

• Crushed if patient is unable to swallow medication whole

• Sugarless gum, hard candy, frequent sips of water for dry mouth

Perform/provide:

• Assistance with ambulation during beginning therapy; drowsiness/dizziness occurs

• Safety measures, including siderails

• Check to see PO medication has been swallowed

Evaluate:

• Therapeutic response: decreased anxiety, restlessness, insomnia

• Mental status: mood, sensorium, affect, sleeping pattern, drowsiness, dizziness

• Physical dependency, withdrawal symptoms: headache, nausea, vomiting, muscle pain, weakness after long-term use

• Suicidal tendencies

Teach patient/family:

• That drug may be taken with food

• Not to be used for everyday stress or used longer than 4 mo, unless directed by physician

• Avoid OTC preparations (cough, cold, hay fever) unless approved by physician

• To avoid driving, activities that require alertness, since drowsiness may ocur

• To avoid alcohol ingestion or other psychotropic medications unless prescribed by physician

• Not to discontinue medication abruptly after long-term use

• To rise slowly or fainting may occur

• That drowsiness might worsen at beginning of treatment

Lab test interferences:

Increase: AST/ALT, serum bilirubin

Decrease: RAIU

False increase: 17-OHCS

Treatment of overdose: Lavage, VS, supportive care

---

oxidized cellulose

Oxycel, Surgicel

Func. class.: Hemostatic

Chem. class.: Cellulose product

Action: Absorbs blood in great quantities

Uses: Hemostasis in surgery, bleeding of tumors (external)

Dosage and routes:

Adult and child: TOP apply using sterile technique as needed, remove after bleeding stops, if possible, or leave in place if needed

Available forms include: TOP knitted fabric

Side effects/adverse reactions:

EENT: Epistaxis, sneezing, burning

INTEG: Burning, stinging, encapsulation

CNS: Headache

Contraindications: Hypersensitivity, large artery hemorrhage, oozing surfaces, implantation in bone deficit

Interactions/incompatibilities: None known

NURSING CONSIDERATIONS

Administer:

• Dry, use only amount needed to control bleeding

• Loosely, remove excess before closure in surgery; irrigate first, then remove using sterile technique

• Using sterile technique

Evaluate:

• Allergy: fever, rash, itching, burning, stinging

• Bleeding: mucous membranes, epistaxis, ecchymosis, petechiae, hematuria, hematemesis

---

*Available in Canada only

Teach patient/family:

• To report any signs of bleeding: gums, under skin, urine, stools, emesis

---

oxtriphylline

(ox-trye'fi-lin)

Choledyl, Theophylline Choline

Func. class.: Spasmolytic

Chem. class.: Choline salt of theophylline

Action: Relaxes smooth muscle of respiratory system by blocking phosphodiesterase, which increases cyclic AMP; 64% theophylline

Uses: Acute bronchial asthma, reversible bronchospasm in chronic bronchitis and COPD

Dosage and routes:

• *Adult and child >12 yr:* PO 200 mg q6h

• *Child 2-12 yr:* PO 4 mg/kg q6h; may be increased to desired response, therapeutic level

Available forms include: Elix 100 mg/5 ml; sol 50 mg/5 ml; tabs 100, 200, 400, 600 mg

Side effects/adverse reactions:

CNS: Anxiety, restlessness, insomnia, dizziness, convulsions, headache, light-headedness

CV: Palpitations, sinus tachycardia, hypotension

GI: Nausea, vomiting, anorexia, diarrhea, bitter taste, dyspepsia, anal irritation (suppositories)

RESP: Increased rate

INTEG: Flushing, urticaria

Contraindications: Hypersensitivity to xanthines, tachydysrhythmias

Precautions: Elderly, CHF, cor pulmonale, hepatic disease, active peptic ulcer disease, diabetes mellitus, hyperthyroidism, hypertension, children

Pharmacokinetics:

IV: Peak 30 min

SOL: Peak 1 hr, metabolized in liver, excreted in urine, breast milk, crosses placenta

Interactions/incompatibilities:

• Do not mix in syringe with other drugs

• Increased action of this drug: cimetidine, erythromycin, troleandomycin

• May increase effects of: anticoagulants

• Cardiotoxicity: beta blockade

NURSING CONSIDERATIONS

Assess:

• Therapeutic blood levels; toxicity may occur with small increase above therapeutic level

• Monitor I&O; diuresis occurs, dehydration may result in elderly or children

• Whether theophylline was given recently

Administer:

• PO after meals to decrease GI symptoms; absorption may be affected

• After meals, hs

• Avoid IM injection; pain occurs

Evaluate:

• Therapeutic response: absence of dyspnea, wheezing

• Respiratory rate, rhythm, depth; auscultate lung fields bilaterally; notify physician of abnormalities

• Allergic reactions: rash, urticaria; if these occur, drug should be discontinued

Teach patient/family:

• To check OTC medications, current prescription medications for ephedrine, which will increase stimulation

• To avoid hazardous activities; dizziness may occur

• On all aspects of drug therapy: dosage, routes, side effects, when to notify the physician

• If GI upset occurs, to take drug with 8 oz water; avoid food; absorption may be decreased

---

italics = common side effects   ***bold italic*** = life threatening reactions

• To remain in bed 15-20 min after rectal suppository is inserted to avoid removal

---

oxybutynin chloride

(ox-i-byoo'ti-nin)

Ditropan

Func. class.: Spasmolytic

Chem. class.: Synthetic tertiary amine

Action: Relaxes smooth muscles in urinary tract

Uses: Antispasmodic for neurogenic bladder

Dosage and routes:

• *Adult:* PO 5 mg bid-tid, not to exceed 5 mg qid

• *Child >5 yr:* PO 5 mg bid, not to exceed 5 mg tid

Available forms include: Sol 5 mg/5 ml; tabs 5 mg

Side effects/adverse reactions:

*HEMA: **Leukopenia, eosinophilia***

CNS: Anxiety, restlessness, dizziness, convulsions, headache, drowsiness, confusion

CV: Palpitations, sinus tachycardia, hypotension

GI: Nausea, vomiting, anorexia, abdominal pain, constipation

GU: Dysuria, retention, hesitancy

INTEG: Urticaria, dermatitis

EENT: Blurred vision, increased intraocular tension, dry mouth, throat

Contraindications: Hypersensitivity, GI obstruction, GI hemorrhage, GU obstruction, glaucoma, severe colitis, myasthenia gravis, unstable CV status in acute hemorrhage

Precautions: Pregnancy, lactation, suspected glaucoma, children <12 yr

Pharmacokinetics: Onset ½-1 hr, peak 3-4 hr, duration 6-10 hr, metabolized by liver, excreted in urine

Interactions/incompatibilities: None known

NURSING CONSIDERATIONS

Evaluate:

• Urinary status: dysuria, frequency, nocturia, incontinence

• Allergic reactions: rash, urticaria; if these occur, drug should be discontinued

Teach patient/family

• To avoid hazardous activities; dizziness may occur

• On all aspects of drug therapy: dosage, routes, side effects, when to notify physician

---

oxycodone HCl

(ox-i-koe'done)

Supeudol*; Combinations—Co-doxy, Percocet,* Percocet-Demi, Percodan, Tylox

Func. class.: Narcotic analgesics

Chem. class.: Opiate, semisynthetic derivative

Controlled Substance Schedule II

Action: Inhibits ascending pain pathways in CNS, increases pain threshold, alters pain perception

Uses: Moderate to severe pain

Dosage and routes:

• *Adult:* REC 1-3 supp/day prn (Supeubol)

• *Child:* PO ¼-½ tab q6h prn (Percodan-Demi)

• *Adult:* PO 1-2 tab q6h prn (Combinations)

Available forms include: Tabs 5 mg; sol 5 mg/5ml

Side effects/adverse reactions:

CNS: Drowsiness, dizziness, confusion, headache, sedation, euphoria

GI: Nausea, vomiting, anorexia, constipation, cramps

GU: Increased urinary output, dysuria

INTEG: Rash, urticaria, bruising, flushing, diaphoresis, pruritus

EENT: Tinnitus, blurred vision, miosis, diplopia

CV: Palpitations, bradycardia, change in B/P
RESP: Respiratory depression
Contraindications: Hypersensitivity, addiction (narcotic)
Precautions: Addictive personality, pregnancy, lactation, increased intracranial pressure, MI (acute), severe heart disease, respiratory depression, hepatic disease, renal disease, child <18 yr
Pharmacokinetics:
PO: Onset 10-15 min, peak ½-1 hr, duration 4-5 hr; detoxified by liver, excreted in urine, crosses placenta, excreted in breast milk
Interactions/incompatibilities:
• Effects may be increased with other CNS depressants: alcohol, narcotics, sedative/hypnotics, antipsychotics, skeletal muscle relaxants

NURSING CONSIDERATIONS
Assess:
• I&O ratio; check for decreasing output; may indicate urinary retention
Administer:
• With antiemetic if nausea, vomiting occur
• When pain is beginning to return; determine dosage interval by patient response
Perform/provide:
• Storage in light-resistant area at room temperature
• Assistance with ambulation
• Safety measures: siderails, night light, call bell within easy reach
Evaluate:
• Therapeutic response: decrease in pain
• CNS changes: dizziness, drowsiness, hallucinations, euphoria, LOC, pupil reaction
• Allergic reactions: rash, urticaria
• Respiratory dysfunction: respiratory depression, character, rash, rhythm; notify physician if respirations are <12/min

• Need for pain medication, physical dependence
Teach patient/family:
• To report any symptoms of CNS changes, allergic reactions
• That physical dependency may result when used for extended periods of time
• Withdrawal symptoms may occur: nausea, vomiting, cramps, fever, faintness, anorexia
Lab test interferences:
Increase: Amylase
Treatment of overdose: Narcan 0.2-0.8 IV, O₂, IV fluids, vasopressors

---

oxymetazoline HCl (nasal)
(ox-i-met-az'oh-leen)
Afrin, Afrin Pediatric Nose Drops, Dristan Long-Lasting, Duramist, Duration, Nostrills, NTZ Long-Acting, Sinex Long-Lasting, St. Joseph's Decongestant for Children
Func. class.: Nasal decongestant
Chem. class.: Sympathomimetic amine

O

Action: Produces vasoconstriction (rapid, long-acting) of arterioles, thereby decreasing fluid exudation, mucosal engorgement
Uses: Nasal congestion
Dosage and routes:
• *Adult and child >6 yr:* INSTILL 2-3 gtts or sprays to each nostril bid
• *Child 2-6 yr:* INSTILL 2-3 gtts or sprays .025% sol bid, not to exceed 5 days
Available forms include: Sol 0.025%, 0.05%
Side effects/adverse reactions:
GI: Nausea, vomiting, anorexia
EENT: Irritation, burning, sneezing, stinging, dryness, rebound congestion
INTEG: Contact dermatitis
CNS: Anxiety, restlessness, trem-

ors, weakness, insomnia, dizziness, fever, headache

Contraindications: Hypersensitivity to sympathomimetic amines

Precautions: Child <6 yr, elderly, diabetes, cardiovascular disease, hypertension, hyperthyroidism, increased ICP, prostatic hypertrophy

Interactions/incompatibilities:

• Hypertension: MAOIs, β-adrenergic blockers

• Hypotension: methyldopa, mecamylamine, reserpine

NURSING CONSIDERATIONS
Administer:

• No more than q4h

• For <4 consecutive days

Perform/provide:

• Environmental humidification to decrease nasal congestion, dryness

• Storage in light-resistant containers; do not expose to high temperatures

Evaluate:

• For redness, swelling, pain in nasal passages

Teach patient/family:

• Stinging may occur for a few applications; drying of mucosa may be decreased by environmental humidification

• To notify physician if irregular pulse, insomnia, dizziness, or tremors occur

• Proper administration to avoid systemic absorption

---

oxymetholone
(ox-i-meth′oh-lone)

Adroyd, Anadrol-50, Anapolon 50*

Func. class.: Androgenic anabolic steroid

Chem. class.: Halogenated testosterone derivative

Action: Increases weight by building body tissue, increases potassium, phosphorus, chloride, and nitrogen levels, increases bone development

Uses: Tissue building after steroid therapy, osteoporosis, aplastic anemia, anemias caused by deficient RBC production

Dosage and routes:

Aplastic anemia

• *Adult and child:* PO 1-5 mg/kg/day, titrated to patient response, not to exceed 3 months

Osteoporosis/tissue building (possible indication)

• *Adult:* PO 5-15 mg/day, not to exceed 30 mg/day or 3 mo

• *Child >6 yr:* PO up to 10 mg/day, not to exceed 1 mo

• *Child <6 yr:* PO 1.25 mg qd-qid, not to exceed 1 mo

Available forms include: Tabs 50 mg

Side effects/adverse reactions:

INTEG: Rash, acneiform lesions, oily hair, skin, flushing, sweating, acne vulgaris, alopecia, hirsutism

CNS: Dizziness, headache, fatigue, tremors, paresthesias, flushing, sweating, anxiety, lability, insomnia

MS: Cramps, spasms

CV: Increased B/P

GU: Hematuria, amenorrhea, vaginitis, decreased libido, decreased breast size, clitoral hypertrophy, testicular atrophy

GI: Nausea, vomiting, constipation, weight gain, *cholestatic jaundice*

EENT: Carpal tunnel syndrome, conjunctival edema, nasal congestion

ENDO: Abnormal GTT

Contraindications: Severe renal disease, severe cardiac disease, severe hepatic disease, hypersensitivity, pregnancy (X), lactation, genital bleeding (abnormal)

Precautions: Diabetes mellitus, CV disease, MI

Pharmacokinetics:
PO: Metabolized in liver, excreted in urine, crosses placenta, excreted in breast milk

Interactions/incompatibilities:
• Increased effects of: oral antidiabetics, oxyphenbutazone
• Increased PT: anticoagulants
• Edema: ACTH, adrenal steroids
• Decreased effects of: insulin

NURSING CONSIDERATIONS

Assess:
• Weight daily, notify physician if weekly weight gain is >5 lb
• B/P q4h
• I&O ratio; be alert for decreasing urinary output, increasing edema
• Growth rate in children since growth rate may be uneven (linear/bone browth) when used for extended period
• Electrolytes: K, Na, Cl, Ca; cholesterol
• Liver function studies: ALT, AST, bilirubin

Administer:
• Titrated dose, use lowest effective dose

Perform/provide:
• Diet with increased calories and protein; decrease sodium if edema occurs
• Supportive drug of anemia

Evaluate:
• Therapeutic response: occurs in 4-6 wk in osteoporosis
• Edema, hypertension, cardiac symptoms, jaundice
• Mental status: affect, mood, behavioral changes, aggression
• Signs of masculinization in female: increased libido, deepening of voice, breast tissue, enlarged clitoris, menstrual irregularities; male: gynecomastia, impotence, testicular atrophy
• Hypercalcemia: lethargy, polyuria, polydipsia, nausea, vomiting, constipation; drug may need to be decreased

• Hypoglycemia in diabetics, since oral anticoagulant action is decreased

Teach patient/family:
• Drug needs to be combined with complete health plan: diet, rest, exercise
• To notify physician if therapeutic response decreases
• Not to discontinue this medication abruptly
• Teach patient all aspects of drug usage, including changes in sex characteristics
• Women to report menstrual irregularities
• That 1-3 mo course is necessary for response in breast cancer
• Procedure for use of buccal tablets (requires 30-60 min to dissolve, change absorption site with each dose; do not eat, drink, chew, or smoke while tablet is in place)

Lab test interferences:
Increase: Serum cholesterol, blood glucose, urine glucose
Decrease: Serum calcium, serum potassium, T_4, T_3, thyroid ^{131}I uptake test, urine 17-OHCS, 17-KS, PBI, BSP

---

oxymorphone HCl

(ox-i-mor-fone)
Numorphan

Func. class.: Narcotic analgesics
Chem. class.: Opiate, semisynthetic phenanthrene derivative

Controlled Substance Schedule II
Action: Inhibits ascending pain pathways in CNS, increases pain threshold, alters pain perception
Uses: Moderate to severe pain
Dosage and routes:
• *Adult:* IM/SC 1-1.5 mg q4-6h prn; IV 0.5 mg q4-6h prn; REC 2.5-5 mg q4-6h prn
Available forms include: Inj SC,

IM, IV 1, 1.5 mg/ml; supp 5 mg

Side effects/adverse reactions:

CNS: Drowsiness, dizziness, confusion, headache, sedation, euphoria

GI: Nausea, vomiting, anorexia, constipation, cramps

GU: Increased urinary output, dysuria

INTEG: Rash, urticaria, bruising, flushing, diaphoresis, pruritus

EENT: Tinnitus, blurred vision, miosis, diplopia

CV: Palpitations, bradycardia, change in B/P

RESP: Respiratory depression

Contraindications: Hypersensitivity, addiction (narcotic)

Precautions: Addictive personality, pregnancy, lactation, increased intracranial pressure, MI (acute), severe heart disease, respiratory depression, hepatic disease, renal disease, child <18 yr

Pharmacokinetics:

SC/IM: Onset 10-15 min, peak 1-½ hr, duration 2-6 hr

IV: Onset 5-10 min, peak 1-½ hr, duration 3-6 hr

REC: Onset 15-30 min, duration 3-6 hr

Metabolized by liver, excreted in urine, crosses placenta

Interactions/incompatibilities:

• Effects may be increased with other CNS depressants: alcohol, narcotics, sedative/hypnotics, antipsychotics, skeletal muscle relaxants

NURSING CONSIDERATIONS

Assess:

• I&O ratio; check for decreasing output; may indicate urinary retention

Administer:

• With antiemetic if nausea, vomiting occur

• When pain is beginning to return; determine dosage interval by patient response

Perform/provide:

• Storage in light-resistant area at room temperature

• Assistance with ambulation

• Safety measures: siderails, night light, call bell within easy reach

Evaluate:

• Therapeutic response: decrease in pain

• CNS changes: dizziness, drowsiness, hallucinations, euphoria, LOC, pupil reaction

• Allergic reactions: rash, urticaria

• Respiratory dysfunction: respiratory depression, character, rate, rhythm; notify physician if respirations are <12/min

• Need for pain medication, physical dependence

Teach patient/family:

• To report any symptoms of CNS changes, allergic reactions

• That physical dependency may result when used for extended periods of time

• Withdrawal symptoms may occur: nausea, vomiting, cramps, fever, faintness, anorexia

Lab test interferences:

Increase: Amylase

Treatment of overdose: Narcan 0.2-0.8 IV, O$_2$, IV fluids, vasopressors

oxyphenbutazone

(ox-i-fen-byoo′ta-zone)

Oxalid

Func. class.: Nonsteroidal

Chem. class.: Pyrazolone derivative

Action: Inhibits prostaglandin synthesis by decreasing an enzyme needed for biosynthesis; possesses analgesic, antiinflammatory, antipyretic properties

Uses: Mild to moderate pain, osteoarthritis, rheumatoid arthritis

Dosage and routes:
Pain
• *Adult:* PO 100-200 mg tid-qid
Acute arthritis
• *Adult:* PO 400 mg, then 100 mg q4h × 4 days or until desired response

Available forms include: Tabs 100 mg

Side effects/adverse reactions:
GI: Nausea, anorexia, vomiting, diarrhea, jaundice, *cholestatic hepatitis,* constipation, flatulence, cramps, dry mouth, peptic ulcer
CNS: Dizziness, drowsiness, fatigue, tremors, confusion, insomnia, anxiety, depression
CV: Tachycardia, peripheral edema, palpitations, dysrhythmias
INTEG: Purpura, rash, pruritus, sweating
GU: Nephrotoxicity: dysuria, hematuria, oliguria, azotemia
HEMA: Blood dyscrasias
EENT: Tinnitus, hearing loss, blurred vision

Contraindications: Hypersensitivity, asthma, severe renal disease, severe hepatic disease
Precautions: Pregnancy, lactation, children, bleeding disorders, GI disorders, cardiac disorders, hypersensitivity to other antiinflammatory agents

Pharmacokinetics:
PO: Peak 2 hr, half-life 3-3½ hr; metabolized in liver, excreted in urine (metabolites), excreted in breast milk

Interactions/incompatibilities:
• May increase action of coumarin, phenytoin, sulfonamides when used with this drug

NURSING CONSIDERATIONS
Assess:
• Renal, liver, blood studies: BUN, creatinine, AST, ALT, Hgb before treatment, periodically thereafter
• Audiometric, ophthalmic exam before, during, after treatment

Administer:
• With food to decrease GI symptoms; best to take on empty stomach to facilitate absorption
Perform/provide:
• Storage at room temperature
Evaluate:
• Therapeutic response: decreased pain, stiffness, swelling in joints, ability to move more easily
• For eye, ear problems: blurred vision, tinnitus (may indicate toxicity)
Teach patient/family:
• To report blurred vision, or ringing, roaring in ears (may indicate toxicity)
• To avoid driving or other hazardous activities if dizziness or drowsiness occurs
• To report change in urine pattern, weight increase, edema, pain increase in joints, fever, blood in urine (indicates nephrotoxicity)
• That therapeutic effects may take up to 1 mo

---

oxyphencyclimine HCl
(ox-i-fen-sye′kli-meen)
Daricon
Func. class.: Gastrointestinal anticholinergic
Chem. class.: Synthetic tertiary amine antimuscarinic

Action: Inhibits muscarinic actions of acetylcholine at postganglionic parasympathetic neuroeffector sites
Uses: Treatment of peptic ulcer disease
Dosage and routes:
• *Adult:* PO 10 mg bid AM and hs or 5 mg bid-tid
Available forms include: Caps 10, 20 mg; tabs 20 mg; syr 10 mg/5 ml; inj IM 10 mg/ml
Side effects/adverse reactions:
CNS: Confusion, stimulation in elderly, headache, insomnia, dizzi-

ness, drowsiness, anxiety, weakness, hallucination

GI: Dry mouth, constipation, paralytic ileus, heartburn, nausea, vomiting, dysphagia, absence of taste

GU: Hesitancy, retention, impotence

CV: Palpitations, tachycardia

EENT: Blurred vision, photophobia, mydriasis, cycloplegia, increased ocular tension

INTEG: Urticaria, rash, pruritus, anhidrosis, fever, allergic reactions

Contraindications: Hypersensitivity to anticholinergics, narrow-angle glaucoma, GI obstruction, myasthenia gravis, paralytic ileus, GI atony, toxic megacolon

Precautions: Hyperthyroidism, coronary artery disease, dysrhythmias, CHF, ulcerative colitis, hypertension, hiatal hernia, hepatic disease, renal disease

Pharmacokinetics:

PO: Onset 1-2 hr, duration 8-12 hr; metabolized by liver, excreted in urine

Interactions/incompatibilities:

• Increased anticholinergic effect: amantadine, tricyclic antidepressants, MAOIs

• Increased effect of: nitrofurantoin

• Decreased effect of: phenothiazines, levodopa

NURSING CONSIDERATIONS

Assess:

• VS, cardiac status: checking for dysrhythmias, increased rate, palpitations

• I&O ratio; check for urinary retention or hesitancy

Administer:

• ½-1 hr ac for better absorption

• Decreased dose to elderly patients; their metabolism may be slowed

• Gum, hard candy, frequent rinsing of mouth for dryness of oral cavity

Perform/provide:

• Storage in tight container protected from light

• Increased fluids, bulk, exercise to patient's lifestyle to decrease constipation

Evaluate:

• Therapeutic response: absence of epigastric pain, bleeding, nausea, vomiting

• GI complaints: pain, bleeding (frank or occult), nausea, vomiting, anorexia

Teach patient/family:

• Avoid driving or other hazardous activities until stabilized on medication

• Avoid alcohol or other CNS depressants; will enhance sedating properties of this drug

• To avoid hot environments, stroke may occur, drug suppresses perspiration

• Use sunglasses when outside to prevent photophobia

---

oxyphenonium bromide

(ox-i-fen-oh'nee-um)

Antrenyl bromide

Func. class.: Gastrointestinal anticholinergic

Chem. class.: Synthetic quaternary ammonium antimuscarinic

Action: Inhibits muscarinic actions of acetylcholine at postganglionic parasympathetic neuroeffector sites

Uses: Treatment of peptic ulcer disease

Dosage and routes:

• *Adult:* PO 10 mg qid × 7 days, then titrated to patient's needs

Available forms include: Tabs 5 mg

Side effects/adverse reactions:

CNS: Confusion, stimulation in elderly, headache, insomnia, dizziness, drowsiness, anxiety, weakness, hallucination

GI: Dry mouth, constipation, paralytic ileus, heartburn, nausea, vomiting, dysphagia, absence of taste

GU: Hesitancy, retention, impotence

CV: Palpitations, tachycardia

EENT: Blurred vision, photophobia, mydriasis, cycloplegia, increased ocular tension

INTEG: Urticaria, rash, pruritus, anhidrosis, fever, allergic reactions

Contraindications: Hypersensitivity to anticholinergics, narrow-angle glaucoma, GI obstruction, myasthenia gravis, paralytic ileus, GI atony, toxic megacolon

Precautions: Hyperthyroidism, coronary artery disease, dysrhythmias, CHF, ulcerative colitis, hypertension, hiatal hernia, hepatic disease, renal disease

Pharmacokinetics:

PO: Onset 30 min, peak 2 hr, duration 4-6 hr; metabolized by liver, excreted in urine (unchanged) half-life 3½ hr

Interactions/incompatibilities:

• Increased anticholinergic effect: amantadine, tricyclic antidepressants, MAOIs

• Increased effect of: nitrofurantoin

• Decreased effect of: phenothiazines, levodopa

NURSING CONSIDERATIONS

Assess:

• VS, cardiac status: checking for dysrhythmias, increased rate, palpitations

• I&O ratio; check for urinary retention or hesitancy

Administer:

• ½-1 hr ac for better absorption

• Decreased dose to elderly patients; their metabolism may be slowed

• Gum, hard candy, frequent rinsing of mouth for dryness of oral cavity

Perform/provide:

• Storage in tight container protected from light

• Increased fluids, bulk, exercise to patient's lifestyle to decrease constipation

Evaluate:

• Therapeutic response: absence of epigastric pain, bleeding, nausea, vomiting

• GI complaints: pain, bleeding (frank or occult), nausea, vomiting, anorexia

Teach patient/family:

• Avoid driving or other hazardous activities until stabilized on medication

• Avoid alcohol or other CNS depressants; will enhance sedating properties of this drug

---

oxytetracycline HCl

(ox-i-tet-ra-sye'kleen)
Dalimycin, Oxlopar, Oxytetraclor, Terramycin, Uri-tet, E.P. mycin
Func. class.: Broad spectrum antibiotic/antiinfective
Chem. class.: Tetracycline

Action: Inhibits protein synthesis, phosphorylation in microorganisms by binding to 30S ribosomal subunits, reversibly binding to 50S ribosomal subunits

Uses: Syphilis, chlamydia trachomatis, gonorrhea, lymphogranuloma venereum

Dosage and routes:

• *Adult:* PO 250 mg q6h; IM 100 mg q8h or 250 mg q12h IV 250-500 mg q6-12h

• *Child >8 yr:* PO 25-50 mg/kg/day in divided doses q6h; IM 15-25 mg/kg/day in divided doses q8-12h; IV 10-20 mg/kg/day in divided doses q12h

Gonorrhea

• *Adult:* PO 1.5 g, then 500 mg qid for a total of 9 g

Chlamydia trachomatis

• *Adult:* PO 100 mg bid × 7 days

Syphilis

• *Adult:* PO 2-3 g in divided doses × 10-15 days

Available forms include: Tabs 250 mg; caps 125, 250 mg, powder for inj IV 250, 500 mg; inj IM 50, 125 mg/ml

Side effects/adverse reactions:

CNS: Fever, headache, paresthesia

HEMA: Eosinophilia, neutropenia, thrombocytopenia, leukocytosis, hemolytic anemia

EENT: Dysphagia, glossitis, decreased calcification of deciduous teeth, abdominal pain, oral candidiasis

GI: Nausea, vomiting, diarrhea, anorexia, enterocolitis, *hepatotoxicity,* flatulence, abdominal cramps, epigastric burning, stomatitis, *pseudomembranous colitis*

CV: Pericarditis

GU: Increased BUN, polyuria, polydipsia, renal failure, nephrotoxicity

INTEG: Rash, urticaria, photosensitivity, increased pigmentation, exfoliative dermatitis, pruritus, angioedema

Contraindications: Hypersensitivity to tetracyclines, children <8 yr

Precautions: Renal disease, hepatic disease, lactation, pregnancy

Pharmacokinetics:

PO: Peak 2-4 hr, half-life 6-9 hr; excreted in urine, bile, feces, in action form, crosses placenta 10%-40% protein bound

Interactions/incompatibilities:

• Decreased effect of this drug: antacids, NaHCO₃, dairy products, alkali products

• Increased effect: anticoagulants

• Decreased effect: penicillins

• Nephrotoxicity: methoxyflurane

NURSING CONSIDERATIONS

Assess:

• I&O ratio

• Blood studies: PT, CBC, AST, ALT, BUN, creatinine

Administer:

• After C&S obtained

• 2 hr before or after laxative or ferrous products, 3 hr after antacid

Perform/provide:

• Storage in tight, light-resistant container at room temperature

Evaluate:

• Therapeutic response: decreased temperature, absence of lesions, negative C&S

• Allergic reactions: rash, itching, pruritus, angioedema

• Nausea, vomiting, diarrhea; administer antiemetic, antacids as ordered

• Overgrowth of infection: increased temperature, malaise, redness, pain, swelling, drainage, perineal itching, diarrhea, changes in cough or sputum

Teach patient/family:

• To avoid sun exposure since burns may occur; sunscreen does not seem to decrease photosensitivity

• Of diabetic to avoid use of Clinistix, Diastix, or Tes-Tape for urine glucose testing

• That all prescribed medication must be taken to prevent superimposed infection

• To avoid milk products

Lab test interferences:

False positive: Urine glucose with Clinistix or Tes-Tape

False increase: Urinary catecholamines

oxytocin, synthetic injection

(ox-i-toe'sin)
Pitocin, Syntocinon, Uteracon
Func. class.: Oxytocic
Chem. class.: Hormone

Action: Directly acts on myofibrils producing uterine contraction, breast stimulation

Uses: Stimulation of labor, induction; missed or incomplete abortion; postpartum bleeding

Dosage and routes:
Stimulation of labor
• *Adult:* IV INF 1 ml/1000 ml D_5W or 0.9% NaCl over 1-2 milli U/min; may increase q15-30 min, not to exceed 20 milli U/min

Incomplete abortion
• *Adult:* IV INF 10 U/500 ml D_5W or 0.9% NaCl given at 20-40 milli U/min

Postpartum bleeding
• *Adult:* IV INF 10-40 U/1000 ml D_5W or 0.9% NaCl given at 20-40 milli U/min

Available forms include: Inj IV 10 U/ml

Side effects/adverse reactions:
CNS: Constipation, hypertension, subarachnoid
GI: Nausea, vomiting
CV: Hypotension, dysrhythmias, increased pulse
GU: Abruptio placentae, decreased uterine blood flow
INTEG: Rash
HEMA: Increased hyperbilirubimia
CV: Bradycardia, tachycardia, PVC
RESP: Anorexia, asphyxia

Contraindications: Hypersensitivity, serum toxemia, cephalopelvic disproportion, fetal distress

Precautions: Cervical/uterine surgery, sepsis (uterine), primipara >35, 1st, 2nd stage of labor

Pharmacokinetics:
IM: Onset 3-7 min, duration 1 hr, half-life 12-17 min
IV: Onset 1 min, duration 30 min, half-life 12-17 min

Interactions/incompatibilities:
• May cause hypertension when used with vasopressors

NURSING CONSIDERATIONS
Assess:
• I&O ratio
• Contraction FHT, B/P, pulse, respiration
• B/P, pulse; watch for changes that may indicate hemorrhage
• Respiratory rate, rhythm, depth; notify physician of abnormalities

Administer:
• By IV infusion
• After having crash cart available on unit (Mg^+SO_4 at bedside)

Evaluate:
• Length, duration of contraction; notify physician of contractions lasting over 1 min or absence of contractions

Teach patient/family:
• To report increased blood loss, abdominal cramps, increased temperature or foul-smelling lochia

oxytocin, synthetic nasal

(ox-i-toe'sin)
Func. class.: Oxytocic hormone

Action: Directly acts on myofibrils producing uterine contraction, breast stimulation

Uses: Postpartum breast engorgement, initial milk let-down

Dosage and routes:
• *Adult:* NAS SPRAY 1 spray into one or both nostrils q2-3 min before breast feeding; NAS DROPS 3 gtts into one or both nostrils q2-3 min before breast feeding

Available forms include: Nas spray 40 U/ml; nas drops

Side effects/adverse reactions:
None
Pharmacokinetics:
Onset 5-10 min, half-life 1 min
Interactions/incompatibilities:
• Hypertension: vasopressors
NURSING CONSIDERATIONS
Assess:
• I&O ratio
• Contraction FHT, B/P, pulse, respiration
• B/P, pulse; watch for changes that may indicate hemorrhage
• Respiratory rate, rhythm, depth; notify physician of abnormalities
Administer:
• By IV infusion
• After having crash cart available on unit (Mg^+SO_4 at bedside)
Evaluate:
• For length, duration of contraction; notify physician of contractions lasting over 1 min or absence of contractions
Teach patient/family:
• To report increased blood loss, abdominal cramps, increased temperature or foul-smelling lochia
• To blow nose before administering
• Rinse dropper with warm water after each use
• Not to over use

---

pancreatin
(pan'kree-a-tin)
Fortezyme*

Func. class.: Digestant
Chem. class.: Pancreatic enzyme concentrate—bovine/porcine

Action: Pancreatic enzyme needed for proper pancreatic functioning
Uses: Exocrine pancreatic secretion insufficiency, cystic fibrosis (digestive aid)
Dosage and routes:
• *Adult:* PO 8000-24,000 USP U ac or with meals

Available forms include: Tab 650, 2000, 12,000 U
Side effects/adverse reactions:
GI: Anorexia, nausea, vomiting, diarrhea, glossitis, anal soreness
GU: Hyperuricuria, hyperuricemia
INTEG: Rash, hypersensitivity
EENT: Buccal soreness
Contraindications: Hypersensitivity to hog protein
Precautions: Pregnancy, lactation
Interactions/incompatibilities:
• Decreased absorption: cimetidine, antacids, oral iron
NURSING CONSIDERATIONS
Assess:
• I&O ratio, watch for increasing urinary output
• Fecal fat, nitrogen, pro-time, calcium during treatment
Administer:
• After antacid or cimetidine; decreased pH inactivates drug
• Whole, not to be crushed, chewed (enteric coated)
• Low fat diet to decrease GI symptoms
Perform/provide:
• Storage in tight container at room temperature
Evaluate:
• For allergy to pork
• For polyuria, polydipsia, polyphagia (may indicate diabetes mellitus)

---

pancrelipase
(pan-kre-li'pase)
Cotazym, Cotazyme-S, Ilozyme, Ku-Zyme HP, Pancrease, Viokase
Func. class.: Digestant
Chem. class.: Pancreatic enzyme—bovine/porcine

Action: Pancreatic enzyme needed for proper pancreatic functioning
Uses: Exocrine pancreatic secretion insufficiency, cystic fibrosis

---

(digestive aid), steatorrhea, pancreatic enzyme deficiency

Dosage and routes:

• *Adult and child:* PO 1-3 caps/tabs ac or with meals, or 1 caps/tab with snack or 1-2 pdr pkt ac

Available forms include: Tab 8000, 11,000, 30,000 U; caps 8000, 30,000 U; enteric coated caps 4000, 5000, 20,000, 25,000 U; powd 16,800 U

Side effects/adverse reactions:

GI: Anorexia, nausea, vomiting, diarrhea

GU: Hyperuricuria, hyperuricemia

Contraindications: Allergy to pork

Precautions: Pregnancy

Interactions/incompatibilities:

• Decreased absorption: cimetidine, antacids, oral iron

NURSING CONSIDERATIONS

Assess:

• I&O ratio, watch for increasing urinary output

• Fecal fat, nitrogen, pro-time during treatment

Administer:

• After antacid or cimetidine; decreased pH inactivates drug

• Powder mixed in prepared fruit for infants, children

• Whole, not crushed or chewed (enteric coated)

• Low fat diet to decrease GI symptoms

• Powder mixed with pureed fruit

Perform/provide:

• Storage in tight container at room temperature

Evaluate:

• For allergy to pork

• For polyuria, polydipsia, polyphagia (may indicate diabetes mellitus)

pancuronium bromide

(pan-kyoo-roe′nee-um)

Pavulon

Func. class.: Neuromuscular blocker (nondepolarizing)

Chem. class.: Synthetic curariform

Action: Inhibits transmission of nerve impulses by binding with cholinergic receptor sites, antagonizing action of acetylcholine

Uses: Facilitation of endotracheal intubation, skeletal muscle relaxation during mechanical ventilation, surgery, or general anesthesia

Dosage and routes:

• *Adult:* IV 0.04-0.1 mg/kg, then 0.01 mg/kg q ½-1 hr

• *Child >10 yr:* IV 0.04-0.1 mg/kg, then ⅕ initial dose q ½-1 hr

Available forms include: Inj IV, IM, 1, 2 mg/ml

Side effects/adverse reactions:

CV: Bradycardia, tachycardia, increased, decreased B/P, ventricular extra systoles

*RESP: Prolonged apnea, **bronchospasm, cyanosis, respiratory depression***

EENT: Increased secretions

MS: Weakness to prolonged skeletal muscle relaxation

INTEG: Rash, flushing, pruritus, urticaria

Contraindications: Hypersensitivity to bromide ion

Precautions: Pregnancy, renal disease, cardiac disease, lactation, children <2 yr, electrolyte imbalances, dehydration, neuromuscular disease, respiratory disease

Pharmacokinetics:

IV: Onset 30-45 sec, peak 3-5 min; metabolized (small amounts), excreted in urine (unchanged), crosses placenta

Interactions/incompatibilities:

• Increased neuromuscular block-

P

ade: aminoglycosides, clindamycin, lincomycin, quinidine, local anesthetics, polymyxin antibiotics, lithium, narcotic analgesics, thiazides, enflurane, isoflurane

• Dysrhythmias: theophylline

• Do not mix with barbiturates in solution or syringe

NURSING CONSIDERATIONS
Assess:

• For electrolyte imbalances (K, Mg), may lead to increased action of this drug

• Vital signs (B/P, pulse, respirations, airway) until fully recovered; rate, depth, pattern of respirations, strength of hand grip

• I&O ratio; check for urinary retention, frequency, hesitancy

Administer:

• Using nerve stimulator by anesthesiologist to determine neuromuscular blockade

• Anticholinesterase to reverse neuromuscular blockade

• By slow IV over 1-2 min (only by qualified persons, usually an anesthesiologist)

• Only slightly discolored solution

Perform/provide:

• Storage in light-resistant area

• Reassurance if communication is difficult during recovery from neuromuscular blockade

Evaluate:

• Therapeutic response: paralysis of jaw, eyelid, head, neck, rest of body

• Recovery: decreased paralysis of face, diaphragm, leg, arm, rest of body

• Allergic reactions: rash, fever, respiratory distress, pruritus; drug should be discontinued

Treatment of overdose: Edrophonium or neostigmine, atropine, monitor VS; may require mechanical ventilation

Lab test interferences:
Decrease: Cholinesterase

papaverine HCl

(pa-pav'er-een)
Cerebid, Cerespan, Lapav, Myobid, Pavabid, Pavacen, Pavadel, Pavasule, Ro-Papav, Vasal, Vasocap, Vasospan, Vazosan

Func. class.: Peripheral vasodilator

Chem. class.: Opium alkaloid (no narcotic activity)

Action: Relaxes all smooth muscle, able to inhibit cyclic nucleotide phosphodiesterase, which increases intracellular cAMP, causing vasodilation

Uses: Arterial spasm resulting in cerebral and peripheral ischemia; myocardial ischemia, associated with vascular spasm; or dysrhythmias; angina pectoris, peripheral, pulmonary embolism; visceral spasm; PVD; ureteral, biliary, GI colic

Dosage and routes:

• *Adult:* PO 60-300 mg 1-5 times day; SUS REL 150-300 mg q8-12 h; IM/IV 30-120 mg q3h prn

Available forms include: Cap time-release 150, 300 mg; tabs 30, 60, 100, 200 mg; tabs time-release 200, 300 mg; inj IM/IV 30 mg/ml

Side effects/adverse reactions:

*CV: **Tachycardia,*** increased B/P

RESP: Increased depth of respirations

CNS: Headache, dizziness, drowsiness, sedation

GI: Nausea, anorexia, abdominal pain, constipation, diarrhea, jaundice, altered liver enzymes, ***hepatotoxicity***

INTEG: Flushing, sweating, rash

*HEMA: **Eosinophilia***

Contraindications: Hypersensitivity, complete AV heart block

Precautions: Cardiac dysrhythmias, glaucoma, pregnancy, lactation, drug dependency, children

Pharmacokinetics:

PO: Onset 30 sec, peak 1-2 hr, duration 3-5 min

SUS REL: Onset erratic

90% bound to plasma proteins, metabolized in liver, excreted in urine (inactive metabolites)

Interactions/incompatibilities:

• Decreased effect of: levodopa

• Increased hypotension: antihypertensives

• Do not add to LR solution, precipitation will occur

NURSING CONSIDERATIONS

Assess:

• B/P, pulse during treatment until stable; take B/P lying, standing; orthostatic hypotension is common

• Hepatic tests: AST, ALT, bilirubin; liver enzymes may increase

Administer:

• With meals to reduce GI upset

• An ordered analgesic if headache develops

• IV over 2 min to decrease hypotension

Perform/provide:

• Storage at room temperature

Evaluate:

• Therapeutic response: ability to walk without pain, increased pulse volume, increased temperature in extremities or orientation, long- and short-term memory

• Hepatic hypersensitivity reaction: nausea, vomiting, jaundice; drug should be discontinued if this occurs

Teach patient/family:

• That medication is not cure, may need to be taken continuously; therapeutic response may not be evident for 2-3 mo

• That it is necessary to quit smoking to prevent excessive vasoconstriction

• To avoid hazardous activities until stabilized on medication; dizziness may occur

• To notify physician if nausea, flushing, sweating, headache, or jaundice occur

Treatment of overdose: Discontinue medication

---

para-aminobenzoic acid

(par-a-a-meen'oo-ben'-zoic)

PABA, Pabagel, Pabanol, Pre-sun

Func. class.: Emollient/protectant

Action: Provides protection by screening harmful burning rays

Uses: Sunburn protection

Dosage and routes:

• *Adult:* TOP apply to skin before sun exposure, reapply after swimming

Available forms include: Lotion 1-24 protection

Side effects/adverse reactions:

INTEG: Contact dermatitis, photocontact dermatitis, irritation

Contraindications: Hypersensitivity, damaged/denuded skin

Interactions/incompatibilities:

None known

NURSING CONSIDERATIONS

Administer:

• To dry skin only; protection is not sufficient when applied to wet skin

• Only to intact skin, never apply to raw, denuded, blistered, or oozing wounds

Evaluate:

• Therapeutic response: absence of sunburn

• Allergic reaction: dermatitis, irritation, discontinue if these occur

• For infection (increased temperature, redness), often bacteria are trapped underneath

Teach patient/family:

• That clothing, swimsuits, towels may be stained

• To follow product direction for application

P

• To reapply if skin becomes wet by swimming, unless directed otherwise on product directions
• To avoid contact with eye area

---

para-aminosalicylate sodium/aminosalicylate sodium

(a-mee-noe-sal-i′si-late)
Parasal Sodium, Pasdium/Nemasol,* P.A.S. Sodium, Rolazid, Teebaconin

Func. class.: Antitubercular
Chem. class.: Sodium salt of PAS

Action: Bactericidal interference with lipid, nucleic acid biosynthesis
Uses: Tuberculosis, as an adjunctive
Dosage and routes:
• *Adult:* PO 14-16 g/day in 3-4 divided doses
• *Child:* PO 240-360 mg/kg/day in 3-4 divided doses
Available forms include: Tabs 0.5, 1 g; powder
Side effects/adverse reactions:
CV: CHF, dysrhythmias
CNS: Headache, anxiety, drowsiness, tremors, *convulsions,* lethargy, depression, confusion, psychosis, aggression
EENT: Blurred vision, optic neuritis, photophobia
HEMA: Megaloblastic anemia, vitamin B_{12}, folic acid deficiency
Contraindications: Hypersensitivity, optic neuritis
Precautions: Pregnancy, renal disease, diabetic retinopathy, cataracts, ocular defects, child <13 yr
Pharmacokinetics:
PO: Peak 1-2 hr, duration 4 hr; metabolized in liver
Interactions/incompatibilities:
• Decreased absorption of: alcohol, diphenhydramine

• Increased action of this drug: probenecid, sulfinpyrazone
• Decreased action of: vitamin B_{12}, folic acid, PABA
• Increased toxicity: salicylates
NURSING CONSIDERATIONS
Assess:
• Temperature, if <101° F drug should be reduced
• Liver studies q wk: ALT, AST, bilirubin
• Renal status before, q mo: BUN, creatinine, output, sp gr, urinalysis
Administer:
• With meals to decrease GI symptoms
• Antiemetic if vomiting occurs
• After C&S is completed; q mo to detect resistance
Evaluate:
• Mental status often: affect, mood, behavioral changes; psychosis may occur
Teach patient/family:
• That compliance with dosage schedule, length is necessary
• That scheduled appointments must be kept or relapse may occur
• Avoid alcohol while taking this drug

---

paraldehyde

(par-al′de-hyde)
Paral

Func. class.: Anticonvulsant
Chem. class.: Cyclic ether

Controlled Substance Schedule IV
Action: CNS depressant; exact mechanism of action is unknown
Uses: Refractory seizures, status epilepticus, sedation, insomnia, alcohol withdrawal, tetanus
Dosage and routes:
Seizures
• *Adult:* IM 5-10 ml, divide 10 ml into 2 inj; IV 0.2-0.4 ml/kg in NS inj

• *Child:* IM 0.15 ml/kg; REC 0.3 ml/kg q4-6h or 1 ml/yr of age, not to exceed 5 ml, may repeat in 1 hr prn; IV 5 ml/90 ml NS inj, begin infusion at 5 ml/hr, titrate to patient response

Alcohol withdrawal

• *Adult:* PO/REC 5-10 ml, not to exceed 60 ml; IM 5 ml q4-6h × 24 hr, then q6h on following days, not to exceed 30 ml

Sedation

• *Adult:* PO/REC 4-10 ml; IM 5 ml; IV 3-5 ml to be used in emergency only

• *Child:* PO/REC/IM 0.15 ml/kg

Tetanus

• *Adult:* IV 4-5 ml or 12 ml by gastric tube q4h diluted with water; IM 5-10 ml prn

Available forms include: Inj IM, IV; oral and rectal liquid

Side effects/adverse reactions:

HEMA: **Thrombocytopenia, agranulocytosis, leukopenia, neutropenia, hemolytic anemia,** increased pro-time

CNS: Stimulation, drowsiness, dizziness, confusion, convulsion, headache, flushing, hallucinations, coma

GI: Foul breath, irritation

GU: Nephrosis

INTEG: Rash, erythema, local pain, sloughing fat necrosis

CV: Pulmonary edema, pulmonary hemorrhage, circulatory respiratory depression, collapse

Contraindications: Hypersensitivity

Precautions: Asthma, hepatic disease, pulmonary disease

Pharmacokinetics:

PO: Onset 10-15 min, peak 1-2 hr, duration 6-8 hr

REC: Onset slow, duration 4-6 hr
Metabolized by liver, excreted by kidneys, crosses placenta, half-life 7.5 hr

Interactions/incompatibilities:

• Increased blood levels of this drug: alcohol, CNS depressants, general anesthetics, disulfiram

• Increase crystallization in kidneys: sulfonamides

NURSING CONSIDERATIONS

Assess:

• VS q30 min after parenteral route

• Blood studies: Hct, Hgb, RBCs, serum folate, vitamin D if on long-term therapy

• Hepatic studies: AST, ALT, bilirubin, creatinine, failure

Administer:

• IM injection in deep large muscle mass to prevent tissue sloughing

• After conservative measures have been tried for insomnia

• Rectal after diluting in cottonseed oil or olive oil as retention enema or 200 ml NS for enema

• Oral with juice or milk to cover taste/smell, decrease GI symptoms

Perform/provide:

• Ventilation of room

Evaluate:

• Mental status: mood, sensorium, affect, memory (long, short)

• Respiratory dysfunction; respiratory depression, character, rate, rhythm; hold drug if respirations are >12/min or if pupils are dilated

Teach patient/family:

• That physical dependency may result when used for extended periods of time

• To avoid driving, other activities that require alertness

• Not to discontinue medication quickly after long-term use, taper over several weeks

Lab test interferences:

False positive: Ketones (serum)(urine), interference, 17-OHCS

P

parathethadione

(par-a-meth-a-dye'one)
Paradione

Func. class.: Anticonvulsant
Chem. class.: Oxazolidinedione

Action: Increases seizure threshold in cortex and basal ganglia; decreases synaptic stimulation to low-frequency impulses

Uses: Refractory absence seizures (partial)

Dosage and routes:
• *Adult:* PO 300 mg tid, may increase by 300 mg/wk, not to exceed 600 mg qid
• *Child >6 yr:* PO 0.9 g/day in divided doses tid or qid
• *Child 2-6 yr:* PO 0.6 g/day in divided doses tid or qid
• *Child <2 yr:* PO 0.3 g/day in divided doses tid or qid

Available forms include: Caps 150, 300 mg; sol 300 mg/ml

Side effects/adverse reactions:
*HEMA: **Thrombocytopenia, agranulocytosis, leukopenia, neutropenia, hemolytic anemia,*** increased pro-time
CNS: Drowsiness, dizziness, fatigue, paresthesia, irritability, headache
GU: Vaginal bleeding, albuminuria, nephrosis, abdominal pain, weight loss
GI: Nausea, vomiting, bleeding gums, abnormal liver function tests
INTEG: Exfoliative dermatitis, rash, alopecia, petechiae, erythema
EENT: Photophobia, diplopia, epistaxis, retinal hemorrhage
CV: Hypertension, hypotension

Contraindications: Hypersensitivity, blood dyscrasias

Precautions: Hepatic disease, renal disease

Pharmacokinetics:
PO: Onset 15-30 min, peak 1-2 hr, duration 4-6 hr
REC: Onset slow, duration 4-6 hr, metabolized by the liver, excreted by the kidneys, crosses placenta, excreted in breast milk, half-life 1-3½ hr

Interactions/incompatibilities:
None known

NURSING CONSIDERATIONS

Assess:
• Blood studies: Hct, Hgb, RBCs, serum folate, vitamin D if on long-term therapy
• Hepatic studies: ALT, AST, bilirubin, creatinine, failure

Administer:
• After diluting oral solution with water
• Oral with juice or milk to cover taste-smell to decrease GI symptoms

Perform/provide:
• Ventilation of room

Evaluate:
• Mental status: mood, sensorium, affect, memory (long, short)

Teach patient/family:
• To avoid driving, other activities that require alertness
• Not to discontinue medication quickly after long-term use; convulsions may result

parathethasone acetate

(par-a-meth'a-sone)
Haldrone

Func. class.: Corticosteroid
Chem. class.: Glucocorticoid, long acting

Action: Decreases inflammation by suppression of migration of polymorphonuclear leukocytes, fibroblasts, reversal to increase capillary permeability and lysosomal stabilization

Uses: Severe inflammation, shock,

adrenal insufficiency, ulcerative colitis

Dosage and routes:
- *Adult:* PO 0.5-6 mg tid-qid
- *Child:* PO 58-800 μg/kg/day in divided doses tid-qid

Available forms include: Tabs 1, 2 mg

Side effects/adverse reactions:
INTEG: Acne, poor wound healing, ecchymosis, petechiae
CNS: Depression, flushing, sweating, headache, mood changes
*CV: Hypotension, **circulatory collapse, thrombophlebitis, embolism,*** tachycardia
*HEMA: **Thrombocytopenia***
MS: Fractures, osteoporosis, weakness
GI: Diarrhea, nausea, abdominal distention, GI hemorrhage, increased appetite, ***pancreatitis***
EENT: Fungal infections, increased intraocular pressure, blurred vision
Contraindications: Psychosis, hypersensitivity, idiopathic thrombocytopenia, acute glomerulonephritis, amebiasis, fungal infections, nonasthmatic bronchial disease, child <2 yr
Precautions: Pregnancy, diabetes mellitus, glaucoma, osteoporosis, seizure disorders, ulcerative colitis, CHF, myasthenia gravis

Pharmacokinetics:
PO: Peak 1-2 hr, duration 2 days
IM: Peak 3-45 hr

Interactions/incompatibilities:
- Decreased action of this drug: cholestyramine, colestipol, barbiturates, rifampin, ephedrine, phenytoin, theophylline
- Decreased effects of: anticoagulants, anticonvulsants, antidiabetics, ambenonium, neostigmine, isoniazid, toxoids, vaccines
- Increased side effects: alcohol, salicylates, indomethacin, amphotericin B, digitalis preparations

- Increased action of this drug: salicylates, estrogens, indomethacin

NURSING CONSIDERATIONS
Assess:
- Potassium, blood sugar, urine glucose while on long-term therapy; hypokalemia and hyperglycemia
- Weight daily, notify physician of weekly gain >5 lb
- B/P q4h, pulse, notify physician if chest pain occurs
- I&O ratio, be alert for decreasing urinary output and increasing edema
- Plasma cortisol levels during long-term therapy (normal level: 138-635 nmol/L SI units when drawn at 8 AM)

Administer:
- Titrated dose, use lowest effective dose
- In one dose in AM to prevent adrenal suppression, avoid SC administration, damage may be done to tissue
- With food or milk to decrease GI symptoms

Perform/provide:
- Assistance with ambulation in patient with bone tissue disease to prevent fractures

Evaluate:
- Therapeutic response: ease of respirations, decreased inflammation
- Infection: increased temperature, WBC, even after withdrawal of medication; drug masks symptoms of infection
- Potassium depletion: paresthesias, fatigue, nausea, vomiting, depression, polyuria, dysrhythmias, weakness
- Edema, hypotension, cardiac symptoms
- Mental status: affect, mood, behavioral changes, aggression

Teach patient/family:
- That ID as steroid user should be carried

P

---

italics = common side effects   ***bold italic*** = life threatening reactions

• To notify physician if therapeutic response decreases; dosage adjustment may be needed
• Not to discontinue this medication abruptly or adrenal crisis can result
• To avoid OTC products: salicylates, alcohol in cough products, cold preparations unless directed by physician
• Teach patient all aspects of drug use, including Cushingoid symptoms
• Symptoms of adrenal insufficiency: nausea, anorexia, fatigue, dizziness, dyspnea, weakness, joint pain

Lab test interferences:
Increase: Cholesterol, sodium, blood glucose, uric acid, calcium, urine glucose
Decrease: Calcium, potassium, T_4, T_3, thyroid ^{131}I uptake test, urine 17-OHCS, 17-KS, PBI
False negative: Skin allergy tests

---

pargyline HCl

(par'gi-leen)
Eutonyl
Func. class.: Antihypertensive
Chem. class.: MAOI

Action: Inhibits monoamine oxidase, decreasing B/P
Uses: Moderate to severe hypertension
Dosage and routes:
• *Adult:* PO 25 mg daily, increase by 10 mg q7 days, not to exceed 200 mg; maintenance dosage: 25-50 mg daily
Available forms include: Tabs 10, 25 mg
Side effects/adverse reactions:
CV: Orthostatic hypotension, tachycardia, chest pain, bradycardia, fluid retention, *CHF*
CNS: Drowsiness, dizziness, seda-tion, headache, depression, insomnia, weakness, fatigue, confusion, blurred vision, EPS
GI: Nausea, vomiting, anorexia, constipation, weight gain
EENT: Dry mouth
GU: Impotence
MS: Arthralgia
MISC: Sweating, increased appetite, hypoglycemia
Contraindications: Hypersensitivity, malignant hypertension, paranoid schizophrenia, severe pulmonary failure, pheochromocytoma, hyperthyroidism, advanced renal failure, children <12 yr
Precautions: Pregnancy (C), lactation, impaired renal function, liver disease, CAD, parkinsonism, diabetes mellitus
Pharmacokinetics:
Excreted in urine, therapeutic response may take 4 days-3 weeks
Interactions/incompatibilities:
• Hypertensive crisis: amphetamine, cyclopent-amide, ephedrine, pseudoephedrine, metaraminol, methylphenidate, phenylpropanolamine, levodopa, methyldopa, reserpine, tryptamine, tyramine foods
• Hypotension and increased sedation: barbiturates, alcohol, narcotics, CNS depressants, antihypertensive agents
• May potentiate effects: doxapram, narcotics, phenothiazines, other psychotropic agents, tricyclic antidepressants

NURSING CONSIDERATIONS
Assess:
• Electrolytes: K, Na, Cl, CO_2
• Renal function studies: catecholamines, BUN, creatinine
• Hepatic function studies: AST, ALT, alk phosphatase
• Weight daily, I&O
• B/P lying, standing before starting treatment

Administer:
• Gum, frequent rinsing of mouth or hard candy for dry mouth
Teach patient/family:
• To report dizziness, palpitations, fainting
• To change position slowly or fainting may occur
• To take drug exactly as pre-scribed
• Not to eat tyramine-rich foods: beer, wine, pickled products, yeast products, aged cheeses, avocados, chocolate
• To avoid all OTC products unless directed by physician
Evaluate:
• Therapeutic response: de-creased B/P
• Nausea, vomiting, diarrhea
• Edema in feet, legs daily
• Skin turgor, dryness of mucous membranes for hydration status
Treatment of overdose: Induce emesis or gastric lavage, support respiration, severe hypertension—administer α-blocker, treat CNS stimulation with IV diazepam, maintain fluid or electrolyte bal-ance

paromomycin sulfate
(par-oh-moe-mye′sin)
Humatin
Func. class.: Amebicide
Chem. class.: Aminoglycoside an-tibiotic

Action: Direct action in intestinal lumen
Uses: Intestinal amebiasis, tape-worms
Dosage and routes:
Intestinal amebiasis
• *Adult and child:* PO 25-35 mg/kg/day in 3 divided doses × 5-10 days pc

Tapeworms
• *Adult:* PO 1 g q15 min × 4 doses
• *Child:* PO 11 mg/kg q15 min × 4 doses
Available forms include: Caps 250 mg
Side effects/adverse reactions:
*HEMA: **Eosinophilia***
INTEG: Rash
CNS: Headache, dizziness
EENT: Ototoxicity
GI: Nausea, vomiting, diarrhea, epigastric distress, anorexia, ste-atorrhea, pruritus ani, hypocholes-terolemia
*GU: **Nephrotoxicity,*** hematuria
Contraindications: Hypersen-sitivity, renal disease, GI ob-struction
Precautions: GI ulcerations
Pharmacokinetics:
PO: Excreted in feces, urine, slowly
Interactions/incompatibilities:
None known
NURSING CONSIDERATIONS
Assess:
• Stools during entire treatment; should be clear at end of therapy, for 1 yr before patient is considered cured
• I&O, stools for number, fre-quency, character
Administer:
• Cleansing enema if ordered be-fore beginning treatment
• PO after meals to avoid GI symp-toms
Perform/provide:
• Storage in tight container
Evaluate:
• Allergic reaction: rash, itching; drug should be discontinued if these occur
• Diarrhea for 2-3 days
Teach patient/family:
• Proper hygiene after BM: hand-washing technique

• Avoid contact of drug with eyes, mouth, nose, other mucous membranes

• Need for compliance with dosage schedule, duration of treatment

Lab test interferences:

Decrease: Serum cholesterol

---

pemoline

(pem'oh-leen)

Cylert

Func. class.: Cerebral stimulant

Chem. class.: Oxazolidinone derivative

Controlled Substance Schedule IV

Action: Increases release of norepinephrine, dopamine in cerebral cortex to reticular activating system.

Uses: Attention deficit disorder with hyperactivity

Dosage and routes:

• *Child >6 yr:* 37.5 mg in AM, increasing by 18.75 mg/wk, not to exceed 112.5 mg/day

Available forms include: Tabs 18.75, 37.5, 75 mg; chewable tabs 37.5 mg

Side effects/adverse reactions:

CNS: Hyperactivity, insomnia, restlessness, dizziness, depression, headache, stimulation, irritability, aggressiveness, hallucination seizures, Gilles de la Tourette's disorder

GI: Nausea, anorexia, diarrhea, abdominal pain, increased liver enzymes

CV: Tachycardia

Contraindications: Hypersensitivity

Precautions: Renal disease, pregnancy (B)

Pharmacokinetics:

PO: Peak 2-4 hr, duration 8 hr, metabolized by liver, excreted by kidneys, half-life 12 hr

Interactions/incompatibilities:

None known

NURSING CONSIDERATIONS

Assess:

• Hepatic function studies: ALT, AST, bilirubin, creatinine

• Child for height, growth rate, since growth retardation occurs

Administer:

• At least 6 hr before hs

• Gum, hard candy, frequent sips of water for dry mouth

Perform/provide:

• Check to see PO medication has been swallowed

Evaluate:

• Mental status: mood, sensorium, affect, stimulation, insomnia, aggressiveness

Teach patient/family:

• To decrease caffeine consumption (coffee, tea, cola, chocolate), which may increase irritability, stimulation

• Avoid OTC preparations unless approved by physician

• To taper off drug over several weeks

• To avoid alcohol ingestion

• To avoid hazardous activities until patient is stabilized on medication

• Therapeutic effect may take 2-4 wk

---

penicillin G benzathine

(pen-i-sill'in)

Bicillin L-A, Megacillin, Permapen

Func. class.: Broad-spectrum antibiotic

Chem. class.: Natural penicillin

Action: Interferes with cell wall replication of susceptible organisms; osmotically unstable cell wall swells, bursts from osmotic pressure

Uses: Respiratory infections, scarlet fever, erysipelas, otitis media, pneumonia, skin and soft tissue infections, gonorrhea; effective for gram-positive cocci *(Staphylococcus, S. pyogenes, S. viridans, S. faecalis, S. bovis, S. pneumoniae)*, gram-negative cocci *(N. gonorrhoeae)*, gram-positive bacilli *(B. anthracis, C. perfringens, C. tetani, C. diphtheriae, L. monocytogenes)*, gram-negative bacilli *(E. coli, P. mirabilis, Salmonella, Shigella, Enterobacter, S. moniliformis)*, spirochetes *(T. pallidum)*, actinomycetes

Dosage and routes:
Early syphilis
• *Adult:* IM 2.4 million U in single dose
Congenital syphilis
• *Child <2 yr:* IM 50,000 U/kg in single dose
Prophylaxis of rheumatic fever, glomerulonephritis
• *Adult and child:* IM 1.2 million U in single dose q month or 600,000 U q 2 wk
Upper respiratory infections (group A streptococcal)
• *Adult:* IM 1.2 million U in single dose, PO 400,000-600,000 U q4-6h
• *Child >27 kg:* IM 900,000 U in single dose
• *Child <27 kg:* IM 300,000-600,000 U in single dose
Available forms include: Inj IM 300,000, 600,000 U/ml; tabs 200,000 U

Side effects/adverse reactions:
HEMA: Anemia, increased bleeding time, *bone marrow depression, granulocytopenia*
GI: Nausea, vomiting, diarrhea, increased AST, ALT, abdominal pain, glossitis, colitis
GU: Oliguria, proteinuria, hematuria, *vaginitis, moniliasis, glomerulonephritis*
CNS: Lethargy, hallucinations, anx-

iety, depression, twitching, *coma, convulsions*
META: Hyperkalemia, hypokalemia, alkalosis, hypernatremia
Contraindications: Hypersensitivity to penicillins; neonates
Precautions: Hypersensitivity to cephalosporins
Pharmacokinetics:
IM: Very slow absorption, duration 21-28 days, half-life 30-60 min, excreted in urine, feces, breast milk, crosses placenta
Interactions/incompatibilities:
• Decreased antimicrobial effect of this drug: tetracyclines, erythromycins
• Increased penicillin concentrations: aspirin, probenecid
NURSING CONSIDERATIONS
Assess:
• I&O ratio; report hematuria, oliguria since penicillin in high doses is nephrotoxic
• Any patient with compromised renal system since drug is excreted slowly in poor renal system function; toxicity may occur rapidly
• Liver studies: AST, ALT
• Blood studies: WBC, RBC, H&H, bleeding time
• Renal studies: urinalysis, protein, blood
• C&S before drug therapy; drug may be taken as soon as culture is taken
Administer:
• On an empty stomach for best absorption
• Drug after C&S has been completed
• Deep IM injection in large muscle masses
Perform/provide:
• Adrenalin, suction, tracheostomy set, endotracheal intubation equipment
• Adequate fluid intake (2000 ml) during diarrhea episodes
• Scratch test to assess allergy, af-

P

---

italics = common side effects   ***bold italic*** = life threatening reactions

ter securing order from physician; usually done when penicillin is only drug of choice

• Storage in tight container; refrigerate injection

Evaluate:

• Therapeutic response: absence of fever, purulent drainage, redness, inflammation

• Bowel pattern before and during treatment

• Skin eruptions after administration of penicillin to 1 wk after discontinuing drug

• Respiratory status: rate, character, wheezing, tightness in chest

• Allergies before initiation of treatment, reaction of each medication; highlight allergies on chart, Kardex

Teach patient/family:

• To take oral penicillin on empty stomach with full glass of water

• Culture may be taken after completed course of medication

• To report sore throat, fever, fatigue; could indicate superimposed infection

• To wear or carry Medic Alert ID if allergic to penicillins

• To notify nurse of diarrhea stools

Lab test interferences:

Decrease: Uric acid

False positive: Urine glucose, urine protein

Treatment of overdose: Withdraw drug, maintain airway, administer epinephrine, aminophylline, O_2, IV corticosteroids for anaphylaxis

penicillin G potassium

Aqueous Penicillin IV, Acrocillin, Benzylpenicillin, Burcillin-G, Deltapen, Falapen,* Megacillin,* P-50,* Pentids, Pfizerpen

Func. class.: Broad-spectrum antibiotic-penicillin

Chem. class.: Natural penicillin

Action: Interferes with cell wall replication of susceptible organisms; osmotically unstable cell wall swells, bursts from osmotic pressure

Uses: Actinomycetes, empyema, gangrene, anthrax, fever, gonorrhea, mastoiditis, meningitis, osteomyelitis, pneumonia, tetanus, urinary tract infections, prophylactically in rheumatic fever; effective for gram-positive cocci *(S. aureus, S. pyogenes, S. viridans, S. faecalis, S. bovis, S. pneumoniae),* gram-negative cocci *(N. gonorrhoeae, N. meningitis),* gram-positive bacilli *(B. anthracis, C. perfringens, C. tetani, C. diphtheriae, L. monocytogenes),* gram-negative bacilli *(Bacteroides, F. nucleatum, P. multocida, S. minor, S. moniliformis),* Spirochetes *(T. pallidum, T. pertenue, B. recurrentis, L. icterohaemorrhagiae),* Actinomycetes

Dosage and routes:

Pneumococcal/streptococcal infections (mild-moderate)

• *Adult:* PO 200,000-500,000 U q6-8h × 10 days (streptococcal infections) or afebrile × 2 days (pneumococcal infections)

• *Child <12 yr:* PO 25,000-90,000 U/kg/day in 3-6 divided doses

Prevention of recurrence of rheumatic fever/chorea

• *Adult:* PO 200,000-250,000 U bid continuously

• *Child <12 yr:* PO 25,000-90,000

U/kg/day in 3-6 divided doses
Vincent's gingivitis/pharyngitis
• *Adult:* PO 200,000-500,000 U q6-8h
Available forms include: Tabs 200,000, 250,000, 400,000, 500,000, 800,000 U; powder for oral sol 200,000, 400,000 U/5 ml
Side effects/adverse reactions:
HEMA: Anemia, increased bleeding time, **bone marrow depression, granulocytopenia**
GI:Nausea, vomiting, diarrhea, increased AST, ALT, abdominal pain, glossitis, colitis
GU: Oliguria, proteinuria, hematuria, *vaginitis, moniliasis,* **glomerulonephritis**
CNS: Lethargy, hallucinations, anxiety, depression, twitching, **coma, convulsions**
META: Hyperkalemia, hypokalemia, alkalosis, hypernatremia
Contraindications: Hypersensitivity to penicillins; neonates
Precautions: Hypersensitivity to cephalosporins
Pharmacokinetics:
PO: Duration 6 hr, peak 1 hr
IM: Peak 12-24 hr, duration 26 days
Metabolized in liver, excreted in feces, breast milk, crosses placenta
Interactions/incompatibilities:
• Decreased antimicrobial effectiveness of this drug: tetracyclines, erythromycins
• Increased penicillin concentrations when used with: aspirin, probenecid
NURSING CONSIDERATIONS
Assess:
• I&O ratio; report hematuria, oliguria since penicillin in high doses is nephrotoxic
• Any patient with compromised renal system since drug is excreted slowly in poor renal system function; toxicity may occur rapidly
• Liver studies: AST, ALT
• Blood studies: WBC, RBC,

H&H, bleeding time
• Renal studies: urinalysis, protein, blood
• C&S before drug therapy; drug may be taken as soon as culture is taken
Administer:
• On an empty stomach for best absorption
• Drug after C&S has been completed
Perform/provide:
• Adrenalin, suction, tracheostomy set, endotracheal intubation equipment
• Adequate fluid intake (2000 ml) during diarrhea episodes
• Scratch test to assess allergy, after securing order from physician; usually done when penicillin is only drug of choice
• Storage in dry, tight container; solution may be stored at room temperature
Evaluate:
• Therapeutic effectiveness: absence of fever, draining wounds
• Bowel pattern before and during treatment
• Skin eruptions after administration of penicillin to 1 wk after discontinuing drug
• Respiratory status: rate, character, wheezing, tightness in chest
• Allergies before initiation of treatment, reaction of each medication; highlight allergies on chart, Kardex
Teach patient/family:
• Aspects of drug therapy, including need to complete course of medication to ensure organism death (10-14 days); culture may be taken after completed course
• To report sore throat, fever, fatigue; could indicate superimposed infection

P

---

italics = common side effects   ***bold italic*** = life threatening reactions

• To wear or carry Medic Alert ID if allergic to penicillins
• To notify nurse of diarrhea stools

Lab test interferences:
Decrease: Uric acid
False positive: Urine glucose, urine protein

Treatment of overdose: Withdraw drug, maintain airway, administer epinephrine, aminophylline, O_2, IV corticosteroids for anaphylaxis

---

penicillin G procaine

Ayercillin,* Crysticillin A.S., Duracillin A.S., Wycillin

Func. class.: Broad-spectrum antibiotic
Chem. class.: Natural penicillin

Action: Interferes with cell wall replication of susceptible organisms; osmotically unstable cell wall swells, bursts from osmotic pressure

Uses: Actinomycetes, empyema, gangrene, anthrax, gonorrhea, mastoiditis, meningitis, osteomyelitis, pneumonia, tetanus, urinary tract infections, prophylactically in rheumatic fever; effective for gram-positive cocci *(S. aureus, S. pyogenes, S. viridans, S. faecalis, S. bovis, S. pneumoniae),* gram-negative cocci *(N. gonorrhoeae, N. meningitidis),* gram-positive bacilli *B. anthracis, C. perfringens, C. tetani, C. diphtheriae, L. monocytogenes),* gram-negative bacilli *(Bacteroides, F. nucleatum, P. multocida, S. minor, S. moniliformis),* Spirochetes *(T. pallidum, T. pertenue, B. recurrentis, L. icterohaemorrhagiae),* Actinomycetes

Dosage and routes:
Moderate to severe infections
• *Adult:* IM 600,000-1.2 million U in single dose

• *Child:* IM 300,000 U in single dose

Gonorrhea
• *Adult and child >12 yr:* IM 4.8 million units in two injections given 30 mins after probenecid 1 gm.

Pneumonia (pneumococcal)
• *Adult and child >12 yr:* IM 300,000-600,000 U q6-12h

Available forms include: Inj IM 300,000, 500,000, 600,000 U/ml

Side effects/adverse reactions:
HEMA: Anemia, increased bleeding time, *bone marrow depression, granulocytopenia*

GI: Nausea, vomiting, diarrhea, increased AST, ALT, abdominal pain, glossitis, colitis

GU: Oliguria, proteinuria, hematuria, *vaginitis, moniliasis, glomerulonephritis*

CNS: Lethargy, hallucinations, anxiety, depression, twitching, *coma, convulsions*

META: Hyperkalemia, hypokalemia, alkalosis, hypernatremia

Contraindications: Hypersensitivity to penicillins, procaine; neonates

Precautions: Hypersensitivity to cephalosporins

Pharmacokinetics:
IM: Peak 1-3 hr, duration 15 hr, excreted in urine

Interactions/incompatibilities:
• Decreased antimicrobial effect of this drug: tetracyclines, erythromycins
• Increased penicillin concentrations: aspirin, probenecid

NURSING CONSIDERATIONS
Assess:
• I&O ratio; report hematuria, oliguria since penicillin in high doses is nephrotoxic
• Any patient with compromised renal system since drug is excreted slowly in poor renal system function; toxicity may occur rapidly
• Liver studies: AST, ALT

• Blood studies: WBC, RBC, H&H, bleeding time

• Renal studies: urinalysis, protein, blood

• C&S before drug therapy; drug may be taken as soon as culture is taken

Administer:

• Drug after C&S has been completed

Perform/provide:

• Adrenalin, suction, tracheostomy set, endotracheal intubation equipment

• Adequate fluid intake (2000 ml) during diarrhea episodes

• Scratch test to assess allergy, after securing order from physician; usually done when penicillin is only drug of choice

• Storage in refrigerator

Evaluate:

• Therapeutic response: absence of fever, purulent drainage, redness, inflammation

• Bowel pattern before and during treatment

• Skin eruptions after administration of penicillin to 1 wk after discontinuing drug

• Respiratory status: rate, character, wheezing, tightness in chest

• Allergies before initiation of treatment, reaction of each medication; highlight allergies on chart, Kardex

Teach patient/family:

• Culture may be taken after completed course of medication

• To report sore throat, fever, fatigue; could indicate superimposed infection

• To wear or carry Medic Alert ID if allergic to penicillins

• To notify nurse of diarrhea stools

Lab test interferences:

Decrease: Uric acid

False positive: Urine glucose, urine protein

Treatment of overdose: Withdraw drug, maintain airway, administer epinephrine, aminophylline, O_2, IV corticosteroids for anaphylaxis

---

penicillin G sodium

Crystipen*

Func. class.: Broad-spectrum antibiotic

Chem. class.: Natural penicillin

Action: Acts by interfering with cell wall replication of susceptible organisms; osmotically unstable cell wall swells and bursts from osmotic pressure

Uses: Actinomycetes, empyema, gangrene, anthrax, gonorrhea, mastoiditis, meningitis, osteomyelitis, pneumonia, tetanus, urinary tract infections, prophylactically in rheumatic fever; effective for gram-positive cocci *(S. aureus, S. pyogenes, S. viridans, S. faecalis, S. bovis, S. pneumoniae)*, gram-negative cocci *(N. gonorrhoeae, N. meningitidis)*, gram-positive bacilli *(B. anthracis, C. perfringens, C. tetani, C. diphtheriae, L. monocytogenes)*, gram-negative bacilli *(Bacteroides, E. nucleatum, P. multocida, S. minor, S. moniliformis)*, Spirochetes *(T. pallidum, T. pertenue, B. recurrentis, L. icterohaemorrhagiae)*, actinomycetes

Dosage and routes:

Moderate to severe infections

• *Adult:* IM/IV 1.2-24 million U in divided doses q4h

• *Child:* IM/IV 25,000-300,000 U in divided doses q4h

Dental surgery prophylaxis for endocarditis

• *Adult:* IM/IV 2 million units ½-1 hr before procedure, then 1 million 6 hr after procedure

Available forms include: Inj IM, IV 5 million U

P

Side effects/adverse reactions:

HEMA: Anemia, increased bleeding time, ***bone marrow depression, granulocytopenia***

GI:Nausea, vomiting, diarrhea, increased AST, ALT, abdominal pain, glossitis, colitis

GU: Oliguria, proteinuria, hematuria, vaginitis, moniliasis, ***glomerulonephritis***

CNS: Lethargy, hallucinations, anxiety, depression, twitching, ***convulsions***

META: Hyperkalemia, hypokalemia, alkalosis, hypernatremia

Contraindications: Hypersensitivity to penicillins; neonates

Precautions: CHF caused by sodium content

Pharmacokinetics:

IM: Peak 1-3 hr, duration 6 hr; excreted in urine

Interactions/incompatibilities:

• Decreased antimicrobial effect of this drug: tetracyclines, erythromycins

• Increased penicillin concentrations: aspirin, probenecid

NURSING CONSIDERATIONS

Assess:

• I&O ratio; report hematuria, oliguria since penicillin in high doses is nephrotoxic

• Any patient with a compromised renal system since drug is excreted slowly in poor renal system function; toxicity may occur rapidly

• Liver studies: AST, ALT

• Blood studies: WBC, RBC, H&H, bleeding time

• Renal studies: urinalysis, protein, blood

• C&S before drug therapy; drug may be taken as soon as culture is taken

Administer:

• Drug after C&S has been completed

Perform/provide:

• Adrenalin, suction, tracheostomy set, endotracheal intubation equipment

• Adequate fluid intake (2000 ml) during diarrhea episodes

• Scratch test to assess allergy, after securing order from physician; usually done when penicillin is only drug of choice

• Storage in tight container; may be stored at room temperature for several days

Evaluate:

• Therapeutic response: absence of fever, purulent drainage, redness, inflammation

• Bowel pattern before, during treatment

• Skin eruptions after administration of penicillin to 1 wk after discontinuing drug

• Respiratory status: rate, character, wheezing, tightness in chest

• Allergies before initiation of treatment, reaction of each medication; highlight allergies on chart, Kardex

Teach patient family:

• Culture may be taken after completed course of medication

• To report sore throat, fever, fatigue; could indicate superimposed infection

• To wear or carry Medic Alert ID if allergic to penicillins

• To notify nurse of diarrhea stools

Lab test interferences:

Decrease: Uric acid

False positive: Urine glucose, urine protein

Treatment of overdose: Withdraw drug, maintain airway, administer epinephrine, aminophylline, O_2, IV corticosteroids for anaphylaxis

penicillin V potassium

Pen-Vee K,* Deltapen-VK, V-cillin K, Veetids, Nadopen-V,* Penbec-V,* PVFK*

Func. class.: Broad-spectrum antibiotic

Chem. class.: Natural penicillin

Action: Interferes with cell wall replication of susceptible organisms; osmotically unstable cell wall swells, bursts from osmotic pressure.

Uses: Effective for gram-positive cocci *(S. aureus, S. pyogenes, S. viridans, S. faecalis, S. bovis, S. pneumoniae)*, gram-negative cocci *(N. gonorrhoeae, N. meningitidis)*, gram-positive bacilli *(B. anthracis, C. perfringens, C. tetani, C. diphtheriae, L. monocytogenes)*, gram-negative bacilli *(S. moniliformis)*, spirochetes *(T. pallidum)*, actinomycetes

Dosage and routes:
Pneumococcal/staphylococcal infections
• *Adult:* PO 250-500 mg q6h
• *Child <12 yr:* PO 25,000-90,000 U/kg/day in 3-6 divided doses (125 mg = 200,000 U)
Streptococcal infections
• *Adult:* PO 125-250 mg q6-8h × 10 days
Prevention of recurrence of rheumatic fever/chorea
• *Adult:* PO 125-250 mg bid continuously
Vincent's infection of oropharynx
• *Adult:* PO 250-500 mg q6-8h
Available forms include: Tabs 125, 250, 500 mg; film-coated tabs 125, 250, 500 mg; powder for oral susp 125, 250 mg/5 ml

Side effects/adverse reactions:
HEMA: Anemia, increased bleeding time, *bone marrow depression, granulocytopenia*

GI: Nausea, vomiting, diarrhea, increased AST, ALT, abdominal pain, glossitis, colitis
GU: Oliguria, proteinuria, hematuria, *vaginitis, moniliasis, glomerulonephritis*
CNS: Lethargy, hallucinations, anxiety, depression, twitching, *coma, convulsions*
META: Hyperkalemia, hypokalemia, alkalosis, hypernatremia
Contraindications: Hypersensitivity to penicillins; neonates
Precautions: Hypersensitivity to cephalosporins
Pharmacokinetics:
PO: Peak 30-60 min, duration 6-8 hr, half-life 30 min, excreted in urine, breast milk
Interactions/incompatibilities:
• Decreased antimicrobial effectiveness of this drug: tetracyclines, erythromycins
• Increased penicillin concentrations when used with: aspirin, probenecid
NURSING CONSIDERATIONS
Assess:
• I&O ratio; report hematuria, oliguria since penicillin in high doses is nephrotoxic
• Any patient with compromised renal system since drug is excreted slowly in poor renal system function; toxicity may occur rapidly
• Liver studies: AST, ALT
• Blood studies: WBC, RBC, H&H, bleeding time
• Renal studies: urinalysis, protein, blood
• C&S before drug therapy; drug may be taken as soon as culture is taken
Administer:
• On an empty stomach for best absorption
• Drug after C&S has been completed
Perform/provide:
• Adrenalin, suction, tracheostomy

P

set, endotracheal intubation equipment
• Adequate fluid intake (2000 ml) during diarrhea episodes
• Scratch test to assess allergy, after securing order from physician; usually done when penicillin is only drug of choice
• Storage in tight container; after reconstituting, refrigerate
Evaluate:
• Therapeutic effectiveness: absence of fever, draining wounds
• Bowel pattern before and during treatment
• Skin eruptions after administration of penicillin to 1 wk after discontinuing drug
• Respiratory status: rate, character, wheezing, tightness in chest
• Allergies before initiation of treatment, reaction of each medication; highlight allergies on chart, Kardex
Teach patient/family:
• Aspects of drug therapy, including need to complete entire course of medication to ensure organism death (10-14 days); culture may be taken after completed course
• To report sore throat, fever, fatigue; could indicate superimposed infection
• To wear or carry Medic Alert ID if allergic to penicillins
• To notify nurse of diarrhea stools
Lab test interferences:
Decrease: Uric acid
False positive: Urine glucose, urine protein
Treatment of overdose: Withdraw drug, maintain airway, administer epinephrine, aminophylline, O_2, IV corticosteroids for anaphylaxis

pentaerythritol tetranitrate

(pen-ta-er-ith'ri-tole)
Desatrate, Duotrate, Nitrin, PETN, Pentraspan, Naptrate, Pentylan, Peritrate, Vasolate
Func. class.: Vasodilatory, coronary
Chem. class.: Nitrate

Action: Decreases preload, afterload; which is responsible for decreasing left ventricular end diastolic pressure, systemic vascular resistance
Uses: Chronic stable angina pectoris, prophylaxis of angina pain
Dosage and routes:
• *Adult:* PO 10-20 mg tid or qid; SUS REL 30-80 mg q12h
Available forms include: Caps ext rel 30, 45, 80 mg; tabs 10, 20, 40 mg; tabs ext rel 80 mg
Side effects/adverse reactions:
CV: Postural hypotension, tachycardia, collapse
GI: Nausea, vomiting
INTEG: Pallor, sweating
CNS: Headache, flushing, dizziness
Contraindications: Hypersensitivity to this drug or nitrites, anemia, increased intracranial pressure, cerebral hemorrhage, acute MI, pregnancy, lactation
Precautions: Postural hypotension, glaucoma
Pharmacokinetics:
PO: Onset 20-60 min, duration 4-5 hr
SUS REL: Duration 12 hr
Metabolized by liver, excreted in urine, half-life 10 min
Interactions/incompatibilities:
• Increased effects: β-blockers, narcotics, tricyclics, diuretics, antihypertensives
• Decreased effects: sympathomimetics

NURSING CONSIDERATIONS
Assess:
• B/P, pulse, respirations during beginning therapy
Administer:
• With 8 oz of water on empty stomach (oral tablet)
Evaluate:
• Pain: duration, time started, activity being performed, character
• Tolerance if taken over long period of time
• Headache, lightheadedness, decreased B/P; may indicate a need for decreased dosage
Teach patient/family:
• That drug may be taken before stressful activity: exercise, sexual activity
• That SL may sting when drug comes in contact with mucous membranes
• To avoid hazardous activities if dizziness occurs
• Stress patient compliance with complete medical regimen
• To make position changes slowly to prevent fainting

---

pentamidine isothionate
(pen-tam′i-deen)
Pentam 300
Func. class.: Antiprotozoal
Chem. class.: Aromatic diamide derivative

Action: Interferes with DNA/RNA synthesis in protozoa
Uses: *Pneumocystis carinii* infections
Dosage and routes:
• *Adult and child:* IV/IM 4 mg/kg/day × 2 wk
Available forms include: Inj IV, IM 300 mg/vial
Side effects/adverse reactions:
CV: Hypotension, ventricular tachycardia, ECG abnormalities
HEMA: Anemia, *leukopenia,* *thrombocytopenia*
INTEG: Sterile abscess, pain at injection site, pruritus, urticaria, rash
*GU: **Acute renal failure***
GI: Nausea, vomiting, anorexia, increased AST, ALT, *acute pancreatitis*
CNS: Disorientation, hallucinations, dizziness
META: Hyperkalemia, hypocalcemia, hypoglycemia
Precautions: Blood dyscrasias, hepatic disease, renal disease, diabetes mellitus, cardiac disease, hypocalcemia
Pharmacokinetics: Excreted unchanged in urine (66%)
Interactions/incompatibilities
• Nephrotoxicity: aminoglycosides, amphotercin B, colistin, cisplatin, methoxyflurane, polymyxin B, vancomycin

NURSING CONSIDERATIONS
Assess:
• Blood studies, blood glucose, CBC, platelets
• I&O ratio; report hematuria, oliguria
• ECG for cardiac dysrhythmias, check B/P
• Any patient with compromised renal system; drug is excreted slowly in poor renal system function; toxicity may occur rapidly
• Liver studies: AST, ALT
• Renal studies: urinalysis, BUN, creatinine; nephrotoxicity may occur
Perform/provide:
• Storage in refrigerator protected from light
Evaluate:
• Therapeutic response: decreased temperature, ability to breath
• Bowel pattern before, during treatment
• Sterile abscess, pain at injection site
• Respiratory status: rate, character, wheezing, dyspnea

• Dizziness, confusion, hallucination

• Allergies before treatment, reaction of each medication; place allergies on chart, Kardex in bright red letters; notify all people giving drugs

Teach patient/family:

•To report sore throat, fever, fatigue, could indicate superimposed infection

---

pentazocine HCl/
pentazocine lactate

(pen-taz′oh-seen)

Talwin Nx

Func. class.: Narcotic analgesic

Chem. class.: Synthetic benzomorphan

Controlled Substance Schedule IV

Action: Inhibits ascending pain pathways in CNS, increases pain threshold, alters pain perception

Uses: Moderate to severe pain

Dosage and routes:

• *Adult:* PO 50-100 mg q3-4h prn, not to exceed 600 mg/day; IV/IM/SC 30 mg q3-4h prn, not to exceed 360 mg/day

Available forms include: SC, IM, IV 30 mg/ml; tabs 50 mg

Side effects/adverse reactions:

CNS: Drowsiness, dizziness, confusion, headache, sedation, euphoria

GI: Nausea, vomiting, anorexia, constipation, cramps

GU: Increased urinary output, dysuria

INTEG: Rash, urticaria, bruising, flushing, diaphoresis, pruritus

EENT: Tinnitus, blurred vision, miosis, diplopia

CV: Palpitations, bradycardia, change in B/P

RESP: Respiratory depression

Contraindications: Hypersensitivity, addiction (narcotic)

Precautions: Addictive personality, pregnancy, lactation, increased intracranial pressure, MI (acute), severe heart disease, respiratory depression, hepatic disease, renal disease, child <18 yr

Pharmacokinetics:

SC/IM: Onset 15-30 min, peak 1-2 hr, duration 2-4 hr

IV: Onset 2-3 min, duration 4-6 hr

Metabolized by liver, excreted by kidneys, crosses placenta

Interactions/incompatibilities:

• Effects may be increased with other CNS depressants: alcohol, narcotics, sedative/hypnotics, antipsychotics, skeletal muscle relaxants

• Do not mix in solutions or syringe with barbiturates

NURSING CONSIDERATIONS

Assess:

• I&O ratio; check for decreasing output; may indicate urinary retention

Administer:

• With antiemetic if nausea, vomiting occur

• When pain is beginning to return; determine dosage interval by patient response

Perform/provide:

• Storage in light-resistant area at room temperature

• Assistance with ambulation

• Safety measures: siderails, night light, call bell within easy reach

Evaluate:

• Therapeutic response: decrease in pain

• CNS changes: dizziness, drowsiness, hallucinations, euphoria, LOC, pupil reaction

• Allergic reactions: rash, urticaria

• Respiratory dysfunction: respiratory depression, character, rate, rhythm; notify physician if respirations are <12/min

---

• Need for pain medication, physical dependence
Teach patient/family:
• To report any symptoms of CNS changes, allergic reactions
• That physical dependency may result when used for extended periods of time
• Withdrawal symptoms may occur: nausea, vomiting, cramps, fever, faintness, anorexia
Lab test interferences:
Increase: Amylase
Treatment of overdose: Narcan 0.2-0.8 IV, O_2, IV fluids, vasopressors

---

pentobarbital/pentobarbital sodium

(pen-toe-bar'bi-tal)
Nebralin/Nembutal sodium, Nova-Rectal,* Penital, Pentogen*
Func. class.: Sedative/hypnotic-barbiturate
Chem. class.: Barbitone, short acting

Controlled Substance Schedule II (USA), Schedule G (Canada)
Action: Depresses activity in brain cells primarily in reticular activating system in brainstem; selectively depresses neurons in posterior hypothalamus, limbic structures
Uses: Insomnia, sedation, preoperative medication, increased intracranial pressure, dental anesthetic
Dosage and routes:
• *Adult:* PO 100-200 mg hs; IM 150-200 mg hs; IV 100 mg initially, then up to 500 mg; REC 120-200 mg hs
• *Child:* IM 3-5 mg, not to exceed 100 mg
• *Child 2 mo-1 yr:* REC 30 mg
• *Child 1-4 yr:* REC 30-60 mg
• *Child 5-12 yr:* REC 60 mg
• *Child 12-14 yr:* REC 60-120 mg
Available forms include: Caps 50,

100 mg; elix 18.2 mg/5 ml; powder, rec supp 30, 60, 120, 200 mg; inj IM, IV 50 mg/ml
Side effects/adverse reactions:
CNS: Lethargy, drowsiness, hangover, dizziness, stimulation in elderly and children, lightheadedness, dependence, CNS depression, mental depression, slurred speech
GI: Nausea, vomiting, diarrhea, constipation
INTEG: Rash, urticaria, pain, abscesses at injection site, angioedema, thrombophlebitis, ***Stevens-Johnson syndrome***
CV: Hypotension, bradycardia
RESP: Depression, apnea, ***laryngospasm, bronchospasm***
*HEMA: **Agranulocytosis, thrombocytopenia, megaloblastic anemia*** (long-term treatment)
Contraindications: Hypersensitivity to barbiturates, respiratory depression, addiction to barbiturates, severe liver impairment, porphyria
Precautions: Anemia, pregnancy (D), lactation, hepatic disease, renal disease, hypertension, elderly, acute/chronic pain
Pharmacokinetics:
PO: Onset 15-30 min, duration 4-6 hr
REC: Onset slow, duration 4-6 hr
Metabolized by liver, excreted by kidneys (metabolites); half-life 15-48 hr
Interactions/incompatibilities:
• Do not mix with other drugs in solution or syringe
• Increased CNS depression: alcohol, MAOIs, sedative, narcotics
• Decreased effect of: oral anticoagulants, corticosteroids, griseofulvin, quinidine
• Increased half-life of doxycycline
NURSING CONSIDERATIONS
Assess:
• VS q 30 min after parenteral route for 2 hr

P

• Blood studies: Hct, Hgb, RBCs, serum folate, vitamin D (if on long-term therapy); pro-time in patients receiving anticoagulants
• Hepatic studies: AST, ALT, bilirubin; if increased, drug is usually discontinued

Administer:
• After removal of cigarettes, to prevent fires
• IM injection in deep large muscle mass to prevent tissue sloughing and abscesses; do not inject more than 5 ml in one site
• After trying conservative measures for insomnia
• After mixing with sterile water for injection, inject within 30 min of preparation
• IV only with resuscitative equipment available, administer at <100 mg/min (only by qualified personnel)
• ½-1 hr before hs for sleeplessness
• On empty stomach for best absorption
• For <14 days since not effective after that; tolerance develops
• Crushed or whole
• Alone, do not mix with other drugs or inject if there is precipitate

Perform/provide:
• Assistance with ambulation after receiving dose
• Safety measure: siderails, nightlight, callbell within easy reach
• Checking to see PO medication has been swallowed
• Storage of suppositories in refrigerator; do not use aqueous solutions that contain precipitate

Evaluate:
• Therapeutic response: ability to sleep at night, decreased amount of early morning awakening if taking drug for insomnia, or decrease in number, severity of seizures if taking drug for seizure disorder
• Mental status: mood, sensorium,

affect, memory (long, short)
• Physical dependency: more frequent requests for medication, shakes, anxiety
• Barbiturate toxicity: hypotension; pulmonary constriction; cold, clammy skin; cyanosis of lips; insomnia; nausea; vomiting; hallucinations; delirium; weakness; mild symptoms may occur in 8-12 hr without drug
• Respiratory dysfunction: respiratory depression, character, rate, rhythm; hold drug if respirations are <12/min or if pupils are dilated
• Blood dyscrasias: fever, sore throat, bruising, rash, jaundice, epistaxis

Teach patient/family:
• That hangover is common
• That drug is indicated only for short-term treatment of insomnia and is probably ineffective after 2 wk
• That physical dependency may result when used for extended periods of time (45-90 days depending on dose)
• To avoid driving or other activities requiring alertness
• To avoid alcohol ingestion or CNS depressants; serious CNS depression may result
• Not to discontinue medication quickly after long-term use; drug should be tapered over 1-2 wk
• To tell all prescribers that a barbiturate is being taken
• That withdrawal insomnia may occur after short-term use; do not start using drug again; insomnia will improve in 1-3 nights
• That effects may take 2 nights for benefits to be noticed
• Alternate measures to improve sleep (reading, exercise several hours before hs, warm bath, warm milk, TV, self-hypnosis, deep breathing)

Lab test interferences:
False increase: Sulfobromophthalein

Treatment of overdose: Lavage, activated charcoal, warming blanket, vital signs, hemodialysis, I&O ratio

---

pentoxifylline

(pen-tox-i′fi-leen)
Trental

Func. class.: Hemorheologic agent
Chem. class.: Dimethylxanthine derivative

Action: Decreases blood viscosity, increases blood flow by increasing flexibility of RBCs; decreases RBC hyperaggregation

Uses: Intermittent claudication related to chronic occlusive vascular disease

Dosage and routes:
• *Adult:* PO 400 mg tid with meals
Available forms include: Tabs, controlled-release 400 mg

Side effects/adverse reactions:
EENT: Blurred vision, earache, increased salivation, sore throat
CNS: Headache, restlessness, anxiety, nervousness, drowsiness, tremors, confusion, insomnia
GI: Nausea, vomiting, anorexia, diarrhea, bloating, belching
INTEG: Rash, pruritus, urticaria, brittle fingernails
CV: Angina, dysrhythmias, palpitation, hypotension, chest pain

Contraindications: Hypersensitivity to this drug or xanthines
Precautions: Pregnancy, angina pectoris, cardiac disease, lactation, children

Pharmacokinetics:
PO: Peak 2-4 hr, half-life ½-1 hr, degradation in liver, excreted in urine

Interactions/incompatibilities:
None known

NURSING CONSIDERATIONS

Assess:
• B/P, respirations of patient taking antihypertensives also
Administer:
• On empty stomach only, to facilitate absorption
Evaluate:
• Therapeutic response: decreased pain, cramping, increased ambulation
Teach patient/family:
• That therapeutic response may take 2-4 wk
• That decreased fats, increased cholesterol, increased exercise, decreased smoking are necessary to correct condition
• To report all severe adverse reactions

---

perphenazine

(per-fen′a-zeen)
Phenazine,* Trilafon

Func. class.: Antipsychotic/neuroleptic
Chem. class.: Phenothiazine-piperidine

Action: Depresses cerebral cortex, hypothalamus, limbic system, which control activity, aggression; blocks neurotransmission produced by dopamine at synapse; exhibits strong α-adrenergic, anticholinergic blocking action; as antiemetic inhibits medullary chemoreceptor trigger zone; mechanism for antipsychotic effects is unclear

Uses: Psychotic disorders, schizophrenia, alcoholism, intractable hiccups, nausea, vomiting

Dosage and routes:
Nausea/vomiting/hiccups/alcoholism
• *Adult and child >12 yr:* IM 5-10 mg prn, max 15 mg in ambulatory patients, 30 mg in hospitalized patients; PO 8-16 mg/day in divided

doses, up to 24 mg; IV not to exceed 5 mg, give diluted or slow IV drip

Psychiatric use in hospitalized patients

• *Adults:* PO 8-16 mg bid-qid, gradually increased to desired dose, not to exceed 64 mg/day; IM 5 mg q6h, not to exceed 30 mg/day

• *Child >12 yr:* PO 6-12 mg in divided doses

Nonhospitalized patients

• *Adult:* PO 4-8 mg tid or 8-32 mg repeat-action bid; IM 5 mg q6h

Available forms include: Tabs 2, 4, 8, 16 mg; conc 16 mg/5ml; inj IM 5 mg/ml; repeat-action tabs 8 mg

Side effects/adverse reactions:

RESP: **Laryngospasm,** dyspnea, **respiratory depression**

CNS: Extrapyramidal symptoms: pseudoparkinsonism, akathisia, dystonia, tardive dyskinesia, seizures, *headache*

HEMA: Anemia, leukopenia, leukocytosis, **agranulocytosis**

INTEG: Rash, photosensitivity, dermatitis

EENT: Blurred vision, glaucoma

GI: Dry mouth, nausea, vomiting, anorexia, constipation, diarrhea, jaundice, weight gain

GU: Urinary retention, urinary frequency, enuresis, impotence, amenorrhea, gynecomastia

CV: Orthostatic hypotension, hypertension, **cardiac arrest,** ECG changes, **tachycardia**

Contraindications: Hypersensitivity, blood dyscrasias, coma, child <12 yr, brain damage, bone marrow depression

Precautions: Pregnancy, lactation, seizure disorders, hypertension, hepatic disease, cardiac disease

Pharmacokinetics:

PO: Onset erratic, peak 2-4 hr

IM: Onset 10 min, peak 1-2 hr, duration 6 hr, occasionally 12-24 hr Metabolized by liver, excreted in urine, crosses placenta, enters breast milk

Interactions/incompatibilities:

• Oversedation: other CNS depressants, alcohol, barbiturate anesthetics

• Toxicity: epinephrine

• Decreased absorption: aluminum hydroxide or magnesium hydroxide antacids

• Decreased effects of: lithium, levodopa

• Increased effects of both drugs: β-adrenergic blockers, alcohol

• Increased anticholinergic effects: anticholinergics

NURSING CONSIDERATIONS

Assess:

• Swallowing of PO medication; check for hoarding or giving of medication to other patients

• I&O ratio; palpate bladder if low urinary output occurs

• Bilirubin, CBC, liver function studies monthly

• Urinalysis is recommended before and during prolonged therapy

Administer:

• Antiparkinsonian agent, after securing order from physician to be used if EPS occur

• Concentrate mixed in water, orange, pineapple, apricot, prune, tomato, grapefruit juice; do not mix with caffeine beverages (coffee, cola), tannics (tea), or pectinates (apple juice) since incompatibility may result; use 60 ml diluent for each 5 ml of concentrate

• Repeat-action tablets whole; do not crush or chew

• IM injection into a large muscle mass

Perform/provide:

• Decreased noise input by dimming lights, avoiding loud noises

• Supervised ambulation until stabilized on medication; do not involve in strenuous exercise program because fainting is possible; patient should not stand still for long periods of time

• Increased fluids to prevent constipation

• Sips of water, candy, gum for dry mouth

• Storage in tight, light-resistant container

Evaluate:

• Therapeutic response: decrease in emotional excitement, hallucinations, delusions, paranoia, reorganization of patterns of thought, speech

• Affect, orientation, LOC, reflexes, gait, coordination, sleep pattern disturbances

• B/P standing and lying; also include pulse, respirations q4h during initial treatment; establish baseline before starting treatment; report drops of 30 mm Hg

• Dizziness, faintness, palpitations, tachycardia on rising

• EPS including akathisia (inability to sit still, no pattern to movements), tardive dyskinesia (bizarre movements of jaw, mouth, tongue, extremities), pseudoparkinsonism (rigidity, tremors, pill rolling, shuffling gait)

• Skin turgor daily

• Constipation, urinary retention daily; if these occur, increase bulk, water in diet

Teach patient/family:

• That orthostatic hypotension occurs frequently, and to rise from sitting or lying position gradually

• To remain lying down after IM injection for at least 30 min

• To avoid hot tubs, hot showers, or tub baths since hypotension may occur

• To avoid abrupt withdrawal of this drug or EPS may result; drugs should be withdrawn slowly

• To avoid OTC preparations (cough, hayfever, cold) unless approved by physician since serious drug interactions may occur; avoid use with alcohol or CNS depressants, increased drowsiness may occur

• To use a sunscreen during sun exposure to prevent burns

• Regarding compliance with drug regimen

• About necessity for meticulous oral hygiene since oral candidiasis may occur

• To report sore throat, malaise, fever, bleeding, mouth sores; if these occur, CBC should be drawn and drug discontinued

• In hot weather, heat stroke may occur; take extra precautions to stay cool

Lab test interferences:

Increase: Liver function tests, cardiac enzymes, cholesterol, blood glucose, prolactin, bilirubin, PBI, cholinesterase, ^{131}I

Decrease: Hormones (blood, urine)

False positive: Pregnancy tests, PKU

False negative: Urinary steroids, 17-OHCS

Treatment of overdose: Lavage if orally injested, provide an airway; *do not induce vomiting*

---

phenacemide

(fe-nass′e-mide)

Phenurone

Func. class.: Anticonvulsant

Chem. class.: Hydantoin

Action: Increases seizure threshold in cortex

Uses: Refractory, generalized tonic-clonic, complex-partial, absence, atypical seizures

Dosage and routes:

• *Adult:* PO 500 mg tid, may in-

crease by 500 mg/wk, not to exceed 5 g/day
• *Child 5-10 yr:* PO 250 mg tid, may increase by 250 mg/wk, not to exceed 1.5 g/day prn
Available forms include: Tabs 500 mg
Side effects/adverse reactions:
*HEMA: **Agranulocytosis, leukopenia, aplastic anemia***
CNS: Drowsiness, dizziness, insomnia, paresthesias, depression, suicidal tendencies, aggression, headache
GI: Anorexia, weight loss, ***hepatitis,*** jaundice, nausea
GU: Nephritis, albuminuria
INTEG: Rash
Contraindications: Hypersensitivity, psychiatric disease, pregnancy
Precautions: Allergies, hepatic disease, renal disease
Pharmacokinetics:
PO: Duration 5 hr, metabolized by liver, excreted by kidneys
Interactions/incompatibilities: None known

NURSING CONSIDERATIONS
Assess:
• Blood, liver function, renal function studies
• Drug level: drug is extremely toxic
Administer:
• With food to decrease GI symptoms
Evaluate:
• Mental status: mood, sensorium, affect, memory (long, short); psychosis is common
• Respiratory depression: respirations <10/min, shallow
• Blood dyscrasias: fever, sore throat, bruising, rash, jaundice
Teach patient/family:
• All aspects of drug therapy: action, dosage side effects, when to notify physician.
• To notify physician if sore throat, fever, rash, fatigue, bleeding,

bruising occur (blood dyscrasia)
• To notify physician if dark urine, jaundice, yellow sclerae, itching occur (liver dysfunction)

---

phenazopyridine HCl
(fen-az-eh-peer'i-deen)
Azogesic, Azo-Pyridon, Baridium, Di-Azo, Diridone, Phenazo,* Phenazodine, Pyridiate, Pyridium, Urodine

Func. class.: Nonnarcotic analgesic
Chem. class.: Azodye

Action: Blocks pain impulses in CNS that occur in response to inhibition of prostaglandin synthesis; antipyretic action results from inhibition of hypothalamic heat-regulating center
Uses: Urinary tract irritation, infection
Dosage and routes:
• *Adult:* PO 100-200 mg tid
• *Child:* PO 100 mg tid
Available forms include: Tabs 100, 200 mg
Side effects/adverse reactions:
*HEMA: **Thrombocytopenia, agranulocytosis, leukopenia, neutropenia, hemolytic anemia***
CNS: Headache
GI: Nausea, vomiting, GI bleeding, diarrhea, heartburn, anorexia, ***hepatic toxicity***
INTEG: Rash, urticaria
*GU: **Renal toxicity***
Contraindications: Hypersensitivity to salicylates
Precautions: Pregnancy
Pharmacokinetics: Metabolized by liver, excreted by kidneys, crosses placenta
Interactions/incompatibilities: None known
NURSING CONSIDERATIONS
Assess:
• Liver function studies: AST,

ALT, bilirubin if patient is on long-term therapy

Administer:

• To patient crushed or whole; chewable tablets may be chewed

• With food or milk to decrease gastric symptoms; give 30 min before or 2 hr after meals

Evaluate:

• Therapeutic response: decrease in pain

• Hepatotoxicity: dark urine, clay-colored stools, yellowing of skin, sclera, itching, abdominal pain, fever, diarrhea if patient is on long-term therapy

• Allergic reactions: rash, urticaria; if these occur, drug may need to be discontinued

Teach patient/family:

• To report any symptoms of hepatotoxicity

• Not to exceed recommended dosage

• To read label on other OTC drugs; many contain aspirin

• Urine may turn red-orange

Treatment of overdose: Methylene blue 1-2 mg/kg IV or 100-200 mg vitamin C PO

---

phendimetrazine tartrate

(fen-dye-me′tra-zeen)

Adipost, Anorex, Bacarate, Bontril, Delcozine, Di-Ap-Trol, Metra Obalan, Obeval, Obezine, Phenazine, Plegine, SPRX 1, SPRX-105, Statobex, Trimstat, Trimtabs

Func. class.: Cerebral stimulant
Chem. class.: Sympathomimetic amine

Controlled Substance Schedule III

Action: Increases release of norepinephrine, dopamine in cerebral cortex to reticular activating system

Uses: Exogenous obesity

Dosage and routes:

Adult: PO 35 mg bid-tid 1 hr ac, not to exceed 70 mg tid

Available forms include: Tabs 35 mg, caps 35 mg

Side effects/adverse reactions:

CNS: Hyperactivity, insomnia, restlessness, dizziness, tremor headache

GI: Nausea, anorexia, dry mouth, diarrhea, constipation, cramps

GU: Dysuria

CV: Palpitations, tachycardia, hypertension

EENT: Blurred vision

Contraindications: Hypersensitivity, hyperthyroidism, hypertension, glaucoma, severe arteriosclerosis, severe cardiovascular disease

Precautions: Drug abuse, anxiety, pregnancy (C)

Pharmacokinetics:

PO: Onset 30 min, peak 1-3 hr, duration 4-20 hr, metabolized by liver, excreted by kidneys, crosses placenta, excreted in breast milk, half-life 10-30 hr

Interactions/incompatibilities:

• Hypertensive crisis: MAOIs or within 14 days of MAOIs

• Increased effect of this drug: acetazolamide, antacids, sodium bicarbonate, ascorbic acid, ammonium chloride, phenothiazines, haloperidol

• Decreased effect of this drug: barbiturates

• Decreased effects of: guanethidine, other antihypertensives

NURSING CONSIDERATIONS

Assess:

• VS, B/P since this drug may reverse antihypertensives; check patients with cardiac disease more often

• CBC, urinalysis, in diabetes: blood sugar, urine sugar; insulin changes may need to be made since eating will decrease

P

• Height, growth rate in children; growth rate may decrease

Administer:

• At least 6 hr before hs to avoid sleeplessness

• For obesity only if patient is on weight reduction program, including dietary changes, exercise; patient will develop tolerance, loss of weight won't occur without additional methods

• Gum, hard candy, frequent sips of water for dry mouth

• If drug is being given for obesity, 1 hr before meals

Perform/provide:

• Check to see PO medication has been swallowed

Teach patient/family:

• To decrease caffeine consumption (coffee, tea, cola, chocolate) which may increase irritability, stimulation

• Avoid OTC preparations unless approved by physician

• To taper off drug over several weeks, or depression, increased sleeping, lethargy will ensue

• To avoid alcohol ingestion

• To avoid hazardous activities until patient is stabilized on medication

• To get needed rest; patients will feel more tired at end of day

Treatment of overdose: Administer fluids, hemodialysis or peritoneal dialysis; antihypertensive for increased B/P; ammonium Cl for increase excretion

---

phenelzine sulfate

(fen'el-zeen)
Nardil

Func. class.: Antidepressant MAOI

Chem. class.: Hydrazine

Action: Increases concentrations of endogenous epinephrine, norepinephrine, serotonin, dopamine in storage sites in CNS by inhibition of MAO; increased concentration reduces depression

Uses: Depression, when uncontrolled by other means

Dosage and routes:

• *Adult:* PO 45 mg/day in divided doses, may increase to 60 mg/day, dose should be reduced to 15 mg/day, not to exceed 90 mg/day

Available forms include: Tabs 15 mg

Side effects/adverse reactions:

HEMA: Anemia

CNS: Dizziness, drowsiness, confusion, headache, anxiety, tremors, stimulation, weakness, hyperreflexia, mania, insomnia, fatigue, weight gain

GI: Constipation, dry mouth, nausea, vomiting, *anorexia,* diarrhea, weight gain

GU: Change in libido, frequency

INTEG: Rash, flushing, increased perspiration

CV: Orthostatic hypotension, hypertension, dysrhythmias, hypertensive crisis

EENT: Blurred vision

ENDO: SIADH-like syndrome

Contraindications: Hypersensitivity to MAOIs, elderly, hypertension, CHF, severe hepatic disease, pheochromocytoma, severe renal disease, severe cardiac disease

Precautions: Suicidal patients, convulsive disorders, severe depression, schizophrenia, hyperactivity, diabetes mellitus, pregnancy (C)

Pharmacokinetics:

Metabolized by liver, excreted by kidneys

Interactions/incompatibilities:

• Increased pressor effects: guanethidine, clonidine, indirect acting sympathomimetics (ephedrine)

• Increased effects of: direct acting sympathomimetics (epinephrine),

alcohol, barbiturates, benzodiaze-pines, CNS depressants
• Hyperpyretic crisis, convulsions, hypertensive episode: tricyclic antidepressants

NURSING CONSIDERATIONS
Assess:
• B/P (lying, standing), pulse; if systolic B/P drops 20 mm Hg hold drug, notify physician
• Blood studies: CBC, leukocytes, cardiac enzymes if patient is receiving long-term therapy
• Hepatic studies: ALT, AST, bilirubin, creatinine; hepatotoxicity may occur

Administer:
• Increased fluids, bulk in diet if constipation, urinary retention occur
• With food or milk or GI symptoms
• Crushed if patient is unable to swallow medication whole
• Dosage hs if over-sedation occurs during day
• Gum, hard candy, or frequent sips of water for dry mouth
• Phentolamine for severe hypertension

Perform/provide:
• Storage in tight container in cool environment
• Assistance with ambulation during beginning therapy since drowsiness/dizziness occurs
• Safety measures including siderails
• Checking to see PO medication swallowed

Evaluate:
• Toxicity: increased headache, palpitation, discontinue drug immediately; prodromal signs of hypertensive crisis
• Mental status: mood, sensorium, affect, memory (long, short); increase in psychiatric symptoms
• Urinary retention, constipation, edema, take weight weekly

• Withdrawal symptoms: headache, nausea, vomiting, muscle pain, weakness

Teach patient/family:
• That therapeutic effects may take 1-4 wk
• To avoid driving or other activities requiring alertness
• To avoid alcohol ingestion, CNS depressants or OTC medications: cold, weight, hay fever, cough syrup
• Not to discontinue medication quickly after long-term use
• To avoid high tyramine foods: cheese (aged), sour cream, beer, wine, pickled products, liver, raisins, bananas, figs, avocados, meat tenderizers, chocolate, yogurt; increase caffeine
• Report headache, palpitation, neck stiffness

Treatment of overdose: Lavage, activated charcoal, monitor electrolytes, vital signs, diazepam IV, $NaHCO_3$

phenmetrazine HCl
(fen-met′ra-zeen)
Preludin

Func. class.: Cerebral stimulant
Chem. class.: Sympathomimetic amine

Controlled Substance Schedule II
Action: Increases release of norepinephrine, dopamine in cerebral cortex to reticular activating system
Uses: Exogenous obesity
Dosage and routes:
• *Adult:* PO 25 mg bid-tid 1 hr ac, not to exceed 75 mg/day; EXT REL 50-75 mg qd in AM
Available forms include: Tabs 25 mg, tabs ext rel 75 mg
Side effects/adverse reactions:
CNS: Hyperactivity, insomnia, restlessness, dizziness, headache
GI: Nausea, anorexia, dry mouth,

constipation, abdominal pain
GU: Impotence, change in libido
CV: Palpitations, tachycardia, hypertension, hypotension
INTEG: Urticaria
EENT: Blurred vision
Contraindications: Hypersensitivity, hyperthyroidism, hypertension, glaucoma, severe arteriosclerosis, angina pectoris, drug abuse, cardiovascular disease
Precautions: Anxiety
Pharmacokinetics:
PO: Onset 15-30 min, peak 2 hr, duration 4 hr
EXT REL: Duration 12 hr, metabolized by liver, excreted by kidneys
Interactions/incompatibilities:
• Hypertensive crisis: MAOIs or within 14 days of MAOIs
• Increased effect of this drug: acetazolamide, antacids, sodium bicarbonate, ascorbic acid, ammonium chloride, phenothiazines, haloperidol
• Decreased effect of this drug: barbiturates
• Decreased effect of: guanethidine, other antihypertensives

NURSING CONSIDERATIONS
Assess:
• VS, B/P since this drug may reverse antihypertensives; check patients with cardiac disease more often
• CBC, urinalysis, in diabetes: blood sugar, urine sugar; insulin changes may need to be made since eating will decrease
• Height, growth rate in children; growth rate may be decreased
Administer:
• At least 6 hr before hs to avoid sleeplessness
• For obesity only if patient is on weight reduction program including dietary changes, exercise; patient will develop tolerance, loss of weight won't occur without additional methods

• Gum, hard candy, frequent sips of water for dry mouth
• If drug is being given for obesity, 1 hr before meals
Perform/provide:
• Check to see PO medication has been swallowed
Evaluate:
• Mental status: mood, sensorium, affect, stimulation, insomnia, aggressiveness
• Physical dependency: should not be used for extended time; dose should be discontinued gradually
• Withdrawal symptoms: headache, nausea, vomiting, muscle pain, weakness
• Drug tolerance after long-term use
• Dosage should not be increased if tolerance develops
Teach patient/family:
• To decrease caffeine consumption (coffee, tea, cola, chocolate), which may increase irritability, stimulation
• Avoid OTC preparations unless approved by physician
• To taper off drug over several weeks, or depression, increased sleeping, lethargy may ensue
• To avoid alcohol ingestion
• To avoid hazardous activities until patient is stabilized on medication
• To get needed rest; patients will feel more tired at end of day
Treatment of overdose: Administer fluids, hemodialysis or peritoneal dialysis; antihypertensive for increased B/P; ammonium Cl for increased excretion

phenobarbital, phenobarbital sodium

(fee-noe-bar'bi-tal)

Bar, Barbita, Eskabarb, Floramine, Gardenal,* Luminal, Orpine, SoluBarb, Stental, Luminal sodium

Func. class.: Anticonvulsant
Chem. class.: Barbiturate

Controlled Substance Schedule IV

Action: Decreases impulse transmission, increases seizure threshold at cerebral cortex level

Uses: All forms of epilepsy, status epilepticus, febrile seizures in children, sedation, insomnia, hyperbilirubinemia, chronic cholestasis

Dosage and routes:

Seizures

• *Adult:* PO 100-200 mg/day in divided doses tid or total dose hs

• *Child:* PO 4-6 mg/kg/day in divided doses q12h, may be given as single dose

Status epilepticus

• *Adult:* IV INF 10 mg/kg, run no faster than 50 mg/min, may give up to 20 mg/kg

• *Child:* IV INF 5-10 mg/kg, may repeat q10-15 min, up to 20 mg/kg, run no faster than 50 mg/min

Insomnia

• *Adult:* PO/IM 100-320 mg

• *Child:* PO/IM 3-6 mg/kg

Sedation

• *Adult:* PO 30-120 mg/day in 2-3 divided doses

• *Child:* PO 6 mg/kg/day in 3 divided doses

Preoperative sedation

• *Adult:* IM 100-200 mg 1-1½ hr before surgery

• *Child:* IM 16-100 mg 1-1½ hr before surgery

Hyperbilirubinemia

• *Neonate:* PO 7 mg/kg/day from days 1-5 after birth

IM 5 mg/kg/day on day 1, then PO on days 2-7 after birth

Chronic cholestasis

• *Adult:* PO 90-180 mg/day in 2-3 divided doses

• *Child <12 yr:* PO 3-12 mg/kg/day in 2-3 divided doses

Available forms include: Caps 16 mg; elix 15, 20 mg/5 ml; tabs 8, 15, 16, 30, 32, 60, 65, 100 mg; inj 30, 60, 65, 130 mg/ml

Side effects/adverse reactions:

CNS: Stimulation, drowsiness, lethargy, hangover headache, flushing, hallucinations, coma

GI: Nausea, vomiting

INTEG: Rash, urticaria, Stevens-Johnsons syndrome, angioedema, local pain, swelling, necrosis, thrombophlebitis

Contraindications: Hypersensitivity to barbiturates, porphyria, hepatic disease, respiratory disease, nephritis, hyperthyroidism, diabetes mellitus, elderly, lactation

Precautions: Anemia

Pharmacokinetics:

PO: Onset 20-60 min, peak 8-12 hr, duration 6-10 hr, metabolized by liver, excreted by kidneys, crosses placenta, excreted in breast milk, half-life 53-118 hr

Interactions/incompatibilities:

• Increased effects: CNS depressants, alcohol chloramphenicol, valproic acid, disulfiram, nondepolarizing skeletal muscle relaxants, sulfonamides

• Increased orthostatic hypotension: furosemide

NURSING CONSIDERATIONS

Assess:

• Blood studies, liver function tests during long-term treatment

• Therapeutic level 15-40 mg/ml

Evaluate:

• Mental status: mood, sensorium, affect, memory (long, short)

• Respiratory depression

---

italics = common side effects   **bold italic** = life threatening reactions

• Blood dyscrasias: fever, sore throat, bruising, rash, jaundice
Teach patient/family:
• All aspects of drug administration: action, dose, route, when to notify physician
Treatment of overdose: Administer calcium gluconate IV

---

phenolphthalein

(fee-nol-thay'leen)

Alophen, Espotabs, Evac-U-Gen, Evac-U-Lax, Ex-Lax, Feen-A-Mint, Phenolax

Func. class.: Laxative, stimulant
Chem. class.: Diphenylmethane

Action: Directly acts on intestine by increasing motor activity; thought to irritate colonic intramural plexus
Uses: Constipation, preparation for bowel surgery or examination
Dosage and routes:
• *Adult:* PO 60-270 mg hs
• *Child >6 yr:* 30-60 mg/day
• *Child 2-5 yr:* 15-20 mg/day
Available forms include: Tabs 60 mg; chew tab 60, 64.8, 80, 90, 97.2 mg; chew gum 97.2 mg; susp 22 mg/5 ml
Side effects/adverse reactions:
INTEG: Rash, urticaria, ***Stevens-Johnson syndrome***
GI: Nausea, vomiting, anorexia, diarrhea
META: Hypokalemia, electrolyte, fluid imbalances
Contraindications: Hypersensitivity, GI obstructions, abdominal pain, nausea/vomiting, fecal impaction
Pharmacokinetics:
PO: Onset 6-8 hr; excreted in feces
Interactions/incompatibilities:
None known
NURSING CONSIDERATIONS
Assess:
• Blood, urine electrolytes if drug

is used often by patient
• I&O ratio to identify fluid loss
Administer:
• Alone for better absorption; do not take within 1 hr of other drugs or within 1 hr of antacids, milk, or cimetidine
• In morning or evening (oral dose)
Evaluate:
• Therapeutic response: decrease in constipation
• Cause of constipation; identify whether fluids, bulk, or exercise is missing from lifestyle
• Cramping, rectal bleeding, nausea, vomiting; if these symptoms occur, drug should be discontinued
Teach patient/family:
• Swallow tabs whole; do not chew
• Not to use laxatives for long-term therapy; bowel tone will be lost
• That normal bowel movements do not always occur daily
• Do not use in presence of abdominal pain, nausea, vomiting
• Notify physician if constipation unrelieved or if symptoms of electrolyte imbalance occur: muscle cramps, pain, weakness, dizziness
• Urine, feces may turn pink
Lab test interferences:
BSP test

---

phenoxybenzamine HCl

(fen-ox-ee-ben'za-meen)

Dibenzyline

Func. class.: Antihypertensive
Chem. class.: α-Adrenergic blocker

Action: α-Adrenergic blocker, which binds to α-adrenergic receptors, dilating peripheral blood vessels, lowers peripheral resistance, lowers blood pressure
Uses: Pheochromocytoma
Dosage and routes:
• *Adult:* PO 10 mg bid, increase by 10 mg qod, not to exceed 60 mg/

day; usual range: 20-40 mg bid-tid

Available forms include: Caps 10 mg

Side effects/adverse reactions:

GI: Dry mouth, nausea, vomiting, diarrhea

CV: Postural hypotension, tachycardia, palpitations

CNS: Dizziness, flushing, drowsiness, sedation, weakness, confusion, headache, malaise

GU: Inhibition of ejaculation

EENT: Nasal congestion, dry mouth, miosis

INTEG: Allergic contact dermatitis

Contraindications: Hypersensitivity, CHF, angina, cerebral vascular insufficiency, coronary arteriosclerosis

Precautions: Severe renal disease, severe pulmonary disease, pregnancy

Pharmacokinetics:

PO: Onset 2 hr, peak 4-6 hr, duration 3-4 days; half-life 24 hr, metabolized in liver, excreted in urine, bile

Interactions/incompatibilities:

• Hypotensive response: epinephrine, antihypertensives

NURSING CONSIDERATIONS

Assess:

• Electrolytes: K, Na, Cl, CO_2

• Weight daily, I&O

• B/P lying, standing before starting treatment, q4h after

Administer:

• Starting with low dose, gradually increasing to prevent side effects

• Gum, frequent rinsing of mouth or hard candy for dry mouth

• With food or milk for GI symptoms

Evaluate:

• Therapeutic response: decreased B/P, increased peripheral pulses

• Nausea, vomiting, diarrhea

• Skin turgor, dryness of mucous membranes for hydration status

Teach patient/family:

• Avoid alcoholic beverages

• To report dizziness, palpitations, fainting

• To change position slowly or fainting may occur

• To take drug exactly as prescribed

• To avoid all OTC products: cough, cold, allergy, unless directed by physician

Treatment of overdose: Administer IV saline, norepinephrine, elevate legs, discontinue drug

---

phenprocoumon

(fen-proe-koo′mon)

Liquamar

Func. class.: Anticoagulant

Chem. class.: Coumarin

Action: Interferes with blood clotting by indirect means; depresses hepatic synthesis of vitamin K-dependent coagulation factors (II, VII, IX, X)

Uses: Deep vein thrombosis, pulmonary emboli, myocardial infarction, rheumatic heart disease, atrial dysrhythmias

Dosage and routes:

• *Adult:* PO 24 mg, then 0.75-6 mg/day titrated to PT level

Available forms include: Tabs 3 mg

Side effects/adverse reactions:

GI: Diarrhea, nausea, vomiting, anorexia, stomatitis, abdominal pain, *hepatitis*

GU: Hematuria

INTEG: Rash, dermatitis, urticaria, alopecia, pruritus

CNS: Fever

HEMA: Hemorrhage, agranulocytosis, leukopenia

Contraindications: Hypersensitivity, hemophilia, leukemia with bleeding, peptic ulcer disease, thrombocytopenic purpura, hepatic

---

disease (severe), renal disease (severe), blood dyscrasias, severe hypertension, subacute bacterial endocarditis, acute nephritis, pregnancy

Precautions: Alcoholism, elderly
Pharmacokinetics:
PO: 48-72 hr; half-life 6½ days
Interactions/incompatibilities:

• Increased action: allopurinol, chloramphenicol, clofibrate amiodarone, diflunisal, heparin, steroids, cimetidine, disulfiram, thyroid, glucagon, metronidazole, quinidine, sulindac, sulfinpyrazone, sulfonamides, tricyclic antidepressants, inhalation anesthetics, salicylates, ethacrynic acid, indomethacin, mefenamic acid, oxyphenbutazones, phenylbutazone, alcohol

• Decreased action: barbiturates, griseofulvin, haloperidol ethchlorvynol, carbamazepine, rifampin, cholestyramine

• Increased or decreased action: chloral hydrate, glutethimide, sulfinpyrazone, triclofos sodium

NURSING CONSIDERATIONS
Assess:

• Blood studies (Hct, platelets, occult blood in stools) q3 mo

• Prothrombin time, which should be 1½-2 × control, PT; often done qd

• B/P, watch for increasing signs of hypertension

Administer:

• At same time each day to maintain steady blood levels

• Alone, do not give with food

• Avoiding all IM injections that may cause bleeding

Perform/provide:

• Storage in tight container

Evaluate:

• Therapeutic response: decrease of deep vein thrombosis

• Bleeding gums, petecchiae, ecchymosis, black tarry stools, hematuria

• Fever, skin rash, urticaria

• Needed dosage change q1-2 wk

Teach patient/family:

• To avoid OTC preparations (aspirin-containing products) that may cause serious drug interactions, unless directed by physician

• That urine may turn orange/red

• Drug may be held during active bleeding (menstruation)

• To use soft-bristle toothbrush to avoid bleeding gums

• To carry a Medic-Alert ID identifying drug taken

• Stress patient compliance

• On all aspects of adjustments: dosage, route, action, side effects, when to notify physician

• To report any signs of bleeding: gums, under skin, urine, stools

• To avoid hazardous activities (football, hockey, skiing) or dangerous work

Lab test interferences:
Increase: T_3 uptake
Decrease: Uric acid
Treatment of overdose:
Administer vitamin K

---

phensuximide
(fen-sux'i-mide)
Milontin

Func. class.: Anticonvulsant
Chem. class.: Succinimide

Action: Inhibits spike, wave formation in absence seizures (petit mal), decreases amplitude, frequency, duration, spread of discharge in minor

Uses: Absence seizures

Dosage and routes:

• *Adult and child:* PO 500 mg-1 g bid or tid

Available forms include: Caps 500 mg

Side effects/adverse reactions:

HEMA: **Agranulocytosis, aplastic anemia, thrombocytopenia, leukocytosis, eosinophilia, pancytopenia**

CNS: Drowsiness, dizziness, fatigue, euphoria, lethargy, anxiety, depression, irritability, insomnia, aggressiveness

GI: Nausea, vomiting, heartburn, anorexia, diarrhea, abdominal pain, cramps, constipation

GU: Vaginal bleeding, **hematuria, renal damage**

INTEG: Urticaria, pruritic erythema, hirsutism, **Stevens-Johnson syndrome**

EENT: Myopia, gum hypertrophy, tongue swelling, blurred vision

Contraindications: Hypersensitivity to succinimide derivatives

Precautions: Lactation, hepatic disease, pregnancy, renal disease

Pharmacokinetics:

PO: Peak 1-4 hr, metabolized by liver, excreted by kidneys, half-life 5-12 hr

Interactions/incompatibilities:

• Antagonist effect: tricyclic antidepressants (imipramine, doxepin)
• Decreased effects of: estrogens, oral contraceptives

NURSING CONSIDERATIONS

Assess:

• Renal studies: urinalysis, BUN, urine creatinine
• Blood studies: CBC, Hct, Hgb, reticulocyte counts q wk for 4 wk then q mo
• Hepatic studies: AST, ALT, bilirubin, creatinine
• Drug levels during initial treatment, therapeutic range (40-80 μg/ml)

Administer:

• With food, milk to decrease GI symptoms

Perform/provide:

• Hard candy, frequent rinsing of mouth, gum for dry mouth

• Assistance with ambulation during early part of treatment; dizziness occurs

Evaluate:

• Mental status: mood, sensorium, affect, behavioral changes; if mental status changes, notify physician
• Eye problems; need for ophthalmic exam before, during, after treatment (slit lamp, fundoscopy, tonometry)
• Allergic reaction: red raised rash; if this occurs, drug should be discontinued
• Blood dyscrasias: fever, sore throat, bruising, rash, jaundice
• Toxicity: bone marrow depression, nausea, vomiting, ataxia, diplopia

Teach patient/family:

• To carry ID card or Medic-Alert bracelet stating drugs taken, condition, physician's name, phone number
• To avoid driving, other activities that require alertness
• To avoid alcohol ingestion, CNS depressants; increased sedation may occur
• Not to discontinue medication quickly after long-term use
• All aspects of drug: action, use, side effects, adverse reactions, when to notify physician
• May color urine pink or red

Lab test interferences:

Increase: Coombs' test

Treatment of overdose: Lavage, activated charcoal, monitor electrolytes, VS

P

---

phentermine HCl

(fen'ter-meen)

Anoxine, Fastin, Ionamin, Parmine, Phentrol, Rolaphent, Wilpowr

Func. class.: Cerebral stimulant
Chem. class.: Sympathomimetic amine

Controlled Substance Schedule IV

Action: Increases release of norepinephrine, dopamine in cerebral cortex to reticular activating system

Uses: Exogenous obesity

Dosage and routes:

• *Adult:* PO 8 mg tid 30 min before meals or 15-30 mg qd

Available forms include: Tabs 8, 15, 30, 37.5 mg; caps 8, 15, 18.75, 30, 37.5 mg; caps time rel 30 mg

Side effects/adverse reactions:

CNS: Hyperactivity, insomnia, restlessness, dizziness

GI: Nausea, anorexia, dry mouth, constipation, unpleasant taste

GU: Impotence, change in libido

CV: Palpitations, tachycardia, hypertension

INTEG: Urticaria

Contraindications: Hypersensitivity, hyperthyroidism, hypertension, glaucoma, severe arteriosclerosis, angina pectoris, cardiovascular disease

Precautions: Anxiety

Pharmacokinetics:

CON REL: Duration 10-14 hr; metabolized by liver, excreted by kidneys

Interactions/incompatibilities:

• Hypertensive crisis: MAOIs or within 14 days of MAOIs

• Increased effect of this drug: acetazolamide, antacids, sodium bicarbonate, ascorbic acid, ammonium chloride, phenothiazines, haloperidol

• Decreased effect of this drug: barbiturates

• Decreased effect of: guanethidine, other antihypertensives

NURSING CONSIDERATIONS

Assess:

• VS, B/P since this drug may reverse antihypertensives Check patients with cardiac disease more often

• CBC, urinalysis, in diabetes: blood sugar, urine sugar; insulin changes may need to be made since eating will decrease

• Height and growth rate in children; growth rate may be decreased

Administer:

• At least 6 hr before hs to avoid sleeplessness

• For obesity only if patient is on weight reduction program including dietary changes, exercise; patient will develop tolerance, and loss of weight won't occur without additional methods

• Gum, hard candy, frequent sips of water for dry mouth

• If drug is being given for obesity, 1 hr before meals

Perform/provide:

• Check to see PO medication has been swallowed

Evaluate:

• Mental status: mood, sensorium, affect, stimulation, insomnia, aggressiveness

• Physical dependency: should not be used for extended periods of time; dose should be discontinued gradually

• Withdrawal symptoms: headache, nausea, vomiting, muscle pain, weakness

• Drug tolerance after long-term use

• Drug should not be increased if tolerance develops

Teach patient/family:

• To decrease caffeine consumption (coffee, tea, cola, chocolate),

---

which may increase irritability, stimulation

• Avoid OTC preparations unless approved by physician

• To taper off drug over several weeks, or depression, increased sleeping, lethargy may ensue

• To avoid alcohol ingestion

• To avoid hazardous activities until patient is stabilized on medication

• To get needed rest; patients will feel more tired at end of day

Treatment of overdose: Administer fluids, hemodialysis or peritoneal dialysis; antihypertensive for increased B/P; ammonium Cl for increase excretion

---

phentolamine mesylate

(fen-tole′a-meen)
Regitine, Rogitine*

Func. class.: Antihypertensive
Chem. class.: α-Adrenergic blocker

Action: α-Adrenergic blocker, binds to α-adrenergic receptors, dilating peripheral blood vessels, lowering peripheral resistances, lowering blood pressure

Uses: Hypertension, pheochromocytoma, prevention, treatment of dermal necrosis following extravasation of norepinephrine or dopamine

Dosage and routes:
Treatment of hypertensive episodes in pheochromocytoma
• *Adult:* 5 mg IV/IM, repeat if necessary
• *Child:* 1 mg IV/IM, repeat if necessary
• *Adult:* 2.5 mg IV, if negative repeat with 5 mg IV
• *Child:* 0.5 mg IV, if negative repeat with 1 mg IV
Prevention, treatment of necrosis
• *Adult:* 5-10 mg/10 ml NS in-

jected into area of norepinephrine extravasation within 12 hr; 10 mg/1000 ml norepinephrine solution is preventive dose

Available forms include: Inj IM, IV 5 mg/ml; tabs 25, 50 mg (only injectable form available in US)

Side effects/adverse reactions:
GI: Dry mouth, nausea, vomiting, diarrhea, abdominal pain
*CV: Hypotension, tachycardia, angina, dysrhythmias, **myocardial infarction***
CNS: Dizziness, flushing, weakness
EENT: Nasal congestion

Contraindications: Hypersensitivity, myocardial infarction, coronary insufficiency, angina

Precautions: Pregnancy (C), lactation

Pharmacokinetics:
IV: Peak 2 min, duration 10-15 min
IM: Peak 15-20 min, duration 3-4 hr
Metabolized in liver, excreted in urine

Interactions/incompatibilities:
• May increase effects of epinephrine, antihypertensives
• Not to be mixed in solution or syringe with any drug except levarterenol

NURSING CONSIDERATIONS
Assess:
• Electrolytes: K, Na, Cl, CO_2
• Weight daily, I&O
• B/P lying, standing before starting treatment, q4h after

Administer:
• Gum, frequent rinsing of mouth or hard candy for dry mouth
• After having vasopressor nearby
• After discontinuing all medication for 24 hr

Evaluate:
• Nausea, vomiting, diarrhea
• Edema in feet, legs daily
• Skin turgor, dryness of mucous membranes for hydration status

P

- Postural hypotension
- Cardiac system: pulse, ECG

Teach patient/family:
- That bedrest is required during treatment, 1 hr after

Treatment of overdose: Administer norepinephrine, discontinue drug

---

phenylbutazone

(fen-ill-byoo'-ta-zone)

Algoverine, Azolid, Butagesic, Butazolidin, Intrabutazone, Malgesic, Neo-Zoline

Func. class.: Nonsteroidal
Chem. class.: Pyrazolone derivative

Action: Inhibits prostaglandin synthesis by decreasing an enzyme needed for biosynthesis; possesses analgesic, antiinflammatory, antipyretic properties

Uses: Mild to moderate pain, osteoarthritis, rheumatoid arthritis

Dosage and routes:

Pain
- *Adult:* PO 100-200 mg tid-qid, then after desired response 100 mg tid-qid, not to exceed 600 mg/day

Acute Arthritis
- *Adult:* PO 400 mg, then 100 mg q4h × 4 days or until desired response

Available forms include: Tabs 100 mg

Side effects/adverse reactions:

GI: Nausea, anorexia, vomiting, diarrhea, jaundice, *cholestatic hepatitis,* constipation, flatulence, cramps, dry mouth, peptic ulcer
CNS: Dizziness, drowsiness, fatigue, tremors, confusion, insomnia, anxiety, depression
CV: Tachycardia, peripheral edema, palpitations, dysrhythmias
INTEG: Purpura, rash, pruritus, sweating
GU: Nephrotoxicity: dysuria, he-

maturia, oliguria, azotemia
HEMA: Blood dyscrasias
EENT: Tinnitus, hearing loss, blurred vision

Contraindications: Hypersensitivity, asthma, severe renal disease, severe hepatic disease

Precautions: Pregnancy, lactation, children, bleeding disorders, GI disorders, cardiac disorders, hypersensitivity to other antiinflammatory agents

Pharmacokinetics:
PO: Peak 2 hr, half-life 3-3½ hr; metabolized in liver, excreted in urine (metabolites) excreted in breast milk

Interactions/incompatibilities:
- May increase action of coumarin, phenytoin, sulfonamides when used with this drug

NURSING CONSIDERATIONS

Assess:
- Renal, liver, blood studies: BUN, creatinine, AST, ALT, Hgb, before treatment, periodically thereafter
- Audiometric, ophthalmic exam before, during, after treatment

Administer:
- With food to decrease GI symptoms; best to take on empty stomach to facilitate absorption

Perform/provide:
- Storage at room temperature

Evaluate:
- Therapeutic response: decreased pain, stiffness, swelling in joints, ability to move more easily
- For eye, ear problems: blurred vision, tinnitus (may indicate toxicity)

Teach patient/family:
- To report blurred vision or ringing, roaring in ears (may indicate toxicity)
- To avoid driving or other hazardous activities if dizziness or drowsiness occurs
- To report change in urine pattern, weight increase, edema, pain in-

crease in joints, fever, blood in urine (indicates nephrotoxicity)

• That therapeutic effects may take up to 1 mo

---

phenylephrine HCl

(fen-ill-ef'rin)

Neo-Synephrine

Func. class.: Adrenergic, direct acting

Chem. class.: Substituted phenyl-ethylamine

Action: Powerful and selective (α1) receptor agonist causing contraction of blood vessels

Uses: Hypotension, paroxysmal supraventricular tachycardia, shock

Dosage and routes:
Hypotension

• *Adult:* SC/IM 2-5 mg, may repeat q10-15 min if needed IV 0.1-0.5 mg, may repeat q10-15 min if needed

PVCs

• *Adult:* IV BOL 0.5 mg given rapidly, not to exceed prior dose by >0.1 mg total dose >1 mg

Shock

• *Adult:* IV INF 10 mg/500 ml D_5W given 100-180 gtts/min, then 40-60 gtts/min titrated to B/P

Available forms include: Inj IV, SC, IM, 1% (10 mg/ml)

Side effects/adverse reactions:

CNS: Headache

CV: Palpitations, tachycardia, hypotension, ectopic beats, angina

GI: Nausea, vomiting

INTEG: Necrosis, tissue sloughing with extravasation, ***gangrene***

Contraindications: Hypersensitivity, ventricular fibrillation, tachydysrhythmias, pheochromocytoma

Precautions: Pregnancy, lactation, arterial embolism, peripheral vascular disease

Pharmacokinetics:

IV: Duration 20-30 min

IM/SC: Duration 45-60 min

Interactions/incompatibilities:

• Do not use within 2 wk of MAOIs, or hypertensive crisis may result

• Dysrhythmias: general anesthetics

• Decreased action of this drug: other β-blockers

• Increase in B/P: oxytocics

• Increased pressor effect: tricyclic antidepressant, MAOIs

• Incompatible with alkaline solutions: Na, HCO_3

NURSING CONSIDERATIONS
Assess:

• I&O ratio

• ECG during administration continuously; if B/P increases, drug is decreased

• B/P and pulse q5 min after parenteral route

• CVP or PWP during infusion if possible

Administer:

• Plasma expanders for hypovolemia

• Parenteral (IV) dose slowly, after reconstituting with 500 ml D_5W or NS

Perform/provide:

• Storage of reconstituted solution if refrigerated for no longer than 24 hr

• Do not use discolored solutions

Evaluate:

• For paresthesias and coldness of extremities, peripheral blood flow may decrease

• Injection site: tissue sloughing if this occurs administer phentolamine mixed with NS

• For therapeutic response: increase B/P with stabilization

Teach patient/family:

• The reason for drug administration

Treatment of overdose: Admin-

P

---

ister an α-blocker, then norepinephrine for severe hypotension

---

phenylephrine HCl

(fen-ill-ef'rin)

AK-Dilate, Isopto Frin, Neo-Synephrine 10% Plain, Neo-Synephrine Viscous, Prefrin

Func. class.: Ophthalmic vasoconstrictor

Chem. class.: Direct sympathomimetic amine

Action: Vasoconstriction of eye arterioles; decreases eye engorgement by stimulation of α-adrenergic receptors

Uses: Topical ocular vasoconstrictor

Dosage and routes:

Eye irritation

• *Adult:* INSTILL 2 gtts of a 0.12%
sol; may repeat q3-4h

Uveitis/glaucoma/surgery

• *Adult and child:* INSTILL 1 gtt
of a 2.5% or 10% sol in upper surface of cornea

Available forms include: Sol 10%,
2.5%, 0.12%

Side effects/adverse reactions:

CNS: Headache, dizziness, weakness

CV: Bradycardia, hypertension,
dysrhythmias, tachycardia, CV
collapse, palpitation

EENT: Stinging, lacrimation,
blurred vision, conjunctival allergy

Contraindications: Hypersensitivity, glaucoma (narrow-angle)

Precautions: Severe hypertension,
diabetes, hyperthyroidism, elderly,
severe arteriosclerosis, cardiac disease, infants, pregnancy

Pharmacokinetics:

INSTILL: Peak 1 hr, duration 0.5-7
hr depending on strength

Interactions/incompatibilities:

• Increased pressor effects:

MAOIs, tricyclic antidepressants

NURSING CONSIDERATIONS

Assess:

• B/P, pulse, systemic absorption
does occur

Perform/provide:

• Storage in tight, light-resistant
container, do not use discolored solutions

Teach patient/family:

• To report change in vision, blurring, loss of sight; breathing trouble, sweating, flushing

• Method of instillation, tilt head
backward, hold dropper over eye,
drop medication inside lower lid,
using pressure on inside corner of
eye hold 1 min, do not touch dropper to eye

• That blurred vision will decrease
with repeated use of drug

• To notify physician if headache,
spots, redness, pain occurs; discontinue use

• To use sunglasses if photophobia
occurs

• To use exactly as prescribed

---

phenylephrine HCl (nasal)

(fen-ill-ef'rin)

Alconefrin, Coricidin Nasal Mist,
Coryzine, Ephrine, Neo-Synephrine Sinarest Nasal Spray, Sino-
phen Intranasal, Vacon

Func. class.: Nasal decongestant
Chem. class.: Sympathomimetic
amine

Action: Produces vasoconstriction
(rapid, long-acting) of arterioles,
thereby decreasing fluid exudation,
mucosal engorgement

Uses: Nasal congestion

Dosage and routes:

• *Adult:* INSTILL 2-3 gtts or
sprays to nasal mucosa bid (0.25%-
1%); TOP apply to nasal mucosa

• *Child 6-12 yr:* INSTILL 2-3 gtts

or sprays (0.25%)

• *Child <6 yr:* INSTILL 2-3 gtts or sprays (0.125%)

Available forms include: Sol 0.125%, 0.16%, 0.2%, 0.25%, 0.5%, 1%; jelly 0.5%

Side effects/adverse reactions:

GI: Nausea, vomiting, anorexia

EENT: Irritation, burning, sneezing, stinging, dryness, rebound congestion

INTEG: Contact dermatitis

CNS: Anxiety, restlessness, tremors, weakness, insomnia, dizziness, fever, headache

Contraindications: Hypersensitivity to sympathomimetic amines

Precautions: Child <6 yr, elderly, diabetes, cardiovascular disease, hypertension, hyperthyroidism, increased ICP, prostatic hypertrophy

Interactions/incompatibilities:

• Hypertension: MAOIs, β-adrenergic blockers

• Hypotension: methyldopa, mecamylamine, reserpine

NURSING CONSIDERATIONS

Administer:

• No more than q4h

• For <4 consecutive days

Perform/provide:

• Environmental humidification to decrease nasal congestion, dryness

• Storage in light-resistant containers; do not expose to high temperatures

Evaluate:

• Redness, swelling, pain in nasal passages

Teach patient/family:

• Stinging may occur for a few applications; drying of mucosa may be decreased by environmental humidification

• To notify physician if irregular pulse, insomnia, dizziness, or tremors occur

• Proper administration to avoid systemic absorption

phenylephrine HCl (optic)

(fen-ill-ef′rin)

Mydfrin, Neo-Synephrine

Func. class.: Mydriatic

Action: Blocks response of iris sphincter muscle, muscle of accommodation of ciliary body to cholinergic stimulation, resulting in dilation, paralysis of accommodation

Uses: Mydriasis, posterior synechia

Dosage and routes:

• *Adult and child:* INSTILL 1 gtt before exam (mydriasis) or 1 gtt of a 10% sol

Available forms include: Sol 2.5%, 10%

Side effects/adverse reactions:

CV: Palpitations, tachycardia

RESP: **Bronchospasm**

EENT: Blurred vision

Contraindications: Hypersensitivity to sympathomimetic amines, narrow-angle glaucoma, dysrhythmias, cardiogenic shock, cerebral arteriosclerosis

Precautions: Elderly, prostatic hypertension, diabetes mellitus, hyperthymus, TB, Parkinson's disease, pregnancy

Pharmacokinetics:

INSTILL: Onset 1 hr, peak 4-8 hr, duration 12-24 hr

Interactions/incompatibilities:

• Dysrhythmias: cyclopropane, halogenated hydrocarbons

• Increased pressor effects: tricyclic antidepressants, antihistamines

NURSING CONSIDERATIONS

Assess:

• Tonometer readings during long-term treatment

• B/P, pulse, respirations

P

---

italics = common side effects   ***bold italic*** = life threatening reactions

Evaluate:
• Allergic reaction: itching, edema of eyelids, eye discharge; drug should be discontinued

Teach patient/family:
• To report change in vision, blurring or loss of sight, trouble breathing, sweating, flushing
• Method of instillation: pressure on lacrimal sac for 1 min, do not touch dropper to eye

---

phenytoin sodium/ phenytoin sodium extended/phenytoin sodium prompt

(fen'i-toy-in)
Dilantin, Dilantin Capsules, Di-Phen, Diphenylan

Func. class.: Anticonvulsant
Chem. class.: Hydantoin

Action: Inhibits spread of seizure activity in motor cortex
Uses: Generalized tonic-clonic seizures, status epilepticus, nonepileptic seizures associated with Reye's syndrome or after head trauma, migraines, trigeminal neuralgia, Bell's palsy, ventricular dysrhythmias uncontrolled by antidysrhythmics

Dosage and routes:
Seizures
• *Adult:* IV loading dose of 900 mg-1.5 g run at 50 mg/min; if patient has received phenytoin, then 100-300 mg run at 50 mg/min; PO loading dose of 900 mg-1.5 g divided tid, then 300 mg/day (extended) or divided tid (extended/prompt)
• *Child:* IV loading dose of 15 mg/kg run at 50 mg/min; if patient has received phenytoin, then 5-7 mg/kg run at 50 mg/min, may repeat in 30 min; PO loading dose of 15 mg/kg divided q8-12h, then 5-7

mg/kg in divided doses q12h
Neuritic pain
• *Adult:* PO 200-400 mg/day
Ventricular dysrhythmias
• *Adult:* PO loading dose 1 g divided over 24 hr, then 500 mg/day × 2 days; IV 250 mg given over 5 min, until dysrhythmias subside or 1 g is given, or 100 mg q15 min until dysrhythmias subside or 1 g is given
• *Child:* PO 3-8 mg/kg or 250 mg/m²/day as single dose or divided in 2 doses; IV 3-8 mg/kg given over several min, or 250 mg/m²/day as single dose or divided in 2 doses

Available forms include: Susp 30, 125 mg/5 ml; tabs, chewable 50 mg; inj 50 mg/ml; caps ext 30, 100 mg; caps prompt 30, 100 mg
Side effects/adverse reactions:
HEMA: Agranulocytosis, leukopenia, aplastic anemia
CNS: Drowsiness, dizziness, insomnia, paresthesias, depression, suicidal tendencies, aggression, headache
GI: Nausea, vomiting, constipation, anorexia, weight loss, *hepatitis,* jaundice
GU: Nephritis, albuminuria
INTEG: Rash
Contraindications: Hypersensitivity, psychiatric disease
Precautions: Allergies, hepatic disease, renal disease
Pharmacokinetics:
PO: Duration 5 hr, metabolized by liver, excreted by kidneys
Interactions/incompatibilities:
• Decreased effects of this drug: alcohol (chronic use), antihistamines, antacids, antineoplastics, CNS depressants, rifampin, folic acid
NURSING CONSIDERATIONS
Assess:
• Blood studies: CBC, platelets q2 wk until stabilized, then q mo ×

12, then q3 mo; discontinue drug if neutrophils are <1600/mm³

Evaluate:

• Mental status: mood, sensorium, affect, memory (long, short)

• Respiratory depression

• Blood dyscrasias: fever, sore throat, bruising, rash, jaundice

Teach patient/family:

• All aspects of drug administration: route, action, dose, when to notify physician

---

physostigmine salicylate/physostigmine sulfate

(fi-zoe-stig'meen)

Isopto Eserine Solution/Eserine Sulfate Ointment, Fisostin, Antilirium, Geneserine

Func. class.: Miotic

Chem. class.: Cholinesterase inhibitor

Action: Increases concentration of acetylcholine at cholinergic transmission sites, thus causing prolonged, exaggerated action; produces constriction of ciliary muscles, iris sphincter, causing iris to be pulled away from anterior chamber angle, aiding in aqueous humor drainage

Uses: Used in treatment of wide-angle glaucoma reversal of anticholinergic or antidepressant poisoning

Dosage and routes:

• *Adult and child:* INSTILL OINT ¼ inch strip of 0.25% oint in conjunctival sac; INSTILL SOL 1-2 gtts of a 0.25%-0.5% sol in conjunctival sac qd-qid

Available forms include: Oint 0.25% (sulfate); sol 0.25% (salicylate)

Side effects/adverse reactions:

CNS: Convulsions, headache

CV: Hypertension, hypotension, bradycardia, irregular pulse

GI: Nausea, vomiting, abdominal cramps

RESP: **Bronchospasm,** dyspnea, pulmonary edema

EENT: Blurred vision, conjunctivitis, allergic reactions, rhinorrhea, salivation, eye, brow pain, lacrimation, twitching of eyelids

Contraindications: Asthma, bronchitis, diabetes mellitus, CV disease, inflammatory disease of iris or ciliary body

Precautions: Epilepsy, parkinsonism, bradycardia

Interactions/incompatibilities:

• Benzalkonium chloride in solution or syringe

NURSING CONSIDERATIONS

Administer:

• Topically to conjunctival sac

• Immediately after reconstituting; discard unused portion

Perform/provide:

• Only clear solutions, never pink or brown

Teach patient/family:

• To report change in vision, blurring or loss of sight, trouble breathing, sweating, flushing

• Method of instillation, including pressure on lacrimal sac for 1 min, not to touch dropper to eye

• That long-term therapy may be required

• That blurred vision will decrease with repeated use of drug

• That drug is often irritating to eye, rarely tolerated for prolonged periods

• That drug may be prescribed for bedtime use to prevent nocturnal rise in ocular tension

• That maximal effect of topical application is reached in 30 min, may last 12-36 hr

• To observe eyes for irritation, development of cataracts

P

---

physostigmine salicylate

(fi-zoe-stig'meen)
Antilirium

Func. class.: Antidote, reversible anticholinesterase
Chem. class.: Tertiary amine

Action: Increases acetylcholine at cholinergic nerve terminals, reverses central, peripheral anticholinergic effects
Uses: Anticholinergic, tricyclic antidepressant poisoning
Dosage and routes:
• *Adult:* PO/IM/IV 0.5-3 mg give 0.5 mg over at least 1 min (IV)
Available forms include: Inj IM, IV 5 mg/ml
Side effects/adverse reactions:
INTEG: Rash, urticaria
CNS: Dizziness, headache, sweating, confusion, weakness, convulsions, incoordination, paralysis
GI: Nausea, diarrhea, vomiting, cramps
CV: Tachycardia
GU: Frequency, incontinence
RESP: Respiratory depression, bronchospasm, constriction
EENT: Miosis, blurred vision, lacrimation
Contraindications: Bradycardia, hypotension, obstruction of intestine, renal system
Precautions: Seizure disorders, bronchial asthma, coronary occlusion, hyperthyroidism, dysrhythmias, peptic ulcer, megacolon, poor GI motility
Pharmacokinetics:
IM/IV/PO: Onset 5 min, duration ½-5 hr; crosses blood-brain barrier, excreted in urine
Interactions/incompatibilities:
• Decreased action of: gallamine, metocurine, pancuronium, tubocurarine, atropine
• Increased action: decamethon-ium, succinylcholine
• Decreased action of this drug: aminoglycosides, anesthetics, procainamide, quinidine
NURSING CONSIDERATIONS
Assess:
• VS; respiration q8h
• I&O ratio; check for urinary retention or incontinence
Administer:
• Only with atropine sulfate available for cholinergic crisis
• Only after all other cholinergics have been discontinued
• Increased doses if tolerance occurs
• With food or milk to decrease GI symptoms
• On empty stomach for better absorption
Perform/provide:
• Storage at room temperature
Evaluate:
• Therapeutic response: LOC—alert
• Bradycardia, hypotension, bronchospasm, headache, dizziness, convulsions, respiratory depression; drug should be discontinued if toxicity occurs
Teach patient/family:
• All aspects of drug: action, side effects, dose, when to notify physician

phytonadione (vitamin K₁)

(fye-toe-na-dye'one)
AquaMEPHYTON, Konakion, Mephyton

Func. class.: Vitamin K₁, fat-soluble vitamin

Action: Needed for adequate blood clotting (factors II, VII, IX, X)
Uses: Vitamin K malabsorption, hypoprothrombinemia, prevention of hypoprothrombinemia caused by oral anticoagulants

Dosage and routes:
Hypoprothrombinemia caused by vitamin K malabsorption
• *Adult:* PO/IM 2-25 mg may repeat or increase to 50 mg
• *Child:* PO/IM 5-10 mg
• *Infants:* PO/IM 2 mg
Hypoprothrombinemia caused by oral anticoagulants
• *Adult:* PO/SC/IM 2.5-10 mg, may repeat 12-48 hr after PO dose or 6-8 hr after SC/IM dose, based on PT
Available forms include: Tabs 5 mg; inj aqueous colloidal IM, IV; inj aqueous dispersion 2, 10 mg/ml, IM only
Side effects/adverse reactions:
CNS: Headache, ***brain damage*** (large doses)
GI: Nausea, decrease liver function tests
*HEMA: **Hemolytic anemia, hemoglobinuria, hyperbilirubinemia***
INTEG: Rash, urticaria
Contraindications: Hypersensitivity, severe hepatic disease, last few weeks of pregnancy, neonates
Pharmacokinetics:
PO/INJ: Metabolized, crosses placenta
Interactions/incompatibilities:
• Decreased action of this drug: antibiotics, cholestyramine, mineral oil
• Decreased action of: oral anticoagulants
NURSING CONSIDERATIONS
Assess:
• Pro-time during treatment (2 sec deviation from control time, bleeding time, and clotting time)
Administer:
• IV only when other routes not possible (deaths have occurred)
Evaluate:
• Therapeutic response: decreased bleeding tendencies, decreased pro-time, decreased clotting time
• Nutritional status: liver (beef), spinach, tomatoes, coffee, asparagus, broccoli, cabbage, lettuce, greens
Teach patient/family
• Not to take other supplements, unless directed by physician
• Necessary foods to be included in diet

pilocarpine HCl/pilocarpine nitrate

(pye-loe-kar'peen)
Adsorbocarpine, Akarpine, Almocarpine, Isopto Carpine, Miocarpine,* Ocusert Pilo, Pilocar, Pilocel, Pilomiotin, P.V. Carpine Liquifilm
Func. class.: Miotic, direct-acting
Chem. class.: Cholinergic agonist

Action: Directly acts on cholinergic receptor sites, induces miosis, spasm of accommodation, fall in intraocular pressure, caused by stimulation of ciliary, pupillary sphincter muscles that cause pulling away of iris from filtration angle, causing outflow of aqueous humor
Uses: Primary glaucoma, early stages of wide-angle glaucoma (less useful in advanced stages), chronic open-angle glaucoma, acute narrow-angle glaucoma before emergency surgery; also used to neutralize mydriatics used during eye exam; may be used alternately with mydriatics to break adhesions between iris and lens
Dosage and routes:
• *Adult and child:* INSTILL SOL 1-2 gtts of 1% or 2% solution in eye q6-8h; INSTILL 20-40 μg/hr (Ocusert) in cul-de-sac of eye
Available forms include: 0.25% to 10% sol; Ocusert Pilo 20, Ocusert Pilo, 40
Side effects/adverse reactions:
CV: Hypotension, tachycardia
*RESP: **Bronchospasm***

GI: Nausea, vomiting, abdominal cramps, diarrhea

EENT: Blurred vision, browache, twitching of eyelids, eye pain with change in focus

Contraindications: Bradycardia, hyperthyroidism, coronary artery disease, obstruction of GI/urinary tracts (or if strength of walls of these structures in question, peptic ulcers), epilepsy, parkinsonism, asthma, pregnancy

Precautions: Bronchial asthma, hypertension

Interactions/incompatibilities: None known

NURSING CONSIDERATIONS
Assess:

• Heart rate, respiratory status, B/P

• Replacement of ocular systems q wk; check system each hs, AM

Administer:

• After shaking vial to mix drug to clear solution, push stopper to mix sterile water with powder

• After cleaning stopper with alcohol

• Excess solution must be wiped away promptly to prevent its flow into lacrimal system, production systemic symptoms

• Atropine should be readily available as antidote

• Immediately after reconstituting; discard unused portion

Perform/provide:

• Protect solution from light

• Store Ocusert systems between 2° and 8° C

Teach patient/family:

• To report change in vision, blurring or loss of sight, trouble breathing, sweating, flushing

• Method of instillation, including pressure on lacrimal sac for 1 min, not to touch dropper to eye

• That long-term therapy may be required

• That blurred vision will decrease

with repeated use of drug

• To discontinue use if local hypersensitivity reaction occurs

• That acuity in dim light will be reduced

• Not to drive while using drug

---

pimozide
(pi'moe-zide)
Orap

Func. class.: Antipsychotic/neuroleptic

Chem. class.: Diphenylbutylpiperidine

Action: Depresses cerebral cortex, hypothalamus, limbic system, which control activity, aggression; blocks neurotransmission produced by dopamine at synapse by blocking CNS dopamine receptors

Uses: Tics in Tourette's disorder

Dosage and routes:

• *Adult and child >12 yr:* PO 1-2 mg qd in divided doses; increase dose qod if needed; maintenance <0.2 mg/kg/day or 10 mg/day, whichever is less, not to exceed 0.3 mg/kg/day or 20 mg/day

Available forms include: Tabs 2, 4, 10 mg

Side effects/adverse reactions:

RESP: ***Laryngospasm,*** dyspnea, ***respiratory depression***

CNS: Extrapyramidal symptoms: pseudoparkinsonism, akathisia, dystonia, tardive dyskinesia, drowsiness, headache, seizures

HEMA: Anemia, leukopenia, leukocytosis, ***agranulocytosis***

INTEG: Rash, photosensitivity, dermatitis, hyperpyrexia

EENT: Blurred vision, cataracts

GI: Dry mouth, nausea, vomiting, anorexia, constipation, diarrhea, jaundice, weight gain

GU: Urinary retention, urinary frequency, enuresis, impotence, amenorrhea, gynecomastia

CV: Orthostatic hypotension, hypertension, *cardiac arrest,* ECG changes, *tachycardia*

Contraindications: Hypersensitivity, CNS depression/coma, parkinsonism, liver disease, blood dyscrasias, renal disease, tics other than Tourette's disorder, cardiac dysrhythmias

Precautions: Child <12 yr, pregnancy (C), lactation, seizure disorders, hypertension, hepatic disease, cardiac disease, renal disease

Pharmacokinetics:

PO: Onset erratic, peak 6-8 hr; metabolized by liver, excreted in urine, half-life 50-55 hr

Interactions/incompatibilities:

• Decreased convulsive threshold: anticonvulsants

• Increased CNS depression: analgesics, sedatives, anxiolytics, alcohol

• Increased QT interval: phenothiazines, tricyclics, antidysrhythmics

NURSING CONSIDERATIONS

Assess:

• For prolonged QT interval

• Those taking anticonvulsants for increased seizure activity

• Swallowing of PO medication; check for hoarding or giving of medication to other patients

• I&O ratio; palpate bladder if low urinary output occurs

• Bilirubin, CBC, liver function studies monthly

• Urinalysis is recommended before and during prolonged therapy

Administer:

• Antiparkinsonian agent, after securing order from physician to be used if EPS occur

Perform/provide:

• Supervised ambulation until stabilized on medication; do not involve in strenuous exercise program because fainting is possible; patient should not stand still for long periods of time

• Increased fluids to prevent constipation

• Sips of water, candy, gum for dry mouth

• Storage in tight, light-resistant container

Evaluate:

• Therapeutic response: decrease in tics

• Affect, orientation, LOC, reflexes, gait, coordination, sleep pattern disturbances

• B/P standing and lying; also include pulse, respirations q4h during initial treatment; establish baseline before starting treatment; report drops of 30 mm Hg

• Dizziness, faintness, palpitations, tachycardia on rising

• EPS including akathisia (inability to sit still, no pattern to movements), tardive dyskinesia (bizarre movements of the jaw, mouth, tongue, extremities), pseudoparkinsonism (rigidity, tremors, pill rolling, shuffling gait)

• Skin turgor daily

• Constipation, urinary retention daily; if these occur increase bulk, water in diet

Teach patient/family:

• That tardive dyskinesia may develop with chronic use

• Not to exceed prescribed dose

• That orthostatic hypotension may occur and to rise from sitting or lying position gradually

• To avoid hot tubs, hot showers, or tub baths since hypotension may occur

• To avoid abrupt withdrawal of this drug or EPS may result; drugs should be withdrawn slowly

• To avoid OTC preparations (cough, hayfever, cold) unless approved by physician since serious drug interactions may occur; avoid use with alcohol or CNS depressants, increased drowsiness may occur

---

italics = common side effects   ***bold italic*** = life threatening reactions

• To avoid hazardous activities if drowsiness or dizziness occurs

• To use a sunscreen during sun exposure to prevent burns

• Regarding compliance with drug regimen

• About necessity for meticulous oral hygiene since oral candidiasis may occur

• To report impaired vision, jaundice, tremors, muscle twitching

• In hot weather, heat stroke may occur; take extra precautions to stay cool

Treatment of overdose: Lavage if orally injested; provide an airway; monitor ECG; *do not induce vomiting*

---

pindolol

(pin'doe-lole)
Visken

Func. class.: Antihypertensive
Chem. class.: Nonselective β-blocker

Action: Competitively blocks stimulation of β-adrenergic receptor within vascular smooth muscle; produces chronotropic, inotropic activity (decreases rate of SA node discharge, increases recovery time), slows conduction of AV node, decreases heart rate, which decreases O_2 consumption in myocardium; also, decreases renin-aldosterone-angiotensin system, at high doses inhibits β-2 receptors in bronchial system

Uses: Mild to moderate hypertension

Dosage and routes:

• *Adult:* PO 5 mg bid, usual dose 15 mg/day (5 mg tid), may increase by 10 mg/day q3-4 wk to a max of 60 mg/day

Available forms include: Tabs 5, 10, 20 mg

Side effects/adverse reactions:

CV: Hypotension, bradycardia, CHF, edema, chest pain, palpitation, claudication, tachycardia, *AV block*

CNS: Insomnia, dizziness, hallucinations, anxiety, fatigue

GI: Nausea, vomiting, *ischemic colitis,* diarrhea, *abdominal pain, mesenteric arterial thrombosis*

INTEG: Rash, alopecia, pruritus, fever

HEMA: Agranulocytosis, thrombocytopenia, purpura

EENT: Visual changes, sore throat, *double vision,* dry burning eyes

GU: Impotence, frequency

RESP: Bronchospasm, dyspnea, cough, rales

MUSC: Joint pain, muscle pain

Contraindications: Hypersensitivity to β-blockers, cardiogenic shock, heart block (2nd, 3rd degree), sinus bradycardia, CHF, cardiac failure, bronchial asthma

Precautions: Major surgery, pregnancy (B), lactation, diabetes mellitus, renal disease, thyroid disease, COPD, well compensated heart failure, CAD, nonallergic bronchospasm

Pharmacokinetics:

PO: Peak 2-4 hr; half-life 3-4 hr, excreted 30%-45% unchanged, 60%-65% is metabolized by liver, excreted in breast milk

Interactions/incompatibilities:

• Increased hypotension, bradycardia: reserpine, hydralazine, methyldopa, prazosin, anticholinergics

• Decreased antihypertensive effects: indomethacin, sympathomimetics

• Increased hypoglycemic effect: insulin

• Decreased bronchodilation: theophyllines

NURSING CONSIDERATIONS

Assess:

• I&O, weight daily

- B/P, pulse q4h; note rate, rhythm, quality
- Apical/radial pulse before administration; notify physician of any significant changes
- Baselines in renal, liver function tests before therapy begins

Administer:
- PO ac, hs, tablet may be crushed or swallowed whole
- Reduced dosage in renal dysfunction

Perform/provide:
- Storage in dry area at room temperature, do not freeze

Evaluate:
- Therapeutic response: decreased B/P after 1-2 wk
- Edema in feet, legs daily
- Skin turgor, dryness of mucous membranes for hydration status

Teach patient/family:
- Take with or immediately after meals
- Not to discontinue drug abruptly, taper over 2 wk, may cause precipitate angina
- Not to use OTC products containing α-adrenergic stimulants (nasal decongestants, OTC cold preparations) unless directed by physician
- To report bradycardia, dizziness, confusion, depression, fever, sore throat, shortness of breath to physician
- To take pulse at home, advise when to notify physician
- To avoid alcohol, smoking, sodium intake
- To comply with weight control, dietary adjustments, modified exercise program
- To carry Medic Alert ID to identify drug you are taking, allergies
- To avoid hazardous activities if dizziness if present
- To report symptoms of CHF: difficult breathing, especially on exertion or when lying down, night cough, swelling of extremities
- Take medication at bedtime to maintain effect of orthostatic hypotension
- Wear support hose to minimize effects of orthostatic hypotension

Lab test interferences:
Increase: Liver function tests, renal function tests

Treatment of overdose: Lavage, IV atropine for bradycardia, IV theophylline for bronchospasm, digitalis, O_2, diuretic for cardiac failure, hemodialysis, hypotension; administer vasopressor (norepinephrine)

---

piperacillin sodium

(pi-per'a-sill-in)
Pipracil*

Func. class.: Broad-spectrum antibiotic
Chem. class.: Extended-spectrum penicillin

Action: Interferes with cell wall replication of susceptible organisms; osmotically unstable cell wall swells and bursts from osmotic pressure

Uses: Respiratory, skin, urinary tract, bone infections, gonorrhea, pneumonia; effective for gram-positive cocci *(S. aureus, S. pyogenes, S. viridans, S. faecalis, S. bovis, S. pneumoniae),* gram-negative cocci *(N. gonorrhoeae, N. meningitidis),* gram-positive bacilli, *C. perfringens, C. tetani,* gram-negative bacilli *(bacteroides, F. nucleatum, E. coli, Klebsiella, P. mirabilis, M. morganii, P. vulgaris, P. rehgesii, Enterobacter, Citrobacter, Bendomonas, P. aeruginosa, Serratia, Acinetobacter, Peptococcus, Peptostreptococcus, Eubacterium)*

Dosage and routes:
Systemic infections

• *Adult and child >12 yr:* IM/IV 100-300 mg/kg in divided doses q4-6h

Prophylaxis of surgical infections
• *Adult:* IV 2g ½-1 hr before procedure, may be repeated during surgery or after surgery

Available forms include: Inj IM, IV 2, 3, 4, 40 g; IV INF 2, 3, 4 g

Side effects/adverse reactions:
HEMA: Anemia, increased bleeding time, *bone marrow depression*
GI: Nausea, vomiting, diarrhea, increased AST, ALT, abdominal pain, glossitis, colitis
GU: Oliguria, proteinuria, hematuria, *vaginitis, moniliasis, glomerulonephritis*
CNS: Lethargy, hallucinations, anxiety, depression, twitching, *coma, convulsions*
META: Hypokalemia

Contraindications: Hypersensitivity to penicillins; neonates
Precautions: Pregnancy (B), hypersensitivity to cephalosporins

Pharmacokinetics:
IM: Peak 30-50 min
IV: Peak 20-30 min
Half-life 0.7-1.33 hr, 0.6-1.35 hr terminal, excreted in urine, bile, breast milk, crosses placenta

Interactions/incompatibilities:
• Decreased antimicrobial effect of this drug: tetracyclines, erythromycins, aminoglycosides IV
• Increased penicillin concentrations: aspirin, probenecid

NURSING CONSIDERATIONS
Assess:
• I&O ratio; report hematuria, oliguria since penicillin in high doses is nephrotoxic
• Any patient with compromised renal system since drug is excreted slowly in poor renal system function; toxicity may occur rapidly
• Liver studies: AST, ALT
• Blood studies: WBC, RBC,

H&H, bleeding time
• Renal studies: urinalysis, protein, blood
• C&S before drug therapy; drug may be taken as soon as culture is taken

Administer:
• Drug after C&S has been completed

Perform/provide:
• Adrenalin, suction, tracheostomy set, endotracheal intubation equipment on unit
• Adequate intake of fluids (2000 ml) during diarrhea episodes
• Scratch test to assess allergy, after securing order from physician; usually done when penicillin is only drug of choice
• Storage at room temperature, reconstituted solution for 24 hr or 7 days refrigerated

Evaluate:
• Therapeutic response: absence of fever, purulent drainage, redness, inflammation
• Bowel pattern before and during treatment
• Skin eruptions after administration of penicillin to 1 wk after discontinuing drug
• Respiratory status: rate, character, wheezing, tightness in chest
• Allergies before initiation of treatment, reaction of each medication; highlight allergies on chart, Kardex

Teach patient/family:
• Culture may be taken after completed course of medication
• To report sore throat, fever, fatigue; could indicate superimposed infection
• To wear or carry Medic Alert ID if allergic to penicillins
• To notify nurse of diarrhea stools
Lab test interferences:
Decrease: Uric acid
False positive: Urine glucose,

urine protein, Coombs'
Treatment of overdose:
Withdraw drug, maintain airway, administer epinephrine, aminophylline, O_2, IV corticosteroids for anaphylaxis

piperazine adipate/ piperazine citrate

(pi′per-a-zeen)

Entacly,* Antepar, Bryrol, Entacyl, Pin-Tega Tabs, Ta-Verm, Vergia,* Vermizine, Vermirex*

Func. class.: Anthelmintic

Action: Causes paralysis in worm, leading to expulsion
Uses: Pinworm, roundworm
Dosage and routes:
Pinworm
• *Adult and child:* PO 65 mg/kg × 7-8 days, not to exceed 2.5 g/day
Roundworm
• *Adult:* PO 3.5 g in single dose × 2 days
• *Child:* PO 75 mg/kg/day in a single dose × 2 days
Available forms include: Tabs 250, 500 mg; syr 500 mg/5ml; powder, oral sol 500 mg
Side effects/adverse reactions:
HEMA: Hemolytic anemia
INTEG: Rash, uriticaria, photosensitivity
RESP: Bronchospasm
CNS: Dizziness, headache, paresthesia, convulsions, fever
EENT: Blurred vision, nystagmus, strabismus, cataracts, rhinorrhea
GI: Nausea, vomiting, anorexia, diarrhea, abdominal cramps
Contraindications: Hypersensitivity, renal disease, hepatic disease, seizures
Precautions: Severe malnutrition, seizure disorders, anemia, pregnancy
Pharmacokinetics:
PO: Excreted in urine (unchanged)

Interactions/incompatibilities:
• May increase extrapyramidal symptoms when used with phenothiazines
NURSING CONSIDERATIONS
Assess:
• Stools during entire treatment, 1, 3 mo after treatment; specimens must be sent to lab while still warm
Administer:
• May be crushed or chewed if unable to swallow whole
• Laxatives if constipated; not needed for drug to work
• Second course after 1 wk off drug, if infection is severe
Perform/provide:
• Storage in tight container at room temperature
Evaluate:
• Therapeutic response: expulsion of worms, 3 negative stool cultures after completion of treatment
• For allergic reaction: rash, itching, urticaria
• For infection in other family members since infection from person to person is common
Teach patient/family:
• Proper hygiene after BM including handwashing technique, tell patient to avoid putting fingers in mouth
• That infected person should sleep alone; do not shake bed linen, change bed linen daily, wash in hot water
• To clean toilet qd with disinfectant (green soap solution)
• Need for compliance with dosage schedule and duration of treatment
• That urine may turn orange or red
• To avoid hazardous activities since drowsiness occurs
• That seizures may recur in patient who is controlled on medication
Lab test interferences:
Decrease: Serum uric acid

P

pipobroman

(pi-poe-brow'man)
Vercyte

Func. class.: Antineoplastic alkylating agent
Chem. class.: Dicarboxylic acid

Action: Alkylates DNA, RNA; inhibits enzymes that allow synthesis of amino acids in proteins; also responsible for cross-linking DNA strands

Uses: Chronic granulocytic leukemia, polycythemia vera

Dosage and routes:
Chronic myelocytic leukemia
• *Adult:* PO 1.5-2.5 mg/kg/day until WBCs drop to 10,000/mm³, then 7-175 mg/day; do not administer if WBCs <3000/mm³ or platelets <150,000/mm³

Polycythemia vera
• *Adult:* PO 1 mg/kg/day × 1 mo, then 1.5-3 mg/kg/day until Hct is 50% to 55%, then 0.1-0.2 mg/kg/day

Available forms include: Tabs 25 mg

Side effects/adverse reactions:
*HEMA: **Thrombocytopenia,** anemia*
GI: Nausea, vomiting, diarrhea, abdominal cramping
INTEG: Rash

Contraindications: Hypersensitivity, bone marrow depression

Precautions: Radiation therapy, children <15 yr, pregnancy (1st trimester)

Pharmacokinetics:
Unknown

Interactions/incompatibilities:
None known

NURSING CONSIDERATIONS

Assess:
• CBC, differential, platelet count weekly; withhold drug if WBC is <4000 or platelet count is <75,000; notify physician of results
• Monitor temperature q4h (may indicate beginning infection)
• Liver function tests before, during therapy (bilirubin, AST, ALT, LDH) as needed or monthly

Administer:
• Medications by oral route if possible; avoid IM, SC, IV routes to prevent infections
• Antacid before oral agent; give drug after evening meal, before bedtime
• Antiemetic 30-60 min before giving drug to prevent vomiting
• Antibiotics for prophylaxis of infection
• Local or systemic drugs for infection

Perform/provide:
• Storage in tight container
• Strict medical asepsis, protective isolation if WBC levels are low
• Special skin care
• Liquid diet, including cola, Jello; dry toast or crackers may be added if patient is not nauseated or vomiting

Evaluate:
• Bleeding: hematuria, guaiac, bruising or petechiae, mucosa or orifices q8h
• Food preferences; list likes, dislikes
• Symptoms indicating severe allergic reaction: rash, urticaria, itching

Teach patient/family:
• Of protective isolation precautions
• To report any complaints or side effects to nurse or physician

piroxicam

(peer-ox′i-kam)
Feldene

Func. class.: Nonsteroidal
Chem. class.: Oxicam derivative

Action: Inhibits prostaglandin synthesis by decreasing an enzyme needed for biosynthesis; possesses analgesic, antiinflammatory, antipyretic properties

Uses: Mild to moderate pain, osteoarthritis, rheumatoid arthritis

Dosage and routes:
• *Adult:* PO 20 qd or 10 mg bid
Available forms include: Caps 10, 20 mg

Side effects/adverse reactions:
GI: Nausea, anorexia, vomiting, diarrhea, jaundice, *cholestatic hepatitis,* constipation, flatulence, cramps, dry mouth, peptic ulcer
CNS: Dizziness, drowsiness, fatigue, tremors, confusion, insomnia, anxiety, depression
CV: Tachycardia, peripheral edema, palpitations, dysrhythmias
INTEG: Purpura, rash, pruritus, sweating
GU: Nephrotoxicity: dysuria, hematuria, oliguria, azotemia
HEMA: Blood dyscrasias
EENT: Tinnitus, hearing loss, blurred vision

Contraindications: Hypersensitivity, asthma, severe renal disease, severe hepatic disease

Precautions: Pregnancy, lactation, children, bleeding disorders, GI disorders, cardiac disorders, hypersensitivity to other antiinflammatory agents

Pharmacokinetics:
PO: Peak 2 hr, half-life 3-3½ hr; metabolized in liver, excreted in urine (metabolites) excreted in breast milk

Interactions/incompatibilities:
• May increase action of coumarin, phenytoin, sulfonamides when used with this drug

NURSING CONSIDERATIONS
Assess:
• Renal, liver, blood studies: BUN, creatinine, AST, ALT, Hgb, before treatment, periodically thereafter
• Audiometric, ophthalmic exam before, during, after treatment

Administer:
• With food to decrease GI symptoms; best to take on empty stomach to facilitate absorption

Perform/provide:
• Storage at room temperature

Evaluate:
• Therapeutic response: decreased pain, stiffness, swelling in joints, ability to move more easily
• For eye, ear problems: blurred vision, tinnitus (may indicate toxicity)

Teach patient/family:
• To report blurred vision or ringing, roaring in ears (may indicate toxicity)
• To avoid driving or other hazardous activities if dizziness or drowsiness occurs
• To report change in urine pattern, weight increase, edema, pain increase in joints, fever, blood in urine (indicates nephrotoxicity)
• That therapeutic effects may take up to 1 mo

plasma protein fraction

Plasmanate, Plasma Plex, Plasmatein, PPF Protenate

Func. class.: Blood derivative
Chem. class.: Human plasma in NaCl

Action: Exerts similar oncotic pressure as human plasma, expands blood volume
Uses: Shock, hypoproteinemia

P

Dosage and routes:
Shock
• *Adult:* IV INF 250-500 ml (12.5-25 g protein), not to exceed 10 ml/min
• *Child:* IV INF 22-33 ml/kg at 5-10 ml/min
Hypoproteinemia
• *Adult:* IV INF 1000-1500 ml qd, not to exceed 8 ml/min
Available forms include: Inj IV 50 mg/ml

Side effects/adverse reactions:
GI: Nausea, vomiting, increased salivation
INTEG: Rash, urticaria, cyanosis
CNS: Fever, chills, headache, paresthesias, flushing
RESP: Altered respirations, dyspnea
CV: Fluid overload, hypotension, erratic pulse
Contraindications: Hypersensitivity, congestive heart failure, severe anemia
Precautions: Decreased salt intake, decreased cardiac reserve, lack of albumin deficiency, hepatic disease, renal disease
Pharmacokinetics:
Metabolized as a protein/energy source
Interactions/incompatibilities:
• Incompatibile with solution with alcohol or norephinephrine
NURSING CONSIDERATIONS
Assess:
• Blood studies: Hct, Hgb; if serum declines, dyspnea, hypoxemia can result
• B/P (decreased) pulse (erratic), respiration
• I&O ratio; urinary output may decrease
• CVP, pulmonary wedge pressure (increases if overload occurs)
Administer:
• IV slowly, prevent fluid overload, dilute with NS for inj or D_5W; may be given undiluted, use infusion pump
• Within 4 hr of opening
Perform/provide:
• Adequate hydration before administration
• Storage—check type of albumin; may need to refrigerate
Evaluate:
• Therapeutic repsonse: increased B/P, decrease edema, increased serum albumin
• Allergy: fever, rash, itching, chills, flushing, urticaria, nausea, vomiting, or hypotension requires discontinuation of infusion; use new lot if therapy reinstituted
• Increased CVP reading: distended neck veins indicate circulatory overload; SOB, anxiety, insomnia, expiratory rales, frothy blood-tinged cough, cyanosis indicate pulmonary overload
Lab test interferences:
False increase: Alk phosphatase

---

plicamycin (mithramycin)
(plik-a-mi′cin)
Mithracin
Func. class.: Antineoplastic, antibiotic
Chem. class.: Crystalline aglycone

Action: Inhibits DNA, RNA, protein synthesis; derived from *Streptomyces plicatus;* replication is decreased by binding to DNA; demonstrates calcium-lowering effect not related to its tumoricidal activity; also acts on osteoclasts and blocks action of parathyroid hormone
Uses: Testicular cancer, hypercalcemia, hypercalciuria, symptomatic treatment of advanced neoplasms
Dosage and routes:
Testicular tumors

• *Adult:* IV 25-30 μg/kg/day × 8-10 days, not to exceed 30 μg/kg/day

Hypercalcemia/hypercalciuria

• *Adult:* IV 25 μg/kg/day × 3-4 days, repeat at intervals of 1 wk

Available forms include: Inj IV 2.5 mg

Side effects/adverse reactions:

META: Decreased serum calcium, phosphorous, potassium

HEMA: **Hemorrhage, thrombocytopenia,** decreased pro-time, WBC count

GI: Nausea, vomiting, anorexia, diarrhea, stomatitis, increased liver enzymes

GU: Increased BUN, creatinine, *proteinuria*

INTEG: Rash, cellulitis, local irritation at injection site

CNS: Drowsiness, weakness, lethargy, headache, flushing, fever, depression

Contraindications: Hypersensitivity, thrombocytopenia, bone marrow depression, bleeding disorders, pregnancy (X)

Precautions: Renal disease, hepatic disease, electrolyte imbalances

Pharmacokinetics: Crosses blood-brain barrier, excreted in urine; little known about pharmacokinetics

Interactions/incompatibilities:

• Increased toxicity: other antineoplastics or radiation

NURSING CONSIDERATIONS

Assess:

• CBC, differential, platelet count weekly; withhold drug if WBC is <4000/mm³ or platelet count is <50,000/mm³; notify physician of results

• Renal function studies: BUN, serum uric acid, urine CrCl, electrolytes before, during therapy

• I&O ratio; report fall in urine output to <30 ml/hr

• Monitor temperature q4h; fever may indicate beginning infection

• Liver function tests before, during therapy: bilirubin, AST, ALT, alk phosphatase prn or monthly

Administer:

• Medications by oral route if possible; avoid IM, SC, IV routes to prevent infections

• Antiemetic 30-60 min before giving drug to prevent vomiting

• Antibiotics for prophylaxis of infection

• Slow IV infusion using 21-, 23-, 25-gauge needle; check for extravasation

• Topical or systemic analgesics for pain

• Transfusion for anemia

• Antispasmodic for GI symptoms

Perform/provide:

• Strict medical asepsis, protective isolation if WBC levels are low

• Liquid diet: carbonated beverages, Jello; dry toast, crackers may be added if patient is not nauseated or vomiting

• Rinsing of mouth tid-qid with water and hydrogen peroxide; brushing of teeth bid-tid with soft brush or cotton-tipped applicators for stomatitis; use unwaxed dental floss

• Warm compresses at injection site for inflammation; check for extravasation

• Usage immediately after mixing

Evaluate:

• Toxicity: facial flushing, epistaxis, increased pro-time, thrombocytopenia; drug should be discontinued

• Bleeding: hematuria, guaiac, bruising or petechiae, mucosa or orifices q8h

• Food preferences; list likes, dislikes

• Inflammation of mucosa, breaks in skin

• Yellowing of skin, sclera, dark urine, clay-colored stools, itchy

P

---

skin, abdominal pain, fever, diarrhea
• Buccal cavity q8h for dryness, sores, ulceration, white patches, oral pain, bleeding, dysphagia
• Local irritation, pain, burning at injection site
• Frequency of stools, characteristics, cramping
• Acidosis, signs of dehydration: rapid respirations, poor skin turgor, decreased urine output, dry skin, restlessness, weakness

Teach patient/family:
• Why protective isolation precautions are necessary
• To report any complaints or side effects to nurse or physician
• To avoid foods with citric acid, hot or rough texture
• To report to physician any bleeding, white spots, ulcerations in the mouth; tell patient to examine mouth qd
• To avoid driving or activities requiring alertness; drowsiness may occur
• To report leg cramps, tingling of fingertips, weakness; may indicate hypokalemia

---

podophyllum resin
(poe-doe-fil′ um)
Podoben

Func. class.: Keratolytic
Chem. class.: Podophyllum derivative

Action: Arrests mitosis by binding to tubulin, protein subunit of spindle microtubules; also interferes with movements of chromosomes

Uses: Venereal warts, keratoses, multiple superficial, epitheliomatoses

Dosage and routes:
Warts
• *Adult:* TOP cover wart, cover with wax paper, bandage for 4-6 hr,

wash, may repeat q wk if needed
Keratoses/epitheliomatoses
• *Adult:* TOP apply qd with applicator, let dry, remove tissue, may reapply if needed

Available forms include: Sol 11.5%, 25%

Side effects/adverse reactions:
HEMA: Thrombocytopenia, leukopenia
INTEG: Irritation of unaffected areas
CNS: Peripheral neuropathy

Contraindications: Hypersensitivity, pregnancy (X)

Interactions/incompatibilities:
• Necrosis of skin: when used with other keratolytic

NURSING CONSIDERATIONS
Assess:
• Platelets, WBC if systemic absorption occurs

Administer:
• Only to affected area, cover normal skin with petrolatum for protection
• Only to small areas or for short periods of time or absorption (systemic) may occur

Evaluate:
• Therapeutic response: decrease in size and amount of lesions
• Allergic reactions: irritation, redness, itching, stinging, burning; drug should be discontinued
• Blood dyscrasias if systemic absorption is suspected: decrease platelets
• CNS toxicity: peripheral neuropathy; drug should be discontinued

Teach patient/family:
• That discomfort will begin after 24 hr, subside in 2-4 days

---

poliovirus vaccine, live, oral, trivalent

Orimune

Func. class.: Vaccine

Action: Produces specific antibodies for poliomyelitis

Uses: Prevention of polio

Dosage and routes:

• *Adult and child >2 yr:* PO 0.5 ml, given q8 wk × 2 doses, then 0.5 ml ½-1 yr after dose 2

• *Infant:* PO 0.5 ml at 2, 4, 18 mo

Available forms include: Oral vaccine

Side effects/adverse reactions:

SYST: Paralysis

Contraindications: Hypersensitivity, active infection, allergy to neomycin/streptomycin, immunosuppression

Precautions: Pregnancy

Interactions/incompatibilities:

• Do not use TB skin test within 6 wk of vaccine

• Do not use within 3 mo of transfusion of whole blood, plasma, or use with immune serum globulin

NURSING CONSIDERATIONS

Administer:

• Only PO

Evaluate:

• For history of allergies, skin conditions (eczema, psoriasis, dermatitis), reactions to vaccinations

• For anaphylaxis: inability to breathe, bronchospasm

polymyxin B sulfate

(pol-i-mix'in)

Aerosporin

Func. class.: Antibacterial

Chem. class.: Polymyxin

Action: Interferes with phospholipids, penetrates cell wall; changes occur immediately in bacterial membrane causing leakage of essential metabolites

Uses: Serious *P. aeruginosa, E. aerogenes, K. pneumoniae, E. coli, H. influenzae* infections or when other antibiotics cannot be used

Dosage and routes:

• *Adult and child:* IV INF 15,000-25,000 U/kg/day in divided doses q12h, or 25,000-30,000 U/kg/day in divided doses q4-8h

P. aeruginosa/H. influenzae

• *Adult and child >2 yr:* INTRATHECAL 50,000 U/day × 3-4 days, then 50,000 U/qod × 2 wk after CSF negative, glucose normal

• *Child <2 yr:* INTRATHECAL 20,000 U/day × 3-4 days, then 25,000 U qod × 2 wk after CSF negative

Available forms include: Inj IV, intrathecal, 500,000 U

Side effects/adverse reactions:

INTEG: Urticaria

CNS: Dizziness, confusion, weakness, drowsiness, paresthesia, slurred speech, *coma, seizures,* headache, stiff neck

RESP: Paralysis

GU: Proteinuria, hematuria, azotemia, leukocyturia

EENT: Blurred vision

SYST: Anaphylaxis

Contraindications: Hypersensitivity, severe renal disease

Precautions: Pregnancy

Pharmacokinetics:

IM: Peak 2 hr, half-life 4½-6 hr, excreted in urine unchanged (60%)

IV: Data not available

Interactions/incompatibilities:

• Increased skeletal muscle relaxation: anesthetics, neuromuscular blockers (tubocurarine decamethonium, succinylcholine, gallamine)

• Increased nephrotoxicity, neurotoxicity: aminoglycosides, sodium

P

citrate, parenteral quinine, parenteral quinidine, polypeptides, antibiotics

• Do not mix in solution or syringe with cephalothin sodium, chloramphenicol sodium succinate, chlorothiazide, heparin, penicillins, tetracyclines, cobalt, magnesium, iron, amphotericin B, nitrofurantoin, prednisolone

NURSING CONSIDERATIONS
Assess:

• I&O ratio; report hematuria, oliguria

• Any patient with compromised renal system; drug is excreted slowly in poor renal system function; toxicity may occur rapidly; monitor BUN, creatinine

• Renal studies: urinalysis, protein, blood

• C&S before drug therapy; drug may be taken as soon as culture is taken; C&S may be done after completion of therapy

Administer:

• IV after reconstituting with 300-500 ml D₅W given over 60-90 min

Perform/provide:

• Intrathecal after reconstituting with 10 ml NS to yield 50,000 U/ml

• Storage in dark area at room temperature

• Do not use procaine HCl in intrathecal injection

• Adrenalin, suction, tracheostomy set, endotracheal intubation equipment on unit

• Adequate intake of fluids (2000 ml) during diarrhea episodes

Evaluate:

• Therapeutic response: absence of fever, purulent drainage, C&S negative

• Skin eruptions, itching; drug should be discontinued

• Respiratory status: rate, character, dyspnea, symptoms of neuromuscular blockade, tightness in chest; discontinue drug if these occur

• Allergies before initiation of treatment, reaction of each medication; place allergies on chart, Kardex in bright red letters; notify all people giving drugs

• For flushing of face, dizziness, disorientation, weakness, paresthesia, blurred vision, slurred speech, restlessness, irritability; indicate neurotoxicity

• For headache, fever, stiff neck; after intrathecal administration, indicate meningeal irritation

Teach patient/family:

• To report sore throat, fever, fatigue; could indicate superimposed infection

Treatment of overdose: Withdraw drug, maintain airway, administer epinephrine, aminophylline, O₂, IV corticosteroids

---

polymyxin B sulfate
(pol-i-mix′in)

Func. class.: Otic
Chem. class.: Antibiotic

Action: Inhibits protein synthesis in susceptible microorganisms
Uses: Acute, chronic otitis externa, otitis media if eardrum is perforated, otomycosis
Dosage and routes:
• *Adult and child:* INSTILL 3-4 gtts tid-qid
Available forms include: Otic sol 10,000 U, usually in combination with hydrocortisone
Side effects/adverse reactions:
EENT: Itching, irritation in ear
INTEG: Rash, urticaria
Contraindications: Hypersensitivity, perforated eardrum
Pharmacokinetics: Not known
Interactions/incompatibilities: None known

NURSING CONSIDERATIONS
Administer:

• After removing impacted cerumen by irrigation

• After cleaning stopper with alcohol

• After restraining child if necessary

• Warming solution to body temperature

Evaluate:

• Therapeutic response: decreased ear pain

• For redness, swelling, pain in ear, which indicates superimposed infection

Teach patient/family:

• Method of instillation using aseptic technique, including not touching dropper to ear

• That dizziness may occur after instillation

---

polymyxin B sulfate (ophthalmic)

(pol-ee-mix'in)

Mycitracin Ophthalmic, Neosporin Ophthalmic, Neotal, Ocumycin

Func. class.: Antiinfective (ophthalmic)

Action: Inhibits bacterial cell wall in organism by preventing amino acids and nucleotides into cell wall

Uses: Infection of eye

Dosage and routes:

• *Adult and child:* INSTILL 1-2 gtts q1h

Available forms include: Only available in combination with bacitracin, neomycin, oxytetracycline

Side effects/adverse reactions:

EENT: Poor corneal wound healing, temporary visual haze, overgrowth of nonsusceptible organisms

Contraindications: Hypersensitivity

Precautions: Antibiotic hypersensitivity

Interactions/incompatibilities: None known

NURSING CONSIDERATIONS
Administer:

• After washing hands, cleanse crusts or discharge from eye before application

Perform/provide:

• Storage at room temperature

Evaluate:

• Therapeutic response: absence of redness, inflammation, tearing

• Allergy: itching, lacrimation, redness, swelling

Teach patient/family:

• To use drug exactly as prescribed

• Not to use eye makeup, towels, washcloths, eye medication of others; reinfection may occur

• That drug container tip should not be touched to eye

• To report itching, increased redness, burning, stinging, swelling; drug should be discontinued

• That drug may cause blurred vision when ointment is applied

---

polythiazide

(pol-i-thye'azide)

Renese

Func. class.: Thiazide diuretic

Chem. class.: Sulfonamide derivative

Action: Acts on distal tubule by increasing excretion of water, sodium, chloride, potassium

Uses: Edema, hypertension

Dosage and routes:

• *Adult:* PO 1-4 mg/day

Available forms include: Tabs 1, 2, 4 mg

Side effects/adverse reactions:

GU: Frequency, polyuria, uremia, glucosuria

CNS: Drowsiness, paresthesia, anxiety, depression, headache, diz-

P

---

ziness, fatigue, weakness

GI: Nausea, vomiting, anorexia, constipation, diarrhea, cramps, pancreatitis, GI irritation, *hepatitis*

EENT: Blurred vision

INTEG: Rash, urticaria, purpura, photosensitivity, fever

META: Hyperglycemia, hyperuricemia, increased creatinine

HEMA: Aplastic anemia, hemolytic anemia, leukopenia, agranulocytosis, thrombocytopenia

CV: Irregular pulse, orthostatic hypotension

ELECT: Hypokalemia, hypercalcemia, hyponatremia, hypochloremia

Contraindications: Hypersensitivity to thiazides or sulfonamides, anuria, renal decompensation

Precautions: Hypokalemia, renal disease, pregnancy, hepatic disease, gout, COPD, lupus erythematosus, diabetes mellitus

Pharmacokinetics:

PO: Onset 2 hr, peak 6 hr, duration 24-48 hr; excreted unchanged by kidneys, crosses placenta, enters breast milk, half-life 26 hr

Interactions/incompatibilities:

• Increased toxicity of: lithium, nondepolarizing skeletal muscle relaxants, digitalis

• Decreased effects of: antidiabetics

• Decreased absorption of thiazides: cholestyramine, colestipol

• Decreased hypotensive response: indomethacin

• Increased action of: quinidine

NURSING CONSIDERATIONS

Assess:

• Weight, I&O daily to determine fluid loss; effect of drug may be decreased if used qd

• Rate, depth, rhythm of respiration, effect of exertion

• B/P lying, standing; postural hypotension may occur

• Electrolytes: potassium, sodium, chloride; include BUN, blood sugar, CBC, serum creatinine, blood pH, ABGs

• Glucose in urine if patient is diabetic

Administer:

• In AM to avoid interference with sleep if using drug as a diuretic

• Potassium replacement if potassium is less than 3.0

• With food, if nausea occurs, absorption may be decreased slightly

Evaluate:

• Improvement in edema of feet, legs, sacral area daily if medication is being used in CHF

• Improvement in CVP q8h

• Signs of metabolic acidosis: drowsiness, restlessness

• Signs of hypokalemia: postural hypotension, malaise, fatigue, tachycardia, leg cramps, weakness

• Rashes, temperature elevation qd

• Confusion, especially in elderly; take safety precautions if needed

Teach patient/family:

• To increase fluid intake 2-3 L/day unless contraindicated; to rise slowly from lying or sitting position

• To notify physician of muscle weakness, cramps, nausea, dizziness

• Drug may be taken with food or milk

• That blood sugar may be increased in diabetics

• Take early in day to avoid nocturia

Lab test interferences:

Increase: BSP retention, calcium, amylase

Decrease: PBI, PSP

Treatment of overdose: Lavage if taken orally, monitor electrolytes, administer dextrose in saline

posterior pituitary
Pituitrin
Func. class.: Pituitary hormone

Action: Stimulates contraction of smooth muscle

Uses: Postoperative ileus, diabetes insipidus, surgical hemostasis

Dosage and routes:
• *Adult:* IM/SC 5-20 units

Available forms include: Inj IM, SC 10, 20 U/ml

Side effects/adverse reactions:
INTEG: Facial pallor

GU: Uterine cramps

EENT: Tinnitus, mydriasis, blurred vision

GI: Increased GI motility, diarrhea

Contraindications: Hypersensitivity, toxemia, hypertension, seizure disorders, advanced arteriosclerosis, cardiac disease

Interactions/incompatibilities:
• Decreased action: lithium, demeclocycline

• Increased action: chlorpropamide

NURSING CONSIDERATIONS
Administer:
• IM if possible

Evaluate:
• Allergic reaction: rash, urticaria, wheezing, fever, nausea, vomiting; drug should be discontinued, administer epinephrine 1:1000

potassium bicarbonate/ potassium acetate/ potassium chloride/ potassium gluconate/ potassium phosphate
K-Lyte, K-Lor, Kaon, Kay Ciel
Func. class.: Electrolyte
Chem. class.: Potassium

Action: Needed for adequate transmission of nerve impulses and cardiac contraction, renal function intracellular ion maintenance

Uses: Prevention and treatment of hypokalemia

Dosage and routes:
Potassium bicarbonate
• *Adult:* PO dissolve 25-50 mEq in water qd-qid

Potassium acetate—hypokalemia
• *Adult and child:* PO 40-100 mEq in divided doses 2-4 days

Hypokalemia (prevention)
• *Adult and child:* PO 20 mEq in divided doses 2-4/days

Potassium chloride
• *Adult:* PO 40-100 mEq in divided doses tid-qid; IV 20 mEq/hr when diluted in 40 mEq/1000 ml, not to exceed 150 mEq

Potassium gluconate
• *Adult:* PO 40-100 mEq in divided doses tid-qid

Potassium phosphate
• *Adult:* IV 1 mEq/hr in sol of 60 mEq/L, not to exceed 150 mEq; PO 40-100 mEq

Available forms include: Tabs for sol 6.5, 25 mEq/inj for prep of IV 2, 4 mEq/caps ext rel 8, 10 mEq; powder for sol 3.3, 5, 6.7, 10, 13.3 mEq; tabs 4, 13.4 mEq; tabs ext rel 6.7, 8, 10 mEq; inj for prep of IV 1.5, 2, 2.4, 3, 3.2 mEq/elix 6.7 mEq; tabs 2, 5 mEq/oral sol 2.375 mEq; inj for prep of IV 4.4, 4.7 mEq

Side effects/adverse reactions:
CNS: Confusion, bradycardia, *cardiac depression, dysrhythmias, arrest, peaking T waves, lowered R and depressed RST, prolonged P-R interval, widened QRS complex*

GI: Nausea, vomiting, cramps, pain, diarrhea

GU: Oliguria

INTEG: Cold extremities, rash

Contraindications: Renal disease (severe), severe hemolytic disease, Addison's disease, hyperkalemia,

P

acute dehydration, extensive tissue breakdown

Precautions: Cardiac disease, potassium sparing diuretic therapy, systemic acidosis

Interactions/incompatibilities:

• Hyperkalemia: potassium sparing, diuretic, or other potassium products

Pharmacokinetics:

PO: Excreted by kidneys and in feces

NURSING CONSIDERATIONS
Assess:

• ECG for peaking T waves, lowered R, depressed RST, prolonged P-R interval, widening QRS complex, hyperkalemia; drug should be reduced or discontinued

• Potassium level during treatment (3.5-5.0 mg/dl is normal level)

• I&O ratio; watch for decreased urinary output, notify physician immediately

Administer:

• Through large-bore needle, to decrease vein inflammation, check for extravasation

• In large vein, avoiding scalp vein in child (IV)

• Slowly by IV route to prevent toxicity, never give IV bolus or IM

Perform/provide:

• Storage at room temperature

Evaluate:

• Therapeutic response: absence of fatigue, muscle weakness, and decrease thirst and urinary output, cardiac changes

• Cardiac status: rate, rhythm, CVP, PWP, PAWP, if being monitored directly

Teach patient/family:

• To add potassium-rich foods to diet: bananas, orange juice, avocados; whole grains, broccoli, carrots, prunes, cocoa after this medication is discontinued

• To avoid OTC products: antacids, salt substitutes, analgesics, vitamin preparations, unless specifically directed by physician

• To report hyperkalemia (lethargy, confusion, diarrhea, nausea, vomiting, fainting, decreased output) or continued hypokalemia (fatigue, weakness, polyuria, polydipsia, cardiac changes)

---

potassium iodide
Potassium Iodide Solution, Strong Iodine Solution, Lugol's Solution
Func. class.: Thyroid hormone antagonist
Chem. class.: Iodine product

Action: Inhibits secretion of thyroid hormone, fosters colloid accumulation in thyroid follicles, decreases vascularity of gland

Uses: Preparation for thyroidectomy, thyrotoxic crisis

Dosage and routes:
Thyrotoxic crisis

• *Adult and child:* PO 1 ml in water tid after meals; IV 2 g as adjunct

Preparation for thyroidectomy

• *Adult and child:* PO 0.1-0.3 ml tid (Strong Iodine Solution) or 5 gtts in water tid pc $\times$ 2-3 wk before surgery (Potassium Iodide Solution)

Available forms include: Solution 5%, 10%, 21 mg/gh; tabs 130, 300 mg; inj IV 10%, 20%

Side effects/adverse reactions:

ENDO: Hypothyroidism, hyperthyroid adenoma

INTEG: Rash, urticaria, angineurotic edema, acne, mucosal hemorrhage, fever

CNS: Headache, confusion, paresthesias

HEMA: **Eosinophilia, lymphedema**

GI: Nausea, diarrhea, vomiting,

---

small bowel lesions, upper gastric pain

MS: Myalgia, arthralgia, weakness

EENT: Metallic taste, stomatitis, salivation, periorbital edema

Contraindications: Hypersensitivity to iodine, hyperkalemia

Precautions: Pregnancy (D), renal disease, pulmonary TB, lactation, cardiac disease, children, Addison's disease

Pharmacokinetics:

PO: Onset 24-48 hr, peak 10-15 days after continuous therapy, uptake by thyroid gland or excreted in urine; crosses placenta

Interactions/incompatibilities:

• Increased action of: lithium, other antithyroid agents

• Increased side effects: potassium agents, K-sparing diuretics

NURSING CONSIDERATIONS

Assess:

• Pulse, B/P, temperature

• I&O ratio; check for edema: puffy hands, feet, periorbit; indicate hypothyroidism

• Weight qd; same clothing, scale, time of day

• T_3, T_4, which is increased; serum TSH, which is decreased; free thyroxine index, which is increased if dosage is too low; discontinue drug 3-4 wk before RAIU

Administer:

• Through straw to prevent tooth discoloration

• With meals to decrease GI upset

• At same time each day, to maintain drug level

• Lowest dose that relieves symptoms

Perform/provide:

• Fluids to 3-4 L/day, unless contraindicated

Evaluate:

• Therapeutic effect: weight gain, decreased pulse, decreased T_4

• Overdose: peripheral edema, heat intolerance, diaphoresis, palpitations, dysrhythmias, severe tachycardia, increased temperature delirium, CNS irritability

• Hypersensitivity: rash, enlarged cervical lymph nodes may indicate drug may need to be discontinued

• Hypoprothrombinemia: bleeding, petechiae, ecchymosis

• Clinical response: after 3 wk should include increased weight, pulse; decreased T_4

Teach patient/family:

• To abstain from breast feeding after delivery

• To take pulse daily

• To keep graph of weight, pulse, mood

• Avoid OTC products that contain iodine

• That seafood, other iodine products may be restricted

• Not to discontinue this medication abruptly; thyroid crisis may occur; stress patient response

• That response may take several months if thyroid is large

• Discontinue drug, notify physician if fever, rash, metallic taste, swelling of throat, burning of mouth, throat, sore gums, teeth, severe GI distress, enlargement of thyroid

Lab test interferences:

Interferes: Urinary 17-OHCS

---

potassium iodide (SSKI)

Pima, Iosat, Thyro-Block

Func. class.: Expectorant

Action: Increases respiratory tract fluid by decreasing surface tension, adhesiveness, which increases removal of mucus

Uses: Bronchial asthma, emphysema, bronchitis, nuclear radiation protection

---

italics = common side effects   ***bold italic*** = life threatening reactions

Dosage and routes:
- *Adult:* PO 0.3-0.6 ml q4-6h
- *Child:* PO 0.25-1 ml saturated sol bid-qid

Radiation protection:
- *Adult:* PO 0.13 ml SSKI before or after initial exposure
- *Infant <1 yr:* Half adult dose

Available forms include: Sol 1 g/ml

Side effects/adverse reactions:
EENT: Burning mouth, throat, eye irritation, swelling of eyelids
GI: Gastric irritation
ENDO: Iodism, goiter, myxedema
RESP: Pulmonary edema
INTEG: Angioedema, rash
CNS: Frontal headache, *CNS depression,* fever, parkinsonism

Contraindications: Hypersensitivity to iodides, pulmonary TB, pregnancy (D), hyperthyroidism, hyperkalemia, acute bronchitis

Precautions: Hypothyroidism, cystic fibrosis, lactation

Pharmacokinetics: Excreted in urine

Interactions/incompatibilities:
- Increased hypothyroid effects: lithium, antithyroid drugs
- Dysrhythmias, hyperkalemia: potassium-sparing diuretics, potassium-containing medication

NURSING CONSIDERATIONS

Administer:
- Decreased dose to elderly patients; their excretion may be slowed
- Diluted water or fruit juice to improve taste, decrease nausea

Perform/provide:
- Storage at room temperature in tight containers
- Increased fluids to liquefy secretions

Evaluate:
- Therapeutic response: absence of cough
- Cough: type, frequency, character including sputum

Teach patient/family:
- Not to use if pregnant
- Symptoms of iodism: eruptions, burning of oral cavity, eye irritation
- Symptoms of hyperthyroidism: CNS depression, fever, glomerulonephritis
- Discontinue, notify physician if fever, rash, metallic taste occur

---

pralidoxime chloride

(pra-li-dox′eem)
Protopam

Func. class.: Cholinesterase reactivator

Chem. class.: Quaternary ammonium oxide

Action: Displaces enzymes at receptor site by reactivation of cholinesterase inhibited by phosphate esters

Uses: Cholinergic crisis in myasthenia gravis, organophosphate poisoning antidote

Dosage and routes:
Cholinergic crisis
- *Adult:* IV 1-2 g, then 250 mg q5 min until desired response

Organophosphate poisoning
- *Adult:* IV INF 1-2 g/dl NS over 15-30 min; PO 1-3 g q5h

Available forms include: Inj IV 600 mg/2 ml; tabs 500 mg

Side effects/adverse reactions:
CNS: Dizziness, headache, drowsiness
GI: Nausea, anorexia
MS: Weakness, muscle rigidity
CV: Tachycardia, hypertension
RESP: Hyperventilation, *laryngospasm*

Contraindications: Hypersensitivity, inorganic phosphates, severe cardiac disease

Precautions: Myasthenia gravis, pregnancy, renal insufficiency

---

Pharmacokinetics:
PO: 2-3 hr
IV: Peak 5-15 min
IM: Peak 10-20 min
Half-life 1½ hr, metabolized in liver, excreted in urine (unchanged)
Interactions/incompatibilities:
None known

NURSING CONSIDERATIONS
Assess:
• B/P, VS, I&O ratio; observe for decreased urinary output for 48-72 hr after poisoning to determine atropine toxicity from poisoning effects
Administer:
• Only with emergency equipment available
• As soon as possible after poisoning; within 4 hr
• Slowly (IV) after dilution with sterile water
• Atropine 2-4 mg IV or IM if cyanosis is present, repeat q5-10 min until toxicity occurs: dry mouth, flushing, tachycardia, delirium, hallucinations
• Only with edrophonium on unit for myasthenia gravis patient
Evaluate:
• Airway, need for assistance with respiration
• Respiratory status: rate, rhythm, characteristics

---

pramoxine HCl (topical)
(pra-mox′-een)
ProctoFoam, Tronolane, Tronothane
Func. class.: Topical anesthetic

Action: Inhibits nerve impulses from sensory nerves, which produces anesthesia
Uses: Pruritus, sunburn, toothache, sore throat, cold sores, oral pain, rectal pain and irritation
Dosage and routes:
• *Adult and child:* TOP apply q3-4h; REC apply 1 full applicator bid-tid and after each BM
Available forms include: Aero, cream, gel, lotion 1%; rec oint 1%; rec or top aero, cream 1%
Side effects/adverse reactions:
INTEG: Rash, irritation, sensitization
Contraindications: Hypersensitivity, infants <1 yr, application to large areas
Precautions: Child <6 yr, sepsis, pregnancy, denuded skin
Interactions/incompatibilities:
None known

NURSING CONSIDERATIONS
Administer:
• After cleansing and drying of affected area
• Rectal aerosol using applicator or tissue
Evaluate:
• Allergy: rash, irritation, reddening, swelling
• Therapeutic response: absence of pain, itching of affected area
• Infection: if affected area is infected, do not apply
Teach patient/family:
• To report rash, irritation, redness, swelling
• How to apply

---

prazepam
(pra′ze-pam)
Centrax
Func. class.: Antianxiety
Chem. class.: Benzodiazepine

Controlled Substance Schedule IV
Action: Depresses subcortical levels of CNS, including limbic system and reticular formation
Uses: Anxiety
Dosage and routes:
• *Adult:* PO 30 mg in divided doses or at hs

Available forms include: Caps 5, 10, 20 mg; tabs 10 mg

Side effects/adverse reactions:

CNS: Dizziness, drowsiness, confusion, headache, anxiety, tremors, stimulation, fatigue, depression, insomnia, hallucinations

GI: Constipation, dry mouth, nausea, vomiting, anorexia, diarrhea

INTEG: Rash, dermatitis, itching

*CV: Orthostatic hypotension, **ECG changes, tachycardia,*** hypotension

EENT: Blurred vision, tinnitus, mydriasis

Contraindications: Hypersensitivity to benzodiazepines, narrow-angle glaucoma, psychosis, pregnancy (D), child <18 yr

Precautions: Elderly, debilitated, hepatic disease, renal disease

Pharmacokinetics:

PO: Peak 6 hr, duration up to 48 hr, metabolized by liver, excreted by kidneys, crosses placenta, breast milk, half-life 30-100 hr

Interactions/incompatibilities:

Decreased effects of this drug: oral contraceptives, rifampin, valproic acid

Increased effects of this drug: CNS depressants, alcohol, cimetidine, disulfiram, oral contraceptives

NURSING CONSIDERATIONS

Assess:

• B/P (lying, standing), pulse; if systolic B/P drops 20 mm Hg, hold drug, notify physician

• Blood studies: CBC

• Hepatic studies: AST, ALT, bilirubin, CrCl

Administer:

• With food or milk for GI symptoms

• Crushed if patient is unable to swallow medication whole

• Gum, hard candy, frequent sips of water for dry mouth

Perform/provide:

• Assistance with ambulation during beginning therapy, since drowsiness/dizziness occurs

• Safety measure including side-rails

Evaluate:

• Mental status: mood, sensorium, affect

• Physical dependency, withdrawal symptoms: headache, nausea, vomiting, muscle pain, weakness after long-term use

• Check to see PO medication has been swallowed

Teach patient/family:

• Not to be used for everyday stress or used longer than 4 mo

• Avoid OTC preparations (cough, cold, hay fever) unless approved by physician

• To avoid driving or other activities that require alertness

• To avoid alcohol ingestion or other psychotropic medications

• Not to discontinue medication quickly after long-term use

Lab test interferences:

Increase: AST, ALT, serum bilirubin, LDH

Decrease: RAIU

False increase: 17-OHCS

Treatment of overdose: Lavage, VS, supportive care

---

praziquantel

(pray-zi-kwon′tel)

Biltricide

Func. class.: Anthelmintic

Chem. class.: Pyrazinoisoquiolone derivative

Action: Causes contraction, paralysis, leading to dislodgement of suckers; they are carried to liver where phagocytosis takes place

Uses: Schistosomiasis, liver flukes, lung flukes, intestinal flukes, tapeworms

Dosage and routes:

• *Adult and child >4 yr:* PO 20

mg/kg q4-6h × 1 day

Available forms include: Tabs 600 mg

Side effects/adverse reactions:

INTEG: Rash, pruritus, urticaria, internal hypertension

CNS: Dizziness, headache, drowsiness, malaise, increased seizure activity, fever, sweating

GI: Nausea, vomiting, anorexia, diarrhea, abdominal pain, increased liver enzymes

Contraindications: Hypersensitivity, lactation

Precautions: Child <4 yr, seizure disorders, pregnancy (B)

Pharmacokinetics:

PO: Peak 1-3 hr, half-life 48-90 min, metabolized by liver (metabolites), excreted in urine, breast milk, CSF

Interactions/incompatibilities: None known

NURSING CONSIDERATIONS

Assess:

• Liver function test: AST, ALT; watch for increase

• Stools during entire treatment, 1, 3 mo after treatment; specimens must be sent to lab while still warm

Administer:

• Corticosteroids as ordered to reduce CNS effects (cerebral cysticerosis)

• Laxatives before treatment to cleanse bowel

• Po with liquids during meals to avoid GI symptoms, not to be chewed

Perform/provide:

• Storage in tight container in cool environment

• To avoid driving or hazardous activities on day of, day after treatment

Evaluate:

• For therapeutic response: expulsion of worms, 3 negative stool cultures after completion of treatment

• For allergic reaction: rash, urticaria, pruritus

• For diarrhea during expulsion of worms

• For CSF reaction: headache, high fever; if these occur, drug should be discontinued, physician notified

Teach patient/family:

• Proper hygiene after BM including handwashing technique, tell patient to avoid putting fingers in mouth

• Need for compliance with dosage schedule, duration of treatment

• To refrain from breast feeding on day of treatment, 72 hr after

Treatment of overdose: Fast-acting laxative

---

prazosin HCl

(pra'zoe-sin)
Minipress

Func. class.: Antihypertensive
Chem. class.: α-Adrenergic blocker

Action: Peripheral blood vessels are dilated, peripheral resistance lowered, reduction in blood pressure results from α-adrenergic receptors being blocked

Uses: Hypertension, refractory CHF, Raynaud's vasospasm

Dosage and routes:

• *Adult:* PO 1 mg bid or tid, increasing to 20 mg qd in divided doses if required, usual range 6-15 mg/day

Available forms include: Caps 1, 2, 5 mg

Side effects/adverse reactions:

CV: Palpitations, orthostatic hypotension, tachycardia, edema, rebound hypertension

CNS: Dizziness, headache, drowsiness, anxiety, depression, vertigo, weakness, fatigue

GI: Nausea, vomiting, diarrhea, constipation, abdominal pain

P

GU: Urinary frequency, incontinence, impotence, priapism
EENT: Blurred vision, epistaxis, tinnitus, dry mouth, red sclera
Contraindications: Hypersensitivity
Precautions: Pregnancy (C), children

Pharmacokinetics:
PO: Onset 2 hr, peak 1-3 hr, duration 6-12 hr; half-life 2-3 hr, metabolized in liver, excreted via bile, feces (>90%), in urine (<10%)

Interactions/Incompatibilities:
• Increased hypotensive effects: β-blockers, nitroglycerin

NURSING CONSIDERATIONS
Assess:
• B/P
• Pulse, jugular venous distention q4h
• BUN, uric acid if on long-term therapy
• Weight daily, I&O

Administer:
• Whole, do not chew or crush tablets

Perform/provide:
• Storage in tight containers in cool environment

Evaluate:
• Edema in feet, legs daily
• Skin turgor, dryness of mucous membranes for hydration status
• Rales, dyspnea, orthopnea q30 min

Teach patient/family:
• Fainting occasionally occurs after 1st dose; do not drive or operate machinery for 4 hr after 1st dose or take 1st dose at bedtime

Treatment of overdose: Administer volume expanders or vasopressors, discontinue drug, place in supine position

prednisolone/prednisolone acetate/prednisolone phosphate/prednisolone tebutate

(pred-niss'oh-lone)
Cortalone, Delta-Cortef, Fernisolone-P/Predoxine/Savacort/Hydeltrasol, PSP-IV/Hydeltra-TBA, Metalone-TBA

Func. class.: Corticosteroid
Chem. class.: Glucocorticoid, immediate acting

Action: Decreases inflammation by suppression of migration of polymorphonuclear leukocytes, fibroblasts, reversal to increase capillary permeability and lysosomal stabilization

Uses: Severe inflammation, immunosuppresion, neoplasms

Dosage and routes:
• *Adult:* PO 2.5-15 mg bid-qid; IM 2-30 mg (acetate, phosphate) q12h; IV 2-30 mg (phosphate) q12h, 2-30 mg in joint or soft tissue (phosphate), 4-40 mg in joint of lesion (tebutate), 0.25-1 ml q wk in joints (acetate-phosphate)

Available forms include: Tabs 5 mg; inj 25, 50, 100 mg/ml acetate; inj 20 mg/ml terbutate; inj 20 mg/ml phosphate; inj 80 mg/ml acetate/phosphate

Side effects/adverse reactions:
INTEG: Acne, poor wound healing, ecchymosis, petechiae
CNS: Depression, flushing, sweating, headache, mood changes
CV: Hypotension, circulatory collapse, thrombophlebitis, embolism, tachycardia
HEMA: Thrombocytopenia
MS: Fractures, osteoporosis, weakness
GI: Diarrhea, nausea, abdominal distention, GI hemorrhage, in-

creased appetite, **pancreatitis**
EENT: Fungal infections, increased intraocular pressure, blurred vision
Contraindications: Psychosis, hypersensitivity, idiopathic thrombocytopenia, acute glomerulonephritis, amebiasis, fungal infections, nonasthmatic bronchial disease, child <2 yr
Precautions: Pregnancy, diabetes mellitus, glaucoma, osteoporosis, seizure disorders, ulcerative colitis, CHF, myasthenia gravis
Pharmacokinetics:
PO: Peak 1-2 hr, duration 2 days
IM: Peak 3-45 hr
Interactions/incompatibilities:
• Decreased action of this drug: cholestyramine, colestipol, barbiturates, rifampin, ephedrine, phenytoin, theophylline
• Decreased effects of: anticoagulants, anticonvulsants, antidiabetics, ambenonium, neostigmine, isoniazid, toxoids, vaccines
• Increased side effects: alcohol, salicylates, indomethacin, amphotericin B, digitalis preparations
• Increased action of this drug: salicylates, estrogens, indomethacin

NURSING CONSIDERATIONS
Assess:
• Potassium, blood sugar, urine glucose while on long-term therapy; hypokalemia and hyperglycemia
• Weight daily, notify physician if weekly gain of >5 lb
• B/P q4h, pulse, notify physician if chest pain occurs
• I&O ratio, be alert for decreasing urinary output and increasing edema
• Plasma cortisol levels during long-term therapy (normal level: 138-635 nmol/L SI units when drawn at 8 AM)
Administer:
• After shaking suspension (parenteral)

• Titrated dose, use lowest effective dose
• IM inj deeply in large mass, rotate sites, avoid deltoid, use 19G needle
• In one dose in AM to prevent adrenal suppression, avoid SC administration, damage may be done to tissue
• With food or milk to decrease GI symptoms
Perform/provide:
• Assistance with ambulation in patient with bone tissue disease to prevent fractures
Evaluate:
• Therapeutic response: ease of respirations, decreased inflammation
• Infection: increased temperature, WBC, even after withdrawal of medication; drug masks symptoms of infection
• Potassium depletion: paresthesias, fatigue, nausea, vomiting, depression, polyuria, dysrhythmias, weakness
• Edema, hypotension, cardiac symptoms
• Mental status: affect, mood, behavioral changes, aggression
Teach patient/family:
• That ID as steroid user should be carried
• To notify physician if therapeutic response decreases; dosage adjustment may be needed
• Not to discontinue this medication abruptly or adrenal crisis can result
• To avoid OTC products: salicylates, alcohol in cough products, cold preparations unless directed by physician
• Teach patient all aspects of drug use, including Cushingoid symptoms
• Symptoms of adrenal insufficiency: nausea, anorexia, fatigue, dizziness, dyspnea, weakness, joint pain

---

italics = common side effects   ***bold italic*** = life threatening reactions

Lab test interferences:

Increase: Cholesterol, sodium, blood glucose, uric acid, calcium, urine glucose

Decrease: Calcium, potassium, T_4, T_3, thyroid ^{131}I uptake test, urine 17-OHCS, 17-KS, PBI

False negative: Skin allergy tests

---

prednisolone acetate (suspension)/predniso-lone sodium phosphate (solution)

(pred-niss'oh-lone)

Econopred, Pred-Forte, Pred Mild, Predulose Ophthalmic/Ak-Pred, Hydelthrasol, Inflamase Forte, Inflamase Ophthalmic, Metreton Ophthalmic

Func. class.: Ophthalmic antiinflammatory

Chem. class.: Analog of hydrocortisone

Action: Decreases inflammation, resulting in decreases in pain, photophobia, hyperemia, cellular infiltration

Uses: Inflammation of eye, lids, conjunctiva, cornea, uveitis, iridocyclitis, allergic condition, burns, foreign bodies

Dosage and routes:

• *Adult and child:* Instill 1-2 gtts into conjunctival sac q1h × 2 days if needed then bid-qid

Available forms include: Susp 0.12%, 0.125%, 1%; sol 0.125%, 0.5%, 1%

Side effects/adverse reactions:

*EENT: **Increased intraocular pressure,** poor corneal wound healing, increased possibility of corneal infections, glaucoma exacerbation, **optic nerve damage,** decreased acuity, visual field

Contraindications: Hypersensitivity, acute superficial herpes sim-

plex, fungal/viral diseases of eye or conjunctiva, active diabetes mellitus, ocular TB, infections of the eye

Precautions: Corneal abrasions, glaucoma

Interactions/incompatibilities: None known

NURSING CONSIDERATIONS

Evaluate:

• Allergic reactions: redness, itching, swelling, lacrimation

• Therapeutic response: absence of swelling, redness, exudate

Administer:

• After shaking

Perform/provide:

• Storage in tight, light-resistant container

Teach patient/family:

• Instillation method: pressure on lacrimal sac for 1 min

• Not to share eye medications with others

---

prednisone

(pred-ni-sone)

Colisone, Deltasone, Meticorten, Orasone, Wojtab

Func. class.: Corticosteroid

Chem. class.: Glucocorticoid, immediate acting

Action: Decreases inflammation by suppression of migration of polymorphonuclear leukocytes, fibroblasts, reversal to increase capillary permeability, and lysosomal stabilization

Uses: Severe inflammation, immunosuppresion, neoplasms, multiple sclerosis

Dosage and routes:

• *Adult:* PO 2.5-15 mg bid-qid, then qd or qod maintenance

• *Child:* PO 0.14-2 mg/kg/day in divided doses qid

Multiple sclerosis

• *Adult:* PO 200 mg/day × 1 wk,

then 80 mg qod × 1 mo
Available forms include: Tabs 1,
2.5, 5, 10, 20, 25, 50 mg; oral sol
5 mg/5 ml; syr 5 mg/5 ml
Side effects/adverse reactions:
INTEG: Acne, poor wound healing,
ecchymosis, petechiae
CNS: Depression, flushing, sweating, headache, mood changes
*CV: Hypotension, **circulatory col-
lapse, thrombophlebitis, embo-
lism,** tachycardia*
*HEMA: **Thrombocytopenia***
MS: Fractures, osteoporosis, weakness
*GI: Diarrhea, nausea, abdominal
distention, GI hemorrhage, increased appetite, **pancreatitis***
EENT: Fungal infections, increased
intraocular pressure, blurred vision
Contraindications: Psychosis, hypersensitivity, idiopathic thrombocytopenia, acute glomerulonephritis, amebiasis, fungal infections, nonasthmatic bronchial disease, child <2 yr
Precautions: Pregnancy, diabetes mellitus, glaucoma, osteoporosis, seizure disorders, ulcerative colitis, CHF, myasthenia gravis
Pharmacokinetics:
PO: Peak 1-2 hr, duration 1-1½ days, half-life 3½-4 days
Interactions/incompatibilities:
• Decreased action of this drug: cholestyramine, colestipol, barbiturates, rifampin, ephedrine, phenytoin, theophylline
• Decreased effects of: anticoagulants, anticonvulsants, antidiabetics, ambenonium, neostigmine, isoniazid, toxoids, vaccines
• Increased side effects: alcohol, salicylates, indomethacin, amphotericin B, digitalis preparations
• Increased action of this drug: salicylates, estrogens, indomethacin
NURSING CONSIDERATIONS
Assess:
• Potassium, blood sugar, urine

glucose while on long-term therapy; hypokalemia and hyperglycemia
• Weight daily, notify physician of weekly gain >5 lb
• B/P q4h, pulse, notify physician if chest pain occurs
• I&O ratio, be alert for decreasing urinary output and increasing edema
• Plasma cortisol levels during long-term therapy (normal level: 138-635 nmol/L SI units when drawn at 8 AM)
Administer:
• Titrated dose, use lowest effective dose
• With food or milk to decrease GI symptoms
Perform/provide:
• Assistance with ambulation in patient with bone tissue disease to prevent fractures
Evaluate:
• Therapeutic response: ease of respirations, decreased inflammation
• Infection: increased temperature, WBC, even after withdrawal of medication; drug masks symptoms of infection
• Potassium depletion: paresthesias, fatigue, nausea, vomiting, depression, polyuria, dysrhythmias, weakness
• Edema, hypotension, cardiac symptoms
• Mental status: affect, mood, behavioral changes, aggression
Teach patient/family:
• That ID as steroid user should be carried
• To notify physician if therapeutic response decreases; dosage adjustment may be needed
• Not to discontinue this medication abruptly or adrenal crisis can result
• To avoid OTC products: salicylates, alcohol in cough products,

---

italics = common side effects   ***bold italic*** = life threatening reactions

cold preparations unless directed by physician

• Teach patient all aspects of drug use, including Cushingoid symptoms

• Symptoms of adrenal insufficiency: nausea, anorexia, fatigue, dizziness, dyspnea, weakness, joint pain

Lab test interferences:

Increase: Cholesterol, sodium, blood glucose, uric acid, calcium, urine glucose

Decrease: Calcium, potassium, T_4, T_3, thyroid ^{131}I uptake test, urine 17-OHCS, 17-KS, PBI

False negative: Skin allergy tests

---

primaquine phosphate

(prim'a-kween)

Func. class.: Antimalarial
Chem. class.: Synthetic 8-aminoquinolone

Action: Action is unknown; thought to destroy exoerythrocytic forms by gametocidal action

Uses: Malaria caused by *Plasmodium vivax*

Dosage and routes:

• *Adult:* PO 15 mg qd × 2 wk

• *Child:* PO 0.3 mg/kg × 2 wk

Available forms include: Tabs 26.3 mg

Side effects/adverse reactions:

INTEG: Pruritus, skin eruptions

CNS: Headache

EENT: Blurred vision, difficulty focusing

GI: Nausea, vomiting, anorexia, cramps

CV: Hypertension

HEMA: Agranulocytosis, granulocytopenia, leukopenia, hemolytic anemia, leukocytosis, mild anemia, *methemoglobinemia*

Contraindications: Hypersensitivity, anemia, lupus erythematosus, methemoglobinemia, porphyria, rheumatoid arthritis, methemoglobin reductase deficiency, G-6-PD deficiency, pregnancy

Pharmacokinetics:

PO: Metabolized by liver (metabolites), half-life 3.7-9.6 hr

Interactions/incompatibilities:

• Toxicity: quinacrine

NURSING CONSIDERATIONS

Assess:

• Ophthalmic test if long-term treatment or drug dosage >150 mg/day

• Liver studies q wk: AST, ALT, bilirubin, if on long-term therapy

• Blood studies, CBC, since blood dyscrasias occur

Administer:

• Before or after meals at same time each day to maintain drug level

Evaluate:

• Allergic reactions: pruritus, rash, urticaria

• Blood dyscrasias: malaise, fever, bruising, bleeding (rare)

• For renal status: dark urine, hematuria, decreased output

• For hemolytic reaction: chills, fever, chest pain, cyanosis; drug should be discontinued immediately

Teach patient/family:

• To report visual problems, fever, fatigue, dark urine, bruising, bleeding; may indicate blood dyscrasias

---

primidone

(pri'mi-done)

Mysoline, Sertan*

Func. class.: Anticonvulsant
Chem. class.: Barbiturate derivative

Action: Raises seizure threshold by conversion of drug to phenobarbital

Uses: Generalized tonic-clonic, complex-partial seizures

Dosage and routes:

• *Adult and child >8 yr:* PO 250 mg/day, may increase by 250 mg/wk, not to exceed 2 g/day in divided doses qid

• *Child <8 yr:* PO 125 mg/day, may increase by 125 mg/wk, not to exceed 1 g/day in divided doses qid

Available forms include: Tabs 50, 250 mg; susp 250 mg/5 ml

Side effects/adverse reactions:

*HEMA: **Thrombocytopenia, leukopenia, neutropenia, eosinophilia, megaloblastic anemia,** serum folate level, lymphadenopathy*

CNS: Stimulation, drowsiness, dizziness, confusion, sedation, headache, flushing, hallucinations, coma, psychosis

GI: Nausea, vomiting, anorexia

INTEG: Rash, edema, alopecia, lupuslike syndrome

EENT: Diplopia, nystagmus

GU: Impotence

Contraindications: Hypersensitivity, porphyria

Precautions: COPD, hepatic disease, renal disease, hyperactive children

Pharmacokinetics:

PO: Peak 4 hr, excreted by kidneys, excreted in breast milk, half-life 3-24 hr

Interactions/incompatibilities:

• Increased blood levels: alcohol, heparin, CNS depressants, isoniazid, phenytoin, phenobarbital

NURSING CONSIDERATIONS

Assess:

• Drug level: therapeutic level 5-10 μg/ml

Evaluate:

• Mental status: mood, sensorium, affect, memory (long, short)

• Respiratory depression

• Blood dyscrasias: fever, sore throat, bruising, rash, jaundice

Teach patient/family:

• All aspects of drug administration: action, route, dose, when to notify physician

---

probenecid

(proe-ben'e-sid)

Benemid, Benn, Benuryl,* Probalan, Probenimead, Robenecid

Func. class.: Uricosuric

Chem. class.: Sulfonamide derivative

Action: Inhibits tubular reabsorption of urates, with increased excretion of uric acids

Uses: Gonorrhea, hyperuricemia in gout, gouty arthritis, adjunct to cephalosporin or penicillin treatment

Dosage and routes:

Gonorrhea

• *Adult:* PO 1 g with 3.5 g ampicillin or 1 g ½ hr before 4.8 mill U of aqueous penicillin G procaine injected into 2 sites IM

Gout/gouty arthritis

• *Adult:* PO 250 mg bid for 1 wk, then 500 mg bid, not to exceed 2 g/day; maintenance: 500 mg/day × 6 mos

Adjunct in penicillin/cephalosporin treatment

• *Adult and child >50 kg:* PO 500 mg qid

• *Child <50 kg:* PO 25 mg/kg, then 40 mg/kg in divided doses qid

Available forms include: Tabs 0.5 g

Side effects/adverse reactions:

CNS: Drowsiness, headache, confusion, stimulation, tremors, *twitching, hyperreflexia, tetany, EEG changes, **convulsions***

CV: Bradycardia

GU: Glycosuria, thirst, frequency, ***nephrotic syndrome***

*GI: Gastric irritation, nausea, vomiting, anorexia, **hepatic necrosis***

INTEG: Rash, pain at infusion site, dermatitis, pruritus, fever

P

META: Acidosis, hypokalemia, hyperchloremia, hyperglycemia
*RESP: **Apnea,*** irregular respirations
Contraindications: Hypersensitivity, severe hepatic disease, blood dyscrasias, severe renal disease, CrC <50 mg/min

Precautions: Pregnancy, severe respiratory disease, lactation, cardiac edema, child <2 yr

Pharmacokinetics:
PO: Peak 2-4 hr, duration 8 hr, half-life 8-10 hr; metabolized by liver, excreted in urine, crosses placenta

Interactions/incompatibilities:
• Increased toxicity: sulfa drugs, dapsone, clofibrate, PAS, indomethacin, rifampin, naproxen, methotrexate, pantothenic acid
• Decreased action of this drug: alcohol, salicylates, nitrofurantoin, diazoxides, diuretics

NURSING CONSIDERATIONS
Assess:
• Uric acid levels (3-7 mg/dl)
• Respiratory rate, rhythm, depth; notify physician of abnormalities
• Electrolytes, CO_2 before, during treatment
• Urine pH, output, glucose during beginning treatment

Administer:
• After meals or with milk if GI symptoms occur
• Increase fluid intake 2-3 L/day to prevent urinary calculi

Perform/provide:
• Low purine diet restricting: organ meats, anchovies, sardines, meat gravy, dried beans, meat extracts

Evaluate:
• Therapeutic response: absence of pain, stiffness in joints
• For CNS symptoms: confusion, twitching, hyperreflexia, stimulation, headache; may indicate overdose

Teach patient/family
• To avoid high purine foods, alcohol, urinary calculi may form
• To avoid OTC preparations (aspirin) unless directed by physician

Lab test interferences:
False positive: Urine glucose
Increase: BSP/urinary PSP
Decrease: Urinary 17-KS

---

probucol

(proe'byoo-kole)
Lorelco
Func. class.: Antilipemic
Chem. class.: Hormone isomer

Action: Inhibits lipolysis, reduces triglyceride synthesis in liver
Uses: Type IV hyperlipidemia, severe hypercholesterolemia when other treatment unsuccessful

Dosage and routes:
Adult: PO 500 mg bid with breakfast, supper
Available forms include: Tabs 250 mg

Side effects/adverse reactions:
GI: Nausea, vomiting, diarrhea, constipation, anorexia
INTEG: Flushing, alopecia, sweating, hyperthermia
CV: Palpitations, dysrhythmias, *myocardial infarction,* prolonged QT interval
EENT: Visual disturbances, ptosis, tinnitus
GU: Menstrual irregularities
CNS: Insomnia, dizziness, palpitations, paresthesias

Contraindications: Hypersensitivity
Precautions: Dysrhythmias, hypertension, angina pectoris, pregnancy (B), lactation, children

Pharmacokinetics:
PO: Excreted in bile/feces
Interactions/incompatibilities:
None known

NURSING CONSIDERATIONS
Assess:
• Renal and hepatic levels, if patient is on long-term therapy

• For signs of vitamin A, D, K deficiency

Administer:

• Drug with meals if GI symptoms occur

Evaluate:

• Therapeutic response: decreased triglycerides, cholesterol levels, (hyperlipidemia), diarrhea, pruritus (excess bile area)

• Bowel pattern daily; increase bulk, water in diet if constipation develops

Teach patient/family:

• Symptoms of hypothrombinemia: bleeding mucous membranes, dark tarry stools, petechiae; report immediately

• That compliance is needed since toxicity may result if doses are missed

• That risk factors should be decreased: high fat diet, smoking, alcohol consumption, absence of exercise

• That OTC preparations should be avoided unless directed by physician

• Birth control should be practiced while on this drug

Lab test interferences:

Increase: Liver function studies, CPK, renal function studies, blood glucose

---

procainamide HCl

(proe-kane-a'mide)
Procan SR, Promaine, Pronestyl, Sub-Quin, Rhythmin
Func. class.: Antidysrhythmic (Class IA)
Chem. class.: Procaine HCl amide analog

Action: Increases electrical stimulation threshold of ventrical, HIS Purkinge system, which stabilizes cardiac membrane

Uses: PVCs, atrial fibrillation, PAT, ventricular tachycardia, atrial dysrhythmias, ventricular tachycardia

Dosage and routes:
Atrial fibrillation/PAT

• *Adult:* PO 1-1.25 g, may give another 750 mg if needed, if no response then 500 mg-1g q2h until desired response

Ventricular tachycardia

• *Adult:* PO 1g; maintenance 50 mg/kg/day given in 3 hr intervals; SUS REL TABS 500 mg-1 g q6h

Other dysrhythmias

• *Adult:* IV BOL 100 mg q5 min, given 25-50 mg/min, not to exceed 1g; then IV INF 2-6 mg/min

Available forms include: Caps 250, 375, 500 mg; tabs 250, 375, 500 mg; tabs sus rel 250, 500, 750 mg; inj IV 100 mg/ml

Side effects/adverse reactions:

CNS: Headache, dizziness, confusion, psychosis, restlessness, irritability

GI: Nausea, vomiting, anorexia, diarrhea

*CV: Hypotension, **heart block, cardiovascular collapse, arrest***

HEMA: SLE syndrome

INTEG: Rash, urticaria, edema, swelling (rare)

Contraindications: Hypersensitivity, severe heart block, supraventricular dysrhythmias

Precautions: Pregnancy, lactation, children, renal disease, liver disease, CHF, respiratory depression, myasthenia gravis

Pharmacokinetics:

PO: Peak 1-2 hr, duration 3 hr (8 hr extended)

IM: Peak 10-60 min, duration 3 hr Half-life 3 hr, metabolized in liver to active metabolites, excreted unchanged by kidneys (60%)

Interactions/incompatibilities:

• Increased effects of neuromus-

P

---

cular blockers when used with this drug
• Increased effects: cimetidine, phenytoin, propranolol, quinidine
• May decrease effects of this drug: barbiturates

NURSING CONSIDERATIONS

Assess:
• ECG continuously to determine increased PR or QRS segments; if these develop, discontinue immediately; watch for increased ventricular ectopic beats, maximum need to rebolus
• IV infusion rate using infusion pump, run at less than 4 mg/min
• Blood levels
• B/P continuously for fluctuations
• I&O ratio, electrolytes (K, Na, Cl)

Administer:
• IM injection in deltoid; aspirate to avoid intravascular administration; check site daily for infiltration or extravasation

Evaluate:
• Malignant hyperthermia: tachypnea, tachycardia, changes in B/P, increased temperature
• Cardiac rate, respiration: rate, rhythm, character, continuously
• Respiratory status: rate, rhythm, lung fields, watch for respiratory depression
• CNS effects: dizziness, confusion, psychosis, paresthesias, convulsions; drug should be discontinued
• Lung fields, bilateral rales may occur in CHF patient
• Increased respiration, increased pulse; drug should be discontinued

procaine HCl

(proe'-kane)
Novocain, Unicaine
Func. class.: Local anesthetic
Chem. class.: Ester

Action: Competes with calcium for sites in nerve membrane that control sodium transport across cell membrane; decreases rise of depolarization phase of action potential

Uses: Spinal anesthesia, epidural, peripheral nerve block, perineum, lower extremities, infiltration

Dosage and routes:
Varies depending on route of anesthesia
Available forms include: Inj 1%, 2%, 10%

Side effects/adverse reactions:
CNS: Anxiety, restlessness, *convulsions, loss of consciousness,* drowsiness, disorientation, tremors, shivering
CV: Myocardial depression, cardiac arrest, dysrhythmias, bradycardia, hypotension, hypertension, fetal bradycardia
GI: Nausea, vomiting
EENT: Blurred vision, tinnitus, pupil constriction
INTEG: Rash, urticaria, allergic reactions, edema, burning, skin discoloration at injection site, tissue necrosis
RESP: Status asthmaticus, respiratory arrest, anaphylaxis

Contraindications: Hypersensitivity, child <12 yr, elderly, severe liver disease

Precautions: Elderly, severe drug allergies

Pharmacokinetics:
Onset 2-5 min, duration 1 hr; metabolized by liver, excreted in urine (metabolites)

Interactions/incompatibilities:
• Dysrhythmias: epinephrine, halothane, enflurane
• Hypertension: MAOIs, tricyclic antidepressants, phenothiazines
• Decreased action of this drug: chloroprocaine

NURSING CONSIDERATIONS
Assess:
• B/P, pulse, respiration during treatment
• Fetal heart tones if drug is used during labor
Administer:
• Only drugs that are not cloudy, do not contain precipitate
• Only with crash cart, resuscitative equipment nearby
• Only drugs without preservatives for epidural or caudal anesthesia
Perform/provide:
• Use of new solution, discard unused portions
Evaluate:
• Therapeutic response: anesthesia necessary for procedure
• Allergic reactions: rash, urticaria, itching
• Cardiac status: ECG for dysrhythmias, pulse, B/P during anesthesia
Treatment of overdose: Airway, O₂, vasopressor, IV fluids, anticonvulsants for seizures

---

procarbazine HCl

(proe-kar'ba-zeen)
Matulane, Natulan*
Func. class.: Antineoplastic, miscellaneous
Chem. class.: Hydrazine derivative

Action: Inhibits DNA, RNA, protein synthesis; has multiple sites of action
Uses: Hodgkin's disease, cancers resistant to other therapy
Dosage and routes:
• *Adult:* PO 2-4 mg/kg/day for first wk; maintain dosage of 4-6 mg/kg/day until platelets and WBC fall; after recovery, 1-2 mg/kg/day
• *Child:* PO 50 mg/day for 7 days, then 100 mg/m² until desired response, leukopenia, or thrombocytopenia occurs; 50 mg/day is maintenance after bone marrow recovery
Available forms include: Caps 50 mg
Side effects/adverse reactions:
HEMA: **Thrombocytopenia, anemia, leukopenia, myelosuppression, bleeding disorders,** purpura, petechiae, epistaxis
GI: Nausea, vomiting, anorexia, diarrhea, constipation, dry mouth, stomatitis
EENT: Retinal hemorrhage, nystagmus, photophobia, diplopia
INTEG: Rash, pruritus, dermatitis, alopecia, herpes, hyperpigmentation
CNS: Headache, dizziness, insomnia, hallucinations, confusion, coma, pain, chills, fever, sweating, paresthesias
RESP: Cough, pneumonitis
Contraindications: Hypersensitivity, thrombocytopenia, bone marrow depression
Precautions: Renal disease, hepatic disease, pregnancy (D), radiation therapy
Pharmacokinetics: Half-life 1 hr; concentrates in liver, kidney, skin; metabolized in liver, excreted in urine
Interactions/incompatibilities:
• Increased CNS depression: barbiturates, antihistamines, narcotics, hypotensive agents, phenothiazines
• Disulfiram-like reaction: ethyl alcohol, MAOIs, tricyclic antidepressants, tyramine foods, sympathomimetic drugs
• Hypertension: guanethidine, le-

P

---

vodopa, methyldopa, reserpine

• Increased hypoglycemia: insulin, oral hypoglycemics

NURSING CONSIDERATIONS
Assess:

• CBC, differential, platelet count weekly; withhold drug if WBC is <4000/mm³ or platelet count is <100,000/mm³; notify physician of these results

• Renal function studies: BUN, serum uric acid, urine CrCl, electrolytes before, during therapy

• I&O ratio, report fall in urine output to <30 ml/hr

• Monitor temperature q4h; fever may indicate beginning infection

• Liver function tests before, during therapy: bilirubin, AST, ALT, alk phosphatase prn or monthly

• CNS changes: confusion, paresthesias, neuropathies, drug should be discontinued

Administer:

• Medications by oral route if possible, avoid IM, SC, IV routes to prevent infections

• Antiemetic 30-60 min before giving drug to prevent vomiting

• Antibiotics for prophylaxis of infection

• Topical or systemic analgesics for pain

• Transfusion for anemia

• Antispasmodic for GI symptoms

Perform/provide:

• Strict medical asepsis and protective isolation if WBC levels are low

• Liquid diet: carbonated beverages, Jello; dry toast, crackers may be added if patient is not nauseated or vomiting

• Storage in tight, light-resistant container in cool environment

Evaluate:

• Toxicity: facial flushing, epistaxis, increased pro-time, thrombocytopenia; drug should be discontinued

• Bleeding: hematuria, guaiac, bruising or petechiae, mucosa or orifices q8h

• Food preferences; list likes, dislikes

• Effects of alopecia on body image; discuss feelings about body changes

• Inflammation of mucosa, breaks in skin

• Yellowing of skin, sclera, dark urine, clay-colored stools, itchy skin, abdominal pain, fever, diarrhea

• Buccal cavity q8h for dryness, sores or ulceration, white patches, oral pain, bleeding, dysphagia

• Local irritation, pain, burning at injection site

• GI symptoms: frequency of stools, cramping

• Acidosis, signs of dehydration: rapid respirations, poor skin turgor, decreased urine output, dry skin, restlessness, weakness

Teach patient/family:

• Why protective isolation precautions are necessary

• To report any complaints, side effects to nurse or physician: cough, shortness of breath, fever, chills, sore throat, bleeding, bruising, vomiting blood, black tarry stools

• That hair may be lost during treatment and wig or hairpiece may make patient feel better; tell patient that new hair may be different in color, texture

• To avoid foods with citric acid, hot or rough texture

• To report any bleeding, white spots, ulcerations in mouth to physician; tell patient to examine mouth qd

• To avoid driving or activities requiring alertness; drowsiness may occur

• That contraceptive measures are recommended during therapy

• Avoid ingestion of alcohol, tyramine-containing foods; cold,

---

hayfever, or weight-reducing products may cause serious drug interactions

---

prochlorperazine edisylate/prochlorperazine maleate

(proe-klor-per'a-zeen)
Compazine, Stemetil*

Func. class.: Antiemetic
Chem. class.: Phenothiazine, piperazine derivative

Action: Acts centrally by blocking chemoreceptor trigger zone, which in turn acts on vomiting center
Uses: Nausea, vomiting
Dosage and routes:
Postoperative nausea/vomiting
• *Adult:* IM 5-10 mg 1-2 hr before anesthesia; may repeat in 30 min; IV 5-10 mg 15-30 min before anesthesia; IV INF 20 mg/L D₅W or NS 15-30 min before anesthesia, not to exceed 40 mg/day
Severe nausea/vomiting
• Adult: PO 5-10 mg tid-qid; SUS REL 15 mg qd in AM or 10 mg q12h; REC 25 mg/bid; IM 5-10 mg; may repeat q4h, not to exceed 40 mg/day
• *Child 18-39 kg:* PO 2.5 mg tid or 5 mg bid; do not exceed 15 mg/day; IM 0.132 mg/kg
• *Child 14-17 kg:* PO/REC 2.5 mg bid-tid, not to exceed 10 mg/day; IM 0.132 mg/kg
• *Child 9-13 kg:* PO/REC 2.5 mg qd-bid, not to exceed 7.5 mg/day; IM 0.132 mg/kg
Available forms include: Oral sol 5 mg/ml; inj 5 mg/ml; tabs 5, 10, 25 mg; caps ext rel 10, 15, 30 mg
Side effects/adverse reactions:
CNS: Euphoria, depression, restlessness, tremor
GI: Nausea, vomiting, anorexia, dry mouth, diarrhea, constipation,

weight loss, metallic taste, cramps
*CV: **Circulatory failure, tachycardia***
*RESP: **Respiratory depression***
Contraindications: Hypersensitivity to phenothiazines, coma, seizure, encephalopathy, bone marrow depression
Precautions: Children <2 yr, pregnancy, elderly
Pharmacokinetics:
PO: Onset 30-40 min, duration 3-4 hr
EX REL: Onset 30-40 min, duration 10-12 hr
REC: Onset 60 min, duration 3-4 hr
IM: Onset 10-20 min, duration 12 hr, metabolized by liver, excreted by kidneys, crosses placenta, excreted in breast milk
Interactions/incompatibilities:
• Decreased effect of this drug: barbiturates, antacids
• Increased anticholinergic action: anticholinergics, antiparkinson drugs, antidepressants
• Do not mix with other drug in syringe or solution
NURSING CONSIDERATIONS
Assess:
• VS, B/P; check patients with cardiac disease more often
Administer:
• IM injection in large muscle mass; aspirate to avoid IV administration
• IV slowly; may cause severe orthostatic hypotension
Evaluate:
• Therapeutic response: absence of nausea, vomiting
• Respiratory status before, during, after administration of emetic; check rate, rhythm, character; respiratory depression can occur rapidly with elderly or debilitated patients
Teach patient/family:
• Avoid hazardous activities, activ-

---

ities requiring alertness; dizziness may occur

---

procyclidine HCl

(proe-sye'kli-deen)

Kemadrin, Procyclid*

Func. class.: Cholinergic blocker
Chem. class.: Tertiary amine

Action: Acts on dopamine receptors in CNS, which decrease involuntary movements

Uses: Parkinson symptoms

Dosage and routes:

• *Adult:* PO 2-2.5 mg tid pc, titrated to patient response, not to exceed 60 mg/day

Available forms include: Tabs 5 mg

Side effects/adverse reactions:

CNS: Confusion, anxiety, restlessness, irritability, delusions, hallucinations, headache, sedation, depression, incoherence, dizziness

EENT: Blurred vision, photophobia, dilated pupils, difficulty swallowing

CV: Palpitations, tachycardia, postural hypotension

GI: Dryness of mouth, constipation, nausea, vomiting, abdominal distress, paralytic ileus

GU: Hesitancy, retention

Contraindications: Hypersensitivity, narrow-angle glaucoma, myasthenia gravis, GI/GU obstruction, child <3 yr

Precautions: Pregnancy, elderly, lactation, tachycardia, prostatic hypertrophy

Pharmacokinetics:

PO: Onset 30-45 mins, duration 4-6 hr

Interactions/incompatibilities:

• Decreased action of: haloperidol, phenothiazines

• Increased anticholinergic effect: alcohol, narcotics, barbiturates, antihistamines, MAOIs, phenothiazines

NURSING CONSIDERATIONS

Assess:

• I&O ratio; retention commonly causes decreased urinary output

Administer:

• With or after meals for GI upset; may give with fluids other than water

• At hs to avoid daytime drowsiness in patient with parkinsonism

Perform/provide:

• Storage at room temperature in tight container

• Hard candy, frequent drinks, sugarless gum to relieve dry mouth

Evaluate:

• Parkinsonism: shuffling gait, muscle rigidity, involuntary movements

• Urinary hesitancy, retention; palpate bladder if retention occurs

• Constipation; increase fluids, bulk, exercise if this occurs

• For tolerance over long-term therapy; dose may need to be increased or changed

• Mental status: affect, mood, CNS depression, worsening of mental symptoms during early therapy

Teach patient/family:

• Not to discontinue this drug abruptly; to taper off over 1 wk

• To avoid driving or other hazardous activities; drowsiness may occur

• To avoid OTC medication: cough, cold preparations with alcohol, antihistamines unless directed by physician

---

progesterone
(proe-jess'ter-one)
Femotrone, Profac-O, Progelan, Progest-50, Progestaject-50, Progestasert

Func. class.: Progestogen
Chem. class.: Progesterone derivative

Action: Inhibits secretion of pituitary gonadotropins, which prevents follicular maturation, ovulation, stimulates growth of mammary tissue, antineoplastic action against endometrial cancer

Uses: Contraception, amenorrhea, premenstrual syndrome, abnormal uterine bleeding

Dosage and routes:
Amenorrhea/uterine bleeding
• Adult: IM 5-10 mg qd × 6-8 doses
Contraception
• Adult: INSERT 1 placed in uterine cavity, active for 1 yr
PMS
• Adult: REC SUPP/VAG SUPP 200-400 mg
Available forms include: Inj IM 25, 50, 100 mg/ml; IU system 38 mg, rec supp, vag supp

Side effects/adverse reactions:
CNS: Dizziness, headache, migraines, depression, fatigue
CV: Hypotension, thrombophlebitis, edema, ***thromboembolism, stroke, pulmonary embolism, myocardial infarction***
GI: Nausea, vomiting, anorexia, cramps, increased weight, ***cholestatic jaundice***
EENT: Diplopia
GU: Amenorrhea, cervical erosion, breakthrough bleeding, dysmenorrhea, vaginal candidiasis, breast changes, *gynecomastia, testicular atrophy, impotence,* endometriosis, ***spontaneous abortion***

INTEG: Rash, urticaria, acne, hirsutism, alopecia, oily skin, seborrhea, purpura, melasma, photosensitivity
META: Hyperglycemia

Contraindications: Breast cancer, hypersensitivity, thromboembolic disorders, reproductive cancer, genital bleeding (abnormal, undiagnosed), cerebral hemorrhage

Precautions: Pregnancy, lactation, hypertension, asthma, blood dyscrasias, gallbladder disease, CHF, diabetes mellitus, bone disease, depression, migraine headache, convulsive disorders, hepatic disease, renal disease, family history of breast or reproductive tract cancer

Pharmacokinetics:
IM: Duration 24 hr
Excreted in urine, feces, metabolized in liver

Interactions/incompatibilities:
None known

NURSING CONSIDERATIONS
Assess:
• Weight daily; notify physician of weekly weight gain >5 lb
• B/P at beginning of treatment and periodically
• I&O ratio; be alert for decreasing urinary output, increasing edema
• Liver function studies: ALT, AST, bilirubin periodically during long-term therapy

Administer:
• Titrated dose; use lowest effective dose
• Oil solution deeply in large muscle mass IM, rotate sites
• In one dose in AM
• With food or milk to decrease GI symptoms
• After warming to dissolve crystals

Perform/provide:
• Storage in dark area

Evaluate:
• Therapeutic response: decrease

P

---

italics = common side effects   ***bold italic*** = life threatening reactions

abnormal uterine bleeding, absence
of amenorrhea
• Edema, hypertension, cardiac
symptoms, jaundice
• Mental status: affect, mood, behavioral changes, depression
• Hypercalcemia
Teach patient/family:
• To avoid sunlight or use sunscreen, photosensitivity can occur
• All aspects of drug usage, including cushingoid symptoms
• To report breast lumps, vaginal
bleeding, edema, jaundice, dark
urine, clay-colored stools, dyspnea, headache, blurred vision, abdominal pain, numbness or stiffness in legs, chest pain; male to
report impotence or gynecomastia
• To report suspected pregnancy
• To monitor blood sugar, if diabetic
Lab test interferences:
Increase: Alk phosphatase, nitrogen (urine), pregnanediol, amino
acids
Decrease: GTT, HDL

---

promazine HCl

(proe'ma-zeen)
Promanyl,* Prozine, Sparine
Func. class.: Antipsychotic/neu-
roleptic
Chem. class.: Phenothiazine, ali-
phatic

Action: Depresses cerebral cortex, hypothalamus, limbic system,
which control activity, aggression;
blocks neurotransmission produced
by dopamine at synapse; exhibits a
strong α-adrenergic, anticholinergic blocking action; as antiemetic,
inhibits medullary chemoreceptor
trigger zone; mechanism for antipsychotic effects is unclear
Uses: Psychotic disorders, schizophrenia, nausea, vomiting, alcohol
withdrawal

Dosage and routes:
Psychosis
• *Adult:* PO 10-200 mg q4-6h, max
dose 1000 mg/day; IM 50-150 mg,
then increased to 300 mg if needed
• *Child >12 yr:* PO 10-25 mg
q4-6h
Nausea/vomiting
• *Adult:* PO 25-50 mg q4-6h; IM
50 mg; IV not recommended, but
may use in concentrations of <25
mg/ml
Available forms include: Tabs 25,
50, 100 mg; syr 10 mg/5ml; inj IV,
IM 25, 50 mg/ml
Side effects/adverse reactions:
RESP: **Laryngospasm,** dyspnea, *re-*
spiratory depression
CNS: Extrapyramidal symptoms:
pseudoparkinsonism, akathisia,
dystonia, tardive dyskinesia,
drowsiness, headache, seizures
HEMA: Anemia, leukopenia, leukocytosis, *agranulocytosis*
INTEG: Rash, photosensitivity, dermatitis
EENT: Blurred vision, glaucoma
GI: Dry mouth, nausea, vomiting,
anorexia, constipation, diarrhea,
jaundice, weight gain
GU: Urinary retention, urinary
frequency, enuresis, impotence,
amenorrhea, gynecomastia
CV: Orthostatic hypotension, hypertension, *cardiac arrest,* ECG
changes, *tachycardia*
Contraindications: Hypersensitivity, blood dyscrasias, coma, child
<12 yr, brain damage, bone mar-
row depression
Precautions: Pregnancy, lactation,
seizure disorders, hypertension, hepatic disease, cardiac disease
Pharmacokinetics:
PO: Onset erratic, peak 2-4 hr
IM: Onset 15 min, peak 1 hr, duration 4-6 hr
Metabolized by liver, excreted in
urine, crosses placenta, enters
breast milk

Interactions/incompatibilities:
• Oversedation: other CNS depressants, alcohol, barbiturate anesthetics
• Toxicity: epinephrine
• Decreased absorption: aluminum hydroxide or magnesium hydroxide antacids
• Decreased effects of: lithium, levodopa
• Increased effects of both drugs: β-adrenergic blockers, alcohol
• Increased anticholinergic effects: anticholinergics

NURSING CONSIDERATIONS
Assess:
• Swallowing of PO medication; check for hoarding or giving of medication to other patients
• I&O ratio; palpate bladder if low urinary output occurs
• Bilirubin, CBC, liver function studies monthly
• Urinalysis is recommended before and during prolonged therapy
Administer:
• Antiparkinsonian agent, after securing order from physician to be used if EPS occur
• Syrup mixed in citrus- or chocolate-flavored drinks
• IM injection into large muscle mass
Perform/provide:
• Decreased noise input by dimming lights, avoiding loud noises
• Supervised ambulation until stabilized on medication; do not involve in strenuous exercise program because fainting is possible; patient should not stand still for long periods of time
• Increased fluids to prevent constipation
• Sips of water, candy, gum for dry mouth
• Storage in tight, light-resistant container
Evaluate:
• Therapeutic response: decrease in emotional excitement, hallucinations, delusions, paranoia, reorganization of patterns of thought, speech
• Affect, orientation, LOC, reflexes, gait, coordination, sleep pattern disturbances
• B/P standing and lying; also include pulse, respirations, q4h during initial treatment; establish baseline before starting treatment; report drops of 30 mm Hg
• Dizziness, faintness, palpitations, tachycardia on rising
• EPS including akathisia (inability to sit still, no pattern to movements), tardive dyskinesia (bizarre movements of jaw, mouth, tongue, extremities), pseudoparkinsonism (rigidity, tremors, pill rolling, shuffling gait)
• Skin turgor daily
• Constipation, urinary retention daily, if these occur increase bulk and water in diet
Teach patient/family:
• That orthostatic hypotension occurs frequently, and to rise from sitting or lying position gradually
• To remain lying down after IM injection for at least 30 min
• To avoid hot tubs, hot showers, or tub baths since hypotension may occur
• To avoid abrupt withdrawal of this drug or EPS may result; drugs should be withdrawn slowly
• To avoid OTC preparations (cough, hayfever, cold) unless approved by physician since serious drug interactions may occur; avoid use with alcohol or CNS depressants, increased drowsiness may occur
• To use a sunscreen during sun exposure to prevent burns
• Regarding compliance with drug regimen
• About EPS and necessity for meticulous oral hygiene since oral

P

candidiasis may occur

• To report sore throat, malaise, fever, bleeding, mouth sores; if these occur, CBC should be drawn and drug discontinued

• In hot weather, heat stroke may occur; take extra precautions to stay cool

Lab test interferences:

Increase: Liver function tests, cardiac enzymes, cholesterol, blood glucose, prolactin, bilirubin, PBI, cholinesterase, ^{131}I

Decrease: Hormones (blood and urine)

False positive: Pregnancy tests, PKU

False negative: Urinary steroids, 17-OHCS

Treatment of overdose: Lavage if orally injested, provide an airway; *do not induce vomiting*

---

promethazine HCl
(proe-meth′a-zeen)

Ganphen, Methazine, Pentazine, Phencen-50, Phenergan, Prorex, Provigan, Remsed, Rolamethazine, Sigazine

Func. class.: Antihistamine, H_1-receptor antagonist

Chem. class.: Phenothiazine derivative

Action: Acts on blood vessels, GI, respiratory system by competing with histamine for H_1-receptor site; decreases allergic response by blocking histamine

Uses: Motion sickness, rhinitis, allergy symptoms, sedation, nausea, preoperative, postoperative sedation

Dosage and routes:

Nausea

• *Adult:* PO/IM 25 mg, may repeat 12.5-25 mg q4-6h

• *Child:* PO/IM 0.5 mg/pd q4-6h

Motion sickness

• *Adult:* PO 25 mg bid

• *Child:* PO/IM/REC 12.5-25 mg bid

Allergy/rhinitis

• *Adult:* PO 12.5 mg qid, or 25 mg hs

• *Child:* PO 6.25-12.5 mg tid or 25 mg hs

Sedation

• *Adult:* PO/IM 25-50 mg hs

• *Child:* PO/IM/REC 12.5-25 mg hs

Sedation (preoperative/postoperative)

• *Adult:* PO/IM/IV 25-50 mg

• *Child:* PO/IM/IV 12.5-25 mg

Available forms include: Tabs 12.5, 25, 50 mg; syr 6.25, 25 mg/5 ml; supp 12.5, 25, 50 mg; inj 25, 50 mg/ml

Side effects/adverse reactions:

CNS: Dizziness, drowsiness, poor coordination, fatigue, anxiety, euphoria, confusion, paresthesia, neuritis

CV: Hypotension, palpitations, tachycardia

RESP: Increased thick secretions, wheezing, chest tightness

HEMA: Thrombocytopenia, agranulocytosis, hemolytic anemia

GI: Dry mouth, nausea, vomiting, anorexia, constipation, diarrhea

INTEG: Rash, urticaria, photosensitivity

GU: Retention, dysuria, frequency

EENT: Blurred vision, dilated pupils, tinnitus, nasal stuffiness, dry nose, throat, mouth, photosensitivity

Contraindications: Hypersensitivity to H_1-receptor antagonist, acute asthma attack, lower respiratory tract disease

Precautions: Increased intraocular pressure, renal disease, cardiac disease, hypertension, bronchial asthma, seizure disorder, stenosed peptic ulcers, hyperthyroidism,

---

prostatic hypertrophy, bladder neck obstruction, pregnancy
Pharmacokinetics:
PO: Onset 20 min, duration 4-6 hr, metabolized in liver, excreted by kidneys, GI tract (inactive metabolites)
Interactions/incompatibilities:
• Increased CNS depression: barbiturates, narcotics, hypnotics, tricyclic antidepressants, alcohol
• Decreased effect of: oral anticoagulants, heparin
• Increased effect of this drug: MAOIs

NURSING CONSIDERATIONS
Assess:
• I&O ratio; be alert for urinary retention, frequency, dysuria; drug should be discontinued if these occur
• CBC during long-term therapy
Administer:
• Coffee, tea, cola (caffeine) to decrease drowsiness
• With meals if GI symptoms occur, absorption may slightly decrease
• Deep IM in large muscle; rotate site
• When used for motion sickness, 30 min before travel
• IV; do not exceed 25 mg/min
Perform/provide:
• Hard candy, gum, frequent rinsing of mouth for dryness
• Storage in tight, light-resistant container; solution, suppositories should be refrigerated
Evaluate:
• Therapeutic response: absence of running or congested nose or rashes
• Respiratory status: rate, rhythm, increase in bronchial secretions, wheezing, chest tightness
• Cardiac status: palpitations, increased pulse, hypotension
Teach patient/family:
• That drug may cause photosensitivity; to avoid prolonged sunlight

• All aspects of drug use; to notify physician if confusion, sedation, hypotension occurs
• To avoid driving or other hazardous activity if drowsiness occurs
• To avoid concurrent use of alcohol or other CNS depressants
Lab test interferences:
False negative: Skin allergy tests
False positive: Urine pregnancy test
Treatment of overdose: Administer ipecac syrup or lavage, diazepam, vasopressors, barbiturates (short-acting)

---

propantheline bromide

(proe-pan'the-leen)
Banlin,* Norpanth, Pro-Banthine, Propanthel,* Robantaline

Func. class.: Gastrointestinal anticholinergic
Chem. class.: Synthetic quarternary ammonium compound

Action: Inhibits muscarinic actions of acetylcholine at postganglionic parasympathetic neuroeffector sites
Uses: Treatment of peptic ulcer disease, irritable bowel syndrome
Dosage and routes:
• *Adult:* PO 15 mg tid ac, 30 mg hs
• *Elderly:* PO 7.5 mg tid ac
Available forms include: Tabs 7.5, 15 mg
Side effects/adverse reactions:
CNS: Confusion, stimulation in elderly, headache, insomnia, dizziness, drowsiness, anxiety, weakness, hallucinations
GI: Dry mouth, constipation, paralytic ileus, heartburn, nausea, vomiting, dysphagia, absence of taste
GU: Hesitancy, retention, impotence
CV: Palpitations, tachycardia
EENT: Blurred vision, photophobia, mydriasis, cycloplegia, in-

P

---

creased ocular tension

INTEG: Urticaria, rash, pruritus, anhidrosis, fever, allergic reactions

Contraindications: Hypersensitivity to anticholinergics, narrow-angle glaucoma, GI obstruction, myasthenia gravis, paralytic ileus, GI atony, toxic megacolon

Precautions: Hyperthyroidism, coronary artery disease, dysrhythmias, CHF, ulcerative colitis, hypertension, hiatal hernia, hepatic disease, renal disease

Pharmacokinetics:

PO: Onset 30-45 min, duration 4-6 hr; metabolized by liver, GI system, excreted in urine, bile

Interactions/incompatibilities:

• Increased anticholinergic effect: amantadine, tricyclic antidepressants, MAOIs

• Increased effect of: nitrofurantoin

• Decreased effect of: phenothiazines, levodopa

NURSING CONSIDERATIONS

Assess:

• VS, cardiac status: checking for dysrhythmias, increased rate, palpitations

• I&O ratio; check for urinary retention or hesitancy

Administer:

• ½-1 hr ac for better absorption

• Decreased dose to elderly patients; their metabolism may be slowed

• Gum, hard candy, frequent rinsing of mouth for dryness of oral cavity

Perform/provide:

• Storage in tight container protected from light

• Increased fluids, bulk, exercise to patient's lifestyle to decrease constipation

Evaluate:

• Therapeutic response: absence of epigastric pain, bleeding, nausea, vomiting

• GI complaints: pain, bleeding (frank or occult), nausea, vomiting, anorexia

Teach patient/family:

• Avoid driving or other hazardous activities until stabilized on medication

• Avoid alcohol or other CNS depressants; will enhance sedating properties of this drug

---

proparacaine HCl

(proe'par-a-caine)

Alcaine, Kainair, Ophthaine, Ophthetic

Func. class.: Ophthalmic anesthetic (short acting)

Chem. class.: Ester

Action: Decreases ion permeability by stabilizing neuronal membrane

Uses: Cataract extraction, tonometry, gonioscopy, removal of foreign bodies, suture removal, glaucoma surgery

Dosage and routes:

Glaucoma surgery/cataract extraction

• *Adult and child:* Instill 1 gtt q5-10 min × 5-7 doses

Tonometry/gonioscopy/suture removal

• *Adult and child:* Instill 1-2 gtts before procedure

Available forms include: Sol 0.5%

Side effects/adverse reactions:

EENT: Blurred vision, stinging, burning, lacrimation, photophobia, conjunctival redness, hemorrhage, iritis, stromal edema, pupil dilation, corneal erosion

INTEG: Contact dermatitis

Contraindications: Hypersensitivity

Precautions: Abnormal levels of plasma esterases, allergies, hyperthyroidism, hypertension, cardiac disease

---

Pharmacokinetics:
Instill: Onset 13-30 sec, duration 15-20 min
Interactions/incompatibilities:
None known
NURSING CONSIDERATIONS
Perform/provide:
• Protective covering for eye
• Storage in tight, light resistant container at room temperature; refrigerate after opening
Teach patient/family:
• To report change in vision, with blurring or loss of sight, trouble breathing, sweating, flushing
• Not to touch or rub eye, which may further damage eye

---

propoxyphene HCl/ propoxyphene napsylate
(proe-pox'i-feen)
Darvon, Dolene, Doraphen, Myospaz, Pargesic-65, Proxagesic, Ropoxy 642,* Darvocet-N, Darvon-N

Func. class.: Narcotic analgesics
Chem. class.: Opiate

Controlled Substance Schedule IV
Action: Inhibits ascending pain pathways in CNS, increases pain threshold, alters pain perception
Uses: Mild to moderate pain
Dosage and routes:
• *Adult:* PO 65 mg q4h prn (HCl)
• *Adult:* PO 100 mg q4h prn (Napsylate)
Available forms include: HCl-tabs 32, 65 mg; napsylate-tabs 100 mg; susp 10 mg/ml
Side effects/adverse reactions:
CNS: Drowsiness, dizziness, confusion, headache, sedation, euphoria
GI: Nausea, vomiting, anorexia, constipation, cramps

GU: Increased urinary output, dysuria
INTEG: Rash, urticaria, bruising, flushing, diaphoresis, pruritus
EENT: Tinnitus, blurred vision, miosis, diplopia
CV: Palpitations, bradycardia, change in B/P
RESP: Respiratory depression
Contraindications: Hypersensitivity, addiction (narcotic)
Precautions: Addictive personality, pregnancy, lactation, increased intracranial pressure, MI (acute), severe heart disease, respiratory depression, hepatic disease, renal disease, child <18 yr
Pharmacokinetics:
PO: Onset 15-30 min, peak 2-3 hr, duration 4-6 hr
REC: Onset slow; duration 4-6 hr
Metabolized by liver, excreted by kidneys (as metabolites), crosses placenta, excreted in breast milk, half-life 30-36 hr (metabolites)
Interactions/incompatibilities:
• Effects may be increased with other CNS depressants: alcohol, narcotics, sedative/hypnotics, antipsychotics, skeletal muscle relaxants
NURSING CONSIDERATIONS
Assess:
• I&O ratio; check for decreasing output; may indicate urinary retention
Administer:
• With antiemetic if nausea, vomiting occur
• When pain is beginning to return; determine dosage interval by patient response
Perform/provide:
• Storage in light-resistant area at room temperature
• Assistance with ambulation
• Safety measures: siderails, night light, call bell within easy reach

P

---

italics = common side effects   ***bold italic*** = life threatening reactions

Evaluate:

• Therapeutic response: decrease in pain

• CNS changes: dizziness, drowsiness, hallucinations, euphoria, LOC, pupil reaction

• Allergic reactions: rash, urticaria

• Respiratory dysfunction: respiratory depression, character, rate, rhythm; notify physician if respirations are <12/min

• Need for pain medication, physical dependence

Teach patient/family:

• To report any symptoms of CNS changes, allergic reactions

• That physical dependency may result when used for extended periods of time

• Withdrawal symptoms may occur: nausea, vomiting, cramps, fever, faintness, anorexia

Lab test interferences:

Increase: Amylase

Treatment of overdose: Narcan 0.2-0.8 IV, O_2, IV fluids, vasopressors

---

propranolol HCl

(proe-pran'oh-lole)

Inderal

Func. class.: Antihypertensive, antianginal

Chem. class.: β-Adrenergic blocker

Action: Decreases preload, afterload, which is responsible for decreasing left ventricular end diastolic pressure, systemic vascular resistance

Uses: Chronic stable angina pectoris, prophylaxis of angina pain

Dosage and routes:

• *Adult:* PO 10-40 mg q6h; IV BOL 0.5-3 mg over 1 mg/min, may repeat in 2 min, dilute 1 mg or less in 10 ml of D_5W or give undiluted over 1 min; IV INT 0.5-3 mg in 50-100 ml NS over 10-15 min

Available forms include: Caps ext rel 80, 120, 160 mg; tabs 10, 20, 40, 60, 80, 90 mg; inj 1 mg/ml

Side effects/adverse reactions:

RESP: Dyspnea, respiratory dysfunction

CV: Bradycardia, hypotension, CHF, palpitations

HEMA: Agranulocytosis, thrombocytopenia

GI: Nausea, vomiting, diarrhea, colitis, constipation, cramps, dry mouth

INTEG: Rash, pruritus, fever

CNS: Depression, hallucinations, dizziness, fatigue, lethargy, paresthesias

EENT: Sore throat, *laryngospasm*

Contraindications: Hypersensitivity to this drug, cardiac failure, cardiogenic shock, 2nd or 3rd degree heart block, bronchospastic disease

Precautions: Diabetes mellitus, pregnancy, renal disease, lactation, CHF, hyperthyroidism, COPD

Pharmacokinetics:

PO: Onset 30 min, peak 1-1½ hr, duration 6 hr

IV: Onset 2 min, peak 15 min, duration 3-6 hr

Half-life 3-5 hr, metabolized by liver, crosses placenta, blood-brain barrier, excreted in breast milk

Interactions/incompatibilities:

• Increased effects of: barbiturates, hypoglycemia, reserpine, levodopa, digitalis, ergots, neuromuscular blocking agents

• Decreased effects: norepinephrine, xanthines, isoproterenol

NURSING CONSIDERATIONS

Assess:

• B/P, pulse, respirations during beginning therapy

• Weight qd, report gain of 5 lb

• I&O ratio, CrCl if kidney damage is diagnosed

• qd, note need to be administered more often

Administer:
• With 8 oz of water on empty stomach (oral tablet)

Evaluate:
• Pain: duration, time started, activity being performed, character
• Tolerance if taken over long period of time
• Headache, lightheadedness, decreased B/P; may indicate a need for decreased dosage

Teach patient/family:
• That drug may be taken before stressful activity: exercise, sexual activity
• That SL may sting when drug comes in contact with mucous membranes
• To avoid hazardous activities if dizziness occurs
• Stress patient compliance with complete medical regimen
• To make position changes slowly to prevent fainting
• Decrease dosage over 2 weeks to prevent cardiac damage

Lab test interferences:
Increase: Serum potassium, serum uric acid, ALT/AST, alk phosphatase, LDH
Decrease: Blood glucose

---

propylthiouracil (PTU)

(proe-pill-thye-oh-yoor′a-sill)
Propyl-Thyracil*
Func. class.: Thyroid hormone antagonist
Chem. class.: Thioamide

Action: Blocks synthesis of T_3, T_4 (triiodothyronine, thyroxine), inhibits organification of iodine
Uses: Preparation for thyroidectomy, thyrotoxic crisis, hyperthyroidism

Dosage and routes:
Thyrotoxic crisis
• *Adult and child:* PO same as hyperthyroidism with iodine and propranolol
Preparation for thyroidectomy
• *Adult*: 600-1200 mg/day
• *Child:* 10 mg/kg/day in divided doses
Hyperthyroidism
• *Adult:* PO 100 mg tid increasing to 300 mg q8h, if condition is severe; continue to euthyroid state, then 100 mg qd-tid
• *Child > 10 yr:* PO 100 mg tid, continue to euthyroid state, then 25 mg tid to 100 mg bid
• *Child 6-10 yr:* PO 50-150 mg in divided doses q8h
Available forms include: Tabs 50 mg

Side effects/adverse reactions:
ENDO: Enlarged thyroid
INTEG: Rash, urticaria, pruritus, alopecia, hyperpigmentation, lupuslike syndrome
GU: Irregular menses, ***nephritis***
CNS: Drowsiness, headache, vertigo, fever, paresthesias, neuritis
*HEMA: **Agranulocytosis, leukopenia, thrombocytopenia, hypothrombinemia, lymphadenopahty***
*GI: Nausea, diarrhea, vomiting, **jaundice, hepatits,** loss of taste*
MS: Myalgia, arthralgia, noctural, muscle cramps

Contraindications: Hypersensitivity, pregnancy (3rd trimester), lactation
Precautions: Infection, bone marrow depression, hepatic disease, pregnancy (1st, 2nd trimester)
Pharmacokinetics:
PO: Onset 30-40 min, duration 2-4 hr, half-life 1-2 hr, excreted in urine, bile, breast milk, crosses placenta
Interactions/incompatibilities:
• Increased anticoagulant effect: heparin, oral anticoagulants

---

italics = common side effects   ***bold italic*** = life threatening reactions

NURSING CONSIDERATIONS
Assess:
• Pulse, B/P, temperature
• I&O ratio; check for edema: puffy hands, feet periorbit; indicate hypothyroidism
• Weight qd; same clothing, scale, time of day
• T_3, T_4, which is increased; serum TSH, which is decreased; free thyroxine index, which is increased if dosage is too low; discontinue drug 3-4 wk before RAIU
• Blood work: CBC for blood dyscrasias: leukopenia, thrombocytopenia, agranulocytosis
Administer:
• With meals to decrease GI upset
• At same time each day, to maintain drug level
• Lowest dose that relieves symptoms
Perform/provide:
• Storage in light-resistant container
• Fluids to 3-4 L/day, unless contraindicated
Evaluate:
• Therapeutic effect: weight gain, decreased pulse, decreased T_4, decreased B/P
• Overdose: peripheral edema, heat intolerance, diaphoresis, palpitations, dysrhythmias, severe tachycardia, increased temperature delirium, CNS irritability
• Hypersensitivity: rash, enlarged cervical lymph nodes, drug may need to be discontinued
• Hypoprothrombinemia: bleeding, petechiae, ecchymosis
• Clinical response: after 3 wk should include increased weight, pulse; decreased T_4
• Bone marrow depression: sore throat, fever, fatigue
Teach patient/family:
• To abstain from breast feeding after delivery
• To take pulse daily

• Report redness, swelling, sore throat, mouth lesions, which indicate blood dyscrasias
• To keep graph of weight, pulse, mood
• Avoid OTC products that contain iodine
• That seafood, other iodine products may be restricted
• Not to discontinue this medication abruptly; thyroid crisis may occur; stress patient response
• That response may take several months if thyroid is large
• Symptoms/signs of overdose: periorbital edema, cold intolerance, mental depression
• Symptoms of inadequate dose: tachycardia, diarrhea, fever, irritability
Lab test interferences:
Increases: Pro-time, AST/ALT, alk phosphatase

---

protamine sulfate
(proe'ta-meen)

Func. class.: Heparin antagonist
Chem. class.: Low molecular weight protein

Action: Produces stable complex when combined with heparin
Uses: Heparin overdose
Dosage and routes:
• *Adult:* IV 1 mg of protamine/78-95 U heparin given, administer slowly 1-3 min; give undiluted to 1%, not to exceed 50 mg/10 min
Available forms include: Inj IV 10, 50, 250 mg/ml
Side effects/adverse reactions:
CV: Hypotension, bradycardia
GI: Nausea, vomiting, anorexia
INTEG: Rash, dermatitis, urticaria, alopecia
CNS: Lassitude
HEMA: Bleeding
Contraindications: Hypersensitivity, hemorrhage

---

*Available in Canada only

Precautions: Cardiovascular disease
Pharmacokinetics:
IV: Onset 5 min, duration 2 hr
Interactions/incompatibilities:
None known

NURSING CONSIDERATIONS
Assess:
• Blood studies (Hct, platelets, occult blood in stools) q 3 mo
• Coagulation tests (APTT, ACT) 15 min after dose, then in several hours
• VS, B/P, pulse of 30 min; plus 3 hr after dose
Administer:
• Over 1-3 min
Evaluate:
• Skin rash, urticaria, dermatitis

---

protriptyline HCl
(proe-trip'te-leen)
Triptil, Vivactil

Func. class.: Antidepressant—tricyclic
Chem. class.: Dibenzocycloheptene—secondary amine

Action: Blocks reuptake of norepinephrine, serotonin into nerve endings, increasing action of norepinephrine, serotonin in nerve cells
Uses: Depression
Dosage and routes:
• *Adult:* PO 15-40 mg/day in divided doses, may increase to 60 mg/day
Available forms include: Tabs 5, 10 mg
Side effects/adverse reactions:
*HEMA: **Agranulocytosis, thrombocytopenia, eosinophilia, leukopenia***
CNS: Dizziness, drowsiness, confusion, headache, anxiety, tremors, stimulation, weakness, insomnia, nightmares, EPS (elderly), increased psychiatric symptoms, paresthesia
GI: Diarrhea, dry mouth, nausea, vomiting, ***paralytic ileus,*** increased appetite, cramps, epigastric distress, jaundice, ***hepatitis,*** stomatitis
*GU: Retention, **acute renal failure***
INTEG: Rash, urticaria, sweating, pruritus, photosensitivity
*CV: Orthostatic hypotension, ECG changes, tachycardia, **hypertension,*** palpitations
EENT: Blurred vision, tinnitus, mydriasis
Contraindications: Hypersensitivity to tricyclic antidepressants, recovery phase of myocardial infarction, convulsive disorders, prostatic hypertrophy
Precautions: Suicidal patients, severe depression, increased intraocular pressure, narrow-angle glaucoma, urinary retention, cardiac disease, hepatic disease, hyperthyroidism, electroshock therapy, elective surgery, pregnancy (C)
Pharmacokinetics:
PO: Onset 15-30 min, peak 24-30 hr, duration 4-6 hr; therapeutic effect 2-3 wk; metabolized by liver, excreted by kidneys, crosses placenta, half-life 54-98 hr
Interactions/incompatibilities:
• Decreased effects of: guanethidine, clonidine, indirect acting sympathomimetics (ephedrine)
• Increased effects of: direct acting sympathomimetics (epinephrine), alcohol, barbiturates, benzodiazepines, CNS depressants
• Hyperpyretic crisis, convulsions, hypertensive episode: MAOI (pargyline [Eutonyl])

NURSING CONSIDERATIONS
Assess:
• B/P (lying, standing), pulse q4h; if systolic B/P drops 20 mm Hg hold drug, notify physician; take vital signs q4h in patients with car-

P

---

diovascular disease

• Blood studies: CBC, leukocytes, differential, cardiac enzymes if patient is receiving long-term therapy

• Hepatic studies: AST, ALT, bilirubin, creatinine

• Weight qwk, appetite may increase with drug

• ECG for flattening of T wave, bundle branch block, AV block, dysrhythmias in cardiac patients

Administer:

• Increased fluids, bulk in diet if constipation, urinary retention occur

• With food or milk for GI symptoms

• Dosage hs if over-sedation occurs during day; may take entire dose hs; elderly may not tolerate once/day dosing

• Gum, hard candy, or frequent sips of water for dry mouth

Perform/provide:

• Storage in tight, light-resistant container at room temperature

• Assistance with ambulation during beginning therapy since drowsiness/dizziness occurs

• Safety measures including siderails, primarily in elderly

• Checking to see PO medication swallowed

Evaluate:

• EPS primarily in elderly: rigidity, dystonia, akathisia

• Mental status: mood, sensorium, affect, suicidal tendencies, increase in psychiatric symptoms: depression, panic

• Urinary retention, constipation; constipation is more likely to occur in children

• Withdrawal symptoms: headache, nausea, vomiting, muscle pain, weakness; do not usually occur unless drug was discontinued abruptly

• Alcohol consumption; if alcohol

is consumed, hold dose until morning

Teach patient/family:

• That therapeutic effects may take 2-3 wk

• Use caution in driving or other activities requiring alertness because of drowsiness, dizziness, blurred vision

• To avoid alcohol ingestion, other CNS depressants

• Not to discontinue medication quickly after long-term use, may cause nausea, headache, malaise

• To wear sunscreen or large hat since photosensitivity occurs

Lab test interferences:

Increase: Serum bilirubin, blood glucose, alk phosphatase

False increase: Urinary catecholamines

Decrease: VMA, 5-HIAA

Treatment of overdose: ECG monitoring, induce emesis, lavage, activated charcoal, administer anticonvulsant

---

povidone-iodine

(poe'vi-done)

ACU-dyne, Aerodine, Betadine, Bridine,* Efo-dine, Mallisol, Proviodine,*

Func. class.: Disinfectant
Chem. class.: Iodophor

Action: Destroys a wide variety of microorganisms by local irritation, germicidal action

Uses: Cleansing wounds, disinfection, preoperative skin preparation removal

Dosage and routes:

• *Adult and child:* SOL Use as needed

Available forms include: Top sol 1.5%, 3%

Side effects/adverse reactions:

*GU: **Renal damage***

META: Metabolic acidosis

INTEG: Irritation

Contraindications: Hypersensitivity to iodine, pregnancy (vaginal antiseptic)

Precautions: Extensive burns

Interactions/incompatibilities:

• Do not use with alcohol or hydrogen peroxide

NURSING CONSIDERATIONS

Perform/provide:

• Storage in tight, light-resistant container

• Bandaging of areas if needed

Evaluate:

• Area of the body involved: irritation, rash, breaks, dryness, scales

Teach patient/family:

• To discontinue use if rash, irritation, or redness occurs

---

pseudoephedrine HCl/ pseudoephedrine sulfate

(soo-doe-e-fed'rin)

Besan, Cenafed, Eltor,* First Sign, Novafed, Robidrine, Sudabid, Sudafed/Afrinol Repetabs

Func. class.: Adrenergic

Chem. class.: Substituted phenylethylamine

Action: Causes increased contractility and heart rate by acting on β-receptors in heart; also, acts on α-receptors, causing vasoconstriction in blood vessels; when larger doses are administered, causes vasodilation in renal, intracerebral, coronary dopaminergic receptors

Uses: Decongestant, nasal congestion

Dosage and routes:

• *Adult:* PO 60 mg q6h; EXT REL 60-120 mg q12h

• *Child 6-12 yr:* PO 30 mg q6h, not to exceed 120 mg/day

• *Child 2-6 yr:* PO 15 mg q6h, not to exceed 60 mg/day

Available forms include: Caps ext rel 120 mg; sol 15 mg, 30 mg/5 ml, 7.5 mg/0.8 ml; tabs 30, 60, 120 mg

Side effects/adverse reactions:

CNS: Tremors, anxiety, insomnia, headache, dizziness, confusion, hallucinations, **convulsions, CNS depression**

EENT: Dry nose, irritation of nose and throat

CV: Palpitations, tachycardia, hypertension, chest pain, **dysrhythmias**

GI: Anorexia, nausea, vomiting

RESP: Depression

Contraindications: Hypersensitivity to sympathomimetics, narrow-angle glaucoma

Precautions: Pregnancy, cardiac disorders, hyperthyroidism, diabetes mellitus, prostatic hypertrophy

Pharmacokinetics:

PO: Onset 15-30 min, duration 4-6 hr, 8-12 hrs (extended release) metabolized in liver, excreted in breast milk

Interactions/incompatibilities:

• Do not use with MAOIs or tricyclic antidepressants, hypertensive crisis may occur

• Decreased effect of this drug: methyldopa, urinary acidifiers, rauwolfia alkaloids

• Increased effect of this drug: urinary alkalizers

NURSING CONSIDERATIONS

Assess:

• I&O ratio

• ECG during administration continuously; if B/P increases, drug is decreased

• B/P and pulse q5 min after parenteral route

• CVP or PWP during infusion if possible

Administer:

• Plasma expanders for hypovolemia

Perform/provide:
• Storage of reconstituted solution if refrigerated for no longer than 24 hr
• Do not use discolored solutions

Evaluate:
• Paresthesias and coldness of extremities, peripheral blood flow may decrease
• Therapeutic response: increased B/P with stabilization

Teach patient/family:
• Reason for drug administration

---

psyllium
(sill'i-um)

Effersyllium Instant Mix, Hydrocil Instant Powder, Konsyl, L.A. Formula, Metamucil, Metamucil Instant Mix, Metamucil Sugar Free, Modance Bulk, Mucillium, Mucilose, Naturacil, Plain Hydrocil, Siblin, Syllact

Func. class.: Laxative, bulk
Chem. class.: Psyllium colloid

Action: Bulk-forming laxative
Uses: Chronic constipation, treatment of ulcerative colitis, irritable bowel syndrome

Dosage and routes:
• *Adult:* PO 5-10 tsps. in 8 oz of water bid or tid, then 8 oz of water or 1 premeasured packet in 8 oz of water bid or tid, then 8 oz of water
• *Child >6 yr:* 5-10 tsps. in 4 oz of water hs

Available forms include: Chew pieces 1.7 g/piece; pdr 309, 390, 430, 450, 486, 500, 600, 630, 654, 672, 791, 919, 950 mg/g, 1 g/g

Side effects/adverse reactions:
GI: Nausea, vomiting, anorexia, diarrhea, cramps

Contraindications: Hypersensitivity, intestinal obstruction, abdominal pain, nausea/vomiting, fecal impaction

Pharmacokinetics: Excreted in feces

NURSING CONSIDERATIONS
Assess:
• Blood, urine electrolytes if drug is used often by patient
• I&O ratio to identify fluid loss

Administer:
• Alone for better absorption; do not take within 1 hr of other drugs or within 1 hr of antacids, milk, or cimetidine
• In morning or evening (oral dose)

Evaluate:
• Therapeutic response: decrease in constipation or decreased diarrhea in colitis
• Cause of constipation; identify whether fluids, bulk, or exercise is missing from lifestyle
• Cramping, rectal bleeding, nausea, vomiting; if these symptoms occur, drug should be discontinued

Teach patient/family:
• That normal bowel movements do not always occur daily
• Do not use in presence of abdominal pain, nausea, vomiting
• Notify physician if constipation unrelieved or if symptoms of electrolyte imbalance occur: muscle cramps, pain, weakness, dizziness

---

pyrantel pamoate
(pi-ran'tel)

Antiminth, Combantrin*

Func. class.: Anthelmintic
Chem. class.: Pyrimidine derivative

Action: Causes paralysis in worm by neuroblockade, caused by stimulation of ganglionic receptors; worms are expelled by normal peristalsis
Uses: Pinworms, roundworms

Dosage and routes:
• *Adult and child >2 yr:* PO 11 mg/kg as single dose, not to exceed

---

1 g; repeat in 2 wk for pinworms
Available forms include: Oral susp
250 mg/5 ml
Side effects/adverse reactions:
INTEG: Rash
CNS: Dizziness, headache, drowsiness, insomnia, fever, weakness
GI: Nausea, vomiting, anorexia, diarrhea, distention, AST
Contraindications: Hypersensitivity
Precautions: Seizure disorders, hepatic disease, dehydration, anemia, child <2 yr, pregnancy (C)
Pharmacokinetics:
PO: Peak 1-3 hr, metabolized in liver, excreted in feces, urine (unchanged/metabolites)
Interactions/incompatibilities:
• Antagonizes effect of drug when used with piperazine
NURSING CONSIDERATIONS
Assess:
• Stools during entire treatment; specimens must be sent to lab while still warm
Administer:
• PO after meals to avoid GI symptoms
• After shaking suspension
Perform/provide:
• Storage in tight, light-resistant containers in cool environment
Evaluate:
• For therapeutic response: expulsion of worms, 3 negative stool cultures after completion of treatment
• For allergic reaction: rash
• For diarrhea during expulsion of worms
Teach patient/family:
• Proper hygiene after BM including handwashing technique; tell patient to avoid putting fingers in mouth
• That infected person should sleep alone; do not shake bed linen, change bed linen qd, wash in hot water
• To clean toilet qd with disinfectant (green soap solution)
• Need for compliance with dosage schedule, duration of treatment
• To drink fruit juice to help expel worms
• To wear shoes, wash all fruits, vegetables well before eating

---

pyrazinamide

(peer-a-zin′a-mide)
Tebrazid*

Func. class.: Antitubercular
Chem. class.: Pyrazinoic acid amine/nicoturimide analog

Action: Bactericidal interference with lipid, nucleic acid biosynthesis
Uses: Tuberculosis, as an adjunctive when other drugs are not feasible
Dosage and routes:
• *Adult:* PO 20-35 mg/kg/day in 3-4 divided doses, not to exceed 3 g/day
Available forms include: Tabs 500 mg
Side effects/adverse reactions:
INTEG: Photosensitivity, urticaria
CNS: Headache
*GI: **Hepatotoxicity,** abnormal liver function tests, peptic ulcer
GU: Urinary difficulty, increased uric acid
HEMA: Hemolytic anemia
Contraindications: Hypersensitivity
Precautions: Pregnancy, child <13 yr
Pharmacokinetics:
PO: Peak 2 hr, half-life 9-10 hr; metabolized in liver, excreted in urine (metabolites/unchanged drug)
Interactions/incompatibilities:
None known
NURSING CONSIDERATIONS
Assess:
• Temperature if <101° F, drug should be reduced

• Liver studies q wk: ALT, AST, bilirubin
• Renal status before, q mo: BUN, creatinine, output, sp gr, urinalysis
Administer:
• With meals to decrease GI symptoms
• After C&S is completed; q mo to detect resistance
Evaluate:
• Hepatic status: decreased appetite, jaundice, dark urine, fatigue
Teach patient/family:
• That compliance with dosage schedule, length is necessary
• That scheduled appointments must be kept or relapse may occur
• Avoid alcohol while taking this drug
Lab test interferences:
Increase: PBI
Decrease: 17-KS

---

pyrethrins/peperonyl butoxide

(peer'e-thrins)
A-200 Pyrinate, Barc, Blue, Pyrin-Aid, Pyrinyl, Rid, TISIT, Triple X

Func. class.: Pediculocide
Chem. class.: Pyrethrin/piperonyl butoxide/petroleum distillate

---

Action: Causes paralysis, death of organism by acting as a contact poison
Uses: Head, body, pubic lice; nits
Dosage and routes:
• *Adult and child:* Apply undiluted to infested area; allow application to remain no longer than 10 min, wash thoroughly with warm water, soap, or shampoo; remove dead lice, eggs with fine-tooth comb; do not exceed 2 consecutive applications within 24 hr
• *Adult and child:* CREAM/LOTION wash area with soap, water; remove visible crusts, apply to skin surfaces, remove with soap, water

in 8-12 hr; may reapply in 1 wk if needed; SHAMPOO using 30 ml, work into lather, rub for 5 min, rinse, dry with towel
Available forms include: Gel, liq, shampoo, cream, lotion
Side effects/adverse reactions:
INTEG: Irritation, pruritus, urticaria, eczema
Contraindications: Hypersensitivity, inflammation of skin, abrasions, or breaks in skin
Precautions: Child/infant, ragweed sensitivity
Pharmacokinetics: Inactivated in GI tract, other data not available
Interactions/incompatibilities: None known

NURSING CONSIDERATIONS
Administer:
• To body areas, scalp only; do not apply to face, lips, mouth, eyes, any mucous membrane, anus, or meatus
• Topical corticosteroids as ordered to decrease contact dermatitis
• Lotions of menthol or phenol to control itching
• Topical antibiotics for infection
Perform/provide:
• Storage in tight container
• Isolation until areas on skin, scalp have cleared and treatment is completed
• Removal of nits by using a fine-tooth comb rinsed in vinegar after treatment
Evaluate:
• Area of body involved, including nits
Teach patient/family:
• To wash all inhabitants' clothing, using insecticide; preventative treatment may be required of all persons living in same house, using lotion or shampoo to decrease spread of infection
• That itching may continue for 4-6 wk
• That drug must be reapplied if

accidently washed off or treatment will be ineffective
• To use externally only

pyridostigmine bromide

(peer-id-oh-stig′meen)
Mestinon, Regonol
Func. class.: Cholinergic
Chem. class.: Tertiary amine carbamate

Action: Inhibits destruction of acetylcholine, which increases concentration at sites where acetylcholine is released; this facilitates transmission of impulses across myoneural junction

Uses: Curare antagonist, myasthenia gravis

Dosage and routes:
Myasthenia gravis
• *Adult:* PO 60-180 mg bid-qid, not to exceed 1.5 g/day; IM/IV ⅟₃₀ of PO dose
Curare antagonist
• *Adult:* 10-30 mg then 0.6-1.2 mg atropine
Available forms include: Tabs 60 mg; tabs sus rel 180 mg; syr 60 mg/5 ml; inj IM/IV 5 mg/ml

Side effects/adverse reactions:
INTEG: Rash, urticaria
CNS: Dizziness, headache, sweating, confusion, weakness, convulsions, incoordination, paralysis
GI: Nausea, diarrhea, vomiting, cramps
CV: Tachycardia
GU: Frequency, incontinence
*RESP: **Respiratory depression, bronchospasm, constriction***
EENT: Miosis, blurred vision, lacrimation

Contraindications: Bradycardia, hypotension, obstruction of intestine, renal system

Precautions: Seizure disorders, bronchial asthma, coronary occlusion, hyperthyroidism, dysrhythmias, peptic ulcer, megacolon, poor GI motility

Phamacokinetics:
PO: Onset 2-4 hr, duration 2½-4 hr
IM/IV/SC: Onset 10-30 min, duration 2½-4 hr
Metabolized in liver, excreted in urine

Interactions/incompatibilities:
• Decreased action: gallamine, metocurine, pancuronium, tubocurarine, atropine
• Increased action: decamethonium, succinylcholine
• Decreased action of this drug: aminoglycosides, anesthetics, procainamide, quinidine

NURSING CONSIDERATIONS

Assess:
• VS, respiration q8h
• I&O ratio; check for urinary retention or incontinence

Administer:
• Only with atropine sulfate available for cholinergic crisis
• Only after all other cholinergics have been discontinued
• Increased doses if tolerance occurs
• Larger doses after exercise or fatigue
• With food or milk to decrease GI symptoms
• On empty stomach for better absorption

Perform/provide:
• Storage at room temperature

Evaluate:
• Therapeutic response: increased muscle strength, hand grasp, improved gait, absence of labored breathing (if severe)
• Bradycardia, hypotension, bronchospasm, headache, dizziness, convulsions, respiratory depression; drug should be discontinued if toxicity occurs

Teach patient/family:
• That drug is not a cure, it only relieves symptoms

P

• All aspects of drug: action, side effects, dose, when to notify physician
• To wear Medic Alert ID specifying myasthenia gravis, drugs taken

---

pyridoxine HCl (vitamin B₆)

(peer-i-dox-een)

Beesix, HexaBetalin, Hexacrest

Func. class.: Vitamin B_6, water soluble

Action: Needed for fat, protein, carbohydrate metabolism; enhances glycogen release from liver and muscle tissue; needed as coenzyme for metabolic transformations of a variety of amino acids

Uses: Vitamin B_6 deficiency associated with inborn errors of metabolism, seizures, isoniazid therapy, or oral contraceptives

Dosage and routes:
Vitamin B₆ deficiency
• *Adult:* PO/IM/IV 10-20 mg qd × 3 wk, then 2-5 mg qd
• *Child:* PO/IM/IV 100 mg until desired response
Inborn errors of metabolism
• *Adult:* IM/IV/PO 600 mg or less qd, then 50 mg qd for life
• *Child:* IM/PO/IV 100 mg, then 2-10 mg IM or 10-100 mg PO qd
Deficiency caused by isoniazid
• *Adult:* PO 100 mg qd × 3 wk, then 50 mg qd
• *Child:* PO dose titrated to patient response
Prevention of deficiency caused by isoniazid
• *Adult:* PO 25-50 mg qd
• *Child:* PO 0.5-1.5 mg qd
• *Infant:* PO 0.1-0.5 mg qd
Available forms include: Tabs 10, 25, 50, 100, 200, 250, 500 mg; tabs time released 500 mg; inj IM-IV 100 mg/ml

Side effects/adverse reactions:
CNS: Paresthesia, flushing, warmth, lethargy (rare with normal renal function)
INTEG: Pain at injection site
Contraindications: Hypersensitivity
Precautions: Pregnancy (increased doses), lactation, children, Parkinson's disease
Pharmacokinetics:
PO/INJ: Half-life 2-3 wk, metabolized in liver, excreted in urine
Interactions/incompatibilities:
• Decreased effects of: levodopa
• Decreased effects of this drug: oral contraceptives, INH, cycloserine, hydralazine, penicillamine
NURSING CONSIDERATIONS
Assess:
• Pyridoxine levels throughout treatment
Evaluate:
• Therapeutic response: absence of nausea, vomiting, anorexia, skin lesions, glossitis, stomatitis, edema, convulsions, restlessness
• Nutritional status: yeast, liver, legumes, bananas, green vegetables, whole grains
Teach patient/family:
• To avoid vitamin supplements unless directed by physician
• To keep out of children's reach
• To increase meat, bananas, potatoes, lima beans, whole grain cereals

---

pyrimethamine

(peer-i-meth'a-meen)

Daraprim, Fansidar (with sulfadoxine)

Func. class.: Antimalarial
Chem. class.: Folic acid antagonist

Action: Inhibits folic acid metabolism in parasite, prevents transmission by stopping growth of fertilized gametes

Uses: Malaria, prophylaxis, toxo-plasmodium vivax

Dosage and routes:

Prophylaxis of malaria

• *Adult:* PO 1 tab q wk or 2 tabs q 2 wk (Fansidar)

• *Child 9-14 yr:* PO ¾ tab q wk or 1½ tabs q 2 wk (Fansidar)

• *Child >10 yr:* PO 25 mg q wk

• *Child 4-10 yr:* PO 12.5 mg q wk

• *Child 4-8 yr:* PO ½ tab q wk or 1 tab q 2 wk (Fansidar)

• *Child <4 yr:* PO ¼ tab q wk or ½ tab q 2 wk (Fansidar)

• *Child <4 yr:* PO 6.25 mg q wk

Acute attacks of malaria

• *Adult:* PO 2-3 tabs as a single dose (Fansidar) alone or with qui-nine or primaquine

• *Child 9-14 yr:* 2 tabs

• *Child 4-8 yr:* 1 tab

• *Child <4 yr:* ½ tab

Toxoplasmosis

• *Adult:* PO 100 mg, then 25 mg qd × 4-5 wk, with 1 g sulfadiazine q6h

• *Child:* PO 1 mg/kg, then 0.25 mg/kg qd × 4-5 wk, with sulfa-diazine 100 mg/kg/day in divided doses q6h

Available forms include: Tabs 25 mg; combo tabs 500 mg

Side effects/adverse reactions:

RESP: **Failure**

INTEG: Skin eruptions, photosen-sitivity

CNS: Stimulation, irritability, ***con-vulsion,*** tremors, ataxia, fatigue

GI: Nausea, vomiting, cramps, an-orexia, diarrhea, atrophic glossitis, gastritis

HEMA: ***Thrombocytopenia, leuko-penia, pancytopenia, megaloblas-tic anemia,*** decreased folic acid, agranulocytosis

Contraindications: Hypersensitiv-ity, chloroquanide-resistant ma-laria, megaloblastic anemia caused by folate deficiency

Precautions: Blood dyscrasias, seizure disorder, pregnancy

Pharmacokinetics:

PO: Peak 2 hr, half-life 111 hr; me-tabolized in liver, highly protein bound, excreted in urine (metabo-lites)

Interactions/incompatibilities:

• Synergestic action: para-amino-benzoic acis or folic acid

NURSING CONSIDERATIONS

Assess:

• Folic acid level, megaloblastic anemia occurs

• Blood studies, CBC, platelets, since blood dyscrasias occur; twice weekly if dosage is increased

Administer:

• Leucovorin IM 3-9 mg/day × 3 days if folic acid deficiency occurs

• Before or after meals at same time each day to maintain drug level to decrease GI symptoms

Perform/provide:

• Storage in tight, light-resistant containers

Evaluate:

• For toxicity: vomiting, anorexia, seizure, blood dyscrasia, glossitis; drug should be discontinued im-mediately

Teach patient/family:

• To report visual problems, fever, fatigue, bruising, bleeding; may in-dicate blood dyscrasias

Treatment of overdose: Gastric lavage, administer short-acting bar-biturate, leucovorin, respiratory support if needed

---

pyrvinium pamoate

(peer-vin'ee-um)

Pamovin,* Povan, Vanquin*

Func. class.: Anthelmintic

Chem. class.: Cyanine dye

Action: Depletes carbohydrates,

---

prevents use of exogenous carbohydrates in worm

Uses: Pinworms

Dosage and routes:

• *Adult and child:* PO 5 mg/kg as
single dose, not to exceed 350 mg;
repeat in 2 wk

Available forms include: Tabs
50 mg

Side effects/adverse reactions:

INTEG: Rash, photosensitivity

CNS: Dizziness

GI: Nausea, vomiting, anorexia,
diarrhea, cramps

Contraindications: Hypersensitivity, intestinal obstruction, GI inflammatory conditions

Precautions: Renal disease, hepatic disease, pregnancy

Pharmacokinetics:

PO: Excreted in feces, urine

Interactions/incompatibilities:
None known

NURSING CONSIDERATIONS

Assess:

• Stools periodically during entire
treatment; specimens must be sent
to lab while still warm

Administer:

• Laxatives if constipated; not
needed for drug to work

• Through straw (emulsion) to
avoid staining teeth

• With fruit juice or milk

Perform/provide:

• Storage protected from light

Evaluate:

• For therapeutic response: expulsion of worms, 3 negative stool cultures after completion of treatment

• For allergic reaction: rash

• For infection in other family
members, since infection from person to person is common

• For diarrhea during expulsion of
worms

Teach patient/family:

• Proper hygiene after BM including handwashing technique; tell pa-

tient to avoid putting fingers in
mouth

• That infected person should sleep
alone; do not shake bed linen,
change bed linen qd, wash in hot
water

• To clean toilet qd with disinfectant (green soap solution)

• Need for compliance with dosage
schedule, duration of treatment

• Stools will stain clothes red if
feces contact clothing

• That follow-up is needed in 5 wk
after end of therapy

---

quinacrine HCl

(kwin'a-kreen)

Atabrine

Func. class.: Anthelmintic

Chem. class.: Acridine dye derivative

Action: Causes worm scolex to de-
tach from GI tract

Uses: Giardiasis, tapeworms (ces-
todiasis), malaria

Dosage and routes:

• *Adult:* PO 100 mg × 5-7 days

• *Child:* PO 7 mg/kg/day in 3 divided doses pc × 5 days, not to
exceed 300 mg/day; may repeat in
2 wk if needed

Available forms include: Tabs
100 mg

Side effects/adverse reactions:

INTEG: Rash, dermatitis, yellow
pigmentation of skin, urticaria

CNS: Dizziness, headache, insomnia, restlessness, confusion, behavioral changes, psychosis, convulsions

EENT: Bad taste, oral irritation, corneal deposits, retinopathy

GI: Nausea, vomiting, anorexia,
diarrhea, cramps, hepatitis

HEMA: Aplastic anemia, agranulocytosis

Contraindications: Hypersensitivity, porphyria, psoriasis

Precautions: Seizure disorders, elderly, psychosis, alcoholism, hepatic disease, depression, child <12 yr, G-6-PD deficiency, pregnancy

Pharmacokinetics:

PO: Peak 8 hr, metabolized by the liver (slowly), excreted primarily in urine, crosses placenta, high protein bindings

Interactions/incompatibilities:

• Increased toxicity: primaquine, hepatotoxic drugs

• Disulfiram-like reaction: alcohol

NURSING CONSIDERATIONS

Assess:

• Stools during entire treatment, collect entire stools × 48 hr, pass through sieve, check for scolex (yellow tapeworms)

• CBC, ophthalmic exam if used for long-term treatment

• Stools 2 wk after last dose for giardiasis

Administer:

• 1-3 mo for malaria

• By duodenal tube for pork tapeworm; prevents vomiting, transportation of parasites into stomach

• Bland liquid diet, no fat, or no-residue 24-48 hr before beginning therapy; patient should be fasting night before, given saline enemas, cleansing enema before beginning therapy (tapeworms only)

• Laxatives before treatment to cleanse bowel

• After meals with fluids for giardiasis, malaria

• In jam or honey to disguise bitter taste of pulverized tablets (children)

Perform/provide:

• Storage in tight containers

Evaluate:

• For therapeutic response: expulsion of worms, 3 negative stool cultures after completion of treatment

• For allergic reaction (rash), visual problems (halos, blurring, inability to focus)

• For infection in other family members since infection from person to person is common

• Mental status: affect, mood, behavioral changes

Teach patient/family:

• Proper hygiene after BM including handwashing technique; tell patient to avoid putting fingers in 235uth

• To clean toilet qd with disinfectant (green soap solution)

• Need for compliance with dosage schedule, duration of treatment

• That skin, urine may turn deep yellow

• To report any visual changes

Lab test interferences:

False positive: Adrenal function tests

Increase: 17-OHCS (Mattingly method)

Treatment of overdose: Induce vomiting

---

quinestrol

(kwin-ess'trole)

Estrovis

Func. class.: Estrogen

Chem. class.: Nonsteroidal synthetic estrogen

Action: Needed for adequate functioning of female reproductive system; affects release of pituitary gonadotropins, inhibits ovulation, promotes adequate calcium use in bone structures

Uses: Menopause, atrophic vaginitis, kraurosis vulvae, female castration, female hypogonadism, primary ovarian failure

Dosage and routes:

• *Adult:* PO 100 μg qd × 1 wk, then 100 μg q wk starting 2 wk after beginning treatment; may increase to 200 μg/wk

Available forms include: Tabs 100 µg

Side effects/adverse reactions:

CNS: Dizziness, headache, migraine, depression

CV: Hypotension, thrombophlebitis, edema, *thromboembolism, stroke, pulmonary embolism, myocardial infarction*

GI: Nausea, vomiting, diarrhea, anorexia, pancreatitis, cramps, constipation, increased appetite, increased weight, cholestatic jaundice

EENT: Contact lens intolerance, increased myopia, astigmatism

GU: Amenorrhea, cervical erosion, breakthrough bleeding, dysmenorrhea, vaginal candidiasis, breast changes, *gynecomastia, testicular atrophy, impotence*

INTEG: Rash, urticaria, acne, hirsutism, alopecia, oily skin, seborrhea, purpura, melasma

META: Folic acid deficiency, hypercalcemia, hyperglycemia

Contraindications: Breast cancer, thromboembolic disorders, reproductive cancer, genital bleeding (abnormal, undiagnosed), pregnancy (X)

Precautions: Hypertension, asthma, blood dyscrasias, gallbladder disease, CHF, diabetes mellitus, bone disease, depression, migraine headache, convulsive disorders, hepatic disease, renal disease, family history of cancer of breast or reproductive tract

Pharmacokinetics:

PO: Degraded in liver, excreted in urine, crosses placenta, excreted in breast milk

Interactions/incompatibilities:

• Decreased action of: anticoagulants, oral hypoglycemics

• Toxicity: tricyclic antidepressants

• Decreased action of this drug: anticonvulsants, barbiturates, phenylbutazone, rifampin

• Increased action of: corticosteroids

NURSING CONSIDERATIONS

Assess:

• Urine glucose in patient with diabetes; increased urine glucose may occur

• Weight daily, notify physician of weekly weight gain >5 lb; if increase, diurectic may be ordered

• B/P q4h, watch for increase caused by water and sodium retention

• I&O ratio, be alert for decreasing urinary output and increasing edema

• Liver function studies, including AST, ALT, bilirubin, alk phosphatase

Administer:

• Titrated dose, use lowest effective dose

• With food or milk to decrease GI symptoms

Evaluate:

• Therapeutic response: absence of breast engorgement, reversal of menopause or decrease in tumor size in prostatic cancer

• Edema, hypertension, cardiac symptoms, jaundice, calcemia

• Mental status: affect mood, behavioral changes, aggression

Teach patient/family:

• To weigh weekly, report gain >5 lb

• To report breast lumps, vaginal bleeding, edema, jaundice, dark urine, clay-colored stools, dyspnea, headache, blurred vision, abdominal pain, numbness or stiffness in legs, chest pain; male to report impotence or gynecomastia

• To avoid sunlight or wear sunscreen; burns may occur

quinethazone

(kwin-eth′a-zone)

Aquamox,* Hydromox

Func. class.: Diuretic

Chem. class.: Thiazide-like; quin-azoline derivative

Action: Acts on distal tubule by increasing excretion of water, sodium, chloride, potassium

Uses: Edema, hypertension

Dosage and routes:

• *Adult:* PO 50-100 mg/day, may need doses up to 150-200 mg/day

Available forms include: Tabs 50 mg

Side effects/adverse reactions:

GU: Frequency, polyuria, uremia, glucosuria

CNS: Drowsiness, paresthesia, anxiety, depression, headache, dizziness, fatigue, weakness

GI: Nausea, vomiting, anorexia, constipation, diarrhea, cramps, pancreatitis, GI irritation, *hepatitis*

EENT: Blurred vision

INTEG: Rash, urticaria, purpura, photosensitivity, fever

META: Hyperglycemia, hyperuricemia, increased creatinine

HEMA: Aplastic anemia, hemolytic anemia, leukopenia, agranulocytosis, thrombocytopenia

CV: Irregular pulse, orthostatic hypotension

ELECT: Hypokalemia, hypercalcemia, hyponatremia, hypochloremia

Contraindications: Hypersensitivity to thiazides or sulfonamides, anuria, renal decompensation

Precautions: Hypokalemia, renal disease, pregnancy, hepatic disease, gout, COPD, lupus erythematosus, diabetes mellitus

Pharmacokinetics:

PO: Onset 2 hr, peak 6 hr, duration 18-24 hr; excreted unchanged by kidneys, crosses placenta, enters breast milk

Interactions/incompatibilities:

• Increased toxicity of: lithium, nondepolarizing skeletal muscle relaxants, digitalis

• Decreased effects of: antidiabetics

• Decreased absorption of thiazides: cholestyramine, colestipol

• Decreased hypotensive response: indomethacin

• Increased action of: quinidine

NURSING CONSIDERATIONS

Assess:

• Weight, I&O daily to determine fluid loss; effect of drug may be decreased if used qd

• Rate, depth, rhythm of respiration, effect of exertion

• B/P lying, standing; postural hypotension may occur

• Electrolytes: potassium, sodium, chloride; include BUN, blood sugar, CBC, serum creatinine, blood pH, ABGs

• Glucose in urine if patient is diabetic

Administer:

• In AM to avoid interference with sleep if using drug as a diuretic

• Potassium replacement if potassium is less than 3.0

• With food, if nausea occurs, absorption may be decreased slightly

Evaluate:

• Improvement in edema of feet, legs, sacral area daily if medication is being used in CHF

• Improvement of CVP q8h

• Signs of metabolic acidosis: drowsiness, restlessness

• Signs of hypokalemia: postural hypotension, malaise, fatigue, tachycardia, leg cramps, weakness

• Rashes, temperature elevation qd

• Confusion, especially in elderly; take safety precautions if needed

Teach patient/family:

• To increase fluid intake 2-3 L/day

---

italics = common side effects   **bold italic** = life threatening reactions

unless contraindicated; to rise slowly from lying or sitting position
• To notify physician of muscle weakness, cramps, nausea, dizziness
• Drug may be taken with food or milk
• That blood sugar may be increased in diabetics
• Take early in day to avoid nocturia

Lab test interferences:
Increase: BSP retention, calcium, amylase
Decrease: PBI, PSP

Treatment of overdose: Lavage if taken orally, monitor electrolytes, administer dextrose in saline

---

quinidine gluconate/ quinidine polygalacturonate/quinidine sulfate

(kwin'i-deen)

Duraquin,* Quinaglute Dura-Tabs, Quinate, Quinatime, Quin-Release/Cardioquin, Cin-Quin, Novoquindin, Quine, Quinidex Extentabs, Quinora

Func. class.: Antidysrhythmic (Class IA)
Chem. class.: Quinine destro isomer

Action: Increases electrical stimulation threshold of ventrical, HIS Purkinge system, which stabilizes cardiac membrane

Uses: PVCs, atrial fibrillation, PAT, ventricular tachycardia, atrial dysrhythmias, ventricular tachycardia

Dosage and routes:
Atrial fibrillation/flutter
• *Adult:* PO 200 mg q2-3h × 5-8 doses, may increase qd until sinus rhythm is restored; to be given only after digitalization

Paroxysmal supraventricular tachycardia
• *Adult:* IM 400-600 mg q2-3h (gluconate)
All other dysrhythmias
• *Adult:* PO 50-200 mg as a test dose, then 200-400 mg q4-6h; IM 600 mg, then 400 mg q2h, after test dose (gluconate); IV INF 800 mg in 40 ml D_5W run at 16 mg/min
• *Child:* PO 2 mg/kg test dose, then 3-6 mg/kg q2-3h × 5 doses
Available forms include: (Gluconate) tabs sus rel 324, 330 mg; inj IM (sulfate) tabs 100, 200, 300 mg; caps 200, 300 mg; tabs sus rel 300 mg; inj IV (polygalacturonate) tabs 275 mg

Side effects/adverse reactions:
CNS: Headache, dizziness, involuntary movement, confusion, psychosis, restlessness, irritability, paresthesias
EENT: Tinnitus, blurred vision, hearing loss
GI: Nausea, vomiting, anorexia, diarrhea
CV: Hypotension, bradycardia, PVCs, *heart block, cardiovascular collapse, arrest*
HEMA: Thrombocytopenia
RESP: Dyspnea, *respiratory depression*
INTEG: Rash, urticaria, edema, swelling

Contraindications: Hypersensitivity, blood dyscrasias, severe heart block

Precautions: Pregnancy, lactation, children, renal disease, liver disease, CHF, respiratory depression, myasthenia gravis

Pharmacokinetics:
PO: Onset 2-3 hr, peak 1-3 hr, duration 6-8 hr; half-life 6-7 hr, metabolized in liver, excreted unchanged by kidneys

Interactions/incompatibilities:
• May increase effects of neuromuscular blockers, digoxin when

used with this drug

• May increase effects when used with: cimetidine, phenytoin, propranolol

• May decrease effects of this drug: barbiturates

NURSING CONSIDERATIONS
Assess:

• ECG continuously to determine increased PR or QRS segments; if these develop, discontinue immediately

• IV infusion rate using infusion pump, run at less than 4 mg/min

• Blood levels (therapeutic level 3-8 mEq/ml)

• B/P continuously for fluctuations
Administer:

• IM injection in deltoid; aspirate to avoid intravascular administration

Evaluate:

• Malignant hyperthermia: tachypnea, tachycardia, changes in B/P, increased temperature

• Cardiac rate, respiration: rate, rhythm, character, continuously

• Respiratory status: rate, rhythm, lung fields for rales

• CNS effects: dizziness, confusion, psychosis, paresthesias, convulsions; drug should be discontinued

• Lung fields, bilateral rales may occur in CHF patient

• Increased respiration, increased pulse; drug should be discontinued
Lab test interferences:

Increase: CPK

Treatment of overdose: O_2, artificial ventilation, ECG, administer dopamine for circulatory depression, administer diazepam or thiopental for convulsions

quinine sulfate
(kwye′nine)

Novoquine,* Quinamm, Quine, Quinite, Quiphile, Strema, Quin-260

Func. class.: Antimalarial
Chem. class.: Cinchoma tree alkaloid

Action: Inhibits parasite replications, transcription of DNA to RNA by forming complexes with DNA of parasite

Uses: *Plasmodium falciparum* malaria, nocturnal leg cramps

Dosage and routes:

• *Adult:* PO 650 mg q8h × 10 days, given with pyrimethamine 25 mg q12h × 3 days, with sulfadiazine 500 mg qid × 5 days; IV INF 600 mg over 1 hr for severe infections q6-8h

Available forms include: Caps 130, 195, 200, 300, 325 mg; tabs 260, 325 mg

Side effects/adverse reactions:

RESP: Dysuria

INTEG: Pruritus, pigmentary changes, skin eruptions, lichen planus–like eruptions, flushing, facial edema, sweating

HEMA: Thrombocytopenia, purpura, hypothrombinemia, hemolysis

CNS: Headache, stimulation, fatigue, irritability, ***convulsion,*** bad dreams, dizziness, fever, confusion, anxiety

EENT: Blurred vision, corneal changes, retinal changes, difficulty focusing, tinnitus, vertigo, deafness, photophobia, diplopia, night blindness

GI: Nausea, vomiting, anorexia, diarrhea, epigastric pain

CV: Angina, dysrhythmias, tachycardia, hypotension, ***acute circulatory failure***

ENDO: Hypoglycemia

Contraindications: Hypersensitivity, G-6-PD deficiency, retinal field changes, pregnancy (X)

Precautions: Blood dyscrasias, severe GI disease, neurologic disease, severe hepatic disease, psoriasis, cardiac dysrhythmias

Pharmacokinetics:

PO: Peak 1-3 hr, metabolized in liver, excreted in urine, half-life 4-5 hr

Interactions/incompatibilities:

• Toxicity: NaHCO₃, acetazolamide

• Decreased absorption: magnesium or aluminum salts

• Increase levels of digoxin, digitoxin, neuromuscular blockers, other anticoagulants

NURSING CONSIDERATIONS

Assess:

• B/P, pulse, if administered IV, watch for hypotension, tachycardia

• Liver studies weekly: ALT, AST, bilirubin

• Blood studies, CBC, since blood dyscrasias occur

Administer:

• By slow IV

• Before or after meals at same time each day to maintain drug level

Perform/provide:

• Storage in tight, light-resistant container

Evaluate:

• For cinchonism: nausea, blurred vision, tinnitus, headache, difficulty focusing

Teach patient/family:

• To avoid OTC preparations: cold preparations, tonic water

Lab test interferences:

Increase: 17-KS

Interference: 17-OHCS

rabies immune globulin, human

Hyperab, Imogam

Func. class.: Immune serum
Chem. class.: IgG

Action: Provides passive immunity; given with HDCV; may be used regardless of time of bite, treatment

Uses: Exposure to rabies

Dosage and routes:

• *Adult and child:* IM 20 IU/kg given at same time as 1st rabies vaccine; infiltrate wound with ½ dose, then administer rest IM

Available forms include: Inj IM 125 IU/ml

Side effects/adverse reactions:

INTEG: Pain at injection site, rash, pruritus

MS: Arthralgia

SYST: Lymphadenopathy, *anaphylaxis*

CNS: Headache, fatigue, malaise

GI: Abdominal pain

Contraindications: Hypersensitivity to equine products

Interactions/incompatibilities:

• Decreased action of this drug: corticosteroids, immunosuppressants

NURSING CONSIDERATIONS

Administer:

• Test dose: dilute drug either with 1:100 or 1:1000 0.9% NaCl for injection, inject 0.1 ml 0.9% NaCl in other arm intradermally, check for wheal 10 mm or > after 10 min; if present, drug should not be used

• Only after epinephrine 1:1000, resuscitative equipment are available

• Only if human immune serum is not available

Evaluate:

• Allergic reactions: dyspnea, rash, pruritus, eruptions

radioactive iodine (sodium iodide) [131]I

Func. class.: Radiopharmaceutical antineoplastic antithyroid

Action: Converted to protein-bound iodine by thyroid gland for use when needed

Uses: Thyroid cancer, hyperthyroidism, thyrotoxicosis, visualization to determine thyroid cancer, diagnostic aid in thyroid function studies

Dosage and routes:
Thyroid cancer
• *Adult:* PO 50-150 mCi, may repeat depending on clinical status
Hyperthyroidism
• *Adult:* PO 4-10 mCi, depending on serum thyroxine level

Available forms include: Caps 1-50, 0.8-100 mCi; oral sol 7.05, 3.5-150 mCi/ml

Side effects/adverse reactions:
ENDO: Hypothyroidism, hyperthyroid adenoma, transient thyroiditis
INTEG: Rash, urticaria, angineurotic edema, acne, mucosal hemorrhage, fever, petechiae, alopecia
CNS: Headache, confusion, paresthesias
*HEMA: **Eosinophilia, lymphedema***
GI: Nausea, diarrhea, vomiting, small bowel lesions, upper gastric pain
MS: Myalgia, arthralgia, weakness
EENT: Metallic taste, stomatitis, salivation, periorbital edema

Contraindications: Recent MI, lactation, large nodular goiter, pregnancy, <30 yr, vomiting/diarrhea, acute hyperthyroidism, use of thyroid drugs

Precautions: Renal disease, cardiac disease

Pharmacokinetics:
PO: Onset 3-6 days, excreted in urine, sweat, feces, crosses placenta, excreted in breast milk, excreted in 56 days

Interactions/incompatibilities:
• May increase action when used with lithium
• Decreased uptake if recent intake of stable iodine, thyroid, antithyroid drugs

NURSING CONSIDERATIONS
Assess:
• Weight qd in same clothing, scale, time of day
• Blood work, including CBC for blood dyscrasias (leukopenia, thrombocytopenia, agranulocytosis)

Administer:
• Only after discontinuing all other thyroid agents × 5-7 days
• After NPO overnight, food delays action
• After menstruation (10 days) or during

Perform/provide:
• Limited contact with patient ½ hr/day for each person
• Adequate rest after treatment
• Fluids to 3-4 L/day for 48 hr after agent is administered to remove agent from body

Evaluate:
• Therapeutic effect: weight gain, decreased pulse, decreased T_4, B/P
• Overdose: peripheral edema, heat intolerance, diaphoresis, palpitations, dysrhythmias, severe tachycardia, increased temperature delirium, CNS irritability
• Hypersensitivity: rash, enlarged cervical lymph nodes; drug may need to be discontinued
• Hypoprothrombinemia: bleeding, petechiae, ecchymosis
• Clinical response: after 3 wk should include increased weight, pulse; decreased T_4
• Bone marrow depression: sore throat, fever, fatigue

R

---

italics = common side effects   ***bold italic*** = life threatening reactions

Teach patient/family:
• To empty bladder often during treatment, avoids radiation of gonads
• Report redness, swelling, sore throat, mouth lesions; indicate blood dyscrasias
• To avoid extended contact with children or spouse for 1 week
• That bathroom may be used by entire family
• Not to take antithyroid agents but propranolol, which decreases hyperthyroid symptoms, until total effects of ^{131}I has taken effect (about 6 wk)
• Avoid coughing, expectorating for 24 hr (saliva and vomiting are highly radioactive for 6-8 hr)

---

ranitidine
(ra-nye' te-deen)
Zantac

Func. class.: Antihistamine — H_2 receptor antagonist

Action: Inhibits histamine at H_2 receptor site in parietal cells, which inhibits gastric acid secretion
Uses: Duodenal ulcer, Zollinger-Ellison syndrome
Dosage and routes:
• *Adult:* PO 150 mg bid; IM 50 mg q6-8h; IV BOL 50 mg diluted to 20 ml over 5 min; IV INT INF 50 mg/100 ml D_5 over 15-20 min
Available forms include: Tabs 150, 300 mg; inj 25 mg/ml IM, IV
Side effects/adverse reactions:
CNS: Headache, sleeplessness, dizziness, confusion, agitation, depression, hallucination
GI: Constipation, abdominal pain, diarrhea, nausea, vomiting, *hepatotoxicity*
GU: Impotence, gynecomastia
CV: Tachycardia, bradycardia, PVCs

EENT: Blurred vision, increased ocular pressure
INTEG: Urticaria, rash, fever, allergic reactions
SYST: **Anaphylaxis**
Contraindications: Hypersensitivity
Precautions: Pregnancy (B), lactation, child <12 yr, hepatic disease, renal disease
Pharmacokinetics:
PO: Peak 2-3 hr, duration 8-12 hr; metabolized by liver, excreted in urine, breast milk, half-life 2-3 hr
Interactions/incompatibilities:
• Decreased action of this drug: antacids

NURSING CONSIDERATIONS
Assess:
• Gastric pH (>5 should be maintained)
• I&O ratio, BUN, creatinine
Administer
• With meals for prolonged drug effect
• Antacids 1 hr before or 1 hr after ranitidine
• IV slowly, bradycardia may occur, give over 30 min
Perform/provide:
• Storage at room temperature
Evaluate:
• Mental status: confusion, dizziness, depression, anxiety, weakness, tremors, psychosis, diarrhea, abdominal discomfort, jaundice; report immediately
• GI complaints: nausea, vomiting, diarrhea, cramps
Teach patient/family:
• That gynecomastia, impotence may occur but are reversible
• Avoid driving or other hazardous activities until patient is stabilized on this medication
• To avoid black pepper, caffeine, alcohol, harsh spices, extremes in temperature of food
• To avoid OTC preparations: aspirin, cough, cold preparations

---

*Available in Canada only

Lab test interferences:
Increase: AST/ALT, alk phosphatase, creatinine, LDH, bilirubin
False positive: Urine protein

---

rauwolfia serpentina

(rah-wool'fee-a)
Raudixin, Raumason, Raupoid, Rausertina, Rauwoldin, Wolfina
Func. class.: Antihypertensive
Chem. class.: Antiadrenergic agent

Action: Inhibits norepinephrine release, depleting norepinephrine stores in adrenergic nerve endings
Uses: Hypertension, as antipsychotic agent
Dosage and routes:
• *Adult:* PO initial 200-400 mg qd or in 2 divided doses, maintenance 50 mg-300 mg qd or in 2 divided doses
Available forms include: Tabs 50, 100 mg
Side effects/adverse reactions:
CV: Bradycardia, chest pain, dysrhythmias
HEMA: Prolonged bleeding time, *thrombocytopenia,* purpura
CNS: Drowsiness, fatigue, lethargy, dizziness, depression, anxiety, headache, increased dreaming, nightmares, convulsions, Parkinson's, EPS (high doses)
GI: Nausea, vomiting, cramps, peptic ulcer, dry mouth, increased appetite, anorexia
INTEG: Rash, alopecia, flushing, warm feeling, pruritus, ecchymosis
EENT: Lacrimation, miosis, blurred vision, ptosis, dry mouth, epistaxis, glaucoma
GU: Impotence, dysuria, nocturia, sodium, water retention, edema, breast engorgement, galactorrhea, gynecomastia
RESP: Bronchospasm, dyspnea, cough, rales
Contraindications: Hypersensitivity, depression/suicidal patients, active peptic ulcer disease, ulcerative colitis, pheochromocytoma, bronchial asthma
Precautions: Pregnancy (C), lactation, seizure disorder
Pharmacokinetics:
PO: Peak 3-6 days, duration 2-6 wk; half-life 50-100 hr, metabolized by liver, excreted in urine, feces, crosses placenta, blood-brian barrier, excreted in breast milk
Interactions/incompatibilities:
• Increased hypotension: diuretics, hypotension, β-blockers, methotrimeprazine
• Dysrhythmias: cardiac glycosides
• Increased cardiac depression: quinidine, procainamide
• Excitation, hypertension: MAOIs
• Increased CNS depression: barbiturates, alcohol, narcotics
• Decreased pressor effects: epinephrine, isoproterenol, norepinephrine
• Decreased pressor effects: ephedrine, amphetamines

NURSING CONSIDERATIONS
Assess:
• Renal function studies in renal impairment (BUN, creatinine)
• Bleeding time, check for ecchymosis, thrombocytopenia, purpura
• I&O in renal disease patient
Evaluate:
• Cardiac status: B/P, pulse, watch for hypotension
• Edema in feet, legs daily; take weight daily
• Skin turgor, dryness of mucous membranes for hydration status
• Symptoms of CHF: edema, dyspnea, wet rales
Teach patient/family:
• To avoid driving, hazardous activities if drowsiness occurs
• Not to discontinue drug abruptly
• Not to use OTC products (cough,

R

---

italics = common side effects   ***bold italic*** = life threatening reactions

cold preparations) unless directed by physician
• To report bradycardia, dizziness, confusion, depression, fever, sore throat
• That impotence, gynecomastia may occur but is reversible
• To rise slowly to sitting or standing position to minimize orthostatic hypotension
• That therapeutic effect may take 2-4 wk

Lab test interferences:
Increase: VMA excretion, 5-HIAA excretion
Interferences: 17-OHCS, 17-KS
Treatment of overdose: Lavage, IV atropine for bradycardia, supportive therapy

---

regular insulin

Beef Regular Iletin II, Humulin R, Iletin Regular,* Novolin R, Pork Regular Iletin II, Regular Iletin I, Regular Pork Insulin, Velosulin

Func. class.: Antidiabetic
Chem. class.: Exogenous unmodified insulin

Action: Decreases blood sugar, increases blood pyruvate, lactate, decreases phosphate, potassium
Uses: Adult-onset diabetes, juvenile diabetes, ketoacidosis
Dosage and routes:
Ketoacidosis
• *Adult:* IV/IM 5-10 U, then 5-10 U/hr until desired response, then switch to SC dose; IV/INF 2-12 U (50 U/500 ml of normal saline)
• *Child:* IV/IM 0.1 U/kg
Replacement
• *Adult:* SC dosage individualized by blood, urine glucose levels, up to qid given ½ hr before meals
Available forms include: IV/IM/ SC inj U 40, U 100

Side effects/adverse reactions:
CNS: Headache, lethargy, tremors, weakness, fatigue, delirium, sweating
CV: Tachycardia, palpitations
EENT: Blurred vision
GI: Hunger, nausea
META: Hypoglycemia
INTEG: Flushing, rash, urticaria, warmth
*SYST: **Anaphylaxis***
Contraindications: Hypersensitivity
Interactions/incompatibilities:
• Increased hypoglycemia: salicylate, alcohol, β-blockers, anabolic steroids, fenfluramine, guanethidine, oral hypoglycemics, MAOIs, tetracycline, clofibrate
• Hyperglycemia: thiazides, thyroid hormones, triamterene, phenothiazines, phenytoin, oral contraceptives, corticosteroids, estrogens, lithium
• Mask signs/symptoms of hypoglycemia: β-blocker
Pharmacokinetics:
SC: Onset 30-60 min, peak 2-3 hr, duration 5-7 hr, half-life 4 hr
IV: Onset 10-30 min, peak 30-60 min, duration 1-2 hr, half-life 3-5 min
Metabolized by liver, muscle, kidneys, excreted in urine
NURSING CONSIDERATIONS
Assess:
• Fasting blood glucose, 2 hr PP (60-100 mg/dl normal fasting level) (70-130 mg/dl-normal 2 hr level)
Administer:
• After warming to room temperature by rotating in palms, to prevent lipodystrophy (from injecting cold insulin)
• ½ hr ac, so peak action coincides with peak sugar level
• Increased doses if tolerance occurs

• Human insulin to those allergic to beef or pork
• IV after diluting with 0.9% NaCl injection

Perform/provide:
• Storage at room temperature for <1 month, refrigerate all other supply, do not use discolored, or cloudy solution
• Rotation of injection sites: abdomen, upper back, thighs, upper arm, buttocks; keep record of sites

Evaluate:
• Therapeutic response: decrease in polyuria, polydipsia, polyphagia, clear sensorium, absence of dizziness, stable gait
• Hypoglycemic/hyperglycemic reaction that can occur soon after meals

Teach patient/family:
• That blurred vision occurs, not to change corrective lens until vision is stabilized 1-2 mo
• To keep insulin, equipment available at all times
• That drug does not cure diabetes, but controls symptoms
• To carry Medic Alert ID as diabetic
• Hypoglycemia reaction: headache, tremors, fatigue, weakness, sweating
• Dosage, route, mixing instructions if any diet restrictions, disease process
• To carry candy or lump sugar to treat hypoglycemia
• Symptoms of ketoacidosis: nausea, thirst, polyuria, dry mouth, decrease B/P, dry, flushed skin, acetone breath, drowsiness, Kussmaul respirations
• That a plan is necessary for diet, exercise; all food on diet should be eaten, exercise routine should not vary
• Urine glucose testing, make sure patient is able to determine glucose, acetone levels, also home blood glucose monitoring
• The pregnant patient to use glucose oxidase reagents
• To avoid OTC drugs unless directed by physician

Lab test interferences:
Increase: VMA
Decrease: Potassium, calcium
Interference: Liver function studies, thyroid function studies
Treatment of overdose: 10%-50% glucose PO if conscious or IV if comatose

---

regular insulin concentrated

Regular (concentrated) Iletin II U-500

Func. class.: Antidiabetic
Chem. class.: Exogenous unmodified insulin

Action: Decreases blood sugar, increases blood pyruvate, lactate, decreases phosphate, potassium
Uses: Treatment of diabetic patients with marked insulin resistance

Dosage and routes:
• *Adult:* SC/IM dosage individualized by blood, urine glucose qd-tid
Available forms include: Inj SC, IM

Side effects/adverse reactions:
CNS: Headache, lethargy, tremors, weakness, fatigue, delirium, sweating
CV: Tachycardia, palpitations
EENT: Blurred vision
GI: Hunger, nausea
META: Hypoglycemia
INTEG: Flushing, rash, urticaria, warmth
*SYST: **Anaphylaxis***
Contraindications: Hypersensitivity

Pharmacokinetics:
SC: Onset 30-60 min, peak 2-5 hr, duration 5-7 hr, half-life 4 hr

R

---

italics = common side effects   ***bold italic*** = life threatening reactions

IV: Onset 10-30 min, peak 30-60 min, duration 1-2 hr, half-life 3-5 min

Metabolized by liver, muscle, kidneys, excreted in urine

Interactions/incompatibilities:

• Increased hypoglycemia: salicylate, alcohol, β-blockers, anabolic steroids, fenfluramine, guanethidine, oral hypoglycemics, MAOIs, tetracycline, clofibrate

• Hyperglycemia: thiazides, thyroid hormones, triamterene, phenothiazines, phenytoin, oral contraceptives, corticosteroids, estrogens, lithium

NURSING CONSIDERATIONS

Assess:

• Fasting blood glucose, 2 hr PP (60-100 mg/dl normal fasting level) (70-130 mg/dl-normal 2 hr level)

Administer:

• After warming to room temperature by rotating in palms, to prevent lipodystrophy from injecting cold insulin

• ½ hr ac, so peak action coincides with peak sugar level

• Increased doses if tolerance occurs

• Human insulin to those allergic to beef or pork

Perform/provide:

• Storage at room temperature for <1 mo, refrigerate all other supply, do not use discolored, or cloudy solution

• Rotation of injection sites: abdomen, upper back, thighs, upper arms, buttocks; keep record of sites

Evaluate:

• Therapeutic response: decrease in polyuria, polydipsia, polyphagia, clear sensorium, absence of dizziness, stable gait

• Hypoglycemic/hyperglycemic reaction that can occur soon after meals

Teach patient/family:

• That blurred vision occurs, not to change corrective lens until vision is stabilized 1-2 mo

• To keep insulin, equipment available at all times

• That drug does not cure diabetes, but controls symptoms

• To carry Medic Alert ID as diabetic

• Hypoglycemia reaction: headache, tremors, fatigue, weakness

• Dosage, route, mixing instructions if any diet restrictions, disease process

• To carry candy or lump sugar to treat hypoglycemia

• Symptoms of ketoacidosis: nausea, thirst, polyuria, dry mouth, decrease B/P, dry, flushed skin, acetone breath, drowsiness, Kussmaul respirations

• That a plan is necessary for diet, exercise; all food on diet should be eaten, exercise routine should not vary

• Urine glucose testing, make sure patient is able to determine glucose, acetone levels

• The pregnant patient to use glucose oxidase reagents

• To avoid OTC drugs unless directed by physician

Lab test interferences:

Increase: VMA

Decrease: Potassium, calcium

Interference: Liver function studies, thyroid function studies

Treatment of overdose: 10%-50% glucose PO if conscious or IV if comatose

---

rescinnamine

(re-sin′a-meen)

Anaprel, Moderil

Func. class.: Antihypertensive

Chem. class.: Antiadrenergic agent

Action: Inhibits norepinephrine re-

lease, depleting norepinephrine stores in adrenergic nerve endings
Uses: Hypertension, as antipsychotic agent
Dosage and routes:
• *Adult:* PO 0.5 mg bid, then 0.25-0.5 mg qd maintenance
Available forms include: Tabs 0.25, 0.5 mg
Side effects/adverse reactions:
CV: Bradycardia, chest pain, dysrhythmias, prolonged bleeding time, thrombocytopenia, purpura
CNS: Drowsiness, fatigue, lethargy, dizziness, depression, anxiety, headache, increased dreaming, nightmares, convulsions, Parkinsonism, EPS (high doses)
GI: Nausea, vomiting, cramps, peptic ulcer, dry mouth, increased appetite, anorexia
INTEG: Rash, purpura, alopecia, flushing, warm feeling, pruritus, ecchymosis
EENT: Lacrimation, miosis, blurred vision, ptosis, dry mouth, epistaxis
GU: Impotence, dysuria, nocturia, sodium, water retention, edema, breast engorgement, galactorrhea, gynecomastia
*RESP: **Bronchospasm,*** dyspnea, cough, rales
Contraindications: Hypersensitivity, depression/suicidal patients, active peptic ulcer disease, ulcerative colitis, ETC
Precautions: Pregnancy, lactation, seizure disorders
Pharmacokinetics:
PO: Peak 3-6 days, duration 2-6 wk; half-life 50-100 hr, metabolized by liver, excreted in urine, feces, crosses placenta, blood-brian barrier, excreted in breast milk
Interactions/incompatibilities:
• Increased hypotension: diuretics, hypotension, β-blockers, methotrimeprazine

• Dysrhythmias: cardiac glycosides
• Increased cardiac depression: quinidine, procainamide
• Excitation, hypertension: MAOIs
• Increased CNS depression: barbiturates, alcohol, narcotics
• Increased pressor effects: epinephrine, isoproterenol, norepinephrine
• Decreased pressor effects: ephedrine, amphetamines
NURSING CONSIDERATIONS
Assess:
• Renal function studies in renal impairment (BUN, creatinine)
• Bleeding time, check for ecchymosis, thrombocytopenia, purpura
• I&O in renal disease patient
Evaluate:
• Cardiac status: B/P, pulse, watch for hypotension
• Edema in feet, legs daily; take weight daily
• Skin turgor, dryness of mucous membranes for hydration status
• Symptoms of CHF: edema, dyspnea, wet rales
Teach patient/family:
• To avoid driving, hazardous activities if drowsiness occurs
• Not to discontinue drug abruptly
• Not to use OTC products (cough, cold preparations) unless directed by physician
• To report bradycardia, dizziness, confusion, depression, fever, sore throat
• That impotence, gynecomastia may occur but is reversible
• To rise slowly to sitting or standing position to minimize orthostatic hypotention
• That therapeutic effects may take 2-4 wk
Lab test interferences:
Increase: VMA excretion, 5-HIAA excretion
Interferences: 17-OHCS, 17-KS
Treatment of overdose: Lavage,

R

---

italics = common side effects   ***bold italic*** = life threatening reactions

IV atropine for bradycardia, supportive therapy

---

reserpine

(re-ser'peen)

Broserpine, Elserpine, Hyperine, Rauserpin, Reserfia,* Serpasil, Serpate, Sertina, Tensin, Zepine

Func. class.: Antihypertensive
Chem. class.: Antiadrenergic agent

Action: Inhibits norepinephrine release, depleting norepinephrine stores in adrenergic nerve endings
Uses: Hypertension; relief in agitated psychotic states unable to tolerate phenothiazines or requiring antihypertensive medication
Dosage and routes:
Hypertension
• *Adult:* PO 0.5 mg qd × 1-2 wk, then 0.1-0.25 mg qd maintenance
• *Child:* PO 0.07 mg/kg or 2 mg/m² given with hydralzine IM q12-24 h
Pyschiatric disorders
• *Adult:* 0.5 mg/day (range 0.1-1 mg)
Available forms include: Tabs 0.1, 0.25, 1 mg; caps-time rel 0.5 mg
Side effects/adverse reactions:
CV: Bradycardia, chest pain, dysrhythmias, prolonged bleeding time, thrombocytopenia, purpura
CNS: Drowsiness, fatigue, lethargy, dizziness, depression, anxiety, headache, increased dreaming, nightmares, convulsions, Parkinsonism, EPS (high doses)
GI: Nausea, vomiting, cramps, peptic ulcer, dry mouth, increased appetite, anorexia
INTEG: Rash, purpura, alopecia, flushing, warm feeling, pruritus, ecchymosis
EENT: Lacrimation, miosis, blurred vision, ptosis, dry mouth, epistaxis
GU: Impotence, dysuria, nocturia, sodium, water retention, edema, breast engorgement, galactorrhea, gynecomastia
*RESP: **Bronchospasm,*** dyspnea, cough, rales
Contraindications: Hypersensitivity, depression/suicidal patients, active peptic ulcer disease, ulcerative colitis, ETC
Precautions: Pregnancy, lactation, seizure disorders
Pharmacokinetics:
PO: Peak 4 hr, duration 2-6 wk; half-life 50-100 hr, metabolized by liver, excreted in urine, feces, crosses placenta, blood-brain barrier, excreted in breast milk
Interactions/incompatibilities:
• Increased hypotension: diuretics, hypotension, β-blockers, methotrimeprazine
• Dysrhythmias: cardiac glycosides
• Increased cardiac depression: quinidine, procainamide
• Excitation, hypertension: MAOIs
• Increased CNS depression: barbiturates, alcohol, narcotics
• Increased pressor effects: epinephrine, isoproterenol, norepinephrine
• Decreased pressor effects: ephedrine, amphetamine
NURSING CONSIDERATIONS
Assess:
• Renal function studies in renal impairment (BUN, creatinine)
• Bleeding time, check for ecchymosis, thrombocytopenia, purpura
• I&O in renal disease patient
Evaluate:
• Cardiac status: B/P, pulse, watch for hypotension
• Edema in feet, legs daily; take weight daily
• Skin turgor, dryness of mucous membranes for hydration status
• Symptoms of CHF: edema, dyspnea, wet rales
Teach patient/family:
• To avoid driving, hazardous ac-

---

tivities if drowsiness occurs
• Not to discontinue drug abruptly
• Not to use OTC products (cough, cold preparations) unless directed by physician
• To report bradycardia, dizziness, confusion, depression, fever, sore throat
• That impotence, gynecomastia may occur but is reversible
• To rise slowly to sitting or standing position to minimize orthostatic hypotension
• That therapeutic effect may take 2-4 wk
Lab test interferences:
Increase: VMA excretion, 5-HIAA excretion
Interferences: 17-OHCS, 17-KS
Treatment of overdose: Lavage, IV atropine for bradycardia, supportive therapy

---

resorcinol/resorcinol monoacetate

(res-or-sin' all)
Euresol, Resorcin
Func. class.: Keratolytic

Action: Corrects abnormal keratinization and causes peeling of skin
Uses: Eczema, acne, seborrhea, psoriasis
Dosage and routes:
• *Adult and child:* Apply as needed depending on condition
Available forms include: Sol 1%, 2%; oint 2%, 10%; paste 45%; lotion 5%; liniment 10%
Side effects/adverse reactions:
INTEG: Irritation, dryness, redness
Contraindications: Hypersensitivity
Interactions/incompatibilities:
None known

NURSING CONSIDERATIONS
Assess:
• Platelets, WBC if systemic absorption occurs
Administer:
• Only to affected area
• Only to small areas or for short periods of time or absorption (systemic) may occur
Evaluate:
• Therapeutic response: decrease in size and amount of lesions
• Allergic reactions: irritation, redness, itching; drug should be discontinued
Teach patient/family:
• That discomfort will begin after 24 hr, subside in 2-4 days
• To avoid contact with eyes, mucous membranes

Rh$_o$ (D) immune globulin, human

Gamulin Rh, HypoRho-D, MICRhoGAM, Mini-Gamulin RH, RHoGAM

Func. class.: Immunizing agent
Chem. class.: IgG

Action: Supresses immune response of non-sensitized Rh$_o$ (D or D$_u$)-negative patients who are exposed to Rh$_o$ (D or D^u)-positive blood
Uses: Prevention of isoimmunization in Rh-negative women exposed to Rh positive blood
Dosage and routes:
Rh exposure/postabortion
• *Adult:* IM 1 vial if fetal packed RBCs <15 ml, or 2 vials if fetal packed RBCs >15 ml; given within 72 hr of delivery or miscarriage
Transfusion error
• *Adult:* IM Give within 72 hr
Available forms include: Inj IM single dose vial

R

Side effects/adverse reactions:
INTEG: Irritation at injection site, fever
CNS: Lethargy
MS: Myalgia
Contraindications: Previous immunization with this drug, Rh₀ (O)-positive/Dᵘ-positive patient
Interactions/incompatibilities: None known
NURSING CONSIDERATIONS
Administer:
• After sending newborn's cord blood to lab after delivery for cross match, type, infant must be Rh-positive, with Rh-negative mother
• IM only in deltoid, aspirate
• Only equal lot numbers of drug, cross-match
• Only MICRhoGAM for abortions
Evaluate:
• Allergic reaction: rash, urticaria, nausea, fever, wheezing
Perform/provide:
• Storage in refrigerator
Teach patient/family:
• How drug works, that drug does not need to be given after subsequent deliveries

---

riboflavin (vitamin B₂)

(rey'boo-flay-vin)
Riobin-50 and others
Func. class.: Vitamin B₂, water soluble

Action: Needed for respiratory reactions by catalyzing proteins
Uses: Vitamin B₂ deficiency or polyneuritis, cheilosis adjunct with thiamin
Dosage and routes:
• *Adult and child >12 yr:* PO 5-50 mg qd
• *Child <12 yr:* PO 2-10 mg qd
Available forms include: Tabs 5, 10, 25, 50, 100 mg

Side effects/adverse reactions:
GU: Yellow discoloration of urine (large doses)
Contraindications: Child <12 yr
Pharmacokinetics:
PO: Half-life 65-85 min, 60% protein-bound, unused amounts excreted in urine (unchanged)
Interactions/incompatibilities:
• Decreased action of: tetracyclines
NURSING CONSIDERATIONS
Administer:
• With food for better absorption
Evaluate:
• Therapeutic response: absence of headache, GI problems, cheilosis, skin lesions, depression, burning, itchy eyes, anemia
• Nutritional status: liver, eggs, dairy products, yeast, whole grain, green vegetables
Teach patient/family:
• That urine may turn bright yellow
• On addition of needed foods that are rich in riboflavin
Lab test interferences:
• May cause false elevations of urinary catecholamines

---

rifampin

(rif'am-pin)
Rifadin, Rimactane, Rofact*
Func. class.: Antitubercular
Chem. class.: Rifamycin B derivative

Action: Inhibits DNA-dependent polymerase, decreases tubercle bacilli replication
Uses: Pulmonary tuberculosis, meningococcal carriers
Dosage and routes:
• *Adult:* PO 600 mg/day as single dose 1 hr ac or 2 hr pc
• *Child >5 yr:* PO 10-20 mg/kg/day as single dose 1 hr ac or 2 hr pc, not to exceed 600 mg/day, with

other antituberculars
Meningococcal carriers
• *Adult:* PO 600 mg bid × 2 days
• *Child >5 yr:* PO 10 mg/kg bid × 2 days, not to exceed 600 mg/dose
Available forms include: Caps 150, 300 mg
Side effects/adverse reactions:
CV: CHF, dysrhythmias
CNS: Headache, anxiety, drowsiness, tremors, *convulsions,* lethargy, depression, confusion, psychosis, aggression
EENT: Blurred vision, optic neuritis, photophobia
HEMA: Hemolytic anemia, thrombocytopenia, leukopenia
Contraindications: Hypersensitivity
Precautions: Pregnancy, child <13 yr
Pharmacokinetics:
PO: Peak 2-3 hr, duration >24 hr, half-life 3 hr; metabolized in liver (active/inactive metabolites), excreted in urine as free drug (30% crosses placenta), excreted in breast milk
Interactions/incompatibilities:
• Decreased action: barbiturates, clofibrate, corticosteroids, dapsone, anticoagulants, antidiabetics, hormones, digoxin, PAS
NURSING CONSIDERATIONS
Assess:
• Temperature, if <101° F drug should be reduced
• Liver studies q wk: ALT, AST, bilirubin
• Renal status before, q mo: BUN, creatinine, output, sp gr, urinalysis
Administer:
• With meals to decrease GI symptoms even though absorption will be decreased
• Antiemetic if vomiting occurs
• After C&S is completed; q mo to detect resistance

Evaluate:
• Mental status often: affect, mood, behavioral changes (psychosis may occur)
• Hepatic status: decreased appetite, jaundice, dark urine, fatigue
Teach patient/family:
• That compliance with dosage schedule, length is necessary
• That scheduled appointments must be kept; relapse may occur
• Avoid alcohol while taking drug
• Urine, feces, saliva, sputum, sweat, tears may be colored red-orange. Soft contact lenses may be permanently stained
Lab test interferences:
Interference: Folate level, vitamin B_{12}, BSP, gall bladder studies

---

ritodrine HCl

(ri′toe-dreen)
Yutopar
Func. class.: Tocolytic, uterine relaxant
Chem. class.: β_2-adrenergic agent

Action: Reduces frequency, intensity of uterine contractions by stimulation of the β_2 receptors in uterine smooth muscle
Uses: Preterm labor
Dosage and routes:
• Adult: IV INF 150 mg/500 ml (0.3 mg/ml) given 0.1 mg/min, increased gradually by 0.05 mg/min q10 min until desired response; PO 10 mg given ½ hr before termination of IV, then 10 mg q2h × 24 hr, then 10-20 mg q4-6h, not to exceed 120 mg/day
Available forms include: Tabs 10 mg; inj 10 mg/ml
Side effects/adverse reactions:
META: Hyperglycemia
CNS: Headache, restlessness, anxiety, nervousness, sweating, chills, drowsiness

R

---

italics = common side effects • ***bold italic*** = life threatening reactions

GI: Nausea, vomiting, anorexia, malaise

CV: Altered maternal, fetal heart tone, B/P, dysrhythmias, palpitation, chest pain

Contraindications: Hypersensitivity, eclampsia, hypertension, dysrhythmias, thyrotoxicosis

Precautions: Cardiac disease

Pharmacokinetics:

PO: Peak ½-1 hr

IV: Peak 1 hr, half-life 6 min, 1½-2½ hr, >10 hr, metabolized in liver, excreted in urine, crosses placenta

Interactions/incompatibilities:

• Pulmonary edema: corticosteroids

• Increased effects of: general anesthetics

NURSING CONSIDERATIONS
Assess:

• Maternal, fetal heart tones during infusion

• Intensity, length of uterine contractions

• Fluid intake to prevent fluid overload; discontinue if this occurs

• Blood glucose in diabetics

Administer:

• Only clear solutions

• After dilutions: 150 mg/500 ml D₅W or NS, give at 0.3 mg/ml

• After infusion pump, or monitor carefully

Perform/provide:

• Positioning of patient in left lateral recumbent position to decrease hypotension, increase renal blood flow

Evaluate:

• Therapeutic response: decreased intensity, length of contraction, absence of preterm labor, decreased B/P

Teach patient/family:

• To remain in bed during infusion

Lab test interferences:

Increase: Blood glucose, free fatty acids, insulin, GTT

Decrease: Potassium

---

salicylamide

(sal-ee-sye'-la-mide)

Artritex,* Lapidar,* Uromide

Func. class.: Nonnarcotic analgesic

Chem. class.: Salicylate derivative

Action: Blocks pain impulses in CNS that occur in response to inhibition of prostaglandin synthesis; antipyretic action results from inhibition of hypothalamic heat-regulating center to produce vasodilation to allow heat dissipation

Uses: Mild to moderate pain

Dosage and routes:

• *Adult:* PO 650 mg qid prn

• *Child:* PO 65 mg/kg/day in 6 divided doses

Available forms include: Tabs 325, 667 mg

Side effects/adverse reactions:

CNS: Stimulation, drowsiness, dizziness, confusion, convulsion, headache, flushing, hallucinations, coma

GI: Nausea, vomiting, GI bleeding, diarrhea, heartburn, anorexia, *hepatitis*

Contraindications: Hypersensitivity, bleeding disorders

Precautions: Anemia

Pharmacokinetics:

PO: Onset 15-30 min, peak 1-2 hr, duration 4-6 hr

REC: Onset slow, duration 4-6 hr, metabolized by liver, excreted by kidneys, crosses placenta, excreted in breast milk, half-life 1-3½ hr

Interactions/incompatibilities:

• Decreased effects of this drug: antacids, steroids, urinary alkalizers

• Increased blood loss: alcohol, heparin

• Increased effects of: anticoagu-

---

lants, insulin, methotrexate

• Decreased effects of: probenecid, spironalactone, sulfinpyrazone, sulfonylamides

• Toxic effects: PABA

• Decreased blood sugar levels: salicylates

NURSING CONSIDERATIONS

Assess:

• Liver function studies: AST, ALT, bilirubin, creatinine if patient is on long-term therapy

• Renal function studies: BUN, urine creatinine if patient is on long-term therapy

• Blood studies: CBC, pro-time if patient is on long-term therapy

• I&O ratio; decreasing output may indicate renal failure (long-term therapy)

Administer:

• To patient crushed or whole; chewable tablets may be chewed

• With food or milk to decrease gastric symptoms; give 30 min before or 2 hr after meals

Teach patient/family:

• To report any symptoms of hepatotoxicity, renal toxicity, visual changes, ototoxicity, allergic reactions (long-term therapy)

• Not to exceed recommended dosage; acute poisoning may result

• To read label on other OTC drugs; many contain aspirin

• That therapeutic response takes 2 wk (arthritis)

• To avoid alcohol ingestion; GI bleeding may occur

Treatment of overdose: Lavage, activated charcoal, monitor electrolytes, VS

---

salicylic acid

Calicylic, Keralyt, Salacid, Salonil

Func. class.: Keratolytic

Action: Corrects abnormal keratinization and causes peeling of skin

Uses: Dandruff, seborrheic dermatitis, psoriasis, multiple superficial epitheliomatoses

Dosage and routes:

• *Adult and child:* Apply as needed, cover at night

Available forms include: Powder, cream 2%, 2.5%, 10%; gel 6%, 17%; oint 25%, 60%; plaster 40%; pledgets 0.5%; shampoo 2%, 4%; solution 0.5%, 13.6%, 17%; stick 2%; susp 2%

Side effects/adverse reactions:

INTEG: Irritation, drying

CNS: Salicylism: hearing loss, tinnitus, dizziness, confusion, headache, hyperventilation

Contraindications: Hypersensitivity

Interactions/incompatibilities: None known

NURSING CONSIDERATIONS

Assess:

• Platelets, WBC if systemic absorption occurs

Administer:

• Only to intact skin, do not use on inflamed, denuded skin

• After wetting skin, wash thoroughly each AM after treatment

• Using an occlusive dressing to increase absorption

Evaluate:

• Therapeutic response: decrease in dandruff, size of lesions

• Salicylism: tinnitus, hearing loss, dizziness, confusion, headache, hyperventilation

• Allergic reactions: irritation, redness

Teach patient/family:

• To avoid contact with eyes, mucous membranes

• To apply lotion if drying occurs

S

salsalate
(sal-sa'late)
Disalcid, Mono-Gesic
Func. class.: Nonnarcotic analgesic
Chem. class.: Salicylate

Action: Blocks pain impulses in CNS that occur in response to inhibition of prostaglandin synthesis; antipyretic action results from inhibition of hypothalamic heat-regulating center

Uses: Mild to moderate pain or fever including arthritis, juvenile rheumatoid arthritis

Dosage and routes:
• *Adult:* PO 1 g bid-qid
Available forms include: Caps 500 mg; tabs 500, 750 mg

Side effects/adverse reactions:
*HEMA: **Thrombocytopenia, agranulocytosis, leukopenia, neutropenia, hemolytic anemia,*** increased pro-time
CNS: Stimulation, drowsiness, dizziness, confusion, convulsion, headache, flushing, hallucinations, coma
GI: Nausea, vomiting, GI bleeding, diarrhea, heartburn, anorexia, *hepatitis*
INTEG: Rash, urticaria, bruising
EENT: Tinnitus, hearing loss
CV: Rapid pulse, pulmonary edema
RESP: Wheezing, hyperpnea
ENDO: Hypoglycemia, hyponatremia, hypokalemia

Contraindications: Hypersensitivity to salicylates, GI bleeding, bleeding disorders, children < 3 yr, pregnancy, lactation, vitamin K deficiency

Precautions: Anemia, hepatic disease, renal disease, Hodgkin's disease

Pharmacokinetics: Metabolized by liver, excreted by kidneys, half-life 1 hr

Interactions/incompatibilities:
• Decreased effects of this drug: antacids, steroids, urinary alkalizers
• Increased blood loss: alcohol, heparin
• Increased effects of: anticoagulants, insulin, methotrexate
• Decreased effects of: probenecid, spironolactone, sulfinpyrazone, sulfonylmides
• Toxic effects: PABA
• Decreased blood sugar levels: salicylates

NURSING CONSIDERATIONS
Assess:
• Liver function studies: AST, ALT, bilirubin, creatinine if patient is on long-term therapy
• Renal function studies: BUN, urine creatinine if patient is on long-term therapy
• Blood studies: CBC, Hct, Hgb, pro-time if patient is on long-term therapy
• I&O ratio; decreasing output may indicate renal failure (long-term therapy)

Administer:
• To patient crushed or whole; chewable tablets may be chewed
• With food or milk to decrease gastric symptoms; give 30 min before or 2 hr after meals
• With full glass of water

Perform/provide:
• Repositioning to decrease pain
• Cool cloth for fever

Evaluate:
• Hepatotoxicity: dark urine, clay-colored stools, yellowing of skin, sclera, itching, abdominal pain, fever, diarrhea if patient is on long-term therapy
• Allergic reactions: rash, urticaria; if these occur, drug may need to be discontinued

• Renal dysfunction: decreased urine output

• Ototoxicity: tinnitus, ringing, roaring in ears; audiometric testing is needed before, after long-term therapy

• Visual changes: blurring, halos, corneal and retinal damage

• Edema in feet, ankles, legs

• Prior drug history; there are many drug interactions

Teach patient/family:

• To report any symptoms of hepatotoxicity, renal toxicity, visual changes, ototoxicity, allergic reactions (long-term therapy)

• Not to exceed recommended dosage; acute poisoning may result

• To read label on other OTC drugs; many contain aspirin

• That therapeutic response takes 2 wk (arthritis)

• To avoid alcohol ingestion; GI bleeding may occur

Lab test interferences:

Increase: Coagulation studies, liver function studies, serum uric acid, amylase, CO_2, urinary protein

Decrease: Serum potassium, PBI, cholesterol

Interfere: Urine catecholamines, pregnancy test

Treatment of overdose: Lavage, activated charcoal, monitor electrolytes, VS

scopolamine (transdermal)

(skoe-pol'-a-meen)
Transderm-Scop

Func. class.: Antiemetic, anticholinergic

Chem. class.: Belladonna alkaloid

Action: Competitive antagonism of acetylcholine at receptor site in eye, smooth muscle, cardiac muscle, glandular cells

Uses: Prevention of motion sickness

Dosage and routes:

• *Adult:* PATCH 1 placed behind ear 4-5 hr before travel

Available forms include: Patch

Side effects/adverse reactions:

CNS: Dizziness, drowsiness, confusion, fatigue

EENT: Blurred vision, altered depth perception, *dilated pupils,* photophobia, *dry mouth*

CV: Bradycardia

Contraindications: Hypersensitivity

Precautions: Children, cardiac disease, elderly

Pharmacokinetics:

PATCH: Onset 15-30 min, duration 72 hr

Interactions/incompatibilities:

• Increased anticholinergic effects: antihistamines, antidepressants

NURSING CONSIDERATIONS:

Teach patient/family:

• To avoid hazardous activities, activities requiring alertness; dizziness may occur

• To wash, dry hands before applying to surface behind ear

• Change patch q72h

• Apply at least 3 hr before traveling

• If blurred vision, severe dizziness, drowsiness occurs, discontinue use, use another type of antiemetic

• To read label of all OTC medications; if any scopolamine is found in product, avoid use

scopolamine hydrobromide

(skoe-pol'a-meen)
Hyoscine, Triptone

Func. class.: Cholinergic blocker

Chem. class.: Belladonna alkaloid

Action: Inhibits acetylcholine at re-

S

ceptor sites in autonomic nervous system, which controls secretions, free acids in stomach; acts on dopamine receptors in CNS, which decrease involuntary movements
Uses: Parkinson symptoms, reduction of secretions before surgery
Dosage and routes:
Parkinson symptoms
• *Adult:* PO 0.5-1 mg tid-qid; IM/SC/IV 0.3-0.6 mg tid-qid diluted using dilution
• *Child:* PO/SC 0.006 mg/kg tid-qid or 0.2 mg/m^2
Preoperatively
• *Adult:* SC 0.4-0.6 mg
Available forms include: Caps 0.25 mg; inj 0.3, 0.4, 0.86, 1 mg/ml
Side effects/adverse reactions:
CNS: Confusion, anxiety, restlessness, irritability, delusions, hallucinations, headache, sedation, depression, incoherence, dizziness
EENT: Blurred vision, photophobia, dilated pupils, difficulty swallowing
CV: Palpitations, tachycardia, postural hypotension
GI: Dryness of mouth, constipation, nausea, vomiting, abdominal distress, paralytic ileus
GU: Hesitancy, retention
Contraindications: Hypersensitivity, narrow-angle glaucoma, myasthenia gravis, GI/GU obstruction, child <3 yr
Precautions: Pregnancy, elderly, lactation, tachycardia, prostatic hypertrophy
Pharmacokinetics:
PO: Peak 1 hr, duration 6 hr
SC/IM: Peak 30-45 min, duration 7 hr
IV: Peak 10-15 min, duration 4 hr
Excreted in urine, bile, feces (unchanged)
Interactions/incompatibilities:
• Increased anticholinergic effect: alcohol, narcotics, antihistamines, phenothiazines

• Do not mix with diazepam, chloramphenicol, pentobarbital, sodium bicarbonate in syringe or solution
NURSING CONSIDERATIONS
Assess:
• I&O ratio; retention commonly causes decreased urinary output
Administer:
• Parenteral dose with patient recumbent to prevent postural hypotension
• Administer with or after meals for GI upset; may give with fluids other than water
• At hs to avoid daytime drowsiness in patient with parkinsonism
• Parenteral dose slowly; keep in bed for at least 1 hr after dose
Perform/provide:
• Storage at room temperature in light-resistant containers
• Hard candy, frequent drinks, sugarless gum to relieve dry mouth
Evaluate:
• Parkinsonism, extrapyramidal symptoms: shuffling gait, muscle rigidity, involuntary movements
• Urinary hesitancy, retention, palpate bladder if retention occurs
• Constipation; increase fluids, bulk, exercise if this occurs
• For tolerance over long-term therapy; dose may need to be increased or changed
• Mental status: affect, mood, CNS depression, worsening of mental symptoms during early therapy
Teach patient/family:
• Not to discontinue this drug abruptly; to taper off over 1 wk
• To avoid driving or other hazardous activities; drowsiness may occur
• To avoid OTC medication: cough, cold preparations with alcohol, antihistamines unless directed by physician

---

*Available in Canada only

scopolamine hydrobromide (optic)

(skoe-pol'a-meen)
Isopto-Hyoscine
Func. class.: Mydriatic
Chem. class.: Synthetic alkaloid

Action: Blocks response of iris sphincter muscle, muscle of accommodation of ciliary body to cholinergic stimulation, resulting in dilation, paralysis of accommodation

Uses: Uveitis, iritis, cycloplegic refraction

Dosage and routes:
• *Adult:* INSTILL 1-2 gtts before refraction or 1-2 gtts qd-tid for iritis or uveitis
• *Child:* INSTILL 1 gtt bid × 2 days before refraction
Available forms include: Sol 0.25%

Side effects/adverse reactions:
CV: Tachycardia
CNS: Confusion, somnolence, flushing, fever
EENT: Blurred vision, photophobia, increased intraocular pressure, irritation, edema

Contraindications: Hypersensitivity, children <6 yr, narrow-angle glaucoma, increased intraocular pressure, infants, pregnancy (C)

Precautions: Children, elderly, hypertension, hyperthyroidism, diabetes

Pharmacokinetics:
INSTILL: Peak 20-30 min, duration 3-7 days

Interactions/incompatibilities:
None known

NURSING CONSIDERATIONS

Evaluate:
• Therapeutic response: decrease in inflammation, cycloplegic refraction
• Eye pain, discontinue use

Teach patient/family:
• To report change in vision, blurring or loss of sight, trouble breathing, sweating, flushing
• Method of instillation: pressure on lacrimal sac for 1 min, do not touch dropper to eye
• That blurred vision will decrease with repeated use of drug
• Not to engage in hazardous activities until able to see
• Wait 5 min to use other drops
• Do not blink more than usual

secobarbital/secobarbital sodium

(see-koe-bar'bi-tal)
Seconal/Secogen Sodium,* Seconal Sodium, Seral*
Func. class.: Sedative/hypnotic-barbiturate
Chem. class.: Barbitone (short acting)

Controlled Substance Schedule II (USA), Schedule G (Canada)

Action: Depresses activity in brain cells primarily in reticular activating system in brainstem; selectively depresses neurons in posterior hypothalamus, limbic structures; able to decrease seizure activity by inhibition of epileptic activity in CNS

Uses: Insomnia, sedation, preoperative medication, status epilepticus, acute tetanus convulsions

Dosage and routes:
Insomnia
• *Adult:* PO/IM 100-200 mg hs
• *Child:* IM 3-5 mg/kg, not to exceed 100 mg, not to inject >5 ml in one site; REC 4-5 mg/kg
Sedation/preoperatively
• *Adult:* PO 200-300 mg 1-2 hr preoperatively
• *Child:* PO 50-100 mg 1-2 hr preoperatively; REC 4-5 mg/kg 1-2 hr preoperatively
Status epilepticus

S

• *Adult and child:* IM/IV 250-350 mg

Acute psychotic agitation

• *Adult and child:* IM/IV 5.5 mg/kg q3-4h

Available forms include: Caps 50, 100 mg; inj IM, IV 50 mg/ml; powder, rec supp 200 mg

Side effects/adverse reactions:

CNS: Lethargy, drowsiness, hangover, dizziness, stimulation in the elderly and children, lightheadedness, dependence, CNS depression, mental depression, slurred speech

GI: Nausea, vomiting, diarrhea, constipation

INTEG: Rash, urticaria, pain, abscesses at injection site, angioedema, thrombophlebitis, *Stevens-Johnson syndrome*

CV: Hypotension, bradycardia

RESP: Depression, apnea, *laryngospasm, bronchospasm*

HEMA: Agranulocytosis, thrombocytopenia, megaloblastic anemia (long-term treatment)

Contraindications: Hypersensitivity to barbiturates, respiratory depression, addiction to barbiturates, severe liver impairment, porphyria

Precautions: Anemia, pregnancy, lactation, hepatic disease, renal disease, hypertension, elderly, acute/chronic pain

Pharmacokinetics:

IM: Onset 10-15 min, duration 4-6 hr

REC: Onset slow, duration 4-6 hr Metabolized by liver, excreted by kidneys (metabolites); half-life 15-40 hr

Interactions/incompatibilities:

• Do not mix with other drugs in solution or syringe

• Increased CNS depression: alcohol, MAOIs, sedative, narcotics

• Decreased effect of these drugs: oral anticoagulants, corticosteroids, griseofulvin, quinidine

• Increased half-life of doxycycline

NURSING CONSIDERATIONS

Assess:

• VS q30 min after parenteral route for 2 hr

• Blood studies: Hct, Hgb, RBCs, serum folate, vitamin D (if on long-term therapy); pro-time in patients receiving anticoagulants

• Hepatic studies: AST, ALT, bilirubin; if increased, the drug is usually discontinued

Administer:

• After removal of cigarettes, to prevent fires

• IM injection in deep large muscle mass to prevent tissue sloughing and abscesses

• After conservative measures have been tried for insomnia

• Within 30 min of mixing with sterile water for injection

• IV only with resuscitative equipment available, administer at <100 mg/min (only by qualified personnel)

• ½-1hr before hs for sleeplessness

• On empty stomach for best absorption

• For <14 days since drug is not effective after that; tolerance develops

• Crushed or whole

• Alone, do not mix with other drugs or inject if there is precipitate

• After cleansing enema if given rectally preoperatively in children

Perform/provide:

• Assistance with ambulation after receiving dose

• Safety measure: siderails, nightlight, callbell within easy reach

• Checking to see PO medication has been swallowed

• Storage of suppositories in refrigerator; do not use aqueous solutions containing precipitate

Evaluate:

• Therapeutic response: ability to

sleep at night, decreased amount of early morning awakening if taking drug for insomnia, or decrease in number, severity of seizures if taking drug for seizure disorder
• Unresolved pain, as drug may cause severe stimulation if pain is present
• Mental status: mood, sensorium, affect, memory (long, short)
• Physical dependency: more frequent requests for medication, shakes, anxiety
• Barbiturate toxicity: hypotension; pulmonary constriction; cold, clammy skin; cyanosis of lips; insomnia; nausea; vomiting; hallucinations; delirium; weakness; mild symptoms may occur in 8-12 hr without drug
• Respiratory dysfunction: respiratory depression, character, rate, rhythm; hold drug if respirations <12/min or if pupils dilated
• Blood dyscrasias: fever, sore throat, bruising, rash, jaundice, epistaxis
• Perianal irritation if rectal forms used

Teach patient/family:
• That hangover is common
• That drug is indicated only for short-term treatment of insomnia and is probably ineffective after 2 wk
• That physical dependency may result when used for extended periods of time (45-90 days depending on dose)
• To avoid driving or other activities requiring alertness
• To avoid alcohol ingestion or CNS depressants; serious CNS depression may result
• Not to discontinue medication quickly after long-term use; drug should be tapered over 1-2 wk
• To tell all prescribers that barbiturate is being taken
• That withdrawal insomnia may

occur after short-term use; do not start using drug again, insomnia will improve in 1-3 nights
• That effects may take 2 nights for benefits to be noticed
• Alternate measures to improve sleep (reading, exercise several hours before hs, warm bath, warm milk, TV, self-hypnosis, deep breathing)

Lab test interferences:
False increase: Sulfobromophthalein

Treatment of overdose: Lavage, activated charcoal, warming blanket, vital signs, hemodialysis, I&O ratio

---

selenium sulfide

(cee-leen'ee-um)
Exsel, Selsun, Sul-Blue
Func. class.: Local antiinfective

Action: Unknown
Uses: Dandruff, seborrhea in scalp
Dosage and routes:
• *Adult and child:* TOP wash hair with 1-2 tsp, leave on 2-3 min; rinse, repeat, use 2 × wk × 2 wk, then 2-3 × wk or as needed
Available forms include: Shampoo 1%, 2.5%
Side effects/adverse reactions:
INTEG: Oiliness of hair/scalp, alopecia, discoloration of hair
Contraindications: Hypersensitivity to sulfur preparations, inflamed skin
Precautions: Infants, pregnancy
Interactions/incompatibilities: None known

NURSING CONSIDERATIONS
Perform/provide:
• Thorough hair rinsing after use
• Storage at room temperature in tight container
Evaluate:
• Toxicity: tremors, perspiration,

pain in abdomen, weakness, anorexia

• Area of body involved, including time involved, what helps or aggravates condition

Teach patient/family:

• To avoid contact with eyes, genital area

• To discontinue use if rash or irritation occurs

• That drug may damage jewelry, remove before application

• That drug is not be taken internally

---

senna

(sin'na)

Black Draught, Senokot, X-Prep

Func. class.: Laxative

Chem. class.: Anthraquinone

Action: Stimulates paristalsis by action on Auerbach's plexis

Uses: Constipation, bowel preparation for surgery or examination

Dosage and routes:

• *Adult:* PO 1-8 tabs (Senokot), ½ to 4 tsps. of granules added to water or juice; REC SUPP 1-2 hs; SYR 1-4 tsps. hs, 7.5-15 ml (Black Draught); ¾ oz dissolved in 2.5 oz liquid given between 2-4 PM the day before procedure (X-Prep)

• *Child >27 kg:* ½ adult dose; do not use Black Draught for children

• *Child 1 mo-1 yr:* SYR 1.25-2.5 ml (Senokot) hs

Available forms include: Supp 625 mg, 30 mg sennosides; powder 662 mg/g, 6, 15 mg sennosides/3g; tabs 8.6 sennosides, 180 mg

Side effects/adverse reactions:

GI: Nausea, vomiting, anorexia, cramps, diarrhea

META: Hypocalcemia, enteropathy, alkalosis, hypokalemia, tetany

Contraindications: Hypersensitivity, GI bleeding, obstruction, CHF, lactation, abdominal pain, nausea/ vomiting, appendicitis, acute surgical abdomen

Pharmacokinetics:

PO: Onset 6-24 hr; metabolized by liver, excreted in feces

Interactions/incompatibilities:

None known

NURSING CONSIDERATIONS

Assess:

• Blood, urine electrolytes if drug is used often by patient

• I&O ratio to identify fluid loss

Administer:

• In morning or evening (oral dose)

Evaluate:

• Therapeutic response: decrease in constipation

• Cause of constipation; identify whether fluids, bulk, or exercise is missing from lifestyle

• Cramping, rectal bleeding, nausea, vomiting; if these symptoms occur, drug should be discontinued

Teach patient/family:

• Not to use laxatives for long-term therapy; bowel tone will be lost

• That normal bowel movements do not always occur daily

• Do not use in presence of abdominal pain, nausea, vomiting

• Notify physician if constipation unrelieved or if symptoms of electrolyte imbalance occur: muscle cramps, pain, weakness, dizziness

---

silver nitrate

Func. class.: Keratolytic

Action: Possesses antiinfective, astringent, caustic properties

Uses: Cauterization of lesions, warts, burns (low concentrations)

Dosage and routes:

• *Adult and child:* Apply by physician

Available forms include: Sticks

Side effects/adverse reactions:

INTEG: Skin discoloration

Contraindications: Hypersensitivity

Interactions/incompatibilities:
• Not to be used with alkalis, phosphates, thimerosol, benzalkonium chloride, halogenated acids

NURSING CONSIDERATIONS

Administer:
• After moistening stick with water
• To burns using a wet dressing (low concentrations 0.125%)

Evaluate:
• Therapeutic response: absence of lesions, healing of burned areas

Perform/provide:
• Storage in cool area

Teach patient/family:
• To avoid contact with clothing or unaffected areas

---

silver nitrate 1% (ophthalmic)

Func. class.: Antiinfective

Action: Inhibits metabolic actions in susceptible organisms
Uses: Prevention, treatment of ophthalmia neonatorum
Dosage and routes:
• *Neonate:* INSTILL 1 gtt into each eye
Available forms include: Sol
Side effects/adverse reactions:
EENT: Redness, discharge, edema, swelling
Contraindications: Hypersensitivity
Precautions: Antibiotic hypersensitivity
Interactions/incompatibilities: None known
NURSING CONSIDERATIONS
Administer:
• After washing hands
Perform/provide:
• Storage at room temperature
Evaluate:
• Allergy: itching, lacrimation, redness, swelling

silver protein, mild

Argyrol S.S., Silvol, Solargentum
Func. class.: Disinfectant
Chem. class.: Silver colloidal compound

Action: Destroys gram-positive, gram-negative organisms
Uses: Eye, nose, throat, swelling, infection
Dosage and routes:
• *Adult and child:* SOL Use as needed
Available forms include: Top sol 5%, 10%, 25%; eyedrops 20%
Side effects/adverse reactions:
INTEG: Irritation, discoloration of tissue
Contraindications: Hypersensitivity
Interactions/incompatibilities: None known
NURSING CONSIDERATIONS
Administer:
• To area to be treated only; do not apply to healthy skin
Perform/provide:
• Storage in tight container
Evaluate:
• Area of body involved: irritation, rash, breaks, dryness, scales

---

silver sulfadiazine (topical)

(sul-fa-dye'a-zeen)
Flamazine, Silvadene
Func. class.: Local antiinfective
Chem. class.: Sulfonamide

Action: Interferes with bacterial cell wall synthesis
Uses: Burns (2nd, 3rd degree)
Dosage and routes:
• *Adult and child:* TOP apply to affected area qd-bid
Available forms include: Cream 10 mg/g

S

---

italics = common side effects   ***bold italic*** = life threatening reactions

Side effects/adverse reactions:
INTEG: Rash, urticaria, stinging, burning, itching
Contraindications: Hypersensitivity, child <2 mo
Precautions: Impaired renal function, pregnancy (C), impaired hepatic function, lactation
Interactions/incompatibilities:
None known

NURSING CONSIDERATIONS
Administer:
• Using aseptic technique
• Enough medication to completely cover burns, keep covered with medication at all times
• After cleansing debris before each application
• Analgesic before application if needed
Perform/provide:
• Storage at room temperature in dry place
Evaluate:
• Allergic reaction: burning, stinging, swelling, redness
• Therapeutic response: development of granulation tissue
Teach patient/family:
• That drug may be continued until graft can be done

---

simethicone

(si-meth'-i-kone)
Mylicon, Ovol,* Silain
Func. class.: Antiflatulet

Action: Disperses, prevents gas pockets in GI system
Uses: Flatulence
Dosage and routes:
• *Adult and child >12 yr:* PO 40-100 mg pc, hs
Available forms include: Chew tabs 40, 80 mg; tabs 50, 60, 95, 125 mg; drops 40 mg/0.6 ml
Side effects/adverse reactions:
GI: Belching, rectal flatus

Contraindications: Hypersensitivity
NURSING CONSIDERATIONS
Evaluate:
• Therapeutic response: absence of flatulence
Teach patient/family:
• That tablets must be chewed

---

sodium bicarbonate

Func. class.: Alkalinizer
Chem. class.: $NaHCO_3$

Action: Orally neutralizes gastric acid, which forms water, NaCl, CO_2; increases plasma bicarbonate, which buffers H^+ ion concentration; reverses acidosis
Uses: Acidosis (metabolic), cardiac arrest, alkalinization (systemic/urinary) antacid
Dosage and routes:
Acidosis
• *Adult and child:* IV INF 2-5 mEq/kg over 4-8 hr depending on CO_2, pH
Cardiac arrest
• *Adult and child:* IV BOL 1 mEq/kg, then 0.5 mEq/kg q10 min, then doses based an ABGs
• *Infant:* IV INF not to exceed 8 mEq/kg/day based on ABGs (4.2% sol)
Alkalinization
• *Adult:* PO 325 mg-2 g qid
• *Child:* PO 12-120 mg/kg/day
Antacid
• *Adult:* PO 300 mg-2 g chewed, taken with water
Available forms include: Tabs 325, 520, 650 mg; powd; inj 4%, 4.2%, 5%, 7.5%, 8.4%
Side effects/adverse reactions:
CNS: Irritability, headache, confusion, stimulation, tremors, *twitching, hyperreflexia, tetany,* weakness, *convulsions*
CV: Irregular pulse, cardiac arrest
GI: Flatulence, belching, disten-

sion, paralytic ileus

META: Alkalosis

RESP: Shallow, slow respirations, cyanosis, apnea

Contraindications: Hypertension, peptic ulcer, renal disease

Precautions: CHF, cirrhosis, toxemia, renal disease

Pharmacokinetics:

PO: Onset 2 min, duration 10 min

IV: Onset 15 min, duration 1-2 hr, excreted in urine

Interactions/incompatibilities:

• Increases effects: amphetamines, mecamylamine, lithium, barbiturates, salicylates, quinine, quinidine, pseudoephedrine

• Do not mix solution with other drugs

NURSING CONSIDERATIONS

Assess:

• Respiratory rate, rhythm, depth, notify physician of abnormalities

• Electrolytes, blood pH, PO_2, HCO_3, during treatment

• Urine pH, urinary output, during beginning treatment

Evaluate:

• Alkalosis: irritability, confusion, twitching, hyperreflexia stimulation, slow respirations, cyanosis, irregular pulse

• Milk-alkali syndrome: confusion, headache, nausea, vomiting, anorexia, urinary stones, hypercalcemia

Teach patient/family:

• To chew antacid tablets and drink 8 oz water

• Not to take antacid with milk, or milk-alkali syndrome may result

• Not to use antacid for more than 2 weeks

Lab tests interferences:

Increase: Urinary urobilinogen

False positive: Urinary protein, blood lactate

sodium biphosphate/ sodium phosphate

Enemeez, Fleet Enema, Phospho-Soda, Saf-tip Phosphate Enema/ Sal-Hepatica

Func. class.: Laxative, saline

Action: Increases water absorption in colon by osmotic action

Uses: Constipation

Dosage and routes:

• *Adult:* PO 5-20 ml with water; POWDER 4 g dissolved in water; SOL 20-46 ml mixed with 4 oz cold water; ENEMA 2-4.5 oz

Available forms include: Powder, sol

Side effects/adverse reactions:

GI: Nausea, cramps, diarrhea

META: Electrolyte, fluid imbalances

Contraindications: Hypersensitivity, rectal fissures, abdominal pain, nausea/vomiting, appendicitis, acute surgical abdomen, ulcerated hemorrhoids

Pharmacokinetics: Excreted in feces

Interactions/incompatibilities: None known

NURSING CONSIDERATIONS

Assess:

• Blood, urine electrolytes if drug is used often by patient

• I&O ratio to identify fluid loss

Administer:

• Alone for better absorption; do not take within 1 hr of other drugs

Evaluate:

• Therapeutic response: decrease in constipation

• Cause of constipation; identify whether fluids, bulk, or exercise is missing from lifestyle

• Cramping, rectal bleeding, nausea, vomiting; if these symptoms occur, drug should be discontinued

S

---

italics = common side effects   ***bold italic*** = life threatening reactions

Teach patient/family:

• Not to use laxatives for long-term therapy; bowel tone will be lost

• That normal bowel movements do not always occur daily

• Do not use in presence of abdominal pain, nausea, vomiting

• Notify physician if constipation unrelieved or if symptoms of electrolyte imbalance occur: muscle cramps, pain, weakness, dizziness

sodium cellulose phosphate

Calcibind, Calcisorb*

Func. class.: Antihypercalcemia
Chem. class.: Phosphorylated cellulose

Action: Decreases hypercalcium by binding with calcium in bowel, facilitates excretion

Uses: Calcium oxalate or calcium phosphate renal stones associated with absorptive hypercalciuria type I

Dosage and routes:

• *Adult:* PO 15 g/day divided between each meal, then 10 g/day when urine Ca <150 mg/day

Available forms include: Powder 2.5 g packets

Side effects/adverse reactions:

GU: Hypomagnesuria, hyperoxaluria

GI: Nausea, anorexia, diarrhea, dyspepsia

MS: Arthralgia

Contraindications: Hypersensitivity, hyperthyroidism, enteric hyperoxaluria, bone disease, hypocalcemia

Precautions: CHF, ascites, liver disease

Pharmacokinetics:
Not known

Interactions/incompatibilities:

• May decrease action of this drug: magnesium preparations

NURSING CONSIDERATIONS
Assess:

• Calcium levels (serum, urinary) throughout treatment

Administer:

• Powder with water, juice; take with meals

• Increase fluids to 3 L/day; urinary output should be >2 L/day

Evaluate:

• Therapeutic response: absence of renal stone formation

Teach patient/family:

• To decrease calcium in diet: dairy products; decrease sodium, citrus fruits in diet; increased excretion of drug will occur; decrease oxalate (chocolate, tea, spinach)

sodium chloride, hypertonic

Adsorbonac Ophthalmic Solution, Hypersal Ophthalmic Solution, Methylcellulose Ophthalmic Solution, Muro Ointment, Sodium Chloride Ointment

Func. class.: Miscellaneous ophthalmic agent

Chem. class.: Hyperosmolar ophthalmic

Action: Reduces corneal edema by osmosis of water through corneal epithelium which is semipermeable

Uses: Reduce corneal edema

Dosage and routes:

• *Adult:* INSTILL 1-2 gtts q3-4h or ointment hs

Available forms include: Sol 2%, 5%; oint 5%

Side effects/adverse reactions:

INTEG: Rash, urticaria

EENT: Stinging

Contraindications: None known

Interactions/incompatibilities:
None known

NURSING CONSIDERATIONS
Perform/provide:

• Storage in tight container

Teach patient/family:
• Method of instillation, including pressure on lacrimal sac for 1 min, and not to touch dropper to eye
• That blurred vision is common with oint

---

sodium fluoride
Fluor-A-Day,* Fluoritabs, Flura-Drops, Karidium, Pediaflor
Func. class.: Trace elements
Chem. class.: Flurideion

Action: Needed for hard tooth enamel, and for resistance to periodontal disease; reduces acid production by dental bacteria
Uses: Prevention of dental caries
Dosage and routes:
• *Adult and child >12 yr:* TOP 10 ml 0.2% sol qd after brushing teeth, rinse mouth for >1 min with sol
• *Child 6-12 yr:* TOP 5 ml 0.2% sol
• *Child >3 yr:* PO 1 mg qd
• *Child <3 yr:* PO 0.5 mg
Available forms include: Tabs chewable 0.25 mg; tabs 0.5, 1 mg, tab effervescent 10 mg; drops 0.125, 0.25, 0.5 mg/ml; rinse supplements 0.2 mg/ml, rinse 0.01%, 0.02%, 0.09%; gel 0.1%, 0.5%, 1.23%
Side effects/adverse reactions:
ACUTE OVERDOSE: Black tarry stools, bloody vomit, diarrhea, decreased respiration, increased salivation, watery eyes
CHRONIC OVERDOSE: Hypocalcemia and tetany, respiratory arrest, sores in mouth, constipation, loss of appetite, nausea, vomiting, weight loss, discoloration of teeth (white, black, brown)
Contraindications: Hypersensitivity, child <6 yr, pregnancy
Pharmacokinetics:
PO: Excreted in urine and feces, crosses placenta, breast milk

Interactions/incompatibilities:
• Avoid use with dairy products
NURSING CONSIDERATIONS
Assess:
• Use in children
Administer:
• Drops after meals with fluids or undiluted tablets, may be chewed; do not swallow whole, may be given with water or juice
Evaluate:
• Therapeutic response: absence of dental caries
• Nutritional status: increase fluoride content of water, decrease carbohydrate snacks, increase fish, tea, mineral water
Teach patient/family:
• To monitor children using gel or rinse, not to be swallowed
• Not to drink, eat, or rinse mouth for at least ½ hr
• Not to use during pregnancy
• To apply after brushing and flossing hs
• Store out of children's reach

---

sodium hypochlorite
Modified Dakin's Solution
Func. class.: Disinfectant

Action: Destroys microorganism
Uses: Cleansing wounds, athlete's foot
Dosage and routes:
• *Adult and child:* SOL use as needed
Available forms include: Top sol 0.5%
Side effects/adverse reactions:
INTEG: Irritation, bleeding at site
Contraindications: Hypersensitivity
NURSING CONSIDERATIONS
Administer:
• New solution each time applied
• Only to skin; application to hair may result in bleaching

---

italics = common side effects   **bold italic** = life threatening reactions

• To area that will not bleed, or clotting may be reduced
Evaluate:
• Area of the body involved: irritation, rash, breaks, dryness, scales

---

sodium lactate

Func. class.: Alkalinizer

Action: Removes lactate and hydrogen, which leads to alkalinization; lactate is converted to CO_2 and water
Uses: Acidosis (metabolic), alkalinization (urinary)
Dosage and routes:
Acidosis
• *Adult:* IV 1/6 molar (167 mEq lactate/L)
Alkalinization
• *Adult:* IV 30 ml of 1/6 molar sol/kg in divided doses
Available forms include: Inj IV
Side effects/adverse reactions:
CNS: Irritability, headache, confusion, stimulation, tremors, *twitching, hyperreflexia, tetany,* weakness, *convulsions*
CV: Irregular pulse, cardiac arrest
GI: Flatulence, belching, distension, paralytic ileus
META: Alkalosis
RESP: Shallow, slow respirations, cyanosis, apnea
Contraindications: Hypertension, peptic ulcer, renal disease
Precautions: CHF, cirrhosis, toxemia, renal disease
Pharmacokinetics:
PO: Onset 2 min, duration 10 min
IV: Onset immediate
Interactions/incompatibilities:
• Increased effects: amphetamines, mecamylamine, lithium, barbiturates, salicylates, quinine, quinidine, pseudoephedrine
• Do not mix solution with other drugs

NURSING CONSIDERATIONS
Assess:
• Respiratory rate, rhythm, depth, notify physician of abnormalities
• Electrolytes, blood pH, PO_2, HCO_3, during treatment
• Urine pH, urinary output, during beginning treatment
Administer:
• IV slowly to avoid pain at infusion site; check for extravasation
Evaluate:
• Alkalosis: irritability, confusion, twitching, hyperreflexia, stimulation, slow respirations, cyanosis, irregular pulse
Lab tests interferences:
Increase: Urinary urobilinogen
False positive: Urinary protein, blood lactate

---

sodium salicylate
Uracel

Func. class.: Nonnarcotic analgesic
Chem. class.: Salicylate

Action: Blocks pain impulses in CNS that occur in response to inhibition of prostaglandin synthesis; antipyretic action results from inhibition of hypothalamic heat-regulating center to produce vasodilation to allow heat dissipation
Uses: Mild to moderate pain or fever including arthritis, juvenile rheumatoid arthritis
Dosage and routes:
• *Adult:* PO 325-650 mg q4-6h prn; IV INF 500 mg over 4-8 hr, not to exceed 1 g/day
Available forms include: Tabs 325, 650 mg; inj IV 100 mg/ml
Side effects/adverse reactions:
HEMA: Thrombocytopenia, agranulocytosis, leukopenia, neutropenia, hemolytic anemia, increased pro-time
CNS: Stimulation, drowsiness, diz-

ziness, confusion, convulsion, headache, flushing, hallucinations, coma

GI: Nausea, vomiting, GI bleeding, diarrhea, heartburn, anorexia, **hepatitis**

INTEG: Rash, urticaria, bruising

EENT: Tinnitus, hearing loss

CV: Rapid pulse, pulmonary edema

RESP: Wheezing, hyperpnea

ENDO: Hypoglycemia, hyponatremia, hypokalemia

Contraindications: Hypersensitivity to salicylates, GI bleeding, bleeding disorders, children < 3 yr, pregnancy, lactation, vitamin K deficiency

Precautions: Anemia, hepatic disease, renal disease, Hodgkin's disease

Pharmacokinetics: Metabolized by liver, excreted by kidneys, crosses placenta, excreted in breast milk

Interactions/incompatibilities:

• Decreased effects of this drug: antacids, steroids, urinary alkalizers

• Increased blood loss: alcohol, heparin

• Increased effects of: anticoagulants, insulin, methotrexate

• Decreased effects of: probenecid, spironolactone, sulfinpyrazone, sulfonylmides

• Toxic effects: PABA

• Decreased blood sugar levels: salicylates

NURSING CONSIDERATIONS

Assess:

• Liver function studies: AST, ALT, bilirubin, creatinine if patient is on long-term therapy

• Renal function studies: BUN, urine creatinine if patient is on long-term therapy

• Blood studies: CBC, Hct, Hgb, pro-time if patient is on long-term therapy

• I&O ratio; decreasing output may

indicate renal failure (long-term therapy)

Administer:

• To patient crushed or whole; chewable tablets may be chewed

• With food or milk to decrease gastric symptoms; give 30 min before or 2 hr after meals

• With full glass of water

Perform/provide:

• Repositioning to decrease pain

• Cool cloth for fever

Evaluate:

• Hepatotoxicity: dark urine, clay-colored stools, yellowing of skin, sclera, itching, abdominal pain, fever, diarrhea if patient is on long-term therapy

• Allergic reactions: rash, urticaria; if these occur, drug may need to be discontinued

• Renal dysfunction: decreased urine output

• Ototoxicity: tinnitus, ringing, roaring in ears; audiometric testing is needed before, after long-term therapy

• Visual changes: blurring, halos, corneal, retinal damage

• Edema in feet, ankles, legs

• Prior drug history; there are many drug interactions

Teach patient/family:

• To report any symptoms of hepatotoxicity, renal toxicity, visual changes, ototoxicity, allergic reactions (long-term therapy)

• Not to exceed recommended dosage; acute poisoning may result

• To read label on other OTC drugs; many contain aspirin

• That therapeutic response takes 2 wk (arthritis)

• To avoid alcohol ingestion; GI bleeding may occur

Lab test interferences:

Increase: Coagulation studies, liver function studies, serum uric acid, amylase, CO_2, urinary protein

S

---

italics = common side effects   ***bold italic*** = life threatening reactions

Decrease: Serum potassium, PBI, cholesterol

Interfere: Urine catecholamines, pregnancy test

Treatment of overdose: Lavage, activated charcoal, monitor electrolytes, VS

---

sodium thiosalicylate

Arthrolate, Nalate, Osteolate, Thiodyne, Thiolate, Thiosal

Func. class.: Nonnarcotic analgesic

Chem. class.: Salicylate

Action: Blocks pain impulses in CNS that occur in response to inhibition of prostaglandin synthesis; antipyretic action results from inhibition of hypothalamic heat-regulating center

Uses: Mild to moderate pain (rheumatic fever, acute gout)

Dosage and routes:
Pain
• *Adult:* IM 50-100 mg qd or qod
Rheumatic fever
• *Adult:* IM 100-150 mg bid
Arthritis
• *Adult:* IM 100 mg/day
Available forms include: Inj IM 50 mg/ml

Side effects/adverse reactions:
*HEMA: **Thrombocytopenia, agranulocytosis, leukopenia, neutropenia, hemolytic anemia,*** increased pro-time

CNS: Stimulation, drowsiness, dizziness, confusion, convulsion, headache, flushing, hallucinations, coma

GI: Nausea, vomiting, GI bleeding, diarrhea, heartburn, anorexia, *hepatitis*

INTEG: Rash, urticaria, bruising
EENT: Tinnitus, hearing loss
CV: Rapid pulse, pulmonary edema
RESP: Wheezing, hyperpnea
ENDO: Hypoglycemia, hyponatremia, hypokalemia

Contraindications: Hypersensitivity to salicylates, GI bleeding, bleeding disorders, children < 3 yr, pregnancy, lactation, vitamin K deficiency

Precautions: Anemia, hepatic disease, renal disease, Hodgkin's disease

Pharmacokinetics:
PO: Onset 15-30 min, peak 1-2 hr, duration 4-6 hr

REC: Onset slow, duration 4-6 hr, Metabolized by liver, excreted by kidneys, crosses placenta, excreted in breast milk, half-life 1-3½ hr

Interactions/incompatibilities:
• Decreased effects of this drug: antacids, steroids, urinary alkalizers
• Increased blood loss: alcohol, heparin
• Increased effects of: anticoagulants, insulin, methotrexate
• Decreased effects of: probenecid, spironolactone, sulfinpyrazone, sulfonylmides
• Toxic effects: PABA
• Decreased blood sugar levels: salicylates

NURSING CONSIDERATIONS
Assess:
• Liver function studies: ALT, AST, bilirubin, creatinine if patient is on long-term therapy
• Renal function studies: BUN, urine creatinine if patient is on long-term therapy
• Blood studies: CBC, Hct, Hgb, pro-time if patient is on long-term therapy
• I&O ratio; decreasing output may indicate renal failure (long-term therapy)
Administer:
• To patient crushed or whole; chewable tablets may be chewed
• With food or milk to decrease gastric symptoms; give 30 min be-

fore or 2 hr after meals
• With full glass of water
Perform/provide:
• Repositioning to decrease pain
• Cool cloth for fever
Evaluate:
• Hepatotoxicity: dark urine, clay-colored stools, yellowing of skin, sclera, itching, abdominal pain, fever, diarrhea if patient is on long-term therapy
• Allergic reactions: rash, urticaria; if these occur, drug may need to be discontinued
• Renal dysfunction: decreased urine output
• Ototoxicity: tinnitus, ringing, roaring in ears; audiometric testing is needed before, after long-term therapy
• Visual changes: blurring, halos, corneal, retinal damage
• Edema in feet, ankles, legs
• Prior drug history; there are many drug interactions
Teach patient/family:
• To report any symptoms of hepatotoxicity, renal toxicity, visual changes, ototoxicity, allergic reactions (long-term therapy)
• Not to exceed recommended dosage; acute poisoning may result
• To read label on other OTC drugs; many contain aspirin
• That therapeutic response takes 2 wk (arthritis)
• To avoid alcohol ingestion; GI bleeding may occur
Lab test interferences:
Increase: Coagulation studies, liver function studies, serum uric acid, amylase, CO_2, urinary protein
Decrease: Serum potassium, PBI, cholesterol
Interfere: Urine catecholamines, pregnancy test
Treatment of overdose: Lavage, activated charcoal, monitor electrolytes, VS

somatotropin (human growth hormone)

(soe-ma-toe-troe'pin)
Asellacrin, Crescormon
Func. class.: Pituitary hormone
Chem. class.: Growth hormone

Action: Stimulates growth
Uses: Pituitary growth hormone deficiency (hypopituitary dwarfism)
Dosage and routes:
• *Child:* IM 2 IU 3 × /wk, less than 48 hr between doses, may give 4 IU if growth is <1 inch/6 mo
Available forms include: Inj IM, IV 2, 4, 10 IU
Side effects/adverse reactions:
GU: Hypercalciuria
INTEG: Rash, urticaria, pain, inflammation at injection site
CNS: Headache, growth of intracranial tumor
ENDO: **Hyperglycemia, ketosis, hypothyroidism**
SYST: **Antibodies to growth hormone**
Contraindications: Hypersensitivity to benzyl-alcohol, closed epiphyses, intracranial lesions
Precautions: Diabetes mellitus, hypothyroidism
Pharmacokinetics:
Half-life 15-60 min, duration 7 days; metabolized in liver
Interactions/incompatibilities:
• Decreased growth: glucocorticosteroids
• Epiphyseal closure: androgens, thyroid hormones
NURSING CONSIDERATIONS
Assess:
• Growth hormone antibodies if patient fails to respond to therapy
• Thyroid function tests: T_3, T_4, T_7, TSH to identify hypothyroidism
Administer:
• IM, rotate injection site
• After reconstituting 10 IU/5 ml

S

---

italics = common side effects   ***bold italic*** = life threatening reactions

bacteriostatic water for injection, do not shake

Perform/provide:

• Storage in refrigerator for <1 mo if reconstituted <1 wk; do not use discolored or cloudy solutions

Evaluate:

• Allergic reaction: rash, itching, fever, nausea, wheezing

• Hypercalciuria: urinary stones, groin, flank pain, nausea, vomiting, frequency, hematuria, chills

• Growth rate of child at intervals during treatment

Teach patient/family:

• All aspects of drug: action, side effects, dose, when to notify physician

---

spectinomycin dihydrochloride

(spek-ti-noe-mye'sin)

Trobicin

Func. class.: Antibiotic, aminoglycoside

Chem. class.: Aminocyclitol

Action: Inhibits bacterial synthesis by binding to 30S subunit on ribosomes

Uses: Gonorrhea

Dosage and routes:

• *Adult:* IM 2-4 g as single dose

Available forms include: Inj IM 2, 4 g

Side effects/adverse reactions:

CNS: Dizziness, chills, fever, insomnia, headache, anxiety

HEMA: Anemia

GI: Nausea, vomiting, increased BUN

GU: Decreased urine output

INTEG: Pain at injection site, urticaria, rash, pruritus, fever

Contraindications: Hypersensitivity, syphilis

Precautions: Pregnancy, infants, children

Pharmacokinetics:

IM: Peak 1-2 hr, duration >8 hr, half-life 1-3 hr, excreted in urine (active form)

Interactions/incompatibilities:

None known

NURSING CONSIDERATIONS

Assess:

• Gonorrhea culture after treatment

• I&O ratio; report decreased output

• Liver studies: AST, ALT, serum alk phosphatase following multiple doses

• Blood studies: Hct, Hgb, BUN if multiple diagnoses given

• Serologic test for syphilis 3 mo after treatment

Administer:

• After shaking vial

• IM in deep muscle mass

• With 20-gauge needle; no more than 5 ml per site

Perform/provide:

• Storage at room temperature; reconstituted solutions should be discarded after 24 hr

Evaluate:

• Therapeutic response: negative gonorrhea culture after treatment

• Allergies before treatment, reaction of each medication

---

spironolactone

(speer'on-oh-lak'tone)

Aldactone

Func. class.: Potassium-sparing diuretic

Chem. class.: Aldosterone antagonist

Action: Competes with aldosterone at receptor sites in renal tubule, resulting in excretion of sodium chloride, water, retention of potassium, phosphate

Uses: Edema, hypertension, diuretic-induced hypokalemia, primary hyperaldosteronism (diagnosis, short-term treatment, long-term treatment)

Dosage and routes:
Edema/hypertension
• *Adult:* PO 25-200 mg/qd in single or divided doses
• *Child:* PO 3.3 mg/kg/day in single or divided doses
Hypokalemia
• *Adult:* PO 25-100 mg/day; if PO, K supplements are unable to be used
Primary hyperaldosteronism
• *Adult:* PO 400 mg/day × 4 days or 4 wk depending on test, then 100-400 mg/day maintenance
Available forms include: Tab 25, 50, 100 mg

Side effects/adverse reactions:
CNS: Headache, confusion, drowsiness, lethargy, ataxia
GI: Diarrhea, cramps, ***hepatic cirrhosis***
INTEG: Rash, pruritus, urticaria
ENDO: Impotence, gynecomastia, irregular menses, amenorrhea, postmenopausal bleeding, hirsutism, deepening voice, breast carcinoma
ELECT: Hyperchloremic metabolic acidosis, hyperkalemia

Contraindications: Hypersensitivity, anuria, severe renal disease, hyperkalemia

Precautions: Dehydration, hepatic disease, pregnancy, lactation, hyponatremia

Pharmacokinetics:
PO: Onset 24-48 hr, peak 48-72 hr; metabolized in liver, excreted in urine, crosses placenta

Interactions/incompatibilities:
• Decreased potassium levels: kayexalate
• Increased action of: antihypertensives, digitalis, lithium
• Increased hyperkalemia: potassium sparing diuretics, potassium products or captopril

NURSING CONSIDERATIONS
Assess:
• Weight, I&O daily to determine fluid loss; effect of drug may be decreased if used qd
Administer:
• In AM to avoid interference with sleep
• With food, if nausea occurs, absorption may be decreased slightly
Evaluate:
• Improvement in edema of feet, legs, sacral area daily if medication is being used in CHF
• Improvement in CVP q8h
• Signs of metabolic acidosis: drowsiness, restlessness
• Rashes, temperature elevation qd
• Confusion, especially in elderly, take safety precautions if needed
• Hydration: skin turgor, thirst, dry mucous membranes
Teach patient/family:
• That drowsiness, ataxia, mental confusion may occur; observe caution in driving
• To notify physician of cramps, diarrhea, lethargy, thirst, headache, skin rash, menstrual abnormalities, deepening voice, breast enlargement
Lab test interferences:
Interfere: 17-OHCS, 17-KS
Treatment of overdose: Lavage if taken orally, monitor electrolytes, administer IV fluids

S

stanozolol

(stan-oh′zoe′lole)
Winstrol
Func. class.: Androgenic anabolic steroid
Chem. class.: Halogenated testosterone derivative

Action: Increases weight by building body tissue, increases potassium, phosphorus, chloride, and ni-

---

trogen levels, increases bone development

Uses: Prevention of hereditary angioedema, aplastic anemia to increase hemoglobin

Dosage and routes:

Aplastic anemia (possibly effective)

• *Adult:* PO 2 mg tid

• *Child 6-12 yr:* PO up to 2 mg tid

• *Child <6 yr:* PO 1 mg bid

Angioedema

• *Adult:* PO 2 mg tid, then decrease q1-3 mo, down to 2 mg qd or q2 days

Available forms include: Tabs 2 mg

Side effects/adverse reactions:

INTEG: Rash, acneiform lesions, oily hair, skin, flushing, sweating, acne vulgaris, alopecia, hirsutism

CNS: Dizziness, headache, fatigue, tremors, paresthesias, flushing, sweating, anxiety, lability, insomnia

MS: Cramps, spasms

CV: Increased B/P

GU: Hematuria, amenorrhea, vaginitis, decreased libido, decreased breast size, clitoral hypertrophy, testicular atrophy

GI: Nausea, vomiting, constipation, weight gain, *cholestatic jaundice*

EENT: Carpal tunnel syndrome, conjunctional edema, nasal congestion

ENDO: Abnormal GTT

Contraindications: Severe renal disease, severe cardiac disease, severe hepatic disease, hypersensitivity, pregnancy (X), lactation, genital bleeding (abnormal)

Precautions: Diabetes mellitus, CV disease, MI

Pharmacokinetics:

PO: Metabolized in liver, excreted in urine, crosses placenta, excreted in breast milk

Interactions/incompatibilities:

• Increased effects of: oral antidiabetics, oxyphenbutazone

• Increased PT: anticoagulants

• Edema: ACTH, adrenal steroids

• Decreased effects of: insulin

NURSING CONSIDERATIONS

Assess:

• Weight daily, notify physician if weekly weight gain is >5 lb

• B/P q4h

• I&O ratio; be alert for decreasing urinary output, increasing edema

• Growth rate in children since growth rate may be uneven (linear/bone browth) when used for extended period

• Electrolytes: K, Na, Cl, Ca; cholesterol

• Liver function studies: ALT, AST, bilirubin

Administer:

• Titrated dose, use lowest effective dose

Perform/provide:

• Diet with increased calories and protein; decrease sodium if edema occurs

• Supportive drug of anemia

Evaluate:

• Therapeutic response: occurs in 4-6 wk in osteoporosis

• Edema, hypertension, cardiac symptoms, jaundice

• Mental status: affect, mood, behavioral changes, aggression

• Signs of masculinization in female: increased libido, deepening of voice, breast tissue, enlarged clitoris, menstrual irregularities; male: gynecomastia, impotence, testicular atrophy

• Hypercalcemia: lethargy, polyuria, polydipsia, nausea, vomiting, constipation; drug may need to be decreased

• Hypoglycemia in diabetics, since oral anticoagulant action is decreased

Teach patient/family:
• Drug needs to be combined with complete health plan: diet, rest, exercise
• To notify physician if therapeutic response decreases
• Not to discontinue this medication abruptly
• Teach patient all aspects of drug usage, including change in sex characteristics
• Women to report menstrual irregularities
• That 1-3 mo course is necessary for response in breast cancer
• Procedure for use of buccal tablets (requires 30-60 min to dissolve, change absorption site with each dose; do not eat, drink, chew, or smoke while tablet is in place)

Lab test interferences:
Increase: Serum cholesterol, blood glucose, urine glucose
Decrease: Serum calcium, serum potassium, T_4, T_3, thyroid ^{131}I uptake test, urine 17-OHCS

---

streptokinase

(strep-toe-kye′nase)
Kabikinase, Streptase
Func. class.: Thrombolytic enzyme
Chem. class.: β-Hemolytic streptococcus filtrate (purified)

Action: Activates conversion of plasminogen to plasmin (fibrinolysin): plasmin is able to dissolve clots (fibrin), fibrinogen, plasma proteins
Uses: Deep vein thrombosis, pulmonary embolism, arterial thrombosis, arterial embolism, arteriovenous cannula occlusion, lysis of coronary artery thrombi after myocardial infarction
Dosage and routes:
Lysis of coronary artery thrombi
• *Adult:* CC 20,000 IU, then 2000

IU/min over 1 hr as IV INF
Arteriovenous cannula occlusion
• *Adult:* IV INF 250,000 IU/2 ml sol into occluded limb of cannula run over 1/2 hr, clamp for 2 hr, aspirate contents, flush with NaCl sol and reconnect
Thrombosis/embolism
• *Adult:* IV INF 250,000 IU over 1/2 hr, then 100,000 IU/hr for 72 hr for deep thrombosis, 100,000 IU/hr over 24-72 hr for pulmonary embolism
Available forms include: Inj IV
Side effects/adverse reactions:
HEMA: Decreased Hct, **bleeding**
INTEG: Rash, urticaria, phlebitis at IV inf site, itching, flushing, headache
CNS: Headache, fever
GI: Nausea
RESP: Altered respirations, SOB, **bronchospasm**
MS: Low back pain
CV: Hypertension, dysrhythmias
EENT: Periorbital edema
Contraindications: Hypersensitivity, active bleeding, intraspinal surgery, neoplasms of the CNS, ulcerative colitis/enteritis, severe hypertension, renal disease, hepatic disease, hypocoagulation, COPD, subacute bacterial endocarditis, rheumatic valvular disease, cerebral embolism/thrombosis/hemorrhage, intraarterial diagnostic procedure or surgery (10 days), recent major surgery
Precautions: Arterial emboli from left side of heart, pregnancy (C)
Pharmacokinetics:
IV: Excreted in bile, urine, half-life <20 min
Interactions/incompatibilities:
• Aspirin, indomethacin, phenylbutazone, anticoagulants, bleeding: potential
NURSING CONSIDERATIONS
Assess:
• VS, B/P, pulse, resp, neuro

S

---

italics = common side effects   **bold italic** = life threatening reactions

signs, temp at least q4h, temp >104° F or indicators of internal bleed, cardiac rhythm following intracoronary administration

Administer:

• As soon as thrombi identified; not useful for thrombi over 1 wk old

• Cryoprecipatate or fresh, frozen plasma if bleeding occurs

• Loading dose at beginning of therapy may require increase loading doses

• Heparin therapy after thrombolytic therapy is discontinued, TT or APTT less than 2 × control (about 3-4 hr)

• After reconstituting with 5 ml of NS or D₅W; do not shake

• About 10% patients have high streptococcal antibody titres requiring increased loading doses

• IV therapy using 0.22 or 0.45 μm filter

Perform/provide:

• Bed rest during entire course of treatment

• Avoidance of invasive procedures: inj, rectal temp

• Treatment of fever with acetaminophen or aspirin

• Pressure for 30 sec to minor bleeding sites; inform physician if this does not attain hemostasis; apply pressure dressing

Evaluate:

• Allergy: fever, rash, itching, chills; mild reaction may be treated with antihistamines

• For bleeding during 1st hr of treatment: hematuria, hematemesis, bleeding from mucous membranes, epistaxis, ecchymosis

• Blood studies (Hct, platelets, PTT, PT, TT, APTT) before starting therapy; PT or APTT must be less than ×2 control before starting therapy TT ot PT q3-4h during treatment

Lab test interferences:

Increase: PT, APTT, TT

---

streptomycin sulfate

(strep-toe-mye′sin)

Func. class.: Antibiotic
Chem. class.: Aminoglycoside

Action: Interferes with protein synthesis in bacterial cell by binding to ribosomal subunit, causing inaccurate peptide sequence to form in protein chain, causing bacterial death

Uses: Sensitive strains of *M. tuberculosis,* nontuberculous infections caused by sensitive strains of *Y. pestus, Brucella, H. influenzae, K. pneumoniae, E. coli, E. aerogenes, S. viridans, F. tularensis*

Dosage and routes:

Tuberculosis

• *Adult:* IM 1g qd × 2-3 mo, then 1 g 2-3 times/week given with other antitubercular drugs

• *Child:* IM 20-40 mg/kg/day in divided doses given with other antitubercular drugs

Streptococcal endocarditis

• *Adult:* IM 1 g q12h × 1 wk with penicillin, then 500 mg bid for 1 wk

Enterococcal endocarditis

• *Adult:* IM 1 g q12h × 2 wk, then 500 mg q12h × 4 wk with penicillin

Available forms include: Inj IM 1, 5 g

Side effects/adverse reactions:

GU: Oliguria, hematuria, renal damage, azotemia, renal failure, nephrotoxicity

CNS: Confusion, depression, numbness, tremors, *convulsions,* muscle twitching, *neurotoxicity*

EENT: Ototoxicity, deafness, visual disturbances

HEMA: Agranulocytosis, thrombocytopenia, leukopenia, eosinophilia, anemia

GI: Nausea, vomiting, anorexia, in-

---

creased ALT, AST, bilirubin, hepatomegaly, *hepatic necrosis,* splenomegaly
CV: Hypotension, myocarditis
INTEG: Rash, burning urticaria, photosensitivity, dermatitis
Contraindications: Severe renal disease, hypersensitivity
Precautions: Neonates, mild renal disease, pregnancy, myasthenia gravis, lactation, hearing deficits, elderly
Pharmacokinetics:
IM: Onset rapid, peak 1-2 hr; plasma half-life 1-3 hr, not metabolized, excreted unchanged in urine, crosses placental barrier
Interactions/incompatibilities:
• Increased ototoxicity, neurotoxicity, nephrotoxicity: other aminoglycosides, amphotericin B, polymyxin, vancomycin, ethacrynic acid, furosemide, mannitol, methoxyflurane, cisplatin, cephalosporins
• Decreased effects of: parenteral penicillins
• Do not mix in solution or syringe: carbenicillin, ticarcillin, amphotericin B, cephalothin, erythromycin, heparin
• Increased effects: nondepolarizing muscle relaxants

NURSING CONSIDERATIONS
Assess:
• Weight before treatment; calculation of dosage is usually done based on ideal body weight, but may be calculated on actual body weight
• I&O ratio, urinalysis daily for proteinuria, cells, casts; report sudden change in urine output
• VS during infusion, watch for hypotension, change in pulse
• IV site for thrombophlebitis including pain, redness, swelling q30 min; change site if needed; apply warm compresses to discontinued site

• Serum peak, drawn at 30-60 min after IV infusion or 60 min after IM injection, trough level drawn just before next dose; blood level should be 2-4 times bacteriostatic level
• Urine pH if drug is used for UTI; urine should be kept alkaline
Administer:
• IM injection in large muscle mass, rotate injection sites
• Drug in evenly spaced doses to maintain blood level
Perform/provide:
• Adequate fluids of 2-3 L/day unless contraindicated to prevent irritation of tubules
• Flush of IV line with NS or D_5W after infusion
• Supervised ambulation, other safety measures with vestibular dysfunction
Evaluate:
• Therapeutic effect: absence of fever, draining wounds, negative C&S after treatment
• Renal impairment by securing urine for CrCl testing, BUN, serum creatinine; lower dosage should be given in renal impairment (CrCl <80 ml/min)
• Deafness by audiometric testing, ringing, roaring in ears, vertigo; assess hearing before, during, after treatment
• Dehydration: high sp gr, decrease in skin turgor, dry mucous membranes, dark urine
• Overgrowth of infection: increased temperature, malaise, redness, pain, swelling, perineal itching, diarrhea, stomatitis, change in cough, sputum
• C&S before starting treatment to identify infecting organism
• Vestibular dysfunction: nausea, vomiting, dizziness, headache; drug should be discontinued if severe
• Injection sites for redness, swell-

S

---

ing, abscesses; use warm compresses at site

Teach patient/family:

• To report headache, dizziness, symptoms of overgrowth of infection, renal impairment

• To report loss of hearing, ringing, roaring in ears, fullness in head

Treatment of overdose: Hemodialysis, monitor serum levels of drug

---

streptozocin

(strep-toe-zoe′sin)

Zanosar

Func. class.: Antineoplastic alkylating agent

Chem. class.: Nitrosourea

Action: Alkylates DNA, RNA; inhibits enzymes that allow synthesis of amino acids in proteins; is also responsible for cross-linking DNA strands

Uses: Metastatic islet cell carcinoma of pancreas

Dosage and routes:

• *Adult:* IV 500 mg/m² × 5 days q6wk until desired response, alternate with 1000 mg/m² qwk × 2 wk, not to exceed 1500 mg/m² in 1 dose

Available forms include: Inj IV 1 g; powder 100 mg/ml

Side effects/adverse reactions:

HEMA: Thrombocytopenia, leukopenia, pancytopenia

CNS: Confusion, depression, lethargy

GI: Nausea, vomiting, diarrhea, weight loss, hepatotoxicity

GU: Azotemia, anuria, hypophosphatemia, glycosuria, renal tubular acidosis

Contraindications: Hypersensitivity

Precautions: Radiation therapy, children, lactation, pregnancy, hepatic disease, renal disease

Pharmacokinetics:

IV: Metabolized by liver, excreted in urine, half-life 5 min, terminal 35-40 min

Interactions/incompatibilities:

• Increased toxicity: neurotoxic agents, other antineoplastics

• Increased action of: doxorubicin

• Decreased effect of this drug: phenytoin

NURSING CONSIDERATIONS

Assess:

• CBC, differential, platelet count weekly; withhold drug if WBC is <4000 or platelet count is <75,000; notify physician of results

• Renal function studies: BUN, serum uric acid, urine CrCl before, during therapy

• I&O ratio; report fall in urine output of 30 ml/hr

• Monitor temperature q4h (may indicate beginning infection)

• Liver function tests before, during therapy (bilirubin, AST, ALT, LDH) as needed or monthly

Administer:

• Medications by oral route; if possible avoid IM, SC, IV routes to prevent infections

• Antiemetic 30-60 min before giving drug to prevent vomiting

• Antibiotics for prophylaxis of infection

• Slow IV infusion using 21-, 23-, 25-gauge needle

• Topical or systemic analgesics for pain

• Local or systemic drugs for infection

Perform/provide:

• Storage protected from light; refrigerate reconstituted solution, stable for 48 hr at room temperature

• Strict medical asepsis, protective isolation if WBC levels are low

• Special skin care

• Liquid diet, including cola, Jello; dry toast or crackers may be added

---

if patient is not nauseated or vomiting
• Warm compresses at injection site for inflammation

Evaluate:
• Bleeding: hematuria, guaiac, bruising or petechiae, mucosa or orifices q8h
• Food preferences; list likes, dislikes
• Inflammation of mucosa, breaks in skin
• Yellowing of skin, sclera, dark urine, clay-colored stools, itchy skin, abdominal pain, fever, diarrhea
• Local irritation, pain, burning, discoloration at injection site
• Symptoms indicating severe allergic reaction: rash, urticaria, itching, flushing

Teach patient/family:
• Of protective isolation precautions
• To report any complaints or side effects to nurse or physician

---

succinylcholine chloride

(suk-sin-ill-koe'leen)
Anectine, Anectine Flo-Pack Powder, Quelicin
Func. class.: Neuromuscular blocker (depolarizing-ultra short)

Action: Inhibits transmission of nerve impulses by binding with cholinergic receptor sites, antagonizing action of acetylcholine
Uses: Facilitation of endotracheal intubation, skeletal muscle relaxation during mechanical ventilation, surgery, or general anesthesia
Dosage and routes:
• *Adult:* IV 25-75 mg, then 2.5 mg/min as needed; IM 2.5 mg/kg, not to exceed 150 mg
• *Child:* IV/IM 1-2 mg/kg, not to exceed 150 mg IM
Available forms include: Inj IM,

IV 20, 50, 100 mg/ml; powder for inj 100, 500 mg/vial, 1 g/vial
Side effects/adverse reactions:
CV: Bradycardia, tachycardia, increased, decreased B/P, *sinus arrest, dysrhythmias*
*RESP: Prolonged apnea, **bronchospasm, cyanosis, respiratory depression***
EENT: Increased secretions, increased intraocular pressure
MS: Weakness, muscle pain, fasciculations, prolonged relaxation
HEMA: Myoglobulinemia
INTEG: Rash, flushing, pruritus, urticaria
Contraindications: Hypersensitivity, malignant hyperthermia, decreased plasma pseudocholinesterase
Precautions: Pregnancy, cardiac disease, severe burns, fractures—fasciculations may increase damage, lactation, children <2 yr, electrolyte imbalances, dehydration, neuromuscular disease, respiratory disease
Pharmacokinetics:
IV: Onset 1 min, peak 2-3 min, duration 6-10 min
IM: Onset 2-3 min
Hydrolyzed in urine (active/inactive metabolites)
Interactions/incompatibilities:
• Increased neuromuscular blockade: aminoglycosides, clindamycin, lincomycin, quinidine, local anesthetics, polymyxin antibiotics, lithium, narcotic analgesics, thiazides, enflurane, isoflurane
• Dysrhythmias: theophylline
• Do not mix with barbiturates in solution or syringe
NURSING CONSIDERATIONS
Assess:
• For electrolyte imbalances (K, Mg); may lead to increased action of this drug
• Vital signs (B/P, pulse, respirations, airway) until fully recovered;

S

---

italics = common side effects   **bold italic** = life threatening reactions

rate, depth, pattern of respirations, strength of hand grip
• I&O ratio; check for urinary retention, frequency, hesitancy
Administer:
• Using nerve stimulator by anesthesiologist to determine neuromuscular blockade
• Anticholinesterase to reverse neuromuscular blockade
• By slow IV over 1-2 min (only by qualified person, usually an anesthesiologist)
• Only slightly discolored solution
Perform/provide:
• Storage in light-resistant area
• Reassurance if communication is difficult during recovery from neuromuscular blockade
Evaluate:
• Therapeutic response: paralysis of jaw, eyelid, head, neck, rest of body
• Recovery: decreased paralysis of face, diaphragm, leg, arm, rest of body
• Allergic reactions: rash, fever, respiratory distress, pruritus; drug should be discontinued
Treatment of overdose: Edrophonium or neostigmine, atropine, monitor VS; may require mechanical ventilation

Side effects/adverse reactions:
CNS: Drowsiness, dizziness
GI: Dry mouth, constipation, nausea, gastric pain, vomiting
INTEG: Urticaria, rash, pruritus
Contraindications: Hypersensitivity
Precautions: Pregnancy (B), lactation, children
Pharmacokinetics:
PO: Duration up to 6 hr
Interactions/incompatibilities:
• Decreased action of: tetracyclines, cimetidine, phenytoin
NURSING CONSIDERATIONS
Assess:
• Gastric pH (>5 should be maintained)
• I&O ratio, BUN, creatinine
Perform/provide:
• Storage at room temperature
Evaluate:
• Therapeutic response: absence of pain, or GI complaints
Teach patient/family:
• Avoid driving or other hazardous activities until patient is stabilized on this medication
• To avoid black pepper, caffeine, alcohol, harsh spices, extremes in temperature of food
• To avoid OTC preparations: aspirin, cough, cold preparations

---

sucralfate

(soo-kral'fate)
Carafate, Sulcrate*

Func. class.: Protectant
Chem. class.: Aluminum hydroxide/sulfated sucrose

Action: Forms a complex that adheres to ulcer site, inhibits pepsin, gastric juice
Uses: Duodenal ulcer
Dosage and routes:
• *Adult:* PO 1 g qid 1 hr ac, hs
Available forms include: Tabs 1 g

sufentanil citrate

(soo-fen'ta-nil)
Sufenta

Func. class.: Narcotic analgesics
Chem. class.: Opiate, synthetic

Controlled Substance Schedule II
Action: Inhibits ascending pain pathways in CNS, increases pain threshold, alters pain perception
Uses: Primary anesthetic, adjunct to general anesthetic
Dosage and routes:
Primary anesthetic
• *Adult:* IV 8-30 μg/kg given with

100% O_2, a muscle relaxant

Adjunct

• *Adult:* IV 1-8 µg/kg given with nitrous oxide/O_2

Available forms include: Inj IV 50 µg/ml

Side effects/adverse reactions:

CNS: Drowsiness, dizziness, confusion, headache, sedation, euphoria

GI: Nausea, vomiting, anorexia, constipation, cramps

GU: Increased urinary output, dysuria

INTEG: Rash, urticaria, bruising, flushing, diaphoresis, pruritus

EENT: Tinnitus, blurred vision, miosis, diplopia

CV: Palpitations, bradycardia, change in B/P

RESP: Respiratory depression

Contraindications: Hypersensitivity, addiction (narcotic)

Precautions: Addictive personality, pregnancy (C), lactation, increased intracranial pressure, MI (acute), severe heart disease, respiratory depression, hepatic disease, renal disease, child <18 yr

Pharmacokinetics:

PO: Onset 15-30 min, peak 1-2 hr, duration 4-6 hr

REC: Onset slow, duration 4-6 hr Metabolized by liver, excreted by kidneys, crosses placenta, excreted in breast milk, half-life 1-3½ hr

Interactions/incompatibilities:

• Effects may be increased with other CNS depressants: alcohol, narcotics, sedative/hypnotics, antipsychotics, skeletal muscle relaxants

NURSING CONSIDERATIONS

Assess:

• I&O ratio; check for decreasing output (may indicate urinary retention)

Administer:

• With antiemetic if nausea, vomiting occur

Perform/provide:

• Storage in light-resistant area at room temperature

• Assistance with ambulation

• Safety measures: siderails, night light, call bell within easy reach

Evaluate:

• Therapeutic response: maintenance of anesthesia

• CNS changes: dizziness, drowsiness, hallucinations, euphoria, LOC, pupil reaction

• Allergic reactions: rash, urticaria

• Respiratory dysfunction: respiratory depression, character, rate, rhythm; notify physician if respirations are <12/min

• Need for pain medication, physical dependence

Teach patient/family:

• To report any symptoms of CNS changes, allergic reactions

• That physical dependency may result when used for extended periods of time

• Withdrawal symptoms may occur: nausea, vomiting, cramps, fever, faintness, anorexia

Lab test interferences:

Increase: Amylase

Treatment of overdose: Narcan 0.2-0.8 IV, O_2, IV fluids, vasopressors

---

sulfacetamide sodium (ophthalmic)

(sul-fa-see'ta-mide)

Bleph-10, Cetamide, Isopto Cetamide, Sodium Sulamyd, Sulf-O

Func. class.: Antiinfective

Action: Inhibits bacterial growth by preventing PABA use, which is necessary for folic acid synthesis

Uses: Conjunctivitis, superficial eye infections

Dosage and routes:

• *Adult and child:* INSTILL 1-2 gtts q2-3h 10%; 1-2 gtts q1-2h

15%; 1 gtt q2h 30%; TOP apply ½-1 inch oint into conjunctival sac qid & hs

Available forms include: Sterile ophth sol 10%, 30%; sterile ophth oint 10%

Side effects/adverse reactions:
EENT: Burning, stinging, swelling

Contraindications: Hypersensitivity

Precautions: Antibiotic hypersensitivity

Interactions/incompatibilities: None known

NURSING CONSIDERATIONS
Administer:
• After washing hands, cleanse crusts or discharge from eye before application

Perform/provide:
• Storage at room temperature

Evaluate:
• Therapeutic response: absence of redness, inflammation, tearing
• Allergy: itching, lacrimation, redness, swelling

Teach patient/family:
• To use drug exactly as prescribed
• Not to use eye makeup, towels, washcloths, eye medication of others; reinfection may occur
• That drug container tip should not be touched to eye
• To report itching, increased redness, burning, stinging; drug should be discontinued
• That drug may cause blurred vision when ointment is applied

---

sulfacytine
(sul-fa-sye′teen)
Renoquid

Func. class.: Antibiotic
Chem. class.: Short-acting sulfonamide

Action: Interferes with bacterial biosynthesis of proteins by competitive antagonism of PABA when adequate levels are maintained

Uses: Urinary tract infections

Dosage and routes:
• *Adult:* PO 500 mg, then 250 mg qid × days

Available forms include: Tabs 250 mg

Side effects/adverse reactions:
SYST: Anaphylaxis

GI: Nausea, vomiting, abdominal pain, stomatitis, *hepatitis,* glossitis, pancreatitis, diarrhea, *enterocolitis*

CNS: Headache, confusion, insomnia, hallucinations, depression, vertigo, fatigue, anxiety, convulsions, drug fever, chills

HEMA: Leukopenia, neutropenia, thrombocytopenia, agranulocytosis, hemolytic anemia

INTEG: Rash, dermatitis, urticaria, *Stevens-Johnson syndrome,* erythema, photosensitivity, pain, inflammation at injection site

GU: Renal failure, toxic nephrosis, increased BUN, creatinine, crystalluria

CV: Allergic myocarditis

Contraindications: Hypersensitivity to sulfonamides, pregnancy at term, child <14 yr

Precautions: Pregnancy (C), lactation, impaired hepatic function, severe allergy, bronchial asthma

Pharmacokinetics:
PO: Rapidly absorbed, peak 2-3 hr; half-life 4 hr, metabolized in liver, excreted in urine (metabolites), breast milk, crosses placenta, protein-binding 86%

Interactions/incompatibilities:
• Decreased absorption of: digoxin, folic acid
• Decreased effectiveness: oral contraceptives
• Increased toxicity: phenothiazines, probenecid
• Increased hypoglycemic response: sulfonylurea agents

• Do not mix with silver preparations
• Increased anticoagulant effects: oral anticoagulants
• Decreased renal excretion of: methotrexate
• Decreased hepatic clearance of: phenytoin

NURSING CONSIDERATIONS
Assess:
• I&O ratio; note color, character, pH of urine if drug administered for urinary tract infections; output should be 800 ml less than intake; if urine is highly acidic, alkalization may be needed
• Kidney function studies: BUN, creatinine, urinalysis if on long-term therapy
• Drug level

Administer:
• With full glass of water to maintain adequate hydration; increase fluids to 2000 ml/day to decrease crystallization in kidneys
• Medication after C&S; repeat C&S after full course of medication completed
• With resuscitative equipment available; severe allergic reactions may occur

Perform/provide:
• Storage in tight, light-resistant containers at room temperature

Evaluate:
• Therapeutic response: absence of pain, fever, C&S negative
• Blood dyscrasias: skin rash, fever, sore throat, bruising, bleeding, fatigue, joint pain
• Allergic reaction: rash, dermatitis, urticaria, pruritus, dyspnea, bronchospasm

Teach patient/family:
• To take each oral dose with full glass of water to prevent crystalluria
• To complete full course of treatment to prevent superimposed infection
• To avoid sunlight or use sunscreen to prevent burns
• To avoid OTC medications, (aspirin, vitamin C) unless directed by physician
• To use alternative contraceptive measures; decreased effectiveness of oral contraceptives may result
• To notify physician if skin rash, sore throat, fever, mouth sores, unusual bruising, bleeding occur

Lab test interferences:
False positive: Urinary glucose test

---

sulfadiazine
(sul-fa-dye′a-zeen)
Microsulfon
Func. class.: Antibiotic
Chem. class.: Sulfonamide

Action: Interferes with bacterial biosynthesis of proteins by competitive antagonism of PABA when adequate levels are maintained

Uses: Urinary tract infections, rheumatic fever prophylaxis, adjunctive in toxoplasmosis

Dosage and routes:
Urinary tract infections
• *Adult:* PO 2-4 g, then 0.5-1 g q6h × 10 days
• *Child:* PO 75 mg/kg, then 150 mg/kg in 4-6 divided doses qd or 2 g/m², then 4 g/m² in 4-6 divided doses qd
Rheumatic fever prophylaxis
• *Child >30 kg:* PO 1 g qd
• *Child <30 kg:* PO 500 mg qd
Available forms include: Tabs 500 mg

Side effects/adverse reactions:
SYST: Anaphylaxis
GI: Nausea, vomiting, abdominal pain, stomatitis, *hepatitis,* glossitis, pancreatitis, diarrhea, *enterocolitis*
CNS: Headache, confusion, insomnia, hallucinations, depression, vertigo, fatigue, anxiety, convul-

S

---

italics = common side effects   ***bold italic*** = life threatening reactions

sions, drug fever, chills

*HEMA: **Leukopenia, neutropenia, thrombocytopenia, agranulocytosis, hemolytic anemia***

INTEG: Rash, dermatitis, urticaria, ***Stevens-Johnson syndrome,*** erythema, photosensitivity, pain, inflammation at injection site

*GU: **Renal failure, toxic nephrosis,*** increased BUN, creatinine, crystalluria

*CV: **Allergic myocarditis***

Contraindications: Hypersensitivity to sulfonamides, pregnancy at term, child <14 yr

Precautions: Pregnancy (C), lactation, impaired hepatic function, severe allergy, bronchial asthma

Pharmacokinetics:

PO: Rapidly absorbed, onset ½ hr, peak 3-6 hr, 30%-50% bound to plasma proteins, half-life 8-10 hr, excreted in urine, breast milk, crosses placenta

Interactions/incompatibilities:

• Decreased absorption of: digoxin, folic acid

• Decreased effectiveness: oral contraceptives

• Increased toxicity: phenothiazines, probenecid

• Increased hypoglycemic response: sulfonylurea agents

• Do not mix with silver preparations

• Increased anticoagulant effects: oral anticoagulants

• Decreased renal excretion of: methotrexate

• Decreased hepatic clearance of: phenytoin

NURSING CONSIDERATIONS

Assess:

• I&O ratio; note color, character, pH of urine if drug administered for urinary tract infections; output should be 800 ml less than intake; if urine is highly acidic, alkalization may be needed

• Kidney function studies: BUN, creatinine, urinalysis if on long-term therapy

• Drug level

Administer:

• With full glass of water to maintain adequate hydration; increase fluids to 2000 ml/day to decrease crystallization in kidneys

• Medication after C&S; repeat C&S after full course of medication completed

• With resuscitative equipment available; severe allergic reactions may occur

Perform/provide:

• Storage in tight, light-resistant containers at room temperature

Evaluate:

• Therapeutic response: absence of pain, fever, C&S negative

• Blood dyscrasias: skin rash, fever, sore throat, bruising, bleeding, fatigue, joint pain

• Allergic reaction: rash, dermatitis, urticaria, pruritus, dyspnea, bronchospasm

Teach patient/family:

• To take each oral dose with full glass of water to prevent crystalluria

• To complete full course of treatment to prevent superimposed infection

• To avoid sunlight or use sunscreen to prevent burns

• To avoid OTC medication (aspirin, vitamin C) unless directed by physician

• To use alternative contraceptive measures; decreased effectiveness of oral contraceptives may result

• To notify physician if skin rash, sore throat, fever, mouth scores, unusual bruising, bleeding occur

Lab test interferences:

False positive: Urinary glucose test

sulfamethizole

(sul-fa-meth'i-zole)
Bursul, Microsul, Sulfasol, Sulfurine, Thiosulfil, Utrasul

Func. class.: Antibiotic
Chem. class.: Sulfonamide

Action: Interferes with bacterial biosynthesis of proteins by competitive antagonism of PABA when adequate levels are maintained
Uses: Urinary tract infections
Dosage and routes:
• *Adult:* PO 0.5-1 g tid-qid
• Child >2 mo: PO 30-45 mg/kg/day in divided doses q6h
Available forms include: Tabs 250, 500 mg
Side effects/adverse reactions:
SYST: Anaphylaxis
GI: Nausea, vomiting, abdominal pain, stomatitis, *hepatitis,* glossitis, pancreatitis, diarrhea, *enterocolitis*
CNS: Headache, confusion, insomnia, hallucinations, depression, vertigo, fatigue, anxiety, convulsions, drug fever, chills
HEMA: Leukopenia, neutropenia, thrombocytopenia, agranulocytosis, hemolytic anemia
INTEG: Rash, dermatitis, urticaria, *Stevens-Johnson syndrome,* erythema, photosensitivity, pain, inflammation at injection site
GU: Renal failure, toxic nephrosis, increased BUN, creatinine, crystalluria
CV: Allergic myocarditis
Contraindications: Hypersensitivity to sulfonamides, pregnancy at term, child <14 yr
Precautions: Pregnancy (C), lactation, impaired hepatic function, severe allergy, bronchial asthma
Pharmacokinetics:
PO: Rapidly absorbed, peak 2 hr, 90% bound to plasma proteins, excreted in urine, breast milk, crosses placenta
Interactions/incompatibilities:
• Decreased absorption of: digoxin, folic acid
• Decreased effectiveness: oral contraceptives
• Increased toxicity: phenothiazines, probenecid
• Increased hypoglycemic response: sulfonylurea agents
• Do not mix with silver preparations
• Increased anticoagulant effects: oral anticoagulants
• Decreased renal excretion of: methotrexate
• Decreased hepatic clearance of: phenytoin
NURSING CONSIDERATIONS
Assess:
• I&O ratio; note color, character, pH of urine if drug administered for urinary tract infections; output should be 800 ml less than intake; if urine is highly acidic, alkalization may be needed
• Kidney function studies: BUN, creatinine, urinalysis if on long-term therapy
• Drug level
Administer:
• With full glass of water to maintain adequate hydration; increase fluids to 2000 ml/day to decrease crystallization in kidneys
• Medication after C&S; repeat C&S after full course of medication completed
• With resuscitative equipment available; severe allergic reactions may occur
Perform/provide:
• Storage in tight, light-resistant containers at room temperature
Evaluate:
• Therapeutic response: absence of pain, fever, C&S negative
• Blood dyscrasias: skin rash, fever, sore throat, bruising, bleeding,

S

fatigue, joint pain

• Allergic reaction: rash, dermatitis, urticaria, pruritus, dyspnea, bronchospasm

Teach patient/family:

• To take each oral dose with full glass of water to prevent crystalluria

• To complete full course of treatment to prevent superimposed infection

• To avoid sunlight or use sunscreen to prevent burns

• To avoid OTC medication (aspirin, vitamin C) unless directed by physician

• To use alternative contraceptive measures; decreased effectiveness of oral contraceptives may result

• To notify physician if skin rash, sore throat, fever, mouth sores, unusual bruising, bleeding occur

Lab test interferences:

False positive: Urinary glucose test

---

sulfamethoxazole

(sul-fa-meth-ox'a-zole)

Gantanol, Urobak

Func. class.: Antibiotic

Chem. class.: Sulfonamide

Action: Interferes with bacterial biosynthesis of proteins by competitive antagonism of PABA when adequate levels are maintained

Uses: Urinary tract infections, lymphogranuloma venereum, systemic infections, trachoma, nocardiosis, toxoplasmosis, malaria, otitis media, meningococcal meningitis

Dosage and routes:

• *Adult:* PO 2 g, then 1 g bid or tid

• *Child >2 mo:* PO 50-60 mg/kg then 25-30 mg/kg bid, not to exceed 75 mg/kg/day

Lymphogranuloma venereum

• Adult: PO 1 g bid × 14 days

Available forms include: Tabs 500 mg, 1 g; oral susp 500 mg/5ml

Side effects/adverse reactions:

*SYST: **Anaphylaxis***

GI: Nausea, vomiting, abdominal pain, stomatitis, **hepatitis,** glossitis, pancreatitis, diarrhea, **enterocolitis**

CNS: Headache, confusion, insomnia, hallucinations, depression, vertigo, fatigue, anxiety, convulsions, drug fever, chills

*HEMA: **Leukopenia, neutropenia, thrombocytopenia, agranulocytosis, hemolytic anemia***

INTEG: Rash, dermatitis, urticaria, **Stevens-Johnson syndrome,** erythema, photosensitivity, pain, inflammation at injection site

*GU: **Renal failure, toxic nephrosis,** increased BUN, creatinine, crystalluria*

*CV: **Allergic myocarditis***

Contraindications: Hypersensitivity to sulfonamides, pregnancy at term, child <14 yr

Precautions: Pregnancy (C), lactation, impaired hepatic function, severe allergy, bronchial asthma

Pharmacokinetics:

PO: Rapidly absorbed, peak 3-4 hr, 50%-70% bound to plasma proteins, half-life 7-12 hr, excreted in urine (unchanged 70%), breast milk, crosses placenta

Interactions/incompatibilities:

• Decreased absorption of: digoxin, folic acid

• Decreased effectiveness: oral contraceptives

• Increased toxicity: phenothiazines, probenecid

• Increased hypoglycemic response: sulfonylurea agents

• Do not mix with silver preparations

• Increased anticoagulant effects: oral anticoagulants

• Decreased renal excretion of: methotrexate

---

*Available in Canada only

• Decreased hepatic clearance of: phenytoin

NURSING CONSIDERATIONS
Assess:

• I&O ratio; note color, character, pH of urine if drug administered for urinary tract infections; output should be 800 ml less than intake; if urine is highly acidic, alkalization may be needed

• Kidney function studies: BUN, creatinine, urinalysis if on long-term therapy

• Drug level

Administer:

• With full glass of water to maintain adequate hydration; increase fluids to 2000 ml/day to decrease crystallization in kidneys

• Medication after C&S; repeat C&S after full course of medication completed

• With resuscitative equipment available; severe allergic reactions may occur

Perform/provide:

• Storage in tight, light-resistant containers at room temperature

Evaluate:

• Therapeutic response: absence of pain, fever, C&S negative

• Blood dyscrasias: skin rash, fever, sore throat, bruising, bleeding, fatigue, joint pain

• Allergic reaction: rash, dermatitis, urticaria, pruritus, dyspnea, bronchospasm

Teach patient/family:

• To take each oral dose with full glass of water to prevent crystalluria

• To complete full course of treatment to prevent superimposed infection

• To avoid sunlight or use sunscreen to prevent burns

• To avoid OTC medication (aspirin, vitamin C) unless directed by physician

• To use alternative contraceptive measures; decreased effectiveness of oral contraceptives may result

• To notify physician if skin rash, sore throat, fever, mouth sores, unusual bruising, bleeding occur

Lab test interferences:

False positive: Urinary glucose test

---

sulfapyridine

(sul-fa-peer′i-deen)
Dagenan*
Func. class.: Antibiotic
Chem. class.: Sulfonamide

Action: Interferes with bacterial biosynthesis of proteins by competitive antagonism of PABA when adequate levels are maintained

Uses: Dermatitis herpetiformis

Dosage and routes:

• *Adult:* PO 500 mg qid until lesions are improved, then decrease dose by 500 mg q3 days until maintenance dose is achieved

Available forms include: Tabs 500 mg

Side effects/adverse reactions:

SYST: Anaphylaxis

GI: Nausea, vomiting, abdominal pain, stomatitis, *hepatitis,* glossitis, pancreatitis, diarrhea, *enterocolitis*

CNS: Headache, confusion, insomnia, hallucinations, depression, vertigo, fatigue, anxiety, convulsions, drug fever, chills

HEMA: Leukopenia, neutropenia, thrombocytopenia, agranulocytosis, hemolytic anemia

INTEG: Rash, dermatitis, urticaria, *Stevens-Johnson syndrome,* erythema, photosensitivity, pain, inflammation at injection site

GU: Renal failure, toxic nephrosis, increased BUN, creatinine, crystalluria

CV: Allergic myocarditis

Contraindications: Hypersensitivity to sulfonamides, pregnancy at

S

---

term, child <14 yr

Precautions: Pregnancy (C), lactation, impaired hepatic function, severe allergy, bronchial asthma

Pharmacokinetics:

PO: Slowly absorbed, peak 5-7 hr, 10%-45% bound to plasma proteins, half-life 7-12 hr, excreted in urine (metabolites 60%), breast milk, crosses placenta

Interactions/incompatibilities:

• Decreased absorption of: digoxin, folic acid

• Decreased effectiveness: oral contraceptives

• Increased toxicity: phenothiazines, probenecid

• Increased hypoglycemic response: sulfonylurea agents

• Do not mix with silver preparations

• Increased anticoagulant effects: oral anticoagulants

• Decreased renal excretion of: methotrexate

• Decreased hepatic clearance of: phenytoin

NURSING CONSIDERATIONS
Assess:

• I&O ratio; note color, character, pH of urine if drug administered for urinary tract infections; output should be 800 ml less than intake; if urine is highly acidic, alkalization may be needed

• Kidney function studies: BUN, creatinine, urinalysis if on long-term therapy

• Drug level

Administer

• With full glass of water to maintain adequate hydration; increase fluids to 2000 ml/day to decrease crystallization in kidneys

• Medication after C&S; repeat C&S after full course of medication completed

• With resuscitative equipment available, severe allergic reactions may occur

Perform/provide:

• Storage in tight, light-resistant containers at room temperature

Evaluate:

• Therapeutic response: absence of pain, fever, C&S negative

• Blood dyscrasias: skin rash, fever, sore throat, bruising, bleeding, fatigue, joint pain

• Allergic reaction: rash, dermatitis, urticaria, pruritus, dyspnea, bronchospasm

Teach patient/family:

• To take each oral dose with full glass of water to prevent crystalluria

• To complete full course of treatment to prevent superimposed infection

• To avoid sunlight or use sunscreen to prevent burns

• To avoid OTC medication (aspirin, vitamin C) unless directed by physician

• To use alternative contraceptive measures; decreased effectiveness of oral contraceptives may result

• To notify physician if skin rash, sore throat, fever, mouth sores, unusual bruising, bleeding occur

Lab test interferences:

False positive: Urinary glucose test

---

sulfasalazine

(sul-fa-sal′a-zeen)

Azulfidine, SAS-500, Salazopyrin*

Func. class.: Antibiotic

Chem. class.: Sulfonamide

Action: Interferes with bacterial biosynthesis of proteins by competitive antagonism of PABA when adequate levels are maintained

Uses: Ulcerative colitis

Dosage and routes:

• *Adult:* PO 3-4 g/day in divided doses; maintenance 1.5-2 g/day in divided doses q6h

• *Child >2 yrs.:* PO 40-60 mg/kg/

day in 3-6 divided doses, then 30 mg/kg/day in 4 doses

Available forms include: Tabs 500 mg; oral susp 250 mg/5ml; enteric-coated tabs 500 mg

Side effects/adverse reactions:

SYST: Anaphylaxis

GI: Nausea, vomiting, abdominal pain, stomatitis, *hepatitis,* glossitis, pancreatitis, diarrhea, *entero-colitis*

CNS: Headache, confusion, insomnia, hallucinations, depression, vertigo, fatigue, anxiety, convulsions, drug fever, chills

HEMA: Leukopenia, neutropenia, thrombocytopenia, agranulocytosis, hemolytic anemia

INTEG: Rash, dermatitis, urticaria, *Stevens-Johnson syndrome,* erythema, photosensitivity, pain, inflammation at injection site

GU: Renal failure, toxic nephrosis, increased BUN, creatinine, crystalluria

CV: Allergic myocarditis

Contraindications: Hypersensitivity to sulfonamides or salicylates, pregnancy at term, child <14 yr

Precautions: Pregnancy (C), lactation, impaired hepatic function, severe allergy, bronchial asthma

Pharmacokinetics:

PO: Rapidly absorbed, peak 1½-6 hr, half-life 5-10 hr, excreted in urine (unchanged), breast milk, crosses placenta

Interactions/incompatibilities:

• Decreased absorption of: digoxin, folic acid
• Decreased effectiveness: oral contraceptives
• Increased toxicity: phenothiazines, probenecid
• Increased hypoglycemic response: sulfonylurea agents
• Do not mix with silver preparations
• Increased anticoagulant effects: oral anticoagulants

• Decreased renal excretion of: methotrexate
• Decreased hepatic clearance of: phenytoin

NURSING CONSIDERATIONS

Assess:

• I&O ratio; note color, character, pH of urine if drug administered for urinary tract infections; output should be 800 ml less than intake; if urine is highly acidic, alkalization may be needed
• Kidney function studies: BUN, creatinine, urinalysis if on long-term therapy
• Drug level

Administer:

• With full glass of water to maintain adequate hydration; increase fluids to 2000 ml/day to decrease crystallization in kidneys
• Medication after C&S; repeat C&S after full course of medication completed
• With resuscitative equipment available; severe allergic reactions may occur
• Total daily dose in evenly spaced doses to help minimize GI intolerance

Perform/provide:

• Storage in tight, light-resistant containers at room temperature

Evaluate:

• Therapeutic response: absence of pain, fever, C&S negative
• Blood dyscrasias: skin rash, fever, sore throat, bruising, bleeding, fatigue, joint pain
• Allergic reaction: rash, dermatitis, urticaria, pruritus, dyspnea, bronchospasm

Teach patient family:

• To take each oral dose with full glass of water to prevent crystalluria
• To complete full course of treatment to prevent superimposed infection
• To avoid sunlight or use sun-

---

italics = common side effects   ***bold italic*** = life threatening reactions

screen to prevent burns
• To avoid OTC medication (aspirin, vitamin C) unless directed by physician
• To use alternative contraceptive measures; decreased effectiveness of oral contraceptives may result
• To notify physician if skin rash, sore throat, fever, mouth sores, unusual bruising, bleeding occur

Lab test intereferences:
False positive: Urinary glucose test

---

sulfinpyrazone

(sul-fin-peer'a-zone)
Antazone, Anturan,* Anturane, Zynol
Func. class.: Uricosuric
Chem. class.: Pyrazolone

Action: Inhibits tubular reabsorption of urates, with increased excretion of uric acid.
Uses: Inhibition of platelet aggregation, gout
Dosage and routes:
Inhibition of platelet aggregation
• *Adult:* PO 200 mg qid
Gout/gouty arthritis
• *Adult:* PO 100-200 mg bid for 1 wk, then 200-400 mg bid, not to exceed 800 mg/day
Available forms include: Tabs 100 mg; caps 200 mg
Side effects/adverse reactions:
CNS: Dizziness, *convulsions, coma*
EENT: Tinnitus
GU: Renal calculi
GI: Gastric irritation, nausea, vomiting, anorexia, hepatic necrosis, GI bleeding
INTEG: Rash, pain at infusion site, dermatitis, pruritus, fever, photosensitivity
HEMA: Agranulocytosis (rare)
RESP: Apnea, irregular respirations
Contraindications: Hypersensitivity to pyrazolone derivatives, severe hepatic disease, blood dyscra-

sias, severe renal disease, CrCl <50 mg/min
Precautions: Pregnancy, lactation
Pharmacokinetics:
PO: Peak 1-2 hr, duration 4-6 hr, half-life 3 hr, metabolized by liver, excreted in urine
Interactions/incompatibilities:
• Increased toxicity: sulfa drugs, dapsone, clofibrate, PAS, indomethacin, rifampin, naproxen, methotrexate, pantothenic acid
NURSING CONSIDERATIONS
Assess:
• Uric acid levels (3-7 mg/dl)
• Respiratory rate, rhythm, depth; notify physician of abnormalities
• Electrolytes, CO_2 before, during treatment
• Urine pH, output, glucose during beginning treatment
Administer:
• With glass of water
• With food for GI symptoms
Evaluate:
• Therapeutic response: absence of pain, stiffness in joints
Lab test interferences:
Increase: PSP, aminohippuric acid

---

sulfisoxazole

(sul-fi-sox'a-zole)
Barazole, Gantrisin, Novosoxazole,* Rosoxol, Soxomide, Urizole
Func. class.: Antibiotic
Chem. class.: Sulfonamide

Action: Interferes with bacterial biosynthesis of proteins by competitive antagonism of PABA when adequate levels are maintained
Uses: Urinary tract, systemic infections; chancroid; trachoma; toxoplasmosis; acute otitis media; meningococcal, *H. influenzae* meningitis
Dosage and routes:
• *Adult:* PO 2-4 g loading dose, then 1-2 g qid

• *Child >2 mo:* PO 75 mg/kg or 2 g/m² loading dose then 150 mg/kg/day or 4 g/m² day in divided doses q6h, not to exceed 6 g/day

Available forms include: Tabs 500 mg; syr, pediatric susp 500 mg/5 ml, inj IM, SC, IV, emul

Side effects/adverse reactions:

*SYST: **Anaphylaxis***

GI: Nausea, vomiting, abdominal pain, stomatitis, ***hepatitis,*** glossitis, pancreatitis, diarrhea, ***enterocolitis***

CNS: Headache, confusion, insomnia, hallucinations, depression, vertigo, fatigue, anxiety, convulsions, drug fever, chills

*HEMA: **Leukopenia, neutropenia, thrombocytopenia, agranulocytosis, hemolytic anemia***

INTEG: Rash, dermatitis, urticaria, ***Stevens-Johnson syndrome,*** erythema, photosensitivity, pain, inflammation at injection site

*GU: **Renal failure, toxic nephrosis,*** increased BUN, creatinine, crystalluria

*CV: **Allergic myocarditis***

Contraindications: Hypersensitivity to sulfonamides, pregnancy at term, child <14 yr

Precautions: Pregnancy (C), lactation, impaired hepatic function, severe allergy, bronchial asthma

Pharmacokinetics:

PO: Rapidly absorbed, peak 2-4 hr, 85% protein bound; half-life 4-7 hr, excreted in urine (70% unchanged), breast milk, crosses placenta

Interactions/incompatibilities:

• Decreased absorption of: digoxin, folic acid

• Decreased effectiveness: oral contraceptives

• Increased toxicity: phenothiazines, probenecid

• Increased hypoglycemic response: sulfonylurea agents

• Do not mix with silver preparations

• Increased anticoagulant effect: oral anticoagulants

• Decreased renal excretion of: methotrexate

• Decreased hepatic clearance of: phenytoin

NURSING CONSIDERATIONS

Assess:

• I&O ratio; note color, character, pH of urine if drug administered for urinary tract infections; output should be 800 ml less than intake; if urine is highly acidic, alkalization may be needed

• Kidney function studies: BUN, creatinine, urinalysis if on long-term therapy

• Drug level

Administer:

• With full glass of water to maintain adequate hydration; increase fluids to 2000 ml/day to decrease crystallization in kidneys

• Medication after C&S; repeat C&S after full course of medication completed

• With resuscitative equipment available; severe allergic reactions may occur

Perform/provide:

• Storage in tight, light-resistant containers at room temperature

Evaluate:

• Therapeutic response: absence of pain, fever, C&S negative

• Blood dyscrasias: skin rash, fever, sore throat, bruising, bleeding, fatigue, joint pain

• Allergic reaction: rash, dermatitis, urticaria, pruritus, dyspnea, bronchospasm

Teach patient/family:

• Take each oral dose with full glass of water to prevent crystalluria

• To complete full course of treatment to prevent superimposed infection

• To avoid sunlight or use sunscreen to prevent burns

S

---

italics = common side effects   ***bold italic*** = life threatening reactions

• To avoid OTC medication (aspirin, vitamin C) unless directed by physician
• To use alternative contraceptive measures; decreased effectiveness of oral contraceptives may result
• To notify physician if skin rash, sore throat, fever, mouth sores, unusual bruising, bleeding occur

Lab test interferences:
False positive: Urinary glucose test

sulfur

Acnomead, Bensulfoid, Liquimat, Transact, Xerac

Func. class.: Keratolytic

Action: Corrects abnormal keratinization and causes peeling of skin
Uses: Acne, scabies, dandruff, seborrheic dermatitis

Dosage and routes:
• *Adult and child:* Apply to affected area bid or more as needed
Available forms include: Powder 33%; tabs for compunding 130 mg; cream 2%; gel 2%, 4%; lotion 2%, 5%

Side effects/adverse reactions:
INTEG: Irritation of unaffected areas

Contraindications: Hypersensitivity, child <2 yr
Interactions/incompatibilities:
None known

NURSING CONSIDERATIONS
Evaluate:
• Allergic reactions: irritation, redness, itching, stinging, burning; drug should be discontinued
Teach patient/family:
• To avoid getting in eyes or mucous membranes
• Not to use with acne preparations
• To discontinue if irritation occurs

sulfurated lime solution

Vlemasque, Vleminckx's solution

Func. class.: Keratolytic

Action: Corrects abnormal keratinization and causes peeling of skin
Uses: Acne, furunculosis, seborrhea

Dosage and routes:
Furunculosis
• *Adult and child:* SOL 30-60 ml to bath, soak 15 min, rinse
Acne vulgaris/seborrhea
• *Adult and child:* 1 pack/1 pt hot water, soak towel, apply to affected area qd for 15-30 min, rinse
Available forms include: Sol 6%
Side effects/adverse reactions:
INTEG: Irritation of unaffected areas

Contraindications: Hypersensitivity, child <2 yr
Interactions/incompatibilities:
None known
Pharmacokinetics:
TOP: Onset 2 hr, peak 8 hr, duration <24 hr

NURSING CONSIDERATIONS
Evaluate:
• Allergic reactions: irritation, redness, itching, stinging, burning; drug should be discontinued
Teach patient/family:
• To avoid getting in eyes or mucous membranes
• Not to use with acne preparations or mercury preparations
• To discontinue if irritation occurs

sulindac

(sul-in'dak)

Clinoril

Func. class.: Nonsteroidal
Chem. class.: Indeneacetic acid derivative

Action: Inhibits prostaglandin syn-

thesis by decreasing an enzyme needed for biosynthesis; possesses analgesic, antiinflammatory, antipyretic properties
Uses: Mild to moderate pain, osteoarthritis, rheumatoid arthritis
Dosage and routes:
Arthritis
• *Adult:* PO 150 mg bid, may increase to 200 mg bid
Bursitis/acute arthritis
• *Adult:* PO 200 mg bid × 1-2 wk, then reduce dose
Available forms include: Tabs 150, 200 mg
Side effects/adverse reactions:
GI: Nausea, anorexia, vomiting, diarrhea, jaundice, *cholestatic hepatitis,* constipation, flatulence, cramps, dry mouth, peptic ulcer
CNS: Dizziness, drowsiness, fatigue, tremors, confusion, insomnia, anxiety, depression
CV: Tachycardia, peripheral edema, palpitations, dysrhythmias
INTEG: Purpura, rash, pruritus, sweating
GU: Nephrotoxicity: dysuria, hematuria, oliguria, azotemia
HEMA: Blood dyscrasias
EENT: Tinnitus, hearing loss, blurred vision
Contraindications: Hypersensitivity, asthma, severe renal disease, severe hepatic disease
Precautions: Pregnancy, lactation, children, bleeding disorders, GI disorders, cardiac disorders, hypersensitivity to other antiinflammatory agents
Pharmacokinetics:
PO: Peak 2 hr, half-life 3-3½ hr; metabolized in liver, excreted in urine (metabolites) excreted in breast milk
Interactions/incompatibilities:
• May increase action of coumarin, phenytoin, sulfonamides when used with this drug

NURSING CONSIDERATIONS
Assess:
• Renal, liver, blood studies: BUN, creatinine, AST, ALT, HgB, before treatment, periodically thereafter
• Audiometric, ophthalmic exam before, during, after treatment
Administer:
• With food to decrease GI symptoms; best to take on empty stomach to facilitate absorption
Perform/provide:
• Storage at room temperature
Evaluate:
• Therapeutic response: decreased pain, stiffness, swelling in joints, ability to move more easily
• For eye, ear problems: blurred vision, tinnitus (may indicate toxicity)
Teach patient/family:
• To report blurred vision or ringing, roaring in ears (may indicate toxicity)
• To avoid driving or other hazardous activities if dizziness or drowsiness occurs
• To report change in urine pattern, weight increase, edema, pain increase in joints, fever, blood in urine (indicates nephrotoxicity)
• That therapeutic effects may take up to 1 mo

suprofen
(soo-proe′fen)
Suprol
Func. class.: Nonsteroidal
Chem. class.: Propionic acid derivative

Action: Inhibits prostaglandin synthesis by decreasing an enzyme needed for biosynthesis; possesses analgesic, antiinflammatory, antipyretic properties
Uses: Mild to moderate pain, osteoarthritis, rheumatoid arthritis

Dosage and routes:

• *Adult:* PO 200 mg q4-6h, not to exceed 800 mg/day

Available forms include: Caps 200 mg

Side effects/adverse reactions:

GI: Nausea, anorexia, vomiting, diarrhea, jaundice, *cholestatic hepatitis,* constipation, flatulence, cramps, dry mouth, peptic ulcer

CNS: Dizziness, drowsiness, fatigue, tremors, confusion, insomnia, anxiety, depression

CV: Tachycardia, peripheral edema, palpitations, dysrhythmias

INTEG: Purpura, rash, pruritus, sweating

GU: *Nephrotoxicity:* dysuria, hematuria, oliguria, azotemia

HEMA: *Blood dyscrasias*

EENT: Tinnitus, hearing loss, blurred vision

Contraindications: Hypersensitivity, asthma, severe renal disease, severe hepatic disease

Precautions: Pregnancy, lactation, children, bleeding disorders, GI disorders, cardiac disorders, hypersensitivity to other antiinflammatory agents

Pharmacokinetics:

PO: Peak 2 hr, half-life 3-3½ hr; metabolized in liver, excreted in urine (metabolites) excreted in breast milk

Interactions/incompatibilities:

• May increase action of coumarin, phenytoin, sulfonamides when used with this drug

NURSING CONSIDERATIONS

Assess:

• Renal, liver, blood studies: BUN, creatinine, AST, ALT, Hgb, before treatment, periodically thereafter

• Audiometric, ophthalmic exam before, during, after treatment

Administer:

• With food to decrease GI symptoms; best to take on empty stomach to facilitate absorption

Perform/provide:

• Storage at room temperature

Evaluate:

• Therapeutic response: decreased pain, stiffness, swelling in joints, ability to move more easily

• For eye, ear problems: blurred vision, tinnitus (may indicate toxicity)

Teach patient/family:

• To report blurred vision or ringing, roaring in ears (may indicate toxicity)

• To avoid driving or other hazardous activities if dizziness or drowsiness occurs

• To report change in urine pattern, weight increase, edema, pain increase in joints, fever, blood in urine (indicates nephrotoxicity)

• That therapeutic effects may take up to 1 mo

---

sutilains

(soo'ti-lains)

Travase

Func. class.: Topical enzyme preparation

Chem. class.: Proteolytic enzyme concentration

Action: Digests necrotic tissue, hemoglobin, exudate that impairs adequate wound healing

Uses: Debridement in decubitus ulcers, severe burns, peripheral vascular ulcers, pyogenic wounds, ulcers secondary to peripheral vascular disease

Dosage and routes:

• *Adult and child:* TOP apply to affected area, ½-inch beyond area to be debrided, cover loosely with wet dressing, reapply tid-qid

Available forms include: Top oint 82,000 casein U/g

Side effects/adverse reactions:

CNS: Pain, paresthesias

INTEG: Bleeding, dermatitis

Contraindications: Hypersensitivity, severe wounds
Precautions: Pregnancy
Pharmacokinetics:
TOP: Onset 1 hr, peak 6 hr, duration 8-12 hr
Interactions/incompatibilities:
• Decreased action: benzalkonium chloride, hexachlorophene, iodine, nitrofurazone, silver nitrate, thimerosal products, detergents

NURSING CONSIDERATIONS
Administer:
• Cover with dressing (loose, wet)
• After putting on gloves to protect healthy skin, wash after application
• After covering healthy skin with protectant such as petrolatum
Perform/provide:
• Refrigeration after use
• Wear gloves
• Thorough cleansing of wound with sterile water with 0.9% NaCl
• Thorough moistening of wound area
• Changing gloves, then applying ointment in thin layer
Evaluate:
• Therapeutic response: clean, pink wound after 5-7 days (burns) or 8-12 days (ulcers)
• Area of body involved, including time involved, what helps or aggravates condition
Teach patient/family:
• To discontinue use if rash, irritation occurs
• To avoid contact with eyes

---

talbutal
(tal'byoo-tal)
Lotusate
Func. class.: Sedative/hypnotic-barbiturate (intermediate acting)
Chem. class.: Barbitone

Controlled Substance Schedule II (USA), Schedule G (Canada)
Action: Depresses activity in brain cells primarily in reticular activating system in brainstem; selectively depresses neurons in posterior hypothalamus, limbic structures
Uses: Insomnia, short-term treatment only
Dosage and routes:
• *Adult:* PO 120 mg hs
Available forms include: Tabs 120 mg
Side effects/adverse reactions:
CNS: Lethargy, drowsiness, hangover, dizziness, stimulation in elderly and children, lightheadedness, dependence, CNS depression, mental depression, slurred speech
GI: Nausea, vomiting, diarrhea, constipation
INTEG: Rash, urticaria, pain, abscesses at injection site, angioedema, thrombophlebitis, ***Stevens-Johnson syndrome***
CV: Hypotension, bradycardia
RESP: Depression, apnea, ***laryngospasm, bronchospasm***
*HEMA: **Agranulocytosis, thrombocytopenia, megaloblastic anemia*** (long-term treatment)
Contraindications: Hypersensitivity to barbiturates, respiratory depression, addiction to barbiturates, severe liver impairment, porphyria
Precautions: Anemia, pregnancy, lactation, hepatic disease, renal disease, hypertension, elderly, acute/chronic pain
Pharmacokinetics:
Onset 30-45 min, duration 4-6 hr; metabolized by liver, excreted by kidneys (metabolites)
Interactions/incompatibilities:
• Increased CNS depression: alcohol, MAOIs, sedative, narcotics
• Decreased effect of: oral anticoagulants, corticosteroids, griseofulvin, quinidine
• Increased half-life of: doxycycline

T

---

italics = common side effects   **bold italic** = life threatening reactions

NURSING CONSIDERATIONS
Assess:

• Blood studies: Hct, Hgb, RBCs, if blood dyscrasias are suspected
• Hepatic studies: AST, ALT, bilirubin, if hepatic damage has occurred

Administer:

• After removal of cigarettes, to prevent fires
• After trying conservative measures for insomnia
• ½-1 hr before hs for sleeplessness
• On empty stomach for best absorption
• For < 14 days since drug is not effective after that, tolerance develops
• Crushed or whole

Perform/provide:

• Assistance with ambulation after receiving dose
• Safety measure: siderails, nightlight, callbell within easy reach
• Checking to see PO medication has been swallowed
• Storage in tight container in cool environment

Evaluate:

• Therapeutic response: ability to sleep at night, decreased amount of early morning awakening
• Mental status: mood, sensorium, affect, memory (long, short)
• Physical dependency: more frequent requests for medication, shakes, anxiety
• Barbiturate toxicity: hypotension; pulmonary constriction; cold, clammy skin; cyanosis of lips; insomnia; nausea; vomiting; hallucinations; delirium; weakness; mild symptoms may occur in 8-12 hr without drug
• Respiratory dysfunction: respiratory depression, character, rate, rhythm; hold drug if respirations are < 12 /min or if pupils are dilated (rare)
• Blood dyscrasias: fever, sore throat, bruising, rash, jaundice, epistaxis (rare)

Teach patient/family:

• That hangover is common
• That drug is indicated only for short-term treatment of insomnia and is probably ineffective after 2 wk
• That physical dependency may result when used for extended periods of time (45-90 days depending on dose)
• To avoid driving or other activities requiring alertness
• To avoid alcohol ingestion or CNS depressants; serious CNS depression may result
• To tell all prescribers that barbiturate is being taken
• That withdrawal insomnia may occur after short-term use; do not start using drug again; insomnia will improve in 1-3 nights
• That effects may take 2 nights for benefits to be noticed
• Alternate measures to improve sleep (reading, exercise several hours before hs, warm bath, warm milk, TV, self-hypnosis, deep breathing)

Lab test interferences:

False increase: Sulfobromophthalein

Treatment of overdose: Lavage, activated charcoal, warming blanket, vital signs, hemodialysis, I&O ratio

tamoxifen citrate
(ta-mox'i-fen)
Nolvadex

Func. class.: Antineoplastic
Chem. class.: Hormone, antiestrogen

Action: Inhibits cell division by binding to cytoplasmic receptors (estrogen receptors); resembles normal cell complex but inhibits DNA synthesis

Uses: Advanced breast carcinoma that has not responded to other therapy

Dosage and routes:
• *Adult:* PO 10-20 mg bid

Available forms include: Tabs 10 mg

Side effects/adverse reactions:

*HEMA: **Thrombocytopenia, leukopenia***

GI: Nausea, vomiting

GU: Vaginal bleeding, pruritus vulvae

INTEG: Rash, alopecia

RESP: Dyspnea

CV: Chest pain

CNS: Hot flashes, headache, lightheadedness

EENT: Ocular lesions, retinopathy, corneal opacity, blurred vision

Contraindications: Hypersensitivity, pregnancy (D)

Precautions: Leukopenia, thrombocytopenia, lactation, cataracts

Pharmacokinetics:

PO: Peak 4-7 hr, half-life 7-14 hr (1 wk terminal), excreted in feces, urine

Interactions/incompatibilities: None known

NURSING CONSIDERATIONS
Assess:
• CBC, differential, platelet count weekly; withhold drug if WBC is <4000 or platelet count is <75,000; notify physician of results
• Pulmonary function tests, chest x-ray films before, during therapy; chest x-ray film should be obtained q2wk during treatment

Administer:
• Medications by oral route; if possible avoid IM, SC, IV routes to prevent infections
• Antacid before oral agent; give drug after evening meal, before bedtime

• Antiemetic 30-60 min before giving drug to prevent vomiting
• Antibiotics for prophylaxis of infection

Perform/provide:
• Strict medical asepsis, protective isolation if WBC levels are low
• Deep breathing exercises with patient tid-qid; place in semi-Fowler's position
• Liquid diet, including cola, Jello; dry toast or crackers may be added if patient is not nauseated or vomiting
• Increase fluid intake to 2-3 L/day to prevent dehydration
• Nutritious diet with iron, vitamin supplements as ordered
• HOB increased to facilitate breathing
• Storage in light-resistant container at room temperature

Evaluate:
• Bleeding: hematuria, guaiac, bruising, petechiae, mucosa or orifices q8h
• Dyspnea, rales, unproductive cough, chest pain, tachypnea, fatigue, increased pulse, pallor, lethargy
• Food preferences; list likes, dislikes
• Effects of alopecia on body image; discuss feelings about body changes
• Edema in feet, joint, stomach pain, shaking
• Symptoms indicating severe allergic reactions: rash, pruritus, urticaria, purpuric skin lesions, itching, flushing

Teach patient/family:
• Of protective isolation precautions
• To report any complaints, side effects to nurse or physician
• That vaginal bleeding, pruritus, hot flashes, ocular lesions can occur, are reversible after discontinuing treatment

T

---

italics = common side effects   ***bold italic*** = life threatening reactions

• To report any changes in breathing, coughing

• That hair may be lost during treatment; a wig or hairpiece may make patient feel better; new hair may be different in color, texture

Lab test interferences:

Increase: Serum Ca

---

temazepam

(te-maz'e-pam)

Restoril

Func. class.: Sedative-hypnotic

Chem. class.: Benzodiazepine

Controlled Substance Schedule IV (USA), Schedule F (Canada)

Action: Produces CNS depression at limbic, thalamic, hypothalamic levels of the CNS; may be mediated by neurotransmitter gamma aminobutyric (GABA); results are sedation, hypnosis, skeletal muscle relaxation, anticonvulsant activity, anxiolytic action

Uses: Insomnia

Dosage and routes:

• *Adult:* PO 15-30 mg hs

Available forms include: Caps 15, 30 mg

Side effects/adverse reactions:

*HEMA: **Leukopenia, granulocytopenia** (rare)*

CNS: Lethargy, drowsiness, daytime sedation, dizziness, confusion, lightheadedness, headache, anxiety, irritability

GI: Nausea, vomiting, diarrhea, heartburn, abdominal pain, constipation

CV: Chest pain, pulse changes

Contraindications: Hypersensitivity to benzodiazepines, pregnancy (X), lactation, intermittent porphyria

Precautions: Anemia, hepatic disease, renal disease, suicidal individuals, drug abuse, elderly, psychosis, child < 15 yr, acute narrow-angle glaucoma, seizure disorders

Pharmacokinetics:

PO: Onset 30-45 min, duration 6-8 hr, half-life 10-20 hr; metabolized by liver, excreted by kidneys, crosses placenta, excreted in breast milk

Interactions/incompatibilities:

• Increased effects of: cimetidine, disulfiram

• Increased or decreased effects of: oral contraceptives

• Increased action of both drugs: alcohol

• Decreased effect of: antacids

NURSING CONSIDERATIONS

Assess:

• Blood studies: Hct, Hgb, RBCs (if on long-term therapy)

• Hepatic studies: AST, ALT, bilirubin (if on long-term therapy)

Administer:

• After removal of cigarettes, to prevent fires

• After trying conservative measures for insomnia

• ½-1 hr before hs for sleeplessness

• On empty stomach fast onset, but may be taken with food if GI symptoms occur

Perform/provide:

• Assistance with ambulation after receiving dose

• Safety measure: siderails, nightlight, callbell within easy reach

• Checking to see PO medication has been swallowed

• Storage in tight container in cool environment

Evaluate:

• Therapeutic response: ability to sleep at night, decreased amount of early morning awakening if taking drug for insomnia

• Mental status: mood, sensorium, affect, memory (long, short)

• Blood dyscrasias: fever, sore throat, bruising, rash, jaundice, epistaxis (rare)

• Type of sleep problem: falling asleep, staying asleep

Teach patient/family:

• To avoid driving or other activities requiring alertness until drug is stabilized

• To avoid alcohol ingestion or CNS depressants; serious CNS depression may result

• That effects may take 2 nights for benefits to be noticed

• Alternate measures to improve sleep: reading, exercise several hours before hs, warm bath, warm milk, TV, self-hypnosis, deep breathing

• That hangover is common in elderly, but less common than with barbiturates

Lab test interferences:

Increase: ALT/AST, serum bilirubin

Decrease: RAI uptake

False increase: Urinary 17-OHCS

Treatment of overdose: Lavage, activated charcoal, monitor electrolytes, vital signs

---

terbutaline sulfate

(ter-byoo′te-leen)

Brethaire, Brethine, Bricanyl

Func. class.: Adrenergic

Chem. class.: Catecholamine

Action: Causes increased contractility and heart rate by acting on β-receptors in heart; also, acts on α-receptors, causing vasoconstriction in blood vessels; when larger doses are administered, causes vasodilation in renal intracerebral, coronary dopaminergic receptors

Uses: Bronchospasm, premature labor

Dosage and routes:

Bronchospasm

• *Adult and child >12 yr:* INH 2 puffs q1 min apart, then q4-6h; PO 2.5-5 mg q8h; SC 0.25 mg q8h

Premature Labor

• *Adult:* IV INF: 0.01 mg/min, increased by 0.005 mg q10 min, not to exceed 0.025 mg/min; SC 0.25 mg q1h; PO 5 mg q4h × 48 hr, then 5 mg q6h as maintenance for above doses

Available forms include: Tabs 2.5, 5 mg; aerosol 0.2 mg/actuation

Side effects/adverse reactions:

CNS: Tremors, anxiety, insomnia, headache, dizziness, stimulation

CV: Palpitations, tachycardia, hypertension, *cardiac arrest*

GI: Nausea

Contraindications: Hypersensitivity to sympathomimetics, narrow-angle glaucoma

Precautions: Pregnancy, cardiac disorders, hyperthyroidism, diabetes mellitus, prostatic hypertrophy

Pharmacokinetics:

PO: Onset ½ hr, duration 4-8 hr

SC: Onset 6-15 min, duration 1½-4 hr

INH: Onset 5-30 min, duration 3-6 hr

Interactions/incompatibilities:

• Increased effects of both drugs: other sympathomimetics

• Decreased action: β-blockers

NURSING CONSIDERATIONS

Assess:

• Respiratory function: vital capacity, forced expiratory volume, ABGs

Administer:

• 2 hr before hs to avoid sleeplessness

Perform/provide:

• Storage at room temperature, do not use discolored solutions

Evaluate:

• Therapeutic response: absence of dyspnea, wheezing

• Tolerance over long-term therapy, dose may need to be increased or changed

Teach patient/family:

• Not to use OTC medications, ex-

T

---

tra stimulation may occur
• Use of inhaler, review package insert with patient
• To avoid getting aerosol in eyes
• To wash inhaler in warm water and dry qd
• On all aspects of drug; avoid smoking, smoke-filled rooms, persons with respiratory infections
Treatment of overdose: Administer an α-blocker, then norepinephrine for severe hypotension

---

terfenadine

(ter-fin'-a-deen)
Seldane

Func. class.: Antihistamine
Chem. class.: Butyrophenone derivative

Action: Acts on blood vessels, GI, respiratory system by competing with histamine for H_1-receptor site; decreases allergic response by blocking histamine
Uses: Rhinitis, allergy symptoms
Dosage and routes:
• *Adult and child >12 yr:* PO 60 mg bid
• *Child <12 yr:* PO 15-30 mg bid
Available forms include: Tabs 60 mg
Side effects/adverse reactions:
CNS: Dizziness, drowsiness, poor coordination
CV: Hypotension, palpitations
RESP: Increased thick secretions
GI: Nausea, vomiting, anorexia, increased liver function tests, dry mouth
INTEG: Rash, urticaria
GU: Retention
Contraindications: Hypersensitivity
Precautions: Pregnancy (C)
Pharmacokinetics:
PO: Peak 1-2 hr, 97% bound to

plasma proteins, half-life is biphasic 3½ hr, 16-23 hr
Interactions/incompatibilities:
None known
NURSING CONSIDERATIONS
Assess:
• I&O ratio; be alert for urinary retention, frequency, dysuria; drug should be discontinued if these occur
• CBC during long-term therapy
Administer:
• Coffee, tea, cola (caffeine) to decrease drowsiness
• With meals if GI symptoms occur; absorption may slightly decrease
• When used for motion sickness, 30 min before travel
Perform/provide:
• Hard candy, gum, frequent rinsing of mouth for dryness
• Storage in tight, light-resistant container
Evaluate:
• Therapeutic response: absence of running or congested nose or rashes
• Respiratory status: rate, rhythm, increase in bronchial secretions, wheezing, chest tightness
• Cardiac status: palpitations, increased pulse, hypotension
Teach patient/family:
• All aspects of drug use; to notify physician if confusion, sedation, hypotension occurs
• To avoid driving or other hazardous activity if drowsiness occurs
Lab test interferences:
False negative: Skin allergy tests
Treatment of overdose: Administer ipecac syrup or lavage, diazepam, vasopressors, barbiturates (short-acting)

---

terpin hydrate

(ter'pin)

Func. class.: Expectorant

Action: Direct action on respiratory tract, which increases fluids, allows for expectoration

Uses: Bronchial secretions

Dosage and routes:

• *Adult:* ELIX 5-10 ml q4-6h

Available forms include: Elix terpin hydrate codeine 10 mg codeine / 85 mg terpin hydrate; elix, plain 85 mg/5 ml

Side effects/adverse reactions:

GI: Nausea, vomiting, anorexia

Contraindications: Hypersensitivity, child <12 yr, lactation, pregnancy

Pharmacokinetics: Not known

Interactions/incompatibilities: None known

NURSING CONSIDERATIONS

Administer:

• With glass of water or food to decrease GI irritation

Perform/provide:

• Storage at room temperature

Evaluate:

• Therapeutic response: absence of thick secretions

• Cough: type, frequency, character including sputum

Teach patient/family:

• Avoid driving, other hazardous activities until patient is stabilized on this medication (if combined with codeine, drowsiness occurs)

• Do not exceed recommended dosage

testolactone

(tess-toe-lak'tone)

Teslac

Func. class.: Antineoplastic

Chem. class.: Hormone, androgen

Action: Acts on adrenal cortex to suppress activity; this drug is a cytotoxic agent that suppresses activity rather than causing cell death

Uses: Advanced breast carcinoma in postmenopausal women

Dosage and routes:

• *Adult:* PO 250 mg qid

Available forms include: Tabs 50 mg

Side effects/adverse reactions:

GI: Nausea, vomiting, anorexia, glossitis

*GU: Urinary retention, **renal failure***

INTEG: Rash, nail changes, facial hair growth

CV: Hypertension, edema

CNS: Paresthesias, dizziness

EENT: Deepening voice

Contraindications: Hypersensitivity, premenopausal women, carcinoma of male breast

Precautions: Renal disease, hypercalcemia, cardiac disease, pregnancy

Pharmacokinetics: None known

Interactions/incompatibilities:

• Enhanced effects of oral anticoagulants

NURSING CONSIDERATIONS

Assess:

• CA$^+$ levels

• B/P q4h, tell patient to rise slowly from sitting or lying down

Administer:

• For at least 3 mo or longer for desired response

Perform/provide:

• Liquid diet, including cola, Jello; dry toast or crackers may be added

T

if patient is not nauseated or vomiting

• Limited calcium intake (dairy products)

Evaluate:

• Food preferences; list likes, dislikes

• Edema in feet, joint, stomach pain, shaking

• Local irritation, pain, burning, discoloration at injection site

• Symptoms indicating severe allergic reaction: rash, pruritus, urticaria, purpuric skin lesions, itching, flushing

• Tingling in hands, face, feet; indication of nephrotoxicity

• Anorexia, nausea, vomiting, constipation, weakness, loss of muscle tone (indicating hypercalcemia)

Teach patient/family:

• To report any complaints, side effects to nurse or physician

Lab test interferences:

Increase: Urinary 17-OHCS

---

testosterone

(tess-toss′ter-one)

Histerone, Malogen, Testoject

Func. class.: Androgenic anabolic steroid

Chem. class.: Halogenated testosterone derivative

Action: Increases weight by building body tissue, increases potassium, phosphorus, chloride, nitrogen levels, increases bone development

Uses: Breast engorgement, breast cancer in postmenopausal women, eunuchoidism, eunuchism, male climacteric

Dosage and routes:

Breast engorgement

• *Adult:* IM 25-50 mg/day × 3-4 days

Breast cancer

• *Adult:* IM 100 mg 3 ×/wk

Male climacteric/eunuchoidism/eunuchism

• *Adult:* IM 10-25 mg 2-5 ×/wk

Available forms include: Inj IM 25, 50, 100 mg/ml

Side effects/adverse reactions:

INTEG: Rash, acneiform lesions, oily hair, skin, flushing, sweating, acne vulgaris, alopecia, hirsutism

CNS: Dizziness, headache, fatigue, tremors, paresthesias, flushing, sweating, anxiety, lability, insomnia

MS: Cramps, spasms

CV: Increased B/P

GU: Hematuria, amenorrhea, vaginitis, decreased libido, decreased breast size, clitoral hypertrophy, testicular atrophy

GI: Nausea, vomiting, constipation, weight gain, *cholestatic jaundice*

EENT: Carpal tunnel syndrome, conjunctival edema, nasal congestion

ENDO: Abnormal GTT

Contraindications: Severe renal disease, severe cardiac disease, severe hepatic disease, hypersensitivity, pregnancy (X), lactation, genital bleeding (abnormal)

Precautions: Diabetes mellitus, CV disease, MI

Pharmacokinetics:

PO: Metabolized in liver, excreted in urine, crosses placenta, excreted in breast milk

Interactions/incompatibilities:

• Increased effects of: oral antidiabetics, oxyphenbutazone

• Increased PT: anticoagulants

• Edema: ACTH, adrenal steroids

• Decreased effects of: insulin

NURSING CONSIDERATIONS

Assess:

• Weight daily, notify physician if weekly weight gain is >5 lb

• B/P q4h

• I&O ratio; be alert for decreasing

urinary output, increasing edema
• Growth rate in children since growth rate may be uneven (linear/bone browth) when used for extended period
• Electrolytes: K, Na, Cl, Ca; cholesterol
• Liver function studies: ALT, AST, bilirubin
Administer:
• Titrated dose, use lowest effective dose
• IM deep into upper outer quadrant of gluteal muscle
Perform/provide:
• Diet with increased calories and protein; decrease sodium if edema occurs
• Supportive drug of anemia
Evaluate:
• Therapeutic response: occurs in 4-6 wk in osteoporosis
• Edema, hypertension, cardiac symptoms, jaundice
• Mental status: affect, mood, behavioral changes, aggression
• Signs of masculinization in female: increased libido, deepening of voice, breast tissue, enlarged clitoris, menstrual irregularities; male: gynecomastia, impotence, testicular atrophy
• Hypercalcemia: lethargy, polyuria, polydipsia, nausea, vomiting, constipation; drug may need to be decreased
• Hypoglycemia in diabetics, since oral anticoagulant action is decreased
Teach patient/family:
• Drug needs to be combined with complete health plan: diet, rest, exercise
• To notify physician if therapeutic response decreases
• Not to discontinue this medication abruptly
• Teach patient all aspects of drug usage, including changes in sex characteristics

• Women to report menstrual irregularities
• That 1-3 mo course is necessary for response in breast cancer
Lab test interferences:
Increase: Serum cholesterol, blood glucose, urine glucose
Decrease: Serum calcium, serum potassium, T_4, T_3, thyroid ^{131}I uptake test, urine 17-OHCS, 17-KS

---

testosterone cypionate/ testosterone enanthate/ testosterone propionate

Andro-Cyp, Andronate, Depotest, Dep-Test, Depo-Testosterone, Duratest/Android-T LA, Andro-LA, Andryl, Delatestryl, Everone, Malogex,* Testostroval-PA/Androlan, Androlin, Testex

Func. class.: Androgenic anabolic steroid
Chem. class.: Halogenated testosterone derivative

Action: Increases weight by building body tissue, increases potassium, phosphorus, chloride, nitrogen levels, increases bone development
Uses: Female breast cancer, eunuchoidism, male climacteric, oligospermia, impotence, osteoporosis
Dosage and routes:
Oligospermia
• *Adult:* IM 100-200 mg q4-6 wk (cypionate or enanthate)
Breast cancer
• *Adult:* IM 50-100 mg 3 × /wk (propionate) or 200-400 mg q2-4 wk (cypionate or enanthate)
Male climacteric/eunuchoidism/eunuchism
• *Adult:* IM 10-25 mg 2-4 × /wk (propionate)
Available forms include: Propionate inj IM 25, 50, 100 mg/ml; en-

T

---

anthate inj IM 100, 200 mg/ml; cypionate inj IM 50, 100, 200 mg/ml

Side effects/adverse reactions:

INTEG: Rash, acneiform lesions, oily hair, skin, flushing, sweating, acne vulgaris, alopecia, hirsutism

CNS: Dizziness, headache, fatigue, tremors, paresthesias, flushing, sweating, anxiety, lability, insomnia

MS: Cramps, spasms

CV: Increased B/P

GU: Hematuria, amenorrhea, vaginitis, decreased libido, decreased breast size, clitoral hypertrophy, testicular atrophy

GI: Nausea, vomiting, constipation, weight gain, *cholestatic jaundice*

EENT: Carpal tunnel syndrome, conjunctional edema, nasal congestion

ENDO: Abnormal GTT

Contraindications: Severe renal disease, severe cardiac disease, severe hepatic disease, hypersensitivity, pregnancy (X), lactation, genital bleeding (abnormal)

Precautions: Diabetes mellitus, CV disease, MI

Pharmacokinetics:

PO: Metabolized in liver, excreted in urine, breast milk; crosses placenta

Interactions/incompatibilities:

• Increased effects of: oral antidiabetics, oxyphenbutazone

• Increased PT: anticoagulants

• Edema: ACTH, adrenal steroids

• Decreased effects of: insulin

NURSING CONSIDERATIONS

Assess:

• Weight daily, notify physician if weekly weight gain is >5 lb

• B/P q4h

• I&O ratio; be alert for decreasing urinary output, increasing edema

• Growth rate in children since growth rate may be uneven (linear/bone growth) used for extended periods of time

• Electrolytes: K, Na, Cl, Ca; cholesterol

• Liver function studies: ALT, AST, bilirubin

Administer:

• Titrated dose; use lowest effective dose

• IM deep into upper outer quadrant of gluteal muscle

Perform/provide:

• Diet with increased calories, protein; decrease sodium if edema occurs

• Supportive drug of anemia

Evaluate:

• Therapeutic response: occurs in 4-6 wk in osteoporosis

• Edema, hypertension, cardiac symptoms, jaundice

• Mental status: affect, mood, behavioral changes, aggression

• Signs of masculinization in female: increased libido, deepening of voice, breast tissue, enlarge clitoris, menstrual irregularities; male: gynecomastia, impotence, testicular atrophy

• Hypercalcemia: lethargy, polyuria, polydipsia, nausea, vomiting, constipation; drug may need to be decreased

• Hypoglycemia in diabetics, since oral anticoagulant action is decreased

Teach patient/family:

• Drug needs to be combined with complete health plan: Diet, rest, exercise

• To notify physician if therapeutic response decreases

• Not to discontinue this medication abruptly

• Teach patient all aspects of drug usage, including changes in sex characteristics

• Women to report menstrual irregularities

• That 1-3 mo course is necessary

---

for response in breast cancer

• Procedure for use of buccal tablets (requires 30-60 min to dissolve, change absorption site with each dose; do not eat, drink, chew, or smoke while tablet is in place)

Lab test interferences:

Increase: Serum cholesterol, blood glucose, urine glucose

Decrease: Serum calcium, serum potassium, T_4, T_3, thyroid ^{131}I uptake test, urine 17-OHCS, 17-KS, PBI

---

tetanus toxoid, adsorbed; tetanus toxoid

Func. class.: Toxoid

Action: Produces specific antibodies to tetanus

Uses: Prevention of tetanus

Dosage and routes:

• *Adult and child:* IM 0.5 ml q4-6 wk × 2 doses, then 0.5 ml 1 yr after dose 2 (adsorbed); SC/IM 0.5 ml q4-8 wk × 3 doses, then 0.5 ml ½-1 yr after dose 3

Available forms include: Inj adsorbed IM 5, 10 LfU/0.5 ml; inj IM, SC 4, 5 LfU/0.5 ml

Side effects/adverse reactions:

GI: Nausea, vomiting, anorexia

INTEG: Skin abscess, urticaria, itching, swelling

CV: Tachycardia, hypotension

SYST: Lymphadenitis, ***anaphylaxis***

CNS: Crying, fretfulness, fever, drowsiness

MS: Osteomyelitis

Contraindications: Hypersensitivity, active infection, poliomyelitis outbreak, immunosuppression

Precautions: Pregnancy

NURSING CONSIDERATIONS

Assess:

• For skin reactions: swelling, rash, urticaria

Administer:

• At least 4 wk apart × 3 doses for children >6 wk old

• Only with epinephrine 1:1000 on unit to treat laryngospasm

• IM only; not to be given SC (vastus lateralis in infants, deltoid in adults)

Evaluate:

• For history of allergies, skin conditions (eczema, psoriasis, dermatitis), reactions to vaccinations

• For anaphylaxis: inability to breathe, bronchospasm

Teach patient/family:

• That doses are given at least 4 wk apart × 3 doses; booster needed at 10 yr intervals

---

tetracaine/tetracaine HCl (topical)

(tet'-ra-cane)

Cetacaine, Pontocaine

Func. class.: Topical anesthetic

Action: Inhibits nerve impulses from sensory nerves, which produces anesthesia

Uses: Pruritus, sunburn, toothache, sore throat, cold sores, oral pain, rectal pain and irritation, control of gagging

Dosage and routes:

• *Adult and child:* TOP apply to affected area 1 oz for adult ¼ oz for child

Available forms include: Sol 2%; aero spray, liq, oint, gel

Side effects/adverse reactions:

INTEG: Rash, irritation, sensitization

Contraindications: Hypersensitivity, infants <1 yr, application to large areas

Precautions: Child <6 yr, sepsis, pregnancy, denuded skin

Interactions/incompatibilities: None known

NURSING CONSIDERATIONS
Administer:

• After cleansing and drying of affected area

Evaluate:

• Allergy: rash, irritation, reddening, swelling

• Therapeutic response: absence of pain, itching of affected area

• Infection: if affected area is infected, do not apply

Teach patient/family:

• To report rash, irritation, redness, swelling

• How to apply solution

---

tetracaine HCl
(tet'-ra-caine)

Pontocaine

Func. class.: Ophthalmic anesthetic

Chem. class.: Ester

Action: Decreases ion permeability by stabilizing neuronal membrane

Uses: Cataract extraction, tonometry, gonioscopy, removal of foreign objects, corneal suture removal, glaucoma surgery

Dosage and routes:

• *Adult and child:* Instill 1-2 gtts before procedure

Available forms include: Sol 0.5%; oint 0.5%

Side effects/adverse reactions:

EENT: Blurred vision, stinging, burning, lacrimation, photophobia, conjunctival redness

INTEG: Contact dermatitis

Contraindications: Hypersensitivity to paraaminobenzoic acid

Precautions: Abnormal levels of plasma esterases, allergies, hyperthyroidism, hypertension, cardiac disease

Pharmacokinetics:

Instill: Onset 13-30 sec, duration 15-20 min

Interactions/incompatibilities:

• Decreases antibacterial action of: sulfonamides

NURSING CONSIDERATIONS
Perform/provide:

• Protective covering for eye

• Storage at room temperature in tight, light resistant container; refrigerate

Teach patient/family:

• To report change in vision, with blurring or loss of sight, trouble breathing, sweating, flushing

• Not to touch or rub eye, which may further damage eye

---

tetracaine HCl
(tet-ra'-kane)

Pontocaine

Func. class.: Local anesthetic

Chem. class.: Ester

Action: Competes with calcium for sites in nerve membrane that control sodium transport across cell membrane; decreases rise of depolarization phase of action potential

Uses: Spinal anesthesia, epidural, peripheral nerve block, perineum, lower extremities

Dosage and routes:

Varies depending on route of anesthesia

Available forms include: Inj 0.2%, 0.3%, 1%; powder

Side effects/adverse reactions:

CNS: Anxiety, restlessness, *convulsions, loss of consciousness,* drowsiness, disorientation, tremors, shivering

CV: Myocardial depression, cardiac arrest, dysrhythmias, bradycardia, hypotension, hypertension, fetal bradycardia

GI: Nausea, vomiting

EENT: Blurred vision, tinnitus, pupil constriction

INTEG: Rash, urticaria, allergic re-

---

actions, edema, burning, skin discoloration at injection site, tissue necrosis

*RESP: **Status asthmaticus, respiratory arrest, anaphylaxis***

Contraindications: Hypersensitivity, child <12 yr, elderly, severe liver disease

Precautions: Elderly, severe drug allergies

Pharmacokinetics:

Onset 15 min, duration 3 hr; metabolized by liver, excreted in urine (metabolites)

Interactions/incompatibilities:

• Dysrhythmias: epinephrine, halothane, enflurane

• Hypertension: MAOIs, tricyclic antidepressants, phenothiazines

• Decreased action of this drug: chloroprocaine

NURSING CONSIDERATIONS

Assess:

• B/P, pulse, respiration during treatment

• Fetal heart tones if drug is used during labor

Administer:

• Only drugs that are not cloudy, do not contain precipitate

• Only with crash cart, resuscitative equipment nearby

• Only drugs without preservatives for epidural or caudal anesthesia

Perform/provide:

• Use of new solution, discard unused portions

Evaluate:

• Therapeutic response: anesthesia necessary for procedure

• Allergic reactions: rash, urticaria, itching

• Cardiac status: ECG for dysrhythmias, pulse, B/P, during anesthesia

Treatment of overdose: Airway, O_2, vasopressor, IV fluids, anticonvulsants for seizures

tetracycline HCl

(tet-ra-sye'kleen)

Achromycin, Bicycline, Cefracycline,* Cycline, Cyclopar, Medicycline,* Neo-Tetrine,* Novotetra,* Panmycin, Sarocycline, Sumycin, Tetracyn, Tetralan, Tetralean,* Trexin, Tetracap

Func. class.: Broad spectrum antibiotic/antiinfective

Chem. class.: Tetracycline

Action: Inhibits protein synthesis and phosphorylation in microorganisms

Uses: Syphilis, chlamydia trachomatis, gonorrhea, lymphogranuloma venereum

Dosage and routes:

• *Adult:* PO 250-500 mg q6h; IM 250 mg/day or 150 mg q12h; IV 250-500 mg q8-12h

• *Child >8 yr:* PO 25-50 mg/kg/day in divided doses q6h; IM 15-25 mg/kg/day in divided doses q8-12h; IV 10-20 mg/kg/day in divided doses q12h

Gonorrhea

• *Adult:* PO 1.5 g, then 500 mg qid for a total of 9 g

Chlamydia trachomatis

• *Adult:* PO 500 mg bid × 7 days

Syphilis

• *Adult:* PO 2-3 g in divided doses × 10-15 days

Available forms include: Oral susp, caps 100, 200, 500 mg; tabs 250, 500 mg; powder for inj

Side effects/adverse reactions:

CNS: Fever, headache, paresthesia

*HEMA: **Eosinophilia, neutropenia, thrombocytopenia, leukocytosis, hemolytic anemia***

EENT: Dysphagia, glossitis, decreased calcification of deciduous teeth, abdominal pain, oral candidiasis

GI: Nausea, vomiting, diarrhea,

T

---

anorexia, enterocolitis, *hepato-toxicity,* flatulence, abdominal cramps, epigastric burning, stomatitis, *pseudomembranous colitis*

CV: Pericarditis

GU: Increased BUN, polyuria, polydipsia, renal failure, nephrotoxicity

INTEG: Rash, urticaria, photosensitivity, increased pigmentation, exfoliative dermatitis, pruritus, angioedema

Contraindications: Hypersensitivity to tetracyclines, children <8 yr
Precautions: Renal disease, hepatic disease, lactation, pregnancy
Pharmacokinetics:

PO: Peak 2-4 hr, duration 6 hr, half-life 6-10 hr; excreted in urine, crosses placenta, excreted in breast milk, 20%-60% protein bound
Interactions/incompatibilities:

• Decreased effect of this drug: antacids, NaHCO₃, dairy products, alkali products

• Increased effect: anticoagulants

• Decreased effect: penicillins

• Nephrotoxicity: methoxyflurane
NURSING CONSIDERATIONS
Assess:

• I&O ratio

• Blood studies: PT, CBC, AST, ALT, BUN, creatinine
Administer:

• After C&S obtained

• 2 hr before or after laxative or ferrous products; 3 hr after antacid
Perform/provide:

• Storage in tight, light-resistant container at room temperature
Evaluate:

• Therapeutic response: decreased temperature, absence of lesions, negative C&S

• Allergic reactions: rash, itching, pruritus, angioedema

• Nausea, vomiting, diarrhea; administer antiemetic, antacids as ordered

• Overgrowth of infection: increased temperature, malaise, redness, pain, swelling, drainage, perineal itching, diarrhea, changes in cough or sputum
Teach patient/family:

• To avoid sun exposure since burns may occur; sunscreen does not seem to decrease photosensitivity

• Of diabetic to avoid use of Clinistix, Diastix, or Tes-Tape for urine glucose testing

• That all prescribed medication must be taken to prevent superimposed infection

• To avoid milk products
Lab test interferences:

False positive: Urine glucose with Clinistix or Tes-Tape

False increase: Urinary catecholamines

---

tetracycline HCl (ophthalmic)

(tet-ra-sye′kleen)
Achromycin Ophthalmic
Func. class.: Antiinfective

Action: Inhibits bacterial cell-wall in organism by preventing amino acids and nucleotides into cell wall
Uses: Infection of eye, ophthalmia neonatorum
Dosage and routes:

• *Adult and child:* INSTILL 1-2 gtts bid-qid as needed
Ophthalmia neonatorum

• *Neonate:* INSTILL 1-2 gtts into each eye immediately after delivery
Available forms include: Oint 1%
Side effects/adverse reactions:

EENT: Poor corneal wound healing, overgrowth of nonsusceptible organisms
Contraindications: Hypersensitivity
Precautions: Antibiotic hypersensitivity

Interactions/incompatibilities:
None known
NURSING CONSIDERATIONS
Administer:
• After washing hands, cleanse crusts or discharge from eye before application
Perform/provide:
• Storage at room temperature
Evaluate:
• Therapeutic response: absence of redness, inflammation, tearing
• Allergy: itching, lacrimation, redness, swelling
Teach patient/family:
• To use drug exactly as prescribed
• Not to use eye make-up, towels, washcloths, or eye medication of others, or reinfection may occur
• That drug container tip should not be touched to eye
• To report itching, increased redness, burning, stinging, swelling; drug should be discontinued
• That drug may cause blurred vision when ointment is applied

---

tetracycline HCl (topical)
(tet-ra-sye'kleen)
Topicycline, Achromycin
Func. class.: Local antiinfective
Chem. class.: Tetracycline

Action: Interferes with microorganism phosphorylation, protein synthesis
Uses: Acne vulgaris
Dosage and routes:
• *Adult and child >12 yr:* TOP apply to affected area bid
Available forms include: Oint 3%; sol 0.22%
Side effects/adverse reactions:
INTEG: Rash, urticaria, stinging, burning
Contraindications: Hypersensitivity
Precautions: Pregnancy, lactation

Interactions/incompatibilities:
None known
NURSING CONSIDERATIONS
Administer:
• Enough medication to completely cover lesions
• After cleansing with soap, water before each application, dry well
Perform/provide:
• Storage at room temperature in dry place
Evaluate:
• Allergic reaction: burning, stinging, swelling, redness
• Therapeutic response: decrease in size, number of lesions
Teach patient/family:
• To apply with glove to prevent further infection
• To avoid use of OTC creams, ointments, lotions unless directed by physician
• To use medical asepsis (hand washing) before, after each application

---

tetrahydrozoline HCl
(tet-ra-hi-droz-o-leen)
Murine Plus, Optigene, Soothe, Visine
Func. class.: Ophthalmic vasoconstrictor
Chem. class.: Direct sympathomimetic amine

Action: Vasoconstriction of eye arterioles; decreases eye engorgement by stimulation of α-adrenergic receptors
Uses: Ocular congestion, irritation, itching
Dosage and routes:
• *Adult and child >2 yr:* INSTILL 1-2 gtts bid or tid
Available forms include: Sol 0.05%
Side effects/adverse reactions:
CNS: Headache, dizziness, weakness

CV: Bradycardia, hypertension, dysrhythmias, tachycardia, CV collapse, palpitation
EENT: Stinging, lacrimation, blurred vision, conjunctival allergy
Contraindications: Hypersensitivity, glaucoma (narrow-angle)
Precautions: Severe hypertension, diabetes, hyperthyroidism, elderly, severe arteriosclerosis, cardiac disease, infants, pregnancy
Pharmacokinetics:
INSTILL: Duration 2-3 hr
Interactions/incompatibilities:
• Increased pressor effects: MAOIs, tricyclic antidepressants
NURSING CONSIDERATIONS
Assess:
• B/P, pulse, systemic absorption does occur
Perform/provide:
• Storage in tight, light-resistant container; do not use discolored solutions
Teach patient/family:
• To report change in vision, blurring, loss of sight; breathing trouble, sweating, flushing
• Method of instillation; tilt head backward, hold dropper over eye, drop medication inside lower lid, using pressure on inside corner of eye hold 1 min, do not touch dropper to eye
• That blurred vision will decrease with repeated use of drug
• To notify physician if headache, spots, redness, pain occurs; discontinue use
• To use sunglasses if photophobia occurs
• To use exactly as prescribed

tetrahydrozoline HCl

(tet-ra-hye-drozz'a-leen)
Tyzine HCl, Tyzine Pediatric

Func. class.: Nasal decongestant
Chem. class.: Sympathomimetic amine

Action: Produces vasoconstriction (rapid, long-acting) of arterioles thereby decreasing fluid exudation, mucosal engorgement
Uses: Nasal congestion
Dosage and routes:
• *Adult and child >6 yr:* INSTILL 2-4 gtts or sprays q4-6h prn
• *Child 2-6 yr:* INSTILL 2-3 gtts q4-6h prn
Available forms include: Sol 0.05%, 0.1%
Side effects/adverse reactions:
GI: Nausea, vomiting, anorexia
EENT: Irritation, burning, sneezing, stinging, dryness, rebound congestion
INTEG: Contact dermatitis
CNS: Anxiety, restlessness, tremors, weakness, insomnia, dizziness, fever, headache
Contraindications: Hypersensitivity to sympathomimetic amines
Precautions: Child <6 yr, elderly, diabetes, cardiovascular disease, hypertension, hyperthyroidism, increased ICP, prostatic hypertrophy
Interactions/incompatibilities:
• Hypertension: MAOIs, β-adrenergic blockers
• Hypotension: methyldopa, mecamylamine, reserpine
NURSING CONSIDERATIONS
Administer:
• No more than q4h
• For <4 consecutive days
Perform/provide:
• Environmental humidification to decrease nasal congestion, dryness
• Storage in light-resistant contain-

ers; do not expose to high temperatures

Evaluate:

• Redness, swelling, pain in nasal passages

Teach patient/family:

• Stinging may occur for several applications; drying of mucosa may be decreased by environmental humidification

• To notify physician if irregular pulse, insomnia, dizziness, or tremors occur

• Proper administration to avoid systemic absorption

---

theophylline, theophylline sodium glycinate

(thee-off'i-lin)

Aquaphyllin, Bronkodyl, Elixophyllin, Slo-Phyllin, Somophyllin-T/ Accurbron, Aerolate, Aquaphyllin, Asmalix, Bronkodyl, Elixicon, Elixomin, Elixophyllin, Lanophyllin, Lixolin, Theolair, Theolixir, Theon, Theophyl, Lodrane, Slo-bid, Slow-Phyllin, Theovent, Theo-Time

Func. class.: Spasmolytic

Chem. class.: Xanthine, ethylenediamine

Action: Relaxes smooth muscle of respiratory system by blocking phosphodiesterase, which increases cyclic AMP

Uses: Bronchial asthma, bronchospasm of COPD, chronic bronchitis

Dosage and routes:

Bronchospasm, bronchial asthma

• *Adult:* PO 100-200 mg q6h, dosage must be individualized; REC 250-500 mg q8-12h

• *Child:* PO 50-100 mg q6h, not to exceed 12 mg/kg/24 hr

COPD, chronic bronchitis

• *Adult:* PO 330-660 mg q6-8h pc (sodium glycinate)

• *Child >12 yr:* PO 220-330 mg q6-8h pc (sodium glycinate)

• *Child 6-12 yr:* PO 330 mg q6-8h pc (sodium glycinate)

• *Child 3-6 yr:* PO 110-165 mg q6-8h pc (sodium glycinate)

• *Child 1-3 yr:* PO 55-110 mg q6-8h pc (sodium glycinate)

Available forms include: Caps 50, 100, 200, 250 mg; tabs 100, 125, 200, 225, 250, 300 mg; tabs time-release 100, 200, 250, 300, 400, 500 mg; caps time-release 50, 65, 100, 125, 130, 200, 250, 260, 300, 400, 500 mg; elix 80, 11.25 mg/ 15 ml; sol 80 mg/15 ml; liq 80, 150, 160 mg/15 ml; susp 300 mg/ 15 ml

Side effects/adverse reactions:

CNS: Anxiety, restlessness, insomnia, dizziness, convulsions, headache, light-headedness

CV: Palpitations, sinus tachycardia, hypotension, other dysrhythmias

GI: Nausea, vomiting, anorexia, diarrhea, bitter taste, dyspepsia, anal irritation (suppositories)

RESP: Increased rate

INTEG: Flushing, urticaria

Contraindications: Hypersensitivity to xanthines, tachydysrhythmias

Precautions: Elderly, CHF, cor pulmonale, hepatic disease, active peptic ulcer disease, diabetes mellitus, hyperthyroidism, hypertension, children, pregnancy (C)

Pharmacokinetics:

IV: Peak 30 min

SOL: Peak 1 hr, metabolized in liver, excreted in urine, breast milk, crosses placenta

Interactions/incompatibilities:

• Increased action of this drug: cimetidine, propranolol, erythromycin, troleandomycin

• May increase effects of: anticoagulants

• Cardiotoxicity: β-blockade

NURSING CONSIDERATIONS

Assess:

• Theophylline blood levels (ther-

T

---

apeutic level is 10-20 µg/ml); toxicity may occur with small increase above 20 µg/ml

• Monitor I&O; diuresis occurs, dehydration may result in elderly or children

• Whether theophylline was given recently

Administer:

• PO after meals to decrease GI symptoms; absorption may be affected

Evaluate:

• Respiratory rate, rhythm, depth; auscultate lung fields bilaterally; notify physician of abnormalities

• Allergic reactions: rash, urticaria; if these occur, drug should be discontinued

Teach patient/family

• To check OTC medications, current prescription medications for ephedrine, which will increase stimulation

• To avoid hazardous activities; dizziness may occur

• On all aspects of drug therapy: dosage, routes, side effects, when to notify the physician

• If GI upset occurs, to take drug with 8 oz water; avoid food, absorption may be decreased

• To remain in bed 15-20 min after rectal suppository is inserted to avoid removal

---

thiabendazole

(thye-a-ben′da-zole)
Mintezol

Func. class.: Anthelmintic
Chem. class.: Benzimadazole derivative

Action: Inhibits enzyme production in worm

Uses: Pinworm, roundworm, threadworm, whipworm, trichinosis, hookworm, cutaneous larva migrans (creeping eruption)

Dosage and routes:

• *Adult and child:* PO 25 mg/kg in 2 doses qd × 2-5 days, not to exceed 3 g/day

Available forms include: Tabs, chew 500 mg; oral susp 500 mg/5 ml

Side effects/adverse reactions:

SYST: Anaphylaxis

GU: Hematuria, nephrotoxicity, enuresis, abnormal smell of urine

INTEG: Rash, pruritus, fever, flushing, convulsions, behavioral changes

CNS: Dizziness, headache, drowsiness

EENT: Tinnitus, blurred vision, xanthopsia

GI: Nausea, vomiting, anorexia, diarrhea, jaundice, liver damage, epigastric distress

CV: Hypotension, bradycardia

Contraindications: Hypersensitivity

Precautions: Severe malnutrition, hepatic disease, renal disease, anemia, severe dehydration, child <14 kg, pregnancy (C)

Pharmacokinetics:

PO: Peak 1-2 hr, metabolized completely by liver, excreted in feces, urine

Interactions/incompatibilities:
None known

NURSING CONSIDERATIONS

Assess:

• Stools periodically during entire treatment

Administer:

• Suspension after shaking

• PO after meals to avoid GI symptoms

Perform/provide:

• Storage in tight containers

Teach patient/family:

• Proper hygiene after BM including handwashing technique; tell patient to avoid putting fingers in mouth

• That infected person should sleep

---

alone; do not shake bed linen, change bed linen qd
• To clean toilet qd with disinfectant (green soap solution)
• Need for compliance with dosage schedule, duration of treatment
• To drink fruit juice to remove mucous that intestinal tapeworms burrow in; aids in expulsion of worms
• To avoid hazardous activities if drowsiness occurs
Treatment of overdose: Induce emesis or gastric lavage

---

thiamine HCl (vitamin B₁)

Apatate Drops, Betaline S, Revitonus, Thia

Func. class.: Vitamin B₁
Chem. class.: Water soluble

Action: Needed for pyruvate metabolism
Uses: Vitamin B₁ deficiency or polyneuritis, cheilosis adjunct with thiamine beriberi, Wernicke-Korsakoff syndrome, pellagra
Dosage and routes:
Beriberi
• *Adult:* IM 10-500 mg tid × 2 wk, then 5-10 mg qd × 1 mo
• *Child:* IM 10-50 mg qd × 4-6 wk
Anemia/alcoholism/pregnancy/pellagra
• *Adult:* PO 100 mg qd
• *Child:* PO 10-50 mg qd in divided doses
Beriberi with cardiac failure
• *Adult and child:* IV 100-500 mg
Wernicke's encephalopathy
• *Adult:* IV 500 mg or less, then 100 mg bid
Available forms include: Tabs 5, 10, 25, 50, 100, 250, 500 mg; inj IM, IV 100, 200 mg/ml
Side effects/adverse reactions:
CNS: Weakness, restlessness
GI: Hemorrhage
CV: Collapse, pulmonary edema

INTEG: Angioneurotic edema, cyanosis, sweating, warmth
SYST: Anaphylaxis
EENT: Tightness of throat
Contraindications: None known
Pharmacokinetics:
PO/INJ: Unused amounts excreted in urine (unchanged)
Interactions/incompatibilities:
None known
NURSING CONSIDERATIONS
Assess:
• Thiamine levels throughout treatment
Administer:
• By IM injection, rotate sites if pain and inflammation occur
• Application of cold may decrease pain
Evaluate:
• Therapeutic response: absence of nausea, vomiting, anorexia, insomnia, tachycardia, paresthesias, depression, muscle weakness
• Nutritional status: yeast, beef, liver, whole grains, legumes
Teach patient/family:
• Necessary foods to be included in diet: yeast, beef, liver, legumes, whole grain

---

thiethylperazine maleate

(thye-eth-il-per′-a-zeen)
Torecan

Func. class.: Antiemetic
Chem. class.: Phenothiazine, piperazine derivative

T

Action: Acts centrally by blocking chemoreceptor trigger zone, which in turn acts on vomiting center
Uses: Nausea, vomiting
Dosage and routes:
• *Adult:* PO/IM/REC 10 mg/qd-tid
Available forms include: Tabs 10 mg; supp 10 mg; inj 5 mg/ml

Side effects/adverse reactions:
CNS: Euphoria, depression, restlessness, tremor, EPS, convulsions
GI: Nausea, vomiting, anorexia, dry mouth, diarrhea, constipation, weight loss, metallic taste, cramps
*CV: **Circulatory failure, tachycardia**,* postural hypotension
*RESP: **Respiratory depression***
Contraindications: Hypersensitivity to phenothiazines, coma, seizure, encephalopathy, bone marrow depression
Precautions: Children <2 yr, pregnancy, elderly
Pharmacokinetics:
PO: Onset 45-60 min
REC: Onset 45-60 min, metabolized by liver, excreted by kidneys, crosses placenta, excreted in breast milk
Interactions/incompatibilities:
• Decreased effect of this drug: barbiturates, antacids
• Increased anticholinergic action: anticholinergics, antiparkinson drugs, antidepressants
• Do not mix with other drug in syringe or solution
NURSING CONSIDERATIONS
Assess:
• VS, B/P; check patients with cardiac disease more often
Administer:
• IM injection in large muscle mass; aspirate to avoid IV administration
Evaluate:
• Therapeutic response: absence of nausea, vomiting
• Respiratory status before, during, after administration of emetic; check rate, rhythm, character; respiratory depression can occur rapidly with elderly or debilitated patients
Teach patient/family:
• Avoid hazardous activities, activities requiring alertness; dizziness may occur

thimerosal

(thye-mer'oh-sal)
Aeroaid Thimerosal, Merthiolate
Func. class.: Disinfectant
Chem. class.: Mercurial

Action: Destroys microorganisms (bacteria, fungi)
Uses: Cleansing wounds, disinfection of skin preoperatively
Dosage and routes:
Adult and child: SOL Apply locally qd-tid
Available forms include: Top sol 0.1%; tinc 0.1%
Side effects/adverse reactions:
INTEG: Irritation, contact dermatitis, erythema
Contraindications: Hypersensitivity to mercurial compounds, external ear wax removal
Interactions/incompatibilities:
• Do not use with acids, heavy metals, permanganate, aluminum salts, iodine
NURSING CONSIDERATIONS
Administer:
• After cleaning wound of all debris if using tincture; do not apply dressing to wet area
Perform/provide:
• Storage in tight, light-resistant container
Evaluate:
• Area of body involved: irritation, rash, breaks, redness, dryness, itching

thioguanine (6-TG)

(thye-oh-gwah'neen)
TG, 6-Thioguanine, Lanvis*
Func. class.: Antineoplastic-antimetabolite
Chem. class.: Purine analog

Action: Interferes with synthesis, utilization of purine nucleotides; effect is related to substitution of ribonucleotides into DNA

Uses: Acute leukemias, chronic granulocytic leukemia, lymphomas, multiple myeloma, solid tumors

Dosage and routes:
• *Adult and child:* PO 2 mg/kg/day, then increase slowly to 3 mg/kg/day after 4 wk

Available forms include: Tabs 40 mg

Side effects/adverse reactions:
*HEMA: **Thrombocytopenia, leukopenia, myelosuppression, anemia***
*GI: Nausea, vomiting, anorexia, diarrhea, stomatitis, **hepatotoxicity,** gastritis, jaundice*
*GU: **Renal failure,** hyperuricemia, oliguria*
INTEG: Rash, dermatitis, dry skin
Contraindications: Prior drug resistance, leukopenia (<2500/mm^3), thrombocytopenia (<100,000/mm^3), anemia

Precautions: Liver disease, pregnancy (D)

Pharmacokinetics: Oral form absorbed only 30%, metabolized in liver, only small amounts excreted in urine (unchanged)

Interactions/incompatibilities:
• Increased toxicity: radiation, other antineoplastics

NURSING CONSIDERATIONS
Assess:
• CBC, differential, platelet count weekly; withhold drug if WBC is <3500/mm^3 or platelet count is <100,000/mm^3; notify physician of these results; drug should be discontinued
• Renal function studies: BUN, serum uric acid, urine CrCl, electrolytes before, during therapy
• I&O ratio; report fall in urine output to <30 ml/hr
• Monitor temperature q4h; fever may indicate beginning infection
• Liver function tests before, dur-

ing therapy: bilirubin, alk phosphatase, AST, ALT
• Bleeding time, coagulation time during treatment

Administer:
• Medications by oral route if possible; avoid IM, SC, IV routes to prevent infections
• Antacid before oral agent; give drug after evening meal before bedtime
• Antiemetic 30-60 min before giving drug to prevent vomiting
• Allopurinol or sodium bicarbonate to maintain uric acid levels, alkalinization of urine
• Antibiotics for prophylaxis of infection
• Topical or systemic analgesics for pain
• Transfusion for anemia

Perform/provide:
• Strict medical asepsis, protective isolation if WBC levels are low
• Liquid diet: carbonated beverage, Jello; dry toast, crackers may be added when patient is not nauseated or vomiting
• Increase fluid intake to 2-3 L/day to prevent urate deposits, calculi formation, unless contraindicated
• Diet low in purines: absence of organ meats (kidney, liver), dried beans, peas to maintain alkaline urine
• Rinsing of mouth tid-qid with water, hydrogen peroxide; brushing of teeth bid-tid with soft brush or cotton-tipped applicators for stomatitis; use unwaxed dental floss
• Nutritious diet with iron, vitamin supplements as ordered
• Storage in tightly closed container in cool environment

Evaluate:
• Bleeding: hematuria, guaiac, bruising, petechiae, mucosa or orifices q8h
• Food preferences; list likes, dislikes

• Hepatotoxicity: yellowing of skin, sclera, dark urine, clay-colored stools, pruritus, abdominal pain, fever, diarrhea

• Buccal cavity q8h for dryness, sores, ulceration, white patches, oral pain, bleeding, dysphagia

• Symptoms indicating severe allergic reaction: rash, urticaria, itching, flushing

Teach patient/family:

• Why protective isolation precautions are needed

• To report any complaints, side effects to nurse or physician: black tarry stools, chills, fever, sore throat, bleeding, bruising, cough, shortness of breath, dark, bloody urine

• To avoid foods with citric acid, hot or rough texture if stomatitis is present

• To report stomatitis: any bleeding, white spots, ulcerations in mouth; tell patient to examine mouth qd, report symptoms

• Contraceptive measures are recommended during therapy

• To drink 10-12 glasses of fluid/day

Lab test interferences:

Increase: Uric acid (blood, urine)

---

thiopental sodium

(thye-oh-pen'tal)
Pentothal

Func. class.: General anesthetic
Chem. class.: Barbiturate

Controlled Substance Schedule III

Action: Acts in reticular-activating system to produce anesthesia

Uses: Short general anesthesia, narcoanalysis, induction anesthesia before other anesthetics

Dosage and routes:
Induction

• *Adult:* IV 210-280 mg or 3-4 ml/kg

General anesthetic

• *Adult:* IV 50-75 mg given at 20-40 sec intervals

Narcoanalysis

• *Adult:* IV 200 mg/min, not to exceed 50 ml/min

Available forms include: Inj IV

Side effects/adverse reactions:

RESP: Respiratory depression, bronchospasm

CNS: Retrograde amnesia, prolonged somnolence

CV: Tachycardia, hypotension, *myocardial depression, dysrhythmias*

EENT: Sneezing, coughing

INTEG: Chills, *shivering,* necrosis, pain at injection site

MS: Muscle irritability

Contraindications: Hypersensitivity, status asthmaticus, hepatic/intermittent porphyrias

Precautions: Severe cardiovascular disease, renal disease, hypotension, liver disease, myxedema, myasthenia gravis, asthma, increased intracranial pressure

Pharmacokinetics:

IV: Onset 30-40 sec; half-life 11½ hr, crosses placenta

Interactions/incompatibilities:

• Increased action: CNS depressants

• Do not mix with atropine or silicone in solution or syringe

NURSING CONSIDERATIONS

Assess:

• VS q3-5 min during IV administration, after dose, q4 hr postoperatively

Administer:

• After preparation with sterile water of 0.9% or 5% dextrose

• Only with crash cart, resuscitative equipment nearby

• IV slowly only

Evaluate:

• Therapeutic response: mainte-

---

nance of anesthesia
• Extravasation, if it occurs use nitroprusside or chloroprocaine to decrease pain, increase circulation
• Dysrhythmias or myocardial depression

thioridazine HCl

(thye-or-rid′ a-zeen)
Mellaril, Millazine, Novoridazine,*
SK Thioridazine
Func. class.: Antipsychotic/neuroleptic
Chem. class.: Phenothiazine, piperidine

Action: Depresses cerebral cortex, hypothalamus, limbic system, which control activity, aggression; blocks neurotransmission produced by dopamine at synapse; exhibits strong α-adrenergic, anticholinergic blocking action; mechanism for antipsychotic effects is unclear
Uses: Psychotic disorders, schizophrenia, behavioral problems in children, alcohol withdrawal, anxiety, major depressive disorders, organic brain syndrome
Dosage and routes:
Psychosis
• *Adult:* PO 50-100 mg tid, max dose 800 mg/day; dose is gradually increased to desired response, then reduced to minimum maintenance
Depression/behavioral problems/ organic brain syndrome
• *Adult:* PO 25 tid, range from 10 mg bid-qid to 50 mg tid-qid
• *Child 2-12 yr:* PO 0.5-3 mg/kg/ day in divided doses
Available forms include: Tabs 10, 15, 25, 50, 100, 150, 200 mg; conc 30, 100 mg/ml; susp 25, 100 mg/ 5 ml
Side effects/adverse reactions:
RESP: Laryngospasm, dyspnea, *respiratory depression*
CNS: Extrapyramidal symptoms

(rare): pseudoparkinsonism, akathisia, dystonia, tardive dyskinesia, seizures, *headache*
HEMA: Anemia, leukopenia, leukocytosis, *agranulocytosis*
INTEG: Rash, photosensitivity, dermatitis
EENT: Blurred vision, glaucoma
GI: Dry mouth, nausea, vomiting, anorexia, constipation, diarrhea, jaundice, weight gain
GU: Urinary retention, urinary frequency, enuresis, impotence, amenorrhea, gynecomastia
CV: Orthostatic hypotension, hypertension, *cardiac arrest,* ECG changes, *tachycardia*
Contraindications: Hypersensitivity, blood dyscrasias, coma, child <2 yr, brain damage, bone marrow depression
Precautions: Pregnancy, lactation, seizure disorders, hypertension, hepatic disease, cardiac disease
Pharmacokinetics:
PO: Onset erratic, peak 2-4 hr; metabolized by liver, excreted in urine, crosses placenta, enters breast milk, half-life 26-36 hr
Interactions/incompatibilities:
• Oversedation: other CNS depressants, alcohol, barbiturate anesthetics
• Toxicity: epinephrine
• Decreased absorption: aluminum hydroxide or magnesium hydroxide antacids
• Decreased effects of: lithium, levodopa
• Increased effects of both drugs: β-adrenergic blockers, alcohol
• Increased anticholinergic effects: anticholinergics
NURSING CONSIDERATIONS
Assess:
• Swallowing of PO medication; check for hoarding or giving of medication to other patients
• I&O ratio; palpate bladder if low urinary output occurs

T

• Bilirubin, CBC, liver function studies monthly
• Urinalysis is recommended before and during prolonged therapy

Administer:
• Antiparkinsonian agent, after securing order from physician to be used if EPS occur
• Concentrate mixed in citrus juices or distilled or acidified tap water

Perform/provide:
• Decreased noise input by dimming lights, avoiding loud noises
• Supervised ambulation until stabilized on medication; do not involve in strenuous exercise program because fainting is possible; patient should not stand still for long periods of time
• Increased fluids to prevent constipation
• Sips of water, candy, gum for dry mouth
• Storage in tight, light-resistant container

Evaluate:
• Therapeutic response: decrease in emotional excitement, hallucinations, delusions, paranoia, reorganization of patterns of thought, speech
• Affect, orientation, LOC, reflexes, gait, coordination, sleep pattern disturbances
• B/P standing and lying; also include pulse and respirations q4h during initial treatment; establish baseline before starting treatment; report drops of 30 mm Hg
• Dizziness, faintness, palpitations, tachycardia on rising
• EPS including akathisia (inability to sit still, no pattern to movements), tardive dyskinesia (bizarre movements of jaw, mouth, tongue, extremities), pseudoparkinsonism (rigidity, tremors, pill rolling, shuffling gait)
• Skin turgor daily

• Constipation, urinary retention daily; if these occur, increase bulk, water in diet

Teach patient/family:
• That orthostatic hypotension occurs frequently, and to rise from sitting or lying position slowly
• To remain lying down after IM injection for at least 30 min
• To avoid hot tubs, hot showers, or tub baths since hypotension may occur
• To avoid abrupt withdrawal of this drug or EPS may result; drugs should be withdrawn slowly
• To avoid OTC preparations (cough, hayfever, cold) unless approved by physician since serious drug interactions may occur; avoid use with alcohol or CNS depressants, increased drowsiness may occur
• To use a sunscreen during sun exposure to prevent burns
• Regarding compliance with drug regimen
• About necessity for meticulous oral hygiene since oral candidiasis may occur
• To report sore throat, malaise, fever, bleeding, mouth sores; if these occur, CBC should be drawn and drug discontinued
• In hot weather, heat stroke may occur; take extra precautions to stay cool

Lab test interferences:
Increase: Liver function tests, cardiac enzymes, cholesterol, blood glucose, prolactin, bilirubin, PBI, cholinesterase, ^{131}I
Decrease: Hormones (blood, urine)
False positive: Pregnancy tests, PKU
False negative: Urinary steroids
Treatment of overdose: Lavage if orally injested, provide an airway; do not induce vomiting

---

*Available in Canada only

thiotepa
(thye-oh-tep'a)
Thiotepa, TSPA

Func. class.: Antineoplastic
Chem. class.: Alkylating agent

Action: Alkylates DNA, RNA; inhibits enzymes that allow synthesis of amino acids in proteins; also responsible for cross-linking DNA strands

Uses: Hodgkin's disease, lymphomas; breast, ovarian, lung, bladder, cancer; neoplastic effusions

Dosage and routes:
• *Adult:* IV 50.2 mg/kg × 5 days, then 0.2 mg/kg q1-3 wk
Neoplastic effusions
• *Adult:* INTRACAVITY 10-15 mg
Bladder cancer
• *Adult:* INSTILL 60 mg/60 ml water instilled in bladder once weekly × 4 wk

Available forms include: Inj 15 mg, powder for inj

Side effects/adverse reactions:
CNS: Dizziness, headache
HEMA: **Thrombocytopenia, leukopenia, pancytopenia**
GI: Nausea, vomiting, anorexia, stomatitis
GU:Hyperuricemia, hematuria, amenorrhea, azoospermia
INTEG: Rash, pruritus

Contraindications: Hypersensitivity

Precautions: Radiation therapy, bone marrow suppression, impaired renal or hepatic function, pregnancy

Pharmacokinetics:
Onset slow, metabolized in liver, excreted in urine

NURSING CONSIDERATIONS
Assess:
• CBC, differential, platelet count weekly; withhold drug if WBC is <4000 or platelet count is <75,000; notify physician of results
• Renal function studies: BUN, serum uric acid, urine CrCl before, during therapy
• I&O ratio, report fall in urine output of 30 ml/hr
• Monitor temperature q4h (may indicate beginning infection)
• Liver function tests before, during therapy (bilirubin, AST, ALT, LDH) as needed or monthly

Administer:
• Medications by oral route; if possible, avoid IM, SC, IV routes to prevent infections
• Antiemetic 30-60 min before giving drug to prevent vomiting
• Allopurinol or sodium bicarbonate to maintain uric acid levels, alkalinization of urine
• Antibiotics for prophylaxis of infection
• Slow IV infusion using 21-, 23-, 25-gauge needle
• Local or systemic drugs for infection

Perform/provide:
• Storage in light-resistant container, refrigerate
• Strict medical asepsis, protective isolation if WBC levels are low
• Special skin care
• Liquid diet, including cola, Jello; dry toast or crackers may be added if patient is not nauseated or vomiting
• Increase fluid intake to 2-3 L/day to prevent urate deposits, calculi formation
• Diet low in purines: organ meats (kidney, liver), dried beans, peas to maintain alkaline urine
• Rinsing of mouth tid-qid with water, hydrogen peroxide; brushing of teeth bid-tid with soft brush or cotton tipped applicators for stomatitis; use unwaxed dental floss
• Warm compresses at injection site for inflammation

italics = common side effects   ***bold italic*** = life threatening reactions

Evaluate:

• Bleeding: hematuria, guaiac, bruising or petechiae, mucosa or orifices q8h

• Food preferences; list likes, dislikes

• Inflammation of mucosa, breaks in skin

• Yellowing of skin, sclera, dark urine, clay-colored stools, itchy skin, abdominal pain, fever, diarrhea

• Buccal cavity q8h for dryness, sores, ulceration, white patches, oral pain, bleeding, dysphagia

• Symptoms indicating severe allergic reaction: rash, pruritus, urticaria, itching, flushing

Teach patient/family:

• Of protective isolation precautions

• That azoospermia or amenorrhea can occur; reversible after discontinuing treatment

• To avoid foods with citric acid, hot or rough texture

• To report any bleeding, white spots or ulcerations in mouth to physician, tell patient to examine mouth qd

• To report any complaints or side effects to nurse or physician

---

thiothixene

(thye-oh-thix′een)

Navane

Func. class.: Antipsychotic/neuroleptic

Chem. class.: Thioxanthene

Action: Depresses cerebral cortex, hypothalamus, limbic system, which control activity, aggression; blocks neurotransmission produced by dopamine at synapse; exhibits strong α-adrenergic, anticholinergic blocking action; mechanism for antipsychotic effects is unclear

Uses: Psychotic disorders, schizophrenia, acute agitation

Dosage and routes:

• *Adult:* PO 2-5 mg bid-qid depending on severity of condition; dose is gradually increased to 15-30 mg if needed; IM 4 mg bid-qid, max dose is 30 mg qd; administer PO dose as soon as possible

Available forms include: Caps 1, 2, 5, 10, 20 mg; conc 5 mg/ml; inj IM 2 mg/ml; powder for inj 5 mg/ml

Side effects/adverse reactions:

*RESP: **Laryngospasm,** dyspnea, **respiratory depression***

CNS: Extrapyramidal symptoms: pseudoparkinsonism, akathisia, dystonia, tardive dyskinesia, seizures, headache

HEMA: Anemia, leukopenia, leukocytosis, ***agranulocytosis***

INTEG: Rash, photosensitivity, dermatitis

EENT: Blurred vision, glaucoma

GI: Dry mouth, nausea, vomiting, anorexia, constipation, diarrhea, jaundice, weight gain

GU: Urinary retention, urinary frequency, enuresis, impotence, amenorrhea, gynecomastia

CV: Orthostatic hypotension, hypertension, ***cardiac arrest,*** ECG changes, ***tachycardia***

Contraindications: Hypersensitivity, blood dyscrasias, child <12 yr, bone marrow depression

Precautions: Pregnancy, lactation, seizure disorders, hypertension, hepatic disease

Pharmacokinetics:

PO: Onset slow, peak 2-8 hr, duration up to 12 hr

IM: Onset 15-30 min, peak 1-6 hr, duration up to 12 hr

Metabolized by liver, excreted in urine, crosses placenta, enters breast milk, half-life 34 hr

Interactions/incompatibilities:

• Oversedation: other CNS depres-

sants, alcohol, barbiturate anesthetics
• Toxicity: epinephrine
• Decreased absorption: aluminum hydroxide or magnesium hydroxide antacids
• Decreased effects of: lithium, levodopa
• Increased effects of both drugs: β-adrenergic blockers, alcohol
• Increased anticholinergic effects: anticholinergics

NURSING CONSIDERATIONS
Assess:
• Swallowing of PO medication; check for hoarding or giving of medication to other patients
• I&O ratio, palpate bladder if low urinary output occurs
• Bilirubin, CBC, liver function studies monthly
• Urinalysis is recommended before and during prolonged therapy

Administer:
• Antiparkinsonian agent, after securing order from physician to be used if EPS occur
• Concentrate mixed in citrus juices or distilled or acidified tap water
• IM injection into large muscle mass

Perform/provide:
• Decreased noise input by dimming lights, avoiding loud noises
• Supervised ambulation until stabilized on medication; do not involve in strenuous exercise program because fainting is possible; patient should not stand still for long periods of time
• Increased fluids to prevent constipation
• Sips of water, candy, gum for dry mouth
• Storage in tight, light-resistant container; place reconstituted solutions at room temperature for up to 48 hr

Evaluate:
• Therapeutic response: decrease in emotional excitement, hallucinations, delusions, paranoia, reorganization of patterns of thought, speech
• Affect, orientation, LOC, reflexes, gait, coordination, sleep pattern disturbances
• B/P standing and lying; also include pulse and respirations q4h during initial treatment; establish baseline before starting treatment; report drops of 30 mm Hg
• Dizziness, faintness, palpitations, tachycardia on rising
• EPS including akathisia (inability to sit still, no pattern to movements), tardive dyskinesia (bizarre movements of jaw, mouth, tongue, extremities), pseudoparkinsonism (rigidity, tremors, pill rolling, shuffling gait)
• Skin turgor daily
• Constipation, urinary retention daily; if these occur, increase bulk, water in diet

Teach patient/family:
• That orthostatic hypotension occurs frequently, and to rise from sitting or lying position gradually
• To remain lying down after IM injection for at least 30 min
• To avoid hot tubs, hot showers, or tub baths since hypotension may occur
• To avoid abrupt withdrawal of this drug or EPS may result; drugs should be withdrawn slowly
• To avoid OTC preparations (cough, hayfever, cold) unless approved by physician since serious drug interactions may occur; avoid use with alcohol or CNS depressants, increased drowsiness may occur
• To use a sunscreen during sun exposure to prevent burns
• Regarding compliance with drug regimen

T

---

italics = common side effects   **bold italic** = life threatening reactions

• About EPS and necessity for meticulous oral hygiene since oral candidiasis may occur

• To report sore throat, malaise, fever, bleeding, mouth sores; if these occur, CBC should be drawn and drug discontinued

• In hot weather, heat stroke may occur; take extra precautions to stay cool

Lab test interferences:

Increase: Liver function tests, cardiac enzymes, cholesterol, blood glucose, prolactin, bilirubin, PBI, cholinesterase, ^{131}I

Decrease: Hormones (blood, urine)

False positive: Pregnancy tests, PKU

False negative: Urinary steroids

Treatment of overdose: Lavage if orally injested, provide an airway; *do not induce vomiting*

---

thrombin

Thrombinar, Thrombostat

Func. class.: Hemostatic

Chem. class.: Bovine prothrombin

Action: Converts fibrinogen to thrombin

Uses: GI hemorrhage, bleeding in dental, plastic, nasal, laryngeal surgery, skin grafting

Dosage and routes:

• *Adult:* TOP apply 100 U/1 ml sterile isotonic NaCl or distilled water in light to moderate bleeding, or 1000-2000 U/ml sterile isotonic NaCl in severe bleeding. Dry area before applying

Available forms include: Powder 1000, 5000, 10,000, 20,000, 50,000 U

Side effects/adverse reactions:

INTEG: Rash, allergic reactions

*HEMA: **Intravascular clotting***

EENT: Epistaxis

Contraindications: Hypersensitiv-

ity to bovine products

Precautions: Pregnancy (C)

Interactions/incompatibilities: None known

NURSING CONSIDERATIONS

Administer:

• Only to dry area

• After preparing with NS, isotonic saline

• After having blood available for transfusion

Perform/provide:

• Storage in refrigerator, use reconstituted solution within 24 hr, discard unused portion

Evaluate:

• For allergic reactions: fever, rash, itching, changes in VS; thrombosis formation

Teach patient/family:

• To report any signs of bleeding: gums, under skin, urine, stools, emesis

---

thyroglobulin

(thye-roe-glob′yoo-lin)

Proloid

Func. class.: Thyroid hormone

Action: Increases metabolic rates, increases cardiac output, O_2 consumption, body temperature, blood volume, growth, development at cellular level

Uses: Hypothyroidism, cretinism, myxedema

Dosage and routes:

Hypothyroidism/myxedema

• *Adult:* PO 15-30 mg qd, increased by 15-30 mg q2 wk until desired response, maintenance dose 60-180 mg qd

• Geriatric: PO 7.5-15 mg qd, double dose q6-8 wk until desired response

Cretinism/juvenile hypothyroidism

• *Child over 1 yr:* PO Up to 180 mg qd, titrated to response

• *Child 4-12 mo:* PO 60-80 mg qd

- *Child 1-4 mo:* PO 15-30 mg qd, may increase q2 wk, titrated to response

Available forms include: Tabs 32, 65, 100, 130, 200 mg

Side effects/adverse reactions:

INTEG: Sweating, alopecia

CNS: Anxiety, insomnia, tremors, headache, heat intolerance, fever, coma, thyroid storm

CV: Tachycardia, palpitations, angina, dysrhythmias, hypertension, CHF

GI: Nausea, diarrhea, increased or decreased appetite, cramps

GU: Menstrual irregularities

Contraindications: Adrenal insufficiency, myocardial infarction, thyrotoxicosis

Precautions: Elderly, angina pectoris, hypertension, ischemia, renal disease, cardiac disease

Pharmacokinetics:

PO: Peak 12-48 hr, half-life 6-7 days

Interactions/incompatibilities:

- Decreased absorption of this drug: colestipol, cholestyramine
- Increased tachycardia: IV phenytoin
- Increased effects of: anticoagulants, sympathomimetics, tricyclic antidepressants
- Toxicity: digitalis preparations, catecholamines

NURSING CONSIDERATIONS

Assess:

- B/P, pulse before each dose
- I&O ratio
- Weight qd in same clothing, using same scale, at same time of day
- Height, growth rate if given to a child
- T_3, T_4, which are decreased, radioimmunoassay of TSH, which is increased, radio uptake, which is decreased if patient is on too low a dose of medication
- Pro-time may require decreased

anticoagulant, check for bleeding, bruising

Administer:

- In AM if possible as a single dose to decrease sleeplessness
- At same time each day to maintain drug level
- Only for hormone imbalances, not to be used for obesity, male infertility, menstrual conditions, lethargy
- Lowest dose that relieves symptoms

Perform/provide:

- Removal of medication 4 wk before RAIU test

Evaluate:

- Therapeutic response: absence of depression, increased weight loss, diuresis, pulse, appetite, absence of constipation, peripheral edema, cold intolerance, pale, cool dry skin, brittle nails, alopecia, coarse hair, menorrhagia, night blindness, paresthesias, syncope, stupor, coma, carotenemia skin, rosy cheeks
- Increased nervousness, excitability, irritability, which may indicate too high dose of medication usually after 1-3 wk of treatment
- Cardiac status: angina, palpitation, chest pain, change in VS

Teach patient/family:

- Hair loss will occur in child, is temporary
- Report excitability, irritability, anxiety, which indicate overdose
- Not to use generic products or switch brands unless approved by physician
- That hypothyroid child will show almost immediate behavior/personality change
- That treatment drug is not to be taken to reduce weight
- To avoid OTC preparations with iodine, read labels
- To avoid iodine food, salt iodin-

T

ized, soy beans, tofu, turnips, some seafood, some bread

Lab test interferences:

Increase: CPK, LDH, AST, PBI, blood glucose

Decrease: TSH, ^{131}I uptake test, uric acid, triglycerides

---

thyroid USP (desiccated)

(thye-roid)

S-P-T, Thyrar, Thyro-Teric

Func. class.: Thyroid hormone

Action: Increases metabolic rates, increases cardiac output, O_2 consumption, body temperature, blood volume, growth, development at cellular level

Uses: Hypothyroidism, cretinism, myxedema

Dosage and routes:

Hypothyroidism

• *Adult:* PO 60 mg qd, increased by 60 mg q30 days until desired response, maintenance dose 60-180 mg qd

• *Geriatric:* PO 7.5-15 mg qd, double dose q6-8 wk until desired response

Cretinism/juvenile hypothyroidism

• *Child over 1 yr:* PO up to 180 mg qd titrated to response

• *Child 4-12 mo:* PO 30-60 mg qd

• *Child 1-4 mo:* PO 15-30 mg qd, may increase q2 wk, titrated to response, maintenance dose 30-45 mg qd

Myxedema

• *Adult:* PO 16 mg qd, double dose q2 wk, not to exceed 120 mg

Available forms include: Tabs 32, 65, 130 mg; tabs enteric coated 32, 65, 130 mg; sugar-coated tabs 32, 65, 130 mg; caps 65, 130, 195, 325 mg

Side effects/adverse reactions:

INTEG: Sweating, alopecia

CNS: Anxiety, insomnia, tremors, headache, heat intolerance, fever, coma, thyroid storm

CV: Tachycardia, palpitations, angina, dysrhythmias, hypertension, CHF

GI: Nausea, diarrhea, increased or decreased appetite, cramps

GU: Menstrual irregularities

Contraindications: Adrenal insufficiency, myocardial infarction, thyrotoxicosis

Precautions: Elderly, angina pectoris, hypertension, ischemia, renal disease, cardiac disease

Pharmacokinetics:

PO: Peak 12-48 hr, half-life 6-7 days

Interactions/incompatibilities:

• Decreased absorption of this drug: colestipol, cholestyramine

• Increased tachycardia: IV phenytoin

• Increased effects of: anticoagulants, sympathomimetics, tricyclic antidepressants

• Toxicity: digitalis preparations, catecholamines

NURSING CONSIDERATIONS

Assess:

• B/P, pulse before each dose

• I&O ratio

• Weight qd in same clothing, using same scale, at same time of day

• Height, growth rate if given to a child

• T_3, T_4, which are decreased, radioimmunoassay of TSH, which is increased, radio uptake, which is decreased if patient is on too low a dose of medication

• Pro-time may require decreased anticoagulant, check for bleeding, bruising

Administer:

• In AM if possible as a single dose to decrease sleeplessness

• At same time each day to maintain drug level

• Only for hormone imbalances, not to be used for obesity, male in-

fertility, menstrual conditions, lethargy
• Lowest dose that relieves symptoms

Perform/provide:
• Removal of medication 4 wk before RAIU test

Evaluate:
• Therapeutic response: absence of depression, increased weight loss, diuresis, pulse, appetite, absence of constipation, peripheral edema, cold intolerance, pale, cool dry skin, brittle nails, alopecia, coarse hair, menorrhagia, night blindness, paresthesias, syncope, stupor, coma, carotenid skin, rosy cheeks
• Increased nervousness, excitability, irritability, may indicate too high dose of medication usually after 1-3 wk of treatment
• Cardiac status: angina, palpitation, chest pain, change in VS

Teach patient/family:
• Hair loss will occur in child, is temporary
• Report excitability, irritability, anxiety; indicates overdose
• Not to use generic products or switch brands unless directed by physician
• That hypothyroid child will show almost immediate behavior/personality change
• That treatment drug is not to be taken to reduce weight
• To avoid OTC preparations with iodine; read labels
• To avoid iodine food, salt-iodinized, soy beans, tofu, turnips, some seafood, some bread

Lab test interferences:
Increase: CPK, LDH, AST, PBI, blood glucose
Decrease: TSH, ^{131}I uptake test, uric acid, triglycerides

thyrotropin (thyroid-stimulating hormone, or TSH)
(thye-roe-troe'pin)
Thytropar
Func. class.: Thyroid hormone
Chem. class.: TSH

Action: Increases uptake of iodine by thyroid gland, increases production of thyroid hormone, increases release of thyroid hormone
Uses: Diagnosis of thyroid cancer, diagnosis of primary/secondary hypothyroidism

Dosage and routes:
Diagnosis of hypothyroidism
• *Adult:* IM/SC 10 Units qd × 1-3 days
Diagnosis of thyroid cancer
• *Adult:* IM/SC 10 IU qd × 3-7 days
Treatment of thyroid cancer
• *Adult:* IM/SC 10 Units qd × 3-8 days
Available forms include: Powder for inj 10 IU/vial

Side effects/adverse reactions:
INTEG: Urticaria
CNS: Headache, fever
CV: Tachycardia, angina, *atrial fibrillation, CHF*
GI: Nausea, vomiting
GU: Menstrual irregularities
SYST: Anaphylactic reactions
Contraindications: Hypersensitivity, coronary thrombosis
Precautions: Angina pectoris, adrenal insufficiency
Pharmacokinetics:
IM/SC: Half-life 35 min
Interactions/incompatibilities:
• Decreased level: levodopa

NURSING CONSIDERATIONS
Administer:
• After dilution with 2 ml sterile saline solution
• Three-day dose schedule for

myxedema (pituitary)

• In combination with ^{131}I to treat thyroid cancer

Treatment of overdose: Discontinue drug, administer supportive care

---

ticarcillin disodium

(tye-kar-sill'in)

Ticaripen,* Ticar

Func. class.: Broad-spectrum antibiotic

Chem. class.: Extended-spectrum penicillin

Action: Interferes with cell wall replication of susceptible organisms; osmotically unstable cell wall swells, bursts from osmotic pressure.

Uses: Respiratory, soft tissue, urinary tract infections, bacterial septicemia; effective for gram-positive cocci *(S. aureus, S. faecalis, S. pneumoniae),* gram-negative cocci *(N. gonorrhoeae),* gram-positive bacilli *(C. perfringens, C. tetani),* gram-negative bacilli *(Bacteroides, F. nucleatum, E. coli, P. mirabilis, Salmonella, M. morganii, P. rettgeri, Enterobacter, P. aeruginosa, Serratia, Peptococcus, Peptostreptococcus, Eubacterium)*

Dosage and routes:

• *Adult:* IV/IM 18 g/day in divided doses q4-6h, infuse over ½-2 hr

• *Child:* IV/IM 200-300 mg/kg/day in divided doses q4-6h

Available forms include: Inj IM, IV 1, 3, 6, 20, 30 g, IV INF 3 g

Side effects/adverse reactions:

HEMA: Anemia, increased bleeding time, *bone marrow depression, granulocytopenia*

GI: Nausea, vomiting, diarrhea, increased AST, ALT, abdominal pain, glossitis, colitis

GU: Oliguria, proteinuria, hema-

turia, *vaginitis, moniliasis, glomerulonephritis*

CNS: Lethargy, hallucinations, anxiety, depression, twitching, *coma, convulsions*

META: Hypokalemia

Contraindications: Hypersensitivity to penicillins; neonates

Precautions: Hypersensitivity to cephalosporins

Pharmacokinetics:

IM: Peak 1 hr, duration 4-6 hr

IV: Peak 30-45 min, duration 4 hr, Half-life 70 min, small amount metabolized in liver, excreted in urine, breast milk

Interactions/incompatibilities:

• Decreased antimicrobial effect of this drug: tetracyclines, erythromycins, aminoglycosides IV

• Increased penicillin concentrations: aspirin, probenecid

NURSING CONSIDERATIONS

Assess:

• I&O ratio; report hematuria, oliguria since penicillin in high doses is nephrotoxic

• Any patient with compromised renal system since drug is excreted slowly in poor renal system function; toxicity may occur rapidly

• Liver studies: AST, ALT

• Blood studies: WBC, RBC, H&H, bleeding time

• Renal studies: urinalysis, protein, blood

• C&S before drug therapy; drug may be taken as soon as culture is taken

Administer:

• Drug after C&S has been completed

Perform/provide:

• Adrenalin, suction, tracheostomy set, endotracheal intubation equipment

• Adequate fluid intake (2000 ml) during diarrhea episodes

• Scratch test to assess allergy, after securing order from physician;

---

usually done when penicillin is only drug of choice

• Storage at room temperature, reconstituted solution for 24 hr or 7 days refrigerated.

Evaluate:

• Therapeutic repsonse: absence of fever, purulent drainage, redness, inflammation

• Bowel pattern before, during treatment

• Skin eruptions after administration of penicillin to 1 wk after discontinuing drug

• Respiratory status: rate, character, wheezing, tightness in chest

• Allergies before initiation of treatment, reaction of each medication; highlight allergies on chart, Kardex

Teach patient/family:

• Culture may be taken after completed course of medication

• To report sore throat, fever, fatigue; could indicate superimposed infection

• To wear or carry Medic Alert ID if allergic to penicillins

• To notify nurse of diarrhea stools

Lab test interferences:

Decrease: Uric acid

False positive: Urine glucose, urine protein

Treatment of overdose: Withdraw drug, maintain airway, administer epinephrine, aminophylline, O_2, IV corticosteroids for anaphylaxis

ticarcillin disodium/ clavulanate potassium

Timentin

Func. class.: Broad-spectrum antibiotic

Chem. class.: Extended-spectrum penicillin

Action: Interferes with cell wall replication of susceptible organisms; osmotically unstable cell wall swells, bursts from osmotic pressure

Uses: Respiratory, soft tissue, and urinary tract infections, bacterial septicemia; effective for gram-positive cocci *(S. aureus, S. faecalis, S. pneumoniae),* gram-negative cocci *(N. gonorrhoeae),* gram-positive bacilli *(C. perfringens, C. tetani),* gram-negative bacilli *(Bacteroides, F. nucleatum, E. coli, P. mirabilis, Salmonella, M. morganii, P. rettgeri, Enterobacter, P. aeruginosa, Serratia, Peptococcus, Peptostreptococcus, Eubacterium)*

Dosage and routes:

• *Adult:* IV INF 1 vial containing ticarcillin 3 g, clavulanate potassium 0.1 g q4-6h, infuse over 30 min

• *Child <60 kg:* 200-300 mg/kg/ day in divided doses q4-6h

Available forms include: Inj IM, IV 3 g; IV INF 3 g

Side effects/adverse reactions:

HEMA: Anemia, increased bleeding time, *bone marrow depression, granulocytopenia*

GI:Nausea, vomiting, diarrhea, increased AST, ALT, abdominal pain, glossitis, colitis

GU: Oliguria, proteinuria, hematuria, (vaginitis, moniliasis), *glomerulonephritis*

*CNS:*Lethargy, hallucinations, anx-

iety, depression, twitching, *coma, convulsions*
META: Hyperkalemia, hypokalemia, alkalosis, hypernatremia
Contraindications: Hypersensitivity to penicillins; neonates
Precautions: Hypersensitivity to cephalosporins
Pharmacokinetics:
IV: Peak 30-45 min, duration 4 hr, half-life 64-68 min
Interactions/incompatibilities:
• Decreased antimicrobial effect of this drug: tetracyclines, erythromycins, aminoglycosides IV
• Increased penicillin concentrations: aspirin, probenecid

NURSING CONSIDERATIONS
Assess:
• I&O ratio; report hematuria, oliguria since penicillin in high doses is nephrotoxic
• Any patient with compromised renal system, since drug is excreted slowly in poor renal system function; toxicity may occur rapidly
• Liver studies: AST, ALT
• Blood studies: WBC, RBC, H&H, bleeding time
• Renal studies: urinalysis, protein, blood
• C&S before drug therapy; drug may be taken as soon as culture is taken

Administer:
• Drug after C&S has been completed
Perform/provide:
• Adrenalin, suction, tracheostomy set, endotracheal intubation equipment
• Adequate fluid intake (2000 ml) during diarrhea episodes
• Scratch test to assess allergy, after securing order from physician; usually done when penicillin is only drug of choice
• Storage at room temperature, reconstituted solution for 24 hr or 7 days refrigerated

Evaluate:
• Therapeutic response: absence of fever, purulent drainage, redness, inflammation
• Bowel pattern before, during treatment
• Skin eruptions after administration of penicillin to 1 wk after discontinuing drug
• Respiratory status: rate, character, wheezing, and tightness in chest
• Allergies before initiation of treatment, reaction of each medication; highlight allergies on chart, Kardex
Teach patient/family:
• Culture may be taken after completed course of medication
• To report sore throat, fever, fatigue; could indicate superimposed infection
• To wear or carry Medic Alert ID if allergic to penicillins
Lab test interferences:
Decrease: Uric acid
False positive: Urine glucose, urine protein
Treatment of overdose: Withdraw drug, maintain airway, administer epinephrine, aminophylline, O_2, IV corticosteroids for anaphylaxis

---

timolol maleate
(tye'moe-lole)
Timoptic Solution
Func. class.: β-Adrenergic blocker
Chem. class.: I-isomer

Action: Releases production of aqueous humor
Uses: Ocular hypertension, chronic open-angle glaucoma, secondary glaucoma, aphakic glaucoma
Dosage and routes:
• *Adult:* INSTILL 1 gtt of 0.25% sol in both eyes bid, then 1 gtt for maintenance, may increase to 1 gtt of 0.5% sol bid if needed

Available forms include: Sol 0.25%, 0.5%

Side effects/adverse reactions:

CNS: Weakness, fatigue, depression, anxiety, headache, confusion

GI: Nausea, anorexia, dyspepsia

EENT: Eye irritation, conjunctivitis, keratitis

INTEG: Rash, urticaria

Contraindications: Hypersensitivity, asthma, 2nd/3rd degree heart block, right ventricular failure, congenital glaucoma (infants)

Pharmacokinetics:

INSTILL: Onset 15-30 min, peak 1-2 h, duration 24 hr

Interactions/incompatibilities:

• Increased effect: propranolol, metoprolol

NURSING CONSIDERATIONS

Teach patient/family:

• To report change in vision, with blurring or loss of sight, trouble breathing, sweating, flushing

• Method of instillation, including pressure on lacrimal sac for 1 min, and not to touch dropper to eye

• That long-term therapy may be required

• That blurred vision will decrease with continued use of drug

---

timolol maleate

(tye′moe-lole)

Blocadren

Func. class.: Antihypertensive

Chem. class.: Nonselective β-blocker

Action: Competitively blocks stimulation of β-adrenergic receptor within vascular smooth muscle; produces chronotropic, inotropic activity (decreases rate of SA node discharge, increases recovery time), slows conduction of AV node, decreases heart rate, which decreases O_2 consumption in myocardium; also, decreases renin-aldosterone-angiotensin system, at high doses inhibits β-2 receptors in bronchial system

Uses: Mild to moderate hypertension, sinus tachycardia, persistent atrial extrasystoles, tachydysrhythmias, prophylaxis of anigina pectoris

Dosage and routes:

Hypertension

• *Adult:* PO 10 mg bid, or 100 mg qd, may increase by 10 mg q2-3 days, not to exceed 60 mg/day

Myocardial infarction

• *Adult:* 10 mg bid

Available forms include: Tabs 5, 10, 20 mg

Side effects/adverse reactions:

CV: Hypotension, bradycardia, **CHF,** edema, chest pain, tachycardia, palpitation, claudication

CNS: Insomnia, dizziness, hallucinations, anxiety

GI: Nausea, vomiting, *ischemic colitis,* diarrhea, *abdominal pain, mesenteric arterial thrombosis*

INTEG: Rash, alopecia, pruritus, fever

HEMA: Agranulocytosis, thrombocytopenia, purpura

EENT: Visual changes, sore throat, *double vision,* dry burning eyes

GU: Impotence, frequency

RESP: Bronchospasm, dyspnea, cough, rales

MUSC: Joint pain, muscle pain

Contraindications: Hypersensitivity to β-blockers, cardiogenic shock, heart block (2nd, 3rd degree), sinus bradycardia, CHF, cardiac failure

Precautions: Major surgery, pregnancy (C), lactation, diabetes mellitus, renal disease, thyroid disease, COPD, well compensated heart failure, CAD, nonallergic bronchospasm

Pharmacokinetics:

PO: Peak 2-4 hr; half-life 3-4 hr, excreted 30%-45% unchanged,

T

60%-65% is metabolized by liver, excreted in breast milk

Interactions/incompatibilities:

• Increased hypotension, bradycardia: reserpine, hydralazine, methyldopa, prazosin, anticholinergics

• Decreased antihypertensive effects: idomethacin

• Increased hypoglycemic effects: insulin

• Decreased bronchodilation: theophyllines

NURSING CONSIDERATIONS
Assess:

• I&O, weight daily

• B/P, pulse q4h; note rate, rhythm, quality

• Apical/radial pulse before administration; notify physician of any significant changes

• Baselines in renal, liver function tests before therapy begins

Administer:

• PO ac, hs, tablet may be crushed or swallowed whole

• Reduced dosage in renal dysfunction

Perform/provide:

• Storage in dry area at room temperature, do not freeze

Evaluate:

• Therapeutic response: decreased B/P after 1-2 wk

• Edema in feet, legs daily

• Skin turgor, dryness of mucous membranes for hydration status

Teach patient/family:

• Take with or immediately after meals

• Not to discontinue drug abruptly, taper over 2 wk, may cause precipitate angina

• Not to use OTC products containing α-adrenergic stimulants (nasal decongestants, cold preparations) unless directed by physician

• To report bradycardia, dizziness, confusion, depression, fever, sore throat, shortness of breath to physician

• To take pulse at home, advise when to notify physician

• To avoid alcohol, smoking, sodium intake

• To comply with weight control, dietary adjustments, modified exercise program

• To carry Medic Alert ID to identify drug you are taking, allergies

• To avoid hazardous activities if dizziness is present

• To report symptoms of CHF: difficult breathing, especially on exertion or when lying down, night cough, swelling of extremities

• Take medication hs to maintain effect of orthostatic hypotension

• Wear support hose to minimize effects of orthostatic hypotension

Lab test interferences:

Increase: Liver function tests, renal function tests

Treatment of overdose: Lavage, IV atropine for bradycardia, IV theophylline for bronchospasm, digitalis, O_2, diuretic for cardiac failure, hemodialysis, administer vasopressor (norepinephrine)

---

tobramycin (ophthalmic)
(toe-bra-mye'sin)
Tobrex

Func. class.: Antiinfective
Chem. class.: Aminoglycoside

Action: Inhibits bacterial cell wall in organism by preventing amino acids and nucleotides into cell wall
Uses: Infection of eye
Dosage and routes:

• *Adult and child:* INSTILL 1-2 gtts q1-4h depending on infection
Available forms include: Oint 0.3%; sol 0.3%

Side effects/adverse reactions:

EENT: Poor corneal wound healing, visual haze, (temporary), over-

---

growth of nonsusceptible organisms

Contraindications: Hypersensitivity

Precautions: Antibiotic hypersensitivity

Interactions/incompatibilities: None known

NURSING CONSIDERATIONS

Administer:

• After washing hands, cleanse crusts or discharge from eye before application

• Apply pressure on lacrimal sac for 1 min

Perform/provide:

• Storage at room temperature

Evaluate:

• Therapeutic response: absence of redness, inflammation, tearing

• Allergy: itching, lacrimation, redness, swelling

Teach patient/family:

• To use drug exactly as prescribed

• Not to use eye make-up, towels, washcloths, or eye medication of others, or reinfection may occur

• That drug container tip should not be touched to eye

• To report itching, increased redness, burning, stinging; drug should be discontinued

• That drug may cause blurred vision when ointment is applied

---

tobramycin sulfate

(toe-bra-mye′sin)

Nebcin

Func. class.: Antibiotic

Chem. class.: Aminoglycoside

Action: Interferes with protein synthesis in bacterial cell by binding to ribosomal subunit, causing inaccurate peptide sequence to form in protein chain, causing bacterial death

Uses: Severe systemic infections of CNS, respiratory, GI, urinary tract, bone, skin, soft tissues caused by *P. aeruginosa, E. coli, Enterobacter, Acinetobacter, Providencia, Citrobacter, Staphylococcus, Proteus, Klebsiella, Serratia*

Dosage and routes:

• *Adult:* IM/IV 3 mg/kg/day in divided doses q8h; may give up to 5 mg/kg/day in divided doses q6-8h

• *Child:* IM/IV 6-7.5 mg/kg/day in 3-4 equally divided doses

• *Neonates <1 wk:* IM up to 4 mg/kg/day in divided doses q12h; IV up to 4 mg/kg/day in divided doses q12h diluted in 50-100 mg NS or D_5W; give over 30-60 min

Available forms include: Inj IM, IV 10, 40 mg/ml; powder for inj 1.2 g; inj 20 mg/2 ml

Side effects/adverse reactions:

GU: Oliguria, hematuria, renal damage, azotemia, renal failure, nephrotoxicity

CNS: Confusion, depression, numbness, tremors, *convulsions,* muscle twitching, *neurotoxicity*

EENT: Ototoxicity, deafness, visual disturbances

HEMA: Agranulocytosis, thrombocytopenia, leukopenia, eosinophilia, anemia

GI: Nausea, vomiting, anorexia, increased ALT, AST, bilirubin, hepatomegaly, *hepatic necrosis,* splenomegaly

CV: Hypotension, myocarditis

INTEG: Rash, burning, urticaria, photosensitivity, dermatitis

Contraindications: Severe renal disease, hypersensitivity

Precautions: Neonates, mild renal disease, pregnancy (B), myasthenia gravis, lactation, hearing deficits

Pharmacokinetics:

IM: Onset rapid, peak 1-2 hr

IV: Onset immediate, peak 1-2 hr

Plasma half-life 1-3 hr, not metabolized, excreted unchanged in urine, crosses placental barrier

T

---

italics = common side effects   ***bold italic*** = life threatening reactions

Interactions/incompatibilities:
• Increased ototoxicity, neurotoxicity, nephrotoxicity: other aminoglycosides, amphotericin B, polymyxin, vancomycin, ethacrynic acid, furosemide, mannitol, methoxyflurane, cisplatin, cephalosporins
• Decreased effects of: parenteral penicillins
• Do not mix in solution or syringe: carbenicillin, ticarcillin, amphotericin B, cephalothin, erythromycin, heparin
• Increased effects: nondepolarizing muscle relaxants

NURSING CONSIDERATIONS
Assess:
• Weight before treatment; calculation of dosage is usually done based on ideal body weight, but may be calculated on actual body weight
• I&O ratio, urinalysis daily for proteinuria, cells, casts; report sudden change in urine output
• VS during infusion, watch for hypotension, change in pulse
• IV site for thrombophlebitis including pain, redness, swelling q30 min, change site if needed; apply warm compresses to discontinued site
• Serum peak, drawn at 30-60 min after IV infusion or 60 min after IM injection, trough level drawn just before next dose; blood level should be 2-4 times bacteriostatic level
• Urine pH if drug is used for UTI; urine should be kept alkaline

Administer:
• IM injection in large muscle mass, rotate injection sites
• Drug in evenly spaced doses to maintain blood level
• Bicarbonate to alkalinize urine if ordered in treating UTI, as drug is most active in an alkaline environment

Perform/provide:
• Adequate fluids of 2-3 L/day unless contraindicated to prevent irritation of tubules
• Flush of IV line with NS or D_5W after infusion
• Supervised ambulation, other safety measures with vestibular dysfunction

Evaluate:
• Therapeutic effect: absence of fever, draining wounds, negative C&S after treatment
• Renal impairment by securing urine for CrCl testing, BUN, serum creatinine; lower dosage should be given in renal impairment (CrCl <80 ml/min)
• Deafness by audiometric testing, ringing, roaring in ears, vertigo; assess hearing before, during, after treatment
• Dehydration: high sp gr, decrease in skin turgor, dry mucous membranes, dark urine
• Overgrowth of infection: increased temperature, malaise, redness, pain, swelling, perineal itching, diarrhea, stomatitis, change in cough, sputum
• C&S before starting treatment to identify infecting organism
• Vestibular dysfunction: nausea, vomiting, dizziness, headache, drug should be discontinued if severe
• Injection sites for redness, swelling, abscesses; use warm compresses at site

Teach patient/family:
• To report headache, dizziness, symptoms of overgrowth of infection, renal impairment
• To report loss of hearing, ringing, roaring in ears, feeling of fullness in head

Treatment of overdose: Hemodialysis, monitor serum levels of drug

---

*Available in Canada only

tocainide HCl

(toe-kay'nide)
Tonocard

Func. class.: Antidysrhythmic
(Class IB)
Chem. class.: Lidocaine analog

Action: Increases electrical stimulation threshold of ventrical, HIS Purkinge system, which stabilizes cardiac membrane

Uses: PVCs, ventricular tachycardia, MI

Dosage and routes:
• *Adult:* PO 400 mg q8h
Available forms include: Tabs 400, 600 mg

Side effects/adverse reactions:
CNS: Headache, dizziness, involuntary movement, confusion, psychosis, restlessness, irritability, paresthesias
EENT: Tinnitus, blurred vision, hearing loss
GI: Nausea, vomiting, anorexia, diarrhea
CV: Hypotension, bradycardia, angina, PVCs, *heart block, cardiovascular collapse, arrest, CHF*
RESP: Dyspnea, *respiratory depression*
INTEG: Rash, urticaria, edema, swelling

Contraindications: Hypersensitivity to amides, blood dyscrasias, severe heart block

Precautions: Pregnancy, lactation, children, renal disease, liver disease, CHF, respiratory depression, myasthenia gravis

Pharmacokinetics:
PO: Peak 1 hr; half-life 10-17 hr, metabolized by liver, excreted in urine

Interactions/incompatibilities:
• May increase effects when used with: propranolol, quinidine

NURSING CONSIDERATIONS

Assess:
• Chest x-ray, pulmonary function test during treatments
• CBC during beginning treatment
• I&O ratio; check for decreasing output
• Blood levels (therapeutic level 4-10 µg/ml)
• B/P continuously for fluctuations
• Lung fields, bilateral rales may occur in CHF patient
• Increased respiration, increased pulse; drug should be discontinued

Evaluate:
• Toxicity: fine tremors, dizziness
• Blood dyscrasias: fatigue, sore throat, fever, bruising, increased temperature
• Cardiac rate, respiration: rate, rhythm, character, continuously

Lab test interferences:
Increase: CPK

Treatment of overdose: O_2, artificial ventilation, ECG, administer dopamine for circulatory depression, administer diazepam or thiopental for convulsions

tolazamide

(tole-az'a-mide)
Tolinase

Func. class.: Antidiabetic
Chem. class.: Sulfonylurea (1st generation)

Action: Causes functioning β-cells in pancreas to synthesize, release insulin, leading to drop in blood glucose levels; stimulation of insulin results in increased insulin binding; this drug not effective if patient lacks functioning β-cells

Uses: Stable adult-onset diabetes mellitus (type II)

Dosage and routes:
• *Adult:* PO 100 mg/day for FBS <200 mg/dl or 250 mg/day for FBS >200 mg/dl; dose should be

titrated to patient response

Available forms include: Tabs 100, 250, 500 mg

Side effects/adverse reactions:

CNS: Headache, weakness, fatigue, lethargy, dizziness, vertigo

GI: Nausea, vomiting, diarrhea, constipation, gas, ***hepatotoxicity, jaundice***

HEMA: ***Leukopenia, thrombocytopenia, agranulocytosis, aplastic anemia, pancytopenia, hemolytic anemia***

INTEG: Rash, (rare) allergic reactions, pruritus, urticaria, eczema, photo-sensitivity, erythema

ENDO: ***Hypoglycemia***

Contraindications: Hypersensitivity to sulfonylureas, juvenile or brittle diabetes, renal disease, hepatic disease

Precautions: Pregnancy, elderly, cardiac disease, thyroid disease, severe hypoglycemic reactions

Pharmacokinetics:

PO: Completely absorbed by GI route; onset 1 hr, peak 4-8 hr, duration 20 hr; half-life 7 hr, metabolized in liver, excreted in urine (metabolites), breast milk, highly protein bound

Interactions/incompatibilities:

• May increase effects when taken with insulin, MAOIs, cimetidine
• Decreased action of this drug: calcium channel blockers, corticosteroids, oral contraceptives, thiazide diuretics, thyroid preparations, estrogens, phenothiazines, phenytoin, rifampin, isoniazide
• Disulfiram-like reaction: alcohol

NURSING CONSIDERATIONS

Administer:

• Drug 30 min before meals

Perform/provide:

• Storage in tight container in cool environment

Evaluate:

• Therapeutic response: decrease in polyuria, polydipsia, polyphagia,

clear sensorium, absence of dizziness, stable gait

• Hypoglycemic/hyperglycemic reaction that can occur soon after meals

Teach patient/family:

• To check for symptoms of cholestatic jaundice (dark urine, pruritus, yellow sclera); if these occur a physician should be notified
• To use a capillary blood glucose test while on this drug
• To test urine glucose levels with Chemstrip approximately 2 hr after each meal
• The symptoms of hypo/hyperglycemia, what to do about each
• That this drug must be continued on a daily basis; explain consequence of discontinuing drug abruptly
• To take drug in morning to prevent hypoglycemic reactions at night
• To avoid OTC medications unless prescribed by a physician
• That diabetes is a life-long illness, drug will not cure disease
• That all food included in diet plan must be eaten in order to prevent hypoglycemia
• To carry a Medic-Alert ID for emergency purposes

Overdose: *Symptoms:* weakness, sweating, coma, lethargy; *Treatment:* 10%-50% glucose solution

---

tolazoline HCl

(toe-laz′a-leen)
Priscoline

Func. class.: Peripheral vasodilator

Chem. class.: Imidazoline derivative

Action: Peripheral vasodilation occurs by direct relaxation on vascular smooth muscle; also has weak α- and β-adrenergic properties

Uses: Persistent pulmonary hypertension of newborn, peripheral vascular disease: Buerger's disease, Raynaud's disease, scleroderma, diabetic arteriosclerosis gangrene

Dosage and routes:
• *Adult:* SC/IM/IV 10-50 mg qid; begin with lower dose and gradually increase until desired response; INTRAART 50-75 mg 1-2 doses, then 2-3 doses/wk
• *Newborn:* IV 1-2 mg/kg via scalp vein; IV INF 1-2 mg/kg/hr

Available forms include: Inj SC, IM, IV 25 mg/ml

Side effects/adverse reactions:
CNS: Paresthesia, headache, dizziness, confusion, hallucinations
*CV: Orthostatic hypotension, angina, **tachycardia**,* dysrhythmias, hypertension, ***cardiovascular collapse***
*RESP: **Pulmonary hemorrhage***
GU: Edema, oliguria, hematuria
GI: Nausea, vomiting, diarrhea, peptic ulcer, ***GI hemorrhage, hepatitis***
INTEG: Flushing, tingling, rash, chills, sweating
*HEMA: **Thrombocytopenia, leukopenia, pancytopenia, agranulocytosis***

Contraindications: Hypersensitivity, CVA, CAD, active peptic ulcer
Precautions: Pregnancy (C)
Pharmacokinetics:
IM/SC: Peak 30-60 min, duration 3-4 hr, excreted in urine, half-life 2 hr

Interactions/incompatibilities:
• Effects may be increased with alcohol, β-blockers, antihypertensive narcotics, tricyclics
• Epinephrine may cause a decrease in B/P with rebound hypertension
• Do not mix in syringe or solution with any other drugs

NURSING CONSIDERATIONS
Assess:
• ABGs, electrolytes, VS in newborn
• B/P, pulse during treatment until stable; take B/P lying, standing; orthostatic hypotension is common
• Hepatic tests: AST, ALT, bilirubin; liver enzymes may increase
• Blood studies: CBC, platelets; watch for thrombocytopenia, agranulocytosis

Administer:
• Ordered analgesic if headache develops
• Intraarterial to patient in supine position
• To patient who is sitting or lying down during treatment

Perform/provide:
• Storage at room temperature

Evaluate:
• Therapeutic response: decrease in pulmonary hypertension or pulse volume, increased temperature in extremities, ability to walk without pain
• Hepatic involvement: nausea, vomiting, jaundice; drug should be discontinued if this occurs
• For bleeding from GI tract: coffee grounds vomitus, increased pulse, pain in upper gastric area
• Affected areas for changes in temperature, color

Teach patient/family:
• To report jaundice, dark urine, joint pain, fatigue, malaise, bruising, easy bleeding, which may indicate blood dyscrasias
• That it is necessary to quit smoking to prevent excessive vasoconstriction if prescribed for PVD
• To avoid hazardous activities until stabilized on medication; dizziness may occur

Treatment of overdose: Administer IV fluids, head-low position

---

italics = common side effects   ***bold italic*** = life threatening reactions

tolbutamide

(tole-byoo'ta-mide)
Mobenol,* Novobutamide,* Orinase, Oramide, Tolbutone*
Func. class.: Antidiabetic
Chem. class.: Sulfonylurea (1st generation)

Action: Causes functioning β-cells in pancreas to synthesize, release insulin, leading to drop in blood glucose levels; stimulation of insulin results in increased insulin binding; this drug is not effective if patient lacks functioning β-cells
Uses: Stable adult-onset diabetes mellitus (type II)
Dosage and routes:
• *Adult:* PO 1-2 g/day in divided doses, titrated to patient response
Available forms include: Tabs 250, 500 mg
Side effects/adverse reactions:
CNS: Headache, weakness, paresthesia
GI: Nausea, fullness, heartburn, *hepatotoxicity, cholestatic jaundice*
HEMA: Leukopenia, thrombocytopenia, agranulocytosis, aplastic anemia, increased AST, ALT, alk phosphatase
INTEG: Rash, allergic reactions, pruritus, urticaria, eczema, photosensitivity, erythema
ENDO: Hypoglycemia
MS: Joint pains
Contraindications: Hypersensitivity to sulfonylureas, juvenile or brittle diabetes, renal disease, hepatic disease
Precautions: Pregnancy, elderly, cardiac disease, thyroid disease, severe hypoglycemic reactions
Pharmacokinetics:
PO: Completely absorbed by GI route; onset 30-60 min, peak 3-5 hr, duration 24 hr; half-life 7 hr,

metabolized in liver, excreted in urine (metabolites), breast milk, 90%-95% is plasma protein bound
Interactions/incompatibilities:
• Adverse effects: oral anticoagulants, hydantoins, salicylates, sulfonamides, non-steroidal antiinflammatories
• Increased effects of this drug: insulin, MAOIs
• Decreased action of this drug: calcium channel blockers, corticosteroids, oral contraceptives, thiazide diuretics, thyroid preparations, estrogens
NURSING CONSIDERATIONS
Administer:
• Drug 30 min before meals
Perform/provide:
• Storage in tight container in cool environment
Evaluate:
• Therapeutic response: decrease in polyuria, polydipsia, polyphagia, clear sensorium, absence of dizziness, stable gait
• Hypoglycemic/hyperglycemic reaction that can occur soon after meals
Teach patient/family:
• To check for symptoms of cholestatic jaundice (dark urine, pruritus, yellow sclera); if these occur a physician should be notified
• To use a capillary blood glucose test while on this drug
• To test urine glucose levels with Chemstrip approximately 2 hr after each meal
• The symptoms of hypo/hyperglycemia, what to do about each
• That this drug must be continued on a daily basis; explain consequence of discontinuing drug abruptly
• To take drug in morning to prevent hypoglycemic reactions at night
• To avoid OTC medications unless prescribed by a physician

• That diabetes is a life-long illness, drug will not cure disease
• That all food included in diet plan must be eaten in order to prevent hypoglycemia
• To carry a Medic-Alert ID for emergency purposes

Lab test interferences:
Decrease: RAIU test
Interfere: Urinary albumin
Overdose: *Symptoms:* Weakness, sweating, coma, lethargy; *Treatment:* 10%-50% glucose solution

---

tolmetin sodium

(tole′met-in)
Tolectin, Tolectin DS
Func. class.: Nonsteroidal
Chem. class.: Pyrrole acetic acid derivative

Action: Inhibits prostaglandin synthesis by decreasing an enzyme needed for biosynthesis; possesses analgesic, antiinflammatory, antipyretic properties
Uses: Mild to moderate pain, osteoarthritis, rheumatoid arthritis
Dosage and routes:
• *Adult:* PO 400 mg tid-qid, not to exceed 2 g/day
• *Child >2 yr:* PO 15-30 mg/kg/day in 3 or 4 divided doses
Available forms include: Caps 400 mg; tabs 200 mg
Side effects/adverse reactions:
GI: Nausea, anorexia, vomiting, diarrhea, jaundice, ***cholestatic hepatitis,*** constipation, flatulence, cramps, dry mouth, peptic ulcer
CNS: Dizziness, drowsiness, fatigue, tremors, confusion, insomnia, anxiety, depression
CV: Tachycardia, peripheral edema, palpitations, dysrhythmias
INTEG: Purpura, rash, pruritus, sweating
GU: ***Nephrotoxicity:*** dysuria, hematuria, oliguria, azotemia

HEMA: ***Blood dyscrasias***
EENT: Tinnitus, hearing loss, blurred vision
Contraindications: Hypersensitivity, asthma, severe renal disease, severe hepatic disease
Precautions: Pregnancy, lactation, children, bleeding disorders, GI disorders, cardiac disorders, hypersensitivity to other antiinflammatory agents
Pharmacokinetics:
PO: Peak 2 hr, half-life 3-3½ hr; metabolized in liver, excreted in urine (metabolites), excreted in breast milk
Interactions/incompatibilities:
• May increase action of coumarin, phenytoin, sulfonamides when used with this drug
NURSING CONSIDERATIONS
Assess:
• Renal, liver, blood studies: BUN, creatinine, AST, ALT, Hgb before treatment, periodically thereafter
• Audiometric, ophthalmic exam before, during, after treatment
Administer:
• With food to decrease GI symptoms; best to take on empty stomach to facilitate absorption
Perform/provide:
• Storage at room temperature
Evaluate:
• Therapeutic response: decreased pain, stiffness, swelling in joints, ability to move more easily
• For eye, ear problems: blurred vision, tinnitus (may indicate toxicity)
Teach patient/family:
• To report blurred vision or ringing, roaring in ears (may indicate toxicity)
• To avoid driving or other hazardous activities if dizziness or drowsiness occurs
• To report change in urine pattern, weight increase, edema, pain increase in joints, fever, blood in

T

---

italics = common side effects   ***bold italic*** = life threatening reactions

urine (indicates nephrotoxicity)
• That therapeutic effects may take up to 1 mo

---

tolnaftate (topical)

(tole-naf'tate)

Aftate, Pitrex, Tinactin

Func. class.: Local antiinfective
Chem. class.: Antifungal

Action: Interferes with fungal DNA replication; binds sterols in fungal cell membrane, which increases permeability, leaking of cell nutrients

Uses: Tinea pedis, tinea cruris, tinea corporis, tinea capitis, tinea unguium, versicolor

Dosage and routes:
• *Adult and child:* TOP apply to affected area bid for 2-6 wk, rub in
Available forms include: Cream, powder, aerosol powder, aerosol liq, gel, sol 1%

Side effects/adverse reactions:
INTEG: Rash, urticaria, stinging

Contraindications: Hypersensitivity

Precautions: Pregnancy, lactation
Interactions/incompatibilities: None known

NURSING CONSIDERATIONS
Administer:
• Aerosol powder after shaking
• Enough medication to completely cover lesions
• After cleansing with soap, water before each application, dry well

Perform/provide:
• Storage at room temperature in dry place, do not puncture or incinerate aerosol container

Evaluate:
• Allergic reaction: burning, stinging, swelling, redness
• Therapeutic response: decrease in size, number of lesions

Teach patient/family:
• To apply with glove to prevent further infection
• To avoid use of OTC creams, ointments, lotions unless directed by physician
• To use medical asepsis (hand washing) before, after each application
• To avoid contact with eyes

---

trace elements (chromium, copper, iodide, manganese, selenium, zinc)

Func. class.: Minerals

Action: Needed for adequate absorption and synthesis of amino acids

Uses: Prevention of trace element deficiency

Dosage and routes:
Chromium
• *Adult:* IV 10-15 µg qd
• *Child:* IV 0.14-0.20 µg/kg/day
Copper
• *Adult:* IV 0.5-1.5 mg/day
• *Child:* IV .05-0.2 mg/kg/day
Iodine
• *Adult:* IV 1 µg/kg/day
Manganese
• *Adult:* IV 1-3 mg/day
Selenium
• *Adult:* 40-120 µg/day
• *Child:* 3 µg/kg/day
Zinc
• *Adult:* IV 2-4 mg/day
• *Child:* IV 0.05 mg/kg/day

Available forms include: Many forms available—see particular elements

Side effects/adverse reactions: None known

Pharmacokinetics: Not known
Interactions/incompatibilities: None known

NURSING CONSIDERATIONS
Assess:
• Trace element levels, notify physician if low copper 0.07-0.15 mg/ml, zinc 0.05-0.15 mg/100 ml, manganese 4-20 µg/100 ml, selenium 0.1-0.19 µg/ml
Administer:
• By IV infusion, often mixed with TPN solution
Evaluate:
• Therapeutic response: absence of element deficiency
• Trace element deficiency if patient is receiving TPN for extended periods of time

---

tranylcypromine sulfate
(tran-ill-sip'roe-meen)
Parnate
Func. class.: Antidepressant-MAOI
Chem. class.: Nonhydrazine

Action: Increases concentrations of endogenous epinephrine, norepinephrine, serotonin, dopamine in storage sites in CNS by inhibition of MAO; increased concentration reduces depression
Uses: Depression, when uncontrolled by other means
Dosage and routes:
• *Adult:* PO 10 mg bid, may increase to 30 mg/day after 2 wk
Available forms include: Tabs 10 mg
Side effects/adverse reactions:
HEMA: Anemia
CNS: Dizziness, drowsiness, confusion, headache, anxiety, tremors, stimulation, weakness, hyperreflexia, mania, insomnia, fatigue, weight gain
GI: Constipation, dry mouth, nausea, vomiting, *anorexia,* diarrhea, weight gain
GU: Change in libido, frequency

INTEG: Rash, flushing, increased perspiration
CV: Orthostatic hypotension, hypertension, dysrhythmias, hypertensive crisis
EENT: Blurred vision
ENDO: **SIADH-like syndrome**
Contraindications: Hypersensitivity to MAOIs, elderly, hypertension, CHF, severe hepatic disease, pheochromocytoma, severe renal disease, severe cardiac disease
Precautions: Suicidal patients, convulsive disorders, severe depression, schizophrenia, hyperactivity, diabetes mellitus, pregnancy (C)
Pharmacokinetics:
Metabolized by liver, excreted by kidneys, crosses placenta, excreted in breast milk
Interactions/incompatibilities:
• Increased pressor effects: guanethidine, clonidine, indirect acting sympathomimetics (ephedrine)
• Increased effects of: direct acting sympathomimetics (epinephrine), alcohol, barbiturates, benzodiazepines, CNS depressants
• Hyperpyretic crisis, convulsions, hypertensive episode: tricyclic antidepressants
NURSING CONSIDERATIONS
Assess:
• B/P (lying, standing), pulse; if systolic B/P drops 20 mm Hg hold drug, notify physician
• Blood studies: CBC, leukocytes, cardiac enzymes if patient is receiving long-term therapy
• Hepatic studies: ALT, AST, bilirubin, creatinine; hepatotoxicity may occur
Administer:
• Increased fluids, bulk in diet if constipation, urinary retention occur
• With food or milk for GI symptoms

---

italics = common side effects   ***bold italic*** = life threatening reactions

• Crushed if patient is unable to swallow medication whole
• Dosage hs if over-sedation occurs during day
• Gum, hard candy, or frequent sips of water for dry mouth
• Phentolamine for severe hypertension

Perform/provide:
• Storage in tight container in cool environment
• Assistance with ambulation during beginning therapy since drowsiness/dizziness occurs
• Safety measures including siderails
• Checking to see PO medication swallowed

Evaluate:
• Toxicity: increased headache, palpitation, discontinue drug immediately; prodromal signs of hypertensive crisis
• Mental status: mood, sensorium, affect, memory (long, short), increase in psychiatric symptoms
• Urinary retention, constipation, edema, take weight weekly
• Withdrawal symptoms: headache, nausea, vomiting, muscle pain, weakness

Teach patient/family:
• That therapeutic effects may take 1-4 wk
• To avoid driving or other activities requiring alertness
• To avoid alcohol ingestion, CNS depressants or OTC medications: cold, weight, hay fever, cough syrup
• Not to discontinue medication quickly after long-term use
• To avoid high tyramine foods: cheese (aged), sour cream, beer, wine, pickled products, liver, raisins, bananas, figs, avocados, meat tenderizers, chocolate, yogurt; increase caffeine
• Report headache, palpitation, neck stiffness

Treatment of overdose: Lavage, activated charcoal, monitor electrolytes, vital signs, diazepam IV, NaHCO₃

---

trazodone HCl

(tray′zoe-done)
Desyrel
Func. class.: Antidepressant—tricyclic-like
Chem. class.: Triazolopyridine

Action: Selectively inhibits serotonin uptake by brain, potentiates behavorial changes
Uses: Depression, enuresis in children

Dosage and routes:
• *Adult:* PO 150 mg/day in divided doses, may be increase by 50 mg/day q3-4d, not to exceed 600 mg/day
Available forms include: Tabs 50, 100 mg

Side effects/adverse reactions:
HEMA: Agranulocytosis, thrombocytopenia, eosinophilia, leukopenia
CNS: Dizziness, drowsiness, confusion, headache, anxiety, tremors, stimulation, weakness, insomnia, nightmares, EPS (elderly), increase in psychiatric symptoms
GI: Diarrhea, dry mouth, nausea, vomiting, *paralytic ileus,* increased appetite, cramps, epigastric distress, jaundice, *hepatitis,* stomatitis
GU: Retention, acute renal failure
INTEG: Rash, urticaria, sweating, pruritus, photosensitivity
CV: Orthostatic hypotension, ECG changes, tachycardia, hypertension, palpitations
EENT: Blurred vision, tinnitus, mydriasis

Contraindications: Hypersensitivity to tricyclic antidepressants, recovery phase of myocardial infarc-

---

tion, convulsive disorders, prostatic hypertrophy

Precautions: Suicidal patients, severe depression, increased intraocular pressure, narrow-angle glaucoma, urinary retention, cardiac disease, hepatic disease, hyperthyroidism, electroshock therapy, elective surgery, pregnancy (C)

Pharmacokinetics:
Metabolized by liver, excreted by kidneys, feces; half-life 4.4-7.5 hr

Interactions/incompatibilities:
• Decreased effects of: guanethidine, clonidine, indirect acting sympathomimetics (ephedrine)
• Increased effects of: direct acting sympathomimetics (epinephrine), alcohol, barbiturates, benzodiazepines, CNS depressants
• **Hyperpyretic crisis, convulsions, hypertensive episode:** MAOI (pargyline [Eutonyl])

NURSING CONSIDERATIONS
Assess:
• B/P (lying, standing), pulse q4h; if systolic B/P drops 20 mm Hg hold drug, notify physician; take vital signs q4h in patients with cardiovascular disease
• Blood studies: CBC, leukocytes, differential, cardiac enzymes if patient is receiving long-term therapy
• Hepatic studies: AST, ALT, bilirubin, creatinine
• Weight qwk, appetite may increase with drug
• ECG for flattening of T wave, bundle branch block, AV block, dysrhythmias in cardiac patients

Administer:
• Increased fluids, bulk in diet if constipation, urinary retention occur
• With food or milk for GI symptoms
• Dosage hs if over-sedation occurs during day; may take entire dose

hs; elderly may not tolerate once/day dosing
• Gum, hard candy, or frequent sips of water for dry mouth

Perform/provide:
• Storage in tight, light-resistant container at room temperature
• Assistance with ambulation during beginning therapy since drowsiness/dizziness occurs
• Safety measures including siderails, primarily in elderly
• Checking to see PO medication swallowed

Evaluate:
• EPS primarily in elderly: rigidity, dystonia, akathisia
• Mental status: mood, sensorium, affect, suicidal tendencies, increase in psychiatric symptoms: depression, panic
• Urinary retention, constipation; constipation is more likely to occur in children
• Withdrawal symptoms: headache, nausea, vomiting, muscle pain, weakness; do not usually occur unless drug was discontinued abruptly
• Alcohol consumption; if alcohol is consumed, hold dose until morning

Teach patient/family:
• That therapeutic effects may take 2-3 wk
• Use caution in driving or other activities requiring alertness because of drowsiness, dizziness, blurred vision
• To avoid alcohol ingestion, other CNS depressants
• Not to discontinue medication quickly after long-term use, may cause nausea, headache, malaise
• To wear sunscreen or large hat since photosensitivity occurs

Lab test interferences:
Increase: Serum bilirubin, blood glucose, alk phosphatase

T

---

italics = common side effects   ***bold italic*** = life threatening reactions

False increase: Urinary catecholamines
Decrease: VMA, 5-HIAA
Treatment of overdose: ECG monitoring, induce emesis, lavage, activated charcoal, administer anticonvulsant

---

tretinoin (vitamin A acid, retinoic acid)

(tret'i-noyn)
Retin-A
Func. class.: Vitamin A acid/acne product
Chem. class.: Tretinoin derivative

Action: Decreases cohesiveness of follicular epithelium, decreases microcomedone formation
Uses: Acne vulgaris (grades 1-3); unlabeled use: skin cancer
Dosage and routes:
• *Adult and child:* TOP cleanse area, apply hs; cover lightly
Available forms include: Top cream 0.1%, 0.05%; top gel 0.025%, 0.01%; top liq 0.05%
Side effects/adverse reactions:
INTEG: Rash, stinging, warmth, redness, erythema, blistering, crusting, peeling, contact dermatitis, hypo/hyperpigmentation
Contraindications: Hypersensitivity
Precautions: Pregnancy (B), lactation, eczema, sunburn
Pharmacokinetics:
TOP: Poor absorption, excreted in urine
Interactions/incompatibilities:
• Increase peeling: medication containing agents such as sulfur, benzoyl peroxide, resorcinol, salicylic acid
• Use with caution medicated or abrasive soaps or cleansers that have drying effect, products with high concentrations of alcohol astringents

NURSING CONSIDERATIONS
Administer:
• Once daily before hs; cover area lightly using gauze
Perform/provide:
• Storage at room temperature
• Washing of hands after application
Evaluate:
• Therapeutic response: decrease in size and number of lesions
• Area of body involved, including time involved, what helps or aggravates condition
Teach patient/family:
• To avoid application on normal skin or getting cream in eyes, nose, or other mucous membranes
• To avoid sunlight or sunlamps
• Treatment may cause warmth, stinging; dryness, peeling will occur
• Cosmetics may be used over drug, do not use shaving lotions
• That rash may occur during first 1-3 wk of therapy
• That drug does not cure condition, only relieves symptoms

---

triamcinolone/triamcinolone acetonide/triamcinolone diacetate/triamcinolone hexacetonide

(trye-am-sin'oh-lone)
Aristocort, Kenacort, Spencort, Tricilone/Azmacort, Kenalog/Amcort/Cenocort Forte, Cino-40, Tracilon, Triam-Forte, Tritoject/Aristospen
Func. class.: Corticosteroid
Chem. class.: Glucocorticoid, immediate-acting

Action: Decreases inflammation by suppression of migration of polymorphonuclear leukocytes, fibroblasts, reversal to increase capillary permeability and lysosomal stabilization

Uses: Severe inflammation, immunosuppresion, neoplasms, asthma (steroid dependent)

Dosage and routes:

• *Adult:* PO 4-48 mg/day in divided doses qd-qid; IM 40 mg q wk (acetonide, or diacetate), 5-48 mg into neoplasms (diacetate, acetonide), 2-40 mg into joint or soft tissue (diacetate, acetonide), 0.5 mg/sq in of affected intralesional skin (hexacetonide), 2-20 mg into joint or soft tissue (hexacetonide)

Asthma

• *Adult:* INH 2 tid-qid, not to exceed 16 INH/day

• *Child 6-12 yr:* INH 1-2 tid-qid, not to exceed 12 INH/day

Available forms include: Tabs 1, 2, 4, 8, 16 mg; syr 2 mg/5 ml, 4 mg/5 ml; inj 25, 40 mg/ml diacetate; inj 10, 40 mg/ml acetonide; inj 20, 5 mg/ml hexacetonide

Side effects/adverse reactions:

INTEG: Acne, poor wound healing, ecchymosis, petechiae

CNS: Depression, flushing, sweating, headache, mood changes

*CV: Hypotension, **circulatory collapse, thrombophlebitis, embolism,** tachycardia

*HEMA: **Thrombocytopenia***

MS: Fractures, osteoporosis, weakness

*GI: Diarrhea, nausea, abdominal distention, GI hemorrhage, increased appetite, **pancreatitis***

EENT: Fungal infections, increased intraocular pressure, blurred vision

Contraindications: Psychosis, hypersensitivity, idiopathic thrombocytopenia, acute glomerulonephritis, amebiasis, fungal infections, nonasthmatic bronchial disease, child <2 yr

Precautions: Pregnancy, diabetes mellitus, glaucoma, osteoporosis,

seizure disorders, ulcerative colitis, CHF, myasthenia gravis

Pharmacokinetics:

PO/IM: Onset 1-2 hr, peak 1-2 hr, 2 days, 1-6 wk (IM), half-life 2-5 hr

Interactions/incompatibilities:

• Decreased action of this drug: cholestyramine, colestipol, barbiturates, rifampin, ephedrine, phenytoin, theophylline

• Decreased effects of: anticoagulants, anticonvulsants, antidiabetics, ambenonium, neostigmine, isoniazid, toxoids, vaccines

• Increased side effects: alcohol, salicylates, indomethacin, amphotericin B, digitalis preparations

• Increased action of this drug: salicylates, estrogens, indomethacin

NURSING CONSIDERATIONS

Assess:

• Potassium, blood sugar, urine glucose while on long-term therapy; hypokalemia and hyperglycemia

• Weight daily, notify physician if weekly gain >5 lb

• B/P q4h, pulse, notify physician if chest pain occurs

• I&O ratio, be alert for decreasing urinary output and increasing edema

• Plasma cortisol levels during long-term therapy (normal level: 138-635 nmol/L SI units when drawn at 8 AM)

Administer:

• After shaking suspension (parenteral)

• Titrated dose, use lowest effective dose

• IM injection deeply in large mass, rotate sites, avoid deltoid, use 19G needle

• In one dose in AM to prevent adrenal suppression, avoid SC administration, damage may be done to tissue

T

• With food or milk to decrease GI symptoms

Perform/provide:

• Assistance with ambulation in patient with bone tissue disease to prevent fractures

Evaluate:

• Therapeutic response: ease of respirations, decreased inflammation

• Infection: increased temperature, WBC, even after withdrawal of medication. Drug masks infections symptoms

• Potassium depletion: paresthesias, fatigue, nausea, vomiting, depression, polyuria, dysrhythmias, weakness

• Edema, hypotension, cardiac symptoms

• Mental status: affect, mood, behavioral changes, aggression

Teach patient/family:

• That ID as steroid user should be carried

• To notify physician if therapeutic response decreases; dosage adjustment may be needed

• Not to discontinue this medication abruptly or adrenal crisis can result

• To avoid OTC products: salicylates, alcohol in cough products, cold preparations unless directed by physician

• Teach patient all aspects of drug use, including Cushingoid symptoms

• Symptoms of adrenal insufficiency: nausea, anorexia, fatigue, dizziness, dyspnea, weakness, joint pain

Lab test interferences:

Increase: Cholesterol, sodium, blood glucose, uric acid, calcium, urine glucose

Decrease: Calcium, potassium, T_4, T_3, thyroid ^{131}I uptake test, urine 17-OHCS, 17-KS, PBI

False negative: Skin allergy tests

triamcinolone acetonide

(trye-am-sin'oh-lone)

Aristocort, Kenalog

Func. class.: Topical corticosteroid

Chem. class.: Synthetic fluorinated agent, group II potency (0.5%), group III potency (0.1%), group IV potency (0.025%)

Action: Possesses antipruritic, antiinflammatory actions

Uses: Psoriasis, eczema, contact dermatitis, pruritus

Dosage and routes:

• *Adult and child:* Apply to affected area bid-qid

Available forms include: Oint 0.025%, 0.1%, 0.5%; cream 0.025%, 0.1%, 0.5%; lotion 0.025%, 0.1%; aerosol 0.2 mg/2 sec; paste 0.1%

Side effects/adverse reactions:

INTEG: Burning, dryness, itching, irritation, acne, folliculitis, hypertrichosis, perioral dermatitis, hypopigmentation, atrophy, striae, miliaria, allergic contact dermatitis, secondary infection

Contraindications: Hypersensitivity to corticosteroids, fungal infections

Precautions: Pregnancy (C), lactation, viral infections, bacterial infections

Interactions/incompatibilities: None known

NURSING CONSIDERATIONS

Assess:

• Temperature; if fever develops, drug should be discontinued

Administer:

• Only to affected areas; do not get in eyes

• Medication, then cover with occlusive dressing (only if prescribed), seal to normal skin, change q12h; use occlusive dressing with extreme caution (group II potency)

• Only to dermatoses; do not use on weeping, denuded, or infected area

Perform/provide:

• Cleansing before application of drug

• Treatment for a few days after area has cleared

• Storage at room temperature

Evaluate:

• Therapeutic response: absence of severe itching, patches on skin, flaking

Teach patient/family:

• To avoid sunlight on affected area; burns may occur

---

triamcinolone acetonide (topical-oral)

(trye-am-sin'oh-lone)

Kenalog in Orabase

Func. class.: Topical anesthetic

Chem. class.: Synthetic fluorinated adrenal corticosteroid

Action: Inhibits nerve impulses from sensory nerves

Uses: Oral pain

Dosage and routes:

• *Adult and child:* TOP press ¼ inch into affected area until film appears, repeat bid-tid

Available forms include: Paste 0.1%

Side effects/adverse reactions:

INTEG: Rash, irritation, sensitization

Contraindications: Hypersensitivity, infants <1 yr, application to large areas, presence of fungal, viral, or bacterial infections of mouth or throat

Precautions: Child <6 yr, sepsis, pregnancy, denuded skin

Interactions/incompatibilities: None known

Administer:

• After cleansing oral cavity

Evaluate:

• Allergy: rash, irritation, reddening, swelling

• Therapeutic response: absence of pain in affected area

• Infection: if affected area is infected, do not apply

Teach patient/family:

• To report rash, irritation, redness, swelling

• How to apply paste

---

triamterene

(trye-am'ter-een)

Dyrenium

Func. class.: Potassium-sparing diuretic

Chem. class.: Pteridine derivative

Action: Acts on distal tubule to inhibit reabsorption of sodium, chloride

Uses: Edema; may be used with other diuretics

Dosage and routes:

• *Adults:* PO 100 mg bid pc, not to exceed 300 mg

Available forms include: Cap 50, 100 mg

Side effects/adverse reactions:

GI: Nausea, diarrhea, vomiting, dry mouth

ELECT: Hyperkalemia, hyponatremia

CNS: Weakness, headache

INTEG: Photosensitivity, rash

*HEMA: **Leukopenia, agranulocytosis, thrombocytopenia, aplastic anemia***

Contraindications: Hypersensitivity, anuria, severe renal disease, severe hepatic disease, hyperkalemia

Precautions: Dehydration, pregnancy, hepatic disease, lactation, CHF, renal disease, cirrhosis

T

Pharmacokinetics:
PO: Onset 2 hr, peak 6-8 hr, duration 12-16 hr; half-life 3 hr; me-. tabolized in liver, excreted in urine

Interactions/incompatibilities:

• Decreased potassium levels: kayexalate

• Enhanced action of: antihypertensives, lithium

• Increased hyperkalemia: other potassium sparing diuretics, potassium products, captopril

• Increased levels: digitalis

NURSING CONSIDERATIONS

Assess:

• Weight, I&O daily to determine fluid loss; effect of drug may be decreased if used qd

• Electrolytes: potassium, sodium, chloride; include BUN, blood sugar, CBC, serum creatinine, blood pH, ABGs

Administer:

• In AM to avoid interference with sleep

• With food if nausea occurs; absorption may be decreased slightly

Evaluate:

• Improvement in edema of feet, legs, sacral area daily if medication is being used in CHF

• Improvement in CVP q8h

• Signs of metabolic acidosis: drowsiness, restlessness

• Rashes, temperature elevation qd

• Confusion, especially in elderly, take safety precautions if needed

• Hydration: skin turgor, thirst, dry mucous membranes

Teach patient/family:

• To take medication after meals for GI upset

• To avoid prolonged exposure to sunlight since photosensitivity may occur

• To notify physician if weakness, headache, nausea, vomiting, dry mouth, fever, sore throat, mouth sores, unusual bleeding or bruising occurs

Lab test interferences:
Interfere: GTT, quinidine serum levels, LDH

Treatment of overdose: Lavage if taken orally, monitor electrolytes, administer IV fluids, dialysis

---

triazolam

(trye-ay'zoe-lam)
Halcion

Func. class.: Sedative-hypnotic
Chem. class.: Benzodiazepine

Controlled Substance Schedule IV (USA), Schedule F (Canada)

Action: Produces CNS depression at limbic, thalamic, hypothalamic levels of CNS; may be mediated by neurotransmitter gamma aminobutyric (GABA); results are sedation, hypnosis, skeletal muscle relaxation, anticonvulsant activity, anxiolytic action

Uses: Insomnia

Dosage and routes:

• *Adult:* PO 0.125-0.5 mg hs

• *Elderly:* PO 0.125-0.25 mg hs

Available forms include: Tabs 0.125, 0.25, 0.5 mg

Side effects/adverse reactions:

*HEMA: **Leukopenia, granulocytopenia** (rare)*

CNS: Headache, lethargy, drowsiness, daytime sedation, dizziness, confusion, lightheadedness, anxiety, irritability

GI: Nausea, vomiting, diarrhea, heartburn, abdominal pain, constipation

CV: Chest pain, pulse changes

Contraindications: Hypersensitivity to benzodiazepines, pregnancy (X), lactation, intermittent porphyria

Precautions: Anemia, hepatic disease, renal disease, suicidal individuals, drug abuse, elderly, psychosis, child < 15 yr, acute narrow-angle glaucoma, seizure disorders

Pharmacokinetics:
PO: Onset 30-45 min, duration 6-8 hr; metabolized by liver, excreted by kidneys (inactive metabolites), crosses placenta, excreted in breast milk; half-life 2-3 hr

Interactions/incompatibilities:
• Increased effects of: cimetidine, disulfiram
• Increased or decreased effects of: oral contraceptives
• Increased action of both drugs: alcohol
• Decreased effect of: antacids

NURSING CONSIDERATIONS
Assess:
• Blood studies: Hct, Hgb, RBCs, if blood dyscrasias are suspected (rare)
• Hepatic studies: AST, ALT, bilirubin if liver damage has occurred

Administer:
• After removal of cigarettes, to prevent fires
• After trying conservative measures for insomnia
• ½-1 hr before hs for sleeplessness
• On empty stomach fast onset, but may be taken with food if GI symptoms occur

Perform/provide:
• Assistance with ambulation after receiving dose
• Safety measure: siderails, nightlight, callbell within easy reach
• Checking to see PO medication has been swallowed
• Storage in tight container in cool environment

Evaluate:
• Therapeutic response: ability to sleep at night, decreased amount of early morning awakening if taking drug for insomnia
• Mental status: mood, sensorium, affect, memory (long, short)
• Blood dyscrasias: fever, sore throat, bruising, rash, jaundice, epistaxis (rare)
• Type of sleep problem: falling asleep, staying asleep

Teach patient/family:
• To avoid driving or other activities requiring alertness until drug is stabilized
• To avoid alcohol ingestion or CNS depressants; serious CNS depression may result
• That effects may take 2 nights for benefits to be noticed
• Alternate measures to improve sleep: reading, exercise several hours before hs, warm bath, warm milk, TV, self-hypnosis, deep breathing
• That hangover is common in elderly, but less common than with barbiturates

Lab test interferences:
Increase: ALT, AST, serum bilirubin
Decrease: RAI uptake
False increase: Urinary 17-OHCS
Treatment of overdose: Lavage, activated charcoal, monitor electrolytes, vital signs

---

trichlormethiazide
(trye-klor-meth-eye′a-zide)
Diureses, Metahydrin, Naqua, Trichlorex

Func. class.: Thiazide diuretic
Chem. class.: Sulfonamide derivative

Action: Acts on distal tubule by increasing excretion of water, sodium, chloride, postassium
Uses: Edema, hypertension
Dosage and routes:
Edema
• *Adult:* PO 1-4 mg/day
Hypertension
• *Adult:* PO 2-4 mg/day
Available forms include: Tabs 2, 4 mg

Side effects/adverse reactions:

GU: Frequency, polyuria, uremia, glucosuria

CNS: Drowsiness, paresthesia, anxiety, depression, headache, dizziness, fatigue, weakness

GI: Nausea, vomiting, anorexia, constipation, diarrhea, cramps, pancreatitis, GI irritation, ***hepatitis***

EENT: Blurred vision

INTEG: Rash, urticaria, purpura, photosensitivity, fever

META: Hyperglycemia, hyperuricemia, increased creatinine

*HEMA: **Aplastic anemia, hemolytic anemia, leukopenia, agranulocytosis, thrombocytopenia***

CV: Irregular pulse, orthostatic hypotension

ELECT: Hypokalemia, hypercalcemia, hyponatremia, hypochloremia

Contraindications: Hypersensitivity to thiazides or sulfonamides, anuria, renal decompensation

Precautions: Hypokalemia, renal disease, pregnancy, hepatic disease, gout, COPD, lupus erythematosus, diabetes mellitus

Pharmacokinetics:

PO: Onset 2 hr, peak 6 hr, duration 24 hr; excreted unchanged by kidneys, crosses placenta, enters breast milk

Interactions/incompatibilities:

• Increased toxicity of: lithium, nondepolarizing skeletal muscle relaxants, digitalis

• Decreased effects of: antidiabetics

• Decreased absorption of thiazides: cholestyramine, colestipol

• Decreased hypotensive response: indomethacin

• Increased action of: quinidine

NURSING CONSIDERATIONS

Assess:

• Weight, I&O daily to determine fluid loss; effect of drug may be decreased if used qd

• Rate, depth, rhythm of respiration, effect of exertion

• B/P lying, standing, postural hypotension may occur

• Electrolytes: potassium, sodium, chloride; include BUN, blood sugar, CBC, serum creatinine, blood pH, ABGs

• Glucose in urine if patient is diabetic

Administer:

• In AM to avoid interference with sleep if using drug as a diuretic

• Potassium replacement if potassium is less than 3.0

• With food, if nausea occurs, absorption may be decreased slightly

Evaluate:

• Improvement in edema of feet, legs, sacral area daily if medication is being used in CHF

• Improvement in CVP q8h

• Signs of metabolic acidosis: drowsiness, restlessness

• Signs of hypokalemia: postural hypotension, malaise, fatigue, tachycardia, leg cramps, weakness

• Rashes, temperature elevation qd

• Confusion, especially in elderly; take safety precautions if needed

Teach patient/family:

• To increase fluid intake 2-3 L/day unless contraindicated; to rise slowly from lying or sitting position

• To notify physician of muscle weakness, cramps, nausea, dizziness

• Drug may be taken with food or milk

• That blood sugar may be increased in diabetics

• Take early in day to avoid nocturia

Lab test interferences:

Increase: BSP retention, calcium, amylase

Decrease: PBI, PSP

Treatment of overdose: Lavage if taken orally, monitor electrolytes, administer dextrose in saline

trientine HCl

(trye-in'-teen)
Cuprid

Func. class.: Heavy metal antagonist

Chem. class.: Chelating agent (thiol compound)

Action: Binds with ions of lead, mercury, copper, iron, zinc to form a water-soluble complex excreted by kidneys

Uses: Wilson's disease

Dosage and routes:
• *Adult:* PO 750-2000 mg in divided doses bid-qid
• *Child:* PO 500-1500 mg in divided doses bid-qid

Available forms include: Caps 125, 250 mg; tabs 250 mg

Side effects/adverse reactions:
HEMA: Anemia, *iron deficiency*
INTEG: Urticaria, fever
SYST: Hypersensitivity

Contraindications: Hypersensitivity

Precautions: Pregnancy

Pharmacokinetics:
PO: Peak 1 hr, metabolized in liver, excreted in urine

Interactions/incompatibilities:
• Decreased action: mineral supplements

NURSING CONSIDERATIONS

Assess:
• Monitor hepatic, renal studies: ALT/AST, alk phosphatase, BUN, creatinine
• Monitor I&O

Administer:
• On an empty stomach, ½-1 hr before meals or 2 hr after meals
• B_6 daily; depleted when this drug is used

Evaluate:
• Therapeutic response: improvement in neurologic, psychiatric symptoms

• Allergic reactions (rash, urticaria); if these occur, drug should be discontinued

Teach patient/family:
• That therapeutic effect may take 1-3 mo

triethanolamine polypeptide oleate-condensate

(trye-than'-oo-la-meen)
Cerumenex

Func. class.: Otic

Action: Emulsifies, disperses ear wax

Uses: Impacted cerumen

Dosage and routes:
• *Adult and child:* INSTILL Fill canal, plug with cotton, wait 15-30 min, flush with warm water

Available forms include: Otic sol 10%

Side effects/adverse reactions:
EENT: Itching, irritation in ear
INTEG: Rash, urticaria

Contraindications: Hypersensitivity, perforated eardrum

Pharmacokinetics: Not known

Interactions/incompatibilities: None known

NURSING CONSIDERATIONS

Administer:
• After restraining child if necessary
• Warming solution to body temperature

Evaluate:
• Therapeutic response: loosened cerumen, ability to hear better

Teach patient/family:
• Method of instillation using aseptic technique, including not touching dropper to ear
• That dizziness may occur after instillation

T

trifluoperazine HCl

(trye-floo-oh-per'a-zeen)
Novoflurazine,* Solazine,* Suprazine, Stelazine, Terfluzine,* Triflurin*

Func. class.: Antipsychotic/neuroleptic
Chem. class.: Phenothiazine, piperazine

Action: Depresses cerebral cortex, hypothalamus, limbic system, which control activity, aggression; blocks neurotransmission produced by dopamine at synapse; exhibits strong α-adrenergic, anticholinergic blocking action; mechanism for antipsychotic effects is unclear

Uses: Psychotic disorders, nonpsychotic anxiety, schizophrenia

Dosage and routes:
Psychotic disorders
• *Adult:* PO 2-5 mg bid, usual range 15-20 mg/day, may require 40 mg/day or more; IM 1-2 mg q4-6h
• *Child:* PO 1 mg qd or bid; IM *not recommended for children,* but 1 mg may be given qd or bid
Nonpsychotic anxiety
• *Adult:* PO 1-2 mg bid, not to exceed 6 mg/day; do not give longer than 12 wk

Available forms include: Tabs 1, 2, 5, 10 mg; conc 10 mg/ml; inj IM 2 mg/ml

Side effects/adverse reactions:
RESP: **Laryngospasm,** dyspnea, **respiratory depression**
CNS: Extrapyramidal symptoms: pseudoparkinsonism, akathisia, dystonia, tardive dyskinesia, seizures, *headache*
HEMA: Anemia, leukopenia, leukocytosis, **agranulocytosis**
INTEG: Rash, photosensitivity, dermatitis
EENT: Blurred vision, glaucoma

GI: Dry mouth, nausea, vomiting, anorexia, constipation, diarrhea, jaundice, weight gain
GU: Urinary retention, urinary frequency, enuresis, impotence, amenorrhea, gynecomastia
CV: Orthostatic hypotension, hypertension, **cardiac arrest,** ECG changes, **tachycardia**

Contraindications: Hypersensitivity, cardiovascular disease, coma, blood dyscrasias, severe hepatic disease, child <6 yr

Precautions: Breast cancer, seizure disorders, pregnancy, lactation

Pharmacokinetics:
PO: Onset rapid, peak 2-3 hr, duration 12 hr
IM: Onset immediate, peak 1 hr, duration 12 hr
Metabolized by liver, excreted in urine, crosses placenta, enters breast milk

Interactions/incompatibilities:
• Oversedation: other CNS depressants, alcohol, barbiturate anesthetics
• Toxicity: epinephrine
• Decreased absorption: aluminum hydroxide or magnesium hydroxide antacids
• Decreased effects of: lithium, levodopa
• Increased effects of both drugs: β-adrenergic blockers, alcohol
• Increased anticholinergic effects: anticholinergics

NURSING CONSIDERATIONS
Assess:
• Swallowing of PO medication; check for hoarding or giving of medication to other patients
• I&O ratio; palpate bladder if low urinary output occurs
• Bilirubin, CBC, liver function studies monthly
• Urinalysis is recommended before and during prolonged therapy

Administer:
• Antiparkinsonian agent, after securing order from physician to be used if EPS occur
• Conc in 60 ml of tomato or fruit juice, milk, orange, carbonated beverage, coffee, tea, water, or semisolid foods (soup, pudding)

Perform/provide:
• Decreased noise input by dimming lights, avoiding loud noises
• Supervised ambulation until stabilized on medication; do not involve in strenuous exercise program because fainting is possible; patient should not stand still for long periods of time
• Increased fluids to prevent constipation
• Sips of water, candy, gum for dry mouth
• Storage in tight, light-resistant container, oral solutions in amber bottles; slight yellowing of inj or conc is common, does not affect potency

Evaluate:
• Therapeutic response: decrease in emotional excitement, hallucinations, delusions, paranoia, reorganization of patterns of thought, speech
• Affect, orientation, LOC, reflexes, gait, coordination, sleep pattern disturbances
• B/P standing and lying; also include pulse, respirations q4h during initial treatment; establish baseline before starting treatment; report drops of 30 mm Hg
• Dizziness, faintness, palpitations, tachycardia on rising
• EPS including akathisia (inability to sit still, no pattern to movements), tardive dyskinesia (bizarre movements of jaw, mouth, tongue, extremities), pseudoparkinsonism (rigidity, tremors, pill rolling, shuffling gait)
• Skin turgor daily

• Constipation, urinary retention daily; if these occur increase bulk, water in diet

Teach patient/family:
• That orthostatic hypotension occurs frequently, and to rise from sitting or lying position gradually
• To remain lying down after IM injection for at least 30 min
• To avoid hot tubs, hot showers, or tub baths since hypotension may occur
• To avoid abrupt withdrawal of this drug or EPS may result; drugs should be withdrawn slowly
• To avoid OTC preparations (cough, hayfever, cold) unless approved by physician since serious drug interactions may occur; avoid use with alcohol or CNS depressants, increased drowsiness may occur
• To use a sunscreen during sun exposure to prevent burns
• Regarding compliance with drug regimen
• About necessity for meticulous oral hygiene since oral candidiasis may occur
• To report sore throat, malaise, fever, bleeding, mouth sores; if these occur, CBC should be drawn and drug discontinued
• In hot weather, heat stroke may occur; take extra precautions to stay cool

Lab test interferences:
Increase: Liver function tests, cardiac enzymes, cholesterol, blood glucose, prolactin, bilirubin, PBI, cholinesterase, ^{131}I
Decrease: Hormones (blood and urine)
False positive: Pregnancy tests, PKU
False negative: Urinary steroids, 17-OHCS
Treatment of overdose: Lavage if orally injested, provide an airway; *do not induce vomiting*

---

italics = common side effects   **bold italic** = life threatening reactions

triflupromazine HCl

(trye-floo-proe'ma-zeen)
Vesprin

Func. class.: Antipsychotic/neuroleptic

Chem. class.: Phenothiazine, aliphatic

Action: Depresses cerebral cortex, hypothalamus, limbic system, which control activity, aggression; blocks neurotransmission produced by dopamine at synapse; exhibits strong α-adrenergic, anticholinergic blocking action; mechanism for antipsychotic effects is unclear

Uses: Psychotic disorders, schizophrenia, acute agitation, nausea, vomiting

Dosage and routes:
Psychosis
• *Adult:* PO 10-50 mg bid-tid depending on severity of condition; dose is gradually increased to desired dose
• *Child >2 yr:* PO 0.5-2 mg/kg/day in 3 divided doses; may increase to 150 mg if needed

Nausea/vomiting
• *Adult:* PO 20-30 mg qd; IV 1-3 mg; IM 5-15 mg, q4h, max 60 mg qd
• *Child >2 yr:* PO/IM 0.2 mg/kg, max 60 mg qd

Acute agitation
• *Adult:* IM 60-150 mg/qd in 3 divided doses
• *Child >2 yr:* IM 0.2-0.25 mg/kg/day in divided doses, max 10 mg/qd

Available forms include: Tabs 10, 25, 50 mg (Canada only); inj IM, IV 10, 20 mg/ml

Side effects/adverse reactions:
RESP: Laryngospasm, dyspnea, *respiratory depression*
CNS: Extrapyramidal symptoms: pseudoparkinsonism, akathisia, dystonia, tardive dyskinesia, drowsiness, headache, seizures
HEMA: Anemia, leukopenia, leukocytosis, *agranulocytosis*
INTEG: Rash, photosensitivity, dermatitis
EENT: Blurred vision, glaucoma
GI: Dry mouth, nausea, vomiting, anorexia, constipation, diarrhea, jaundice, weight gain
GU: Urinary retention, urinary frequency, enuresis, impotence, amenorrhea, gynecomastia
CV: Orthostatic hypotension, hypertension, *cardiac arrest,* ECG changes, *tachycardia*

Contraindications: Hypersensitivity, blood dyscrasias, coma, child <2 yr, brain damage, bone marrow depression

Precautions: Pregnancy, lactation, seizure disorders, hypertension, hepatic disease, cardiac disease

Pharmacokinetics:
PO: Onset erratic, peak 2-4 hr, duration 4-6 hr
IM: Onset 15-30 min, peak 15-20 min, duration 4-6 hr
Metabolized by liver, excreted in urine and feces, crosses placenta, enters breast milk

Interactions/incompatibilities:
• Oversedation: other CNS depressants, alcohol, barbiturate anesthetics
• Toxicity: epinephrine
• Decreased absorption: aluminum hydroxide or magnesium hydroxide antacids
• Decreased effects of: lithium, levodopa
• Increased effects of both drugs: β-adrenergic blockers, alcohol
• Increased anticholinergic effects: anticholinergics

NURSING CONSIDERATIONS
Assess:
• Swallowing of PO medication; check for hoarding or giving of medication to other patients

- I&O ratio; palpate bladder if low urinary output occurs
- Bilirubin, CBC, liver function studies monthly
- Urinalysis is recommended before and during prolonged therapy

Administer:

- Antiparkinsonian agent, after securing order from physician to be used if EPS occur
- IM injection into large muscle mass

Perform/provide:

- Decreased noise input by dimming lights, avoiding loud noises
- Supervised ambulation until stabilized on medication; do not involve in strenuous exercise program because fainting is possible; patient should not stand still for long periods of time
- Increased fluids to prevent constipation
- Sips of water, candy, gum for dry mouth
- Storage in tight, light-resistant container

Evaluate:

- Therapeutic response: decrease in emotional excitement, hallucinations, delusions, paranoia, reorganization of patterns of thought, speech
- Affect, orientation, LOC, reflexes, gait, coordination, sleep pattern disturbances
- B/P standing and lying; also include pulse, respirations q4h during initial treatment; establish baseline before starting treatment; report drops of 30 mm Hg
- Dizziness, faintness, palpitations, tachycardia on rising
- EPS including akathisia (inability to sit still, no pattern to movements), tardive dyskinesia (bizarre movements of jaw, mouth, tongue, extremities), pseudoparkinsonism (rigidity, tremors, pill rolling, shuffling gait)

- Skin turgor daily
- Constipation, urinary retention daily; if these occur increase bulk, water in the diet

Teach patient/family:

- That orthostatic hypotension occurs frequently, and to rise from sitting or lying position gradually
- To remain lying down after IM injection for at least 30 min
- To avoid hot tubs, hot showers, or tub baths since hypotension may occur
- To avoid abrupt withdrawal of this drug or EPS may result; drugs should be withdrawn slowly
- To avoid OTC preparations (cough, hayfever, cold) unless approved by physician since serious drug interactions may occur; avoid use with alcohol or CNS depressants, increased drowsiness may occur
- To use sunscreen during sun exposure to prevent burns
- Regarding compliance with drug regimen
- About necessity for meticulous oral hygiene since oral candidiasis may occur
- To report sore throat, malaise, fever, bleeding, mouth sores; if these occur, CBC should be drawn and drug discontinued
- In hot weather, heat stroke may occur; take extra precautions to stay cool

Lab test interferences:

Increase: Liver function tests, cardiac enzymes, cholesterol, blood glucose, prolactin, bilirubin, PBI, cholinesterase, ^{131}I

Decrease: Hormones (blood and urine)

False positive: Pregnancy tests, PKU

False negative: Urinary steroids

Treatment of overdose: Lavage if orally injested, provide an airway; *do not induce vomiting*

T

---

italics = common side effects   **bold italic** = life threatening reactions

trifluridine (ophthalmic)

(trye-flure'i-deen)

Viroptic Ophthalmic Solution

Func. class.: Antiviral

Chem. class.: Pyrimidine nucleoside

Action: Inhibits viral DNA synthesis and replication

Uses: Primary keratoconjunctivitis, recurring epithelial keratitis

Dosage and routes:

• *Adult and child:* INSTILL 1 gtt q2h, not to exceed 9 gtts/day, until corneal epithelium is regrown, then 1 gtt q4h × 1 wk

Available forms include: Sol 1%

Side effects/adverse reactions:

EENT: Burning, stinging, swelling, photophobia

Contraindications: Hypersensitivity

Precautions: Antibiotic hypersensitivity

Interactions/incompatibilities: None known

NURSING CONSIDERATIONS

Administer:

• After washing hands, cleanse crusts or discharge from eye before application

Perform/provide:

• Storage in refrigerator

Evaluate:

• Therapeutic response: absence of redness, inflammation, tearing

• Allergy: itching, lacrimation, redness, swelling

Teach patient/family:

• To use drug exactly as prescribed

• Not to use eye make-up, towels, washcloths, or eye medication of others, or reinfection may occur

• That drug container tip should not be touched to eye

• To report itching, increased redness, burning, stinging; drug should be discontinued

trihexyphenidyl HCl

(trye-hex-ee-fen'i-dill)

Aparkane,* Aphen, Artane, Hexaphen, Novohexidyl,* T.H.P., Trihexane, Trihexidyl

Func. class.: Cholinergic blocker

Chem. class.: Synthetic tertiary amine

Action: Acts on dopamine receptors in CNS, which decrease involuntary movements

Uses: Parkinson symptoms (drug-induced)

Dosage and routes:

• *Adult:* PO 1 mg, then 2 mg q3-5 days to a total of 6-10 mg/day

Available forms include: Tabs 2, 5 mg; caps sus-rel 5 mg; elix 2 mg/5 ml

Side effects/adverse reactions:

CNS: Confusion, anxiety, restlessness, irritability, delusions, hallucinations, headache, sedation, depression, incoherence, dizziness

EENT: Blurred vision, photophobia, dilated pupils, difficulty swallowing

CV: Palpitations, tachycardia, postural hypotension

GI: Dryness of mouth, constipation, nausea, vomiting, abdominal distress, paralytic ileus

GU: Hesitancy, retention

Contraindications: Hypersensitivity, narrow-angle glaucoma, myasthenia gravis, GI/GU obstruction, child <3 yr

Precautions: Pregnancy, elderly, lactation, tachycardia, prostatic hypertrophy

Pharmacokinetics:

PO: Onset 1 hr, peak 2-3 hr, duration 6-12 hr, excreted in urine

Interactions/incompatibilities:

• Increased anticholinergic effects: alcohol, narcotics, barbiturates, antihistamines, MAOIs, phenothiazines, amantadine

NURSING CONSIDERATIONS
Assess:
• I&O ratio; retention commonly causes decreased urinary output
Administer:
• With or after meals for GI upset; may give with fluids other than water
• At hs to avoid daytime drowsiness in patient with parkinsonism
Perform/provide:
• Storage at room temperature in light resistant containers
• Hard candy, frequent drinks, sugarless gum to relieve dry mouth
Evaluate:
• Parkinsonism: shuffling gait, muscle rigidity, involuntary movements
• Urinary hesitancy, retention; palpate bladder if retention occurs
• Constipation; increase fluids, bulk, exercise if this occurs
• For tolerance over long-term therapy; dose may need to be increased or changed
• Mental status: affect, mood, CNS depression, worsening of mental symptoms during early therapy
Teach patient/family:
• Not to discontinue this drug abruptly; to taper off over 1 wk
• To avoid driving or other hazardous activities; drowsiness may occur
• To avoid OTC medications: cough, cold preparations with alcohol, antihistamines unless directed by physician

trilostane

(trye-loss-tane)
Modrastane

Func. class.: Antineoplastic
Chem. class.: Hormone, adrenal steroid inhibitor

Action: Inhibits DNA, RNA, protein synthesis; derived from *Streptomyces verticillus;* replication is decreased by binding to DNA, which causes strand splitting; drug is phase specific in G_2, M phases
Uses: Metastatic breast cancer, adrenal cancer, suppression of adrenal function in Cushing's syndrome
Dosage and routes:
• *Adult:* PO 30 mg qid, may increase q3-4d up to 480 mg/day
Available forms include: Caps 30, 60 mg
Side effects/adverse reactions:
*HEMA: **Thrombocytopenia, leukopenia, myelosuppression, anemia***
*GI: Nausea, vomiting, anorexia, **hepatotoxicity***
GU: Hirsutism
INTEG: Rash, pruritus
CV: Hypotension, tachycardia
CNS: Dizziness, headache
Contraindications: Hypersensitivity, hypothyroidism
Precautions: Renal disease, hepatic disease, respiratory disease, pregnancy
Pharmacokinetics: Half-life 13 hr, metabolized in liver, excreted in urine, crosses placenta
Interactions/incompatibilities:
None known
NURSING CONSIDERATIONS
Assess:
• CBC, differential, platelet count weekly; withhold drug if WBC is <4000 or platelet count is <75,000; notify physician of results
• Renal function studies: BUN, se-

T

rum uric acid, urine CrCl, electrolytes before, during therapy
• I&O ratio; report fall in urine output of 30 ml/hr
• Monitor temperature q4h (may indicate beginning infection)
• Liver function tests before, during therapy (bilirubin, AST, ALT, LDH) as needed or monthly
• RBC, Hct, Hgb since these may be decreased

Administer:
• Medications by oral route; if possible avoid IM, SC, IV routes to prevent infections
• Antacid before oral agent, give drug after evening meal, before bedtime
• Antiemetic 30-60 min before giving drug to prevent vomiting
• Antibiotics for prophylaxis of infection
• Local or systemic drugs for infection

Perform/provide:
• Strict medical asepsis, protective isolation if WBC levels are low
• Special skin care
• Liquid diet, including cola, Jello; dry toast or crackers may be added if patient is not nauseated or vomiting
• Nutritious diet with iron, vitamin supplements as ordered

Evaluate:
• Bleeding: hematuria, guaiac, bruising, petechiae, mucosa or orifices q8h
• Food preferences; list likes, dislikes
• Edema in feet, joint, stomach pain, shaking
• Inflammation of mucosa, breaks in skin
• Yellowing of skin, sclera, dark urine, clay-colored stools, itchy skin, abdominal pain, fever, diarrhea
• Symptoms indicating severe allergic reactions: rash, pruritus, urticaria, purpuric skin lesions, itching, flushing

Teach patient/family:
• To report any complaints, side effects to nurse or physician
• That masculinization can occur, is reversible after discontinuing treatment

trimeprazine tartrate

(trye-mep′ra-zeen)
Panectyl,* Temaril
Func. class.: Antihistamine
Chem. class.: Phenothiazine analog, H_1-receptor antagonist

Action: Acts on blood vessels, GI, respiratory system by competing with histamine for H_1-receptor site; decreases allergic response by blocking histamine
Uses: Pruritus
Dosage and routes:
• *Adult:* PO 2.5 mg qid; TIME-REL 5 mg bid
• *Child 3-12 yr:* PO 2.5 mg tid or hs
• *Child 6 mo-1 yr:* PO 1.25 mg tid or hs
Available forms include: Tabs 2.5 mg; spans 5 mg; syr 2.5 mg/5 ml
Side effects/adverse reactions:
CNS: Dizziness, drowsiness, poor condition, fatigue, anxiety, euphoria, confusion, paresthesia, neuritis
CV: Hypotension, palpitations, tachycardia
RESP: Increased thick secretions, wheezing, chest tightness
*HEMA: **Thrombocytopenia, agranulocytosis, hemolytic anemia***
GI: Dry mouth, nausea, vomiting, anorexia, constipation, diarrhea
INTEG: Rash, urticaria, photosensitivity
GU: Retention, dysuria, frequency

EENT: Blurred vision, dilated pupils, tinnitus, nasal stuffiness, dry nose, throat, mouth

Contraindications: Hypersensitivity to H₁-receptor antagonist, acute asthma attack, lower respiratory tract diseases

Precautions: Increased intraocular pressure, renal disease, cardiac disease, hypertension, bronchial asthma, seizure disorder, stenosed peptic ulcers, hyperthyroidism, prostatic hypertrophy, bladder neck obstruction, pregnancy (C)

Pharmacokinetics: Not known

Interactions/incompatibilities:

• Increased CNS depression: barbiturates, narcotics, hypnotics, tricyclic antidepressants, alcohol

• Decreased effect of: oral anticoagulants, heparin

• Increased effect of this drug: MAOIs

NURSING CONSIDERATIONS

Assess:

• I&O ratio; be alert for urinary retention, frequency, dysuria; drug should be discontinued if these occur

• CBC during long-term therapy

Administer:

• Coffee, tea, cola (caffeine) to decrease drowsiness

• With meals if GI symptoms occur; absorption may slightly decrease

• Sustained-release formulation only to adults

Perform/provide:

• Hard candy, gum, frequent rinsing of mouth for dryness

• Storage in tight container at room temperature

Evaluate:

• Therapeutic response: decreased itching associated with pruritus

• Respiratory status: rate, rhythm, increase in bronchial secretions, wheezing, chest tightness

• Cardiac status: palpitations, increased pulse, hypotension

Teach patient/family:

• All aspects of drug use; to notify physician if confusion, sedation, hypotension occurs

• To avoid driving or other hazardous activity if drowsiness occurs

• To avoid concurrent use of alcohol or other CNS depressants

Lab test interferences:

False negative: Skin allergy tests

Treatment of overdose: Administer ipecac syrup or lavage, diazepam, vasopressors, barbiturates (short-acting)

---

trimethadione

(trye-meth-a-dye′one)
Tridione

Func. class.: Anticonvulsant
Chem. class.: Oxazolidinedione

Action: Increases seizures in cortex, basal ganglia; decreases synaptic stimulation to low-frequency impulses

Uses: Refractory absence seizures

Dosage and routes:

• *Adult:* PO 300 mg tid, may increase by 300 mg/wk, not to exceed 600 mg qid

• *Child:* PO 20-50 mg/kg/day, may increase by 150-300 mg/wk

Available forms include: Caps 300 mg; chew tabs 150 mg; sol 200 mg/5 ml; oral sol 40 mg/ml

Side effects/adverse reactions:

HEMA: **Thrombocytopenia, agranulocytosis, leukopenia, neutropenia, hemolytic anemia,** increased pro-time

CNS: Drowsiness, dizziness, fatigue, paresthesia, irritability, headache

GU: Vaginal bleeding, albuminuria, nephrosis, abdominal pain, weight loss

T

GI: Nausea, vomiting, bleeding
gums, abnormal liver function tests
INTEG: Exfoliative dermatitis, rash,
alopecia, petechiae, erythema
EENT: Photophobia, diplopia, epi-
staxis, retinal hemorrhage
CV: Hypertension, hypotension
Contraindications: Hypersensitiv-
ity, blood dyscrasias
Precautions: Hepatic disease, re-
nal disease
Pharmacokinetics:
PO: Peak 30 min-2 hr, excreted by
kidneys, half-life 6-13 days
Interactions/incompatibilities:
None known
NURSING CONSIDERATIONS
Assess:
• Blood studies: Hct, Hgb, RBCs,
serum folate, vitamin D if on long-
term therapy
• Hepatic studies: AST, ALT, bili-
rubin, creatinine, failure
Administer:
• After diluting oral solution with
water
• Oral with juice or milk to cover
taste/smell; decreases GI symp-
toms
Perform/provide:
• Ventilation of room
Evaluate:
• Mental status: mood, sensorium,
affect, memory (long, short)
• Rash, alopecia, convulsions; dis-
continue drug if these occur
Teach patient/family:
• That physical dependency may
result when used for extended pe-
riods
• To avoid driving, other activities
that require alertness
• Not to discontinue medication
quickly after long-term use; convulsions may result

trimethaphan camsylate
(trye-meth′a-fan)
Arfonad

Func. class.: Antihypertensive
Chem. class.: Ganglionic blocker

Action: Occupies receptor site,
prevents acetylcholine from attaching to postsynaptic nerve endings
in sympathetic, parasympathetic
ganglia
Uses: Hypertensive emergencies,
production of controlled hypotension during surgery
Dosage and routes:
• *Adult:* IV INF dilute 500 mg in
500 ml of 5% dextrose injection,
run at 3-4 mg/ml, adjust to maintain B/P at desired rate; range 0.3-
6.0 mg/min
• *Child:* 50-150 µg/kg/min
Available forms include: Inj IV 50
mg/ml
Side effects/adverse reactions:
CV: Orthostatic hypotension, angina, tachycardia, edema
*GI: Nausea, vomiting, anorexia,
dry mouth, diarrhea,* constipation
CNS: Headache, agitation, weakness, restlessness
INTEG: Rash, urticaria, pruritus
*RESP: **Respiratory arrest***
EENT: Blurred vision, diplopia, pupillary dilation
GU: Urinary retention
Contraindications: Uncorrected
respiratory insufficiency, hypersensitivity, pregnancy (C), hypovo-
lemic shock, glaucoma
Precautions: Elderly, debilitated,
allergic individuals, cardiac disease, degenerative CNS disease,
hepatic disease, renal disease, diabetes mellitus, Addison's disease,
children
Pharmacokinetics:
IV: Onset 1-2 min, duration up to

30 min; excreted in urine, crosses placenta

Interactions/incompatibilities:

• Effects may be increased by diuretics, antihypertensives, anesthetics

• Do not mix with any drug in syringe or solution

NURSING CONSIDERATIONS

Assess:

• Electrolytes: K, Na, Cl, CO_2

• Renal function studies: BUN, creatinine

• B/P, other VS throughout treatment

• Weight daily, I&O

• ECG throughout treatment if there is a history of cardiac problems

Administer:

• IV infusion by microdrip regulator

• Diluted solution only (50 mg of drug/500 ml of D_5)

Perform/provide:

• Artificial ventilation equipment nearby

• Use of only freshly prepared solution

Evaluate:

• Therapeutic effect: decreased B/P, primarily systolic B/P

• Nausea, vomiting, diarrhea

• Edema in feet, legs daily

• Skin turgor, dryness of mucous membranes for hydration status

• Constipation: number of stools, consistency, give stool softener if ordered or increase bulk in diet if constipation occurs, or antidiarrheal for diarrhea

• Respiratory dysfunction: bronchospasm, wheezing, tachypnea, respiratory arrest

• Signs of peripheral vascular collapse

Teach patient/family:

• That lying in bed is needed during infusion

Treatment of overdose: Administer vasopressors, phenylephrine, discontinue drug

trimethobenzamide

(trye-meth-oh-ben′za-mide)

Spengan, Ticon, Tigan

Func. class.: Antiemetic

Chem. class.: Ethanolamine derivative

Action: Acts centrally by blocking chemoreceptor trigger zone, which in turn acts on vomiting center

Uses: Nausea, vomiting, prevention of postoperative vomiting

Dosage and routes:

Postoperative vomiting

• *Adult:* IM/REC 200 mg before or during surgery; may repeat 3 hr after

Discontinuing anesthesia

• *Child 13-40 kg:* PO/REC 100-200 mg tid-qid

• *Child <13 kg:* PO/REC 100 mg tid-qid

Nausea/vomiting

• *Adult:* PO 250 mg tid-qid; IM/REC 200 mg tid-qid

Available forms include: Caps 100, 250 mg; supp 100, 200 mg; inj IM 100 mg/ml

Side effects/adverse reactions:

CNS: Drowsiness, restlessness, headache, dizziness, insomnia, confusion, nervousness, tingling, vertigo, EPS

GI: Nausea, anorexia, diarrhea, vomiting, constipation

CV: Hypertension, hypotension, palpitation

INTEG: Rash, urticaria, fever, chills, flushing

EENT: Dry mouth, blurred vision, diplopia, nasal congestion, photosensitivity

Contraindications: Hypersensitivity to narcotics, shock

Precautions: Children, cardiac dysrhythmias, elderly, asthma, pregnancy, prostatic hypertrophy, bladder-neck obstruction, narrow-angle glaucoma, stenosing peptic ulcer, pyloroduodenal obstruction

Pharmacokinetics:

PO: Onset 20-40 min, duration 3-4 hr

IM: Onset 15 min, duration 2-3 hr, metabolized by liver, excreted by kidneys

Interactions/incompatibilities:

• Increased effect: CNS depressants

• May mask ototoxic symptoms associated with antibiotics

NURSING CONSIDERATIONS

Assess:

• VS, B/P; check patients with cardiac disease more often

Administer:

• IM injection in large muscle mass; aspirate to avoid IV administration

• Tablets may be swallowed whole, chewed, allowed to dissolve

Evaluate:

• Signs of toxicity of other drugs or masking of symptoms of disease: brain tumor, intestinal obstruction

• Observe for drowsiness, dizziness

Teach patient/family:

• Avoid hazardous activities, activities requiring alertness; dizziness may occur; instruct patient to request assistance with ambulation

• Avoid alcohol, other depressants

---

trimethoprim

(trye-meth'oh-prim)

Proloprim, Trimpex

Func. class.: Urinary antiinfective

Chem. class.: Folate antagonist

Action: Prevents bacterial synthesis by blocking enzyme reduction of dihyodrofolic acid

Uses: *E.coli, P. mirabilis, Klebsi-*

ella, Enterobacter urinary tract infections

Dosage and routes:

• *Adult:* PO 100 mg q12h

Available forms include: Tabs 100, 200 mg

Side effects/adverse reactions:

INTEG: Exfoliative dermatitis, pruritus, rash

HEMA: Thrombocytopenia, leukopenia, neutropenia, megaloblastic anemia (rare)

GI: Nausea, vomiting, abdominal pain, abnormal taste, increased AST, ALT, bilirubin, creatinine

CNS: Fever

Contraindications: Hypersensitivity, CrCl <15 ml/min, renal disease, hepatic disease, megaloblastic anemia

Precautions: Folate deficiency, pregnancy, lactation, fragile X chromosome, children <12 yr old, infants <2 mo

Pharmacokinetics:

PO: Peak 1-4 hr, half-life 8-11 hr, metabolized in liver, excreted in urine (unchanged 60%), breast milk, crosses placenta

Interactions/incompatabilities:

• Decreased action of: phenytoin

NURSING CONSIDERATIONS

Assess:

• Nocturia; may indicate drug resistance

• AST/ALT, BUN, bilirubin, creatinine, urine cultures

• C&S before drug therapy; drug may be taken as soon as culture is taken

Administer:

• With full glass of water

Perform/provide:

• Storage in tight, light-resistant container

• Adequate intake of fluids (2000 ml) to decrease bacteria in bladder

Evaluate:

• Therapeutic response: absence of pain in bladder area, negative C&S

• Skin eruptions

• Allergies before treatment, reaction of each medication; place allergies on chart, Kardex in bright red letters; notify all people giving drugs

Teach patient/family:

• Aspects of drug therapy: need to complete entire course of medication to ensure organism death (10-14 days); culture may be taken after completed course of medication

• That drug must be taken in equal intervals around clock to maintain blood levels

• To notify nurse of nausea, vomiting

---

trimipramine maleate

(tri-mip′ra-meen)
Surmontil
Func. class.: Antidepressant—tricyclic
Chem. class.: Tertiary amine

Action: Selectively inhibits serotonin uptake by brain; potentiates behavioral changes

Uses: Depression, enuresis in children

Dosage and routes:

• *Adult:* PO 75 mg/day in divided doses, may be increased to 200 mg/day

• *Child >6 yr:* 25 mg hs, may increase to 50 mg in children <12 yr or 75 mg in children >12 yr

Available forms include: Caps 25, 50, 100 mg

Side effects/adverse reactions:

HEMA: Agranulocytosis, thrombocytopenia, eosinophilia, leukopenia

CNS: Dizziness, drowsiness, confusion, headache, anxiety, tremors, stimulation, weakness, insomnia, nightmares, EPS (elderly), increase in psychiatric symptoms

GI: Diarrhea, dry mouth, nausea, vomiting, *paralytic ileus,* increased appetite, cramps, epigastric distress, jaundice, *hepatitis,* stomatitis

*GU: Retention, **acute renal failure***

INTEG: Rash, urticaria, sweating, pruritus, photosensitivity

*CV: Orthostatic hypotension, ECG changes, tachycardia, **hypertension,*** palpitations

EENT: Blurred vision, tinnitus, mydriasis

Contraindications: Hypersensitivity to tricyclic antidepressants, recovery phase of myocardial infarction, convulsive disorders, prostatic hypertrophy

Precautions: Suicidal patients, severe depression, increased intraocular pressure, narrow-angle glaucoma, urinary retention, cardiac disease, hepatic disease, hyperthyroidism, electroshock therapy, elective surgery, pregnancy (C)

Pharmacokinetics:

Metabolized by liver, excreted by kidneys, steady state 2-6 days; half-life 7-30 hr

Interactions/incompatibilities:

• Decreased effects of: guanethidine, clonidine, indirect acting sympathomimetics (ephedrine)

• Increased effects of: direct acting sympathomimetics (epinephrine), alcohol, barbiturates, benzodiazepines, CNS depressants

• Hyperpyretic crisis, convulsions, hypertensive episode: MAOI (pargyline [Eutonyl])

NURSING CONSIDERATIONS

Assess:

• B/P (lying, standing), pulse q4h; if systolic B/P drops 20 mm Hg hold drug, notify physician; take vital signs q4h in patients with cardiovascular disease

• Blood studies: CBC, leukocytes, differential, cardiac enzymes if patient is receiving long-term therapy

T

• Hepatic studies: AST, ALT, bilirubin, creatinine
• Weight qwk, appetite may increase with drug
• ECG for flattening of T wave, bundle branch block, AV block, dysrhythmias in cardiac patients

Administer:

• Increased fluids, bulk in diet if constipation, urinary retention occur
• With food or milk for GI symptoms
• Dosage hs if over-sedation occurs during day; may take entire dose hs; elderly may not tolerate once/day dosing
• Gum, hard candy, or frequent sips of water for dry mouth

Perform/provide:

• Storage in tight, light-resistant container at room temperature
• Assistance with ambulation during beginning therapy since drowsiness/dizziness occurs
• Safety measures, including siderails primarily in elderly
• Checking to see PO medication swallowed

Evaluate:

• EPS primarily in elderly: rigidity, dystonia, akathisia
• Mental status: mood, sensorium, affect, suicidal tendencies, increase in psychiatric symptoms: depression, panic
• Urinary retention, constipation; constipation is more likely to occur in children
• Withdrawal symptoms: headache, nausea, vomiting, muscle pain, weakness; do not usually occur unless drug was discontinued abruptly
• Alcohol consumption; if alcohol is consumed, hold dose until morning

Teach patient/family:

• That therapeutic effects may take 2-3 wk

• Use caution in driving or other activities requiring alertness because of drowsiness, dizziness, blurred vision
• To avoid alcohol ingestion, other CNS depressants
• Not to discontinue medication quickly after long-term use, may cause nausea, headache, malaise
• To wear sunscreen or large hat since photosensitivity occurs

Lab test interferences:

Increase: Serum bilirubin, blood glucose, alk phosphatase
False increase: Urinary catecholamines
Decrease: VMA, 5-HIAA

Treatment of overdose: ECG monitoring, induce emesis, lavage, activated charcoal, administer anticonvulsant

---

tripelennamine HCl

(tri-pel-een′a-meen)
PBZ-SR, Pelamine, Pyribenzamine, Ro-Hist

Func. class.: Antihistamine
Chem. class.: Ethylenediamine derivative

Action: Acts on blood vessels, GI, respiratory system, by competing with histamine for H_1-receptor site; decreases allergic response by blocking histamine

Uses: Rhinitis, allergy symptoms

Dosage and routes:

• *Adult:* PO 25-50 mg q4-6h, not to exceed 600 mg/day; TIME-REL 100 mg bid-tid, not to exceed 600 mg/day
• *Child >5 yr:* TIME-REL 50 mg q8-12hr, not to exceed 300 mg/day
• *Child <5 yr:* PO 5 mg/kg/day in 4-6 divided doses, not to exceed 300 mg/day

Available forms include: Tab 25, 50 mg; time-rel tab 100 mg; elix 37.5 mg/5 ml

Side effects/adverse reactions:

CNS: Dizziness, drowsiness, poor coordination, fatigue, anxiety, euphoria, confusion, paresthesia, neuritis

CV: Hypotension, palpitations, tachycardia

RESP: Increased thick secretions, wheezing, chest tightness

*HEMA: **Thrombocytopenia, agranulocytosis, hemolytic anemia***

GI: Dry mouth, nausea, vomiting, anorexia, constipation, diarrhea

INTEG: Rash, urticaria, photosensitivity

GU: Retention, dysuria, frequency

EENT: Blurred vision, dilated pupils, tinnitus, nasal stuffiness, dry nose, throat, mouth

Contraindications: Hypersensitivity to H_1-receptor antagonist, acute asthma attack, lower respiratory tract disease

Precautions: Increased intraocular pressure, renal disease, cardiac disease, hypertension, bronchial asthma, seizure disorder, stenosed peptic ulcers, hyperthyroidism, prostatic hypertrophy, bladder/neck obstruction, pregnancy

Pharmacokinetics:

PO: Onset 15-30 min, duration 4-6 hr, detoxified in liver, excreted by kidneys

Interactions/incompatibilities:

• Increased CNS depressants: barbiturates, narcotics, hypnotics, tricyclic antidepressants, alcohol

• Decreased effect of: oral anticoagulants, heparin

• Increased effect of this drug: MAOIs

NURSING CONSIDERATIONS

Assess:

• I&O ratio; be alert for urinary retention, frequency, dysuria; drug should be discontinued if these occur

• CBC during long-term therapy

Administer:

• Coffee, tea, cola (caffeine) to decrease drowsiness

• With meals if GI symptoms occur; absorption may slightly decrease

• Time-release formulation to adults only

Perform/provide:

• Hard candy, gum, frequent rinsing of mouth for dryness

• Storage in tight container at room temperature

Evaluate:

• Therapeutic response: decrease itching associated with pruritus

• Respiratory status: rate, rhythm, increase in bronchial secretions, wheezing, chest tightness

• Cardiac status: palpitations, increased pulse, hypotension

Teach patient/family:

• All aspects of drug use; to notify physician if confusion, sedation, hypotension occurs

• To avoid driving or other hazardous activity if drowsiness occurs

• To avoid concurrent use of alcohol or other CNS depressants

Lab test interferences:

False negative: Skin allergy test

False positive: Urine pregnancy tests

Treatment of overdose: Administer ipecac syrup or lavage, diazepam, vasopressors, barbiturates (short-acting)

T

triprolidine HCl

(trye-proe′li-deen)

Actidil, Bayidyl

Func. class.: Antihistamine

Chem. class.: Alkylamine, H_1-receptor antagonist

Action: Acts on blood vessels, GI,

---

italics = common side effects   ***bold italic*** = life threatening reactions

respiratory system, by competing with histamine for H_1-receptor site; decreases allergic response by blocking histamine

Uses: Rhinitis, allergy symptoms

Dosage and routes:
• *Adult:* PO 2.5 mg tid-qid
• *Child >6 yr:* PO 1.25 mg tid-qid
• *Child 4-6 yr:* PO 0.9 mg tid-qid
• *Child 2-4 yr:* PO 0.6 mg tid-qid
• *Child 4 mo-2 yr:* 0.3 mg tid-qid
Available forms include: Tab 2.5 mg; syr 1.25 mg/5 ml

Side effects/adverse reactions:

CNS: Dizziness, drowsiness, poor coordination, fatigue, anxiety, euphoria, confusion, paresthesia, neuritis

CV: Hypotension, palpitations, tachycardia

RESP: Increased thick secretions, wheezing, chest tightness

*HEMA: **Thrombocytopenia, agranulocytosis, hemolytic anemia***

GI: Dry mouth, nausea, vomiting, anorexia, constipation, diarrhea

INTEG: Rash, urticaria, photosensitivity

GU: Retention, dysuria, frequency

EENT: Blurred vision, dilated pupils, tinnitus, nasal stuffiness, dry nose, throat, mouth

Contraindications: Hypersensitivity to H_1-receptor antagonist, acute asthma attack, lower respiratory tract disease

Precautions: Increased intraocular pressure, renal disease, cardiac disease, hypertension, bronchial asthma, seizure disorder, stenosed peptic ulcers, hyperthyroidism, prostatic hypertrophy, bladder/neck obstruction, pregnancy (C)

Pharmacokinetics:

PO: Onset 20-60 min, duration 8-12 hr, detoxified in liver, excreted by kidneys (metabolites/free drug), half-life 20-24 hr

Interactions/incompatibilities:
• Increased CNS depressants: barbiturates, narcotics, hypnotics, tricyclic antidepressants, alcohol
• Decreased effect of: oral anticoagulants, heparin
• Increased effect of this drug: MAOIs

NURSING CONSIDERATIONS

Assess:
• I&O ratio; be alert for urinary retention, frequency, dysuria; drug should be discontinued if these occur
• CBC during long-term therapy

Administer:
• Coffee, tea, cola (caffeine) to decrease drowsiness
• With meals if GI symptoms occur; absorption may slightly decrease
• Time-release formulation to adults only

Perform/provide:
• Hard candy, gum, frequent rinsing of mouth for dryness
• Storage in tight container at room temperature

Evaluate:
• Therapeutic response: decreased itching associated with pruritus
• Respiratory status: rate, rhythm, increase in bronchial secretions, wheezing, chest tightness
• Cardiac status: palpitations, increased pulse, hypotension

Teach patient/family:
• All aspects of drug use; to notify physician if confusion, sedation, hypotension occurs
• To avoid driving or other hazardous activity if drowsiness occurs
• To avoid concurrent use of alcohol or other CNS depressants while taking this drug

Lab test interferences:

False negative: Skin allergy tests

Treatment of overdose: Administer ipecac syrup or lavage, diazepam, vasopressors, barbiturates (short-acting)

---

troleandomycin

(troe-lee-an-doe-mye'sin)
TAO

Func. class.: Antibacterial, macrolide
Chem. class.: Oleandomycin derivative

Action: Inhibits cell wall bacterial synthesis by binding to 50S subunit of ribosome
Uses: *P. pneumonia* or group A β-hemolytic streptococcal respiratory infections
Dosage and routes:
• *Adult:* PO 250-500 mg q6h
• *Child:* PO 6.6-11 mg/kg q6h
Available forms include: Caps 250 mg
Side effects/adverse reactions:
*SYST: **Anaphylaxis***
INTEG: Urticaria, rash
GI: Nausea, vomiting, rectal burning, esophagitis, abdominal cramps, ***cholangiolytic hepatitis***
Contraindications: Hypersensitivity, minor infections
Precautions: Hepatic disease, pregnancy
Pharmacokinetics:
PO: Peak 2 hr, duration >12 hr, metabolized in liver, excreted in urine (active drug 25%) and bile
Interactions/incompatibilities:
• Increased ischemic reactions: ergotamine preparations
• Increased theophylline levels: theophylline
• Increased action of: carbamazepine
NURSING CONSIDERATIONS
Assess:
• Liver studies: AST, ALT
• C&S before drug therapy; drug may be taken as soon as culture is

taken; C&S may be taken after treatment
Perform/provide:
• Storage at room temperature
• Adrenalin, suction, tracheostomy set, endotracheal intubation equipment on unit
Evaluate:
• Jaundice, fever, nausea, vomiting, right upper quadrant pain indicating cholangiolytic hepatitis; drug should be discontinued
Teach patient/family:
• To take oral drug on empty stomach with full glass of water
• Aspects of drug therapy: need to complete entire course of medication to ensure organism death (10 days); culture may be taken after completed course of medication
• To report sore throat, fever, fatigue; could indicate superimposed infection
• That drug must be taken in equal intervals around clock to maintain blood levels
Lab test interferences:
False increase: Urinary 17-KS, 17-OHCS

---

tromethamine

(troe-meth'a-meen)
Tham, Tham-E
Func. class.: Alkalinizer
Chem. class.: Amine

Action: Proton acceptor which corrects acidosis by combining with hydrogen ions to form bicarbonate and buffer; acts as diuretic (osmotic)
Uses: Acidosis (metabolic)
Dosage and routes:
• *Adult:* 0.3 M required = kg of weight × HCO_3 deficit (mEq/L)
• *Child:* Same as above given over 3-6 hr, not to exceed 40 ml/kg
Available forms include: Inj IV 36 mg/ml, powd for inj IV 36 g

T

---

italics = common side effects   ***bold italic*** = life threatening reactions

Side effects/adverse reactions:
CNS: Irritability, headache, confusion, stimulation, tremors, *twitching, hyperreflexia, tetany,* weakness, *convulsions*
CV: Irregular pulse, *cardiac arrest*
GI: Flatulence, belching, distention, paralytic ileus
META: Alkalosis
RESP: Shallow, slow respirations, cyanosis, *apnea*
Contraindications: Hypersensitivity, anuria, uremia
Precautions: Severe respiratory disease/respiratory depression, pregnancy, cardiac edema, renal disease, infants
Pharmacokinetics:
IV: Excreted in urine
Interactions/incompatibilities:
None known
NURSING CONSIDERATIONS
Assess:
• Respiratory rate, rhythm, depth, notify physician of abnormalities that may indicate acidosis
• Electrolytes, chloride CO_2, before, during treatment
• Urine pH, urinary output, urine glucose during beginning treatment
• I&O ratio, report large increase or decrease
Administer:
• PO with meals if GI symptoms occur
• IV slowly to avoid pain at infusion site and toxicity
• After diluting solutions to 2.14% IV
• With glass of water for expectorant
Evaluate:
• CNS symptoms: confusion, twitching, hyperreflexia, stimulation, headache, which may indicate ammonia toxicity
Teach patient/family:
• To increase K + in diet: bananas, oranges, cantaloupe, honeydew, spinach, potatoes, dried fruit

tropicamide (optic)

(troe-pik′a-mide)
Mydriacyl
Func. class.: Mydriatic, cycloplegia, anticholingeric
Chem. class.: Belladonna alkaloid

Action: Blocks response of sphincter muscle of iris and ciliary body dilatation and paralysis of accommodation
Uses: Fundus exam, cycloplegic refraction
Dosage and routes:
• *Adult and child:* INSTILL 1-2 gtts of 1% sol, repeat in 5 min (refraction) or 1-2 gtts of 0.5% sol 15-20 min before exam (fundus examination)
Available forms include: Sol 0.5%, 1%
Side effects/adverse reactions:
SYST: Tachycardia, confusion, hallucinations, emotional changes in children, fever, flushing, dry skin, dry mouth, abdominal discomfort (infants: bladder distention, irregular pulse, *respiratory depression*)
Contraindications: Hypersensitivity, infants <3 mo, local or systemic glaucoma, conjunctivitis
Pharmacokinetics:
INSTILL: Peak 30-40 min, (mydriasis), 60-180 min, (cycloplegia), duration 6-12 days
Interactions/incompatibilities:
None known
NURSING CONSIDERATIONS
Evaluate:
• Eye pain, discontinue use
Teach patient/family:
• To report change in vision, with blurring or loss of sight, trouble breathing, sweating, flushing
• Method of instillation, including pressure on lacrimal sac for 1 min, and not to touch dropper to eye
• That blurred vision will decrease

with repeated use of drug
• Not to engage in hazardous activities until able to see
• Wait 5 min to use other drops
• Do not blink more than usual
• Dark glasses may be worn if photophobia occurs

---

tubocurarine chloride

(too-boe-kyoo-ar'een)
Tubarine*

Func. class.: Neuromuscular blockers
Chem. class.: Curare alkaloid

Action: Inhibits transmission of nerve impulses by binding with cholinergic receptor sites, antagonizing action of acetylcholine
Uses: Facilitation of endotracheal intubation, skeletal muscle relaxation during mechanical ventilation, surgery, or general anesthesia
Dosage and routes:
• *Adult:* IV BOL 0.4-0.5 mg/kg, then 0.08-0.10 mg/kg 20-45 min after 1st dose if needed for prolonged procedures
Available forms include: Inj IV 3 mg/ml, 20 U/ml
Side effects/adverse reactions:
CV: Bradycardia, tachycardia, increased, decreased B/P
*RESP: Prolonged apnea, **bronchospasm, cyanosis, respiratory depression***
EENT: Increased secretions
INTEG: Rash, flushing, pruritus, urticaria
Contraindications: Hypersensitivity
Precautions: Pregnancy, cardiac disease, lactation, children <2 yr, electrolyte imbalances, dehydration, neuromuscular disease, respiratory disease
Pharmacokinetics:
IV: Onset 15 sec, peak 2-3 min, duration ½-1½ hr; half-life 1-3 hr, de-

graded in liver, kidney (minimally), excreted in urine (unchanged) crosses placenta
Interactions/incompatibilities:
• Increased neuromuscular blockade: aminoglycosides, clindamycin, lincomycin, quinidine, local anesthetics, polymyxin antibiotics, lithium, narcotic analgesics, thiazides, enflurane, isoflurane
• Dysrhythmias: theophylline
• Do not mix with barbiturates in solution or syringe
NURSING CONSIDERATIONS
Assess:
• For electrolyte imbalances (K, Mg); may lead to increased action of this drug
• Vital signs (B/P, pulse, respirations, airway) until fully recovered; rate, depth, pattern of respirations, strength of hand grip
• I&O ratio; check for urinary retention, frequency, hesitancy
Administer:
• Using nerve stimulator by anesthesiologist to determine neuromuscular blockade
• Anticholinesterase to reverse neuromuscular blockade
• By slow IV over 1-2 min (only by qualified person, usually an anesthesiologist)
• Only slightly discolored solution
Perform/provide:
• Storage in light-resistant area
• Reassurance if communication is difficult during recovery from neuromuscular blockade
Evaluate:
• Therapeutic response: paralysis of jaw, eyelid, head, neck, rest of body
• Recovery: decreased paralysis of face, diaphragm, leg, arm, rest of body
• Allergic reactions: rash, fever, respiratory distress, pruritus; drug should be discontinued
Treatment of overdose: Edro-

phonium or neostigmine, atropine, monitor VS; may require mechanical ventilation

undecylenic acid (topical)

(un-dek'-sye-lin-ik)
Cruex, Desenex, NP-27, Ting, Unde-Jen

Func. class.: Local antiinfective
Chem. class.: Antifungal

Action: Interferes with fungal DNA replication
Uses: Tinea cruris pedis
Dosage and routes:
• *Adult and child:* TOP apply to affected areas bid
Available forms include: Powder, oint, cream, liq, foam, soap
Side effects/adverse reactions:
INTEG: Rash, urticaria, stinging, burning
Contraindications: Hypersensitivity
Precautions: Pregnancy, lactation
Interactions/incompatibilities:
None known
NURSING CONSIDERATIONS
Administer:
• Enough medication to completely cover lesions
• After cleansing with soap, water before each application, dry well
Perform/provide:
• Storage at room temperature in dry place
Evaluate for:
• Allergic reaction: burning, stinging, swelling, redness
• Therapeutic response: decrease in size, number of lesions
Teach patient/family:
• To apply with glove to prevent further infection
• To avoid use of OTC creams, ointments, lotions unless directed by physician
• To use medical asepsis (hand washing) before, after each application

uracil mustard

(yoor'a-sill)
Func. class.: Antineoplastic alkylating agent
Chem. class.: Nitrogen mustard

Action: Alkylates DNA, RNA; inhibits enzymes that allow synthesis of amino acids in proteins; also responsible for cross-linking DNA strands
Uses: Hodgkin's disease, lymphomas; cervix, ovarian, lung cancer; chronic lymphocytic, myelocytic leukemia; reticulum cell sarcoma, mycosis fungoides; polycythemia vera
Dosage and routes:
• *Adult:* PO 1-2 mg/day × 3 mo or desired response, then 1 mg/day for 3 out of 4 wk until desired response or 3-5 mg × 7 days, not to exceed total dose of 0.5 mg/kg then 1 mg/day until desired response, then 1 mg/day 3 out of 4 wk
Available forms include: Caps 1 mg
Side effects/adverse reactions:
*HEMA: **Thrombocytopenia, leukopenia,** anemia*
*GI: Nausea, vomiting, diarrhea, **hepatotoxicity***
GU: Amenorrhea, azoospermia
INTEG: Alopecia, dermatitis, pruritus, rash
Contraindications: Severe thrombocytopenia/leukopenia, hypersensitivity
Precautions: Radiation therapy, pregnancy
Pharmacokinetics:
Excreted unchanged in urine
Interactions/incompatibilities:
• Increased toxicity when used with antineoplastics, radiation

NURSING CONSIDERATIONS
Assess:
• CBC, differential, platelet count weekly; withhold drug if WBC is <4000 or platelet count is <75,000; notify physician of results
• Renal function studies: BUN, serum uric acid, urine CrCl before, during therapy
• I&O ratio; report fall in urine output of 30 ml/hr
• Monitor temperature q4h (may indicate beginning infection)
• Liver function tests before, during therapy (bilirubin, AST, ALT, LDH) as needed or monthly

Administer:
• Medications by oral route if possible; avoid IM, SC, IV routes to prevent infections
• Antacid before oral agent; give drug after evening meal, before bedtime
• Antiemetic 30-60 min before giving drug to prevent vomiting
• Antibiotics for prophylaxis of infection
• Topical or systemic analgesics for pain
• Local or systemic drugs for infection

Perform/provide:
• Storage in tight container at room temperature
• Strict medical asepsis, protective isolation if WBC levels are low
• Special skin care
• Liquid diet, including cola, Jello; dry toast or crackers may be added if patient is not nauseated or vomiting
• Increase fluid intake to 2-3 L/day to prevent urate deposits, calculi formation

Evaluate:
• Bleeding: hematuria, guaiac, bruising or petechiae, mucosa or orifices q8h

• Food preferences; list likes, dislikes
• Yellowing of skin, sclera, dark urine, clay-colored stools, itchy skin, abdominal pain, fever, diarrhea
• Effects of alopecia on body image; discuss feelings about body changes
• Inflammation of mucosa, breaks in skin
• Symptoms indicating severe allergic reaction: rash, pruritus, urticaria, itching
• Check for tartrazine dye allergy

Teach patient/family:
• Of protective isolation precautions
• To report any complaints or side effects to nurse or physician
• That azoospermia, amenorrhea can occur; are reversible after discontinuing treatment
• That hair may be lost during treatment; a wig or hairpiece may make patient feel better; new hair may be different in color, texture
• To avoid foods with citric acid, hot or rough texture

---

urea

(yoor-ee′a)
Ureaphil, Carbamex*

Func. class.: Diuretic, osmotic
Chem. class.: Carbonic acid diamide salt

Action: Increases osmotic pressure by inhibiting reabsorption of sodium, potassium, chloride; increases water in extracellular compartment by increasing blood plasma osmolality
Uses: To decrease intracranial pressure, intraocular pressure
Dosage and routes:
• *Adult:* IV 1-1.5 g/kg of a 30% sol over 1-3 hr

• *Child >2 yr:* IV 0.5-1.5 g/kg up to 4 ml/min
• *Child <2 yr:* IV 0.1 g/kg up to 4 ml/min

Available forms include: Inj IV 4 g/150 ml

Side effects/adverse reactions:

CNS: Dizziness, headache, disorientation, fever

GI: Nausea, vomiting

INTEG: Venous thrombosis, phlebitis, extravasation

CV: Postural hypotension

Contraindications: Severe renal disease, active intracranial bleeding, marked dehydration, liver failure

Precautions: Hepatic disease, renal disease, pregnancy

Pharmacokinetics:

IV: Onset ½-1 hr, peak 1 hr, duration 3-10 hr, (diuresis) 5-6 hr (intraocular pressure); half-life 1 hr, excreted in urine, crosses placenta, excreted in breast milk

Interactions/incompatibilities:

• Incompatible with whole blood, in solution or syringe with any other drug or solution

• Increased renal excretion of: lithium

NURSING CONSIDERATIONS
Assess:

• Weight, I&O daily to determine fluid loss; effect of drug may be decreased if used qd

• Rate, depth, rhythm of respiration, effect of exertion

• B/P lying, standing, postural hypotension may occur

• Electrolytes: potassium, sodium, chloride; include BUN, blood sugar, CBC, serum creatinine, blood pH, ABGs

Administer:

• IV slowly over 1-2½ hr, do not exceed 4 ml/min

Evaluate:

• Improvement in edema of feet, legs, sacral area daily if medication is being used in CHF

• Improvement in CVP q8h

• Signs of metabolic acidosis: drowsiness, restlessness

• Signs of hypokalemia: postural hypotension, malaise, fatigue, tachycardia, leg cramps, weakness

• Temperature elevation, signs of extravasation qd

• Confusion, especially in elderly, take safety precautions if needed

• Hydration: skin turgor, thirst, dry mucous membranes

Teach patient/family:

• That drug will cause diuresis in ½ hr

Treatment of overdose: Lavage if taken orally, monitor electrolytes, administer IV fluids, monitor BUN

---

urokinase

(yoor-oh-kin'ase)

Abbokinase, Win-Kinase

Func. class.: Thrombolytic enzyme

Chem. class.: β-Hemolytic streptococcus filtrate (purified)

Action: Promotes thrombolysis by acting directly on endogenous fibrinolytic system to change plasminogen to plasmin

Uses: Venous thrombosis, pulmonary embolism, arterial thrombosis, arterial embolism, arteriovenous cannula occlusion, lysis of coronary artery thrombi after myocardial infarction

Dosage and routes:

Lysis of pulmonary emboli

• *Adult:* IV 4400 IU/kg/hr × 12-24 hr not to exceed 200 ml; then IV heparin, then anticoagulants

Coronary artery thrombosis

• *Adult:* INSTILL 6000 IU/min into occluded artery for 1-2 hr after giving IV bol of heparin 2500-10,000 U

Venous catheter occlusion

• *Adult:* INSTILL 5000 IU into line, wait 5 min, then aspirate, repeat aspiration attempts q5min × ½ hr; if occlusion has not been removed, then cap line and wait ½-1 hr then aspirate; may need 2nd dose if still occluded

Available forms include: Inj

Side effects/adverse reactions:

*HEMA: Decreased Hct, **bleeding***

INTEG: Rash, urticaria, phlebitis at IV infusion site, itching, flushing, headache

CNS: Headache, fever,

GI: Nausea

RESP: Altered respirations, SOB, ***bronchospasm***

MS: Low back pain

CV: Hypertension, dysrhythmias

EENT: Periorbital edema

Contraindications: Hypersensitivity, active bleeding, intraspinal surgery, neoplasms of CNS, ulcerative colitis/enteritis, severe hypertension, renal disease, hepatic disease, hypocoagulation, COPD, subacute bacterial endocarditis, rheumatic valvular disease, cerebral embolism/thrombosis/hemorrhage, intraarterial diagnostic procedure or surgery (10 days), recent major surgery

Precautions: Arterial emboli from left side of heart, pregnancy (B)

Pharmacokinetics:

IV: Half-life 10-20 min, small amounts excreted in urine

Interactions/incompatibilities:

• Aspirin, indomethacin, phenylbutazone, anticoagulants, bleeding: potential

NURSING CONSIDERATIONS

Assess:

• VS, B/P, pulse, resp, neuro signs, temp at least q4h, temp >104° F or indicators of internal bleed, cardiac rhythm following intracoronary administration

Administer:

• Using infusion pump, terminal filter (0.45 μm or smaller)

• Reconstitute only with sterile water for injection (not bacteriostatic water), and roll (not shake) to enhance reconstitution

• As soon as thrombi identified; not useful for thrombi over 1 wk old

• Cryoprecipitate or fresh, frozen plasma if bleeding occurs

• Loading dose at beginning of therapy may require increased loading doses

• Heparin therapy after thrombolytic therapy is discontinued, TT or APTT less than 2 times control (about 3-4 hr)

• After reconstituting with 5 ml of NS or D_5W; do not shake

• About 10% patients have high streptococcal antibody titres, requiring increased loading doses

• IV therapy using 0.22 or 0.45 μm filter

• Store in refrigerator; use immediately after reconstitution

Perform/provide:

• Bed rest during entire course of treatment

• Avoidance of invasive procedures: inj, rectal temp

• Treatment of fever with acetaminophen or aspirin

• Pressure for 30 sec to minor bleeding sites; inform physician if hemostasis not attained, apply pressure dressing

Evaluate:

• Allergy: fever, rash, itching, chills; mild reaction may be treated with antihistamines

• Bleeding during 1st hr of treatment (hematuria, hematemesis, bleeding from mucous membranes, epistaxis, ecchymosis)

• Blood studies (Hct, platelets, PTT, PT, TT, APTT) before starting therapy; PT or APTT must be less than 2 × control before starting therapy TT ot PT q3-4h during treatment

U

---

italics = common side effects   ***bold italic*** = life threatening reactions

Lab test interferences:
Increase: PT, APTT, TT

---

valproate sodium/valproate sodium—valproic acid/valproic acid
(val-proe'ate)
Depakene Syrup/Depakote/Depakene

Func. class.: Anticonvulsant
Chem. class.: Carboxylic acid derivative

Action: Increases levels of gamma-aminobutyric acid (GABA) in brain
Uses: Simple, complex absence, mixed, tonic-clonic seizures
Dosage and routes:
• *Adult and child:* PO 15 mg/kg/day divided in 2-3 doses, may increase by 5-10 mg/kg/day q wk, not to exceed 30 mg/kg/day in 2-3 divided doses
Available forms include: Caps 250 mg; tabs 125, 250, 500 mg; syr 250 mg/5 ml
Side effects/adverse reactions:
HEMA: Thrombocytopenia, leukopenia, lymphocytosis, increased pro-time
CNS: Sedation, drowsiness, dizziness, headache, incoordination, paresthesia, depression, hallucinations, behavioral changes, tremors
GI: Nausea, vomiting, constipation, diarrhea, heartburn, anorexia, cramps, *hepatic failure, pancreatitis, toxic hepatitis*
INTEG: Rash, alopecia, bruising
GU: Enuresis, irregular menses
Contraindications: Hypersensitivity
Precautions: MI (recovery phase), hepatic disease, renal disease, Addison's disease, pregnancy, lactation

Pharmacokinetics:
PO: Onset 15-30 min, peak 1-4 hr, duration 4-6 hr
REC: Onset slow, duration 4-6 hr
Metabolized by liver, excreted by kidneys, feces, crosses placenta, excreted in breast milk, half-life 6-16 hr
Interactions/incompatibilities:
• Increased effects: CNS depressants
• Increased toxicity: salicylates, warfarin, sulfinpyrazone
NURSING CONSIDERATIONS
Assess:
• Blood studies: Hct, Hgb, RBCs, serum folate, vitamin D if on long-term therapy
• Hepatic studies: AST, ALT, bilirubin, creatinine, failure
• Blood levels: therapeutic level 50-100 μg/ml
Administer:
• Tablets or capsules whole
• Elixir alone; do not dilute with carbonated beverage
Evaluate:
• Mental status: mood, sensorium, affect, memory (long, short)
• Respiratory dysfunction: respiratory depression, character, rate, rhythm; hold drug if respirations are <12/min or if pupils are dilated
Teach patient/family:
• That physical dependency may result when used for extended periods
• To avoid driving, other activities that require alertness
• Not to discontinue medication quickly after long-term use; convulsions may result

vancomycin HCl

(van-koe-mye'sin)
Vancocin

Func. class.: Antibacterial
Chem. class.: Tricyclic glucopeptide

Action: Inhibits cell wall bacterial synthesis

Uses: Resistant staphylococcal infections, pseudomembranous colitis, staphylococcal enterocolitis, endocarditis prophylaxis for dental procedures

Dosage and routes:
Serious staphylococcal infections
• *Adult:* IV 500 mg q6h or 1 g q12h
• *Child:* IV 44 mg/kg/day divided q6h
• *Neonates:* IV 10 mg/kg q12h
Pseudomembranous/staphylococcal enterocolitis
• *Adult:* PO 500 mg q6h × 7-10 days
• *Child:* PO 44 mg/kg/day divided q6h
Endocarditis prophylaxis
• *Adult:* IV 1 g over 1 hr, 1 hr before dental procedure
Available forms include: Pulvules 125, 250 mg; powder for oral sol 1, 10 g; powder for inj IV 500 mg, 1 g

Side effects/adverse reactions:
*CV: **Cardiac arrest, vascular collapse***
*EENT: **Ototoxicity, permanent deafness,** tinnitus*
*HEMA: **Leukopenia, eosinophilia, neutropenia***
*GI: **Nausea***
RESP: Wheezing, dyspnea
*SYST: **Anaphylaxis***
*GU: **Nephrotoxicity,** increased BUN, creatinine, albumin, **fatal uremia***
INTEG: Chills, fever, rash, thrombophlebitis at injection site, urticaria, pruritus, necrosis

Contraindications: Hypersensitivity, decreased hearing

Precautions: Renal disease, pregnancy, lactation, elderly, neonates

Pharmacokinetics:
Peak 1 hr, through 12 hr, half-life 6-8 hr, excreted in urine (active form), crosses placenta

Interactions/incompatibilities:
• Ototoxicity or nephrotoxicity: aminoglycosides, cephalosporins, colistin, polymyxin, bacitracin, cisplatin
• Do not mix in solution or syringe with alkaline solutions; check product information

NURSING CONSIDERATIONS

Assess:
• I&O ratio; report hematuria, oliguria since nephrotoxicity may occur
• Any patient with compromised renal system; drug is excreted slowly in poor renal system function; toxicity may occur rapidly
• Blood studies: WBC
• C&S before drug therapy; drug may be taken as soon as culture is taken
• Auditory function during, after treatment
• B/P during administration; sudden drop may indicate Redman's syndrome

Administer:
• After reconstitution with 10 ml sterile water for injection 500 mg/100 ml; further dilution is needed for IV
• Infuse over 60 min; avoid extravasation

Perform/provide:
• Storage at room temperature for up to 2 wk after reconstitution
• Adrenalin, suction, tracheostomy set, endotracheal intubation equipment on unit; anaphylaxis may occur

• Adequate intake of fluids (2000 ml) to prevent nephrotoxicity

Evaluate:

• Therapeutic response: absence of fever, sore throat

• Hearing loss, ringing, roaring in ears; drug should be discontinued

• Skin eruptions

• Respiratory status: rate, character, wheezing, tightness in chest

• Allergies before treatment, reaction of each medication; place allergies on chart, Kardex in bright red letters; notify all people giving drugs

Teach patient/family:

• Aspects of drug therapy: need to complete entire course of medication to ensure organism death (7-10 days); culture may be taken after completed course of medication

• To report sore throat, fever, fatigue; could indicate superimposed infection

• That drug must be taken in equal intervals around clock to maintain blood levels

---

vasopressin (antidiuretic hormone)/vasopressin tannate

(vay-soe-press'in)

Pitressin Synthetic/Pitressin Tannate

Func. class.: Pituitary hormone

Chem. class.: Lysine vasopressin

Action: Promotes reabsorption of water by action on renal tubular epithelium

Uses: Diabetes insipidus (nonnephrogenic/nonpsychogenic), abdominal distention postoperatively, intraarterial upper GI hemorrhage

Dosage and routes:

Diabetes insipidus

• *Adult:* IM/SC 5-10 units bid-qid as needed; IM/SC 2.5-5 units q2-3 days (Pitressin Tannate) for chronic therapy

• *Child:* IM/SC 2.5-10 units bid-qid as needed; IM/SC 1.25-2.5 units q2-3 days (Pitressin Tannate) for chronic therapy

Abdominal distention

• *Adult:* IM 5 units, then q3-4h, increasing to 10 units if needed (aqueous)

GI hemorrhage

• *Adult:* INTRAARTERIAL 100 U/500 ml 0.9% saline at 200-400 units/min

Available forms include: Inj IM, SC 20, 5 U/ml (tannate)

Side effects/adverse reactions:

EENT: Nasal irritation, congestion, rhinitis

CNS: Drowsiness, headache, lethargy, flushing

GU: Vulval pain

GI: Nausea, heartburn, cramps

CV: Increased B/P

Contraindications: Pregnancy, childbearing-age women

Precautions: CAD

Pharmacokinetics:

NASAL: Onset 1 hr, duration 3-8 hr, half-life 15 min; metabolized in liver, kidneys, excreted in urine

Interactions/incompatibilities: None known

NURSING CONSIDERATIONS

Assess:

• Pulse, B/P, when giving drug IV or IM

• I&O ratio, weight daily, check for edema in extremities, if water retention is severe, diuretic may be prescribed

Evaluate:

• Therapeutic response: absence of severe thirst, decreased urine output, osmolality

• Water intoxication: lethargy, behavioral changes, disorientation, neuromuscular excitability

Teach patient/family:

• All aspects of drug: action, side

effects, dose, when to notify physician

---

vecuronium bromide

(vek-yoo-roe'nee-um)

Norcuron

Func. class.: Neuromuscular blocker

Action: Inhibits transmission of nerve impulses by binding with cholinergic receptor sites, antagonizing action of acetylcholine

Uses: Facilitation of endotracheal intubation, skeletal muscle relaxation during mechanical ventilation, surgery, or general anesthesia

Dosage and routes:

• *Adult and child >9 yr:* IV BOL 0.08-0.10 mg/kg, then 0.010-0.015 mg/kg for prolonged procedures

Available forms include: IV 10 mg/5 ml

Side effects/adverse reactions:

CV: Bradycardia, tachycardia, increased, decreased B/P

*RESP: Prolonged apnea, **bronchospasm, cyanosis, respiratory depression***

EENT: Increased secretions

INTEG: Rash, flushing, pruritus, urticaria

Contraindications: Hypersensitivity

Precautions: Pregnancy, cardiac disease, lactation, children <2 yr, electrolyte imbalances, dehydration, neuromuscular disease, respiratory disease

Pharmacokinetics:

IV: Onset 15 min, peak 3-5 min, duration 45-60 min; half-life 65-75 min, not metabolized, excreted in feces, crosses placenta

Interactions/incompatibilities:

• Increased neuromuscular blockade: aminoglycosides, clindamycin, lincomycin, quinidine, local anesthetics, polymyxin antibiotics, lithium, narcotic analgesics, thiazides, enflurane, isoflurane

• Dysrhythmias: theophylline

• Do not mix with barbiturates in solution or syringe

NURSING CONSIDERATIONS

Assess:

• For electrolyte imbalances (K, Mg); may lead to increased action of this drug

• Vital signs (B/P, pulse, respirations, airway) until fully recovered; rate, depth, pattern of respirations, strength of hand grip

• I&O ratio; check for urinary retention, frequency, hesitancy

Administer:

• Using nerve stimulator by anesthesiologist to determine neuromuscular blockade

• Anticholinesterase to reverse neuromuscular blockade

• By slow IV over 1-2 min (only by qualified person, usually an anesthesiologist)

• Only slightly discolored solution

Perform/provide:

• Storage in light-resistant area

• Reassurance if communication is difficult during recovery from neuromuscular blockade

Evaluate:

• Therapeutic response: paralysis of jaw, eyelid, head, neck, rest of body

• Recovery: decreased paralysis of face, diaphragm, leg, arm, rest of body

• Allergic reactions: rash, fever, respiratory distress, pruritus; drug should be discontinued

Treatment of overdose: Edrophonium or neostigmine, atropine, monitor VS; may require mechanical ventilation

---

italics = common side effects   ***bold italic*** = life threatening reactions

verapamil HCl

(ver-ap′-a-mill)
Calan, Isoptin

Func. class.: Calcium channel blocker

Action: Inhibits calcium ion influx across cell membrane during cardiac depolarization; produces relaxation of coronary vascular smooth muscle, dilates coronary arteries

Uses: Chronic stable angina pectoris, vasospastic angina

Dosage and routes:

• *Adult:* PO 80 mg tid or qid, increase gwk; IV BOL 5-10 mg over 2 min, repeat if necessary; maintenance dose 2-10 mg according to prothrombin time

• *Child 0-1 yr:* IV BOL 0.1-0.2 mg/kg over 2 min with ECG monitoring, repeat if necessary in 30 min

• *Child 1-15 yr:* IV BOL 0.1-0.3 mg/kg, repeat in 30 min, not to exceed 10 mg in a single dose

Available forms include: Tabs 80, 120, 240 mg; inj 2.5 mg/ml

Side effects/adverse reactions:

CV: Dysrhythmia, edema, CHF, bradycardia, hypotension, palpitations

GI: Nausea, vomiting, diarrhea, gastric upset, constipation, increased liver function studies

GU: Nocturia, polyuria, *acute renal failure*

INTEG: Rash, pruritus, flushing, photosensitivity

CNS: Headache, fatigue, drowsiness, dizziness, anxiety, depression, weakness, insomnia, confusion

Contraindications: Sick sinus syndrome, 2nd or 3rd degree heart block, hypotension less than 90 mm Hg systolic

Precautions: CHF, hypotension, hepatic injury, pregnancy, lactation, children, renal disease

Pharmacokinetics:

IV: Onset 3 min, duration 10-20 min

PO: Onset variable, peak 3-4 hr, duration 17-24 hr, half-life (biphasic) 4 min, 2-5 hr (terminal)

Metabolized by liver, excreted in urine (96% as metabolites)

Interactions/incompatibilities:

• Increased effects of: barbiturates, hypoglycemia, reserpine, levodopa, digitalis, ergots, neuromuscular blocking agents

• Decreased effects: norepinephrine, xanthines, isoproterenol

NURSING CONSIDERATIONS

Assess:

• Blood levels (therapeutic levels: 0.025-0.1 μg/ml)

Administer:

• Before meals, hs

Evaluate:

• Therapeutic response: decreased anginal pain

• Cardiac status: B/P, pulse, respiration, ECG

Teach patient/family:

• How to take pulse before taking drug; record or graph should be kept

• To avoid hazardous activities until stabilized on drug, dizziness is no longer a problem

• To limit caffeine consumption

• To avoid OTC drugs unless directed by a physician

• Stress patient compliance to all areas of medical regimen: diet, exercise, stress reduction, drug therapy

Lab test interferences:

Increase: Liver function tests

Treatment of overdose: Defibrillation, atropine for AV block, vasopressor for hypotension

vidarabine (ophthalmic)

(vye-dare'a-been)

Vira-A Ophthalmic

Func. class.: Antiviral
Chem. class.: Purine nucleoside

Action: Inhibits viral DNA synthesis by blocking DNA polymerase

Uses: Herpes simplex, encephalitis, herpes zoster

Dosage and routes:

• *Adult and child:* TOP ½ inch oint into conjunctival sac q3h × 5 days

Available forms include: Oint 3%

Side effects/adverse reactions:

EENT: Burning, stinging, photophobia, pain, temporary visual haze

Contraindications: Hypersensitivity

Precautions: Antibiotic hypersensitivity

Interactions/incompatibilities: None known

NURSING CONSIDERATIONS

Administer:

• After washing hands, cleanse crusts or discharge from eye before application

Perform/provide:

• Storage at room temperature

Evaluate:

• Therapeutic response: absence of redness, inflammation, tearing

• Allergy: itching, lacrimation, redness, swelling

Teach patient/family:

• To use drug exactly as prescribed

• Not to use eye makeup, towels, washcloths, or eye medication of others, or reinfection may occur

• That drug container tip should not be touched to eye

• To report itching, increased redness, burning, stinging, drug should be discontinued

• That drug may cause blurred vision when ointment is applied

vidarabine monohydrate

(vye-dare'a-been)

Vira-A

Func. class.: Antibacterial, antiviral
Chem. class.: Purine nucleoside

Action: Inhibits bacterial/viral replication by preventing DNA synthesis

Uses: Herpes simplex virus encephalitis, hepatitis B, varicella-zoster encephalomyelitis

Dosage and routes:

• *Adult and child:* IV INF 15 mg/kg/day × 10 days; infuse over 12-24 hr

Available forms include: Inj IV 200 mg/ml

Side effects/adverse reactions:

CNS: Psychosis, hallucinations, dizziness, weakness, tremors, *fatal metabolic encephalopathy,* confusion, malaise

GU: SIADH

HEMA: **Anemia, thrombocytopenia, neutropenia**

GI: *Nausea, vomiting, anorexia, diarrhea,* weight loss

INTEG: Pain, thrombophlebitis at injection site

Contraindications: Hypersensitivity

Precautions: Renal disease, liver disease, lactation, pregnancy

Pharmacokinetics: Crosses blood-brain barrier, excreted by kidneys (metabolites), crosses placenta, half-life 1½-3 hr

Interactions/incompatibilities:

• Increased neurologic side effects: allopurinol

NURSING CONSIDERATIONS

Assess:

• Liver studies: AST, ALT

• Blood studies: WBC, RBC, Hct, Hgb, platelets

V

---

italics = common side effects   ***bold italic*** = life threatening reactions

• Renal studies: urinalysis, protein, blood

• C&S before drug therapy; drug may be taken as soon as culture is taken; C&S may be taken after therapy

Administer:

• Using in-line filter with mean pore diameter of 0.45 mm or less

• Shake solution; dilute to 450 mg/L IV fluid

• At constant rate over 12-24 hr

Evaluate:

• Therapeutic response: decreased amount of lesion, itching

• Bowel pattern before, during treatment

• Fluid overload; drug requires large volume to stay in solutions

• Weakness, tremors, confusion, dizziness, psychosis; if these occur, drug might need to be decreased or discontinued

---

vinblastine sulfate (VLB)

(vin-blast'een)

Velban, Velbe*

Func. class.: Antineoplastic
Chem. class.: Vinca rosea alkaloid

Action: Inhibits mitotic activity, arrests cell cycle at metaphase; inhibits RNA synthesis, blocks cellular use of glutamic acid needed for purine synthesis

Uses: Breast, testicular cancer, lymphomas, neuroblastoma, Hodgkin's non-Hodgkin's lymphomas, mycosis fungoides, histiocytosis

Dosage and routes:

• *Adult and child:* IV 0.1 mg/kg or 3.7 mg/m^2 q wk or q2 wk, not to exceed 0.5 mg/kg or 18.5 mg/m^2 q wk in adults

Available forms include: Inj IV, powder 10 mg for 10 ml IV inj

Side effects/adverse reactions:

HEMA: Thrombocytopenia, leuko-

penia, myelosupppression, anemia

GI: Nausea, vomiting, anorexia, stomatitis, constipation, abdominal pain, *hepatotoxicity*

GU: Urinary retention, *renal failure*

INTEG: Rash, alopecia, photosensitivity

RESP: Fibrosis, pulmonary infiltrate

CV: Tachycardia, orthostatic hypotension, *convulsions*

CNS: Paresthesias, peripheral neuropathy, depression, headache

Contraindications: Hypersensitivity, infants, pregnancy (1st trimester)

Precautions: Renal disease, hepatic disease

Pharmacokinetics: Half-life (triphasic) 35 min, 53 min, 19 hr, metabolized in liver, excreted in urine, feces, crosses blood-brain barrier

Interactions/incompatibilities:

• May increase action of methotrexate

• Do not use with radiation

• Synergism may occur with bleomycin

NURSING CONSIDERATIONS

Assess:

• CBC, differential, platelet count weekly, withhold drug if WBC is <4000 or platelet count is <75,000; notify physician of results

• Pulmonary function tests, chest X-ray studies before, during therapy; chest X-ray film should be obtained q2 wk during treatment

• Renal function studies: BUN, serum uric acid, urine CrCl, electrolytes before, during therapy

• I&O ratio, report fall in urine output of 30 ml/hr

• Monitor temperature q4h; may indicate beginning infection

• Liver function tests before, during therapy (bilirubin, AST, ALT,

LDH) as needed or monthly
• RBC, Hct, Hgb since these may
be decreased

Administer:
• Medications by oral route if possible; avoid IM, SC, IV routes to prevent infections
• Antacid before oral agent; give drug after evening meal before bedtime
• Antiemetic 30-60 min before giving drug to prevent vomiting
• Allopurinol or sodium bicarbonate to maintain uric acid levels, alkalinization of urine
• Antibiotics for prophylaxis of infection
• IV infusion using 21-, 23-, 25-gauge needle; administer by slow IV infusion
• Topical or systemic analgesics for pain
• Local or systemic drugs for infection
• Transfusion for anemia
• Antispasmodic

Perform/provide:
• Strict medical asepsis, protective isolation if WBC levels are low
• Special skin care
• Deep-breathing exercises with patient 3-4 × day; place in semi-Fowler's position
• Liquid diet: cola, Jell-O; dry toast or crackers may be added if patient is not nauseated or vomiting
• Increase fluid intake to 2-3 L/day to prevent urate deposits, calculi formation
• Diet low in purines: organ meats (kidney, liver), dried beans, peas to maintain alkaline urine
• Rinsing of mouth 3-4 × day with water, hydrogen peroxide
• Brushing of teeth 2-3 × day with soft brush or cotton-tipped applicators for stomatitis; use unwaxed dental floss
• Warm compresses at injection site for inflammation
• Nutritious diet with iron, vitamin supplements
• HOB increased to facilitate breathing

Evaluate:
• Bleeding: hematuria, guaiac, bruising or petechiae, mucosa of orifices q8h
• Dyspnea, rales, unproductive cough, chest pain, tachypnea, fatigue, increased pulse, pallor, lethargy
• Food preferences; list likes, dislikes
• Effects of alopecia on body image; discuss feelings about body changes
• Edema in feet, joint pain, stomach pain, shaking
• Inflammation of mucosa, breaks in skin
• Yellowing of skin and sclera, dark urine, clay-colored stools, itchy skin, abdominal pain, fever, diarrhea
• Buccal cavity q8h for dryness, sores or ulceration, white patches, oral pain, bleeding, dysphagia
• Local irritation, pain, burning, discoloration at injection site
• Symptoms indicating severe allergic reaction: rash, pruritus, urticaria, purpuric skin lesions, itching, flushing
• Frequency of stools and characteristics: cramping, acidosis; signs of dehydration: rapid respirations, poor skin turgor, decreased urine output, dry skin, restlessness, weakness

Teach patient/family:
• Of protective isolation precautions
• To report any complaints or side effects to the nurse or physician
• That impotence or amennorrhea can occur, are reversible after discontinuing treatment
• To report any changes in breathing or coughing

V

---

italics = common side effects   ***bold italic*** = life threatening reactions

• That hair may be lost during treatment, a wig or hairpiece may make patient feel better; tell patient that new hair may be different in color, texture

• To avoid foods with citric acid, hot or rough texture

• To report any bleeding, white spots or ulcerations in mouth to physician; tell patient to examine mouth qd

---

vincristine sulfate
(vin-kris´teen)
Oncovin
Func. class.: Antineoplastic
Chem. class.: Vinca alkaloid

Action: Inhibits mitotic activity, arrests cell cycle at metaphase; inhibits RNA synthesis, blocks cellular use of glutamic acid needed for purine synthesis

Uses: Breast, lung cancer, lymphomas, neuroblastoma, Hodgkin's disease, acute lymphoblastic and other leukemias, rhabdomyosarcoma, Wilm's tumor, osteogenic and other sarcomas

Dosage and routes:

• *Adult:* IV 1-2 mg/m²/wk, not to exceed 2 mg

• *Child:* IV 1.5-2 mg/m²/wk, not to exceed 2 mg

Available forms include: Inj IV 1 mg/ml

Side effects/adverse reactions:

*HEMA: **Thrombocytopenia, leukopenia, myelosuppression, anemia***

*GI: Nausea, vomiting, anorexia, stomatitis, constipation, paralytic ileus, abdominal pain, **hepatotoxicity***

CV: Orthostatic hypotension

CNS: Decreased reflexes, numbness, weakness, motor difficulties, CNS depression, cranial nerve paralysis

Contraindications: Hypersensitivity, infants, pregnancy (1st trimester)

Precautions: Renal disease, hepatic disease, hypertension, neuromuscular disease

Pharmacokinetics: Half-life (triphasic) 0.85 min, 7.4 min, 164 min, metabolized in liver, excreted in bile, feces, crosses placental barrier, crosses blood-brain barrier

Interactions/incompatibilities:

• May increase action of methotrexate

• Do not use with radiation

• May increase neurotoxicity when used with other peripheral nervous system drugs

NURSING CONSIDERATIONS
Assess:

• CBC, differential, platelet count weekly; withhold drug if WBC is <4000 or platelet count is <75,000; notify physician of results

• Renal function studies: BUN, serum uric acid, urine CrCl, electrolytes before, during therapy

• I&O ratio, report fall in urine output of 30 ml/hr

• Monitor temperature q4h; may indicate beginning infection

• Liver function tests before, during therapy (bilirubin, AST, ALT, LDH) as needed or monthly

• RBC, Hct, Hgb since these may be decreased

Administer:

• Medications by oral route if possible; avoid IM, SC, IV routes to prevent infections

• Antiemetic 30-60 min before giving drug to prevent vomiting

• Antibiotics for prophylaxis of infection

• IV infusion using 21-, 23-, 25-gauge needle; administer by slow IV infusion

• Topical or systemic analgesics for pain

- Local or systemic drugs for infection
- Transfusion for anemia
- Antispasmodic

Perform/provide:

- Strict medical asepsis, protective isolation if WBC levels are low
- Special skin care
- Liquid diet: cola, Jell-O; dry toast or crackers may be added if patient is not nauseated or vomiting
- Rinsing of mouth 3-4 × day with water, hydrogen peroxide
- Brushing of teeth 2-3 × day with soft brush or cotton-tipped applicators for stomatitis; use unwaxed dental floss
- Warm compresses at injection site for inflammation
- Nutritious diet with iron, vitamin supplements

Evaluate:

- Bleeding: hematuria, guaiac, bruising or petechiae, mucosa of orifices q8h
- Dyspnea, rales, unproductive cough, chest pain, tachypnea, fatigue, increased pulse, pallor, lethargy
- Food preferences; list likes, dislikes
- Effects of alopecia on body image, discuss feelings about body changes
- Edema in feet, joint pain, stomach pain, shaking
- Inflammation of mucosa, breaks in skin
- Yellowing of skin and sclera, dark urine, clay-colored stools, itchy skin, abdominal pain, fever, diarrhea
- Buccal cavity q8h for dryness, sores or ulceration, white patches, oral pain, bleeding, dysphagia
- Local irritation, pain, burning, discoloration at injection site
- Symptoms indicating severe allergic reaction: rash, pruritus, ur-

ticaria, purpuric skin lesions, itching, flushing

- Frequency of stools, characteristics: cramping, acidosis; signs of dehydration: rapid respirations, poor skin turgor, decreased urine output, dry skin, restlessness, weakness

Teach patient/family:

- Of protective isolation precautions
- To report any complaints or side effects to nurse or physician
- To report any bleeding, white spots or ulcerations in mouth to physician; tell patient to examine mouth qd

---

vindesine sulfate

(vin-dis'een)
DAVA, Eldisine

Func. class.: Antineoplastic
Chem. class.: Vinca alkaloid

Action: Inhibits mitotic activity, arrests cell cycle at metaphase; inhibits RNA synthesis, blocks cellular use of glutamic acid needed for purine synthesis

Uses: Breast, non-small-cell lung cancer; acute lymphoblastic, malignant melanoma; lymphosarcoma

Dosage and routes:

- *Adult:* IV 3-4 mg/m^2 q7-14 days; IV INF 1.2-1.5 mg/m^2/day × 5 days q3 wk

Available forms include: Inj IV 5 mg

Side effects/adverse reactions:

HEMA: ***Thrombocytopenia, leukopenia, myelosuppression, anemia, neutropenia***

GI: Nausea, vomiting, anorexia, constipation, stomatitis, ***hepatotoxicity,*** parlytic ileus, abdominal pain

CV: Chest pain

CNS: Neuritis, dizziness

Contraindications: Hypersensitiv-

ity, infants, pregnancy (1st trimester)

Precautions: Renal disease, hepatic disease

Pharmacokinetics: Half-life 3 min, 100 min >20 hr, metabolized in liver, excreted in urine, crosses placental barrier

Interactions/incompatibilities:

• May increase action of methotrexate

• Do not use with radiation

NURSING CONSIDERATIONS
Assess:

• CBC, differential, platelet count weekly; withhold drug if WBC is <4000 or platelet count is <75,000; notify physician of results

• Renal function studies: BUN, serum uric acid, urine CrCl, electrolytes before, during therapy

• I&O ratio, report fall in urine output of 30 ml/hr

• Monitor temperature q4h; may indicate beginning infection

• Liver function tests before, during therapy (bilirubin), AST, ALT, LDH) as needed or monthly

• RBC, Hct, Hgb since these may be decreased

Administer:

• Medications by oral route if possible; avoid IM, SC, IV routes to prevent infections

• Antiemetic 30-60 min before giving drug to prevent vomiting

• Antibiotics for prophylaxis of infection

• IV infusion using 21-, 23-, 25-gauge needle; administer by slow IV infusion

• Topical or systemic analgesics for pain

• Local or systemic drugs for infection

• Transfusion for anemia

• Antispasmodic

Perform/provide:

• Strict medical asepsis, protective isolation if WBC levels are low

• Special skin care

• Liquid diet: cola, Jell-O; dry toast or crackers may be added if patient is not nauseated or vomiting

• Rinsing of mouth 3-4 × day with water, hydrogen peroxide

• Brushing of teeth 2-3 × day with soft brush or cotton-tipped applicators for stomatitis; use unwaxed dental floss

• Warm compresses at injection site for inflammation

• Nutritious diet with iron, vitamin supplements

• HOB increased to facilitate breathing

Evaluate:

• Bleeding: hematuria, guaiac, bruising or petechiae, mucosa of orifices q8h

• Dyspnea, rales, unproductive cough, chest pain, tachypnea, fatigue, increased pulse, pallor, lethargy

• Food preferences; list likes, dislikes

• Effects of alopecia on body image, discuss feelings about body changes

• Edema in feet, joint pain, stomach pain, shaking

• Inflammation of mucosa, breaks in skin

• Yellowing of skin and sclera, dark urine, clay-colored stools, itchy skin, abdominal pain, fever, diarrhea

• Buccal cavity q8h for dryness, sores or ulceration, white patches, oral pain, bleeding, dysphagia

• Local irritation, pain, burning, discoloration at injection site

• Symptoms indicating severe allergic reaction: rash, pruritus, urticaria, purpuric skin lesions, itching, flushing

• Frequency of stools, characteristics: cramping, acidosis; signs of dehydration: rapid respirations, poor skin turgor, decreased urine output, dry skin, restlessness, weakness

Teach patient/family:

• Of protective isolation precautions

• To report any complaints or side effects to nurse or physician

• That hair may be lost during treatment, a wig or hairpiece may make patient feel better; tell patient that new hair may be different in color, texture

• To avoid foods with citric acid, hot or rough texture

• To report any bleeding, white spots or ulcerations in mouth to physician; tell patient to examine mouth qd

---

vitamin A

Acon, Afaxin, Aquasol A, Natola

Func. class.: Vitamin, fat soluble
Chem. class.: Retinol

Action: Needed for normal bone and teeth development, visual dark adaptation, skin disease, mucosa tissue repair, assists in production of adrenal steroids, cholesterol, RNA

Uses: Vitamin A deficiency

Dosage and routes:

• *Adult and child >8 yr:* PO 100,000-500,000 IU qd 3 days, then 50,000 qd × 2 wk; dose based on severity of deficiency; maintenance 10,000-20,000 IU for 2 mo

• *Child 1-8 yr:* IM 17,500-35,000 IU qd × 10 days

• *Infants <1 yr:* IM 7500-15,000 IU × 10 days

Maintenance

• Child 4-8 yr: IM 15,000 IU qd × 2 mo

• Child <4 yr: IM 10,000 IU qd × 2 mo

Available forms include: Caps

10,000, 25,000, 50,000 IU; drops 5,000 IU; inj 50,000 IU/ml

Side effects/adverse reactions:

GI: Nausea, vomiting, anorexia, abdominal pain, ***jaundice***

CNS: Headache, increased intracranial pressure, intracranial hypertension, lethargy, malaise

EENT: Gingivitis, papillaedema, exophthalmos, inflammation of tongue and lips

INTEG: Drying of skin, pruritus, increased pigmentation, night sweats, alopecia

MS: Arthraglia, retarded growth, hard areas on bone

META: Hypomenorrhea, hypercalcemia

Contraindications: Hypersensitivity to vitamin A, malabsorption syndrome (PO)

Precautions: Lactation, impaired renal function

Pharmacokinetics:

PO/INJ: Stored in liver, kidneys, fat; excreted (metabolites) in urine, feces

Interactions/incompatibilities:

• Decreased absorption of this drug: mineral oil

• Increased levels of this drug: corticosteroids

NURSING CONSIDERATIONS

Administer:

• With food (PO) for better absorption

Evaluate:

• Nutritional status: yellow and dark green vegetables, yellow/orange fruits, vitamin A fortified foods, liver, egg yolks

• Vitamin A deficiency: decreased growth, night blindness, dry, brittle nails, hair loss, urinary stones, increased infection

• Therapeutic response: increased growth rate, weight; absence of dry skin and mucous membranes, night blindness

---

italics = common side effects   ***bold italic*** = life threatening reactions

Teach patient/family:
• Not to use mineral oil while taking this drug
• To notify a physician of nausea, vomiting, lip cracking, loss of hair, headache
• Not to take more than the prescribed amount

Lab test interferences:
False increase: Bilirubin, serum cholesterol

Treatment of overdose: Discontinue drug

vitamin A, D ointment

A&D, Balmex, Caldesene, Clocream, Comfortine, Desitin, Primaderm

Func. class.: Emollient/protectant

Action: Prevents irritation of surgical areas by preventing evaporation of moisture

Uses: Irritation, sunburn, dry, chapped skin, diaper rash

Dosage and routes:
• *Adult:* TOP apply to skin several times/day

Available forms include: Oint

Side effects/adverse reactions:
INTEG: Rash, irritation

Contraindications: Raw, denuded, blistered, oozing wounds

Interactions/incompatibilities: None known

NURSING CONSIDERATIONS

Administer:
• Only to intact skin, never apply to raw, denuded, blistered, or oozing wounds

Perform/provide:
• Skin cleansing at least qd or more often if needed

Evaluate:
• Therapeutic response: absence of itching, irritation, burning
• Skin condition: irritation, rash
• For infection (increased temper-

ature, redness), often bacteria are trapped underneath

Teach patient/family:
• To report color changes on skin, redness, increased temperature, which may indicate infection

vitamin D (cholecalciferol, vitamin D₃ or ergocalciferol, vitamin D₂)

Calciferol, Deltalin, Drisodol, Radiostol,* Radiostol Forte*

Func. class.: Vitamin D
Chem. class.: Fat soluble

Action: Needed for regulation of calcium, phosphate levels, normal bone development, parathyroid activity, neuromuscular functioning

Uses: Vitamin D deficiency, rickets, renal osteodystrophy, hypoparathyroidism, hypophosphatemia, psoriasis, rheumatoid arthritis

Dosage and routes:
• *Adult:* PO/IM 12,000 IU qd, then increased to 500,000 IU/day
• *Child:* PO/IM 1500/5000 IU qd × 2-4 wk, may repeat after 2 wk or 600,000 IU as single dose

Hypoparathyroidism
• *Adult and child:* PO/IM 200,000 IU given with 4 g calcium tab

Available forms include: Tabs 400, 1000, 50,000 IU; caps 25,000, 50,000; liq 8000 IU/ml; inj 500,000 IU/ml, 500,000 IU/5 ml IM

Side effects/adverse reactions:
GI: Nausea, vomiting, anorexia, cramps, diarrhea, constipation, metallic taste, dry mouth
CNS: Fatigue, weakness, drowsiness, convulsion, headache
GU: Polyuria, nocturia, hematuria, albuminuria, *renal failure*
CV: Hypertension, dysrhythmias
MS: Decreased bone growth, early joint pain, early muscle pain

INTEG: Pruritus, photophobia
Contraindications: Hypersensitivity, hypercalcemia, renal dysfunction, hyperphosphatemia
Precautions: Cardiovascular disease, renal calculi
Pharmacokinetics:
PO/INJ: Half-life 7-12 hr, stored in liver, duration 2 mo, excreted in bile (metabolites) and urine
Interactions/incompatibilities:
• Decreased effects of this drug: cholestyramine, colestipol, phenobarbital, phenytoin
• Increased toxicity: diuretics (thiazides), antacids

NURSING CONSIDERATIONS

Assess:
• Vitamin D levels q2 wk during treatment
• Ca, PO$_4$, Mg, BUN, alk phosphatase, urine Ca, creatinine
Administer:
• IM injection in deep muscle mass, administer slowly
Evaluate:
• Therapeutic response: absence of rickets/osteomalacia, adequate calcium/phosphate levels, decrease in bone pain
• Nutritional status: egg yolk, fortified dairy products, cod, halibut
Teach patient/family:
• Necessary foods to be included in diet
• To avoid vitamin supplements unless directed by physician
• To keep doctor's appointments since line between therapeutic and toxic doses is narrow
• To report weakness, lethargy, headache, anorexia, loss of weight
• Nausea, vomiting, abdominal cramps, diarrhea, constipation, excessive thirst, polyuria, muscle and bone pain

vitamin E

Aquasol E, Daltose,* E-Ferol, Eprolin, Hy-E-Plex, Kell-E, Lethopherol, Maxi-E, Pertropin, Tocopher-Caps, Tocopherol

Func. class.: Vitamin E
Chem. class.: Fat soluble

Action: Needed for digestion and metabolism of polyunsaturated fats, decreased platelet aggregation, decreases blood clot formation, promotes normal growth, and development of muscle tissue
Uses: Vitamin E deficiency, impaired fat absorption, hemolytic anemia in premature neonates, prevention of retrolental fibroplasia, sickle cell anemia, supplement in malabsorption syndrome
Dosage and routes:
• *Adult:* PO/IM 60-75 IU qd, not to exceed 300 IU/day
• *Child:* PO/IM 1 mg/0.6 g of dietary fat
Available forms include: Caps 50, 100, 200, 400, 500, 600, 1000 IU; 74, 165, 294, 331 mg; tabs 200, 400 IU; 331 mg; drops 50 mg/ml
Side effects/adverse reactions:
META: Altered metabolism of hormones, thyroid, pituitary, adrenal, altered immunity
MS: Weakness
CNS: Headache, fatigue
GI: Nausea, cramps, diarrhea
GU: Gonadal dysfunction
CV: Increased risk thrombophlebitis
EENT: Blurred vision
INTEG: Sterile abscess, contact dermatitis
Contraindications: None significant
Pharmacokinetics:
PO: Metabolized in liver, excreted in bile

V

---

italics = common side effects **bold italic** = life threatening reactions

Interactions/incompatibilities:
• Increased action of: oral anticoagulants

NURSING CONSIDERATIONS
Assess:
• BUN, creatinine
• Vitamin E levels during treatment
• CBC; hemolytic anemia may occur

Administer:
• Topically to moisturize dry skin
Evaluate:
• Therapeutic response: absence of hemolytic anemia, adequate vitamin E levels, improvement in skin lesions, decreased edema
• Nutritional status: wheat germ, dark green leafy vegetables, nuts, eggs, liver, vegetable oils, dairy products, cereals

Teach patient/family:
• Necessary foods to be included in diet
• To avoid vitamin supplements unless directed by physician

---

warfarin sodium
(war'far-in)
Coufarin, Coumadin, Panwarfin, Warfilone Sodium,* Warnerin*
Func. class.: Heparin antagonist

Action: Interferes with blood clotting by indirect means; depresses hepatic synthesis of vitamin K-dependent coagulation factors (II, VII, IX, X)

Uses: Pulmonary emboli, deep vein thrombosis, myocardial infarction, rheumatic heart disease, atrial dysrhythmias

Dosage and routes:
• *Adult:* PO 10-15 mg × 3 days, then titrated to PT qd or 40-60 mg qd, then 2-10 mg qd titrated to PT level not to exceed 50 mg/10 min
Available forms include: Tabs 2, 2.5, 5, 7.5, 10 mg; inj 50 mg/2 ml

Side effects/adverse reactions:
GI: Diarrhea, nausea, vomiting, anorexia, stomatitis, cramps, *hepatitis*
GU: Hematuria
INTEG: Rash, dermatitis, urticaria, alopecia, pruritus
CNS: Fever
HEMA: Hemorrhage, agranulocytosis, leukopenia

Contraindications: Hypersensitivity, hemophilia, leukemia with bleeding, peptic ulcer disease, thrombocytopenic purpura, hepatic disease (severe), renal disease (severe), severe hypertension, subacute bacterial endocarditis, acute nephritis, blood dyscrasias, pregnancy

Precautions: Alcoholism, elderly
Pharmacokinetics:
PO: Onset 24 hr, peak ½-3 days, duration 3-5 days, half-life ½-3 days; metabolized in liver, excreted in urine/feces (active/inactive metabolites), crosses placenta

Interactions/incompatibilities:
• Increased action: allopurinol, chloramphenicol, clofibrate, amiodarone, diflunisal, heparin, steroids, cimetidine, disulfiram, thyroid, glucagon, metronidazole, quinidine, sulindac, sulfinpyrazone, sulfonamides, tricyclic antidepressants, inhalation anesthetics, salicylates, ethacrynic acids, indomethacin, mefenamic acid, oxyphenbutazones, phenylbutazone
• Decreased action: barbiturates, griseofulvin, haloperidol, ethchlorvynol, carbamazepine, rifampin, cholestyramine
• Increased or decreased action: chloral hydrate, glutethimide, sulfinpyrazone, triclofos sodium, alcohol

NURSING CONSIDERATIONS
Assess:
• Blood studies (Hct, platelets, occult blood in stools) q 3 mo

• Prothrombin time, which should be 1½-2 × control, PT; often done qd

• B/P, watch for increasing signs of hypertension

Administer:

• At same time each day to maintain steady blood levels

• Alone, do not give with food

• Avoiding all IM injections that may cause bleeding

Perform/provide:

• Storage in tight container

Evaluate:

• Therapeutic response: decrease of deep vein thrombosis

• Bleeding gums, petecchiae, ecchymosis, black tarry stools, hematuria

• Fever, skin rash, urticaria

• Needed dosage change q 1-2 wk

Teach patient/family:

• To avoid OTC preparations that may cause serious drug interactions unless directed by physician

• That urine may turn orange/red

• Drug may be held during active bleeding (menstruation)

• To use soft-bristle toothbrush to avoid bleeding gums

• To carry a Medic-Alert ID identifying drug taken

• Stress patient compliance

• On all aspects of adjustments: dosage, route, action, side effects, when to notify physician

• To report any signs of bleeding: gums, under skin, urine, stools

• To avoid hazardous activities (football, hockey, skiing) or dangerous work

Lab test interferences:

Increase: T_3 uptake

Decrease: Uric acid

Treatment of overdose: Administer vitamin K

xylometazoline HCl (nasal)

(xye-loe-met-az'oh-leen)

Neo-Synephrine II, Otrivin, Sine-Off Nasal Spray, Sinex-LA

Func. class.: Nasal decongestant

Chem. class.: Sympathomimetic amine

Action: Dilates arterioles of nasal membrane, which decreases congestion

Uses: Nasal congestion

Dosage and routes:

• *Adult and child >12 yr:* INSTILL 2-3 gtts or 2 sprays q8-10h (0.1%)

• *Child <12 yr:* INSTILL 2-3 gtts or 1 spray q8-10h (0.05%)

Available forms include: Sol 0.05%, 0.1%

Side effects/adverse reactions:

EENT: Irritation, burning, sneezing, stinging, dryness, rebound congestion

INTEG: Contact dermatitis

Contraindications: Hypersensitivity to sympathomimetic amines

Pharmacokinetics:

INSTILL: Onset 5-10 min, duration 5-6 hr

Interactions/incompatibilities:

None known

NURSING CONSIDERATIONS

Administer:

• No more than q4h

• For <4 consecutive days

Perform/provide:

• Environmental humidification to decrease nasal congestion, dryness

• Storage in light-resistant containers; do not expose to high temperatures

Evaluate:

• Redness, swelling, pain in nasal passages

---

italics = common side effects   ***bold italic*** = life threatening reactions

Teach patient/family:
• To avoid contamination of container
• Stinging may occur for a few applications; drying of mucosa may be decreased by environmental humidification
• To notify physician if irregular pulse, insomnia, dizziness, or tremors occur
• Proper administration to avoid systemic absorption

---

zidovudine (formerly azidothymidine or AZT)

(zid-oo′-vue-dine)
Retrovir

Func. class.: Antiviral
Chem. class.: Thymidine analog

Action: Inhibits replication of HLV virus by interfering with transcription of RNA and DNA
Uses: Symptomatic HLV infections (AIDS, ARC), confirmed *P. carinii* pneumonia, or absolute CD4 lymphocytes of <200/mm₃

Dosage and routes:
• *Adult:* PO 200 mg q4h, may need to stop treatment if severe bone marrow depression occurs, and restart after bone marrow recovery
Available forms include: Caps 100 mg

Side effects/adverse reactions:
*HEMA: **Granulocytopenia, anemia***
CNS: Fever, headache, malaise, diaphoresis, dizziness, insomnia, paresthesia, somnolence, chills, tremor, twitching, anxiety, confusion, depression, lability, vertigo, loss of mental acuity
GI: Nausea, vomiting, diarrhea, anorexia, cramps, dyspepsia, constipation, dysphagia, flatulence, rectal bleeding, mouth ulcer
RESP: Dyspnea
EENT: Taste change, hearing loss, photophobia

INTEG: Rash, acne, pruritus, urticaria
MS: Myalgia, arthralgia, muscle spasm
GU: Dysuria, polyuria, frequency, hesitancy
Contraindications: Hypersensitivity
Precautions: Granulocyte count <1000/mm₃ or Hgb <9.5 g/dl, pregnancy (C), lactation, children, severe renal disease, severe hepatic function
Pharmacokinetics:
PO: Rapidly absorbed from GI tract, peak ½-1½ hr, metabolized in liver (inactive metabolites), excreted by kidneys
Interactions/incompatibilities:
• Toxicity: amphotericin B, dapsone, flucytosine, adriamycin, interferon vincristine, vinblastine, pentamidine, probenecid, experimental nucleoside analogues
• Granulocytopenia: acetaminophen, aspirin, indomethacin

NURSING CONSIDERATIONS
Assess:
• Blood counts q2 wk, watch for decreasing granulocytes, Hgb; if low, therapy may need to be discontinued and restarted after hematologic recovery; blood transfusions may be required
Administer:
• By mouth, capsules should be swallowed whole
• Trimethoprim-sulfamethoxazole, pyrimethamine, or acyclovir as ordered to prevent opportunistic infections; if these drugs are given, watch for neurotoxicity
Perform/provide:
• Storage in cool environment, protect from light
Evaluate:
• Blood dyscrasias (anemia, granulocytopenia): bruising, fatigue, bleeding, poor healing

---

*Available in Canada only

Teach patient/family:
• Drug is not cure for AIDS, but will control symptoms
• To call physician if sore throat, swollen lymph nodes, malaise, fever occur since other infections may occur
• That even with drug administration, patient is still infective and may pass AIDS virus on to others
• That follow-up visits must be continued since serious toxicity may occur, blood counts must be done q2 wk
• That drug must be taken q4h around clock even during night
• That serious drug interactions may occur if OTC products are ingested, check with physician first if taking aspirin, acetaminophen, indomethacin
• That other drugs may be necessary to prevent other infections

zinc gelatin

Dome-Paste, Unna's Boot
Func. class.: Emollient/protectant

Action: Reduced irritation by decreasing friction
Uses: Lesions, injuries on arms, legs
Dosage and routes:
• *Adult:* TOP wrap wet bandage, remove in 7 days
Available forms include: Gel
Side effects/adverse reactions:
None known
Interactions/incompatibilities:
None known
NURSING CONSIDERATIONS
Administer:
• Zinc boot; to remove, soak in warm water, unwind outer bandage
• In direction of the hair follicle growth
• Using open technique, do not cover with tight dressing

Perform/provide:
• Skin cleansing after removal (1 wk)
Evaluate:
• Therapeutic response: healing of lesions on arms, legs
• Area for vasoconstriction, check color, temperature in extremities
• For infection (increased temperature, redness), often bacteria are trapped underneath
Teach patient/family:
• Not to bathe with zinc boot on leg

zinc sulfate

Eye-Sed Ophthalmic, Op-Thal-Zin
Func. class.: Ophthalmic vasoconstrictor
Chem. class.: Zinc product

Action: Vasoconstriction occurs by action on conjunctiva
Uses: Ocular congestion, irritation, itching
Dosage and routes:
• *Adult and child >2 yr:* INSTILL 1-2 gtts bid or tid
Available forms include: Sol 0.217%, 0.25%
Side effects/adverse reactions:
EENT: Eye irritation, burning
Contraindications: Hypersensitivity
Precautions: Narrow-angle glaucoma, pregnancy
Interactions/incompatibilities:
None known
NURSING CONSIDERATIONS
Perform/provide:
• Storage in tight container
Teach patient/family:
• To report change in vision, or irritation
• Method of instillation; tilt head backward, hold dropper over eye, drop medication inside lower lid,

Z

using pressure on inside corner of eye hold 1 min, do not touch dropper to eye

---

zinc sulfate

Orazinc

Func. class.: Trace element

Action: Needed for adequate healing, bone and joint development (23% zinc)

Uses: Prevention of zinc deficiency

Dosage and routes:
• *Adult:* PO 200-220 mg tid
• *Child:* PO 0.3 mg/kg/day

Available forms include: Tabs 110, 200, 220 mg; caps 110, 220 mg

Side effects/adverse reactions:
GI: Nausea, vomiting, cramps, heartburn, ulcer formation

OVERDOSE: Diarrhea, rash, dehydration, restlessness

Pharmacokinetics: Not known

Interactions/incompatibilities: None known

NURSING CONSIDERATIONS

Assess:
• Zinc levels during treatment

Administer:
• With meals to decrease gastric upset; avoid dairy products

Evaluate:
• Therapeutic response: absence of zinc deficiency

Teach patient/family:
• That element will need to be taken for 2 mo to be effective
• To immediately report nausea, diarrhea, rash, severe vomiting, restlessness

Appendixes

appendix a

Abbreviations

ā	before	BM	bowel movement
aa	of each	BMR	basal metabolism rate
AB	abortion	B/P	blood pressure
abd	abdomen	BPH	benign prostatic hypertrophy
ABGs	arterial blood gases	BS	blood sugar
ac	before meals	BSP	bromsulphalein
ACE	angiotensin-converting enzyme	BUN	blood urea nitrogen
ad lib	as desired	Bx	biopsy
ADA	American Diabetes Association	c̄	with
ADH	antidiuretic hormone	cap	capsules
AKA	also known as	C	Celsius (centigrade)
ALT	alanine aminotransferase, serum	Ca	cancer
AMA	against medical advice	CAD	coronary artery disease
amb	ambulation	cath	catheterization or catheterize
ANA	antinuclear antibodies	CC	chief complaint
ant	anterior	cc	cubic centimeter
AP	anterior-posterior	CBC	complete blood count
APTT	activated partial thromboplastin time	CHF	congestive heart failure
AROM	active range of motion	cm	centimeter
ASA	acetylsalicylic acid, aspirin	CNS	central nervous system
ASAP	as soon as possible	CO_2	carbon dioxide
AST	aspartate aminotransferase, serum	c/o	complains of
ASHD	arteriosclerotic heart disease	COPD	chronic obstructive pulmonary disease
AV	atrioventricular	CPAP	continuous positive airway pressure
BAL	blood alcohol level	CPK	creatinine phosphokinase
bid	twice a day		

CPR	cardiopulmonary resuscitation
CrCl	creatinine clearance
C section	cesarean section
CSF	cerebrospinal fluid
CVA	cerebrovascular accident
CVP	central venous pressure
D&C	dilatation and curettage
DM	diabetes mellitus
DOA	dead on arrival
DOB	date of birth
dr	dram
dsg	dressing
D₅W	5% glucose in distilled water
dx	diagnosis
ECG	electrocardiogram (EKG)
EDTA	ethylenediaminetetraacetic acid
EEG	electroencephalogram
EENT	ear, eye, nose, and throat
elix	elixir
ESR	erythrocyte sedimentation rate
F	Farenheit
FBS	fasting blood sugar
FHT	fetal heart tones
FIo₂	inspired oxygen concentration
FSH	follicle-stimulating hormone
fx	fracture
g	gram
gal	gallon
gr	grain
GTT	glucose tolerance test
gtt	drop
GI	gastrointestinal
GU	genitourinary
Gyn	gynecology
H	hypodermically
H & H	hematocrit and hemoglobin
Hct	hematocrit
HDCV	human diploid cell rabies vaccine
Hgb	hemoglobin
H₂O	water
HOB	head of bed
HR	heart rate
hr	hour
hs	at bedtime
Hx	history
IgG	immunoglobulin G
IM	intramuscular
INH	inhalation
inj	injection
IPPB	intermittent positive pressure breathing
I&O	intake and output
IUD	intrauterine contraceptive device
IV	intravenous
IVAC	intravenous controller
IVP	intravenous pyelogram
IVPB	intravenous piggyback
K	potassium
Kg	kilogram
L or l	left
L	liter
lat	lateral
lb	pound
LDH	lactic dehydrogenase
LE	lupus erythematosus
LH	luteinizing hormone
liq	liquid
LLQ	left lower quadrant
LMP	last menstrual period
LOC	loss of consciousness
LR	lactated Ringer's solution
LUQ	left upper quadrant
M	meter
m	minim

m²	square meter
MAOI	monoamine oxidase inhibitor
MCA	motorcycle accident
mEq	milliequivalent
mg	milligram
μg	microgram
MI	myocardial infarction
min	minute
mixt	mixture
ml	milliliter
mm	millimeter
mo	month
MRC	medical research council
MVA	motorvehicle accident
Na	sodium
NC	nasal cannula
neg	negative
NKA	no known allergies
noc	night
NPO	nothing by mouth (Lat. *nulla per os*)
NS	normal saline
NV	neurovascular
O₂	oxygen
OBS	organic brain syndrome
OD	right eye
OOB	out of bed
OR	operating room
ORIF	open reduction, internal fixation
OS	left eye
os	mouth
OTC	over the counter
OU	each eye
oz	ounce
p̄	after
p	pulse
P56	plasma-lyte 56
Paco₂	arterial carbon dioxide tension (pressure)

Pao₂	arterial oxygen tension (pressure)
PBI	protein-bound iodine
PAT	paroxysmal atrial tachycardia
PCN	penicillin
PE	physical examination
PEEP	positive end expiratory pressure
PERRLA	pupils equal, round, react to light and accommodation
pH	hydrogen ion concentration
PO	by mouth
postop	postoperatively
PP	post prandial
preop	preoperatively
prep	preparation
prn	as needed
pro-time, PT	prothrombin time
PTT	partial thromboplastin time
PVC	premature ventricular contraction
q	every
qAM	every morning
qd	every day
qh	every hour
qid	four times a day
qod	every other day
qPM	every night
qs	quantity sufficient
qt	quart
q2h	every 2 hours
q3h	every 3 hours
q4h	every 4 hours
q6h	every 6 hours
q12h	every 12 hours
R	respirations, rectal
r	right
RAIU	radioactive iodine uptake

RBC(s)	red blood count or cell(s)	**tinc**	tincture
REM	rapid eye movement	**TPN**	total parenteral nutrition
RLQ	right lower quadrant	**TPR**	temperature, pulse, respirations
R/O	rule out		
ROM	range of motion	**top**	topical
RUQ	right upper quadrant	**TSH**	thyroid-stimulating hormone
Rx	therapy, treatment, or prescription		
s̄	without	**tsp**	teaspoon
SAN	sinoatrial node	**U**	unit
SC	subcutaneous	**UA**	urinalysis
sig	label	**UV**	ultraviolet
SIMV	synchronous intermittent mandatory ventilation	**vag**	vaginal
		VD	veneral disease
		VMA	vanillylmandelic acid
SL	sublingual	**VO**	verbal order
SOB	short of breath	**vol**	volume
sol	solution	**VS**	vital signs
ss	one half	**WBC**	white blood count
stat	at once	**wk**	week
surg	surgical	**WNL**	within normal limits
Sx	symptoms	**wt**	weight
supp	suppository	**yr**	year
syr	syrup	**>**	greater than
T	temperature	**<**	less than
T&A	tonsillectomy and adenoidectomy	**=**	equal
		≠	not equal
tab	tablet	**↑**	increase
TAH	total abdominal hysterectomy	**↓**	decrease
		2°	secondary
tbsp	tablespoon	**°**	degree
temp	temperature	**%**	percent
tid	three times daily	**@**	at

appendix b

Formulas for drug calculations

Surface area rule:

$$\text{Child dose} = \frac{\text{Surface area (m}^2)}{1.73\text{m}^2} \times \text{Adult dose}$$

Calculating strength of a solution:

Solution Strength: *Desired Solution:*

$$\frac{x}{100} = \frac{\text{Amount of drug desired}}{\text{Amount of finished solution}}$$

Calculating flow rate for IV:

$$\text{Rate of Flow} = \frac{\text{Amount of fluid} \times \text{Administration set calibration}}{\text{Running time}}$$

$$\frac{x}{1} = \frac{\text{(ml) (gtt/min)}}{\text{min}}$$

Calculation of medication dosages:

Formula method:

$$\frac{\text{Amount ordered}}{\text{Amount on hand}} \times \text{Vehicle}$$

$$= \text{Number of tablets, capsules, or amount of liquid}$$

Vehicle is the drug form or amount of liquid containing the dosage. Amounts used in calculation by formula must be in same system.

Ratio—proportion method:

1 tablet: tablet in mg on hand:: x tablet order in mg
                Know or have:: Want to know or order

Multiply means and extremes, divide both sides by known amount to get X. Amounts used in equation must be in same system.

Dimensional analysis method:

Order in mg $\times \dfrac{1 \text{ tablet or capsule}}{\text{What 1 tablet or capsule is in mg}}$

= Tablets or capsules to be given

If amounts are in different systems:

Order in mg $\times \dfrac{1 \text{ tablet or capsule}}{\text{What 1 tablet or capsule is in g}} \times \dfrac{1}{1000 \text{ mg}}$

= Tablets or capsules to be given

appendix c

Bibliography

Drug Information 87: Bethesda, 1987, American Hospital Formulary Service.

Dorr, R., and Fritz, W.: Cancer chemotherapy handbook, New York, 1986, Elsevier Science Publishing Co.

Facts and Comparisons: Philadelphia, updated monthly, J.B. Lippincott Co.

Goodman, A., and others: Goodman and Gilman's The pharmacological basis of therapeutics, New York, 1985, Macmillan Publishing Co.

Goth, A.: Medical pharmacology, St. Louis, 1984, The C.V. Mosby Co.

Krogh, C.M.E., editor: Compendium of pharmaceuticals and specialties, ed. 21, Ottawa, 1986, Canadian Pharmaceutical Assoc.

Mediphor Editorial Group: Drug interaction facts, Philadelphia, updated quarterly, J.B. Lippincott Co.

Pagliaro, A.M., and Pagliaro, L.A.: Pharmacologic aspects of nursing care, St. Louis, 1986, The C.V. Mosby Co.

Shinn, A., editor: Evaluations of drug interactions, St. Louis, 1985, The C.V. Mosby Co.

appendix d

Combination products

Aceta with Codeine, Empracet with Codeine Phosphate 30 mg No. 3, Tylenol with Codeine No. 3: acetaminophen 300 mg with codeine phosphate 30 mg

Achromycin Intramuscular: tetracycline HCl 100 mg with procaine HCl 40 mg

Achromycin Intramuscular: tetracycline HCl 250 mg with procaine HCl 40 mg

Aethralgen: salicylamide 250 mg with acetaminophen 250 mg

Alazide, Spironazide, Spirozide: spironolactone 25 mg with hydrochlorothiazide 25 mg

Aldactazide 25/25: spironolactone 25 mg with hydrochlorothiazide 25 mg

Aldactazide 50/50: spironolactone 50 mg with hydrochlorothiazide 50 mg

Aldoclor-15: methyldopa 250 mg with chlorothiazide 15 mg

Aldoclor-150: methyldopa 250 mg with chlorothiazide 150 mg

Aldoclor-250: methyldopa 250 mg with chlorothiazide 250 mg

Aldoril-15, Methyldopa and Hydrochlorothiazide Tablets 250 mg/15 mg: methyldopa 250 mg with hydrochlorothiazide 15 mg

Aldoril-25, Methyldopa and Hydrochlorothiazide Tablets 250 mg/25 mg: methyldopa 250 mg with hydrochlorothiazide 25 mg

Aldoril D30, Alodopa-H-30, Methyldopa and Hydrochlorothiazide Tablets 500 mg/30 mg: methyldopa 500 mg with hydrochlorothiazide 30 mg

Aldoril D50, Alodopa-H-50, Methyldopa and Hydrochlorothiazide Tablets 500 mg/50 mg: methyldopa 500 mg with hydrochlorothiazide 50 mg

Amaphen with Codeine No. 3: acetaminophen 325 mg with butalbital 50 mg, caffeine 40 mg, codeine phosphate 30 mg

Ambenyl: diphenhydramine HCl 12.5 mg/5 ml with codeine phosphate 10 mg/5 ml

Anacin: aspirin 400 mg with caffeine 32 mg

Anexsia: hydrocodone bitartrate 7 mg with aspirin 325 mg

Anexsia with Codeine, Empirim with Codeine 30 mg No. 3: codeine 30 mg with aspirin 325 mg

Anodynos-DHC, DIA-Gesic:

acetaminophen 150 mg with aspirin 230 mg, caffeine 30 mg, hydrocodone bitartrate 5 mg

Antrocol: atropine sulfate 0.195 mg with phenobarbital 16 mg

Antrocol Elixir: atropine sulfate 0.039 mg/ml with phenobarbital 3 mg/ml

A.P.C. with Codeine No. 3 Tabloid: aspirin 227 mg with caffeine 32 mg, codeine phosphate 30 mg, phenacetin 162 mg

A.P.C. with Codeine No. 4 Tabloid: aspirin 227 mg with caffeine 32 mg, codeine phosphate 60 mg, phenobarbital 162 mg

Apresazide 25/25, Aprozide 25/25, Hydralazine 25/25, Hydralazine-Thiazide 25/25: hydralazine HCl 25 mg with hydrochlorothiazide 25 mg

Apresazide 50/50, Aprozide 50/50, Hydralazine 50/50, Hydralazine-Thiazide 50/50: hydralazine HCl 50 mg with hydrochlorothiazide 50 mg

Apresazide 100/50, Aprozide 100/50, Hydralazine 100/50, Hydralazine-Thiazide 100/50: hydralazine HCl 100 mg with hydrochlorothiazide 50 mg

Apresodex, Apresoline-Esidrix, Hydralazine-Thiazide: hydralazine HCl 25 mg with hydrochlorothiazide 15 mg

Aralen Phosphate with Primaquine Phosphate: chloroquine phosphate 300 mg (of chloroquine) with primaquine phosphate 45 mg (of primaquine)

A.S.A. and Codeine Compound No. 3 Pulvules: codeine 30 mg with aspirin 380 mg, caffeine 30 mg

Ascriptin with Codeine No. 2: aspirin 325 mg with codeine phosphate 15 mg, buffers

Ascriptin with Codeine No. 3: aspirin 325 mg with codeine phosphate 30 mg, buffers

Atropine, Demerol Injection: meperidine HCl 50 mg/ml with atropine sulfate 0.4 mg/ml

Atropine, Demerol Injection: meperidine HCl 75 mg/ml with atropine sulfate 0.4 mg/ml

Axotal: aspirin 650 mg with butalbital 50 mg

Azo-Gamazole, Azo Gantanol, Azo-Sulfamethoxazole: sulfamethoxazole 500 mg with phenazopyridine HCl 100 mg

Azo-Gantrisin, Azo-Gulfasin, Azo-Sulfisocon, Azo-Sulfamethoxazole: sulfisoxazole 500 mg with phenazopyridine HCl 50 mg

B-A-C: aspirin 650 mg with butalbital 50 mg, caffeine 40 mg, buffers

B-A-C No. 3: aspirin 325 mg with butalbital 50 mg, caffeine 40 mg, codeine phosphate 30 mg, buffers

BC Powder: aspirin 650 mg with caffeine 32 mg, salicylamide 195 mg

Bancap: acetaminophen 325 mg with butalbital 50 mg

Bancap HC, Dolacet, Hydrocet, Zydone: hydrocodone bitartrate 5 mg with acetaminophen 500 mg

Barbidonna: belladonna alkaloids, atropine sulfate 0.025 mg, hyoscyamine sulfate 0.1286 mg, phenobarbital 16 mg, scopolamine hydrobromide 0.0074 mg

Barbidonna Elixir: belladonna alkaloids, atropine sulfate 0.034 mg/5 ml, hyoscyamine sulfate 0.0174 mg/5 ml, phenobarbital 21.6 mg/ml, scopolamine hydrobromide 0.01 mg/5 ml

Barbidonna No. 2: belladonna alkaloids, atropine sulfate 0.025 mg, hyoscyamine sulfate 0.1286 mg, phenobarbital 32 mg, scopolamine hydrobromide 0.0074 mg

Bayer Children's Cold Medicine, St. Joseph's Cold Tablets for Children: phenylpropanolamine HCl 3.125 mg with aspirin 81 mg

Bayer Cold Syrup for Children: dextromethorphan hydrobromide 7.5 mg/5 ml with phenylpropanolamine HCl 9 mg/5 ml

Belap, Pheno-Bella: belladonna extract 10.8 mg (0.135 mg of alkaloids of belladonna leaf) with phenobarbital 16.2 mg

Belladenal-S: levorotatory belladonna alkaloids malates 0.25 mg (of levorotatory belladonna alkaloids) with phenobarbital 50 mg

Bellalphen, Donnatal, Hyosophen: belladonna alkaloids atropine sulfate 0.0194 mg, hyoscyamine sulfate 0.1037 mg, phenobarbital 16.2 mg, scopolamine hydrobromide 0.0065 mg

Bellergal: ergotamine tartrate 0.3 mg with levorotatory belladonna alkaloids malates 0.1 mg (of levorotatory belladonna alkaloids), phenobarbital 20 mg

Bellergal-S: ergotamine tartrate 0.6 mg with levorotatory belladonna alkaloids malates 0.2 mg (of lavorotatory belladonna alkaloids 40 mg)

Benadryl: diphenhydramine HCl 25 mg with pseudoephedrine HCl 60 mg

Benylin: diphenhydramine HCl 12.5 mg/5 ml with pseudoephedrine HCl 30 mg/5 ml

Benylin DM: dextromethorphan hydrobromide 5 mg/5 ml with guaifenesin 100 mg/5 ml

Bexophene, Darvon Compound-65 Pulvules, Dolene Compound-65, Doxaphene Compound, Propoxyphene-AC, Propoxyphene Compound-65, SK-65: propoxyphene HCl 65 mg with aspirin 389 mg, caffeine 32.4 mg

Bicillin C-R: 150,000 units (of penicillin G) per ml with penicillin G benzathine 150,000 units (of penicillin G) per ml

Bicillin C-R: penicillin G procaine 300,000 units (of penicillin G) per ml with penicillin G benzathine 300,000 units (of penicillin G) per ml

Bicillin C-R 900/300: penicillin G procaine 150,000 units (of penicillin G) per ml with penicillin G benzathine 450,000 units (of penicillin G) per ml

B&O Suprettes No. 15A: powdered opium 30 mg with

belladonna extract 16.2 mg (equivalent to belladonna alkaloids 0.21 mg)

B&O Suprettes No. 16A: powdered opium 60 mg with belladonna extract 16.2 mg (equivalent to belladonna alkaloids 0.21 mg)

Bromo-seltzer Granules: acetaminophen 325 mg/capful measure with citric acid 2.224 g/capful measure, sodium bicarbonate 2.871 g/capful measure

Butibel: belladonna extract 15 mg (0.187 mg of alkaloids of belladonna leaf) with butabarbital sodium 15 mg

Butibel Elixir: belladonna extract 15 mg (0.187 mg of alkaloids of belladonna leaf) with butabarbital sodium 15 mg

Cafatine, Cafergot, Caffeien-Ergotamine, Ercaf, Lanatrate: ergotamine tartrate 1 mg with caffeine 100 mg

Cafatine PB, Cafergot, Caferate-PB, Ergo-Caff with Phenobarbital, Migergot PB: ergotamine tartrate 2 mg with caffeine 100 mg, levorotatory belladonna alkaloids malates 0.25 mg (of levorotatory belladonna alkaloids), phenobarbital 60 mg

Cafergot: ergotamine tartrate 1 mg with caffeine 100 mg, levorotatory alkaloids malates 0.125 mg (of levorotatory belladonna alkaloids), phenobarbital sodium 30 mg

Cafergot, Wigraine: ergotamine tartrate 2 mg with caffeine 100 mg

Caladryl: diphenhydramine HCl 1% with calamine 8%, camphor 0.1%

Calcidrine Syrup: codeine 8.4 mg/5 ml with calcium iodide anhydrous 152 mg/5 ml

Cantri, Vagilia: sulfisoxazole 10% with allantoin 2%, aminacrine HCl 0.2%

Capital and Codeine: codeine 30 mg with acetaminophen 325 mg

Capital with Codeine: acetaminophen 120 mg/5 ml with codeine 12 mg/5 ml

Capozide 25/15: captopril 25 mg with hydrochlorothiazide 15 mg

Capozide 25/25: captopril 25 mg with hydrochlorothiazide 25 mg

Capozide 50/15: captopril 50 mg with hydrochlorothiazide 15 mg

Capozide 50/25: captopril 50 mg with hydrochlorothiazide 25 mg

Carisoprodol Compound, Soprodol Compound, Soma Compound, Soprodol Compound: risoprodol 200 mg with aspirin 325 mg

CDP Plus, Clindex, Clinoxide, Clipoxide, Librax, Lidox, Lidoxide: clidinium bromide 2.5 mg with chlordiazepoxide HCl 5 mg

Chardonna-2: belladonna extract 15 mg (0.187 mg of alkaloids of belladonna leaf) with phenobarbital 15 mg

Cherapas, Hydroserpine Plus, Ser-A-Gen, Ser-Ap-Es, Sera-

thide, Serpazide, Tri-Hydroserpine, Unipres: reserpine 0.1 mg with hydralazine HCl 25 mg, hydrochlothiazide 15 mg

Children's Hold 4 Hour: dextromethorphan hydrobromide 3.75 mg with phenylpropanolamine HCl 6.25 mg

Chlorofon-F, Chlorzone Forte, Paracet Forte, Parafon Forte, Zoxaphen: chlorzoxazone 250 mg with acetaminophen 300 mg

Chloroserp-250, Chloroserpine-250, Diupres-250: reserpine 0.125 mg with chlorothiazide 250 mg

Chloroserp-500, Chloropserpine-500, Diupres-500: reserpine 0.125 mg with chlorothiazide 500 mg

Clindex, Clinoxide, Clipoxide, Librax, Lidox: chlordiazepoxide HCl 5 mg with clidinium bromide 2.5 mg

Co-Gesic, Damacet-P, Duradyne, Hy-Phen, Norcet, Vicodin: hydrocodone bitartrate 5 mg with acetaminophen 500 mg

Codalan No. 1: acetaminophen 500 mg with caffeine 30 mg, codeine phosphate 8 mg

Codalan No. 2: acetaminophen 500 mg with caffeine 30 mg, codeine phosphate 15 mg

Codalan No. 3: acetaminophen 500 mg with caffeine 30 mg, codeine phosphate 30 mg

Codxym, Percodan, Roxiprin: oxycodone HCl 4.5 mg, oxycodone terephthalate 0.38 mg with aspirin 325 mg

Combipres 0.1 mg: clonidine HCl 0.1 mg with chlorthalidone 15 mg

Combipres 0.2 mg: clonidine HCl 0.2 mg with chlorthalidone 15 mg

Combipres 0.3 mg: clonidine HCl 0.3 mg with chlorthalidone 15 mg

Comtrex: dextromethorphan hydrobromide 10 mg with acetaminophen 325 mg, chlorpheniramine maleate 2 mg, phenylpropanolamine hydrochloride 12.5 mg

Comtrex: dextromethorphan hydrobromide 3.3 mg/5 ml with acetaminophen 108.3 mg/5 ml, chlorpheniramine maleate 0.67 mg/5 ml, phenylpropanolamine HCl 4.2 mg/5 ml

Conar Expectorant: dextromethorphan hydrobromide 15 mg/5 ml with guaifenesin 100 mg/5 ml, phenylephrine HCl 10 mg/5 ml

Conar: dextromethorphan hydrobromide 15 mg with acetaminophen 300 mg, guaifenesin 100 mg, phenylephrine HCl 10 mg

Conar Syrup: dextromethorphan hydrobromide 15 mg/5 ml with phenylephrine HCl 10 mg/5 ml

Congespirin: phenylpropanolamine HCl 6.25 mg/5 ml with acetaminophen 130 mg/5 ml

Congespirin, Aspirin-Free: acetaminophen 81 mg with phenylephrine HCl 81 mg

Contac Jr.: dextromethorphan hydrobromide 5 mg/5 ml with acetaminophen 160 mg/5 ml, pseudoephedrine HCl 15 mg/ 5 ml

Contac Severe Cold Formula, Nyquil Nighttime Cold Medicine, Nytime Cold Medicine, Quiet Nite: dextromethorphan hydrobromide 5 mg/5 ml with acetaminophen 167 mg/5 ml, doxylamine succinate 1.25 mg/ 5 ml, pseudoephedrine HCl 10 mg/5 ml

Copavin Pulvules: codeine sulfate 15 mg with papaverine HCl 15 mg

Corzide 40/5: bendroflumethiazide 5 mg with nadolol 4 mg

Corzide 80/5: bendroflumethiazide 5 mg with nadolol 40 mg

CoTylenol: dextromethorphan hydrobromide 5 mg/5 ml with acetaminophen 108.3 mg/5 ml, chlorpheniramine maleate 0.67 mg/5 ml, pseudoephedrine HCl 10 mg/5 ml

CoTylenol Cold Medication Tablets: dextromethorphan hydrobromide 15 mg with acetaminophen 325 mg, chlorpheniramine maleate 2 mg, pseudoephedrine HCl 30 mg

Cremacoat 3: dextromethorphan hydrobromide 6.7 mg/5 ml with guaifenesin 66.7 mg/5 ml, phenylpropanolamine HCl 12.5 mg/5 ml

Cremacoat 4: dextromethorphan hydrobromide 6.7 mg/5 ml with doxylamine succinate 2.5 mg/5 ml, phenylpropanolamine HCl 12.5 mg/5 ml

Damason-P: hydrocodone bitartrate 5 mg with aspirin 224 mg, caffeine 32 mg

Darvocet-N 50, Propoxyphene Napsylate with Acetaminophen Tablets: acetaminophen 325 mg with propoxyphene napsylate 50 mg

Darvocet-N 100, Doxapap-N, Propacet 100: propoxyphene napsylate 100 mg with acetaminophen 650 mg

Darvon Compound Pulvules: aspirin 389 mg with caffeine 32.4 mg propoxyphene HCl 32 mg

Darvon Compound-65 Pulvules, Dolene Compound-65, SK-65-Compound: aspirin 389 mg with caffeine 32.4 mg, propoxyphene HCl 65 mg

Darvon with A.S.A. Pulvules: aspirin 325 mg with propoxyphene HCl 65 mg

Darvon-N and A.S.A.: aspirin 325 mg with propoxyphene napsylate 100 mg

Deconex: phenylpropanolamine HCl 18 mg with acetaminophen 325 mg

Demerol APAP: acetaminophen 300 mg with meperidine HCl 50 mg

Demi-Regroton: chlorthalidone 25 mg with reserpine 0.125 mg

Deprol: meprobamate 400 mg with benactyzine HCl 1 mg

Dihydrocodeine Compound Modified, Synalgos: aspirin 356.4 mg with caffeine 30 mg and dihydrocodeine bitartrate 16 mg

Dilantin with Phenobarbital Kapseals: Phenytoin Sodium 100 mg with Phenobarbital 32 mg

COMBINATION PRODUCTS

Dilantin with Phenobarbital Kapseals: phenobarbital 16 mg with phenytoin sodium 100 mg

Dimetane-DX Cough Syrup: dextromethorphan hydrobromide 10 mg/5 ml with brompheniramine maleate 2 mg/5 ml, pseudoephedrine HCl 30 mg/5 ml

Diurese, Matatensin No. 4, Trichlormethiazide with Reserpine Tablets, Trichlortensin: trichlormethiazide 4 mg with reserpine 0.1 mg

Diutensen: methyclothiazide 2.5 mg with cryptenamine tannates 2 mg (of cryptenamine)

Diutensen: reserpine 0.1 mg with methyclothiazide 2.5 mg

Diutensin-R: methyclothiazide 25 mg with reserpine 0.1 mg

Diutrim: phenylpropanolamine HCl 75 mg with benzocaine 9 mg, carboxymethylcellulose 75 mg

Dolene AP-65: acetaminophen 650 mg with propoxyphene HCl 65 mg

Donnatal: belladonna alkaloids atropine sulfate 0.0194 mg, hyoscyamine sulfate 0.1037 mg, phenobarbital 32.4 mg, scopolamine hydrobromide 0.0065 mg

Donnatal Elixir, Hyosophen Elixir: belladonna alkaloids atropine sulfate 0.0194 mg/5 ml, hyoscyamine sulfate 0.1037 mg/5 ml, phenobarbital 16.2 mg/5 ml, scopolamine hydrobromide 0.0065/5 ml

Donnatal Extentabs: belladonna alkaloids atropine sulfate 0.0582 mg, hyoscyamine sulfate 0.3111 mg, phenobarbital 48.6 mg, scopolamine hydrobromide 0.0195 mg

Donnatal, Hyosophen: belladonna alkaloids atropine sulfate 0.0194 mg, hyoscyamine sulfate 0.1037 mg, phenobarbital 16.2 mg, scopolamine hydrobromide 0.0065 mg

Dorcol Children's Cough Syrup: dextromethorphan hydrobromide 5 mg/5 ml with guaifenesin 50 mg/5 ml, pseudoephedrine HCl 15 mg/5 ml

DUO-Medihaler: isoproterenol HCl 160 μg/metered spray with phenylephrine bitartrate 240 μg/metered spray

Ebdecon, Phenapap No. 2: acetaminophen 325 mg with phenylpropanolamine HCl 25 mg

Empirin with Codeine 15 mg No. 2: codeine 15 mg with aspirin 325 mg

Empirin with Codeine 60 mg No. 4: aspirin 325 mg with codeine phosphate 60 mg

Empracet with Codeine Phosphate 60 mg No. 4, Tylenol with Codeine No. 4: acetaminophen 300 mg with codeine phosphate 60 mg

Endecon, Phenapap No. 2: phenylpropanolamine HCl 25 mg with acetaminophen 325 mg

Enduronyl, Eserdine Forte, Methyclothiazide and Deserpidine Tablets 5 mg/0.5 mg, Methy-Deserpidine Forte, Methy-Deserpidine Strong: methyclothiazide 5 mg with deserpidine 0.5 mg

Enduronyl, Eserdine, Methy-chlothiazide, Deserpidine Tablets 5 mg/0.25 mg: deserpidine 0.25 mg with methychlothiazide 5 mg

Epromate, Equagesic, Equazine-M, Hepto-M, Mepro Compound, Meprogesic, Micranin: meprobamate 200 mg with aspirin 325 mg

Equagesic, Equazine-M, Mepro-Analgesic, Mepor Compound, Micrainin: aspirin 325 mg with meprobamate 200 mg

Esgic, Fioricet: acetaminophen 325 mg with butalbital 50 mg, caffeine 40 mg

Esimil: guanethidine monosulfate 10 mg (equivalent to guanethidine sulfate 8.4 mg) with hydrochlorothiazide 25 mg

Eutron Filmtab: pargyline HCl 25 mg with methyclothiazide 5 mg

Excedrin: acetaminophen 194 mg with aspirin 227 mg, caffeine 33 mg, buffers

Excedrin: aspirin 250 mg with acetaminophen 250 mg, caffeine 65 mg

Excedrin P.M.: acetaminophen 500 mg with diphenhydramine citrate 38 mg

Femguard, Sulfa-Gyn, Sultrin, Sulfa, Trysul: miscellaneous sulfonamide-sulfonamide sulfabenzamide 3.7%, sulfacetamide 2.85%, sulfiazole 3.42%, and urea 0.64%

Fiorinal: aspirin 325 mg with butalbital 50 mg, caffeine 40 mg

Fiorinal with Codeine No. 1: aspirin 325 mg with butalbital 50 mg, caffeine 40 mg, codeine phosphate 7.5 mg

Fiorinal with Codeine No. 2: aspirin 325 mg with butalbital 50 mg, caffeine 40 mg, and codeine phosphate 15 mg

Fiorinal with Codeine No. 3: aspirin 325 mg with butalbital 50 mg, caffeine 40 mg, codeine phosphate 30 mg

Firgesic, Ursinus Inlay Tablets: aspirin 325 mg with pseudoephedrine HCl 30 mg

G-1: acetaminophen 500 mg with butalbital 50 mg, caffeine 40 mg

G-2: acetaminophen 500 mg with butalbital 50 mg, codeine phosphate 15 mg

G-3, Sedapap No. 3: codeine 30 mg with acetaminophen 500 mg, butalbital 50 mg

G-3: acetaminophen 500 mg with butalbital 50 mg, codeine phosphate 30 mg

Gemnisyn: acetaminophen 325 mg with aspirin 325 mg

Goody's Headache Powder: acetaminophen 260 mg with aspirin 520 mg, caffeine 32.5 mg

Hybephen: belladonna alkaloids atropine sulfate 0.0233 mg, hyoscyamine sulfate 0.1277 mg, phenobarbital 15 mg, scopolamine hydrobromide 0.0094 mg

Hydro-Fluserpine No 1, Hydropine, Salazide-Demi, Salutensin-Demi: reserpine 0.125 mg with hydroflumethiazide 25 mg

Hydro-Fluserpine No. 2, Hydropine H.P., Salazide, Salutensin: hydroflumethiazide 50 mg with reserpine 0.125 mg

Hydrogesic: hydrocodone bitartrate 7.5 mg with acetaminophen 650 mg

Hydromox R: quinethazone 50 mg with reserpine 0.125 mg

Hydropres-25, Hydro-Reserpine-25, Hydroserp, Hydroserpine No. 1, Hydrosine 25 mg, Mallopress: reserpine 0.125 mg with hydrochlorothiazide 25 mg

Hydropres-50, Hydro-Reserpine-50, Hydroserp, Hydroserpine No. 2, Hydrosine 50 mg, Hydrotensin, Hydroserpalan: reserpine 0.125 mg with hydrochlorothiazide 50 mg

Inderide 40/25, Propranolol HCl, Hydrochlorothiazide Tablets 40/25: propranolol HCl 40 mg with hydrochlorothiazide 25 mg

Inderide 80/25, Propranolol HCl, Hydrochlorothiazide Tablets 80/25: propranolol HCl 80 mg with hydrochlorothiazide 25 mg

Inderide LA 80/50: propranolol HCl 80 mg with hydrochlorothiazide 50 mg

Inderide LA 120/50: propranolol HCl 120 mg with hydrochlorothiazide 50 mg

Inderide LA 160/50: propranolol HCl 160 mg with hydrochlorothiazide 50 mg

INH: isoniazid 1 tablet, isoniazid 300 mg

Iophen DM, Tussi-Organidin DM: dextromethorphan hydrobromide 10 mg/5 ml with iodinated glycerol 30 mg/5 ml

Kinesed: belladonna alkaloids atropine sulfate 0.02 mg, hyoscyamine sulfate 0.12 mg, phenobarbital 16 mg, scopolamine hydrobromide 0.007 mg

Levsin with Phenobarbital Tablets, Anaspaz: hyoscyamine sulfate 0.125 mg with phenobarbital

Levsinex with Phenobarbital Elixir: hyoscyamine sulfate 0.125 mg/5 ml with phenobarbital 15 mg/5 ml

Levsinex with Phenobarbital Timecaps: hyoscyamine sulfate 0.375 mg with phenobarbital 45 mg

Levsin-PB: hyoscyamine sulfate 0.125 mg/ml with phenobarbital 15 mg/ml

Lopressor HCT 50/25: metoprolol tartrate 50 mg with hydrochlorothiazide 25 mg

Lopressor HCT 100/25: metoprolol tartrate 100 mg with hydrochlorothiazide 25 mg

Lopressor HCT 100/50: metoprolol tartrate 100 mg with hydrochlorothiazide 50 mg

Maximum Strength Anacin: aspirin 500 mg with caffeine 32 mg

Maximum Strength Midol for Cramps: aspirin 500 mg with caffeine 32.4 mg, cinnamedrine HCl 14.9 mg

Mediqueall: dextromethorphan hydrobromide 15 mg with pseudoephedrine HCl 30 mg

Menrium 5-2: chlordiazepoxide

5 mg with esterified estrogens 0.2 mg

Menrium 5-4: chlordiazepoxide 5 mg with esterified estrogens 0.4 mg

Menrium 10-4: chlordiazepoxide 10 mg with esterified estrogens 0.4 mg

Mepergan: meperidine HCl 25 mg/ml with promethazine HCl 25 mg/ml

Mepergan Fortis: meperidine HCl 50 mg with promethazine HCl 25 mg

Metatensin No. 2: reserpine 0.1 mg with trichlormethiazide 2 mg

Midol Caplets: aspirin 454 mg with caffeine 32.4 mg, cinnamedrine HCl 14.9 mg

Midol PMS Caplets: acetaminophen 500 mg with pamabrom 25 mg, pyrilamine maleate 15 mg

Milprem-200, PMB 200: meprobamate 200 mg with conjugated estrogens 0.45 mg

Milprem-400, PMB 400: meprobamate 400 mg with conjugated estrogens 0.45 mg

Minizide 1: prazosin HCl 1 mg (of prazosin) with polythiazide 0.5 mg

Minizide 2: prazosin HCl 2 mg (of prazosin) with polythiazide 0.5 mg

Minizide 5: prazosin HCl 5 mg (of prazosin) with polythiazide 0.5 mg

Morphine, Atropine Sulfate Injection: morphine sulfate 16 mg/ml with atropine sulfate 0.4 mg/ml

Myapap with Codeine, Tylenol with Codeine: acetaminophen 120 mg/5 ml with codeine phosphate 12 mg/5 ml

Mysteclin F: amphotericin B 25 mg/5 ml with tetracycline equivalent to tetracycline HCl 25 mg/5 ml

Mysteclin-F: amphotericin B 50 mg with tetracycline equivalent to tetracycline HCl 250 mg

Mysteclin-F: tetracycline equivalent to 125 mg tetracycline HCl per 5 ml with amphotericin B 25 mg/5 ml

Mysteclin-F: tetracycline equivalent to 350 mg tetracycline HCl with amphotericin B 50 mg/5 ml

Mysteclin-F Syrup: tetracycline equivalent to 125 mg tetracycline HCl per 5 ml with amphotericin B 25 mg/5 ml

Naldecon-DX Adult: dextromethorphan hydrobromide 15 mg/5 ml with guaifenesin 200 mg/5 ml, phenylpropanolamine HCl 18 mg/5 ml

Naldecon-DX Children's Syrup: dextromethorphan hydrobromide 7.5 mg/5 ml with guaifenesin 100 mg/5 ml, phenylpropanolamine HCl 9 mg/5 ml

Naldegisic: acetaminophen 325 mg with pseudoephedrine HCl 15 mg

Naturetin with K 5 mg: bendroflumethiazide 5 mg with potassium chloride 500 mg

Neosporin G.U. Irrigant: polymyxin B sulfate 200,000 units (of polymyxin B)

Norgesic: orphenadrine citrate 25 mg with aspirin 385 mg, caffeine 30 mg

Norgesic Forte: orphenadrine citrate 50 mg with aspirin 770 mg, caffeine 60 mg

Novahistine Cough and Cold Formula: dextromethorphan hydrobromide 10 mg/5 ml with chlorpheniramine maleate 2 mg/5 ml, pseudoephedrine HCl 30 mg/5 ml

Opium and Belladonna: powdered opium 60 mg with belladonna extract 15 mg (equivalent to belladonna alkaloids 0.2 mg)

Oreticyl 25: deserpidine 0.125 mg with hydrochlorothiazide 25 mg

Oreticyl 50: deserpidine 0.125 mg with hydrochlorothiazide 50 mg

Oreticyl Forte: deserpidine 0.25 mg with hydrochlorothiazide 50 mg

Ornex: phenylpropanolamine HCl 12.5 mg with acetaminophen 325 mg

Orthoxicol Cough Syrup: dextromethorphan hydrobromide 10 mg/5 ml with methoxyphenamine HCl 17 mg/5 ml

Oxymycin, Terramycin Intramuscular Solution: oxytetracycline 50 mg/ml with lidocaine 2%

Pamprin: acetaminophen 325 mg with pamabrom 25 mg, pyrilamine maleate 12.5 mg

Pamprin Maximum Cramp Relief: acetaminophen 500 mg with pamabrom 25 mg, pyrilamine maleate 15 mg

Pathibamate-200: meprobamate 200 mg with tridihexethyl chloride 25 mg

Pathibamate-400: meprobamate 400 mg with tridihexethyl chloride 25 mg

Pediacare 3: dextromethorphan hydrobromide 5 mg/5 ml with chlorpheniramine maleate 1 mg/5 ml, pseudoephedrine HCl 15 mg/5 ml

Pediacare 3 Chewable Tablets: dextromethorphan hydrobromide 2.5 mg with chlorpheniramine maleate 0.5 mg, pseudophedrine HCl 7.5 mg

Pediazole: erythromycin ethlysuccinate 200 mg (of erythromycin) per 5 ml with sulfisoxazole acetyl 600 mg (of sulfisoxazole) per 5 ml

Penntuss: codeine polistirex equivalent to codeine 10 mg/5 ml with chlorpheniramine polistirex equivalent to chlorpheniramine maleate 4 mg/5 ml

Percodan-Demi: aspirin 325 mg with oxycodone HCl 2.25 mg, oxycodone terephthalate 0.19 mg

Percogesic: acetaminophen 325 mg with phenyltoloxamine citrate 30 mg

Persistin: salsalate 487.5 mg with aspirin 162.5 mg

Phenaphen with Codeine No. 2: acetaminophen 325 mg with codeine phosphate 15 mg

Phenaphen with Codeine No.

2, Proval No. 3: codeine 30 mg with acetaminophen 325 mg

Phenaphen with Codeine No. 3, Proval No. 2: acetaminophen 325 mg with codeine phosphate 30 mg

Phenaphen with Codeine No. 4: acetaminophen 325 mg with codeine phosphate 60 mg

Phenaphen-650 with Codeine: acetaminophen 650 mg with codeine phosphate 30 mg

Phenergan: promethazine HCl 6.25 mg/5 ml with phenylephrine HCl 5 mg/5 ml

Phenergan-D: promethazine HCl 6.25 mg with pseudoephedrine HCl 60 mg

Phenergan VC Syrup, Promethazine HCl VC: promethazine HCl 6.25 mg/5 ml with phenylephrine HCl 5 mg/5 ml

Phenergan with Dextromethorphan: dextromethorphan hydrobromide 15 mg/5 ml with promethazine HCl 6.35 mg/5 ml

Phrenilin: acetaminophen 325 mg with butalbital 50 mg, caffeine 40 mg

Phrenilin Forte: acetaminophen 650 mg with butalbital 50 mg

Phrenilin with Codeine No. 3: acetaminophen 325 mg with butalbital 50 mg, codeine phosphate 30 mg

Propoxyphene HCl/65, Wygesic: acetaminophen 650 mg with propoxyphene HCl 65 mg

Prunicodeine: terpin hydrate 29 mg/5 ml with codeine sulfate 10 mg/5 ml

Rautrax: rauwolfia 50 mg with flumethiazide 400 mg, potassium chloride 400 mg

Rautrax-N: bendroflumethiazide 4 mg with rauwolfia serpentina 50 mg, potassium chloride 400 mg

Rauzide: bendroflumethiazide 4 mg with rauwolfia serpentina 50 mg

Regroton: reserpine 0.25 mg with chlorthalidone 50 mg

Renese: reserpine 0.25 mg with polythiazide 2 mg

Rifamate: isoniazid 150 mg with rifampin 300 mg

Rimactane: isoniazid 2 capsules, rifampin 300 mg

Rimactane: rifampin 1 tablet, isoniazid 300 mg

Rimactane: rifampin 2 capsules, isoniazid 300 mg

Robaxisal, Robomol/ASA: methocarbamol 400 mg with aspirin 325 mg

Robitussin-DM: dextromethorphan hydrobromide 15 mg/5 ml with guaifenesin 100 mg/5 ml

Roxicet: oxycodone HCl 5 mg/5 ml with acetaminophen 325 mg/5 ml

S-A-C: salicylamide 230 mg with acetaminophen 150 mg, caffeine 30 mg

Salimeth Forte: salicylamide 600 mg with acetaminophen 250 mg

S.B.P.: secobarbital sodium 50 mg with butabarbital sodium 30 mg, phenobarbital 15 mg

Serpasil-Apresoline HCl No. 1: hydralazine HCl 25 mg with reserpine 0.1 mg

Serpasil-Apresoline HCl No.

2: hydralazine HCl 25 mg with reserpine 0.2 mg

Serpasil-Esidrix No. 1: reserpine 0.1 mg with hydrochlorothiazide 25 mg

Serpasil-Esidrix No. 2: reserpine 0.1 mg with hydrochlorothiazide 50 mg

Sine-Aid: acetaminophen 325 mg with pseudoephedrine HCl 30 mg

Sine-Aid Extra Strength Caplets, Tylenol Sinus Maximum Strength Caplets: acetaminophen 500 mg with pseudoephedrine HCl 30 mg

Sine-Off Extra Strength, Sinutab: acetaminophen 500 mg with pseudoephedrine HCl 30 mg

Sinubid: acetaminophen 600 mg with phenylpropanolamine HCl 100 mg, phenyltoloxamine citrate 66 mg

Sinutab Maximum Nighttime: acetaminophen 167 mg/5 ml with diphenhydramine HCl 8.3 mg/5 ml, pseudoephedrine HCl 10 mg/5 ml

Sinutab II Maximum, Tylenol maximum strength sinus: acetaminophen 500 mg with pseudoephedrine HCl 30 mg

SK-APAP with Codeine, Tylenol with Codeine No. 2: codeine 5 mg with acetaminophen 300 mg

Soma Compound with Codeine: codeine 16 mg with aspirin 325 mg, carisoprodol 200 mg

Somines Pain Relief: acetaminophen 500 mg with diphenhydramine HCl 25 mg

Spec-T: Phenylpropanolamine 10.5 mg with Benzocaine 10 mg, Phenylephrine HCl 5 mg

Spec-T Sore Throat Cough Suppressant: dextromethorphan hydrobromide 10 mg with benzocaine 10 mg

Sudafed Cough Syrup: dextromethorphan hydrobromide 5 mg/5 ml with guaifenesin 100 mg/5 ml, pseudoephedrine HCl 15 mg/5 ml

Sultrin: miscellaneous sulfonamide-sulfonamide sulfabenzamide 184 mg, sulfacetamide 143.75 mg, sulfathiazole 172.5 mg, urea 31.83 mg

Talacen: pentazocine HCl 25 mg (of pentazocine) with acetaminophen 650 mg

Talwin Compound Caplets: aspirin 325 mg with pentazocine HCl 12.5 mg (of pentazocine)

Tenoretic 50: atenolol 50 mg with chlorthalidone 25 mg

Tenoretic 100: atenolol 100 mg with chlorthalidone 25 mg

Terpin Hydrate and Codeine: terpin hydrate 85 mg/5 ml with dextromethorphan hydrobromide 10 mg/5 ml (with alcohol 39%-44%)

Terramycin Intramuscular Solution: oxytetracycline 125 mg/ml with lidocaine 2%

T-Gesic: hydrocodone bitartrate 5 mg with acetaminophen 325 mg, butalbital 30 mg, caffeine 40 mg

Timolide 10/25: timolol ma-

leate 10 mg with hydrochlorothiazide 25 mg

Trendar: acetaminophen 325
mg with pamabrom 25 mg

Triaminic-DM Cough Formula: dextromethorphan hydrobromide 10 mg/5 ml with
phenylpropanolamine HCl 12.5
mg/5 ml

Triaminicol: dextromethorphan
hydrobromide 10 mg/5 ml with
chlorpheniramine maleate 2 mg/5
ml, phenylpropanolamine HCl
12.5 mg/5 ml

Trigesic: aspirin 230 mg with
acetaminophen 125 mg, caffeine 30 mg

Tuinal 50 mg Pulvules: secobarbital sodium 25 mg with
amobarbital sodium 25 mg

Tuinal 100 mg Pulvules: secobarbital sodium 50 mg with
amobarbital sodium 50 mg

Tuinal 200 mg Pulvules: secobarbital sodium 100 mg with
amobarbital sodium 100 mg

Tylenol with Codeine No. 1:
acetaminophen 300 mg with codeine phosphate 7.5 mg

Tylenol with Codeine No. 2:
acetaminophen 300 mg with codeine phosphate 15 mg

Tylenol with Codeine No. 3:
acetaminophen 300 mg with codeine phosphate 30 mg

Tylenol with Codeine No. 4:
acetaminophen 300 mg with codeine phosphate 60 mg

Tylox: acetaminophen 500 mg
with oxycodone HCl 5 mg

Urobiotic-250: oxytetracycline
HCl 250 mg (of oxytetracycline) with phenazopyridine

HCl 50 mg, sulfamethizole
250 mg

Vanquish Caplets: aspirin 227
mg with acetaminophen 194
mg, caffeine 30 mg, buffers

Vaseretic 10-25: enalapril maleate 10 mg with hydrochlorothiazide 25 mg

Vicks Childrens Cough Syrup:
dextromethorphan hydrobromide
3.5 mg/5 ml with guaifenesin
25 mg/5 ml

Vicks Cough Silencers: dextromethorphan hydrobromide
2.5 mg with benzocaine 1 mg

Vicks Daycare: dextromethorphan hydrobromide 10 mg with
acetaminophen 325 mg, guaifenesin 100 mg, pseudoephedrine
HCl 30 mg

Vicks Daycare: dextromethorphan hydrobromide 3.3 mg/5
ml with acetaminophen 108.3
mg/5 ml, guaifenesin 33.3 mg/
5 ml, pseudoephedrine HCl 10
mg/5 ml

**Vicks Formula 44 Cough
Control Discs:** dextromethorphan hydrobromide 5 mg with
benzocaine 1.25 mg

**Vicks Formula 44 Cough
Mixture:** dextromethorphan
hydrobromide 15 mg/5 ml
with doxylamine succinate 3.75
mg/5 ml

Vicks Formula 44D: dextromethorphan hydrobromide 10 mg/
5 ml with guaifenesin 66.7 mg/
5 ml, pseudoephedrine HCl 20
mg/5 ml

Vicks Formula 44M: dextromethorphan hydrobromide 7.4
mg/5 ml with acetaminophen

125 mg/5 ml, guaifenesin 50 mg/5 ml, pseudoephedrine HCl 15 mg/5 ml

Westrim-1: phenylpropanolamine HCl 25 mg with benzocaine 5 mg, methylcellulose 300 mg

Wyanoids: belladonna extract 15 mg (0.19 mg of alkaloids of belladonna leaf) with ephedrine 3 mg

Ziradyl: diphenhydramine HCl 2% with zinc oxide 2%

Index

INDEX

INDEX

Controlled substance chart

Drugs	United States	Canada
Heroin, LSD, peyote, marijuana, mescaline	Schedule I	Schedule H
Opium (morphine, meperidine), amphetamines, cocaine, short-acting barbiturates (secobarbital)	Schedule II	Schedule G
Chorphentermine, glutethimide, mazindol, paregoric, phendimetrazine	Schedule III	Schedule F
Chloral hydrate, chlordiazepoxide, diazepam, meprobamate, phenobarbital	Schedule IV	Schedule F
Antidiarrheals with opium, antitussives	Schedule V	

FDA pregnancy categories

A No risk demonstrated to the fetus in any trimester

B No adverse effects in animals, no human studies available

C Only given after risks to the fetus are considered; animal studies have shown adverse reactions, no human studies available

D Definite fetal risks, may be given in spite of risks if needed in life-threatening conditions

X Absolute fetal abnormalities; not to be used anytime in pregnancy